Radiology Review
Manual

Second Edition

Radiology Review Manual

Second Edition

Wolfgang Dähnert, M.D.

Department of Radiology
Good Samaritan Regional Medical Center
Phoenix, Arizona

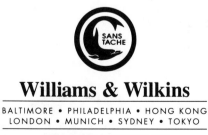

Williams & Wilkins

BALTIMORE • PHILADELPHIA • HONG KONG
LONDON • MUNICH • SYDNEY • TOKYO

A WAVERLY COMPANY

Editor: Timothy H. Grayson
Project Manager: Raymond E. Reter
Copy Editor: Klemie Bryte
Designer: Wilma E. Rosenberger

Accurate indications, adverse reactions, and dosage schedules for drugs are provided in this book, but it is possible that they may change. The reader is urged to review the package information data of the manufacturers of the medications mentioned.

Printed in the United States of America

Library of Congress Cataloging-in-Publication Data

Dähnert, Wolfgang.
   Radiology review manual / Wolfgang Dähnert.—2nd ed.
     p. cm.
   Includes bibliographical references and index.
   ISBN 0-683-02340-3
   1.Radiology, Medical—Outlines, syllabi, etc. 2. Diagnosis,
Radioscopic—Outlines, syllabi, etc. I. Title.
   [DNLM: 1. Radiology—outlines. WN 18 D131r]
RC78. D29 1993
616.07'57—dc20
DNLM / DLC
for Library of Congress
                            92–49039
                               CIP

                    93 94 95 96
          1 2 3 4 5 6 7 8 9 10

*"Nothing in the world can take the place of persistence.
Talent will not; nothing is more common than unsuccessful men
with talent. Genius will not; unrewarded genius is almost a proverb.
Education will not; the world is full of educated derelicts.
Persistence and determination alone are omnipotent."*

Calvin Coolidge 1872–1933
Vice President 1921–1923
President 1923–1929

To my dear wife Sue,
to our children Mathias and Patrick
who mean so much to me

About the Author

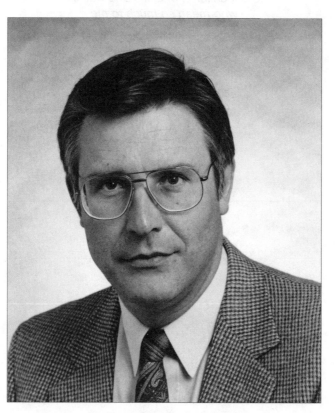

Wolfgang Dähnert, M.D.

Wolfgang Dähnert was born in Hamburg, Germany. He studied medicine at the universities of Düsseldorf and Mainz, where he graduated in 1975. After internship and a short surgical residency he enrolled in a 4-year radiology residency program at the Johannes-Gutenberg University in Mainz and received his German certification for radiology in 1982. In 1984 he started a 2-year fellowship in ultrasound and computed tomography at the Johns Hopkins Hospital in Baltimore and was appointed Clinical Instructor at the same institution in 1986. During his Hopkins years he sat for the FLEX exam, and the radiology specialty exam with the American Board of Radiology. During these three years the foundation of *Radiology Review Manual* was laid. Between 1987 and 1989 he worked as Assistant Professor of Radiology in ultrasound at Thomas Jefferson Hospital in Philadelphia. During these three years *Radiology Review Manual* was taken to fruition. Since December of 1989 he has been associated with Clinical Diagnostic Radiology & Nuclear Medicine, a large subspecialized radiology group practice in Phoenix, Arizona, providing radiology service to Good Samaritan Regional Medical Center, a tertiary care hospital, and the Children's Hospital of Phoenix.

PREFACE TO SECOND EDITION

The success of the first edition of *Radiology Review Manual* has surpassed the expectation of the author and publisher. Its litmus test has been the impressive number of volumes sold. Foreign stamps on my mail attest to the appeal this book has to radiologists in other parts of the world. *Radiology Review Manual* has found a place on the desk tops and work stations of many radiologists, even those outside the primary target group of radiology residents. Some academic teachers consult with *Radiology Review Manual* to become familiar with their residents' study guide or to prepare for irritating challenges brought forth by a sagacious resident. I hope the ensuing discussions intensified the mutual learning process.

I am most grateful for the many notes thanking me for the outline between the green cover. The positive reinforcement has spurred my efforts to improve the contents for the second edition. Almost all sections have been refurnished and refurbished over the past two years. The additions largely reflect my personal needs that arose in the wake of my professional switch from academics into private practice. For example, you will notice expansion of the ENT section and many new entries in the CNS section. The dreadful printer's devil had been on the lurk in the first edition. It is hoped that now most typographical errors have been zapped. Mnemonics (which I personally abhor) have been expanded by request. Some of the pearls of several other excellent textbooks have been added: Barkovich AJ: *Pediatric Neuroimaging*; Harnsberger HR: *Handbooks in Radiology, Head and Neck Imaging*; Margulis AR, Burhenne HJ: *Alimentary Tract Radiology*; Megibow AJ, Balthazar EJ: *Computed Tomography of the Gastrointestinal Tract*; Mittelstaedt CA: *Abdominal Ultrasound*; Newton TH, Hasso AN, Dillon WP: *Computed Tomography of the Head and Neck in Modern Neuroradiology*; Resnick D, Niwayama G: *Diagnosis of Bone and Joint Disorders*; Romero R, Pilu G, Jeanty P, Ghidini A, Hobbins JC: *Prenatal Diagnosis of Congenital Anomalies*; Tabár L, Dean PB: *Teaching Atlas of Mammography*. However, the most significant sources are the journals dedicated to imaging as well as syllabi from various CME courses. As a result, *Radiology Review Manual* has grown by many pages. Unfortunately, we have come to the point where size and handiness cross. I could not bring myself to sacrifice or discard some of its contents.

As author, it is my prerogative not to follow every recommendation offered. There are differences in opinion about the proper place and task of this book. As before, this edition will not deal with the physics of magnetic resonance imaging, ultrasound and Doppler, CT scanning, or radiography. You have to draw the line somewhere! Some board candidates requested a separate pediatric section. Separation of pediatrics, however, would violate the book's organization by organ system. Also, it would add many pages with double entries, as many pediatric diseases extend their relevance into adulthood. My key argument remains: the examination covers all topics on the very same day. Thus, there is no need for sequestering pediatrics — unless you are conditioned.

My thanks to my colleague Ross Levatter for his thorough review of the section on nuclear medicine, and to those of you who have taken the time to drop me a note or speak to me personally. This feedback has been the life support for this second edition and the vital ingredient for growth and restructure — signs of a live organism.

Phoenix, October 1992

Toward the end of an intensive 4-year training program, the resident in radiology is usually well-equipped to prove his/her diagnostic ability. Although most residency programs prepare well for the written and oral examination, the board candidate who rests comfortably on the accumulated knowledge has yet to be born. Faced with the large amount of material to be reviewed in a short period of time, residents often find themselves in a state of mental paralysis, which is soon overcome and replaced by frantic study activity.

In preparation for the exam, of course, hundreds of books can be found in the department's library and many have, hopefully, been read during the residency program. But day and night wouldn't be enough to go through just a fraction of these in the little time that remains. There are those textbooks that are especially popular to review certain topics. Naturally, they are checked out when you need them, and few residents have the resources to purchase them. The multi-volume books covering every aspect of a subspecialty rest in peace. Who has the time now to read them from cover to cover?

It has struck me as peculiar that I was unable to find a comprehensive review textbook to help me prepare for the exam, in contrast to most other subspecialties for which such material is available. Instead, I joined the ranks of previous generations of examinees going through the same routine: the typical study room is crammed with handouts, review articles, various textooks, ACR syllabi, hand-written notes taken during lectures, etc. All this is seasoned by mountains of photocopies containing hand- or type-written reports from previous exams diligently prepared by returning board candidates, which often enough provide more questions than answers. All these resources are organized into various piles and commonly spread on the floor for lack of desk top space. It is a formidable task indeed trying to look up some minutia, probably unimportant and irrelevant for one's performance, but seemingly so vital at that particular moment. Valuable time is wasted thumbing through piles of paper in an effort to track down trivia. How frustrating an experience to come up empty-handed. More precious time is lost organizing lists of differential diagnosis or etiologies into memorable groups and categories, possibly acronyms or other mnemonics. In short, much of one's effort is directed toward the task of collecting and hunting rather than digesting. Every 3rd or 4th year resident is doing over again those things that generations of board candidates have gone through — but their collections and recollections have never been passed on in a readily available and organized fashion.

Radiology Review Manual was created in preparation for the specialty exam as the "book under the pillow." It served me as a quick review on a large number of topics. In its original concept, generated as computer printouts in file format, it represents a very personal choice and includes topics that were unfamiliar to me or with which I had struggled. However, I learned that my choices were appropriate for many examinees.

I have to credit the idea to publish this material to several residents who urged me to do so. Over the years, this material has been continuously changed, upgraded and expanded — even as we speak. Our voluminous field of diagnostic radiology makes it necessary to use a short-hand style for the sake of conserving space and thus provides only an extract of information, a quintessence if you will. This may, at times, jeopardize the full meaning of statements when taken out of context. It should be kept in mind that this book is not intended for the novice and that it requires familiarity with the subject of radiology and the background information of major textbooks. In addition, it provides such a density of information that it is quite unsuitable to be read from cover to cover.

How to use this book:
The organization of this book has caused a major headache as any topic can be looked at from various points of view. I have selected just one of many possibilities to avoid redundancy. The material is presented in a manner that is in keeping with the topics of the current board exam. Unfortunately, this grouping is inconsistent, sectioning off by age (Pediatric Radiology) and image modality (Nuclear Medicine, Ultrasound). In order to avoid repitition, pediatric entities are subsumed within organ systems. Ultrasound and Nuclear Medicine are used from head to heel and consequently are mentioned in all body sections. However, Nuclear Medicine is additionally treated in a separate section when emphasis is on technique and functional aspects not covered elsewhere. A section on ear, nose, and throat topics is placed at the end of the section on CNS disorders. The skull and spine are dealt with as the first part of the CNS section.

The organization within the individual chapters follows the practical approach of reading films. The initial step of film interpretation is the description of radiologic patterns which serves to identify categories in which they belong. Therefore, radiologic patterns for differential diagnoses are found in the first portion of a chapter. Once the diagnostic possibilities have been reviewed in brief outline, one can look up detailed information about a disease entity in the last segment of a chapter. The disease entities are presented in alphabetical order. Both these segments are separated by a few pages of functional, anatomic, or embryologic aspects. Occasionally, important clinical signs and their differential diagnoses are included in the first portion of a chapter.

The backbone of the book is disease entities, radiological symptoms, as well as lists of differential diagnosis. Disease entities are headed by their most commonly used name with other designations listed below. As a radiologic diagnosis should be entertained in context with its probability to be correct, percentages in regard to frequency of signs and symptoms are included liberally, often giving the lowest and the highest number found in the literature. The truth may be somewhere in between for a non-selected patient population. Arbitrary choices have been made in situations when different or contradictory results are found in the literature — unfortunately, an occurrence not at all infrequent.

Lists of differential diagnoses can be presented in many fashions. There is no right or wrong way, but there certainly is a chaotic versus an organized approach. An orderly thought process portrays familiarity with a problem. Examinees have always felt that "nailing" the diagnosis is secondary, but including it in one's consideration is paramount to a successful exam. Accordingly, an attempt is made to categorize differential diagnostic considerations or etiologies of certain diseases in a manner digestible for recapitulation. It is common experience that this is not always possible, satisfactory, or complete.

A table of contents and abbreviations used throughout the book are found in front. A user-friendly index, which selectively refers to those pages with significant information concludes the manual. Notice that most systemic diseases will be mentioned in more than one chapter with some unavoidable redundancy. However, emphasized are those manifestations of the disease that occur within the organ under which it is listed. The index also includes so-called "buzz words" that are miraculously attached to diseases.

Radiology Review Manual is not exclusive to the near-term resident. It has continued to refresh my memory bank for years beyond the specialty exam. In fact, the stimulus to go through with this project has been the challenge found in daily practice as well as my encounters in teaching residents and fellow radiologists. Just as the cases presented in the oral exam apply to the real world of a radiologist, so do the topics in this book. Thus, I can recommend it to any practicing radiologist. I sincerely hope that *Radiology Review Manual* will serve its users in the same manner it has helped me in preparation for the board exam and beyond this scope in daily practice and teaching.

Acknowledgement:
The information contained herein has been gathered over several years and stems from various sources. Data from numerous radiological articles and textbooks are incorporated and anecdotal contributions can no longer be traced. I realize, in retrospect, that this may present a problem when certain statements appear unlikely and their verification has to be left to the user. For my defense, I can only say that I have tried to extract all data as diligently as possible. I would like to acknowledge the input of numerous teachers, residents, fellows, past and present board candidates at the Johns Hopkins Hospital, Baltimore, and Thomas Jefferson University Hospital, Philadelphia.

The following textbooks have been particularly helpful and deserve mention: Burgener FA, Kormano M: *Differential Diagnosis in Conventional Radiology*; Chapman S, Nakielny R: *Aids to Radiological Differential Diagnosis*; Davidson AJ: *Radiology of the Kidney*; Eideken J: *Roentgen Diagnosis of Diseases of Bone*; Fraser RG, Pare JAP: *Diagnosis of Diseases of the Chest*; Gedgaudas E, Moller JH, Castaneda-Zuniga WR, Amplatz K: *Cardiovascular Radiology*; Kadir S: *Diagnostic Angiography*; Kirks DR: *Practical Pediatric Imaging*; Reed JC: *Chest Radiology: Plain Film Patterns and Differential Diagnosis*; Reeder MM, Felson B: *Gamuts in Radiology*; Sanders RC, James AE: *Ultrasonography in Obstetrics and Gynecology*; Swischuk LE: *Plain Film Interpretation in Congenital Heart Disease*; Taveras JM, Ferrucci JT: *Radiology – Diagnosis – Imaging – Intervention*

I am particularly indebted to the following individuals for reviewing the separate sections of this book: Christopher Canino, Thomas Chang, Adam E. Flanders, Keith Haidet, Charles Intenzo, David Karasick, Stephen Karasick, Alfred B. Kurtz, Esmond M. Mapp, Joel Raichlen, Paul Spirn, Robert M. Steiner, and C. Amy Wilson.

Phoenix, September 1990

I would appreciate any comments and suggestions which you feel would improve *Radiology Review Manual*. Your input is of value to me and will be considered in future editions.

Wolfgang Dähnert, M.D.
c/o Williams & Wilkins
428 East Preston Street
Baltimore, MD 21202

CONTENTS

√	radiologic sign		demonstration project		coagulation
•	clinical sign, symptom	BCG	bacille Calmette-Guérin	DIDA	diethyl iminodiacetic acid
=	equals, is	BE	barium enema	DIL	drug-induced lupus
@	at anatomic location of	BIDA	butyl iminodiacetic acid		erythematosus
/	or, per	BIH	benign intracranial	DIP	desquamative interstitial
+	and, plus, with		hypertension		pneumonia
±	with or without	BKG	background	DIP	distal interphalangeal
<	less than	BP	blood pressure	DISH	diffuse idiopathic skeletal
>	more than, over	BPD	biparietal diameter		hyperostosis
Δ	nota bene	BPH	benign prostatic hyperplasia	DISIDA	diisopropyl iminodiacetic acid
		bpm	beats per minute	DIT	diiodotyrosine
ABC	aneurysmal bone cyst	BSA	body surface area	DMSA	dimercaptosuccinic acid
AC	abdominal circumference	Bx	biopsy	DTPA	diethylenetriamine pentaacetic
ACA	anterior cerebral artery				acid
ACE	angiotensin I-converting	Ca	calcium	DVT	deep vein thrombosis
	enzyme	CAD	coronary artery disease	Dx	diagnosis
ACom	anterior communicating artery	CAM	cystic adenomatoid		
ACTH	adrenocorticotropic hormone		malformation	EAC	external auditory canal
ADH	antidiuretic hormone	CBD	common bile duct	ECA	external carotid artery
AFP	alpha-fetoprotein	CC	craniocaudad	ECD	endocardial cushion defect
AICA	anterior inferior cerebellar	CCA	common carotid artery	ECF	extracellular fluid
	artery	CCAM	congenital cystic adenomatoid	ECG	electrocardiogram
AIDS	acquired immune deficiency		malformation	ECHO	echocardiogram
	syndrome	CCK	cholecystokinin	ED	end-diastole
ALL	acute lymphoblastic leukemia	CECT	contrast-enhanced computed	EDV	end-diastolic volume
AMA	antimitochondrial antibody		tomography	EEG	electroencephalogram
AML	acute myeloblastic leukemia	CHD	common hepatic duct	EF	ejection fraction
AML	angiomyolipoma	CHD	congenital heart defect	EFW	estimated fetal weight
aML	anterior mitral valve leaflet	CHF	congestive heart failure	EG	eosinophilic granuloma
ANA	antinuclear antibodies	CLL	chronic lymphatic leukemia	eg	exempli gratia
Angio	angiography	CMC	carpometacarpal	EHDP	ethylene
ANT	anterior	CML	chronic myelogenous leukemia		hydroxydiphosphonate
Ao	aorta	CMV	cytomegalovirus	ERC	endoscopic retrograde
AP	anteroposterior	CNS	central nervous system		cholangiography
APUD	amine precursor uptake and	CO	carbon monoxide	ES	end-systole
	decarboxylation	CoA	coarctation of aorta	esp.	especially
APVR	anomalous pulmonary	COPD	chronic obstructive pulmonary	ESR	erythrocyte sedimentation rate
	venous return		disease	ESV	end-systolic volume
ARA-C	arabinoside C	CPA	cerebellopontine angle		
ARDS	acute respiratory distress	CPPD	calcium pyrophosphate	F	female
	syndrome		dihydrate	FDA	Federal Drug Administration
AS	aortic stenosis	CPR	cardiopulmonary resuscitation	FDG	fluorodeoxyglucose
ASA	acetylsalicylic acid	CRT	cathode ray tube	FEV	forced expiratory volume
ASD	atrial septal defect	CSF	cerebrospinal fluid	FIGO	Fédération Internationale de
ASH	asymmetric septal hypertrophy	CST	contraction stress test		Gynécologie et d'Obstétrique
aTL	anterior tricuspid valve leaflet	CT	cardiothoracic ratio	FISP	fast imaging with steady-state
ATN	acute tubular necrosis	CT	computed tomography		precession
AV	arteriovenous	CVA	cerebrovascular accident	FLASH	fast low-angle shot
AV	atrioventricular	CWP	coal worker's pneumoconiosis	FN	false negative
AVF	arteriovenous fistula	Cx	complication	FNH	follicular nodular hyperplasia
AVM	arteriovenous malformation	CXR	chest X-ray	FP	false positive
AVN	avascular necrosis			FRC	functional residual capacity
AVNA	atrioventricular node artery	DCIS	ductal carcinoma in situ	FS	fractional shortening
		DDx	differential diagnosis	FSH	follicle stimulating hormone
Ba	barium	DES	diethylstilbestrol	FWHM	full-width at half-maximum
BCDDP	breast cancer detection	DIC	disseminated intravascular		

GA	gestational age	IUD	intrauterine device	MFH	malignant fibrous histiocytoma
GB	gallbladder	IUGR	intrauterine growth retardation	MIBG	metaiodobenzylguanidine
GBS	group B streptococcus	IV	intravenous	MID	multi-infarct dementia
Gd	gadolinium	IVC	inferior vena cava	MIT	monoiodotyrosine
GE	gastroesophageal	IVH	intraventricular hemorrhage	ML	middle lobe
GER	gastroesophageal reflux	IVP	intravenous pyelogram	MLCN	multilocular cystic nephroma
GFR	glomerular filtration rate	IVS	intraventricular septum	MLO	mediolateral oblique
GI	gastrointestinal			MMAA	mini-microaggregated albumin colloid
GMRH	germinal matrix related hemorrhage	KCC	Kulchitzky cell carcinoma	MMFR	maximal midexpiratory flow rate
GN	glomerulonephritis	L	left	MPS	mucopolysaccharidosis
GRE	gradient refocused echo	L-DOPA	3-(3,4-dihydroxyphenyl)-levo-alanin	MR	magnetic resonance
GU	genitourinary	LA	left atrium	MS-AFP	maternal serum α-fetoprotein
		LAD	left anterior descending	MTP	metatarsophalangeal
Hb	hemoglobin	LAO	left anterior oblique	MUGA	multiple gated acquisition
HC	head circumference	LAT	lateral	MV	mitral valve
hCG	human chorionic gonadotropin	LATS	long-acting thyroid stimulating	Myelo	myelography
HD	Hodgkin disease	LAV	lymphadenopathy-associated virus		
HIAA	hydroxyindole acetic acid			N.B.	nota bene
HIDA	hepatic 2,6-dimethyl iminodiacetic acid	LCA	left coronary artery	NBS	National Bureau of Standards
HIP	health insurance plan	LCIS	lobular carcinoma in situ	NEC	necrotizing enterocolitis
Histo	histology	LCX	left circumflex coronary artery	NECT	non-enhanced computed tomography
HIV	human immunodeficiency virus	LDH	lactate dehydrogenase	NHL	non-Hodgkin lymphoma
HL	Hodgkin lymphoma	LE	lupus erythematosus	NPH	normal pressure hydrocephalus
HOCM	hypertrophic obstructive cardiomyopathy	LES	lower esophageal sphincter	NPH	nucleus pulposus herniation
HPT	hyperparathyroidism	LGA	large for gestational age	npl	neoplasm
HRCT	high-resolution CT	LH	luteinizing hormone	NST	non-stress test
HSA	human serum albumin	LIP	lymphocytic interstitial pneumonitis	NTD	neural tube defect
HSE	herpes simplex encephalitis	LL	lower lobes	NUC	nuclear medicine
HSG	hysterosalpingography	LLL	left lower lobe		
HSV	herpes simplex virus	LLQ	left lower quadrant	OB-US	obstetrical ultrasound
HTLV	human T-cell lymphotropic virus	Lnn	lymph nodes	OCG	oral cholecystogram
HU	Hounsfield unit	LPA	left pulmonary artery	OCVM	occult vascular malformation
HWP	hepatic wedge pressure	LPO	left posterior oblique	OHP	orthogonal-hole test pattern
Hx	history	LSD	lysergic acid diethylamide	OHSS	ovarian hyperstimulation syndrome
		LUL	left upper lobe	OIH	orthoiodohippurate
IAC	internal auditory canal	LUQ	left upper quadrant		
ICA	internal carotid artery	LV	left ventricle	P	phosphorus
IDA	iminodiacetic acid	LVET	left ventricular ejection time	PA	posteroanterior
IDM	infant of diabetic mother	LVFT$_2$	left ventricular slow filling time	PA	pulmonary artery
IDP	iminodiphosphonate	LVOT	left ventricular outflow tract	PAC	premature atrial contraction
ie	id est	LVT$_1$	left ventricular fast filling time	PAH	para-aminohippurate
IHSS	idiopathic hypertrophic subaortic stenosis	M	male	PAP	primary atypical pneumonia
IM	intramuscular	MA	menstrual age	PAP	pulmonary alveolar proteinosis
IMA	inferior mesenteric artery	MAA	macroaggregated albumin	PAPVR	partial anomalous pulmonary venous return
In	indium	MAG	mercaptoacetyltriglycine	PAS	periodic acid Schiff
IPF	idiopathic pulmonary fibrosis	MAI	Mycobacterium avium intracellulare	Path	pathology
IPH	idiopathic pulmonary hemosiderosis	MCA	middle cerebral artery	PAVM	pulmonary arteriovenous malformation
		MCDK	multicystic dysplastic kidney		
IR	inversion recovery	MCK	multicystic kidney	PBF	pulmonary blood flow
IRP	international reference preparation	MCP	metacarpophalangeal	PCA	posterior cerebral artery
		MDP	methylene diphosphonate	PCAVC	persistent complete atrioventricular canal
IS	ileosacral, international standard	MEA	multiple endocrine adenomas		
		MEN	multiple endocrine neoplasms	PCKD	polycystic kidney disease

PCom	posterior communicating artery	PVR	pulse volume recording	SV	stroke volume
PCP	Pneumocystis carinii pneumonia	R	right	SVC	superior vena cava
PCWP	pulmonary capillary wedge pressure	RA	rheumatoid arthritis	T1WI	T1 weighted image
		RA	right atrium	T2WI	T2 weighted image
PD	posterior descending artery	RAO	right anterior oblique	TAPVR	total anomalous pulmonary venous return
PDA	patent ductus arteriosus	RBC	red blood cell		
PE	pulmonary embolism	RCA	right coronary artery	TB	tuberculosis
PEEP	positive end expiratory pressure	RCC	renal cell carcinoma	TBG	thyroxin binding globulin
		RDS	respiratory distress syndrome	TBPA	thyroxin binding prealbumin
PEP	preejection period	RES	reticuloendothelial system	TCC	transitional cell carcinoma
PET	positron emission tomography	RIND	reversible ischemic neurologic deficit	TDLU	terminal ductal lobular unit
pHPT	primary hyperparathyroidism			TE	tracheo-esophageal fistula
PICA	posterior inferior cerebellar artery	RISA	radioiodine serum albumin	TGA	transposition of great arteries
		RLL	right lower lobe	tHPT	tertiary hyperparathyroidism
PIE	pulmonary infiltrate with eosinophilia	RLQ	right lower quadrant	TIA	transitory ischemic attack
		RML	right middle lobe	TLC	total lung capacity
PIE	pulmonary interstitial emphysema	ROC	receiver operating characteristic	TN	true negative
				TOF	tetralogy of Fallot
PIOPED	prospective investigation of pulmonary embolus detection	ROI	region of interest	TORCH	toxoplasmosis, rubella, cytomegalovirus, herpes virus
		RPA	right pulmonary artery		
PIP	proximal interphalangeal	RPF	renal plasma flow	TP	true positive
PIPIDA	paraisopropyl iminodiacetic acid	RPO	right posterior oblique	TR	repetition time
		RTA	renal tubular acidosis	TRH	thyrotropin releasing hormone
PLES	parallel-line-equal spacing	RUL	right upper lobe	TRV	transverse
PM	photomultiplier	RV	residual volume	TSH	thyroid stimulating hormone
PMF	progressive massive fibrosis	RV	right ventricle	TURP	transurethral resection of prostate
PML	progressive multifocal leukoencephalopathy	RVOT	right ventricular outflow tract		
		Rx	therapy	TV	tidal volume
pML	posterior mitral valve leaflet				
PMN	polymorphonuclear	S/P	status post	UGI	upper gastrointestinal series
PMT	photomultiplier tube	SAE	subcortical arteriosclerotic encephalopathy	UIP	usual interstitial pneumonia
PNET	primitive neuroectodermal tumor			UL	upper lobe
		SAG	sagittal	UPJ	ureteropelvic junction
POST	posterior	SAM	systolic anterior motion of mitral valve	US	ultrasound
PPG	photoplethysmography			USP XX	United States Pharmacopeia, 20th edition
PPLO	pleuropneumonia-like organism	SANA	sinoatrial node artery		
ppm	posterior papillary muscle	SBE	subacute bacterial endocarditis	UTI	urinary tract infection
PS	pulmonary stenosis	SD	standard deviation	UVJ	ureterovesical junction
PSS	progressive systemic sclerosis	SE	spin echo		
PTC	percutaneous transhepatic cholangiography	SGA	small for gestational age	VC	vital capacity
		sHPT	secondary hyperparathyroidism	VIP	vasoactive intestinal peptides
PTH	parathyroid hormone	SIJ	sacroiliac joint	VMA	vanillylmandelic acid
pTL	posterior tricuspid valve leaflet	SFA	superficial femoral artery	V/Q	ventilation perfusion
PTU	propylthiouracil	SLE	systemic lupus erythematosus	VS	interventricular septum
PVC	polyvinyl chloride	SMA	superior mesenteric artery	VSD	ventricular septal defect
PVE	periventricular echogenicity	SMV	superior mesenteric vein		
PVH	pulmonary venous hypertension	Sn	stannum	WBC	white blood cells
		SONK	spontaneous osteonecrosis of knee	WDHA	watery diarrhea, hypokalemia, achlorhydria
PVL	periventricular leukomalacia				
PVNS	pigmented villonodular synovitis	S/P	status post	WDHH	watery diarrhea, hypokalemia, hypochlorhydria
		SPECT	single photon emission		
PYP	pyrophosphate	STIR	short tau inversion recovery	XGP	xanthogranulomatous pyelonephritis

DIFFERENTIAL DIAGNOSIS OF MUSCULOSKELETAL DISORDERS

Differential-diagnostic gamut of bone disorders

Conditions to be considered = "dissect bone disease with a DIATTOM"

Dysplasia + **D**ystrophy
Infection
Anomalies of development
Tumor + tumorlike conditions
Trauma
Osteochondritis + ischemic necrosis
Metabolic disease

DYSPLASIA   = disturbance of bone growth
DYSTROPHY   = disturbance of nutrition

BONE SCLEROSIS
Constitutional sclerosing bone disease
1. Engelmann-Camurati disease
2. Infantile cortical hyperostosis
3. Melorheostosis
4. Osteopathia striata
5. Osteopetrosis
6. Osteopoikilosis
7. Pachydermoperiostosis
8. Pyknodysostosis
9. Van Buchem disease
10. Williams syndrome

Diffuse osteosclerosis
mnemonic: "MARBLE"
Myelosclerosis, **M**astocytosis, **M**etabolic: hypervitaminosis D, fluorosis, hypothyroidism, phosphorus poisoning
Anemia (sickle cell)
Renal osteodystrophy
Blastic metastases
Lymphoma
Enigmas: Paget disease, osteopetrosis, melorheostosis, pyknodysostosis, tuberous sclerosis

Solitary osteosclerotic lesion
A. DEVELOPMENTAL
   1. Bone island
B. VASCULAR
   1. Old bone infarct
   2. Aseptic / ischemic / avascular necrosis
C. HEALING BONE LESION
   (a) <u>trauma</u>: Callus formation
   (b) <u>benign tumor</u>: fibrous cortical defect / nonossifying fibroma, brown tumor; bone cyst
   (c) <u>malignant tumor</u>: lytic metastasis after radiation, chemo-, hormone therapy
D. INFECTION / INFLAMMATION
   (low-grade chronic infection / healing infection)
   1. Osteoid osteoma

2. Chronic / healed osteomyelitis: bacterial, tuberculous, fungal
3. Sclerosing osteomyelitis of Garré
4. Granuloma
5. Brodie abscess
E. BENIGN TUMOR
   1. Osteoma
   2. Ossifying fibroma
   3. Enchondroma / osteochondroma
   4. Osteoblastoma
F. MALIGNANT TUMOR
   1. Osteoblastic metastasis (prostate, breast)
   2. Lymphoma
   3. Sarcoma: osteo-, chondro-, Ewing sarcoma
G. OTHERS
   1. Sclerotic phase of Paget disease
   2. Fibrous dysplasia

Multiple osteosclerotic lesions
A. FAMILIAL
   1. Osteopoikilosis
   2. Enchondromatosis = Ollier disease
   3. Melorheostosis
   4. Multiple osteomas: associated with Gardner syndrome
   5. Osteopetrosis
   6. Pyknodysostosis
   7. Osteopathia striata
   8. Chondrodystrophia calcificans congenita = congenital stippled epiphyses
   9. Multiple epiphyseal dysplasia = Fairbank disease
B. SYSTEMIC DISEASE
   1. Mastocytosis = urticaria pigmentosa
   2. Tuberous sclerosis

Dense metaphyseal bands
mnemonic: "**H**eavy **C**retins **S**ift **S**currilously through **R**ickety **S**ystems"
Heavy metal poisoning (lead, bismuth, phosphorus)
Cretinism
Syphilis, congenital
Scurvy
Rickets (healed)
Systemic illness
also: normal variant; methotrexate therapy

mnemonic: "DENSE LINES"
D-vitamin intoxication
Elemental arsenic, bismuth, phosphorus
Normal variant
Systemic illness
Estrogen to mother during pregnancy
Leukemia, **L**ead poisoning
Infection (TORCH), **I**diopathic hypercalcemia

Never forget rickets
Early hypothyroidism
Scurvy, **S**ickle cell disease

Bone-within-bone appearance
= endosteal new bone formation
1. Normal
   (a) thoracic + lumbar vertebrae (in infants)
   (b) growth recovery lines (after infancy)
2. Infantile cortical hyperostosis (Caffey)
3. Sickle cell disease / thalassemia
4. Congenital syphilis
5. Osteopetrosis / oxalosis
6. Radiation
7. Acromegaly
8. Paget disease

OSTEOPENIA
= decrease in bone density
Categories: 1. Osteoporosis = decreased osteoid
                    production
              2. Osteomalacia = undermineralization of
                    osteoid
              3. Hyperparathyroidism
              4. Multiple myeloma / diffuse metastases

Osteoporosis
= reduced bone mass of normal composition secondary
   to (a) osteoclastic resorption (85%) (trabecular,
   endosteal, intracortical, subperiosteal) (b) osteocytic
   resorption (15%)
Incidence: 7% of all women between ages 35 – 40
               years; 1 in 3 women > age 65 years
Etiology:
A. <u>Congenital disorders</u>
   1. Osteogenesis imperfecta (the only
      osteoporosis with bending)
   2. Homocystinuria
B. <u>Idiopathic</u> (bone loss begins earlier + proceeds
   more rapidly in women)
   1. Juvenile osteoporosis: <20 years
   2. Adult osteoporosis: 20 – 40 years
   3. Postmenopausal osteoporosis: >50 years
   4. Senile osteoporosis: >60 years
      progressively decreasing bone density at a rate
      of 8% in females; 3% in males
C. <u>Nutritional disturbances</u>
   scurvy; protein deficiency (malnutrition, nephrosis,
   chronic liver disease, alcoholism, anorexia
   nervosa, kwashiorkor, starvation), calcium
   deficiency
D. <u>Endocrinopathy</u>
   Cushing disease, hypogonadism (Turner
   syndrome, eunuchoidism), hyperthyroidism,
   hyperparathyroidism, acromegaly, Addison
   disease, diabetes mellitus, pregnancy
E. <u>Renal osteodystrophy</u>
   decrease / same / increase in spinal trabecular
   bone; rapid loss in appendicular skeleton
F. <u>Immobilization</u> = disuse osteoporosis

Scurvy
Prot. def.
Calc. def.

G. <u>Collagen disease, rheumatoid arthritis</u>
H. <u>Bone marrow replacement</u>
   infiltration by lymphoma / leukemia, multiple
   myeloma, diffuse metastases, marrow hyperplasia
   secondary to hemolytic anemia
I. <u>Drug therapy</u>
   heparin (15,000 – 30,000 U for >6 months),
   methotrexate, corticosteroids, vitamin A
J. <u>Radiation therapy</u>
K. <u>Localized osteoporosis</u>
   Sudeck dystrophy, transient osteoporosis of hip,
   regional migratory osteoporosis of lower
   extremities

• serum calcium, phosphorus, alkaline phosphatase
  frequently normal
• hydroxyproline may be elevated during acute stage
Technique:
(1) Single photon absorptiometry
     measures primarily cortical bone of appendicular
     bones, single-energy I-125 radioisotope source
     Site: distal radius (= wrist bone density), os
             calcis
     Dose: 2 – 3 mrem; Precision: 1 – 3%
(2) Dual photon absorptiometry
     radioactive energy source with two photon peaks;
     should be reserved for patients < 65 years of age
     because of interference from osteophytosis +
     vascular calcifications
     Site: vertebrae, femoral neck
     Dose: 5 – 10 mrem; Precision: 2 – 4%
(3) Quantitative computed tomography
     high-turnover cancellous bone + low-turnover
     compact bone can be measured separately
     Site: vertebrae L1 – L3, other sites
     (a) single energy: 300 – 500 mrem;
                          6 – 25% precision
     (b) dual energy : 750 – 800 mrem;
                          5 – 10% precision
(4) Dual energy radiography = quantitative digital
     radiography = dual energy x-ray absorptiometry
     x-ray tube produces a two-peak energy spectrum
     Site: vertebrae, femoral neck
     Dose: <3 mrem; Precision:1 – 2%
Δ radiographs are insensitive prior to bone loss of 25
  – 30%
Δ bone scans do NOT show a diffuse increase in
  activity

Location: axial skeleton (lower dorsal + lumbar spine),
            proximal humerus, neck of femur, wrist, ribs
√ decreased number + thickness of trabeculae
√ cortical thinning (endosteal + intracortical resorption)
√ juxtaarticular osteopenia with trabecular bone
  predominance
√ delayed fracture healing with poor callus formation
  (DDx: abundant callus formation in osteogenesis
  imperfecta + Cushing syndrome)
@ Spine
  √ diminished radiographic density

To read Vit D metabolism.

√ vertical striations (= marked thinning of transverse trabeculae with relative accentuation of vertical trabeculae along lines of stress)
√ prominence of endplates
√ "picture framing" (= accentuation of cortical outline with preservation of external dimensions secondary to endosteal + intracortical resorption)
√ compression deformities with protrusion of intervertebral discs
   √ biconcave vertebrae
   √ Schmorl nodes
   √ wedging
   √ decreased height of vertebrae
√ absence of osteophytes

Cx: (1) compression fractures of lower dorsal + lumbar spine
       (2) complete fractures of extremities (ribs, hips, wrists)

Rx: calcitonin, sodium fluoride, diphosphonates, parathyroid hormone supplements, estrogen replacement

Osteomalacia

= accumulation of excessive amounts of uncalcified osteoid with bone softening + insufficient mineralization of osteoid due to
(a) high remodeling rate: excessive osteoid formation + normal / little mineralization
(b) low remodeling rate: normal osteoid production + diminished mineralization

Etiology:

diet   (1) dietary deficiency of vitamin D_3 + lack of solar irradiation
metabolism   (2) deficiency of metabolism of vitamin D:
      — chronic renal tubular disease
      — chronic administration of phenobarbital (alternate liver pathway)
      — diphenylhydantoin (interferes with vitamin D action on bowel)
absorption   (3) decreased absorption of vitamin D:
      — malabsorption syndromes (most common)
      — partial gastrectomy (self-restriction of fatty foods)
↓ *depo.* Ca^{++} (4) decreased deposition of calcium in bone
      — diphosphonates (for treatment of Paget disease)

Histo: excess of osteoid seams + decreased appositional rate

• bone pain / tenderness
• muscular weakness
• serum calcium slightly low / normal
• decreased serum phosphorus
• elevated serum alkaline phosphatase

√ uniform osteopenia
√ fuzzy indistinct trabecular detail of endosteal surface

Looser's zones.

√ thin cortices of long bone
√ coarsened frayed trabeculae decreased in number + size
√ bone deformity from softening: hourglass thorax, bowing of long bones, buckled / compressed pelvis
√ increased incidence of fractures, biconcave vertebral bodies
√ mottled skull
√ pseudofractures - *Looser's zones*

Localized osteopenia

1. Disuse atrophy
   Etiology: local immobilization secondary to
         (1) fracture (more pronounced distal to fracture site)
         (2) neural paralysis
         (3) muscular paralysis
2. Reflex sympathetic dystrophy = Sudeck dystrophy
3. Regional migratory osteoporosis, transient osteoporosis of hip
4. Osteolytic tumor
5. Lytic phase of Paget disease
6. Inflammation: rheumatoid arthritis, osteomyelitis, tuberculosis
7. Early phase of bone infarct and hemorrhage
8. Burns + frostbite

Transverse lucent metaphyseal lines

mnemonic: "LINING"
Leukemia
Illness, systemic (rickets, scurvy)
Normal variant
Infection, transplacental (congenital syphilis)
Neuroblastoma metastases
Growth lines

OSTEOLYSIS

1. Acroosteolysis
2. Massive osteolysis
3. Essential osteolysis   *Gorham's disease.*
4. Ainhum disease

Familial idiopathic acroosteolysis
terminal + more proximal

= HAJDU-CHENEY SYNDROME
rare bizarre entity of unknown etiology;
may be unilateral

• fingernails remain intact; sensory changes + plantar ulcers rare

√ pseudoclubbing of fingers + toes with osteolysis of terminal + more proximal phalanges
√ multiple skeletal anomalies: genu varum / valgum, hypoplasia of proximal end of radius, subluxation of radial head, scaphocephaly, wide sutures, persistent metopic suture, Wormian bones, basilar impression, poorly developed sinuses, kyphoscoliosis, severe osteoporosis + fractures at multiple sites (esp. of spine), protrusio acetabuli

Acquired acroosteolysis   *Distal + middle*
Causes:

Burns; frostbite; electric shock; PVC; syringomyelia; diabetes; congenital insensitivity to pain; leprosy; Raynaud disease; thrombangitis obliterans; collagen disease; sarcoidosis; psoriasis; yaws; Ehlers-Danlos syndrome; HPT; Kaposi sarcoma; progeria; pyknodysostosis; pachydermoperiostosis

mnemonic: "PETER's DIAPER SPLASH"
Psoriasis, **P**orphyria
Ehlers-Danlos syndrome
Thrombangitis obliterans
Ergot therapy
Raynaud disease
Diabetes, **D**ermatomyositis, **D**ilantin therapy
Injury (burns, frostbite)
Arteriosclerosis
PVC worker
Epidermolysis bullosa
Rheumatoid arthritis, **R**eiter syndrome
Sarcoidosis
Progeria, **P**yknodysostosis
Leprosy, **L**esch-Nyhan syndrome
Absence of pain
Scleroderma
Hyperparathyroidism

√ lytic destructive process involving distal + middle phalanges
√ NO periosteal reaction
√ epiphyses resist osteolysis until late

Frayed metaphyses
mnemonic: "CHARMS"
Congenital infections (rubella, syphilis)
Hypophosphatasia
Achondroplasia
Rickets
Metaphyseal dysostosis
Scurvy

PERIOSTEAL REACTION
1. Trauma, hemophilia
2. Infection
3. Inflammatory: arthritis
4. Neoplasm
5. Congenital: physiologic in newborn
6. Metabolic: hypertrophic osteoarthropathy, thyroid acropachy, hypervitaminosis A
7. Vascular: venous stasis

Solid periosteal reaction
= reaction to periosteal irritant
√ even + uniform thickness >1 mm
√ persistent + unchanged for weeks
Patterns:
(a) thin: eosinophilic granuloma, osteoid osteoma
(b) dense undulating: vascular disease
(c) thin undulating: pulmonary osteoarthropathy

(d) dense elliptical: osteoid osteoma; long-standing malignant disease (with destruction)
(e) cloaking: storage disease; chronic infection

Interrupted periosteal reaction
= pleomorphic, rapidly progressing process undergoing constant change
(a) lamellated = "onion skin": acute osteomyelitis; malignant tumor (osteosarcoma, Ewing sarcoma)
(b) perpendicular = "sunburst": osteosarcoma; Ewing sarcoma; chondrosarcoma; fibrosarcoma; leukemia; metastasis; acute osteomyelitis
(c) amorphous: malignancy (deposits may represent extension of tumor / periosteal response); osteosarcoma
(d) Codman triangle: hemorrhage; malignancy (osteosarcoma, Ewing sarcoma); acute osteomyelitis; fracture

Symmetric periosteal reaction in adulthood   *VHP FT*
1. Vascular insufficiency (lower extremity)
2. Hypertrophic osteoarthropathy
3. Pachydermoperiostosis
4. Thyroid acropachy
5. Fluorosis

Periosteal reaction in childhood
(a) benign
   1. Physiologic (up to 35%): symmetric involvement of diaphyses during first 1 – 6 months of life
   2. Battered child syndrome
   3 Infantile cortical hyperostosis <6 months of age
   4. Hypervitaminosis A
   5. Scurvy
   6. Osteogenesis imperfecta
   7. Congenital syphilis
(b) malignant
   1. Multicentric osteosarcoma
   2. Metastases from neuroblastoma + retinoblastoma
   3. Acute leukemia

mnemonic: "SCALP"
Scurvy, **S**yphilis
Caffey disease, **C**hild abuse   *Cong. syphilis*
Accident, **A**-hypervitaminosis
Leukemia
Physiologic, *Battered baby & OI*

BONE TUMOR
Age incidence of malignant bone tumors
80% of bone tumors are correctly determined on the basis of age alone!

Age (years)	Tumor
0.1	Neuroblastoma
0.1 – 10	Ewing tumor in tubular bones (diaphysis)

Average Age for Occurrence of Benign and Malignant Bone Tumors

10 – 30	Osteosarcoma (metaphysis); Ewing tumor in flat bones
30 – 40	Reticulum cell sarcoma (similar histology to Ewing tumor); fibrosarcoma; malignant giant cell tumor (similar histology to fibrosarcoma); parosteal sarcoma; lymphoma
>40	Metastatic carcinoma; multiple myeloma; chondrosarcoma

SARCOMAS BY AGE:
mnemonic: "**E**very **O**ther **R**unner **F**eels **C**rampy **P**ain **O**n **M**oving"

Ewing sarcoma	0 – 10 years
Osteogenic sarcoma	10 – 30 years
Reticulum cell sarcoma	20 – 40 years
Fibrosarcoma	20 – 40 years
Chondrosarcoma	40 – 50 years
Parosteal sarcoma	40 – 50 years
Osteosarcoma	60 – 70 years
Metastases	60 – 70 years

ROUND CELL TUMORS:
arise in midshaft; osteolytic; reactive new bone formation; no tumor new bone
mnemonic: "LEMON"
Leukemia, **L**ymphoma
Ewing sarcoma, **E**osinophilic granuloma
Multiple myeloma
√ **O**steomyelitis   mimics RC Tumors.
Neuroblastoma

MALIGNANCY WITH SOFT-TISSUE INVOLVEMENT
mnemonic: "**M**y **M**other **E**ats **C**hocolate **F**udge **O**ften"
Metastasis
Myeloma
Ewing sarcoma
Chondrosarcoma
Fibrosarcoma
Osteosarcoma

Tumor matrix
Cartilage-forming tumors
A. BENIGN
    1. Enchondroma
    2. Parosteal chondroma
    3. Chondroblastoma
    4. Chondromyxoid fibroma
    5. Osteochondroma
B. MALIGNANT
    1. Chondrosarcoma
√   centrally located ring-like / flocculent / fleck-like radiodensities

Bone-forming tumors
A. BENIGN
    1. Osteoma
    2. Osteoid osteoma
    3. Osteoblastoma
    4. Ossifying fibroma
B. MALIGNANT
    1. Osteogenic sarcoma
√   inhomogeneous / homogeneous radiodense collections of variable size + extent

Fibrous connective tissue tumors
A. BENIGN
    1. Nonossifying fibroma
    2. Periosteal desmoid = avulsive cortical irregularity
    3. Desmoplastic fibroma
B. MALIGNANT
    1. Fibrosarcoma

BENIGN FIBROUS BONE LESIONS
  (a) cortical
    1. Benign cortical defect
    2. Avulsion cortical irregularity
  (b) medullary
    1. Herniation pit
    2. Nonossifying fibroma
    3. Ossifying fibroma
    4. Congenital generalized fibromatosis
  (c) corticomedullary
    1. Nonossifying fibroma
    2. Ossifying fibroma
    3. Fibrous dysplasia
    4. Cherubism
    5. Desmoplastic fibroma
    6. Fibromyxoma

Tumors of histiocytic origin
A. LOCALLY AGGRESSIVE
    1. Giant cell tumor
    2. Benign fibrous histiocytoma
B. MALIGNANT
    1. Malignant fibrous histiocytoma

Tumors of fatty tissue origin
A. BENIGN
    1. Intraosseous lipoma
    2. Parosteal lipoma
B. MALIGNANT
    1. Intraosseous liposarcoma

Tumors of vascular origin
<1% of all bone tumors
A. BENIGN
    1. Hemangioma
    2. Glomus tumor
    3. Lymphangioma
    4. Cystic angiomatosis
    5. Hemangiopericytoma
B. MALIGNANT
    1. Malignant hemangiopericytoma
    2. Angiosarcoma = hemangioendothelioma
       Metastatic sites: lung, brain, lymph nodes, other bones

Tumors of neural origin
A. BENIGN
1. Solitary neurofibroma
2. Neurilemoma
B. MALIGNANT
1. Neurogenic sarcoma = malignant schwannoma

Pattern of bone destruction
A. Geographic bone destruction:
Indicative of slow-growing usually benign tumor
√ well-defined smooth / irregular margin
√ short zone of transition

B. Moth-eaten bone destruction
Indicative of more rapid growth as in malignant bone tumor / osteomyelitis
√ less well-defined / demarcated lesional margin
√ longer zone of transition
mnemonic: "H LEMMON"
Histiocytosis X
Lymphoma
Ewing sarcoma
Metastasis
Multiple myeloma
Osteomyelitis
Neuroblastoma

C. Permeative bone destruction
Aggressive bone lesion with rapid growth potential (eg, Ewing sarcoma)
√ poorly demarcated lesion imperceptibly merging with uninvolved bone
√ long zone of transition

D. Size of lesion
Primary malignant tumors are larger than benign tumors
E. Elongated lesion   *CARE*
√ greatest lesional diameter is >1 1/2 times the least diameter
CARE → { Ewing sarcoma, reticulum cell sarcoma, chondrosarcoma, angiosarcoma

Tumor position in transverse plane
A. CENTRAL MEDULLARY LESION
1. Enchondroma   *SE*
2. Solitary bone cyst
B. ECCENTRIC MEDULLARY LESION   *OCQ*
1. Giant cell tumor
2. Osteogenic sarcoma, chondrosarcoma, fibrosarcoma
3. Chondromyxoid fibroma
C. CORTICAL LESION   *ON*
1. Nonossifying fibroma
2. Osteoid osteoma
D. PAROSTEAL / JUXTACORTICAL LESION
1. Juxtacortical chondroma   *JOP.*
2. Osteochondroma
3. Parosteal osteogenic sarcoma

Tumor position in longitudinal plane
A. EPIPHYSEAL LESION
1. Chondroblastoma   *GIC*
2. Intraosseous ganglion
3. Giant cell tumor (originating in metaphysis)
mnemonic: "DELCO"
Degenerative
Enchondroma
Lipoma
Cyst, **C**hondroblastoma
Osteomyelitis
B. METAPHYSEAL LESION
1. Nonossifying fibroma   *CM BOOS*
2. Chondromyxoid fibroma
3. Solitary bone cyst
4. Osteochondroma
5. Brodie abscess
6. Osteogenic sarcoma, chondrosarcoma
C. DIAPHYSEAL LESION
1. Round cell tumor (eg, Ewing sarcoma)
2. Nonossifying fibroma
3. Solitary bone cyst   *RSNA OFE*
4. Aneurysmal bone cyst
5. Enchondroma
6. Osteoblastoma
7. Fibrous dysplasia
mnemonic: "FEMALE"
Fibrous dysplasia
Eosinophilic granuloma
Metastasis
Adamantinoma
Leukemia, **L**ymphoma
Ewing sarcoma

Tumor-like conditions
1. Solitary bone cyst
2. Juxtaarticular ("synovial") cyst
3. Aneurysmal bone cyst
4. Nonossifying fibroma; cortical defect; cortical desmoid
5. Eosinophilic granuloma
6. Reparative giant cell granuloma
7. Fibrous dysplasia (monostotic; polyostotic)
8. Myositis ossificans
9. "Brown tumor" of hyperparathyroidism
10. Massive osteolysis

INTRAOSSEOUS LESION

Bubbly bone lesion   *Soap bubble appearance*
mnemonic: "FOG MACHINES"
Fibrous dysplasia, **F**ibrous cortical defect
Osteoblastoma
Giant cell tumor
Myeloma (plasmacytoma), **M**etastases from kidney, thyroid, breast
Aneurysmal bone cyst / **A**ngioma
Chondromyxoid fibroma, **C**hondroblastoma
Histiocytosis X, **H**yperparathyroid brown tumor, **H**emophilia

Infection (Brodie abscess, echinococcus,
  coccidioidomycosis)
Nonossifying fibroma
Enchondroma, **E**pithelial inclusion cyst
Simple unilocular bone cyst

Infectious bubbly lesion
1. Brodie abscess (Staph. aureus)
2. Coccidioidomycosis
3. Echinococcus
4. Atypical mycobacterium
5. Cystic tuberculosis

Blow out lesion
A. METASTASES
   Carcinoma of thyroid, kidney, breast
B. PRIMARY BONE TUMOR
   1. Fibrosarcoma
   2. Multiple myeloma (sometimes)
   3. Aneurysmal bone cyst
   4. Hemophilic pseudotumor

Nonexpansile unilocular well-demarcated bone defect
1. Fibrous cortical defect
2. Nonossifying fibroma
3. Simple unicameral bone cyst
4. Giant cell tumor
5. Brown tumor of HPT
6. Eosinophilic granuloma
7. Enchondroma
8. Epidermoid inclusion cyst
9. Posttraumatic / degenerative cyst
10. Pseudotumor of hemophilia
11. Intraosseous ganglion
12. Histiocytoma
13. Arthritic lesion
14. Endosteal pigmented villonodular synovitis
15. Fibrous dysplasia
16. Infectious lesion

Nonexpansile multilocular well-demarcated bone defect
1. Aneurysmal bone cyst
2. Giant cell tumor
3. Fibrous dysplasia
4. Simple bone cyst

Expansile unilocular well-demarcated bone defect
1. Simple unicameral bone cyst
2. Enchondroma
3. Aneurysmal bone cyst
4. Juxtacortical chondroma
5. Nonossifying fibroma
6. Eosinophilic granuloma
7. Brown tumor of HPT

Poorly demarcated osteolytic lesion without periosteal reaction
A. NONEXPANSILE
   1. Metastases from any primary
   2. Multiple myeloma
   3. Hemangioma
B. EXPANSILE
   1. Chondrosarcoma
   2. Giant cell tumor
   3. Metastasis from kidney / thyroid

Poorly demarcated osteolytic lesion + periosteal reaction
1. Osteomyelitis
2. Ewing sarcoma
3. Osteosarcoma

Mixed sclerotic and lytic lesion
A. WITH SEQUESTRUM
   1. Osteomyelitis
B. WITHOUT SEQUESTRUM
   1. Osteomyelitis
   2. Tuberculosis
   3. Ewing sarcoma
   4. Metastasis
   5. Osteosarcoma

Marked sclerosis surrounding osteolysis - *O'penia* ✓
1. Osteoid osteoma
2. Benign osteoblastoma
3. Chronic osteomyelitis
4. Tuberculosis

Trabeculated bone lesion
1. Giant cell tumor: delicate thin trabeculae
2. Chondromyxoid fibroma: coarse thick trabeculae
3. Nonossifying fibroma: loculated
4. Aneurysmal bone cyst: delicate, horizontally oriented trabeculae
5. Hemangioma: striated radiating trabeculae

Lytic lesion on both sides of joint
mnemonic: "SAC"
   Synovioma
   Angioma
   Chondroid lesion

Multiple lytic lesions
mnemonic: "FEEMHI"
   Fibrous dysplasia
   Enchondromas
   Eosinophilic granuloma
   Metastases, **M**ultiple myeloma
   Hyperparathyroidism (brown tumors), **H**emangiomas
   Infection

DWARFISM
Micromelic dwarfism
= disproportionate shortening of entire leg
A. Mild micromelic dwarfism
  1. Jeune syndrome
  2. Ellis-van Creveld syndrome
      = chondroectodermal dysplasia
  3. Diastrophic dwarfism
B. Mild bowed micromelic dwarfism
  1. Camptomelic dysplasia
  2. Osteogenesis imperfecta, type III
C. Severe micromelic dwarfism
  1. Thanatophoric dysplasia
  2. Homozygous achondroplasia
  3. Osteogenesis imperfecta, type II
  4. Achondrogenesis
  5. Hypophosphatasia
  6. Short-rib polydactyly syndrome

Acromelic dwarfism
= distal shortening (hands, feet)
  1. Asphyxiating thoracic dysplasia

Mesomelic dwarfism
= shortening of intermediate segments (radius + ulna or tibia + fibula)
  1. Langer syndrome: autosomal recessive
  2. Nievergelt syndrome: autosomal dominant
  3. Reinhardt syndrome: autosomal dominant
  4. Robinow syndrome: autosomal dominant
  5. Werner syndrome: autosomal dominant

Rhizomelic dwarfism
= shortening of proximal segments (humerus, femur)
  1. Heterozygous achondroplasia
  2. Chondrodysplasia punctata, rhizomelic type

Lethal dwarfism
  1. Achondrogenesis
  2. Thanatophoric dwarfism
  3. Achondroplasia (homozygous)
  4. Osteogenesis imperfecta (congenital)
  5. Chondrodysplasia punctata (recessive)

Nonlethal dwarfism
  1. Achondroplasia (heterozygous)
  2. Asphyxiating thoracic dysplasia
  3. Chondroectodermal dysplasia
  4. Chondrodysplasia punctata
  5. Spondyloepiphyseal dysplasia (congenital)
  6. Diastrophic dwarfism
  7. Metatrophic dwarfism
  8. Hypochondroplasia

Late onset dwarfism
  1. Spondyloepiphyseal dysplasia tarda
  2. Multiple epiphyseal dysplasia
  3. Pseudoachondroplasia
  4. Metaphyseal chondrodysplasia

  5. Dyschondrosteosis
  6. Cleidocranial dysplasia
  7. Progressive diaphyseal dysplasia

Osteochondrodysplasia
A. Failure of
  (a) articular cartilage: spondyloepiphyseal dysplasia
  (b) ossification center: multiple epiphyseal dysplasia
  (c) proliferating cartilage: achondroplasia
  (d) spongiosa formation: hypophosphatasia
  (e) spongiosa absorption: osteopetrosis
  (f) periosteal bone: osteogenesis imperfecta
  (g) endosteal bone: idiopathic osteoporosis
B. Excess of
  (a) articular cartilage: dysplasia epiphysealis hemimelica
  (b) hypertrophic cartilage: enchondromatosis
  (c) spongiosa: multiple exostosis
  (d) periosteal bone: progressive diaphyseal dysplasia
  (e) endosteal bone: hyperphosphatemia

LIMB REDUCTION ANOMALIES
Amelia   = absence of limb
Hemimelia   = absence of distal parts
Phocomelia = proximal reduction with distal parts attached to trunk

Aplasia / hypoplasia of radius
mnemonic: "**The Furry Cat Hit My Dog**"
  Thrombocytopenia absent radius syndrome
  Fanconi anemia
  Cornelia de Lange syndrome
  Holt-Oram syndrome
  Myositis ossificans progressiva (thumb only)
  Diastrophic dwarfism

Pubic bone maldevelopment
mnemonic: "**CHIEF**"
  Cleidocranial dysostosis
  Hypospadia, epispadia
  Idiopathic
  Extrophy of bladder
  F for syringomyelia

BONE OVERGROWTH
Bone overdevelopment
  1. Marfan syndrome
  2. Klippel-Trenaunay syndrome
  3. Macrodystrophia lipomatosa

Erlenmeyer flask deformity
= expansion of distal end of long bones, usually femur
  1. Gaucher disease, Niemann-Pick disease
  2. Rickets
  3. Anemias
  4. Fibrous dysplasia

5. Osteopetrosis
6. Heavy metal poisoning
7. Metaphyseal dysplasia
8. Down syndrome
9. Achondroplasia
10. Rheumatoid arthritis

mnemonic: "TOP DOG"
　Thalassemia
　Osteopetrosis
　Pyle disease
　Diaphyseal aclasis
　Ollier disease
　Gaucher disease

JOINTS
Signs of arthritis
Prevalence of arthritis: 15% of population in United
　　　　　　　　　　　　　States
Conventional X-ray:
　√ narrowing of radiologic joint space
　　(a) uniform = inflammatory arthritis
　　(b) nonuniform = degenerative arthritis
　√ evidence of disease on both sides of joint:
　　√ osteopenia
　　√ subchondral sclerosis
　　√ erosion
　　√ subchondral cyst formation
　　√ malalignment
　√ joint effusion
　√ joint bodies
NUC:
　√ increase in regional blood flow (active disease)
　√ distribution of disease
MR:
　√ irregularity + narrowing of articular cartilage
　√ joint effusion
　√ Gd-DTPA enhancement of synovium (active
　　disease)

Classification of arthritides
A. BACTERIAL ARTHRITIS
　1. Tuberculous
　2. Pyogenic
　3. Lyme arthritis
B. ARTHRITIS OF COLLAGEN / COLLAGEN-LIKE
　　DISEASE
　1. Rheumatoid arthritis
　2. Ankylosing spondylitis
　3. Psoriatic arthritis
　4. Rheumatic fever
　5. Sarcoidosis
C. BIOCHEMICAL ARTHRITIS
　1. Gout
　2. Chondrocalcinosis
　3. Ochronosis
　4. Hemophilic arthritis
D. DEGENERATIVE JOINT DISEASE = Osteoarthritis
E. TRAUMATIC
　1. Secondary osteoarthritis

2. Neurotrophic arthritis
3. Pigmented villonodular synovitis
F. ARTHRITIS OF INFLAMMATORY BOWEL
　　DISEASE
　1. Ulcerative colitis (in 10 – 20%)
　2. Crohn disease (in 5%)
　　peripheral arthritis increases with colonic disease
　3. Whipple disease (in 60 – 90% transient
　　intermittent polyarthritis: sacroiliitis, spondylitis)
　Δ Resection of diseased bowel is associated with
　　regression of arthritic symptomatology!

SPONDYLOARTHRITIS + HLA-B 27
HISTOCOMPATIBILITY COMPLEX
positive testing in:
1. Ankylosing spondylitis 95%
2. Reiter disease 80%
3. Psoriatic spondylitis 70%
4. Arthropathy of inflammatory bowel disease 70%
5. Normal population 10%

Articular disorders of the hand + wrist
1. Osteoarthritis = degenerative joint disease
　= abnormal stress with minor + major traumatic
　　episodes
　target areas:　　DIP, PIP, 1st CMC,
　　　　　　　　　　trapezioscaphoid
　√ sclerosis + osteophytes
2. Erosive osteoarthritis = inflammatory osteoarthritis
　Age:　predominantly middle-aged /
　　　　　postmenopausal women
　• acute inflammatory episodes
　target areas:　DIP, PIP, 1st CMC,
　　　　　　　　　trapezioscaphoid
　√ subchondral "gull wing" erosions
　√ rare ankylosis
3. Psoriatic arthritis
　= rheumatoid variant / seronegative
　　spondyloarthropathy; peripheral manifestation in
　　monarthritis / asymmetric oligoarthritis / symmetric
　　polyarthritis
　target areas:　all hand + wrist joints (commonly
　　　　　　　　　distal)
　√ "mouse ears" marginal erosions
　√ new bone formation
4. Rheumatoid arthritis
　= synovial proliferative granulation tissue = pannus
　target areas:　　PIP, MCP, all wrist joints, ulnar
　　　　　　　　　　styloid
　√ marginal poorly defined erosions
　√ joint deformities
5. Gouty arthritis
　• monosodium urate crystals in synovial fluid
　• asymptomatic periods from months to years
　target areas:　　commonly CMC + all hand joints
　√ development of chronic tophaceous gout
　√ well-defined erosions with overhanging edge
　　(often periarticular)
　√ joint space narrowing

6. Calcium pyrophosphate dihydrate crystal deposition
   disease = CPPD
   target areas: MCP, radiocarpal
   √ chondrocalcinosis
   √ "degenerative changes" in unusual locations
   √ no erosions
7. SLE
   = myositis, symmetric polyarthritis, deforming
   nonerosive arthropathy, osteonecrosis
   target areas: PIP, MCP
   √ reversible deformities
8. Scleroderma = progressive systemic sclerosis
   (PSS)
   target areas: DIP, PIP, 1st CMC
   √ tuft resorption
   √ soft tissue calcifications

Arthritis with periostitis
1. Juvenile rheumatoid arthritis
2. Psoriatric arthritis
3. Reiter syndrome
4. Infectious arthritis

Arthritis with demineralization
mnemonic: "HORSE"
Hemophilia
Osteomyelitis
Rheumatoid arthritis, **R**eiter disease
Scleroderma
Erythematosus, systemic lupus

Arthritis without demineralization
1. Gout
2. Neuropathic arthropathy
3. Psoriasis
4. Reiter disease
5. Pigmented villonodular synovitis

Premature osteoarthritis
mnemonic: "COME CHAT"
Calcium pyrophosphate dihydrate arthropathy
Ochronosis
Marfan syndrome
Epiphyseal dysplasia
Charcot joint = neuroarthropathy
Hemophilic arthropathy
Acromegaly
Trauma

Arthritis of interphalangeal joint of great toe
1. Psoriatic arthritis
2. Reiter disease
3. Gout
4. Degenerative joint disease

Ankylosis of interphalangeal joints
mnemonic: "S - Lesions"
1. P**s**oriatic arthritis
2. Ankylo**s**ing spondylitis

3. Ero**s**ive osteoarthritis
4. **S**till disease

Loose intraarticular bodies
1. Osteochondrosis dissecans
2. Synovial osteochondromatosis
3. Chip fracture from trauma
4. Degenerative joint disease
5. Neuropathic arthropathy

Synovial disease with decreased signal intensity
= hemosiderin deposition
1. Pigmented villonodular synovitis
2. Rheumatoid arthritis
3. Hemophilia

Sacroiliitis
Anatomy:
   only anterior inferior aspect of sacroiliac apposition
   is covered with cartilage (1 mm thick hyalin cartilage
   on iliac side, 3 – 5 mm thick fibrous cartilage on
   sacral side); 2 – 5 mm normal joint width
Positioning: Ferguson view = AP projection with 23°
   angulation towards head
A. BILATERAL SYMMETRICAL:
   1. Ankylosing spondylitis
      √ small regular erosion = loss of definition of
        white cortical line on iliac side
      √ ankylosis
      √ ossification of intraosseous ligaments
   2. Rheumatoid arthritis (in late stages)
      √ joint space narrowing without reparation
      √ osteoporosis
      √ ankylosis may occur
   3. Deposition arthropathy: gout, CPPD,
      ochronosis, acromegaly
      √ slow loss of cartilage
      √ subchondral reparative bone + osteophytes
   4. Enteropathic
B. BILATERAL ASYMMETRICAL:
   1. Psoriatric arthritis
      √ large + extensive erosive + reparative process
      √ occasional ankylosis
   2. Reiter syndrome
   3. Juvenile rheumatoid arthritis
C. UNILATERAL:
   1. Infection
   2. Osteoarthritis from abnormal mechanical stress
      √ irregular narrowing of joint space with
        subchondral bone repair
      √ osteophytes at anterosuperior / -inferior
        aspect of joint (may resemble ankylosis)
DDx: Hyperparathyroidism
      √ subchondral bone resorption on iliac side
        resembling erosion + widening of joint

Protrusio acetabuli
= acetabular floor bulging into pelvis
√ crossing of medial + lateral components of pelvic
  "teardrop"

A. UNILATERAL
1. Tuberculous arthritis
2. Trauma
3. Fibrous dysplasia
B. BILATERAL
1. Rheumatoid arthritis
2. Paget disease
3. Osteomalacia

mnemonic: "PROT"
Paget disease
Rheumatoid arthritis
Osteomalacia (HPT)
Trauma

Subchondral cyst
= SYNOVIAL CYST = SUBARTICULAR PSEUDOCYST
= NECROTIC PSEUDOCYST = GEODES
Etiology: bone necrosis allows pressure-induced
intrusion of synovial fluid into subchondral
bone; in conditions with synovial
inflammation
Causes: (1) Osteoarthritis (2) Rheumatoid arthritis
(3) Osteonecrosis (4) CPPD
√ size of cyst usually 2 – 35 mm
√ may be large + expansile (especially in CPPD)
DDx: (1)   Giant cell tumor
(2)   Pigmented villonodular synovitis
(3)   Metastasis
(4)   Intraosseous ganglion
(5)   Hemophilia

Chondrocalcinosis
mnemonic: "WHIP A DOG"
Wilson disease
Hemochromatosis, **H**emophilia, **H**ypothyroidism,
1° **H**yperparathyroidism (15%), **H**ypophosphatasia,
Familial **H**ypomagnesemia
Idiopathic (aging)
Pseudogout (CPPD)
Arthritis (rheumatoid, postinfectious, traumatic,
degenerative), **A**myloidosis, **A**cromegaly
Diabetes mellitus
Ochronosis
Gout

Enthesopathy
Enthesis = osseous attachment of tendon composed
of 4 zones, ie, tendon itself + unmineralized
fibrocartilage + mineralized fibrocartilage + bone
Cause:
1. Degenerative disorder
2. Seronegative arthropathies: ankylosing
spondylitis, Reiter disease, psoriatic arthritis
3. Diffuse idiopathic skeletal hyperostosis
4. Acromegaly
5. Rheumatoid arthritis (occasionally)

Location: at site of tendon + ligament attachment

√ bone proliferation (enthesophyte)
√ calcification of tendon + ligament
√ erosion

EPIPHYSIS
Stippled epiphyses
1. Normal variant
2. Avascular necrosis
3. Hypothyroidism
4. Chondrodysplasia punctata
5. Multiple epiphyseal dysplasia
6. Spondyloepiphyseal dysplasia
7. Hypoparathyroidism
8. Down syndrome
9. Trisomy 18
10. Fetal warfarin syndrome
11. Homocystinuria (distal radial + ulnar epiphyses =
pathognomonic)
12. Zellweger cerebrohepatorenal syndrome

Epiphyseal overgrowth
1. Juvenile rheumatoid arthritis
2. Hemophilia
3. Healed Legg-Perthes disease
4. Tuberculous arthritis
5. Pyogenic arthritis (chronic)
6. Fungal arthritis
7. Epiphyseal dysplasia hemimelica
8. Fibrous dysplasia of epiphysis
9. Winchester syndrome

Ring epiphysis
1. Severe osteoporosis
2. Healing rickets
3. Scurvy

Epiphyseolysis
= SLIPPED EPIPHYSIS (zone of maturing
hypertrophic cartilage affected, not zone of
proliferation)

1. Idiopathic / juvenile epiphyseolysis
Age: 12 – 15 years (? puberty-related hormonal
dysregulation)
• adiposogenital type; tall stature
2. Renal osteodystrophy
3. Hyperparathyroidism in chronic renal disease
4. Hypothyroidism
5. Radiotherapy

Tibiotalar slanting
= downward slanting of medial tibial plafond
1. Hemophilia
2. Still disease
3. Sickle cell disease
4. Epiphyseal dysplasia
5. Trauma

TRAUMA
Trauma in childhood
1. Greenstick fracture
   = incomplete fracture of soft growing bone with intact periosteum
2. Bowing fracture
3. Traumatic epiphyseolysis
4. Battered child syndrome
5. Epiphyseal plate injury

Pseudarthrosis in long bones
1. Nonunion of fracture
2. Fibrous dysplasia
3. Neurofibromatosis
4. Osteogenesis imperfecta
5. Congenital: clavicular pseudarthrosis

Excessive callus formation
1. Steroid therapy / Cushing syndrome
2. Neuropathic arthropathy
3. Osteogenesis imperfecta
4. Congenital insensitivity to pain
5. Paralysis
6. Renal osteodystrophy
7. Multiple myeloma

WRIST & HAND

Resorption of terminal tufts
A. TRAUMA
   1. Amputation
   2. Burns, electric injury
   3. Frostbite
   4. Vinyl chloride poisoning
B. NEUROPATHIC
   1. Congenital indifference to pain
   2. Syringomyelia
   3. Myelomeningocele
   4. Diabetes mellitus
   5. Leprosy
C. COLLAGEN-VASCULAR DISEASE
   1. Scleroderma
   2. Dermatomyositis
   3. Raynaud disease
D. METABOLIC
   1. Hyperparathyroidism
E. INHERITED
   1. Familial acroosteolysis
   2. Pyknodysostosis
   3. Progeria = Werner syndrome
   4. Pachydermoperiostosis
F. OTHERS
   1. Sarcoidosis
   2. Psoriatic arthropathy
   3. Epidermolysis bullosa

Carpal angle
= angle of 130° formed by tangents to proximal row of carpal bones

A. DECREASED CARPAL ANGLE (<124°)
   1. Turner syndrome
   2. Hurler syndrome
   3. Morquio syndrome
   4. Madelung deformity
B. INCREASED CARPAL ANGLE (>139°)
   1. Down syndrome
   2. Arthrogryposis
   3. Bone dysplasia with epiphyseal involvement

Metacarpal sign
= tangent between 4th + 5th metacarpals intersects 3rd metacarpal = shortening of 4th metacarpal
1. Idiopathic
2. Gonadal dysgenesis: Turner syndrome, Klinefelter syndrome
3. Pseudo- and Pseudopseudohypoparathyroidism
4. Ectodermal dysplasia = Cornelia de Lange syndrome
5. Hereditary multiple exostoses
6. Peripheral dysostosis
7. Basal cell nevus syndrome
8. Melorheostosis

mnemonic: "**P**ing **P**ong **I**s **T**ough **T**o **T**each"
Pseudohypoparathyroidism
Pseudopseudohypoparathyroidism
Idiopathic
Trauma
Turner syndrome
Trisomy 13–18

Brachydactyly
= shortening / broadening of metacarpals ± phalanges
1. Idiopathic
2. Trauma
3. Osteomyelitis
4. Arthritis
5. Turner syndrome
6. Osteochondrodysplasia
7. Pseudohypoparathyroidism, Pseudopseudohypoparathyroidism
8. Mucopolysaccharidoses
9. Cornelia de Lange syndrome
10. Basal cell nevus syndrome
11. Hereditary multiple exostoses

Syndactyly
= osseous ± cutaneous fusion of digits
1. Apert syndrome
2. Carpenter syndrome
3. Down syndrome
4. Neurofibromatosis
5. Poland syndrome
6. Others

Polydactyly
Frequently associated with:
1. Carpenter syndrome
2. Ellis-van Creveld syndrome

3. Meckel-Gruber syndrome
4. Polysyndactyly syndrome
5. Short rib-polydactyly syndrome
6. Trisomy 13

Clinodactyly
= curvature of finger in mediolateral plane
1. Normal variant
2. Down syndrome
3. Multiple dysplasia
4. Trauma, arthritis, contractures

Lucent lesion in finger
A. BENIGN TUMOR
1. Giant cell tumor
2. Aneurysmal bone cyst
3. Brown tumor
4   Hemophilic pseudotumor
5. Epidermoid inclusion cyst
6   Glomus tumor
7. Solitary bone cyst
8. Osteoblastoma
9. Enchondroma
B. MALIGNANT TUMOR
1. Osteosarcoma
2. Fibrosarcoma
3. Metastasis from lung, breast, malignant melanoma

mnemonic: "GAMES PAGES"
Glomus tumor
Arthritis (gout, rheumatoid)
Metastasis (lung, breast)
Enchondroma
Simple cyst (inclusion)
Pancreatitis
Aneurysmal bone cyst
Giant cell tumor
Epidermoid
Sarcoid

Acroosteosclerosis
= focal opaque areas + endosteal thickening
1. Incidental in middle-aged women
2. Rheumatoid arthritis
3. Sarcoidosis
4. Scleroderma
5. Systemic lupus erythematosus
6. Hodgkin disease
7. Hematologic disorders

Fingertip calcifications
1. Scleroderma / CREST syndrome
2. Raynaud disease
3. Systemic lupus erythematosus
4. Dermatomyositis
5. Calcinosis circumscripta universalis
6. Hyperparathyroidism

RIBS

Rib lesions
A. BENIGN RIB LESION
1. Healing fracture
    (a) cough fractures: 4 – 9th rib in anterior axillary line
    (b) fatigue fracture: 1st rib (from carrying a heavy back pack)
2. Fibrous dysplasia (most common benign lesion)
    √ predominantly posterior location
3. Enchondroma: at costochondral / costovertebral junction
4. Osteochondroma: at costochondral / costovertebral junction
5. Eosinophilic granuloma
6. Osteomyelitis

B. MALIGNANT RIB LESION
1. Metastasis (most common malignant lesion)
2. Multiple myeloma
3. Chondrosarcoma
4. Osteosarcoma
5. Ewing sarcoma
6. Malignant lymphoma

Rib notching on inferior margin
A. VASCULAR
    (a) Aorta: coarctation, thrombosis
    (b) Subclavian artery: Blalock-Taussig shunt
    (c) Pulmonary artery: pulmonary stenosis, tetralogy of Fallot, absent pulmonary artery
    (d) AV fistula
    (e) Superior vena cava obstruction
B. NEUROGENIC
1. Intercostal neuroma
2. Neurofibromatosis
3. Poliomyelitis / quadriplegia / paraplegia
C. OSSEOUS
1. Hyperparathyroidism
2. Thalassemia
3. Melnick-Needles syndrome

Rib notching on superior margin
1. Rheumatoid arthritis
2. Scleroderma
3. Systemic lupus erythematosus
4. Hyperparathyroidism
5. Restrictive lung disease
6. Marfan syndrome

Ribbon ribs
1. Osteogenesis imperfecta
2. Neurofibromatosis

Bulbous enlargement of costochondral junction
1. Rachitic rosary
2. Scurvy
3. Achondroplasia

Wide ribs
1. Marrow hyperplasia (anemias)
2. Fibrous dysplasia
3. Paget disease
4. Achondroplasia
5. Mucopolysaccharidoses

Expansile rib lesion
mnemonic: "THELMA"
 Tuberculosis
 Hematopoiesis
 Eosinophilic granuloma, **E**wing sarcoma,
  Enchondroma
 Leukemia, **L**ymphoma
 Myeloma, **M**etastases
 Aneurysmal bone cyst

Short ribs
1. Achondroplasia
2. Achondrogenesis
3.. Thanatophoric dysplasia
4. Asphyxiating thoracic dysplasia
5. Mesomelic dwarfism
6. Short rib-polydactyly syndrome
7. Spondyloepiphyseal dysplasia
8. Enchondromatosis
9. Chondroectodermal dysplasia (Ellis-van Creveld)

Dense ribs
1. Osteopetrosis
2. Mastocytosis
3. Fluorosis

Hyperlucent ribs
1. Osteopetrosis
2. Cushing disease
3. Acromegaly
4. Scurvy

CLAVICLE
Absence of outer end of clavicle
1. Rheumatoid arthritis
2. Hyperparathyroidism
3. Posttraumatic osteolysis
4. Metastasis / multiple myeloma
5. Cleidocranial dysplasia

Penciled distal end of clavicle
mnemonic: "SHIRT Pocket"
 Scleroderma
 Hyperparathyroidism
 Infection
 Rheumatoid arthritis
 Trauma
 Progeria

Destruction of medial end of clavicle
mnemonic: "MILERS"
 Metastases

Infection
Lymphoma
Eosinophilic granuloma
Rheumatoid arthritis
Sarcoma

FOOT
Clubfoot
= Talipes equinovarus (talipes = inversion of foot along long axis; equinus = plantar flexion of ankle; metatarsus varus = lateral deviation of metatarsals)
1. Arthrogryposis multiplex congenita
2. Chondrodysplasia punctata
3. Neurofibromatosis
4. Spina bifida
5. Myelomeningocele

Vertical talus
= "Rocker-bottom foot"
√ vertically oriented talus with increased lateral talocalcaneal angle
√ dorsal navicular displacement
√ heel equinus
√ rigid deformity
Associated with: Arthrogryposis multiplex congenita; spina bifida; trisomy 13–18

Heel pad thickening
= heel pad thickening >25 mm (normal <21 mm)
mnemonic: "MAD COP"
 Myxedema
 Acromegaly
 Dilantin therapy
 Callous
 Obesity
 Peripheral edema

SOFT TISSUE CALCIFICATION
Metastatic calcification
= deposit of calcium salts in previously normal tissue
 (1) as a result of elevation of Ca x P product above 60 – 70
 (2) with normal Ca x P product after renal transplant
Location: lung (alveolar septa, bronchial wall, vessel wall), kidney, gastric mucosa, heart, peripheral vessels
Causes:
 (a) Skeletal deossification
  1. 1° HPT
  2. Ectopic HPT production (lung / kidney tumor)
  3. Renal osteodystrophy + 2° HPT
  4. Hypoparathyroidism
 (b) Massive bone destruction
  1. Widespread bone metastases
  2. Plasma cell myeloma
  3. Leukemia
 (c) Increased intestinal absorption
  1. Hypervitaminosis D
  2. Milk-alkali syndrome

3. Excess ingestion / IV administration of calcium salts
4. Prolonged immobilization
5. Sarcoidosis
(d) Idiopathic hypercalcemia

Dystrophic calcification
= in presence of normal serum Ca + P levels secondary to local electrolyte / enzyme alterations in areas of tissue injury

(a) Metabolic disorder without hypercalcemia
1. Renal osteodystrophy with 2° HPT
2. Hypoparathyroidism
3. Pseudohypoparathyroidism
4. Pseudopseudohypoparathyroidism
5. Gout
6. Pseudogout = chondrocalcinosis
7. Ochronosis = alkaptonuria
8. Diabetes mellitus
(b) Connective tissue disorder
1. Scleroderma
2. Dermatomyositis
3. Systemic lupus erythematosus
(c) Trauma
1. Neuropathic calcifications
2. Frostbite
3. Myositis ossificans progressiva
4. Calcific tendinitis / bursitis
(d) Infestation
1. Cysticercosis
2. Dracunculosis (guinea worm)
3. Loiasis
4. Bancroft filariasis
5. Hydatid disease
6. Leprosy
(e) Vascular disease
1. Atherosclerosis
2. Media sclerosis (Mönckeberg)
3. Venous calcifications
4. Tissue infarction (eg, myocardial infarction)
(f) Miscellaneous
1. Ehlers-Danlos syndrome
2. Pseudoxanthoma elasticum
3. Werner syndrome = progeria
4. Calcinosis (circumscripta, universalis, tumoral calcinosis)
5. Necrotic tumor

Soft tissue ossification
= formation of trabecular bone
1. Myositis ossificans progressiva / circumscripta
2. Paraosteoarthropathy
3. Soft tissue osteosarcoma
4. Parosteal osteosarcoma
5. Posttraumatic periostitis = periosteoma
6. Surgical scar
7. Severely burned patient

Generalized calcinosis
(a) Collagen vascular disorders
1. Scleroderma
2. Dermatomyositis
(b) Idiopathic tumoral calcinosis
(c) Idiopathic calcinosis universalis

Interstitial calcinosis
Calcinosis circumscripta
1. Acrosclerosis: granular deposits around joints of fingers + toes, fingertips
2. Scleroderma: acrosclerosis + absorption of ends of distal phalanges
3. Dermatomyositis: extensive subcutaneous deposits
4. Varicosities: particularly in calf
5. 1° Hyperparathyroidism: infrequently periarticular calcinosis
6. Renal osteodystrophy with 2° hyperparathyroidism: extensive vascular deposits even in young individuals
7. Hypoparathyroidism: occasionally around joints; symmetrical in basal ganglia
8. Vitamin D intoxication: periarticular in rheumatoid arthritis (putty-like); calcium deposit in tophi

Calcinosis universalis
Progressive disease of unknown origin
Age: children + young adults
√ plaque-like calcium deposits in skin + subcutaneous tissues; sometimes in tendons + muscles
√ NO true bone formation

FAT-CONTAINING SOFT-TISSUE MASSES
A. BENIGN LIPOMATOUS TUMORS
1. Lipoma
2. Intra- / intermuscular lipoma
3. Synovial lipoma
4. Lipoma arborescens = diffuse synovial lipoma
5. Neural fibrolipoma = fibrolipomatous tumor of nerve
6. Macrodystrophia lipomatosa
B. LIPOMA VARIANTS
1. Lipoblastoma (exclusively in infancy + early childhood
2. **Lipomatosis** = diffuse overgrowth of mature adipose tissue infiltrating through the soft tissues of affected extremity / trunk
3. **Hibernoma** = rare benign tumor of brown fat; often in peri- / interscapular region, axilla, thigh, chest wall
√ marked hypervascularity
C. MALIGNANT LIPOMATOUS TUMOR
1. Liposarcoma
D. OTHER FAT-CONTAINING TUMORS
1. Hemangioma
2. Elastofibroma
E. LESIONS MIMICKING FAT-CONTAINING TUMORS
1. Myxoid tumors: intramuscular myxoma, extraskeletal myxoid chondrosarcoma, myxoid malignant fibrous histiocytoma

2. Neural tumors: neurofibroma, neurilemoma, malignant schwannoma
   √ 73% have tissue attenuation less than muscle
3. Hemorrhage

FIXATION DEVICES
Internal fixation devices
A. Screws
1. Cortical screw = threaded over entire length, shallow closely spaced threads, blunt tip
2. Cancellous screw = wide thread diameter with varying length of smooth shank between head + threads
3. Malleolar screw = partially threaded
4. Interference screw = short, fully threaded, cancellous thread pattern, self-tapping tip, recessed head
5. Cannulated screw = hollow screw inserted over guide pin
6. Herbert screw = cannulated screw threaded on both ends with different pitches, no screw head
B. Washer
1. Flat washer = increase surface area over which force is distributed
2. Serrated washer = spiked edges used for affixing avulsed ligaments
C. Plates
— Compression plate = used for compression of stable fractures
— Neutralization plate = protects fracture from bending, rotation + axial-loading forces
— Buttress plate = support of unstable fractures in compression / axial loading

1. Straight plate
   (a) straight plate with round holes
   (b) dynamic compression plate = oval holes
   (c) tubular plate = thin pliable plate with concave inner surface
   (d) reconstruction plate = thin pliable plate to allow bending, twisting, contouring
2. Special plates
   T-shaped, L-shaped, Y-shaped, cloverleaf, spoon, cobra, condylar blade plate, dynamic compression screw system
D. Staples
   Fixation = bone = epiphyseal = fracture staples with smooth / barbed surface
   — Coventry = stepped osteotomy staple
   — stone = table staple
E. Wires
1. K wire = unthreaded segments of extruded wire of variable thickness
2. Cerclage wiring = wire placed around bone
3. Tension band wiring = figure-of-eight wire placed on tension side of bone

External fixation devices
= smooth / threaded pins / wires attached to an external frame
   (a) unilateral pin = enters bone only from one side
      1. Steinman pin = large-caliber wire with pointed tip

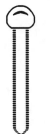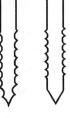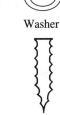

Cortical   Cancellous   Malleolar   Herbert   Interference

Screws

Washer

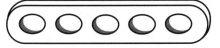

Dynamic compression plate

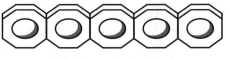

Malleable reconstruction plate

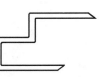

Fixation staples   Table staple   Coventry staple

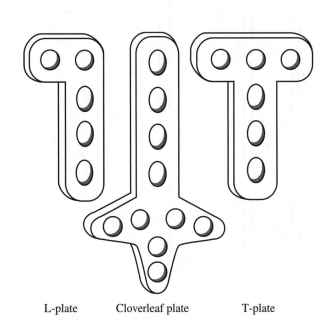

L-plate   Cloverleaf plate   T-plate

2. Rush pin = smooth intramedullary pin
3. Schanz screw = pin threaded at one end to engage cortex, smooth at other end to connect to external fixation device
4. Knowles pin (for femoral neck fracture)
(b) transfixing pin = pass through extremity supported by external fixation device on both ends

Intramedullary fixation devices

(a) nail = driven into bone without reaming
(b) rod = solid / hollowdevice with blunted tip driven into reamed channel
(c) interlocking nail = accessory pins / screws / deployable fins placed to prevent rotation
1. Rush pin = beveled end + hooked end
2. Ender nail = oval in cross section
3. Sampson rod = slightly curved rigid rod with fluted surface
4. Küntscher nail = clover-leaf in cross section with rounded tip

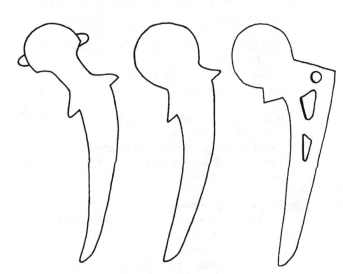

Charnley-Mueller   Thompson   Austin-Moore

Hip prosthesis

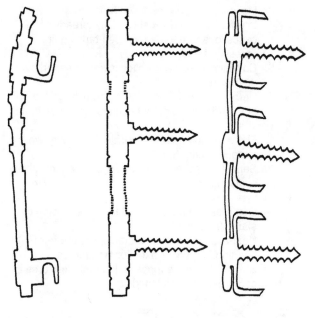

Harrington rod   Dunn rod   Dwyer cable

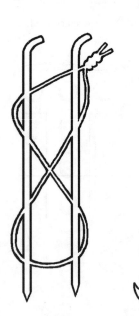

Pins + figure-of-eight band wiring   Rush pin   Blade plate

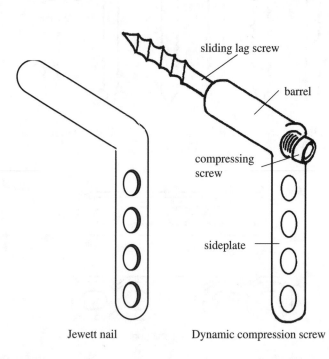

sliding lag screw
barrel
compressing screw
sideplate

Jewett nail   Dynamic compression screw

ANATOMY AND METABOLISM OF BONE

Calcium
A. 99% in bone
B. serum calcium
 (a) protein-bound fraction (albumin)
 (b) ionic (pH-dependent) 3% as calcium citrate / phosphate in serum
Absorption: facilitated by vitamin D
Excretion : related to dietary intake; >500 mg/24 hours = hypercalciuria

Phosphorus
Absorption: requires sodium; decreased by aluminum hydroxide gel in gut
Excretion : increased by estrogen, parathormone decreased by vitamin D, growth hormone, glucocorticoids

Parathormone
Major stimulus: low levels of serum calcium ions
 (action requires vitamin D presence)
Target organs:
 (a) BONE: increase in osteocytic + osteoclastic activity mobilizes calcium + phosphate = bone resorption
 (b) KIDNEY: (1) increase in tubular reabsorption of calcium
 (2) decrease in tubular reabsorption of phosphate (+ amino acids) = phosphate diuresis
 (c) GUT: increased absorption of calcium + phosphorus

Major function: • increase of serum calcium levels
 • increase in serum alkaline phosphatase (50%)

Vitamin D Metabolism
required for
 (1) adequate calcium absorption from gut
 (2) synthesis of calcium-binding protein in intestinal mucosa
 (3) parathormone effects (stimulation of osteoclastic + osteocytic resorption of bone)

Biochemistry:
 inactive form of vitamin D_3 present through diet / exposure to sunlight; vitamin D_3 is converted into 25-OH-vitamin D_3 by liver and then converted into 1,25-OH vitamin D_3 (= hormone) by kidney
 Stimulus for conversion: (1) hypophosphatemia
 (2) PTH elevation
Action:
 (a) INTESTINE: (1) increased absorption of calcium from bowel
 (2) increased absorption of phosphate from distal small bowel
 (b) BONE: (1) proper mineralization of osteoid
 (2) mobilization of calcium + phosphate (potentiates parathormone action)
 (c) KIDNEY: (1) increased absorption of calcium from renal tubule
 (2) increased absorption of phosphate from renal tubule

Calcitonin
secreted by parafollicular cells of thyroid
Major stimulus: increase in serum calcium
Target organs:
 (a) BONE: (1) inhibits parathormone-induced osteoclasis by reducing number of osteoclasts
 (2) enhances deposition of calcium phosphate; responsible for sclerosis in renal osteodystrophy
 (b) KIDNEY: inhibits phosphate reabsorption in renal tubule
 (c) GUT: increases excretion of sodium + water into gut
Major function: decreases serum calcium + phosphate

	PTH ACTION		NET EFFECT	
Principal:	(1) phosphate diuresis (2) resorption of Ca + P from bone		(1) Serum:	increase in Ca decrease in P
Secondary:	(3) resorption of Ca from gut (4) reabsorption of Ca from renal tubule		(2) Urine:	increase in Ca increase in P

Occurrence of bone centers at elbow

mnemonic: "CRITOE"

Capitellum	1 year	(<1 year)
Radial head	5 years	(3 – 6 years)
Internal humeral epicondyle	7 years	(5 – 7 years, last to fuse)
Trochlea	10 years	(9 – 10 years)
Olecranon	10 years	(6 – 10 years)
External humeral epicondyle	12 years	(9 – 13 years)

Rotator cuff muscles

mnemonic: "SITS"

Supraspinatus
Infraspinatus
Teres minor
Subscapularis

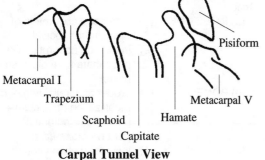

Carpal Tunnel View

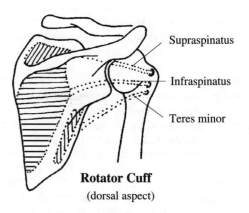

Rotator Cuff
(dorsal aspect)

Muscle Attachments of Thigh

	Origin	*Insertion*
Gracilis	inferior pubic ramus	pes anserinus
Semimembranosus	ischial tuberosity	medial tibial condyle
Semitendinosus	ischial tuberosity	pes anserinus
Biceps femoris		
— long head:	ischial tuberosity	fibular head
— short head:	lateral linea aspera	fibular head
Adductor		
— longus	superior pubic ramus	medial linea aspera
— magnus	inferior pubic ramus	medial linea aspera
Sartorius	anterior superior iliac spine	pes anserinus
Quadriceps		
— rectus	anterior inferior iliac spine	patellar tendon
— vastus lateralis	greater trochanter	patellar tendon
— vastus medialis	medial intertrochanteric line	patellar tendon
Iliopsoas		
— iliacus	ilium	lesser trochanter
— psoas	lumbar spine	lesser trochanter
Tensor fasciae latae	anterior superior iliac spine	anterolateral tibia

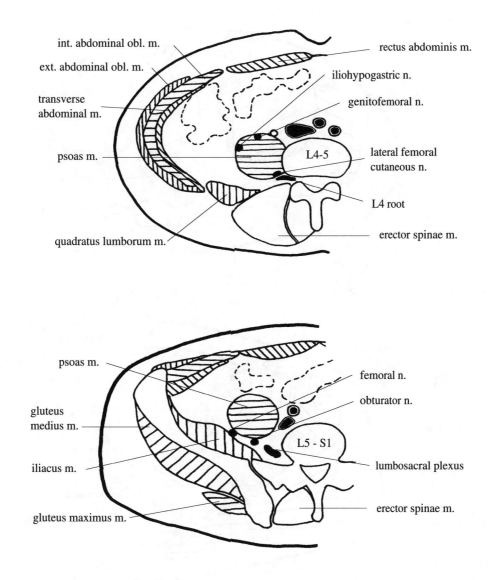

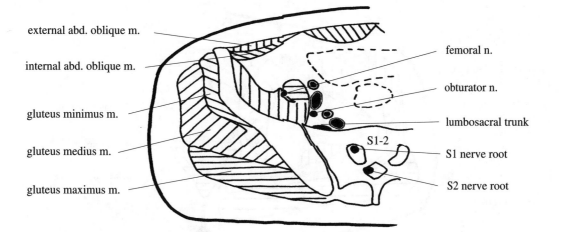

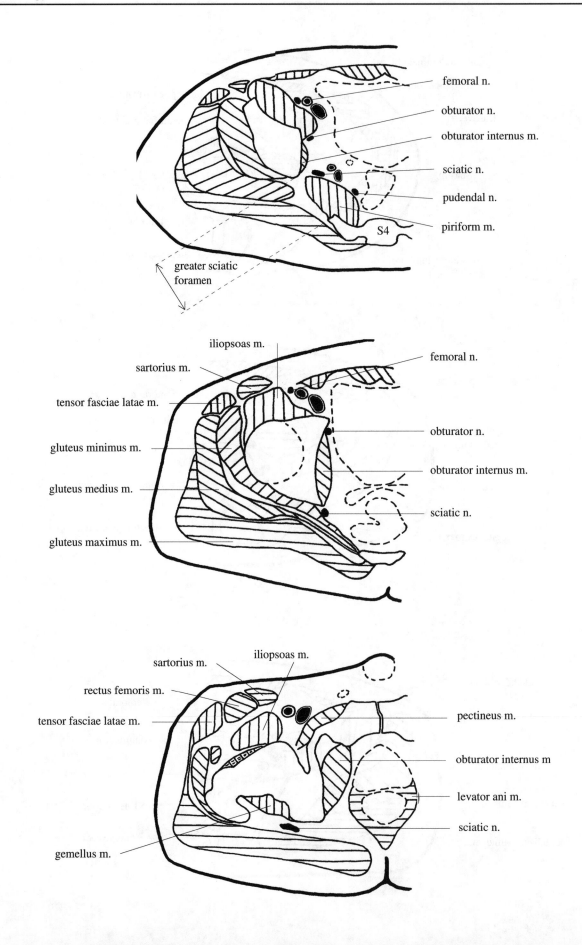

femoral n.

obturator n.

obturator internus m.

sciatic n.

pudendal n.

piriform m.

S4

greater sciatic
foramen

iliopsoas m.

sartorius m.

tensor fasciae latae m.

gluteus minimus m.

gluteus medius m.

gluteus maximus m.

femoral n.

obturator n.

obturator internus m.

sciatic n.

sartorius m.

iliopsoas m.

rectus femoris m.

tensor fasciae latae m.

pectineus m.

obturator internus m

levator ani m.

sciatic n.

gemellus m.

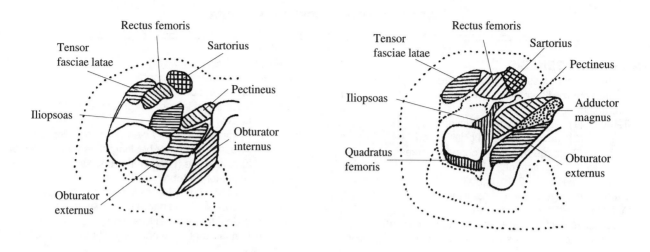

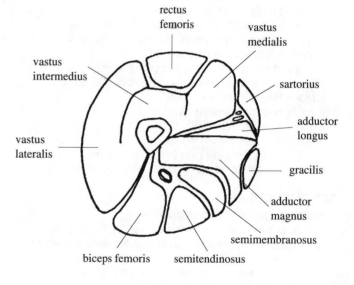

Cross-section through right thigh

BONE AND SOFT TISSUE DISORDERS

ACHONDROGENESIS

= autosomal recessive lethal chondrodystrophy characterized by extreme micromelia, short trunk, large cranium

TRIAD: (1) severe short limb dwarfism
          (2) lack of vertebral calcification
          (3) large head with normal / decreased calvarial ossification

Birth prevalence: 2.3:100,000
Path: disorganization of cartilage

A. TYPE I = Parenti-Fraccaro
   defective enchondral + membranous ossification
- √ complete lack of ossification of calvarium + spine + pelvis
- √ absent sacrum + pubic bone
- √ extremely short long bones without bowing, especially femur, radius, ulna
- √ thin ribs with multiple fractures (frequent)

B. TYPE II = Langer-Saldino
   defective enchondral ossification only
- √ good ossification of skull vault
- √ nonossification of lower lumbar vertebrae + sacrum
- √ short + stubby horizontal ribs without fractures
- often subcutaneous edema
- √ irregular flared metaphyses (esp. humerus)
- √ short trunk with narrow chest + protruding abdomen
- √ redundant soft tissues
- √ polyhydramnios (common)
- √ increase in HC:AC ratio

Prognosis: lethal often in utero / within few hours or days after birth (respiratory failure)
DDx: often confused with thanatophoric dwarfism

ACHONDROPLASIA

Heterozygous Achondroplasia

= autosomal dominant / sporadic (80%) disease with quantitatively defective endochondral bone formation; related to advanced paternal age; prototype of rhizomelic dwarfism; epiphyseal maturation + ossification unaffected

Incidence: 1:26,000 – 66,000 births, most common nonlethal bone dysplasia; M<F

- normal intelligence + motor function
- neurologic defects
- classically circus dwarfs
- @ Skull
  - receding bridge of nose (hypoplastic base of skull)
  - brachycephaly with enlarged bulging forehead (nonprogressive hydrocephalus)
  - relative prognathism
  - √ large calvarium with frontal bossing
  - √ broad mandible
  - √ shortened base of skull + small foramen magnum
  - √ communicating hydrocephalus caused by obstruction of basal cisterns + aqueduct secondary to small foramen magnum

- @ Chest & Spine
  - protuberant abdomen
  - prominent buttocks
  - √ squaring of inferior scapular margin
  - √ narrow chest
  - √ hypoplastic bullet- / wedge-shaped vertebra
    = rounded anterior beaking of vertebra in upper lumbar spine (DDx: Hurler disease)
  - √ posterior vertebral scalloping
  - √ narrowing of spinal canal (ventrodorsal + interpediculate space) in lumbar spine
  - √ wide intervertebral foramina
  - √ lumbar angular kyphosis (gibbus) + sacral lordosis
- @ Pelvis
  - rolling gait from backward tilt of pelvis and hip joints
  - √ square-shaped flat nonflared pelvic bones with tombstone configuration
  - √ flattened iliac wings ("champagne glass")
  - √ horizontal acetabula (decreased acetabular angle)
  - √ small sacrosciatic notch
- @ Extremities
  - trident hand = separation of 2nd + 3rd digit and inability to approximate 3rd + 4th finger
  - √ predominantly rhizomelic shortness of long bones (femur, humerus)
  - √ "trumpet" appearance with short long bones but normal metaphyseal width
  - √ limb bowing
  - √ "ball-in-socket" epiphysis = broad V-shaped metaphysis in which epiphysis is incorporated
  - √ high position of fibular head (fibula less short)
  - √ short ulna with thick proximal + slender distal end
  - √ brachydactyly (uniform length of short bones) + divergent fingers

OB-US (>27th week GA):
- √ shortening of proximal long bones
- √ increased BPD, HC, HC:AC ratio
- √ decreased FL:BPD ratio
- √ normal mineralization, no fractures
- √ normal thorax + normal cardiothoracic ratio

Cx: (1) Hydrocephalus + syringomyelia (small foramen magnum)
      (2) Recurrent ear infection (poorly developed facial bones)
      (3) Crowded dentition + malocclusion
      (4) Neurologic complications (spinal cord compression)
DDx: various mucopolysaccharidoses

Homozygous Achondroplasia

= hereditary autosomal dominant disease with severe features of achondroplasia (disproportionate limb shortening, more marked proximally than distally)

√ large skull with short base + small face
√ short ribs with flared ends
√ hypoplastic vertebral bodies
√ decreased interpedicular distance
√ short squared innominate bones
√ flattened acetabular roof
√ small sciatic notch
√ short limb bones with flared metaphyses
√ short broad widely spaced tubular bones of hand
Prognosis: often stillborn; lethal in neonatal period
(from respiratory failure)
DDx: thanatophoric dysplasia

ACROCEPHALOSYNDACTYLY
= syndrome characterized by (1) increased height of skull
vault due to generalized craniosynostosis (= acro-
cephaly, oxycephaly) (2) syndactyly of fingers / toes
Type I : Apert syndrome = acrocephalosyndactyly
Type II : Vogt cephalosyndactyly
Type III : Acrocephalosyndactyly with asymmetry of skull
+ mild syndactyly
Type IV : Wardenburg type
Type V : Pfeiffer type

ACROOSTEOLYSIS, FAMILIAL
dominant inheritance
Age: onset in 2nd decade; M:F = 3:1
• sensory changes in hands + feet
• destruction of nails
• joint hypermobility
• swelling of plantar of foot with deep wide ulcer + ejection
of bone fragments
@ Skull
√ Wormian bones
√ craniosynostosis
√ basilar impression
√ protuberant occiput
√ resorption of alveolar processes + loss of teeth
@ Spine
√ spinal osteoporosis ± fracture
√ kyphoscoliosis + progressive decrease in height

ACROMEGALY
Etiology: excess growth hormone due to eosinophilic
adenoma / hyperplasia
• gigantism in children (DDx: **Soto syndrome** of cerebral
gigantism = large skull, mental retardation, cerebral
atrophy, advanced bone age)
√ osseous enlargement (phalangeal tufts, vertebrae)
√ flared ends of long bone
√ cystic changes in carpals, femoral trochanters
√ osteoporosis
@ Hand
• spade-like hand
√ widening of terminal tufts
@ Skull
√ prognathism (= elongation of mandible) in few cases
√ sellar enlargement + erosion
√ enlargement of paranasal sinuses: large frontal
sinuses (75%)

√ calvarial hyperostosis (especially inner table)
√ enlarged occipital protuberance
@ Vertebrae
√ posterior scalloping in 30% (secondary to pressure
of enlarged soft tissue)
√ anterior new bone
√ loss of disc space (weakening of cartilage)
@ Soft tissue
√ heel pad >25 mm
@ Joints
√ premature osteoarthritis (commonly knees)

ACTINOMYCOSIS
Types: (1) cervicofacial (poor oral hygiene, common)
(2) lungs (hematogenous / inhalation)
(3) ileocecal (after rupture / surgery of appendix)
• draining cutaneous sinuses
Location: predilection for thorax + spine
@ Mandible
√ destruction of mandible (most frequently involved)
around tooth socket without new bone formation,
spread to soft tissues at angle of jaw + into neck
@ Vertebra
√ destruction of vertebra with preservation of disc +
small paravertebral abscess without calcification
(DDx to tuberculosis: disc destroyed, large abscess
with calcium)
√ thickening of cervical vertebrae around margins
@ Tubular bones of hands
√ destructive lesion of mottled permeating type
√ cartilage destruction + subarticular erosive defects
in joints (simulating TB)
√ destruction / thickening of ribs + pleuritis
@ Abdomen
Initially localized to cecum / appendix
√ ulcerations with abscess (containing yellow sulphur
granules)
√ abscesses in liver, retroperitoneum, psoas muscles,
chronic sinus in groin

ADAMANTINOMA
= (MALIGNANT) ANGIOBLASTOMA = locally aggressive
/ malignant lesion
Histo: pseudoepithelial cell masses with peripheral
columnar cells in a palisade pattern with varying
amounts of fibrous stroma; areas of squamous /
tubular / alveolar / vessel transformation;
prominent vascularity; resembles ameloblastoma
of the jaw
Age: 25 – 50 years, commonest in 3rd – 4th decade
• frequently history of trauma
• local swelling ± pain
Location: middle 1/3 of tibia (90%), fibula, ulna, carpals,
metacarpals, humerus, shaft of femur
√ eccentric round osteolytic lesion with sclerotic margin,
may have additional foci in continuity with major lesion
(CHARACTERISTIC)
√ may show mottled density
√ bone expansion frequent
√ often multiple

Prognosis: tendency to recur after local excision; after several recurrences pulmonary metastases may develop

DDx: fibrous dysplasia (possibly related)

AINHUM DISEASE
= DACTYLOLYSIS SPONTANEA

ainhum = fissure, saw, sword

Etiology: unknown

Histo: hyperkeratotic epidermis with fibrotic thickening of collagen bundles below; chronic lymphocytic inflammatory reaction may be present; arterial walls may be thickened with narrowed vessel lumina

Incidence: up to 2%

Age: usually in males in 4th + 5th decades; blacks (West Africa) + their American descendants; M > F

- deep soft tissue groove forming on medial aspect of plantar surface of proximal phalanx with edema distally
- painful ulceration may develop

Location: mostly 5th / 4th toe (rarely finger); near interphalangeal joint; mostly bilateral

√ sharply demarcated progressive bone resorption of distal / middle phalanx with tapering of proximal phalanx to complete autoamputation (after an average of 5 years)

√ osteoporosis

Rx: early surgical resection of groove with Z plasty

DDx: (1) Neuropathic disorders (diabetes, leprosy, syphilis)
    (2) Trauma (burns, frostbite)
    (3) Acroosteolysis from inflammatory arthritis, infection, polyvinyl chloride exposure
    (4) Congenitally constricting bands in amniotic band syndrome

AMYLOIDOSIS
= accumulation + infiltration of a chemically diverse group of protein polysaccharides in body tissues; tends to form around capillaries + endothelial cells of larger blood vessels causing ultimately vascular obliteration with infarction

- rubbery soft tissue swelling
√ periarticular soft tissue swelling (amyloid deposited in synovium, joint capsule, tendons, ligaments)
√ subluxation of proximal humerus + femoral neck
√ osteoporosis
√ coarse trabecular pattern (DDx: sarcoidosis)
√ solitary osteolytic lesion (secondary invasion + erosion of articular bone) in ribs, olecranon, coronoid process
√ pathologic fractures may occur (vertebral fracture)

PRIMARY AMYLOIDOSIS
In 10 – 15% of multiple myeloma; may precede development of multiple myeloma; sporadic, familial; predominantly connective tissue involvement
- progressive cardiac failure
- bone pain
- periarticular soft tissue swelling + stiffness (shoulders, hips, fingers)

- Bence Jones protein (without myeloma)

Location:

heart (90%)	GI tract (70%)	tongue (40%)
spleen (40%)	liver (35%)	lungs (30%)
skin + subcutis (25%)		

SECONDARY AMYLOIDOSIS
In chronic suppurative disease of lungs / skeleton; chronic inflammatory disease of GI tract (ulcerative colitis); lymphoproliferative disorders (multiple myeloma, Waldenström, heavy chain disease); rheumatoid arthritis, amyloidosis of aging; long-term hemodialysis

Location: spleen, liver, kidneys, GI tract

ANEURYSMAL BONE CYST
= expansile lesion of bone containing thin-walled blood-filled cystic cavities; name derived from roentgen appearance

Etiology:
  (a) primary nonneoplastic lesion (2/3)
  (b) arising in preexisting bone tumor (1/3):
     giant cell tumor (39%), angioma, osteoblastoma, chondroblastoma, telangiectatic osteosarcoma, solitary bone cyst, fibrous dysplasia, xanthoma, chondromyxoid fibroma, nonossifying fibroma, metastatic carcinoma

Histo:
"intraosseous arteriovenous malformation" with honey-combed spaces filled with blood + lined by granulation tissue / osteoid; areas of free hemorrhage; sometimes multi-nucleated giant cells

Types:
  1. INTRAOSSEOUS ABC
    = primary cystic / telangiectatic tumor of giant cell family, originating in bone marrow cavity, slow expansion of cortex; rarely related to history of trauma
  2. EXTRAOSSEOUS ABC
    = posttraumatic hemorrhagic cyst; originating on surface of bones, erosion through cortex into marrow

Age: peak age 16 years (range 10 – 30 years) in 75% <20 years; F > M

- pain of relatively acute onset with rapid increase of severity over 6 – 12 weeks
- ± history of trauma
- neurologic signs (radiculopathy to quadriplegia) if in spine

Location:
  (a) spine (30%) with slight predilection for posterior elements + lumbar spine, cervical spine (22%); involvement of vertebral body (40%); may involve two contiguous vertebrae (25%)
  (b) long bones: eccentric in metaphysis of femur, tibia, humerus, fibula; pelvis

√ purely lytic eccentric radiolucency
√ aggressive expansile ballooning lesion of "soap-bubble" pattern + thin internal trabeculations
√ rapid progression within 6 weeks to 3 months
√ sclerotic inner portion

√ almost invisible thin cortex (CT shows integrity)
√ tumor respects epiphyseal plate
√ no periosteal reaction (except when fractured)
CT:
  √ may show fluid-fluid levels due to blood layering
MR:
  √ multiple cysts of different signal intensity representing different stages of blood by-products
Bone scan:
  √ increased uptake

Cx: (1) pathologic fracture (frequent)
    (2) extradural block with paraplegia
DDx: (1) Giant cell tumor (particularly in spine)
     (2) Hemorrhagic cyst (end of bone / epiphysis, not expansile)
     (3) Enchondroma
     (4) Metastasis (renal cell + thyroid carcinoma)
     (5) Plasmacytoma
     (6) Condro- and fibrosarcoma
     (7) Fibrous dysplasia
     (8) Hemophilic pseudotumor
     (9) Hydatid cyst

ANKYLOSING SPONDYLITIS
= chronic inflammatory disease primarily affecting spine
Age: young men; M:F = 15:1; caucasians:blacks = 3:1
Associated with: (1) ulcerative colitis, regional enteritis
                   (2) iritis in 25%
                   (3) aortic insufficiency + atrioventricular conduction defect
• HLA-B 27 positive in 96%
Location: bilateral + asymmetric; hips + shoulders (80%), small peripheral joints (50%)

@ HAND (30%)
  Target area: MCP, PIP, DIP
  √ exuberant osseous proliferation
  √ osteoporosis, joint space narrowing, osseous erosions (deformities less striking than in rheumatoid arthritis)
@ SACROILIAC / SYMPHYSIS PUBIS
  √ initially sclerosis of joint margins primarily on iliac side (bilateral + symmetric)
  √ later irregularities + widening of joint (cartilage destruction)
@ SPINE
  √ straightening / squaring of anterior vertebral margins = osteitis of anterior corners
  √ reactive sclerosis of corners of vertebral bodies
  √ asymmetric erosions of laminar + spinous process at level of lumbar spine
  √ ossification of annulus fibrosus (NOT anterior longitudinal ligament)
  √ apophyseal + costovertebral ankylosis
  √ marginal syndesmophyte formation = thin vertical radiodense spicules
  √ "bamboo" spine = undulating contour of ligamentous calcifications; prone to fracture resulting in pseudarthrosis

√ periostitic "whiskering": ischial tuberosity, iliac crest, ischiopubic rami, greater femoral trochanter, external occipital protuberance, calcaneus
√ dorsal arachnoid diverticula in lumbar spine with erosion of posterior elements (Cx: cauda equina syndrome)
√ atlantoaxial subluxation
@ CHEST
  √ bilateral upper lobe pulmonary fibrosis (1%)
@ CARDIOVASCULAR
  1. Aortitis (5%) of ascending aorta ± aortic valve insufficiency

√ temporomandibular joint space narrowing, erosions, osteophytosis

ANTERIOR TIBIAL BOWING
= WEISMANN-NETTER SYNDROME = congenital painless nonprogressive bilateral anterior leg bowing
Age: beginning in early childhood
• may be accompanied by mental retardation, goiter, anemia
√ anterior bowing of tibia + fibula, bilaterally, symmetrically at middiaphysis
√ thickening of posterior tibial + fibular cortices
√ minor radioulnar bowing
√ kyphoscoliosis
√ extensive dural calcification
DDx: Luetic saber shin (bowing at lower end of tibia + anterior cortical thickening)

APERT SYNDROME
Autosomal dominant; may be mentally retarded
@ Skull
  √ oxycephalic skull + flat occiput
  √ hypertelorism + bilateral exophthalmus
  √ underdeveloped paranasal sinuses
  √ underdeveloped maxilla with prognathism
  √ high pointed arch of palate
  √ prominent vertical crest in middle of forehead (increased intracranial pressure)
  √ V-shaped anterior fossa due to elevation of lateral margins of lesser sphenoid
  √ sella may be enlarged
  √ cervical spine may be fused
@ Hand & feet
  √ fusion of distal portions of phalanges, metacarpals / carpals (2nd, 3rd + 4th digit)
  √ absence of middle phalanges
  √ missing / supernumerary carpal / tarsal bones
  √ pseudarthroses

ARTERIOVENOUS FISTULA OF BONE
Etiology: (a) acquired (usually gunshot wound)
            (b) congenital
Location: lower extremity most frequent
√ soft tissue mass
√ presence of large vessels
√ phleboliths (DDx: long-standing varicosity)
√ accelerated bone growth

√ cortical osteolytic defect (= pathway for large vessels into medulla)

√ increased bone density

ARTHROGRYPOSIS

= ARTHROGRYPOSIS MULTIPLEX CONGENITA

= nonprogressive congenital syndrome complex characterized by poorly developed + contracted muscles, deformed joints with thickened periarticular capsule and intact sensory system

Etiology:
congenital / acquired defect of motor unit (anterior horn cells, nerve roots, peripheral nerves, motor endplates, muscle) early in fetal life with immobilization of joints at various stages in their development

Cause: ? neurotropic agents, toxic chemicals, hard drugs, hyperthermia, neuromuscular blocking agents, mytotic abnormalities, mechanical immobilization

Incidence: 0.03% of newborn infants; 5% risk of recurrence in sibling

Path: diminution in size of muscle fibers + fat deposits in fibrous tissue

Associated with: (1) neurogenic disorders (90%)
(2) myopathic disorders
(3) skeletal dysplasias
(4) intrauterine limitation of movement (myomata, amniotic band, twin, oligohydramnios)
(5) connective tissue disorders

Distribution: all extremities (46%), lower extremities only (43%), upper extremities only (11%); symmetrical; peripheral joints >> proximal joints

• club foot
• congenital dislocation of hip
• claw hand
• diminished muscle mass
• skin webs
√ flexion + extension contractures
√ osteopenia ± pathologic fractures
√ congenital dislocation of hip
√ carpal coalition
√ vertical talus
√ calcaneal valgus deformity

ASPHYXIATING THORACIC DYSPLASIA

= JEUNE DISEASE = autosomal recessive disorder

Incidence: 100 cases

Associated with: renal anomalies (hydroureter), PDA

• reduced thoracic mobility (abdominal breathing) + frequent pulmonary infections
• progressive renal failure + hypertension

@ Chest
√ markedly narrow + elongated bell-shaped chest
√ normal size of heart leaving little room for lungs
√ horizontal clavicles at level of 6th cervical vertebra
√ short horizontal ribs + irregular bulbous costochondral junction

@ Pelvis
√ trident pelvis (retardation of ossification of triradiate cartilage)
√ small iliac bone flared + shortened in cephalocaudal diameter ("wine glass" pelvis)
√ short ischial + pubic bones
√ reduced acetabular angle
√ prematue ossification of capital femoral epiphysis
@ Extremities
√ rhizomelic brachymelia (humerus, femur) = long bones shorter + wider than normal
√ metaphyseal irregularity
√ postaxial hexadactyly
√ shortening of distal phalanges + cone-shaped epiphyses in hands + feet
@ Kidneys
√ enlarged kidneys with linear streaking on nephrogram
OB-US:
√ proportionate shortening of long bones
√ small thorax with decreased circumference
√ increased cardiothoracic ratio
√ occasionally polydactyly
√ polyhydramnios
Prognosis: neonatal death in 80% (respiratory failure + infections)
DDx: Ellis-van Creveld syndrome

AVASCULAR NECROSIS

= AVN = OSTEONECROSIS = ASEPTIC NECROSIS

= consequence of interrupted blood supply to bone with death of cellular elements

Histo:
(a) cellular ischemia leading to death of hematopoietic cells (in 6 – 12 hours), osteocytes (in 12 – 48 hours) + lipocytes (in 2 – 5 days)
(b) necrotic debris in intertrabecular spaces + proliferation and infiltration by mesenchymal cells + capillaries
(c) mesenchymal cells differentiate to osteoblasts on the surface of dead trabeculae synthesizing new bone layers + resulting in trabecular thickening

Pathogenesis:
(1) obstruction of extra- and intraosseous vessels by embolism, thrombosis, external compression
(2) cumulative stress from cytotoxic factors

Causes:
mnemonic: "PLASTIC RAGS"
Pancreatitis, **P**regnancy
Legg-Perthes disease, **L**upus erythematosus
Alcoholism, **A**therosclerosis
Steroids
Trauma (hip fracture / dislocation)
Idiopathic (Legg-Perthes disease), **I**nfection
Caisson disease, **C**ollagen disease (SLE)
Rheumatoid arthritis, **R**adiation
Amyloid
Gaucher disease
Sickle cell disease
NO predisposing factors in 25%

Location: hip (most common)

Avascular Necrosis of Hip
Involvement of one hip increases risk to contralateral
hip to 70%!
Age: 20 – 50 years
- hip / groin / thigh / knee pain
- limited range of motion

Plain film (limited in detection of early disease / severity
of disease):
Grade 0 = normal / mild degenerative changes
Grade I = barely detectable trabecular mottling
Grade II = focal sclerosis / trabecular rarefaction in
femoral head
Grade III = mild alteration in femoral head contour +
normal joint space
Grade IV = profound flattening of femoral head
Grade V = narrowing of joint space + acetabular
involvement

NUC (80 – 85% sensitivity):
Δ Bone marrow imaging (with radiocolloid) more
sensitive than bone imaging (with diphosphonates)
Δ More sensitive than plain films in early AVN
(evidence of ischemia seen as much as 1 year
earlier)
Δ Less sensitive than MR
Technique: imaging improved with double counts,
pin-hole collimation
√ <u>early</u>: cold = photopenic defect (interrupted blood
supply)
√ <u>late</u>: increased uptake (capillary infiltration + new
bone synthesis)
CT (utilized for staging of known disease):
√ staging upgrades in 30% compared with plain films
Stage I = no abnormalities
Stage IIA = focal sclerosis + osteopenia
Stage IIB = distinct sclerosis + osteoporosis + early
crescent sign
Stage IIIA = subchondral undermining + cyst
formation
Stage IIIB = alteration in femoral head contour /
subchondral fracture
Stage IV = marked collapse of femoral head +
significant acetabular involvement

MR (90 – 100% sensitivity for symptomatic disease):
Prevalence of clinically occult disease: 6%
√ cleft of low-signal intensity on T1WI + high signal
intensity on T2WI (= subchondral fracture), esp. in
anterosuperior portion of femoral head
√ large irregular areas of decreased signal intensity
extending into femoral neck
√ low-intensity band / ring (= mesenchymal + fibrous
repair tissue, amorphous cellular debris, thickened
trabecular bone) on T1WI
√ central area of high signal intensity (= necrotic bone
+ marrow not invaded by capillaries +
mesenchymal tissue) on T1WI

Cx: collapse of femoral head in 3 – 5 years with joint
destruction if left untreated
Rx: core decompression / osteotomy (for grade 0 –
II), arthroplasty / arthrodesis / total hip
replacement (for grade >III)

BASAL CELL NEVUS SYNDROME
= GORLIN SYNDROME = syndrome of autosomal
dominant inheritance characterized by (1) multiple
cutaneous basal cell carcinomas (2) jaw cysts
(3) ectopic calcifications (4) skeletal anomalies
- nevoid basal cell carcinomas (nose, mouth, chest, back)
at mean age of 19 years; after puberty aggressive,
may metastasize
- pitlike defects in palms + soles
Associated with: high incidence of medulloblastoma in
children
√ multiple mandibular + maxillary cysts (dentigerous cysts
+ ectopic dentition)
√ anomalies of upper 5 ribs: bifid, fused, dysplastic
√ bifid spinous processes, spina bifida
√ scoliosis (cervical + upper thoracic)
√ hemivertebrae + block vertebrae
√ Sprengel deformity (scapula elevated, hypoplastic,
bowed)
√ brachydactyly
√ calcification of falx
√ ectopic calcifications of subcutaneous tissue, ovaries,
sacrotuberous ligaments, mesentery
√ bony bridging of sella turcica

BATTERED CHILD SYNDROME
= CAFFEY-KEMPE SYNDROME = CHILD ABUSE =
PARENT / INFANT TRAUMATIC STRESS SYNDROME
= NONACCIDENTAL TRAUMA
Most common cause of serious intracranial injuries in
children <1 year of age; 3rd most common cause of
death in children after sudden infant death syndrome +
true accidents
Incidence: 5 – 10% of children seen in emergency
rooms
Age: usually <2 years
- skin burns, bruising, lacerations, hematomas

@ Skeletal Trauma (50 – 80%)
Site: multiple ribs, sternum, costochondral /
costovertebral separation, clavicles, scapula,
skull, vertebral compression, tibia, metacarpus
√ multiple asymmetric fractures in different stages of
repair
√ separation of distal epiphysis
√ marked irregularity + fragmentation of metaphyses
(DDx: osteochondritis stage of congenital syphilis;
infractions of scurvy)
√ "bucket-handle" fracture = avulsion of an arcuate
metaphyseal fragment overlying the lucent
epiphyseal cartilage
√ corner fracture secondary to sudden twisting motion
of extremity around knee, elbow, distal tibia, fibula,
radius, ulna

√ isolated spiral fracture (15%) secondary to external rotatory force applied to femur / humerus

√ extensive periosteal reaction from subperiosteal hemorrhage (DDx: scurvy, copper deficiency)

√ exuberant callus formation at fracture sites

√ cortical hyperostosis extending to epiphyseal plate (DDx: not in infantile cortical hyperostosis)

√ avulsion fracture of ligamentous insertion; frequently seen without periosteal reaction

@ Head trauma (13 – 25%)

Most common cause of death + physical disability

(1) Impact injury with translational force: skull fracture (flexible calvaria + meninges decrease likelihood of skull fractures), subdural hematoma, brain contusion, cerebral hemorrhage, infarction, generalized edema

(2) Whiplash injury with rotational force: shearing injuries + associated subarachnoid hemorrhage

• bulging fontanelles, convulsions

Skull film (associated fracture in 1%):

√ linear fracture > comminuted fracture > diastases (conspicuously absent)

CT:

√ subdural hemorrhage (most common): interhemispheric location most common

√ subarachnoid hemorrhage

√ epidural hemorrhage (uncommon)

√ cerebral edema (focal, multifocal, diffuse)

√ acute cerebral contusion as ovoid collection of intraparenchymal blood with surrounding edema

MR: more sensitive in identifying hematomas of differing ages

√ white matter shearing injuries as areas of prolonged T1 + T2 at corticomedullary junction, centrum semiovale, corpus callosum

@ Viscera (3%)

√ small bowel / gastric rupture

√ traumatic pancreatic pseudocyst

√ lacerations of lung / liver / spleen / kidney

Cx: (1) Brain atrophy (up to 100%)
    (2) Infarction (50%)
    (3) Subdural hygroma
    (4) Encephalomalacia
    (5) Porencephaly

BENIGN CORTICAL DEFECT

= developmental intracortical bone defect

Age: usually 1st – 2nd decade; uncommon in boys <2 years of age; uncommon in girls <4 years of age

• asymptomatic

Site: metaphysis of long bone

√ well-defined intracortical round / oval lucency

√ usually <2 cm long

√ sclerotic margins

Cx: pathologic / avulsion fracture following minor trauma (infrequent)

Prognosis:

(1) Spontaneous healing resulting in sclerosis / disappearance

(2) Ballooning of endosteal surface of cortex = fibrous cortical defect

(3) Medullary extension resulting in nonossifying fibroma

BLASTOMYCOSIS

= NORTH AMERICAN BLASTOMYCOSIS

Organism: Blastomyces dermatitidis

Primary lesions usually in skin with direct extension into bone; occasionally hematogenous spread (resembles actinomycosis)

√ marked destruction ± surrounding sclerosis

√ multiple osseous lesions are frequent

√ vertebral bodies + intervertebral discs are destroyed (similar to tuberculosis)

√ lytic skull lesions + soft tissue abscess

BLOUNT DISEASE

= TIBIA VARA

= avascular necrosis of medial tibial condyle

Age: >6 years

• limping, lateral bowing of leg

√ medial tibial condyle enlarged + deformed (DDx: Turner syndrome)

√ irregularity of metaphysis (medially + posteriorly prolonged with beak)

BONE INFARCT

Etiology:

A. Occlusion of vessel:

(a) Thrombus: thromboembolic disease, sickle cell anemia (SS + SC hemoglobin), polycythemia rubra vera

(b) Fat: pancreatitis (intramedullary fat necrosis from circulating lipase), alcoholism

(c) Gas: caisson disease, astronauts

B. Vessel wall disease:

1. Arteritis: SLE, rheumatoid arthritis, polyarteritis nodosa, sarcoidosis

2. Arteriosclerosis

C. Vascular compression by deposition of:

(a) fat: corticosteroid therapy (eg, renal transplant, Cushing disease)

(b) blood: trauma (fractures + dislocations)

(c) inflammatory cells: osteomyelitis, infection, histiocytosis X

(d) edema: radiation therapy, hypothyroidism, frostbite

(e) substances: Gaucher disease (vascular compression by lipid-filled histiocytes), gout

D. Others: idiopathic, hypopituitarism, pheochromocytoma (microscopic thrombotic disease), osteochondroses

Medullary Infarction

Nutrient artery is the sole blood supply for diaphysis!

Location: distal femur, proximal tibia, iliac wings, ribs, humeri

(a) Acute phase:
   √ NO radiographic changes without cortical involvement
   √ area of rarefaction
   √ bone marrow scan: diminished uptake in medullary RES for long period of time
   √ bone scan: photon-deficient lesion within 24 – 48 hours; increased uptake after collateral circulation established
(b) Healing phase: (complete healing / fibrosis / calcification)
   √ demarcation by zone of serpiginous / linear calcification + ossification parallel to cortex
   √ dense bone indicating revascularization

Cortical Infarction
Requires compromise of
   (a) nutrient artery and (b) periosteal vessels
Age: particularly in childhood where periosteum is easily elevated by edema
√ avascular necrosis = osteonecrosis
√ osteochondrosis dissecans
Cx: (1) Growth disturbances
   √ cupped / triangular / coned epiphyses
   √ "H-shaped" vertebral bodies
   (2) Fibrosarcoma (most common), malignant fibrous histiocytoma, benign cysts
   (3) Osteoarthritis

BONE ISLAND
= ENOSTOSIS = COMPACT ISLAND = FOCAL SCLEROSIS = SCLEROTIC BONE ISLAND = CALCIFIED MEDULLARY DEFECT
• asymptomatic
Age: any age; grows more rapidly in children
Histo: nest of compacted trabeculae of mature lamellar bone
Location: ilium, ribs, femur, humerus, phalanges (not in skull)
√ round solitary density of trabeculated bone <2 cm in size
√ "brush" border margins = sharply demarcated with thorny radiations
√ may show activity on bone scan
√ may demonstrate slow growth
Prognosis: may increase to 8 – 12 cm over years (40%); may decrease / disappear

BRUCELLAR OSTEOMYELITIS
Organism: small Gram-negative nonencapsulated coccobacilli
Location: commonest site of involvement is reticuloendothelial system; spine > long bones
√ sharply demarcated lesion with little sclerosis (resembling TB)
DDx: fibrous dysplasia, benign tumor, osteoid osteoma

BURKITT LYMPHOMA
Endemic in areas with malaria: tropical Africa, New Guinea

Age: <10 years of age
Path: resemblance to Hodgkin disease
Location: mandible (first), maxilla; multifocal (10%); soft tissues: abdominal lymph nodes, ovaries, kidneys
@ Mandible / maxilla
   √ grossly destructive lesion, spicules of bone growing at right angles
   √ large soft tissue mass
@ Other skeleton
   √ reminiscent of Ewing tumor / reticulum cell sarcoma
   √ lamellated periosteal reaction around major long bones
Prognosis: long-term survival in 50%

CAISSON DISEASE
= DECOMPRESSION SICKNESS = THE BENDS
Etiology:
during too rapid decompression = reduction of surrounding pressure (ascent from dive, exit from caisson / hyperbaric chamber, ascent to altitude) nitrogen bubbles form (nitrogen more soluble in fat of panniculus adiposus, spinal cord, brain, bones containing fatty marrow)
• "the bends" = local pain in knee, elbow, shoulder, hip
• neurologic symptoms (paresthesia, major cerebral / spinal involvement)
• "chokes" = substernal discomfort + coughing (embolization of pulmonary vessels)
Location: mostly in long tubular bones of lower extremity (distal end of shaft + epiphyseal portion); symmetrical lesions
√ early: area of rarefaction
√ healing phase: irregular new bone formation with greater density
√ peripheral zone of calcification / ossification
√ ischemic necrosis of articular surface with secondary osteoarthritis

CALCIUM PYROPHOSPHATE DIHYDRATE DEPOSITION DISEASE
= CPPD = PSEUDOGOUT = FAMILIAL CHONDROCALCINOSIS
Types:
   1. Osteoarthritic form (50%)
   2. Pseudogout = acute synovitis (20%)
   3. Rheumatoid form (5%)
   4. Neuropathic arthropathy
   5. Asymptomatic with tophaceous pseudogout (common)
M:F = 3:2
• calcium pyrophosphate crystals in synovial fluid + within leukocytes (characteristic weakly positive birefringent diffraction pattern)
Location:
   (a) knee (especially meniscus + cartilage of patellofemoral joint)
   (b) wrist (triangular fibrocartilage in distal radioulnar joint bilaterally)
   (c) pelvis (sacroiliac joint, symphysis)

(d) spine (annulus fibrosis of lumbar intervertebral disc; NEVER in nucleus pulposus as in ochronosis)

(e) shoulder, hip, elbow, ankle, acromioclavicular joint

√ polyarticular chondrocalcinosis (in fibro- and hyaline cartilage)

√ involvement of tendons, bursae, pinnae of the ear

√ pyrophosphate arthropathy resembles osteoarthritis: joint space narrowing, subchondral eburnation, cyst formation

√ numerous intraarticular bodies (fragmentation of subchondral bone)

CALVÉ-KÜMMEL-VERNEUIL DISEASE
= VERTEBRAL OSTEOCHONDROSIS = VERTEBRA PLANA = avascular necrosis of vertebral body

Age: 2 – 15 years

√ uniform collapse of vertebral body into flat thin disc

√ increased density of vertebra

√ neural arches NOT affected

√ discs are normal with normal intervertebral disc space

√ intravertebral vacuum cleft sign (PATHOGNOMONIC)

DDx: Eosinophilic granuloma, metastatic disease

CAMPOMELIC DYSPLASIA
= sporadic / autosomal recessive dwarfism

Incidence: 0.05:10,000 births

Associated with:
1. Hydrocephalus (23%)
2. Congenital heart disease (30%): VSD, ASD, Tetralogy, AS
3. Hydronephrosis (30%)

• pretibial dimple

√ macrocephaly, cleft palate, micrognathia (90 – 99%)

@ Chest & Spine
   √ hypoplastic scapulae (92%)
   √ narrow bell-shaped chest
   √ hypoplastic vertebral bodies + nonmineralized pedicles (especially lower cervical spine)

@ Pelvis
   √ vertically narrowed iliac bones
   √ vertical inclination of ischii
   √ wide symphysis
   √ narrow iliac bones with small wings
   √ shallow acetabulum

@ Extremities (lower extremity more severely affected)
   √ dislocation of hips + knees
   √ anterior bowing (= campo) of long bones: marked in tibia + moderate in femur
   √ hypoplastic fibula
   √ small secondary ossification center of knee
   √ small primary ossification center of talus
   √ club foot

OB-US:
   √ bowing of tibia + femur
   √ decreased thoracic circumference
   √ hypoplastic scapulae
   √ ± cleft palate

Prognosis: death usually <5 months of age (within first year in 97%) due to respiratory insufficiency

CARPENTER SYNDROME
= ACROCEPHALOPOLYSYNDACTYLY

autosomal recessive

• retardation   • hypogonadism

√ patent ductus arteriosus

√ acro(oxy)cephaly

√ polysyndactyly

CHONDROBLASTOMA
= CODMAN TUMOR = CARTILAGE-CONTAINING GIANT CELL TUMOR = BENIGN CHONDROBLASTOMA; occurs before cessation of enchondral bone growth

Incidence: 1% of primary bone neoplasms (700 cases in world literature)

Age: peak in 2nd decade (range of 8 – 59 years); 5 – 25 years (88%); M:F = 2:1

Histo: polyhedral chondroblasts + multinucleated giant cells = epiphyseal chondromatous giant cell tumor (resembles chondromyxoid fibroma)

• mild joint pain, tenderness, swelling, limitation of motion

Location: proximal femur + greater trochanter (23%), distal femur (20%), proximal tibia (17%), proximal humerus (17%), tarsal bones; 2/3 lower extremity, 50% about knee; may occur in apophyses (minor + greater trochanter, patella, greater tuberosity of humerus), near triradiate cartilage of innominate bone

Site: eccentric medullary, subarticular location with open growth plate; tumor growth may continue to involve metaphysis

√ oval / round radiolucency usually 1 – 4 cm in diameter

√ well-defined sclerotic margin, may be lobulated

√ punctate / irregular calcifications in 25 – 50%

√ no periosteal reaction / joint involvement

√ periostitis of adjacent metaphysis / diaphysis (30%)

Rx: curettage

DDx: (1) Ischemic necrosis of femoral head (may be indistinguishable, more irregular configuration)

(2) Giant cell tumor (usually larger + less well demarcated, not calcified, older age group)

(3) Chondromyxoid fibroma

CHONDRODYSPLASIA PUNCTATA
= CONGENITAL STIPPLED EPIPHYSES
= DYSPLASIA EPIPHYSEALIS PUNCTATA
= CHONDRODYSTROPHIA CALCIFICANS CONGENITA
= proportional / mesomelic dwarfism

Etiology: peroxisomal disorder characterized by fibroblast plasmalogen deficiency

Incidence: 1:110,000 births

A. AUTOSOMAL RECESSIVE CHONDRODYSPLASIA PUNCTATA = RHIZOMELIC TYPE

Associated with: CHD (common)

• flat face
• congenital cataracts
• ichthiotic skin thickening
• mental retardation

- cleft palate
√ multiple small punce calcifications of varying size
in epiphyses (knee, hip, shoulder, wrist), in base of
skull, in posterior elements of vertebrae, in
respiratory cartilage and soft tissues (neck, rib
ends) before appearance of ossification centers
√ prominent symmetrical shortening of femur +
humerus (rarely all limbs symmetrically affected)
√ congenital dislocation of hip
√ flexion contractures of extremities
√ club feet
√ metaphyseal splaying of proximal tubular bones (in
particular about knee)
√ thickening of diaphyses
√ prominent vertebral + paravertebral calcifications
√ coronal clefts in vertebral bodies
Prognosis: death usually <1 year of age
DDx: Zellweger syndrome
B. CONRADI-HÜNERMANN DISEASE
= NONRHIZOMELIC TYPE
more common milder nonlethal variety;
autosomal dominant
- normal intelligence
√ more widespread but milder involvement as above
Prognosis: survival often into adulthood
Cx: respiratory failure (severe underdevelopment of
ribs), tracheal stenosis, spinal cord compression
DDx: (1) Cretinism (may show epiphyseal
fragmentation, much larger calcifications within
epiphysis)
(2) Warfarin embryopathy
(3) Zellweger syndrome

CHONDROECTODERMAL DYSPLASIA
= ELLIS-VAN CREVELD SYNDROME = MESODERMAL
DYSPLASIA
= autosomal recessive acromesomelic dwarfism
Incidence: 120 cases; in inbred Amish communities
Associated with: congenital heart disease in 50% (single
atrium, ASD, VSD)

- ectodermal dysplasia:
  - absent / hypoplastic brittle spoon-shaped nails
  - irregular + pointed teeth, partial anodontia, teeth may
    be present at birth
  - scant / fine hair
- obliteration of maxillary mucobuccal space (thick frenula
  between alveolar mucosa + upper lip)
- strabismus
- genital malformations: epispadia, hypospadia,
  hypoplastic external genitalia, undescended testicles
√ hepatosplenomegaly
√ accelerated skeletal maturation
√ normal spine
@ Skull
  √ Wormian bones
  √ cleft lip
@ Chest
  √ long narrow thorax in AP + transverse dimensions
  √ horizontal ribs + elevated clavicles
@ Pelvis
  √ small flattened ilia
  √ trident shape of acetabulum with indentation in roof +
    bony spur (almost pathognomonic)
  √ acetabular + tibial exostoses
@ Extremities
  √ thickening + shortening of all long bones, more severe
    in forearms + lower legs (radius + tibia > humerus +
    femur)
  √ excessive shortening of fibula
  √ widening of proximal tibial shaft + delayed
    development of tibial plateau
  √ dislocation of radial head (due to shortening of ulna)
  √ carpal / tarsal coalition = frequent fusion of two / more
    carpal (hamate + capitate) + tarsal bones
  √ supernumerary carpal bones
  √ hypoplasia / absence of terminal phalanges + cone-
    shaped epiphyses
  √ postaxial polydactyly common (usually finger, rarely
    toe) ± syndactyly of hands + feet
  √ carpal fusion (after complete ossification)

	Classification of Chondromalacia Patellae	
Grade	Arthroscopic pathology	T1WI of MRI
1	softening + swelling of articular cartilage	focal hypointense areas not extending to cartilage surface / subcondral bone
2	blistering of articular cartilage producing deformity of surface	focal hypointense areas extending to cartilage surface with preservation of sharp cartilage margins
3	surface irregularity + cartilage fibrillation with minimal extension to subchondral bone ("brush-border sign")	focal hypointense areas extending to articular surface but not to osseous surface; loss of sharp dark margin between articular cartilage of patella + trochlea
4	ulceration with exposure of subchondral bone	focal hypointense areas extending from subchondral bone to cartilage surface; cartilage thinned to subchondral bone

OB-US:
√ proportional shortening of long bones
√ small thorax with decreased circumference
√ increased cardiothoracic ratio
√ ASD
√ polydactyly

Prognosis: death within first month of life in 33%
(due to respiratory / cardiac complications)
DDx: Asphyxiating thoracic dysplasia (difficult distinction);
rhizomelic achondroplasia

CHONDROMALACIA PATELLAE
= pathologic softening of patellar cartilage
Cause: trauma, tracking abnormality of patella
• anterior knee pain
• asymptomatic (incidental athroscopic diagnosis)

CHONDROMYXOID FIBROMA
Rare benign cartilaginous tumor; initially arising in cortex
Incidence: <1% of all bone tumors
Histo: chondroid + fibrous + myxoid tissue (related to
chondroblastoma); may be mistaken for
chondrosarcoma
Age: peak 2nd – 3rd decade (range of 5 – 79 years)
M:F = 1:1
• slowly progressive local pain, swelling, restriction of
motion

Location:
  (a) long bones (60%): about knee (50%), proximal
      tibia (82% of tibial lesions), distal femur (71% of
      femoral lesions), fibula
  (b) short tubular bones of hand + feet (20%)
  (c) flat bones: pelvis, ribs (classic but uncommon)
Site: eccentric, metaphyseal (47 – 53%), metadiaphyseal
      (20 – 43%), metaepiphyseal (26%), diaphyseal (1 –
      10%), epiphyseal (3%)
√ expansile ovoid lesion with radiolucent center + oval
  shape at each end of lesion
√ long axis parallel to long axis of host bone (1 – 10 cm in
  length and 4 – 7 cm in width)
√ geographic bone destruction (100%)
√ well-defined sclerotic margin (86%)
√ expanded shell = bulged + thinned overlying cortex
  (68%)
√ partial cortical erosion (68%)
√ scalloped margin (58%)
√ septations (57%) may mimic trabeculations
√ stippled calcifications within tumor in advanced lesions
  (7%)
√ NO periosteal reaction (unless fractured)

Prognosis: 25% recurrence rate following currettage
Cx: malignant degeneration distinctly unusual
DDx: (1) Aneurysmal bone cyst (2) Simple bone cyst
       (3) Nonossifying fibroma (4) Fibrous dysplasia
       (5) Enchondroma (6) Chondroblastoma
       (7) Eosinophilic granuloma (8) Fibrous cortical
       defect (9) Giant cell tumor

CHONDROSARCOMA
A. PRIMARY CHONDROSARCOMA
B. SECONDARY CHONDROSARCOMA
   as a complication of a preexisting skeletal
   abnormality such as
   1. Osteochondroma
   2. Enchondroma
   3. Parosteal chondroma

Peripheral Chondrosarcoma
= EXOSTOTIC CHONDROSARCOMA = malignant
degeneration of hereditary multiple exostoses and
rarely of a solitary exostosis (beginning in
cartilaginous cap of osteochondroma)
Peak age: 5th – 6th decade; M:F = 1.5:1
• asymptomatic / pain + swelling

Location: pelvis, scapula, sternum, ribs, ends of
          humerus / femur, skull, facial bones
√ unusually large soft tissue mass attached to bone
√ flocculent / streaky chondroid calcification
  (CHARACTERISTIC)
√ dense radiopaque center with streaks radiating to
  periphery (not marginated)
√ thickening of cortex at site of attachment
√ late destruction of bone
DDx:
  (1) Osteochondroma (densely calcified with multiple
  punctate calcifications) (2) Parosteal osteosarcoma
  (more homogeneous density of calcified osteoid)

Central Chondrosarcoma
= ENDOSTEAL CHONDROSARCOMA = 3rd most
common primary bone tumor (1st multiple myeloma,
2nd osteosarcoma)
Histo: arises from chondroblasts (tumor osteoid is
         never formed)
Age: median 45 years; 50% >40 years; 10% in
       children (rapidly fatal); M:F = 2:1
• hyperglycemia as paraneoplastic syndrome (85%)

Location: neck of femur, pubic rami, proximal humerus,
          ribs, skull (sphenoid bone, cerebellopontine
          angle, mandible), sternum
Site: central + meta- / diaphysis
√ expansile osteolytic lesion 1 – several cm in size
√ short transition zone ± sclerotic margin (well defined
  from host bone)
√ ± small irregular punctate / snowflake type of
  calcification; single / multiple
√ late: loss of definition + break through cortex
√ endosteal cortical thickening, sometimes at a distance
  from the tumor
√ presence of large soft tissue mass
DDx: benign enchondroma, osteochondroma,
       osteosarcoma, fibrosarcoma

Clear Cell Chondrosarcoma
Low grade malignancy, usually mistaken for
chondroblastoma (may be related)

Histo: small lobules of tissue composed of cells with centrally filled vesicular nuclei surrounded by large clear cytoplasm

Age: 19 – 68 years, predominantly after epiphyseal fusion

Location: proximal femur, proximal humerus, proximal ulna, lamina vertebrae (5%); pubic ramus

Site: epiphysis
√ single lobulated oval / round sharply marginated lesion of 1 – 2 cm in size
√ surrounding increased bone density
√ aggressive rapid growth over 3 cm
√ may contain calcifications
√ bone often enlarged
√ indistinguishable from conventional chondrosarcoma / chondroblastoma (slow growth over years)

CLEIDOCRANIAL DYSOSTOSIS
= CLEIDOCRANIAL DYSPLASIA = MUTATIONAL DYSOSTOSIS
= delayed ossification of midline structures (particularly of membranous bone)
Autosomal dominant
@ Skull
• large head
√ diminished / absent ossification of skull (in early infancy)
√ Wormian bones
√ widened fontanelles + sutures with delayed closure
√ persistent metopic suture
√ brachycephaly + prominent bossing
√ large mandible
√ high narrow palate (± cleft)
√ hypoplastic paranasal sinuses
√ delayed / defective dentition
@ Chest
√ hypoplasia / absence (10%) of clavicles (defective development usually of lateral portion, R > L (DDx: congenital pseudarthrosis of clavicle)
√ thorax may be narrowed + bell-shaped
√ supernumerary ribs
√ incompletely ossified sternum
√ hemivertebrae, spondylosis (frequent)
@ Pelvis
√ delayed ossification of bones forming symphysis pubis (DDx: bladder extrophy)
√ hypoplastic iliac bones
@ Extremities
√ radius short / absent
√ elongated second metacarpals
√ pseudoepiphyses of metacarpal bases
√ short hypoplastic distal phalanges of hand
√ pointed terminal tufts
√ coned epiphyses
√ coxa vara = deformed / absent femoral necks
√ accessory epiphyses in hands + feet (common)
OB-US:
√ cephalopelvic disproportion (large fetal head + narrow birth canal of affected maternal pelvis) necessitates cesarean section

COCCIDIOIDOMYCOSIS
Endemic in southern California + southern Arizona (San Joaquin Valley)
(1) primary / respiratory phase: usually asymptomatic; erythema nodosum in 5%
(2) secondary phase: disseminated infection from bronchial ulceration in 10 – 20%
Histo: granulomatous bone lesions

Location: most frequent site at end of bone / bony prominences of tibial tubercle, ankle, acromion, medial end of clavicle, spine, ribs, pelvis
√ focal areas of destruction, formation of cavities (early) followed by sclerosis of surrounding bone (later) = bubbly bone lesion
√ proliferation of overlying periosteum
√ joints generally not infected
√ destruction of vertebra with preservation of disc space
√ psoas abscess indistinguishable from tuberculosis, may calcify
√ soft tissue abscesses common

CONGENITAL DYSPLASIA OF HIP
= DEVELOPMENTAL DYSPLASIA OF HIP (DDH)
Etiology:
abnormal ligamentous laxity; maternal estrogen effect not inactivated by immature fetal liver; hyperflexion of breech presentation results in shortening of iliopsoas muscle (breech:vertex = 6:1); heredity (6% risk for subsequent sibling of normal parents, 36% risk for subsequent sibling of one affected parent; 12% risk for patient's own children)
Incidence: 1.3:1000 newborns

Increased risk: infants born in breech position, with skull-molding deformities, neuromuscular disorders (eg, myelodysplasia), congenital torticollis, foot deformities (metatarsus adductus, clubfoot), family history of CHD
Increased prevalence: females, firstborns, pregnancy with oligohydramnios
Age: most dislocations probably occur after birth; M:F = 1:8; caucasians > blacks

Classification:
Type 1 = DISLOCATABLE UNSTABLE HIP
Incidence: 0.25 – 0.85% of all newborn infants; 2/3 are firstborns
√ slight increase in femoral anteversion
√ mild marginal abnormalities in acetabular cartilage
√ early labral eversion
Prognosis: 60% will become stable after 1 week; 88% will become stable by age of 2 months
Type 2 = SUBLUXED HIP
√ loss of femoral head sphericity
√ increased femoral anteversion
√ early labral inversion
√ shallow acetabulum
Type 3 = DISLOCATED HIP
√ accentuated flattening of femoral head
√ shallow acetabulum

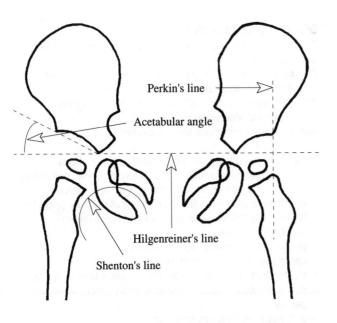

Perkin's line

Acetabular angle

Hilgenreiner's line

Shenton's line

√ limbus formation (= inward growth + hypertrophy of labrum)
- positive Ortolani test = reduction of proximal femur into the acetabulum by progressive abduction
- positive Barlow test = displacement of proximal femur by progressive adduction with hip flexed

Location: left:right:bilateral = 11:1:4

Radiologic lines:
1. Line of Hilgenreiner
    = line connecting superolateral margins of triradiate cartilages

2. Acetabular angle / index
    = angle that lies between Hilgenreiner's line and a line drawn from most superolateral ossified edge of acetabulum to superolateral margin of triradiate cartilage
    √ >30° strongly suggests dysplasia
3. Perkin's line
    = vertical line to Hilgenreiner's line through the lateral rim of acetabulum
4. Shenton's line
    = line drawn between medial border of femur neck + superior border of obturator foramen

AP pelvic radiograph:
√ line drawn along axis of femoral shaft will not pass through upper edge of acetabulum but intersect the anterior-superior iliac spine (during Barlow maneuver)
√ femoral shaft above horizontal line drawn through the Y-synchondroses
√ apex of metaphysis lateral to edge of acetabulum
√ eccentric position of femoral epiphysis (position estimated by a circle drawn with a diameter equivalent to width of femoral neck)
√ proximal + lateral migration of femoral neck adjacent to ilium
√ acetabular dysplasia = shallow incompletely developed acetabulum
√ development of false acetabulum
√ interrupted discontinuous arc of Shenton's line
√ femoral ossific nucleus / medial beak of femoral metaphysis outside inner lower quadrant of coordinates established by Hilgenreiner's + Perkin's lines

Sonographic Hip Types

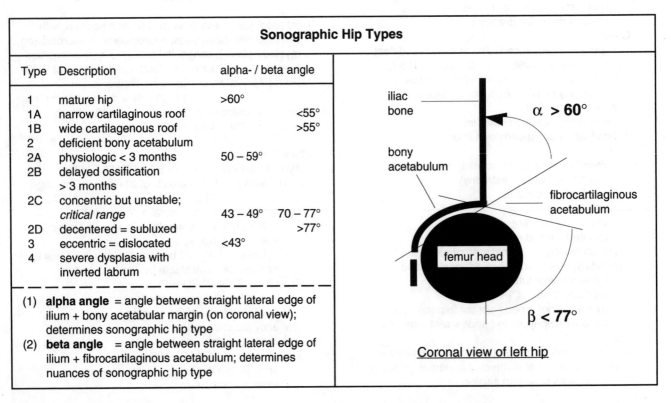

Type	Description	alpha- / beta angle	
1	mature hip	>60°	
1A	narrow cartilaginous roof		<55°
1B	wide cartilagenous roof		>55°
2	deficient bony acetabulum		
2A	physiologic < 3 months	50 – 59°	
2B	delayed ossification > 3 months		
2C	concentric but unstable; *critical range*	43 – 49°	70 – 77°
2D	decentered = subluxed		>77°
3	eccentric = dislocated	<43°	
4	severe dysplasia with inverted labrum		

(1) **alpha angle** = angle between straight lateral edge of ilium + bony acetabular margin (on coronal view); determines sonographic hip type
(2) **beta angle** = angle between straight lateral edge of ilium + fibrocartilaginous acetabulum; determines nuances of sonographic hip type

iliac bone

bony acetabulum

$\alpha > 60°$

fibrocartilaginous acetabulum

femur head

$\beta < 77°$

Coronal view of left hip

√ proximal migration of femur = unilateral shortening of vertical distance from femoral ossific nucleus / femoral metaphysis to Hilgenreiner's line
√ delayed ossification of femoral epiphysis (usually evident between 2nd and 8th month of life)
US (practical only up to 8 – 10 months of age):
√ direct visualization of unossified femoral head
√ femoral head position at rest in neutral position: normal / subluxed = decentered / dislocated = eccentric
√ hip instability under motion + stress maneuvers: normal / lax = subluxable / subluxed / dislocatable = unstable / dislocated reducible / dislocated irreducible
  Δ subluxability up to 6 mm is normal in newborns (still under influence of maternal hormones); decreasing to 3 mm by 2nd day of life
  Δ examination should be performed >1 – 2 weeks of age!
√ dislocatable (= concentric but unstable) hip can be pushed out of hip joint (Barlow positive)
√ posterior + superior dislocation of head against ilium
√ dislocated (= eccentric) hip can be reduced (Ortolani positive)
√ hypoechoic femoral head not centered over triradiate cartilage between pubis + ischium (on transverse view)
√ increased amount of soft-tissue echoes ("pulvinar") between femoral head and acetabulum
√ cartilaginous acetabular labrum interposed between head and acetabulum (inverted labrum)
√ disparity in presence + size of ossific nucleus
√ disparity in size of femoral head
√ wavy contour of bony acetabulum with only slight curvature
√ delayed ossification of acetabular corner
√ equator sign = <50% of femoral head lies medial to line drawn along iliac bone (on coronal view); 58% to 33% coverage is indeterminate, <33% coverage is abnormal
√ abnormally acute alpha angle (= angle between straight lateral edge of ilium bony acetabular margin)
  Δ 4° – 6° interobserver variation!
Prognosis:
  alpha-angle <50° at birth / 50° - 59° after 3 months indicates significant risk for dislocation without treatment; follow-up in 4-week intervals
Rx:
  (1) flexion-abduction-external rotation brace (Pavlik harness) / splint / spica cast
  (2) femoral varus osteotomy
  (3) pelvic (Salter) / acetabular rotation
  (4) increase in acetabular depth (Pemberton)
  (5) medialization of femoral head (Chiari)

CONGENITAL GENERALIZED FIBROMATOSIS
= INFANTILE MULTIPLE FIBROMATOSIS
= rare disorder of fibroblastic origin
Type 1: <u>CONGENITAL GENERALIZED FIBROMATOSIS</u>
  Involvement of bone + visceral organs (lungs, intestines, liver, pancreas, kidney)

Age: lesions present at birth / first 4 months with progressive growth
√ multiple focal fibrous lesions anywhere in the body
Prognosis: 80% die within 4 months
Type 2: <u>CONGENITAL DIFFUSE FIBROMATOSIS</u> = CONGENITAL MULTIPLE FIBROMATOSIS
  Predominant involvement of bone, no visceral involvement (occasionally colon)
  Prognosis: good, spontaneous regression may occur
Location: bilateral, symmetric
Site: metaphyseal in long bones
√ destructive bone lesions with smooth margins 0.5 – 1.0 cm in size
√ well-defined sclerotic margin occasionally
√ any bone may be involved
DDx: (1) Letterer-Siwe disease (skin lesions)
  (2) Neurofibromatosis (multiple masses)
  (3) Osseous hemangiomas / lymphangiomatosis / lipomatosis
  (4) Metastatic neuroblastoma

CONGENITAL INSENSITIVITY TO PAIN WITH ANHYDROSIS
= rare autosomal recessive disorder presumably on the basis of abnormal neural crest development
Age: presenting at birth
Incidence: 15 reported cases
Path: absence of dorsal + sympathetic ganglia, deficiency of neural fibers <6 μm in diameter + disproportionate number of fibers of 6 – 10 μm in diameter

• history of painless injuries + burns (DDx: familial dysautonomia, congenital sensory neuropathy, hereditary sensory radicular neuropathy, acquired sensory neuropathy, syringomyelia)
• abnormal pain + temperature perception
• burns, bruises, infections are common
• biting injuries of fingers, lips, tongue
• absence of sweating
• mental retardation
CRITERIA: (1) defect must be present at birth
  (2) general insensitivity to pain
  (3) general mental / physical retardation
√ epiphyseal separation in infancy (epiphyseal injuries result in growth problems)
√ metaphyseal fractures in early childhood
√ diaphyseal fractures in late childhood
√ Charcot joints = neurotrophic joints (usually weight-bearing joints) with effusions + synovial thickening
√ ligamentous laxity
√ bizarre deformities + gross displacement + considerable hemorrhage (unnoticed fractures + dislocations)
√ osteomyelitis + septic arthritis may occur + progress extensively
DDx (1) sensory neuropathies (eg, diabetes mellitus)
  (2) hysteria (3) syphilis (4) mental deficiency
  (5) syringomyelia (6) organic brain disease

CORNELIA DE LANGE SYNDROME

= Amsterdam dwarfism
- mental retardation (IQ <50)
- hirsutism; hypoplastic genitalia
- feeble growling cry
- high forehead; short neck
- arched palate
- bushy eyebrows meeting in midline + long curved eyelashes
- small nose with depressed bridge; upward tilted nostrils; excessive distance between nose + upper lip
√ small + brachycephalic skull
√ hypoplasia of long bones (upper extremity more involved)
√ forearm bones may be absent
√ short radius + elbow dislocation
√ thumbs placed proximally (hypoplastic 1st metacarpal)
√ short phalanges + clinodactyly of 5th finger

CORTICAL DESMOID

= AVULSIVE CORTICAL IRREGULARITY
= PERIOSTEAL / SUBPERIOSTEAL DESMOID
= SUBPERIOSTEAL / CORTICAL ABRASION
= SUBPERIOSTEAL CORTICAL DEFECT
= rare fibrous lesion of the periosteum
Age: peak 14 – 16 years (range of 3 – 17 years); M:F = 3:1
Histo: shallow defect filled with proliferating fibroblasts, multiple small fragments of resorbing bone (microavulsions) at tendinous insertions
- no localizing signs / symptoms
Location: posteromedial aspect of medial femoral epicondyle along medial ridge of linea aspera at attachment of adductor magnus aponeurosis; 1/3 bilateral
√ area of cortical thickening
√ 1 – 2 cm irregular, shallow, concave saucer-like crater with sharp margin
√ lamellated periosteal reaction
√ localized cortical hyperostosis proximally (healing phase)
CAVE: may be confused with a malignant tumor (osteosarcoma) / osteomyelitis

CRI-DU-CHAT SYNDROME

= deletion of short arm of 5th chromosome (5 p)
- generalized dwarfism due to marked growth retardation
- failure to thrive
- peculiar high-pitched cat cry (hypoplastic larynx)
- antimongoloid palpebral fissures
- strabismus
- profound mental retardation
- round facies
- low set ears
Associated with: congenital heart disease (obtain CXR!)
√ agenesis of corpus callosum
√ microcephaly
√ hypertelorism
√ small mandible
√ faulty long bone development

√ short 3rd, 4th, 5th metacarpals
√ long 2nd, 3rd, 4th, 5th proximal phalanges
√ horseshoe kidney
Dx: made clinically

CROUZON DISEASE

= CRANIOFACIAL SYNOSTOSIS = Apert syndrome without syndactyly
- parrot-beak nose
- strabismus
- deafness
- mental retardation
- dental abnormalities
√ acro(oxy)cephaly (premature craniosynostosis)
√ hypertelorism + exophthalmus
√ hypoplastic maxilla (relative prominence of mandible)

CUSHING SYNDROME

√ most often axial osteoporosis
√ stippled calvarium
√ demineralized dorsum sellae
Cx: (1) pathologic fractures of vertebrae + ribs with excessive callus formation
      (2) aseptic necrosis of hips
      (3) bone infarcts
      (4) delayed skeletal maturation in children

CYSTIC ANGIOMATOSIS

= LYMPHANGIOMATOSIS / HEMANGIOMATOSIS
Histo: endothelial lined cysts in bone
Age: peak 10 – 15 years; range of 3 months – 55 years
Location: long bones, skull, flat bones
√ multiple osteolytic metaphyseal lesions of 1 – 2 mm to several cm with fine sclerotic margins + relative sparing of medullary cavity
√ may show overgrowth of long bone
√ endosteal thickening
√ sometimes associated with soft tissue mass ± phleboliths
√ chylous pleural effusion suggests fatal prognosis
DDx: (other polyostotic diseases as) histiocytosis X, fibrous dysplasia, metastases, Gaucher disease, congenital fibromatosis, neurofibromatosis, enchondromatosis, Maffucci syndrome

DERMATOMYOSITIS

= POLYMYOSITIS = damaged chondroitin sulfate no longer inhibiting calcification
Histo: atrophy of muscle bundles followed by edema and coagulation necrosis; mucoid degeneration with round cell infiltrates concentrated around blood vessels
Age: 4th – 6th decade, F > M
@ Skeleton
√ linear + confluent calcifications in soft tissues (extremities, hands, abdominal wall, chest wall, axilla, inguinal region)
√ pointing of terminal tufts
√ rheumatoid-like arthritis (rare)
√ "floppy-thumb" sign

@ Chest
  √ disseminated pulmonary infiltrates (reminiscent of scleroderma)
@ Myocardium
  √ changes similar to skeletal muscle
@ GI tract
  √ atony + dilatation of esophagus
  √ atony of small intestines + colon
ACUTE FORM
  • fever, joint pain, lymphadenopathy, splenomegaly, subcutaneous edema
  Prognosis: death within a few months
CHRONIC FORM
  • low-grade fever, muscular aches + pains, muscle weakness, edema, skin erythema
Cx: high incidence of malignant neoplasms in GI tract, lung, kidney, ovary, breast

DESMOPLASTIC FIBROMA
= INTRAOSSEOUS DESMOID TUMOR
= rare locally aggressive benign neoplasm of bone with borderline malignancy resembling soft tissue desmoids / musculoaponeurotic fibromatosis
Incidence: 107 cases in world literature
Histo: intracellular collagenous material in fibroblasts with small nuclei
Age: mean of 21 years (range 15 months to 75 years); in 90% <30 years; M:F = 1:1
  • slowly progressive pain + local tenderness
  • palpable mass
Location: mandible (26%), ilium (14%), >50% in long bones (femur [14%], humerus [11%], radius [9%], tibia [7%], clavicle), scapula, vertebra, calcaneus
Site: central meta- / diaphyseal (if growth plate open); may extend into epiphysis with subarticular location (if growth plate closed)
√ geographic (96%) / moth-eaten (4%) bone destruction without matrix mineralization
√ narrow (96%) / poorly defined (4%) zone of transition
√ no marginal sclerosis (94%)
√ residual columns of bone with "pseudotrabeculae" are CLASSIC (91%)
√ bone expansion (89%); may grow to massive size (simulating aneurysmal bone cyst / metastatic renal cell carcinoma)
√ breach of cortex + soft-tissue mass (29%)

Cx: pathologic fracture (9%)
Prognosis: 52% rate of local recurrence
Rx: wide excision
DDx:
  (1) Giant cell tumor (round rather than oval, may extend into epiphysis + subchondral bone plate)
  (2) Fibrous dysplasia (occupies longer bone, contains mineralized matrix, often with sclerotic rim)
  (3) Aneurysmal bone cyst (eccentric blowout appearance rather than fusiform)
  (4) Chondromyxoid fibroma (eccentric with delicate marginal sclerosis + scalloped border)

DIASTROPHIC DYSPLASIA
= DIASTROPHIC DWARFISM = EPIPHYSEAL DYSOSTOSIS
= autosomal recessive severe rhizomelic dwarfism secondary to generalized disorder of cartilage followed by fibrous scars + ossifications
  • diastrophic = "twisted" habitus
  • "cauliflower ear" = ear deformity from inflammation of pinna
  • laryngomalacia
  • lax + rigid joints with contractures
  • normal intellectual development

@ Axial skeleton
  √ cleft palate (25%)
  √ cervical spina bifida occulta
  √ hypoplasia of odontoid
  √ severe progressive kyphoscoliosis of lumbar spine (not present at birth)
  √ narrowed interpedicular space in lumbar spine
  √ short + broad bony pelvis
  √ posterior tilt of sacrum
@ Extremities
  √ severe micromelia (predominantly rhizomelic = humerus + femur shorter than distal long bones
  √ widened metaphysis
  √ flattened epiphysis (retardation of epiphyseal ossification) with invagination of ossification centers into distal ends of femora
  √ multiple joint flexion contractures (notably of major joints)
  √ dislocation of one / more large joints (hip, elbow), lateral dislocation of patella
  √ coxa vara (common)
  √ medially bowed metatarsals
  √ clubfoot = severe talipes equinovarus
  √ ulnar deviation of hands
  √ oval + hypoplastic 1st metacarpal bone + abducted proximally positioned thumb = "hitchhiker's thumb" (CHARACTERISTIC)
  √ bizarre carpal bones with supernumerary centers
  √ widely spaced fingers
OB-US:
  √ proportionately shortened long bones
  √ hitchhiker thumb
  √ clubfeet
  √ joint contractures
  √ abnormal spinal curvature
Prognosis: death in infancy (due to abnormal softening of tracheal cartilage)

DIFFUSE IDIOPATHIC SKELETAL HYPEROSTOSIS
= DISH = FORESTIER DISEASE = ANKYLOSING HYPEROSTOSIS
= common ossifying diathesis characterized by bone proliferation at sites of tendinous + ligamentous attachment (enthesis)
Etiology:
  (1) may be caused by altered vitamin A metabolism (elevated plasma levels of unbound retinol)

(2) long-term ingestion of retinoid derivates for dermatologic disorders (eg, Accutane®); ? hypertrophic variant of spondylosis deformans
Age: >50 years; M > F
- pain, tenderness in extraspinal locations
- restricted motion of vertebral column
- hyperglycemia
- positive HLA-B27 in 34%

Location: lower thoracic > lower cervical > entire lumbar spine
√ anterior + lateral right-sided syndesmophytes of vertebral column (not on left because of aorta)
√ disc spaces well preserved, no apophyseal ankylosis, no sacroiliitis
√ flowing ossification along anterior / anterolateral aspect of at least 4 contiguous vertebral bodies
√ "whiskering" at iliac crest, ischial tuberosity, trochanters
√ spurs of olecranon process of ulna + calcaneus (plantar + posterior surface) + anterior surface of patella
√ broad osteophytes at lateral acetabular edge, inferior portions of sacroiliac joints, superior aspect of symphysis pubis
√ ossification of iliolumbar + sacrotuberous + sacroiliitic ligaments (high probability for presence of spinal DISH, DDx: fluorosis)
√ ossification of coracoclavicular ligament, patellar ligament, tibial tuberosity, interosseous membranes
√ increased incidence of hyperostosis frontalis interna
DDx: (1) Fluorosis (increased skeletal density)
(2) Acromegaly (posterior scalloping, skull features)
(3) Ankylosing spondylitis (squaring of vertebral bodies, coarser syndesmophytes, sacroiliitis, apophyseal alteration)

DISLOCATION
Shoulder Dislocation
Glenohumeral joint dislocations make up >50% of all dislocations
A. <u>ANTERIOR / SUBCORACOID SHOULDER DISLOCATION</u> (96%)
Mechanism: external rotation + abduction; 40% recurrent
Age: in younger individuals
May be associated with:
√ fracture of greater tuberosity (15%)
√ Bankart lesion = fracture of inferior glenoid rim (detachment of labrum)
√ fracture of anterior rim of glenoid
√ Hill-Sachs defect (50%) = depression fracture of posterolateral surface of humeral head (impaction against glenoid rim)
B. <u>POSTERIOR SHOULDER DISLOCATION</u> (2 – 4%)
in patients with convulsive disorders /electric shock therapy
√ rim sign (66%) = distance between medial border of humeral head + anterior glenoid rim <6 mm

May be associated with:
√ trough sign (75%) = "reverse Hill-Sachs" = compression fracture of anteromedial humeral head (tangential Grashey view of glenoid!)
√ fracture of posterior glenoid rim
√ avulsion fracture of lesser tuberosity
C. <u>ANTEROINFERIOR SHOULDER DISLOCATION</u> = LUXATIO ERECTA
rare type with extremity held over head in fixed position
Mechanism: severe hyperabduction of arm resulting in impingement of humeral head against acromion
√ humeral articular surface faces inferiorly
Cx: rotator cuff tear; fracture of acromion ± inferior glenoid fossa ± greater tuberosity; neurovascular injury

Wrist Dislocation
Mechanism: fall on outstretched hand
Incidence: 10% of all carpal injuries

A. <u>LUNATE DISLOCATION</u>
B. <u>PERILUNATE DISLOCATION</u>
2 – 3 times more common than lunate dislocation accompanied by fracture in 75% (= transscaphoid perilunate dislocation)
√ most commonly dorsal dislocation
C. <u>ROTARY SUBLUXATION OF SCAPHOID</u>
Mechanism: acute dorsiflexion of wrist; may be associated with rheumatoid arthritis
= tearing of interosseous ligaments of lunate, scaphoid, capitate
√ gap >4 mm between scaphoid + lunate (PA radiograph)
√ foreshortening of scaphoid
√ ring sign of distal pole of scaphoid
D. <u>MIDCARPAL DISLOCATION</u>

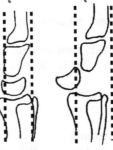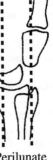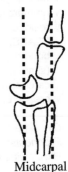

Normal   Lunate Dislocation   Perilunate Dislocation   Midcarpal Dislocation

DOWN SYNDROME
= MONGOLISM = TRISOMY 21 (95% nondisjunction, 5% translocation)
- mental retardation
- characteristic facies
- hypotonia in infancy
- Simian crease

@ Skull
- √ hypotelorism
- √ persistent metopic suture (40 – 79%) after age 10
- √ hypoplasia of sinuses + facial bones
- √ microcrania (brachycephaly)
- √ delayed closure of sutures + fontanelles
- √ dental abnormalities (underdeveloped tooth No. 2)
- √ flat-bridged nose

@ Axial skeleton
- √ atlantoaxial subluxation (25%)
- √ anterior scalloping of vertebral bodies
- √ "squared vertebral bodies" = centra high and narrow = positive lateral lumbar index (ratio of horizontal to vertical diameters of L2)

@ Chest
- √ Congenital heart disease (40%): endocardial cushion defect
- √ hypersegmentation of manubrium = 2 – 3 ossification centers (90%)
- √ gracile ribs; 11 pairs of ribs (25%)

@ Pelvis
- √ flaring of iliac wings (decreased iliac angle + index) = "Mickey Mouse ears" / "elephant ears"
- √ flattening of acetabular roof (decreased acetabular angle)
- √ tapering of ischial rami

@ Extremities
- √ metaphyseal flaring
- √ clinodactyly (50%); widened space between first two digits of hands + feet
- √ hypoplastic and triangular middle + distal phalanges of 5th finger = acromicria (DDx: normal individuals, cretins, achondroplastic dwarfs)
- √ pseudoepiphyses of 1st + 2nd metacarpals

@ Gastrointestinal
- √ umbilical hernia
- √ "double bubble" sign = duodenal atresia / stenosis / annular pancreas
- √ tracheo-esophageal fistula
- √ anorectal anomalies
- √ Hirschsprung disease

OB-US:
- *Incidence:*   1:800 births
- low alpha-fetoprotein (20 – 30%)
- advanced maternal age
  - Δ in 1:385 livebirths for women >35 years of age
  - Δ 20% of fetuses with Down syndrome are born to mothers >35 years of age
  - Δ 80% of fetuses with Down syndrome are born to mothers <35 years of age

- √ occipital-nuchal skin thickening >6 mm (in 40 – 70%) on transcerebellar diameter view (69% positive predictive value in 2nd trimester, 0.1% false- positives)
- √ cystic hygroma
- √ ratio of measured-to-expected femur length ≤ 0.91 (sensitivity 40%, specificity 95%); not acceptable as screening procedure (positive predictive value of 0.33%, false positive rate of 5%)

- √ elevated BPD / femur ratio (secondary to short femur)
- √ hypoplasia of middle phalanx of 5th digit resulting in inward curve (60%)
- √ VSD / complete AV canal (50%)
- √ double bubble of duodenal atresia (8%), not apparent before 22 weeks GA
- √ omphalocele
- √ hyperechogenic bowel at <20 weeks GA
- √ mild cerebral ventricular dilatation
- √ IUGR

Cx: leukemia (increased frequency 3 – 20 x)

DYSCHONDROSTEOSIS
= LÉRI-LAYANI-WEILL SYNDROME = mesomelic long bone shortening (forearm + leg); autosomal dominant
M:F = 1:4
- limited motion of elbow + wrist
- √ bilateral Madelung deformity
  - √ radial shortening in relation to ulna
  - √ bowing of radius laterally + dorsally
  - √ dorsal subluxation of distal end of ulna
  - √ carpal wedging between radius + ulna (due to triangular shape of distal radial epiphysis + underdevelopment of ulna)
- *DDx:* Pseudo-Madelung deformity (from trauma / infection)

DYSPLASIA EPIPHYSEALIS HEMIMELICA
= TREVOR DISEASE = TARSOEPIPHYSEAL ACLASIS
= eccentric usually medial epiphyseal cartilaginous overgrowth of one / more epiphyses; spontaneous occurrence
Age: 2 – 4 years; M>F
May be associated with hemihypertrophy
- limitation of joint mobility (due to localized painless mass)
Location: localized to tarsus, carpus, knee, ankle; occasionally generalized
- √ osteochondroma-like growth from one side of epiphysis
Cx: genu valgum
DDx: osteochondroma

ECHINOCOCCUS OF BONE
Occurs occasionally in the U.S.; usually in foreign-born individuals; bone involvement in 1%
Histo: no connective tissue barrier; daughter cysts extend directly into bone
@ Pelvis, sacrum, rarely long tubular bones
- √ round / irregular regions of rarefaction
- √ multiloculated lesion (bunch of grapes)
- √ no sharp demarcation (DDx: chondroma, giant cell tumor) with secondary infection
  - √ thickening of trabeculae with generalized perifocal condensation
  - √ cortical breakthrough with soft tissue mass
@ Vertebra
- √ sclerosis without pathologic fracture
- √ intervertebral discs not affected

√ vertebral lamina often involved
√ frequently involvement of adjacent ribs

EHLERS-DANLOS SYNDROME
= group of autosomal dominant diseases of connective tissue characterized by abnormal collagen synthesis
Types: 10 types have been described which differ clinically, biochemically and genetically
Age: present at birth; predominantly in males
• hyperelasticity of skin
• fragile brittle skin with gaping wounds and poor healing
• molluscoid pseudotumors over pressure points
• hyperextensibility of joints
• joint contractures with advanced age
• bleeding tendency (fragility of blood vessels)
• blue sclera, microcornea, myopia, keratoconus, ectopia lentis
√ multiple ovoid calcifications (2 – 10 mm) in subcutis / in fatty cysts ("spheroids"), most frequently in periarticular areas of legs
√ ectopic bone formation
√ hemarthrosis (particularly in knee)
√ malalignment / subluxation / dislocation of joints on stress radiographs
√ recurrent dislocations (hip, patella, shoulder, radius, clavicle)
√ precocious osteoarthrosis (predominantly in knees)
√ ulnar synostosis
√ kyphoscoliosis
√ spondylolisthesis
√ spina bifida occulta
√ diaphragmatic hernia
√ aneurysm of great vessels, aortic dissection, tortuosity of arch, ectasia of pulmonary arteries
√ ectasia of gastrointestinal tract
AORTOGRAPHY CONTRAINDICATED!
(Cx following arteriography: aortic rupture, hematomas)

ELASTOFIBROMA
= benign tumorlike lesion forming as a reaction to mechanical friction
Incidence: in 24% of women + 11% of men >55 years (autopsy study)
Age: elderly; M:F = 1:2
Histo: enlarged irregular serrated elastic hypereosinophilic fibers, collagen, scattered fibroblasts, occasional lobules of adipose tissue
• asymptomatic
• may remain clinically inapparent
Location: between inferior margin of scapula + posterior chest wall; bilateral in 25%
√ inhomogeneous poorly defined lesion of soft-tissue attenuation similar to muscle
√ well-defined intermediate-signal intensity lesion with interlaced areas of fat-intensity signal on T1WI + T2WI

ENCHONDROMA
= benign cartilaginous growth in medullary cavity; bones preformed in cartilage are affected (NOT skull)
Age: 10 – 30 years; M:F = 1:1

Histo: lobules of hyaline cartilage
• usually asymptomatic, painless swelling
Location: (frequently multiple = enchondromatosis)
   (a) in 40% small bones of wrists + hand (most frequent tumor here), distal + mid aspects of metacarpals, proximal / middle phalanges
   (b) femur, tibia, humerus, radius, ulna, foot, rib
Site: central + diaphyseal, epiphysis only affected after closure of growth plate
√ oval / round lucency near epiphysis with fine marginal line
√ scalloped endosteum
√ ground glass appearance
√ calcification: pinhead, stippled, flocculent, "rings and arcs" pattern
√ bulbous expansion of bone with thinning of cortex
√ Madelung deformity = bowing deformities of limb, discrepant length
√ NO cortical breakthrough / periosteal reaction
Cx: (1) pathologic fracture
     (2) malignant degeneration in long bone enchondromas in 15 – 20%
DDx:
   (1) Epidermoid inclusion cyst (phalangeal tuft, Hx of trauma, more lucent)
   (2) Unicameral bone cyst (rare in hands, more radiolucent)
   (3) Giant cell tumor of tendon sheath (commonly erodes bone, soft tissue mass outside bone)
   (4) Fibrous dysplasia (rare in hand, mostly polyostotic)
   (5) Bone infarct
   (6) Chondrosarcoma

ENCHONDROMATOSIS
= OLLIER DISEASE = DYSCHONDROPLASIA
= MULTIPLE ENCHONDROMATOSIS = nonhereditary failure of cartilage ossification
Age: early childhood presentation
• growth disparity with leg / arm shortening
• hand + feet deformity
Location: predominantly unilateral monomelic distribution
   (a) localized (b) regional (c) generalized
√ rounded masses / columnar streaks of decreased density from epiphyseal plate into diaphysis of long bones = cartilaginous rests
√ bony spurs pointing toward the joint (DDx: exostosis points away from it)
√ cartilaginous areas show punctate calcifications with age
√ associated with dwarfing of the involved bone due to impairment of epiphyseal fusion
√ club-like deformity of metaphyseal region
√ cartilaginous metaphyseal expansion with cortical expansion + thinning + breakthrough
√ bowing deformities of limb bones
√ discrepancy in length = Madelung deformity (radius, ulna)
√ small bones of feet + hands: aggressive deforming tumors that may break through cortex secondary to tendency to continue to proliferate

√ fan-like radiation of cartilage from center to crest of ilium
Cx: sarcomatous transformation (in 25 – 50%): osteosarcoma (young adults); chondro- / fibrosarcoma (in older patients)

MAFFUCCI SYNDROME
= nonhereditary enchondromatosis + multiple soft-tissue cavernous hemangiomas
Age: generally not before puberty
• multiple nodules particularly on digits + extremities (cavernous hemangiomas)
• normal intelligence
Location: unilateral involvement / marked asymmetry; distinct predilection for hands + feet
√ phleboliths may be present
√ striking tendency for enchondromata to be very large projecting into soft tissues
√ growth disturbance of long bones (common)
Cx: malignant transformation even higher than in Ollier disease

ENGELMANN-CAMURATI DISEASE
= PROGRESSIVE DIAPHYSEAL DYSPLASIA
= ENGELMANN DISEASE = RIBBING DISEASE (as forme fruste)
Autosomal dominant
Age: 5 – 25 years, M > F
• neuromuscular dystrophy = delayed walking (18 – 24 months) with wide-based waddling gait; often misdiagnosed as muscular dystrophy / poliomyelitis
• weakness + easy fatigability
• bone pain + tenderness usually in midshaft of long bones
• underdevelopment of muscles secondary to malnutrition
• NORMAL laboratory values

Location: usually symmetrical; NO involvement of hands, feet, ribs, scapulae
@ Skull (initially affected)
   √ amorphous increase in density at base of skull
@ Long bones (bilateral symmetrical distribution)
   √ fusiform enlargement of diaphyses with cortical thickening (endosteal + periosteal accretion of mottled new bone) and progressive obliteration of medullary cavity; symmetrical involvement
   √ progression of lesions along long axis of bone toward either end
   √ abrupt demarcation of lesions (metaphyses + epiphyses spared)
   √ relative elongation of extremities
√ NORMAL epiphyses + metaphyses
√ hands + feet UNAFFECTED
DDx:
   (1) Chronic osteomyelitis (single bone)
   (2) Hyperphosphatasemia (high alkaline phosphatase levels)
   (3) Paget disease (age, new bone formation, increased alkaline phosphatase)
   (4) Infantile cortical hyperostosis (fever; mandible, rib, clavicles; regresses, <1 year of age)

   (5) Fibrous dysplasia (predominantly unilateral, subperiosteal new bone)
   (6) Osteopetrosis (very little bony enlargement)
   (7) Vitamin A poisoning

EPIDERMOID INCLUSION CYST
= INTRAOSSEOUS KERATIN CYST = IMPLANTATION CYST
Age: 2nd – 4th decade; M > F
Histo: stratified squamous epithelium, keratin, cholesterol crystals (soft white cheesy contents)
• history of trauma (implantation of epithelium under skin with secondary bone erosion)
• asymptomatic

Location: superficially situated bones such as calvarium (typically in frontal / parietal bone), phalanx (usually terminal tuft of middle finger), L > R hand, occasionally in foot
√ well-defined round osteolysis with sclerotic margin
√ cortex frequently expanded + thinned
√ NO calcifications / periosteal reaction / soft tissue swelling
√ pathologic fracture often without periosteal reaction
DDx: (a) in finger: glomus tumor, enchondroma (rare in terminal phalanx)
         (b) in skull: infection, metastasis (poorly defined), eosinophilic granuloma (beveled margin)

EPIPHYSEOLYSIS OF FEMORAL HEAD
= SLIPPED CAPITAL FEMORAL EPIPHYSIS; Salter-Harris type I epiphyseal injury
Age: in overweight adolescent males
Etiology: trauma, renal osteodystrophy, rickets, childhood irradiation, growth hormone therapy
• knee / hip pain
Location: usually unilateral
√ widening of epiphyseal plate + slight irregularity of margins
√ irregularity + rarefaction of metaphysis of femoral neck
√ blurring of junction between metaphysis and epiphysis
√ posteromedial displacement (frog-leg view!)

ESSENTIAL OSTEOLYSIS
Progressive slow bone-resorptive disease
Histo: proliferation + hyperplasia of smooth muscle cells of synovial arterioles
√ progressive osteolysis of carpal + tarsal bones
√ thinned pointed proximal ends of metacarpals + metatarsals
√ elbows show same type of destruction
√ bathyrocephalic depression of base of skull
DDx:
   (1) Massive osteolysis = Gorham disease (local destuction of contiguous bones, usually not affecting hands / feet) (2) Tabes dorsalis (3) Leprosy
   (4) Syringomyelia (5) Scleroderma (6) Raynaud disease
   (7) Regional post-traumatic osteolysis (8) Ulcero-mutilating acropathy (9) Mutilating forms of rheumatoid arthritis (10) Acrodinia mutilante (nonhereditary)

EWING SARCOMA
= EWING TUMOR = 4 – 10% of all bone tumors (less common than osteo- / chondrosarcoma); most common malignant bone tumor in children

Histo:
small round cells, uniformly sized + solidly packed (DDx: lymphoma, osteosarcoma, myeloma, neuroblastoma, carcinoma, eosinophilic granuloma) invading medullary cavity and entering subperiosteum via Haversian canals producing periostitis, soft tissue mass, osteolysis; glycogen granules present (DDx to reticulum cell sarcoma); absence of alkaline phosphatase (DDx to osteosarcoma)

Age: peak 15 years (range 5 months – 54 years); in 30% <10 years; in 39% 11 – 15 years; in 31% >15 years; in 50% <20 years; in 95% 4 – 25 years; M:F = 2:1; caucasians in 96%
- severe localized pain
- soft tissue mass
- fever, leukocytosis, anemia (in early metastases) simulating infection

Location:
femur (25%), pelvis-ilium (14%), tibia (11%), humerus (10%), fibula (8%), ribs (6%)
- (a) long bones in 60%:
  metadiaphysis (44%), middiaphysis (33%), metaphysis (15%), metaepiphyseal (6%), epiphyseal (2%); usually no involvement of epiphysis as tumor originates in medullary cavity with invasion of Haversian system
- (b) flat bones in 40%: pelvis, scapula, skull, vertebrae (sacrum > lumbar > thoracic > cervical spine); ribs (in 7% > age 10; in 30% < age 10)

Δ >20 years of age predominantly in flat bones
Δ <20 years of age predominantly in cylindrical bones (tumor derived from red marrow)
√ 8 – 10 cm long lytic lesion in shaft of long bone (62% lytic, 23% mixed density, 15% dense)
√ mottled "moth-eaten" destructive permeative lesion (72%) (late finding)
√ penetration into soft tissue (55%) with preservation of tissue planes (DDx: osteomyelitis with diffuse soft tissue swelling)
√ early fusiform lamellated "onion-skin" periosteal reaction (53%) / spiculated = "sunburst" / "hair-on-end" (23%), Codman triangle
√ cortical thickening (16%)
√ cortical destruction (18%)
√ ± cortical sequestration
√ reactive sclerotic new bone (30%)
√ bone expansion (12%)
√ Ewing sarcoma of rib: disproportionately large inhomogeneous soft tissue mass with large intrathoracic + minimal extrathoracic component

Metastases to: lung + bones
in 11 – 30% at time of diagnosis,
in 40 – 45% within 2 years of diagnosis
Cx: pathologic fracture (5 – 14%)
Prognosis: 60% 5-year survival

DDx:
(1) Multiple myeloma (older age group)
(2) Osteomyelitis (duration of pain <2 weeks)
(3) Eosinophilic granuloma (solid periosteal reaction)
(4) Osteosarcoma (ossification in soft tissue, near age 20, no lamellar periosteal reaction)
(5) Reticulum cell sarcoma (clinically healthy, between 30 and 50 years, no glycogen)
(6) Neuroblastoma (< age 5)
(7) Anaplastic metastatic carcinoma (>30 years of age)

EXTRAMEDULLARY HEMATOPOIESIS
Causes: prolonged erythrocyte deficiency due to
(1) destruction of RBC:
congenital hemolytic anemia, sickle cell anemia, idiopathic severe anemia, erythroblastosis fetalis
(2) inability of normal blood-forming organs to produce erythrocytes: myelofibrosis, polycythemia, leukemia, Hodgkin disease, carcinomatosis
- absence of pain, bone erosion, calcification
Sites: in areas of fetal erythropoiesis = liver, spleen, adrenal, heart, thymus, lung, lymph nodes, renal pelvis, gastrointestinal lymphatics, dura mater (falx cerebri and over brain convexity)
@ Chest:
√ paraspinal masses with round + lobulated margins between T8 and T12, may be bilateral
√ extramedullary hematopoiesis may compress cord

FANCONI ANEMIA
= autosomal recessive disease with severe hypoplastic anemia + skin pigmentation + skeletal and urogenital anomalies
- skin pigmentation (melanin deposits) in 74% (trunk, axilla, groin, neck)
- anemia onset between 17 months and 22 years of age
- bleeding tendency (pancytopenia)
- hypogonadism (40%)
- microphthalmia (20%)
√ slight / moderate dwarfism
√ minimal microcephaly
√ renal anomalies (30%): renal aplasia, ectopia, horseshoe kidney
√ anomalies of radial component of upper extremity (strongly suggestive): absent / hypoplastic / supernumerary thumb; hypoplastic / absent radius; absent / hypoplastic navicular / greater multangular bone
Prognosis: fatal within 5 years after onset of anemia; patient's family shows high incidence of leukemia

FARBER DISEASE
= DISSEMINATED LIPOGRANULOMATOSIS
Histo: foam cell granulomas; lipid storage of neuronal tissue (accumulation of ceramide + gangliosides)
- hoarse weak cry
- swelling of extremities; generalized joint swelling
- subcutaneous + periarticular granulomas

- intermittent fever, dyspnea
- lymphadenopathy
√ capsular distension of multiple joints (hand, elbow, knee)
√ juxtaarticular bone erosions from soft tissue granulomas
√ subluxation / dislocation
√ disuse / steroid deossification
Prognosis: death from respiratory failure within 2 years

FIBROCHONDROGENESIS
= autosomal recessive lethal short-limb skeletal dysplasia
Incidence: 5 cases
√ severe micromelia + broad dumbbell-shaped metaphyses
√ flat + clefted pear-shaped vertebral bodies
√ short + cupped ribs
√ frontal bossing
√ low set abnormally formed ears
Prognosis: stillbirth / death shortly after birth
DDx: (1) Thanatophoric dysplasia
          (2) Metatropic dysplasia
          (3) Spondyloepiphyseal dysplasia

FIBROSARCOMA
Incidence: 4% of all primary bone neoplasm
Etiology:
   A. PRIMARY FIBROSARCOMA (70%)
   B. SECONDARY FIBROSARCOMA (30%)
      1. following radiotherapy of giant cell tumor / lymphoma / breast cancer
      2. underlying benign lesion: Paget disease (common); giant cell tumor, bone infarct, osteomyelitis, desmoplastic fibroma, enchondroma, fibrous dysplasia (rare)
      3. dedifferentiation of low grade chondrosarcoma

Histo: spectrum of well to poorly differentiated fibrous tissue proliferation; will not produce osteoid / chondroid / osseous matrix
Age: predominantly in 3rd – 5th decade (range of 8 – 88 years); M:F = 1:1
Metastases to: lung, lymph nodes
- localized painful mass
Location: tubular bones in young, flat bones in older patients; femur (40%), tibia (16%) (about knee in 30 – 50%), jaw, pelvis (9%); rare in small bones of hand + feet or spinal column
Site: eccentric at diaphyseal-metaphyseal junction into metaphysis; intramedullary / periosteal

   A. CENTRAL FIBROSARCOMA
   =   intramedullary
   √   well-defined lucent bone lesion
   √   thin expanded cortex
   √   aggressive osteolysis with geographic / ragged / permeative bone destruction + wide zone of transition
   √   occasionally large osteolytic lesion with cortical destruction, periosteal reaction + soft-tissue invasion

√ sequestration of bone may be present (DDx: eosinophilic granuloma, bacterial granuloma)
√ sparse periosteal proliferation (uncommon)
√ intramedullary discontinuous spread
√ no calcification
DDx: malignant fibrous histiocytoma, myeloma, telangiectatic osteosarcoma, lymphoma, desmoplastic fibroma, osteolytic metastasis
   B. PERIOSTEAL FIBROSARCOMA
   = rare tumor arising from periosteal connective tissue
   Location: long bones of lower extremity, jaw
   √   contour irregularity of cortical border
   √   periosteal reaction with perpendicular bone formation may be present
   √   rarely extension into medullary cavity

Cx: pathologic fracture (uncommon)
Prognosis: 20% 10-year survival
DDx: (1) Osteolytic osteosarcoma (2nd – 3rd decade)
          (2) Chondrosarcoma (usually contains characteristic calcifications)
          (3) Aneurysmal bone cyst (eccentric blown-out appearance with rapid progression)
          (4) Malignant giant cell tumor (begins in metaphysis extending towards joint)

FIBROUS CORTICAL DEFECT
Incidence: 30% of children; M:F = 2:1
Age: peak age of 7 – 8 years (range of 2 – 10 years); mostly before epiphyseal closure
Histo: fibrous tissue from periosteum invading underlying cortex
- asymptomatic
Location: metaphyseal cortex of long bone; posterior medial aspect of distal femur, proximal tibia, proximal femur, proximal humerus, ribs, ilium, fibula
√ round when small, average diameter of 1 – 2 cm
√ oval, extending parallel to long axis of host bone
√ cortical thinning + expansion may occur
√ smooth, well-defined / scalloped margins
√ larger lesions are multilocular
√ involution over 2 – 4 years
Prognosis:
   (a) potential to grow and encroach on the medullary cavity leading to non-ossifying fibroma
   (b) bone islands in the adult may be residue of incompletely involuted cortical defect

FIBROUS DYSPLASIA
= LICHTENSTEIN-JAFFE DISEASE
= benign fibro-osseous developmental anomaly of the mesenchymal precursor of bone, manifested as a defect in osteoblastic differentiation and maturation
Age: 1st – 2nd decade (highest incidence between 3 and 15 years), 75% before age 30; progresses until growth ceases; M=F
Histo: medullary cavity replaced by myxofibrous + woven-bone trabeculae containing spindle cells and fluid-filled cysts

Types:

A. <u>MONOSTOTIC FORM</u> (70 – 80%)
- mostly asymptomatic

Location: ribs (28%), proximal femur (23%), craniofacial bones (10 – 25%)

B. <u>POLYOSTOTIC FORM</u> (20 – 30%)

Age: mean age of 8 years

Location: unilateral predominance (uncommon)
- 2/3 symptomatic by age 10
- leg pain, limp, pathologic fracture (75%)
- abnormal vaginal bleeding (25%)

Location: femur (91%), tibia (81%), pelvis (78%), foot (73%), ribs, skull and facial bones (50%), upper extremities, lumbar spine (14%), clavicle (10%), cervical spine (7%)

√ leg length discrepancy (70%)
√ shepherd's crook deformity (35%)
√ facial asymmetry
√ tibial bowing
√ rib deformity

C. CRANIOFACIAL FORM = <u>LEONTIASIS OSSEA</u>

Incidence: in 10 – 25% of monostotic form / in 50% of polyostotic form / isolated
- cranial asymmetry
- facial deformity
- exophthalmus
- visual impairment

Location: sphenoid, frontal, maxillary, ethmoid bones > occipital, temporal bones

√ unilateral overgrowth of facial bones + calvarium (NO extracranial lesions)

Cx: neurologic deficit secondary to narrowed cranial foramina (eg, blindness)

D. <u>CHERUBISM</u> (special variant)
= autosomal dominant disorder of variable penetrance

Age: childhood; more severe in males

√ symmetric involvement of mandible + maxilla

Prognosis: regression after adolescence

May be associated with
(a) endocrine disorders:
— precocious puberty in girls
— hyperthyroidism
— hyperparathyroidism
— acromegaly
— diabetes mellitus
— Cushing syndrome
(b) soft-tissue myxoma (rare): typically multiple intramuscular lesions

VARIANT: **McCune-Albright Syndrome** (10%)
(1) polyostotic unilateral fibrous dysplasia
(2) "coast of Maine" café-au-lait spots (35%)
(3) endocrine dysfunction: precocious puberty in females (20%), hyperthyroidism

- swelling + tenderness
- limp, pain (± pathologic fracture)
- increased alkaline phosphatase

- advanced skeletal + somatic maturation (early)
- coast of Maine café-au-lait spots = yellowish to brownish patches of cutaneous pigmentation with irregular / serrated border, predominantly on back of trunk (30 – 50%), often ipsilateral to bone lesions (DDx: "coast of California" spots of neurofibromatosis)

Common location: rib cage (30%), craniofacial bones (calvarium, mandible) (25%), femoral neck + tibia (25%), pelvis

Site: metaphysis is primary site with extension into diaphysis (rarely entire length of bone)

√ normal bone architecture altered + remodelled
√ lesions in medullary cavity: radiolucent / ground glass / increased density
√ trabeculated appearance due to reinforced subperiosteal bone ridges in wall of lesion
√ expansion of bones (ribs, skull, long bones)
√ well-defined sclerotic margin of reactive bone = rind
√ endosteal scalloping with thinned / lost cortex (ribs, long bones)
√ lesion may undergo calcification + enchondral bone formation = fibrocartilaginous dysplasia
√ increased activity on bone scan during early perfusion + on delayed images

@ Skull
- skull deformity with cranial nerve compromise
- proptosis

Location: frontal bone > sphenoid bone; hemicranial involvement (DDx: Paget disease is bilateral)

√ sclerotic skull base, may narrow neural foramina (visual + hearing loss)
√ widened diploic space with displacement of outer table, inner table spared (DDx: Paget disease, inner table involved)
√ obliteration of sphenoid + frontal sinuses due to encroachment by fibrous dysplastic bone
√ inferolateral displacement of orbit
√ sclerosis of orbital plate + small orbit + hypoplasia of frontal sinuses (DDx: Paget disease, meningioma en plaque)
√ occipital thickening
√ cystic calvarial lesions, commonly crossing sutures
√ mandibular cystic lesion (very common) = osteocementoma, ossifying fibroma

@ Pelvis + Ribs
√ cystic lesions (extremely common)
√ protrusio acetabuli

@ Extremities
- short stature as adult / dwarfism
√ premature fusion of ossification centers
√ epiphysis rarely affected before closure of growth plate
√ bowing deformities + discrepant limb length (tibia, femur)
√ "shepherd's crook" deformity of femoral neck = coxa vara
√ pseudarthrosis in infancy = osteofibrous dysplasia (DDx: neurofibromatosis)

Cx:
(1) Transformation into osteo- / chondro- / fibrosarcoma or malignant fibrous histiocytoma (0.5 – 1%, more often in polyostotic form)
• increasing pain
√ enlarging soft-tissue mass
√ previously mineralized lesion turns lytic
(2) Pathologic fractures

DDx:
(1) HPT (chemical changes, generalized deossification, subperiosteal resorption)
(2) Neurofibromatosis (rarely osseous lesions, cystic intraosseous neurofibroma rare, café-au-lait spots smooth, familial disease)
(3) Paget disease (mosaic pattern histologically, radiographically identical to monostotic cranial lesion)
(4) Osteofibrous dysplasia (almost exclusively in tibia of infants, monostotic, lesion begins in cortex)
(5) Nonossifying fibroma
(6) Simple bone cyst
(7) Giant cell tumor (no sclerotic margin)
(8) Enchondromatosis
(9) Eosinophilic granuloma
(10) Osteoblastoma
(11) Hemangioma
(12) Meningioma

FIBROUS HISTIOCYTOMA
Benign Fibrous Histiocytoma
Incidence: 0.1% of all bone tumors
Histo: interlacing bundles of fibrous tissue in storiform pattern (whorled / woven) interspersed with mono- / multinucleated cells resembling histiocytes, benign giant cells, and lipid-laden macrophages; resembles nonossifying fibroma / fibroxanthoma
Age: 23 – 60 years
• localized intermittently painful soft-tissue swelling
Location: long bone, pelvis, vertebra (rare)
Site: typically in epiphysis / epiphyseal equivalent
√ well-defined radiolucent lesion with septae / soap-bubble appearance / no definable matrix
√ may have reactive sclerotic rim
√ narrow transition zone (= nonaggressive lesion)
√ no periosteal reaction
Rx: curettage
DDx: nonossifying fibroma (childhood / adolescence, asymptomatic, eccentric metaphyseal location)

Atypical Benign Fibrous Histiocytoma
Histo: "atypical aggressive" features = mitotic figures present
√ lytic defect with irregular edges
Prognosis: may metastasize

FOCAL FIBROCARTILAGINOUS DYSPLASIA OF TIBIA
Associated with tibia vara
Age: 9 – 28 months
Histo: dense hypocellular fibrous tissue resembling tendon with lacuna formation
• slight shortening of affected leg

Location: insertion of pes anserinus (= tendinous insertion of gracilis, sartorius, semitendinous muscles) distal to proximal tibial physis; unilateral involvement
√ unilateral tibia vara
√ well-defined elliptic obliquely oriented lucent defect in medial tibial metadiaphyseal cortex
√ sclerosis along lateral border of lesion
√ absence of bone margin superomedially
Rx: brace
Prognosis: resolution in 1 – 4 years
DDx:
(1) Unilateral Blount disease (typically bilateral in infants, varus angulation of upper tibia, decreased height of medial tibial metaphysis, irregular physis)
(2) Chondromyxoid fibroma, eosinophilic granuloma, osteoid osteoma, osteoma, fibroma, chondroma (not associated with tibia vara, soft-tissue mass)

FRACTURE
NUC:
Typical time course:
1. Acute phase (3 – 4 weeks)
abnormal in 80% <24 hours, in 95% <72 hours
Δ elderly patients show delayed appearance of positive scan
√ broad area of increased tracer uptake (wider than fracture line)
2. Subacute phase (2 – 3 months) = time of most intense tracer accumulation
√ more focal increased tracer uptake corresponding to fracture line
3. Chronic phase (1 – 2 years)
√ slow decline in tracer accumulation
√ in 65% normal after 1 year; >95% normal after 3 years

Return to normal:
Δ non-weight-bearing bone returns to normal more quickly than weight-bearing bone
Δ rib fractures return to normal most rapidly
Δ complicated fractures with orthopedic fixation devices take longest to return to normal
1. Simple fractures : 90% normal by 2 years
2. Open reduction / fixation : <50% normal by 3 years
3. Delayed union : slower than normal for type of fracture
4. Nonunion : persistent intense uptake in 80%
5. Complicated union (true pseudarthrosis, soft tissue interposition, impaired blood supply, presence of infection)
√ intense uptake at fracture ends
√ decreased uptake at fracture site
6. Vertebral compression fractures: 60% normal by 1 year; 90% by 2 years; 97% by 3 years

Stress fracture

A. INSUFFICIENCY FRACTURE = normal physiologic stress applied to bone with abnormal elastic resistance / deficient mineralization

Cause:
1. Osteoporosis
2. Rheumatoid arthritis
3. Osteomalacia / rickets
4. Paget disease
5. Hyperparathyroidism
6. Renal osteodystrophy
7. Radiation therapy
8. Steroid-induced osteopenia

Location: lower extremity, sacrum, ilium, pubic bone

B. FATIGUE FRACTURE = abnormal muscular stress applied to bone with normal elastic resistance
1. **Clay shoveler's fracture**: spinous process of lower cervical / upper thoracic spine
2. **Clavicle**: postoperative (radical neck dissection)
3. **Coracoid process of scapula**: trap shooting
4. **Ribs**: carrying heavy pack, golf, coughing
5. **Distal shaft of humerus**: throwing ball
6. **Coronoid process of ulna**: pitching ball, throwing javelin, pitchfork work, propelling wheelchairs
7. **Hook of hamate**: swinging golf club / tennis raquet / baseball bat
8. **Spondylolysis** = pars interarticularis of lumbar vertebrae: ballet, lifting heavy objects, scrubbing floors
9. **Femoral neck**: ballet, long-distance running
10. **Femoral shaft**: ballet, marching, long-distance running, gymnastics
11. **Obturator ring of pelvis**: stooping, bowling, gymnastics
12. **Patella**: hurdling
13. **Tibial shaft**: ballet, jogging
14. **Fibula**: long-distance running, jumping, parachuting
15. **Calcaneus**: jumping, parachuting, prolonged standing, recent immobilization
16. **Navicular**: stomping on ground, marching, prolonged standing, ballet
17. **Metatarsal** (commonly 2nd MT): marching, stomping on ground, prolonged standing, ballet, postoperative bunionectomy
18. **Sesamoids of metatarsal**: prolonged standing

X-Ray:
(a) compression fracture in cancellous bone (notoriously difficult to detect)
(b) distraction fracture in compact bone
√ sclerosis due to trabecular compression + callus formation
√ lucency through cortex / focal area of sclerosis (early)
√ solid thick lamellar periosteal + endosteal reaction (later)

MR:
Signal intensity pattern consistent with edema in soft tissue adjacent to fracture + in subperiosteal space.
√ diminished marrow signal intensity on T1WI
√ increased marrow signal intensity on T2WI

NUC:
√ positive bone scan 3 – 4 weeks prior to radiographic abnormality
√ focal fusiform area of increased tracer accumulation with extension into medullary space on radionuclide angiogram, blood pool image, and delayed image

DDx:
(1) Shin splints
√ long linear uptake on posteromedial (soleus muscle) / anterolateral (tibialis anterior muscle) tibial cortex on delayed images from stress to periosteum at muscle insertion site
(2) Osteoid osteoma (eccentric, without periosteal reaction)
(3) Chronic sclerosing osteomyelitis (dense, sclerotic, involving entire circumference)
(4) Osteomalacia (looser zones, smudged appearance of trabeculae)
(5) Osteogenic sarcoma (metaphyseal, aggressive periosteal reaction)
(6) Ewing tumor (lytic destructive appearance)

Epiphyseal Plate Injury

Mechanism: 80% shearing force; 20% compression
Resistance to trauma: ligament > bone > physis

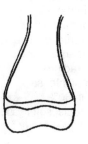 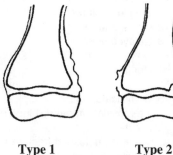 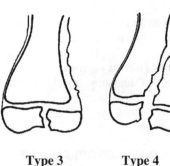 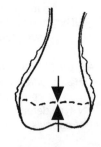

| normal | Type 1 | Type 2 | Type 3 | Type 4 | Type 5 |

Salter-Harris classification of epiphyseal plate injuries

<u>Salter-Harris classification</u> (considering probability of growth disturbance)

Type 1 (5 – 6%)
= slip of epiphysis due to shearing force separating epiphysis from physis
√ growth plate involvement only
(includes: apophyseal avulsion, slipped capital femoral epiphysis)
Prognosis: good

Type 2 (50 – 75%)
= shearing force splits growth plate, fracture line extends into metaphysis
Prognosis: good

Type 3 (8%)
= intra-articular fracture
√ epiphysis split vertically
Prognosis: fair (imprecise reduction leads to alteration in linearity of articular plane)

Type 4 (8 – 12%)
√ fracture involves metaphysis + physis + epiphysis
Prognosis: guarded (germinal cells of physis usually injured)

Type 5 (1%)
= crush injury with injury to vascular supply
√ no fracture line (diagnosis difficult + often made retrospectively)
Prognosis: poor (impairment of growth)

mnemonic: "SALTR"

Slip of physis	= type I
Above physis	= type II
Lower than physis	= type III
Through physis	= type IV
Rammed physis	= type V

Cx:
(1) progressive angular deformity from segmental arrest of germinal zone growth
(2) limb length discrepancy from total cessation of growth
(3) articular incongruity from disruption of articular surface

Apophyseal injury
Physis under secondary ossification center is weakest part
Mechanism: avulsive force
Location: tibial tubercle, ischial apophysis, lesser trochanter of femur, anterior superior + anterior inferior iliac spine, iliac crest

Hand fracture
Bennett Fracture
Mechanism: forced abduction of thumb
√ intraarticular fracture / dislocation of base of 1st metacarpal
√ small fragment of 1st metacarpal continues to articulate with trapezium
√ lateral retraction of 1st metacarpal shaft by abductor pollicis longus

Rx: anatomic reduction important, difficult to keep in anatomic alignment
Cx: pseudarthrosis

Boxer's Fracture
Mechanism: direct blow with clenched fist
√ transverse fracture of distal metacarpal (usually 5th)

Gamekeeper's Thumb
= SKIER'S THUMB
Mechanism: hyperextension of ulnar collateral ligament in 1st MCP (faulty handling of ski pole)
√ disruption of ulnar collateral ligament of 1st MCP joint
√ stress examination necessary to document ligamentous disruption

Navicular Fracture
Mechanism: fall on outstretched hand
Location: 80% through waist of navicular bone
Cx: avascular necrosis of proximal fragment (blood supply derived from distal part)

Rolando Fracture
√ comminuted intraarticular fracture through base of thumb
Prognosis: worse than Bennett's fracture (difficult to reduce)

Forearm fracture
Barton Fracture
Mechanism: fall on outstretched hand
√ intraarticular oblique fracture of dorsal lip of distal radius
√ carpus dislocates with distal fragment up and back on radius

Chauffer Fracture
Mechanism: acute dorsiflexion + abduction of hand
√ triangular fracture of radial styloid process

Colles Fracture
Most common fracture in this region
Mechanism: fall on outstretched hand
√ radial fracture in distal 2 cm ± ulnar styloid fracture
√ dorsal displacement of distal fragment
√ "silver-fork" deformity
Cx: posttraumatic arthritis
Rx: anatomic reduction important
Significant postreduction deformity:
1. Residual positive ulnar variance >5 mm indicates unsatisfactory outcome in 40%
2. Dorsal angulation of palmar tilt >15° decreases grip strength + endurance in >50%

Galeazzi Fracture
Mechanism: fall on outstretched hand with elbow flexed

√ radial fracture in distal third + subluxation /
dislocation of distal radioulnar joint

√ dorsal angulation

√ ulnar plus variance (= radial shortening) of >10 mm
implies complete disruption of interosseous
membrane = complete instability of radioulnar joint

Cx: (1)   high incidence of nonunion, delayed union,
malunion (unstable fracture)

       (2)   limitation of pronation / supination

Smith Fracture
= REVERSE COLLES FRACTURE

Mechanism: hyperflexion with fall on back of hand

√ distal radial fracture

√ ventral displacement of fragment

√ radial deviation of hand

√ "garden spade" deformity

Cx: altered function of carpus

Monteggia Fracture
Mechanism: fall on outstretched hand with elbow
flexed

√ anteriorly angulated proximal ulnar fracture +
anterior dislocation of radiohumeral joint

√ may have associated wrist injury

Cx: nonunion, limitation of motion at elbow, nerve
abnormalities

REVERSE MONTEGGIA FRACTURE = dorsally
angulated proximal ulnar fracture + posterior
dislocation of radial head

Pelvic fracture
Malgaigne Fracture
Mechanism: direct trauma

• shortening of involved extremity

√ vertical fractures through one side of pelvic ring

(1) superior to acetabulum

(2) inferior to acetabulum

(3) ± sacroiliac dislocation / fracture

Bucket Handle Fracture
√ double vertical fracture through superior and inferior
pubic rami + sacroiliac joint dislocation on
contralateral side

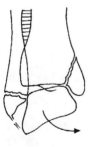 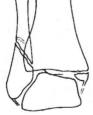 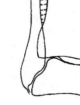

supination-   **supination-**   **pronation-**
adduction   **abduction**   **external rotation**

Knee fracture
Segond Fracture
Mechanism: external rotation + varus stress causing
excessive tension of the lateral
capsular ligament

Associated with: lesion of anterior cruciate ligament
(75 – 100%), meniscal tear (67%)

√ cortical avulsion fracture of proximal lateral tibia
immediately distal to lateral plateau

Foot fracture
Ankle Fracture
Incidence: ankle injuries account for 10% of all
emergency room visits; 85% of all ankle
sprains involve lateral ligaments

Ligamentous connections at ankle:

(a) binding tibia + fibula
1. anterior inferior tibiofibular ligament
(= tibiofibular syndesmosis)
2. posterior inferior tibiofibular ligament
3. transverse tibiofibular ligament
4. interosseous membrane

(b) lateral malleolus
85% of all ankle sprains involve these
ligaments:
1. anterior talofibular ligament
2. posterior talofibular ligament
3. calcaneofibular ligament

(c) medial malleolus = deltoid ligament with
1. navicular portion
2. sustentaculum portion
3. talar portion

A. SUPINATION-ADDUCTION
= INVERSION-ADDUCTION INJURY

Mechanism: (1) avulsive forces affect lateral
ankle structures

(2) impactive forces secondary to
talar shift stress medial structures

√ sprain / rupture of lateral collateral ligament

√ transverse avulsion of malleolus sparing
tibiofibular ligaments

√ oblique fracture of medial malleolus ± posterior lip
fracture

B. SUPINATION-ABDUCTION
= EVERSION / EXTERNAL ROTATION

Mechanism: (1) avulsive forces on medial
structures

(2) impacting forces on lateral
structures (talar impact)

√ lateral subluxation of talus

√ oblique / spiral fracture of lateral malleolus

√ partial disruption of tibiofibular ligament

√ sprain / rupture / avulsion of deltoid ligament

√ transverse fracture of medial malleolus

(a) **Pott Fracture**
√ fracture of fibula above an intact tibiofibular
ligament

(b) **Dupuytren Fracture**
√ fracture of fibula above a disrupted tibiofibular
ligament

C. PRONATION-EXTERNAL ROTATION
= EVERSION + EXTERNAL ROTATION
√ tear of tibiofibular ligament / avulsion of anterior tubercle (Tillaux-Chaput) / avulsion of posterior tubercle (Volkmann)
√ tear of interosseous membrane = lateral instability
√ fibular fracture higher than ankle joint (Maisonneuve fracture if around knee)

Jones Fracture

Mechanism: plantar flexion + inversion (stepping off a curb)
√ transverse avulsion fracture of base of 5th metatarsal (insertion of peroneus brevis tendon)

Lisfranc Fracture

Mechanism: metatarsal heads fixed and hindfoot forced plantarwards and into rotation
√ fracture / dislocation of tarsometatarsal joints

Calcaneal Fracture

Incidence: most commonly fractured tarsal bone; 60% of all tarsal fractures; 2% of all fractures in the body; commonly bilateral
Mechanism: fall from heights
May be associated with   lumbar vertebral fracture
Age: 95% in adults, 5% in children
—   adulthood: intraarticular (75%), extraarticular (25%)
—   childhood: extraarticular (63 – 92%)
Classification:
(a) Extraarticular fracture of calcaneal tuberosity: beak type, vertical, horizontal, medial avulsion
(b) Intraarticular fracture
—   subtalar joint involvement: undisplaced, displaced, comminuted
—   calcaneocuboid joint involvement
√ apex of lateral talar process does not point to "crucial angle" of Gissane
√ Boehler angle decreased below 28° – 40°

FREIBERG DISEASE

= osteochondrosis of head of 2nd metatarsal
Age: 10 – 15 years; girls
√ compression of 2nd metatarsal head

FROSTBITE

Cause: cessation of circulation secondary to cellular aggregates + thrombi forming as a result of exposure to low temperatures below -13° Celsius (usually cold air)
• firm white numb areas in cutis (separation of epidermal-dermal interface)
√ thumb commonly spared (protected by clenched fist)
CHILD
√ fragmentation / premature fusion / destruction of distal phalangeal epiphyses
√ secondary infection, articular cartilage injury, joint space narrowing, sclerosis, osteophytosis of DIP
√ shortening + deviation / deformity of fingers

ADULT
√ osteoporosis (4 – 10 weeks after injury)
√ acromutilation (secondary to osteomyelitis + surgical removal) + tuftal resorption (result of soft-tissue loss)
√ small round punched-out areas near edge of joint
√ periostitis
Angio:
√ vasospasm, stenosis, occlusion
Rx: selective angiography with intraarterial reserpine

GANGLION

= cystic tumor-like lesion usually attached to a tendon sheath
Origin: synovial herniation / tissue degeneration
• uni- / multilocular swelling
Location: hand, wrist, foot
Site: arise from tendon, muscle, semilunar cartilage
√ soft-tissue mass with surface bone resorption
√ periosteal new bone formation
√ arthrography may demonstrate communication with joint / tendon sheath
Rx: steroid injection may improve symptomatology

INTRAOSSEOUS GANGLION
= subchondral radiolucent lesion
• mild localized pain
Age: middle age
Path: uni- / multilocular cyst surrounded by fibrous lining + containing gelatinous material
Location: epiphysis of long bone (medial malleolus, femoral head) / subarticular flat bone (acetabulum)
√ well-demarcated solitary 0.6 – 6 cm lytic lesion
√ sclerotic margin
√ NO communication with joint
DDx: posttraumatic / degenerative cyst

GARDNER SYNDROME

= autosomal dominant syndrome characterized by (1) osteomas (2) soft tissue tumors (3) colonic polyps

Location of osteomas: paranasal sinuses; outer table of skull (frequent); mandible (at angle)
√ endosteal cortical thickening / osteomas in any bone
√ may have solid periosteal cortical thickening
√ osteomas / exostoses may protrude from periosteal surface
√ wavy cortical thickening of superior aspect of ribs
√ polyps: colon, stomach, duodenum, ampulla of Vater, small intestine
Cx: high incidence of carcinoma of duodenum / ampulla of Vater

GAUCHER DISEASE

= rare autosomal recessive disorder / dominant (in a few), common among Ashkenazi Jews
Etiology: deficiency of lysosomal hydrolase acid ß-glycosidase leads to accumulation of glucosyl ceramide within cells of RES

Histo: bone-marrow aspirate shows Gaucher cells (kerasin-laden histiocytes)

Types:
(1) rapidly fatal infantile form: 1 – 12 months
   • early onset of significant hepatosplenomegaly
   • severe progressive neurologic symptoms
(2) juvenile form: 2 – 6 years
   • mild neurologic involvement
(3) adult form (most common form)
   pulmonary involvement / hepatic failure may lead to early death
• hepatosplenomegaly, impairment of liver function, ascites
• anemia, leukopenia, thrombocytopenia (hypersplenism)
• hemochromatosis (yellowish-brown pigmentation of conjunctiva + skin)
• dull bone pain; bone involvement in 75%

Location: distal femur, pelvis, other long bones
√ generalized osteopenia (decrease in trabecular bone density)
√ striking cortical thinning + bone widening
√ Erlenmeyer flask deformity of distal femur
√ numerous sharply circumscribed lytic lesions resembling metastases / multiple myeloma (marrow replacement)
√ periosteal reaction = cloaking
√ weakening of subchondral bone + degenerative arthritis
√ bone infarction in long bone metaphyses (common)
√ H-shaped / "step-off" / biconcave "fish-mouth" vertebra
@ Spleen
   √ multiple nodular lesions of low-attenuation without enhancement on CT / hypoechoic or hyperechoic on US (= clusters of RES cells laden with glucosyl ceramide)

Cx: Δ >90% have orthopedic complications at some time
(1) pathologic fractures + compression fractures of vertebrae
(2) aseptic necrosis of femoral head, humeral head, wrist, ankle (common)
(3) osteomyelitis (increased incidence)
(4) myelosclerosis in long-standing disease
Prognosis: highly variable clinical course

GIANT CELL REPARATIVE GRANULOMA
= GIANT CELL REACTION
Histo: numerous giant cells in exuberant fibrous matrix, osteoid formation, areas of hemorrhage
Peak age: 2nd + 3rd decade (range from childhood to 76 years); M:F = 1:1
Location: mandible, maxilla, small bones of hand + feet
• pain + mass in affected bone
√ expansile lytic defect with thinning of overlying cortex
√ periosteal reaction may be present
√ soft tissue swelling / extension beyond cortex
√ no matrix calcification
Cx: pathologic fracture
Rx: curettage (50% recurrence rate) / local excision

DDx: (1) Enchondroma (same location, matrix calcification)
(2) Aneurysmal bone cyst (rare in small bones of hand + feet, typically prior to epiphyseal closure)
(3) Giant cell tumor (more aggressive appearance)
(4) Infection (clinical)
(5) Brown tumor of HPT (periosteal bone resorption, abnormal Ca + P levels)

GIANT CELL TUMOR
= OSTEOCLASTOMA = probably arise from zone of intense osteoclastic activity in skeletally immature patients
Incidence: 4.2% of all primary bone tumors; 21% of benign skeletal tumors
Histo: multinucleated giant cells within fibroid stroma (giant cells characteristic of all reactive bone disease, seen in pigmented villonodular synovitis, benign chondroblastoma, nonosteogenic fibroma, chondromyxoid fibroma, fibrous dysplasia)
Age: in 98.3% after (in 1.7% before) epiphyseal plate fusion; 14% < age 20; 70 – 80% between 20 and 40 years; M:F = 1:1
• tenderness + pain at affected site

Location:
(a) 85% in long bones
   — lower extremity (50 – 60% about knee): distal end of femur > proximal end of tibia
   — upper extremity (away from elbow): distal end of radius > proximal end of humerus
(b) 15% in flat bones: pelvis, sacrum near SIJ (common, 2nd only to chordoma), spine (5%), rib (anterior / posterior end), skull
Site: eccentric in metaphysis of long bones, adjacent to / in ossified epiphyseal line, subarticular if epiphyseal plate is fused (MOST TYPICAL)
√ expansile solitary radiolucent lesion ("soap bubble"), large at diagnosis
√ conspicuous peripheral trabeculae without tumor matrix
√ no sclerosis / periosteal reaction (aggressive rapid growth) in absence of fracture
√ may break through bone cortex with cortical thinning, soft tissue invasion (25%), pathologic fracture (5%)
√ destruction of vertebral body with secondary invasion of posterior elements
√ may cross joint space (exceedingly rare)

Cx: 15% malignant within first 5 years (M:F = 3:1); metastases to lung
DDx: (1) Aneurysmal bone cyst (in posterior elements of spine with invasion of vertebral body)
(2) Brown tumor of HPT (lab values)
(3) Cartilage tumor: chondroblastoma, enchondroma (not epiphyseal), chondromyxoid fibroma, chondrosarcoma
(4) Bone abscess
(5) Hemangioma
(6) Fibrous dysplasia

GLOMUS TUMOR OF BONE

= rare benign lesion composed of cells derived from neuromyoarterial glomus

Age: most in 4 – 5th decade
- painful

Location: distal aspect of terminal phalanx of finger
√ resembles enchondroma

GOUT

= deposition of positively birefringent monosodium urate monohydrate crystals in poorly vascularized tissues (synovial membranes, articular cartilage, ligaments, bursae) leading to destruction of cartilage

Age: >40 years; males (in women gout may occur after menopause)

Causes:
A. Idiopathic Gout
   Incidence: 0.3%; M:F = 20:1
   (1) Overproduction of uric acid (phosphoribosyl transferase deficiency)
   (2) Abnormality of renal urate excretion
B. Secondary Gout
   rarely cause for radiographically apparent disease
   (1) Myeloproliferative disorders + sequelae of their treatment: polycythemia vera, leukemia, lymphoma, multiple myeloma
   (2) Blood dyscrasias
   (3) Endocrinologic: myxedema, hyperparathyroidism
   (4) Chronic renal failure
   (5) Enzyme defects: glycogen storage disease
   (6) Vascular: myocardial infarction, hypertension
   (7) Lead poisoning

Stages:
(1) asymptomatic hyperuricemia
(2) acute monarticular gout
(3) polyarticular gout
(4) large multiple urate deposits

Location:
(a) joints: hands + feet (1st MTP joint most commonly affected = podagra), elbow, wrist (carpometacarpal compartment especially common), knee, shoulder, hip, sacroiliac joint (15%, unilateral)
(b) ear > bones, tendon, bursa
Involvement of hip + spine is rare

Δ Radiologic features usually not seen until 6 – 12 years after initial attack
Δ Radiologic features present in 50% of inflicted patients
√ calcific deposits in gouty tophi in 50% (sodium urate crystals not radiopaque, only after calcium deposition)
√ juxtaarticular lobulated soft-tissue masses (hands + feet)
√ "punched-out" lytic bone lesion = "mouse / rat bite" from erosion of long-standing soft-tissue tophus
√ "overhanging margin" = elevated osseous spicule in sites of tophus formation associated with erosion of adjacent bone (in intra- and extraarticular locations) (HALLMARK)
√ erosion of joint margins (resembling rheumatoid arthritis) but with sclerosis
√ round / oval subarticular cysts up to 3 cm
√ preservation of joint space (important clue!)
√ absence of periarticular demineralization (DDx: rheumatoid arthritis)
√ cartilage destruction (late)
√ periarticular swelling
√ chondrocalcinosis (menisci, articular cartilage of knee) resulting in secondary osteoarthritis
√ bilateral effusion of bursae olecrani (PATHOGNOMONIC)
√ aural calcification
√ ischemic necrosis of femoral / humeral heads
√ bone infarction due to deposits at vascular basement membrane (DDx: bone island)

Coexisting disorders:
1. Psoriasis
2. Glycogen storage disease Type I
3. Hypo- and hyperparathyroidism
4. Down syndrome
5. Lesch-Nyhan syndrome (choreaatetosis, spasticity, mental retardation, self-mutilation of lips + fingertips)
Δ NOT associated with rheumatoid arthritis!
Rx: colchicine, allopurinol

HEMANGIOENDOTHELIAL SARCOMA

= ANGIOSARCOMA = HEMANGIOENDOTHELIOMA
= HEMANGIOEPITHELIOMA

Histo: irregular anastomosing vascular channels lined by one / several layers of atypical anaplastic endothelial cells

Age: 4th – 5th decade; M:F = 2:1
- history of trauma / irradiation

Location: femur, tibia, humerus, pelvis, skull; multicentric lesions in 30% often with regional distribution (less aggressive)
√ eccentric lesion in metaphysis of long bones
√ osteolytic aggressively destructive area with indistinct margins (high grade)
√ well-demarcated margins with scattered bony trabeculae (low grade)
√ osteoblastic area in vertebrae, contiguous through several vertebrae

Metastases to: lung (early)
Prognosis: 26% 5-year survival rate
DDx: Aneurysmal bone cyst, poorly differentiated fibrosarcoma, highly vascular metastasis, alveolar rhabdomyosarcoma

HEMANGIOMA OF BONE

Incidence: 10%
Histo: mostly cavernous; capillary type is rare
Age: 4th – 5th decade; M:F = 1:2
Location: (a) vertebral body in lower thoracic / upper lumbar spine
          (b) calvarium with predilection for frontal bone

@ Vertebra (30%)
   Incidence: in 5 – 11% of autopsies
   Histo: abnormal vascular channels interspersed in fatty matrix

Age: >40 years; female
√ "accordion" / "corduroy" / "honeycomb" vertebra
    = exaggerated vertical trabeculae (also in multiple
    myeloma, lymphoma, metastasis)
√ posterior bulge of cortex
√ extraosseous extension beyond bony lesion (with
    cord compression)
√ paravertebral soft tissue extension
MR:
    √ mottled pattern of increased intensity on
        T1WI + T2WI (CHARACTERISTIC)
Cx: vertebral collapse (unusual), spinal cord
        compression
@ Calvarium
    √ <4 cm round osteolytic lesion
    √ sunburst appearance without definite margin
    √ may occur in diploe, producing palpable lump
        secondary to widening of diploe
@ Flat bones & long bones (rare)
    ribs, clavicle, mandible, zygoma, nasal bones,
    metaphyseal ends of long bones (frequently capillary
    type of hemangioma)

HEMANGIOMA OF SOFT TISSUE
= broad spectrum of benign neoplasms that closely
  resemble normal blood vessels at histologic
  examination
Nonvascular elements: fat, smooth muscle, fibrous
                        tissue, thrombus, bone
Categories:
    (1) Cavernous hemangioma = large-caliber vessels
    (2) Capillary hemangioma = small-caliber vessels

√ nonspecific soft-tissue mass
√ may contain phleboliths (SPECIFIC)
√ may contain such large amounts of fat as to be
    indistinguishable from lipoma
CT:
    √ poorly defined mass with attenuation similar to muscle
    √ areas of decreased attenuation approximating
        subcutaneous fat
MR:
    √ poorly marginated mass isointense to muscle on
        T1WI
    √ areas with increased signal intensity (fat)
    √ well-marginated markedly hyperintense mass on
        T2WI (increased free water content in stagnant blood)
    √ linear areas of decreased signal (fibrofatty septa)

HEMANGIOPERICYTOMA
= borderline tumor with benign / locally aggressive /
  malignant behavior (counterpart of glomus tumor)
Age: 4th – 5th decade
Location: lower extremities, vertebrae, pelvis, skull (dura
            similar to meningioma)
√ osteolytic lesions in metaphysis of long / flat bone
√ subperiosteal large blowout lesion (similar to
    aneurysmal bone cyst)
Angio:
    √ displacement of main artery

√ pedicle of tumor feeder arteries
√ spider-shaped arrangement of vessels encircling
    tumor
√ small corkscrew arteries
√ dense tumor stain

HEMOCHROMATOSIS
1. PRIMARY HEMOCHROMATOSIS
   = autosomal recessive / indeterminate inheritance
     (abnormal iron-loading gene) in thalassemia,
     sideroblastic anemia
2. SECONDARY HEMOCHROMATOSIS
   = excessive iron absorption in anemias, myelofibrosis,
     portocaval shunt, exogenous administration of iron,
     porphyria cutanea tarda, beer brewed in iron vessels
     + deposition of excessive iron in liver, pancreas,
     spleen, GI tract, kidney, gonads, heart, endocrine
     glands (pituitary, hypothalamus)
Age: > age 40 years; M:F = 10:1 (females protected by
        menstruation)
• cirrhosis
• "bronzed diabetes"
• congestive heart failure
• skin pigmentation
• hypogonadism
• arthritic symptoms (30%)
• increase in serum iron
@ Skeleton
   Site: most commonly in hands (metacarpal heads,
           particularly 2nd + 3rd MCP joints), carpal +
           proximal interphalangeal joints, knees, hips
   √ generalized osteoporosis
   √ small subchondral cystlike rarefactions with fine rim
       of sclerosis (metacarpal heads)
   √ arthropathy in 50% with iron deposition in synovium
   √ uniform joint space narrowing
   √ enlargement of metacarpal heads
   √ eventually osteophyte formation
   √ chondrocalcinosis in >60%, knees most commonly
       affected
       (a) calcium pyrophosphate deposition (inhibition of
             pyrophosphatase enzyme within cartilage which
             hydrolyzes pyrophosphate to soluble
             orthophosphate)
       (b) calcification of triangular cartilage of wrist,
             menisci, annulus fibrosus, ligamentum flavum,
             symphysis pubis, Achilles tendon, plantar fascia
@ Brain
   MRI:
       √ marked loss in signal intensity of anterior lobe of
           pituitary gland (iron deposition)
Cx: hepatoma (in 30%)
Prognosis: death from CHF (30%), death from hepatic
              failure (25%)
DDx: (1) Pseudogout (no arthropathy)
        (2) Psoriatic arthritis (skin + nail changes)
        (3) Osteoarthritis (predominantly distal joints in
              hands)
        (4) Rheumatoid arthritis
        (5) Gout (may also have chondrocalcinosis)

HEMOPHILIA

= X-linked deficiency / functional abnormality of coagulation factor VIII (= hemophilia A) in >80% / factor IX (= hemophilia B = Christmas disease)

Incidence: 1:10,000 males

@ Hemarthrosis (most common)

Histo: hypertrophic synovial membrane with pannus formation that erodes cartilage, loss of subchondral bone plate, formation of subarticular cysts

- tense red warm joint with decreased range of motion (muscle spasm)
- fever, elevated WBC (DDx: septic arthritis)

Location: in knee, ankle, elbow

√ soft tissue swelling of joint

√ enlargement of epiphysis (secondary to synovial hyperemia)

√ thinning of joint cartilage (particularly patella) secondary to cartilage destruction

√ erosion of articular surface with multiple subcondral cysts

√ superimposed degenerative joint disease

√ "squared" patella

√ widening of intercondylar notch

√ medial "slanting" of tibiotalar joint

√ juxtaarticular osteoporosis

@ Hemophilic pseudotumor (1 – 2%)

= posthemorrhagic cystic swelling within muscle + bone characterized by pressure necrosis + destruction

(a) juvenile form = usually multiple intramedullary expansile lesions without soft tissue mass in small bones of hand / feet (before epiphyseal closure)

(b) adult form = usually single intramedullary expansile lesion with large soft tissue mass in ilium / femur

(c) soft tissue involvement of retroperitoneum (psoas muscle), bowel wall, renal collecting system

√ mixed cystic expansile lesion

√ bone erosion + pathologic fracture

CT:

√ sometimes encapsulated mass containing areas of low attenuation + calcifications

MR:

√ hemorrhage of varying age

N.B.: Needle aspiration / biopsy / excision may cause fistulae / infection / uncontrolled bleeding!

Rx: palliative radiation therapy (destroys vessels prone to bleed) + transfusion of procoagulation factor concentrate

HEREDITARY HYPERPHOSPHATASIA

= "JUVENILE PAGET DISEASE" = rare autosomal recessive disease with sustained elevation of serum alkaline phosphatase, especially in individuals of Puerto Rican descent

Histo: rapid turnover of lamellar bone without formation of cortical bone; immature woven bone is rapidly laid down, but simultaneous rapid destruction prevents normal maturation

Age: 1st – 3rd year; usually stillborn

- rapid enlargement of calvarium + long bones
- dwarfism
- cranial nerve deficit (blind, deaf)
- hypertension
- frequent respiratory infections
- pseudoxanthoma elasticum
- elevated akaline phosphatase

√ deossification = decreased density of long bones with coarse trabecular pattern

√ metaphyseal growth deficiency

√ wide irregular epiphyseal lines (resembling rickets in childhood), persistent metaphyseal defects (40% of adults)

√ bowing of long bones + fractures with irregular callus

√ widened medullary canal with cortical thinning (cortex modeled from trabecular bone)

√ skull greatly thickened with wide tables, cotton wool appearance

√ vertebra plana

OB-US: √ diagnosis suspected in utero in 20%

Cx: pathologic fractures; vertebra plana universalis

DDx: (1) Osteogenesis imperfecta
(2) Polyostotic fibrous dysplasia
(3) Paget disease (> age 20, not generalized)
(4) Pyle disease (spares midshaft)
(5) van Buchem syndrome (only diaphyses > age 20, NO long bone bowing)
(6) Engelmann syndrome (lower limbs)

HEREDITARY MULTIPLE EXOSTOSES

= DIAPHYSEAL ACLASIS

Inheritance: autosomal dominant (unaffected female may be carrier)

Age: discovered between 2 and 10 years; M:F = 2:1

Path: ectopic cartilaginous rest in metaphysis + defect in periosteum; cap of hyaline cartilage; often bursa formation over cap

- usually painless mass near joints
- tendons, blood vessels, nerves may be impaired
- mechanical limitation of joint movement

Location: multiple + usually bilateral; common sites are knee, elbow, scapula, pelvis, ribs

Site: metaphyses of long bones near epiphyseal plate (distance to epiphyseal line increases with growth)

√ cortex + cancellous bone of exostosis contiguous to host bone

√ slope on epiphyseal side + right angle on diaphyseal side of stalk = points away from joint + toward center of of shaft

√ occasionally small punctate calcifications in cartilaginous cap

√ shortening of 4th + 5th metacarpals

√ supernumerary fingers / toes

√ Madelung / reversed Madelung deformity = radius usually longer + bowed

√ occasionally results in disproportionate shortening of an extremity, radioulnar synostosis, dislocation of radial head

Prognosis: exostosis begins in childhood; stops growing
      when nearest epiphyseal center fuses
Cx:
  (1) Cord compression secondary to involvement of
      posterior spinal elements
  (2) Malignant transformation to chondrosarcoma in
      <5%; iliac bone commonest site; growth with
      irregularity of outline + fuzziness; sudden painful
      growth spurt

HEREDITARY SPHEROCYTOSIS
= autosomal dominant congenital hemolytic anemia
Age: anemia begins in early infancy to late adulthood
- rarely severe anemia
- jaundice
- spherocytes in peripheral smear
√ bone changes rare (due to mild anemia); long bones
  rarely affected
√ widening of diploe with displacement + thinning of outer
  table
√ hair-on-end appearance
Rx: splenectomy corrects anemia even though
     spherocytemia persists
     √ improvement in skeletal alterations following
       splenectomy

HERNIATION PIT
= CONVERSION DEFECT
= localized bone erosion caused by herniated synovium
  from adjacent joint
Histo: fibroalveolar tissue
Age: usually in older individuals
- asymptomatic
- no clinical significance
Location: superolateral aspect of proximal femoral neck
Site: subcortical
√ well-circumscribed round lucency
√ usually <1 cm in diameter
√ reactive thin sclerotic border

HISTIOCYTOSIS X
= LANGERHANS CELL HISTIOCYTOSIS
Path: influx of eosinophilic leukocytes simulating
     inflammation; reticulum cells accumulate
     cholesterol + lipids (= foam cells); sheets or
     nodules of histiocytes may fuse to form giant
     cells, cytoplasm contains Langerhans bodies

Letterer-Siwe Disease
  = acute disseminated, fulminant form of histiocytosis X
  Incidence: 1: 2,000,000; 10% of histiocytosis X
  Age: several weeks after birth to 2 years
  Path: generalized involvement of reticulum cells; may
      be confused with leukemia
  - hemorrhage, purpura
  - severe progressive anemia
  - intermittent fever
  - failure to grow
  √ hepatosplenomegaly + lymphadenopathy
  @ Bone involvement (50%):

√ widespread multiple lytic lesions; "raindrop" pattern
  in calvarium
Prognosis: 70% mortality rate

Hand-Schüller-Christian Disease
= chronic disseminated form of histiocytosis X
  (15 – 40%) in 10% characterized by a triad of
  (1) exophthalmus
  (2) diabetes insipidus
  (3) lytic skull lesions
Path: proliferation of histiocytes, may simulate Ewing
     sarcoma
Age at onset: 5 – 10 years (range from birth to 40
         years); M:F = 1:1
- diabetes insipidus (30 – 50%) often with large lytic
  lesion in sphenoid bone
- otitis media with mastoid + inner ear invasion
- exophthalmus (33%), sometimes with orbital wall
  destruction
- generalized eczematoid skin lesions (30%)
- ulcers of mucous membranes
@ Bone
  √ osteolytic skull lesions with overlying soft tissue
    nodules
  √ "geographic skull" = ovoid / serpiginous
    destruction of large area
  √ "floating teeth" with mandibular involvement
  √ destruction of petrous ridge + mastoids + sella
    turcica
@ Orbit
  √ diffuse orbital disease with multiple osteolytic bone
    lesions
@ Soft tissue
  √ hepatosplenomegaly (rare) with scattered
    granuloma
  √ lymphadenopathy (may be massive)
@ Lung
  √ cyst + bleb formation with spontaneous
    pneumothorax (25%)
  √ ill-defined diffuse nodular infiltration often
    progressing to fibrosis + honeycomb lung
Prognosis: spontaneous remissions + exacerbations

Eosinophilic Granuloma
= most benign variety of histiocytosis X (60 – 80%)
  localized to bone
Age: 5 – 10 years (highest frequency); range 2 – 30
     years; <20 years (in 75%); M:F = 3:2
Path: bone lesions arise within medullary canal
     (RES)
- eosinophilia in blood + CSF
Location: monostotic involvement in 50 – 75%;
      calvarium > mandible > spine > ribs > large
      long bones
@ Skull (50%)
  - intractable otitis media with chronically draining
    ear (temporal bone involvement)
  Site: diploic space of parietal bone (most
      commonly involved) + temporal bone (petrous
      ridge, mastoid)

√ round / ovoid punched-out lesion with serrated + beveled edge

√ sharply marginated without sclerotic rim (DDx: epidermoid with bone sclerosis)

√ sclerotic margin during healing phase (50%)

√ "hole-within-hole" appearance = uneven involvement of inner + outer table

√ "button sequestrum" = central bone density within lytic lesion

√ soft tissue mass overlying the lytic process in calvarium (often palpable)

√ destructive lesion near mastoid antrum (resembling cholesteatoma)

√ infiltration of mandible

√ isodense homogeneously enhancing mass in hypothalamus / pituitary gland

@ Orbit
  √ benign focal mass ± infiltration of orbital bones

@ Axial skeleton (25%)
  √ "vertebra plana" = "coin on edge" = Calvé disease (6%) = collapse of vertebra (most commonly thoracic); preserved disc space; rare involvement of posterior elements; no kyphosis; most common cause of vertebra plana in children
  √ lytic lesion in supraacetabular region

@ Proximal long bones (15%)
  • painful bone lesion
  Site: mostly diaphyseal, epiphyseal lesions are uncommon
  √ expansile lytic lesion with ill-defined / sclerotic edges
  √ erosion of cortex + soft tissue mass
  √ laminated periosteal reaction (frequent), may show interruptions
  √ may appear rapidly within 3 weeks
  √ lesions respect joint space + growth plate

@ Lung involvement (20%)
  Incidence: 0.05 to 0.5 / 100,000 annually
  Age: peak between 20 and 40 years
  √ 3 – 10 mm nodules
  √ reticulonodular pattern with predilection for apices
  √ may develop into honeycomb lung
  √ recurrent pneumothoraces (25%)
  √ rib lesions with fractures (common)
  √ pleural effusion, hilar adenopathy (unusual)
NUC:
  √ negative bone scans in 35% (radiographs more sensitive)

√ bone lesions generally not Ga-67 avid

√ Ga-67 may be helpful for detecting nonosseous lesions

Prognosis: excellent with spontaneous resolution of bone lesions in 6 – 18 months

HOLT-ORAM SYNDROME

Autosomal dominant; M < F

Associated with CHD: secundum type ASD (most common), VSD, persistent left SVC, tetralogy, coarctation

• intermittent cardiac arrhythmia
• bradycardia (50 – 60/min)

Location: upper extremity only involved; symmetry of lesions is the rule; left side may be more severely affected

√ aplasia / hypoplasia of radial structures: thumb, 1st metacarpal, carpal bones, radius

√ "fingerized" hypoplastic thumb / triphalangeal thumb

√ slender elongated hypoplastic carpals + metacarpals

√ hypoplastic radius; absent radial styloid

√ shallow glenoid fossa (voluntary dislocation of shoulder common)

√ hypoplastic clavicula

√ high arched palate

√ cervical scoliosis

√ pectus excavatum

HOMOCYSTINURIA

Autosomal recessive disorder

Etiology: cystathionine B synthetase deficiency results in defective methionine metabolism with accumulation of homocystine + homocysteine in blood and urine; causes defect in collagen / elastin structure

• thromboembolic phenomena due to stickiness of platelets
• ligamentous laxity
• downward dislocation of lens (DDx: upward dislocation in Marfan syndrome)
• mild / moderate mental retardation
• crowding of maxillary teeth and protrusion of incisors
• malar flush

√ arachnodactyly in 1/3 (DDx: Marfan syndrome)

√ microcephaly

√ enlarged paranasal sinuses

√ osteoporosis of vertebrae (biconcave / flattened / widened vertebrae)

	Marfan syndrome	Homocystinuria
Inheritance:	autosomal dominant	autosomal recessive
Biochemical defect:	not known	cystathionine synthetase
Osteoporosis:	no	yes
Spine:	scoliosis	biconcave vertebrae
Lens dislocation:	upward	downward
Arachnodactyly:	100%	33%

√ scoliosis
√ pectus excavatum / carinatum (75%)
√ osteoporosis of long bones (75%) with bowing + fractures
√ children: metaphyseal cupping (50%); enlargement of ossification centers in 50% (knee, carpal bones); epiphyseal calcifications (esp. in wrist, resembling phenylketonuria); delayed ossification
√ Harris lines = multiple growth lines
√ genu valgum, coxa valga, coxa magna, pes cavus
√ premature vascular calcifications

Prognosis: death from occlusive vascular disease / minor vascular trauma

HYPERPARATHYROIDISM

Age: middle age; M:F = 1:3
Histo: decreased bone mass secondary to increased number of osteoclasts, increased osteoid volume (defect in mineralization), slightly increased number of osteoblasts

A. BONE RESORPTION
   (a) subperiosteal: radial margins of middle phalanges, phalangeal tufts, proximal tibial shaft medially, femoral neck medially, humeral neck, upper margins of ribs in midclavicular line, lamina dura of skull and teeth
   (b) subchondral = pseudowidening of joint space: acromioclavicular joint, sternoclavicular joint, sacroiliac joint, symphysis pubis, Schmorl nodes
   (c) intracortical: scalloped inner surface + tunneling of cortex
   (d) trabecular = granular deossification with indistinct + coarse trabecular pattern, ground glass appearance, salt and pepper skull
   (e) subligamentous: ischial + humeral tuberosity, greater + lesser trochanter, inferior surface of calcaneus, inferior aspect of distal clavicle

B. BONE SOFTENING
   √ basilar impression of skull
   √ wedged vertebrae, kyphoscoliosis, biconcave vertebral deformities
   √ bowing of long bones
   √ slipped capital femoral epiphysis

C. BROWN TUMOR
   More frequent in 1° HPT
   Location: jaw, pelvis, rib, metaphyses of long bones, facial bones
   √ expansile lytic well-marginated cystlike lesion = osteoclastoma (DDx: giant cell tumor)
   √ destruction of midportions of distal phalanges with telescoping

D. OSTEOSCLEROSIS
   More frequent in 2° HPT
   √ "rugger jersey spine" = sclerosis of vertebral endplates; skull; metaphyses

E. SOFT-TISSUE CALCIFICATION
   More frequent in 2° HPT; metastatic calcification when Ca x P product >70 mg/dl
   (a) cornea, viscera (lung, stomach, kidney)
   (b) periarticular in hip, knee, shoulder, wrist
   (c) arterial wall (resembling diabetes mellitus)
   (d) Chondrocalcinosis (15 – 18%) = calcification of hyaline / fibrous cartilage in menisci, wrist, shoulder, hip, elbow

F. EROSIVE ARTHROPATHY
   • asymptomatic
   √ simulates rheumatoid arthritis with preserved joint spaces

Sequelae:
1. Renal stones / nephrocalcinosis (70%)
2. Increased osteoblastic activity (25%)
   • increased alkaline phosphatase
   (a) osteitis fibrosa cystica
       √ subperiosteal bone resorption + cortical tunneling
       √ brown tumors (primary HPT)
   (b) bone softening
       √ fractures
3. Peptic ulcer disease (increased gastric secretion from gastrinoma)
4. Calcific pancreatitis
5. Soft tissue calcifications (2° HPT)
6. Marginal joint erosions + subarticular collapse (DIP, PIP, MCP)

Primary Hyperparathyroidism

= pHPT = 1° HPT = intrinsic abnormality of parathyroid gland featuring
   (1) brown tumor
   (2) chondrocalcinosis (20 – 30%)
Δ requires surgical Rx
Incidence: 25 / 100,000 per year; incidence of bone lesions in HPT is 25 – 40%
Etiology:
   (a) Parathyroid adenoma (87%): single (80%); multiple (7%)
   (b) Parathyroid hyperplasia (10%): chief cell (5%); clear cell (5%)
   (c) Parathyroid carcinoma (3%)
Histo: increased number of osteoclasts, increased osteoid volume (defect in mineralization), slightly increased osteoblasts = decreased bone mass
Age: 3rd – 5th decade; M:F = 1:3
Associated with:
   (a) Wermer syndrome = MEA I (+ pituitary adenoma + pancreatic islet cell tumor)
   (b) Sipple syndrome = MEA II (+ medullary thyroid carcinoma + pheochromocytoma)
   • elevation of serum calcium + decrease in serum phosphate (30%)
   • increase in serum alkaline phosphatase (50%)
   • increase in parathyroid hormone (100%)
   • hypotonicity of muscles, weakness, constipation, difficulty in swallowing, duodenal / gastric peptic ulcer disease (secondary to hypercalcemia)
   • polyuria, polydypsia (hypercalciuria + hyperphosphaturia)

- renal colic + renal insufficiency (nephrocalculosis + nephrocalcinosis)
- rheumatic bone pain + tenderness (particularly at site of brown tumor), pathologic fracture secondary to brown tumor

X-ray (skeletal involvement in 20%):
- √ thin cortices with lacy cortical pattern (subperiosteal bone resorption)
- √ brown tumor (particularly in jaw + long bones)
- √ osteitis cystica fibrosa (= intertrabecular fibrous connective tissue)

NUC:
- √ normal bone scan in 80%
- √ foci of abnormal uptake: calvarium (especially periphery), mandible, sternum, acromioclavicular joint, lateral humeral epicondyles, hands
- √ increased uptake in brown tumors
- √ extraskeletal uptake: cornea, cartilage, joint capsules, tendons, periarticular areas, lungs, stomach
- √ normal renal excretion [except in stone disease / calcium nephropathy (10%)]

Secondary Hyperparathyroidism

= sHPT = 2° HPT = diffuse / adenomatous hyperplasia of all four parathyroid glands as a compensatory mechanism in any state of hypocalcemia featuring (1) soft-tissue calcifications (2) osteosclerosis
Δ requires medical Rx
Etiology:
(a) renal osteodystrophy (renal insufficiency + osteomalacia / rickets)
(b) calcium deprivation, maternal hypoparathyroidism, pregnancy, hypovitaminosis D
(c) rise in serum phosphate leading to decrease in calcium by feedback mechanism
NUC:
- √ "superscan" in 2° HPT:
  - √ absent kidney sign
  - √ increased bone-to-soft tissue uptake ratio
  - √ increased uptake in calvarium, mandible, acromioclavicular region, sternum, vertebrae, distal third of long bones, ribs

Tertiary Hyperparathyroidism

= tHPT = 3° HPT = development of autonomous PTH adenoma in patients with chronically overstimulated hyperplastic parathyroid glands (renal insufficiency);
Δ requires surgical Rx

Clue: (a) intractable hypercalcemia
(b) inability to control osteomalacia by vitamin D administration

Ectopic Parathormone Production

= pseudohyperparathyroidism as paraneoplastic syndrome in bronchogenic carcinoma + renal cell carcinoma

HYPERTROPHIC OSTEOARTHROPATHY

= HYPERTROPHIC PULMONARY OSTEOARTHROPATHY
Etiology: (1) Release of vasodilators which are not metabolized by lung
(2) Increased flow through AV shunts
(3) Reflex peripheral vasodilation (vagal impulses)
(4) Hormones: estrogen, growth hormone, prostaglandin

A. THORACIC CAUSES
(a) malignant tumor (0.7 – 12%): bronchogenic carcinoma, mesothelioma, lymphoma, pulmonary metastasis from osteogenic sarcoma, melanoma, renal cell carcinoma, breast cancer
(b) benign tumor: benign pleural fibroma, tumor of ribs, thymoma, esophageal leiomyoma, pulmonary hemangioma, pulmonary congenital cyst
(c) chronic infection / inflammation: pulmonary abscess, bronchiectasis, blastomycosis, TB (very rare); cystic fibrosis, interstitial fibrosis
(d) congenital heart disease
B. EXTRATHORACIC CAUSES
(a) GI tract: ulcerative colitis, amebic + bacillary dysentery, intestinal TB, Whipple disease, Crohn disease, gastric ulcer, bowel lymphoma, gastric carcinoma

	HypoPT	PseudoHypoPT	PseudopseudoHypoPT
Serum-Ca	down	down	norm
Serum-P	up	up	norm
AlkaPhos	down/norm	down/norm	norm

Response to PTH-Injection	norm / HypoPT	PseudoHypoPT
Urine-AMP	up	norm
Urine-P	up	norm
Plasma-AMP	up	norm

(b) liver disease: biliary + alcoholic cirrhosis, posthepatic cirrhosis, chronic active hepatitis, bile duct carcinoma, benign bile duct stricture, amyloidosis, liver abscess

(c) undifferentiated nasopharyngeal carcinoma, pancreatic carcinoma, chronic myelogenous leukemia

- burning pain, painful swelling of limbs, and stiffness of joints: ankles (88%), wrists (83%), knees (75%), elbows (17%), shoulders (10%), fingers (7%)
- peripheral neurovascular disorders: local cyanosis, areas of increased sweating, paresthesia, chronic erythema, flushing + blanching of skin
- hypocratic fingers + toes (clubbing)
- hypertrophy of extremities (soft tissue swelling)

Location: tibia + fibula (75%), radius + ulna (80%), proximal phalanges (60%), femur (50%), metacarpus + metatarsus (40%), humerus + distal phalanges (25%), pelvis (5%); unilateral (rare)

Site: in diametaphyseal regions
√ periosteal proliferation of new bone, at first smooth then undulating + rough, most conspicuous on concavity of long bones (dorsal + medial aspects)
√ regression of periosteal reaction after thoracotomy
√ soft tissue swelling ("clubbing") of distal phalanges

Bone scan (reveals changes with greater clarity):
    √ symmetric diffusely increased uptake along cortical margins of diaphysis + metaphysis of tubular bones of the extremities with irregularities
    √ increased periarticular uptake (= synovitis)
    √ scapular involvement in 2/3
    √ mandible ± maxilla abnormal in 40%

HYPERVITAMINOSIS A

Age: usually infants + children
- anorexia, irritability
- loss of hair, dry skin, pruritus, fissures of lips
- jaundice, enlargement of liver
√ separation of cranial sutures secondary to hydrocephalus (coronal > lambdoid) in children <10 years of age, may appear within a few days
√ symmetrical solid periosteal new bone formation along shafts of long + short bones (ulna, calvicle)
√ premature epiphyseal closure + thinning of epiphyseal plates
√ accelerated growth
√ tendinous, ligamentous, pericapsular calcifications
√ changes usually disappear after cessation of vitamin A ingestion
DDx: Infantile cortical hyperostosis (mandible involved)

HYPERVITAMINOSIS D

= excessive ingestion of vitamin D (large doses act like parathormone)
- loss of appetite, drowsiness, headaches
- polyuria, polydipsia, renal damage
- anemia
- diarrhea
- convulsions

- excessive phosphaturia (parathormone decreases tubular absorption)
- hypercalcemia + hypercalciuria
√ deossification
√ widening of provisional zone of calcification
√ cortical + trabecular thickening
√ alternating bands of increased + decreased density near / in epiphysis (zone of provisional calcification)
√ vertebra outlined by dense band of bone + adjacent radiolucent line within
√ dense calvarium
√ metastatic calcinosis in (a) arterial walls (between age 20 and 30) (b) kidneys = nephrocalcinosis (c) periarticular tissue (putty-like) (d) premature calcification of falx cerebri (most consistent sign!)

HYPOPARATHYROIDISM

Etiology:
A. Idiopathic Hypoparathyroidism
    = rare condition of unknown cause
    - round face, short dwarf-like, obese
    - mental retardation
    - cataracts
    - dry scaly skin, atrophy of nails
    - dental hypoplasia (delayed tooth eruption, impaction of teeth, supernumerary teeth)
B. Secondary Hypoparathyroidism
    = accidental removal / damage to parathyroid glands in thyroid surgery / radical neck dissection (5%); I-131 therapy (rare); external beam radiation; hemorrhage; infection; thyroid carcinoma; hemochromatosis (iron deposition)
- tetany = neuromuscular excitability (numbness, cramps, carpopedal spasm, laryngeal stridor, generalized convulsions)
- hypocalcemia + hyperphosphatemia
- normal / low serum alkaline phosphatase
√ premature closure of epiphyses
√ hypoplasia of tooth enamel + dentine; blunting of roots
√ generalized increase in bone density in 9%
    √ localized thickening of skull
    √ sacroiliac sclerosis
    √ band-like density in metaphysis of long bones (25%), iliac crest, vertebral bodies
    √ thickened lamina dura (inner table) + widened diploe
    √ deformed hips with thickening + sclerosis of femoral head + acetabulum
@ Soft tissue
    √ intracranial calcifications in basal ganglia, choroid plexus, occasionally in cerebellum
    √ calcification of spinal and other ligaments
    √ subcutaneous calcifications
    √ ossification of muscle insertions
    √ ectopic bone formation

HYPOPHOSPHATASIA

= autosomal recessive congenital disease with low activity of serum-, bone-, liver-alkaline phosphatase resulting in poor mineralization (deficient generation of bone crystals)

Incidence: 1:100,000
Histo: indistinguishable from rickets
- phosphoethanolamine in urine as precursor of alkaline phosphatase
- normal serum calcium + phosphorus
A. GROUP I = neonatal = congenital lethal form
  √ marked demineralization of calvarium ("caput membranaceum" = soft skull)
  √ lack of calcification of metaphyseal end of long bones
  √ streaky irregular spotty margins of calcification
  √ cupping of metaphysis
  √ angulated shaft fractures with abundant callus formation
  √ short poorly ossified ribs
  √ poorly ossified vertebrae (especially neural arches)
  √ small pelvic bones
  OB-US:
    √ high incidence of intrauterine fetal demise
    √ increased echogenicity of falx (enhanced sound transmission secondary to poorly mineralized calvarium)
    √ poorly mineralized short bowed tubular bones + multiple fractures
    √ poorly mineralized spine
    √ short poorly ossified ribs
    √ polyhydramnios
  Prognosis: death within 6 months
B. GROUP II = juvenile severe form
  onset of symptoms within weeks to months
  - moderate / severe dwarfism
  - delayed weight bearing
  √ resembles rickets
  √ separated cranial sutures; craniostenosis in 2nd year
  Prognosis: 50% mortality
C. GROUP III = adult mild form
  recognized later in childhood / adolescence / adulthood
  - dwarfism
  √ clubfoot, genu valgum
  √ demineralization of ossification centers (at birth / 3 – 4 months of age)
  Prognosis: excellent; after 1 year no further progression
D. GROUP IV = latent form
  heterozygous state
  - normal / borderline levels of alkaline phosphatase
  - patients are small for age
  - disturbance of primary dentition
  √ bone fragility + healed fractures
  √ enlarged chondral ends of ribs
  √ metaphyseal notching of long bones
  √ Erlenmeyer flask deformity of femur

HYPOTHYROIDISM
= CRETINISM
A. Childhood:
  √ delayed skeletal maturation (appearance + growth of ossification centers, epiphyseal closure)
  √ fragmented stippled epiphyses
  √ wide sutures / fontanelles with delayed closure
  √ delayed dentition

√ delayed / decreased pneumatization of sinuses + mastoids
√ hypertelorism
√ dense vertebral margins
√ demineralization
√ hypoplastic phalanges of 5th finger
B. Adulthood:
  √ calvarial thickening / sclerosis
  √ wedging of dorsolumbar vertebral bodies
  √ coxa vara with flattened femoral head
  √ premature atherosclerosis
No skeletal changes with adult onset!

INFANTILE CORTICAL HYPEROSTOSIS
= CAFFEY DISEASE
= uncommon self-limiting proliferative bone disease of infancy; sporadic (rare) / autosomal dominant with variable expression + incomplete penetrance; remission + exacerbations are common
Age: <6 months, reported in utero; M:F = 1:1
- sudden hard extremely tender soft tissue swellings over bone
- irritability, fever
Location: mandible (80%) > clavicle > ulna + others (except phalanges + vertebrae)
Site: hyperostosis affects diaphysis of tubular bones asymmetrically, epiphyses spared
√ massive periosteal new bone formation + perifocal soft tissue swelling
√ "double exposed" ribs
√ bone expansion with remodeling of old cortex
Prognosis: usually complete recovery by 30 months
Rx: mild analgesics, steroids

CHRONIC INFANTILE HYPEROSTOSIS
  Disease may persist or recur intermittently for years
  √ bowing deformities, osseous bridging, diaphyseal expansion
  - delayed muscular development, crippling deformities
DDx: (1) Periostitis of prematurity (2) Healing rickets (3) Scurvy (uncommon <4 months of age) (4) Hypervitaminosis A (rarely <1 year of age) (5) Syphilis (focal destruction) (6) Child abuse (7) Prostaglandin administration (usually following 4 – 6 weeks of therapy) (8) Osteomyelitis (9) Leukemia (10) Neuroblastoma (11) Kinky hair syndrome (12) Hereditary hyperphosphatasia

IRON DEFICIENCY ANEMIA
Age: infants affected
Causes:
  (1) inadequate iron stores at birth (2) deficient iron in diet (3) impaired gastrointestinal absorption of iron (4) excessive iron demands from blood loss (5) polycythemia vera (6) cyanotic CHD
√ widening of diploe + thinning of tables with sparing of occiput (no red marrow)
√ hair-on-end appearance of skull
√ osteoporosis in long bones (most prominent in hands)
√ absence of facial bone involvement

JACCOUD ARTHROPATHY

After subsidence of frequent severe attacks of rheumatic fever

Path: periarticular fascial + tendon fibrosis without synovitis

• rheumatic valve disease

Location: primarily involvement of hands; occasionally in great toe

√ muscular atrophy

√ periarticular swelling of small joints of hands + feet

√ ulnar deviation + flexion of MCP joints most marked in 4th + 5th finger

√ NO joint narrowing / erosion

JUVENILE APONEUROTIC FIBROMA

Rare benign fibrous tumor

Histo: cellular dense fibrous tissue with focal chondral elements infiltrating adjacent structures (= cartilaginous tumor)

Age: children + adolescents; male preponderance

Location: deep palmar fascia of hand + wrist

√ soft tissue mass overlying inflamed bursa (often mistaken for calcified bursitis)

√ stippled calcifications

√ interosseous soft tissue mass of forearm + wrist

√ bone erosion may occur

DDx: Synovial sarcoma, chondroma, fibrosarcoma, osteosarcoma, myositis ossificans

KAPOSI SARCOMA

Histo: simulates malignant angioma

Associated with: AIDS

Location: lower extremities

√ lytic cortical lesion

√ subcutaneous nodules

KIENBÖCK DISEASE

= LUNATOMALACIA

= avascular necrosis of lunate bone

Predisposed: individuals engaged in manual labor with repeated / single episode of trauma

Age: 20 - 40 years

Associated with ulna minus variant (short ulna) in 75%

• progressive pain + soft-tissue swelling of wrist

Location: uni- > bilateral (usually right hand)

√ initially normal radiograph

√ fracture / osteonecrosis of lunate

√ increased density + altered shape + collapse of lunate

Cx: scapholunate separation, ulnar deviation of triquetrum, degenerative joint disease in radiocarpal / midcarpal compartments

Rx: ulnar lengthening / radial shortening, lunate replacement

KLINEFELTER SYNDROME

47,XXY (rarely XXYY) chromosomal abnormality

Incidence: 1:750 live births (probably commonest chromosomal aberration)

• testicular atrophy (hyalinization of seminiferous tubules) = small / absent testes, sterility (azoospermia)

• eunuchoid constitution: gynecomastia; paucity of hair on face + chest; female pubic escutcheon

• mild mental retardation

• high level of urinary gonadotropins + low level of 17-ketosteroids after puberty

Δ NO distinctive radiological findings!

√ may have delayed bone maturation

√ failure of frontal sinus to develop

√ small bridged sella turcica

√ ± scoliosis, kyphosis

√ ± coxa valga

√ ± metacarpal sign (short 4th metacarpal)

√ accessory epiphyses of 2nd metacarpal bilaterally

47,XXX = SUPERFEMALE SYNDROME

• usually over 6 feet tall; subnormal intelligence; frequently antisocial behavior

KLIPPEL-TRENAUNAY SYNDROME

= sporadic disease of equal sex distribution characterized by a triad of:

(1) port-wine nevus = unilateral flat cutaneous capillary hemangioma often in dermatomal distribution on affected limb; may fade in 2nd – 3rd decade

(2) varicose veins on lateral aspect of affected limb; usually ipsilateral to hemangioma

(3) limb overgrowth (especially during adolescent growth spurt)

Associated with:

— polydactyly, syndactyly, clinodactyly, congenital dislocation of hip

— hemangiomas of colon / bladder (3 – 10%)

— spinal hemangiomas + AVMs

— hemangiomas in liver / spleen

— lymphangiomas of limb

Location: lower extremity (10 – 15 x more common than upper extremity); bilateral in <5%

√ increased metatarsal / metacarpal + phalangeal size

√ cortical thickening

√ valveless lateral venous channels

√ punctate calcifications (phleboliths) in pelvis (bowel wall, urinary bladder)

DDx:

(1) **Parkes-Weber Syndrome** (similar triad + arteriovenous fistula)

(2) Neurofibromatosis (café-au-lait spots, axillary freckling, cutaneous neurofibromas, macrodactyly secondary to plexiform neurofibromas, wavy cortical reaction, early fusion of growth plate, limb hypertrophy not as extensive / bilateral)

(3) Beckwith-Wiedemann syndrome (aniridia, macroglossia, cryptorchidism, Wilms tumor, broad metaphyses, thickened long bone cortex, advanced bone age, periosteal new bone formation, hemihypertrophy)

(4) Macrodystrophia lipomatosis (hyperlucency of fat, distal phalanges most commonly affected, overgrowth ceases with puberty, usually limited to digits)

(5) Maffucci syndrome (cavernous hemangiomas, soft tissue hypertrophy, phleboliths, multiple enchondromas)

KÖHLER DISEASE
= avascular necrosis of tarsal scaphoid
Age: 3 – 10 years; boys
√ irregular outline
√ fragmentation
√ disc-like compression in AP direction
√ increased density
√ joint space maintained
√ decreased / increased uptake on radionuclide study

LAURENCE-MOON-BIEDL SYNDROME
• retardation
• obesity
• hypogonadism
√ craniosynostosis
√ polysyndactyly

LEAD POISONING
= PLUMBISM
Path: lead concentrates in metaphyses of growing bones (distal femur > both ends of tibia > distal radius) leading to failure of removal of calcified cartilaginous trabeculae in provisional zone
• loss of appetite, vomiting, constipation, abdominal cramps
• peripheral neuritis (adults), meningoencephalitis (children)
• anemia
• lead line at gums (adults)

√ bands of increased density at metaphyses of tubular bones (only in growing bone)
√ lead lines may persist
√ clubbing if poisoning severe (anemia)
√ bone-in-bone apppearance

DDx: (1) Healed rickets
(2) Normal increased density in infants <3 years of age

LEGG-PERTHES-CALVÉ DISEASE
= COXA PLANA = idiopathic avascular necrosis of femoral head in children; one of the most common sites of AVN; 10% bilateral
Age: (a) 4 – 7 years: more frequent in females
(b) adulthood: **Chandler disease**
Cause:
trauma 30% (subcapital fracture, epiphyseolysis, esp. posterior dislocation), closed reduction of congenital hip dislocation, prolonged interval between injury and reduction
Pathophysiology:
femoral head blood supply insufficient (epiphyseal plate acts as a barrier in ages 4 – 10; ligamentum teres vessels become nonfunctional; blood supply is from medial circumflex artery + lateral epiphyseal artery only

Stages:
Stage I = histologic + clinical diagnosis without radiographic findings
Stage II = sclerosis ± cystic changes with preservation of contour + surface of femoral head
Stage III = loss of structural integrity of femoral head
Stage IV = in addition loss of structural integrity of acetabulum
• 1 week – 6 months (mean 2.7 months) duration of symptoms prior to initial presentation

NUC (may assist in early diagnosis):
√ decreased uptake (early) in femoral head = interruption of blood supply
√ increased uptake (late) in femoral head =
(a) revascularization + bone repair
(b) degenerative osteoarthritis
√ increased acetabular activity with associated degenerative joint disease
X-RAY:
Early signs:
√ femoral epiphysis smaller than on contralateral side (96%)
√ sclerosis of femoral head epiphysis (sequestration + compression) (82%)
√ slight widening of joint space due to thickening of cartilage, failure of epiphyseal growth, presence of joint fluid, joint laxity (60%)
√ ipsilateral bone demineralization (46%)
√ alteration of pericapsular soft tissue outline due to atrophy of ipsilateral periarticular soft tissues (73%)
√ rarefaction of lateral + medial metaphyseal areas of neck
√ NEVER destruction of articular cortex as in bacterial arthritis
Late signs:
√ delayed osseous maturation of a mild degree
√ "radiolucent crescent line" of subchondral fracture = small archlike subcortical lucency (32%)
√ subcortical fracture on anterior articular surface (best seen on frog-leg view)
√ femoral head fragmentation
√ femoral neck cysts (from intramedullary hemorrhage in response to stress fractures)
√ loose bodies (only found in males)
√ coxa plana = flattened collection of sclerotic fragments (over 18 months)
√ coxa magna = remodeling of femoral head to become wider + flatter in mushroom configuration to match widened metaphysis + epiphyseal plate
CT:
√ "asterisk" sign = remodeled compact trabecular bone
MR:
√ "double-line" sign (80%) = sclerotic non-signal rim producing line between necrotic + viable bone edged by a hyperintense rim of granulation tissue
√ fluid within fracture plane
√ central low-signal intensity region = "asterisk" sign
Cx: severe degenerative joint disease in early adulthood

LEPROSY
= HANSEN DISEASE
Organism: Mycobacterium leprae
Types:
(1) lepromatous: in cutis, mucous membranes, viscera
(2) neural: enlarged indurated nodular nerve trunks; anesthesia, muscular atrophy, neurotrophic changes
(3) mixed form
Osseous changes in 15 – 54% of patients:

SPECIFIC SIGNS
Location: center of distal end of phalanges / eccentric
√ ill-defined areas of decalcification, reticulated trabecular pattern, small rounded osteolytic lesions, cortical erosions
√ joint spaces preserved
√ healing phase: complete resolution / bone defect with sclerotic rim + endosteal thickening
√ nasal spine absorption + destruction of maxilla, nasal bone, alveolar ridge
√ enlarged nutrient foramina in claw-like hand
√ erosive changes of ungual tufts
NONSPECIFIC SIGNS
√ soft tissue swelling; calcification of nerves
√ contractures / deep ulcerations
√ neurotrophic joints (distal phalanges in hands, MTP in feet, Charcot joints in tarsus)

LEUKEMIA OF BONE
A. CHILDHOOD
Histo: almost always acute lymphoblastic leukemia
• arthritic symptoms (may be confused with acute rheumatic fever / rheumatoid arthritis)
• fever, elevated sedimentation rate
• splenomegaly, occasionally lymphadenopathy
Skeletal manifestations in 50%:
√ multiple small clearly defined ovoid / spheroid osteolytic lesions (destruction of spongiosa, later cortex) in 30 – 60%
√ coarse trabeculation of spongiosa (due to destruction of finer trabeculae)
√ diffuse demineralization of long bones + spine (leukemic infiltrates + catabolic protein / mineral metabolism) in 30%
√ periosteal reaction: smooth / lamellated / sunburst pattern (cortical penetration by sheets of leukemic cells into subperiosteum) in 12 – 25%
√ transverse radiolucent metaphyseal bands around large joints (tibia, femur, proximal humerus, distal radius + ulna) in 10 – 20%; become dense after treatment
√ horizontal / curvilinear bands in vertebral bodies + edges of iliac crest
√ multiple biconcave / partially collapsed vertebrae (14%)
√ osteosclerotic lesions (late in disease due to reactive osteoblastic proliferation)
√ mixed lesions (lytic + bone-forming) in 18%
Dx: sternal marrow / peripheral blood smear

Cx: proliferation of leukemic cells in marrow leads to extraskeletal hematopoiesis
DDx: metastatic neuroblastoma

B. ADULTHOOD
Death usually occurs before skeletal abnormalities manifest
√ osteoporosis
√ solitary radiolucent foci (vertebral collapse)
√ permeating radiolucent mottling (proximal humerus)

LIPOBLASTOMA
= postnatal proliferation of mesenchymal cells with a spectrum of differentiation ranging from prelipoblasts (spindle cells) to mature adipocytes
Path: immature adipose tissue separated by septa into multiple lobules
Histo: uni- and multivacuolated lipoblasts interspersed between spindle / stellate mesenchymal cells; suspended in myxoid stroma
Age: <3 years of age; M:F = 2:1
Location: subcutaneous tissue of extremities, neck, trunk, perineum, retroperitoneum
√ fatty tumor with enhancing soft-tissue component
DDx: liposarcoma (extremely rare in children)

LIPOMA OF BONE
= INTRAOSSEOUS LIPOMA
Radiographic appearance similar to unicameral bone cyst (infarcted lipoma = unicameral bone cyst ?)
Age: any; M:F = 1:1
May be associated with: hyperlipoproteinemia
Location: calcaneus, extremities (proximal femur > tibia, fibula, humerus), skull, ribs
Site: metaphysis
√ expansile radiolucent lesion + thinned cortex
√ may contain clump of calcification centrally (= dystrophic calcification from fat necrosis)
√ loculated / septated appearance (trabeculae)

LIPOMA OF SOFT TISSUE
Most common mesenchymal tumor composed of mature adipose tissue
Histo: mature fat cells (adipocytes) that are uniform in size + shape, occasionally have fibrous connective tissue as septations; fat unavailable for systemic metabolism
• stable size after initial period of discernible growth
Age: 5th – 6th decade
Location:
(a) superficial = subcutaneous lipoma (more common)
(b) deep lipoma in retroperitoneum, chest wall, deep soft tissue of hands + feet
multiple in 5 – 7% (up to several hundred tumors)
√ mass of fat opacity / density / intensity identical to subcutaneous fat
√ cortical thickening (with adjacent parosteal lipoma)
CT:
√ well-defined + homogeneous tumor with low attenuation coefficient (-65 to -120 HU)

√ no enhancement following IV contrast material
MR:
  √ signal intensity characteristics similar to subcutaneous fat: hyperintense on T1WI + T2WI
  √ differentiation from other lesions by fat suppression technique

Benign Mesenchymoma
= long-standing lipoma with chondroid + osseous metaplasia

Infiltrating Lipoma
= INTRAMUSCULAR LIPOMA = relatively common benign lipomatous tumor extending between muscle fibers that become variably atrophic
Peak age: 5 – 6th decade; M>F
Location: thigh (50%), shoulder, upper arm

Lipoma Arborescens
= DIFFUSE SYNOVIAL LIPOMA = lipomalike lesion composed of hypertrophic synovial villi distended with fat, probably reactive process to chronic synovitis
Location: knee; monarticular
Frequently associated with
  degenerative joint disease, chronic rheumatoid arthritis, prior trauma

Neural Fibrolipoma
= FIBROLIPOMATOUS HAMARTOMA OF NERVE
Age: early adulthood
• soft slowly enlarging mass
• pain, tenderness, decreased sensation, paresthesia
Location: volar aspect of hand, wrist, forearm
+ macrodactyly (in 1/3) = **macrodystrophia lipomatosa**

LIPOSARCOMA
Malignant tumor of mesenchymal origin with bulk of tumor tissue differentiating into adipose tissue
Incidence: 12 – 18% of all malignant soft-tissue tumors; 2nd most common soft-tissue sarcoma in adults (after malignant fibrous histiocytoma)
Age: 5th – 6th decade
Histo: (a) well-differentiated
  (b) myxoid in 40 – 50% (most common): proliferating fibroblasts, plexiform capillary pattern, myxoid matrix, fat amount <10%
  (c) round cell = poorly differentiated myxoid
  (d) pleomorphic
• usually painless mass (may be painful in 10 – 15%)

Location: trunk (42%), lower extremity (41%), upper extremity (11%), head + neck (6%); particularly in thigh + retroperitoneum
Spread: hematogenous to lung, visceral organs; myxoid liposarcoma shows tendency for serosal + pleural surfaces, subcutaneous tissue, bone
√ nonspecific soft-tissue mass (frequently fat is radiologically not detectable)
√ inhomogeneous mass with soft-tissue + fatty components

√ enhancement after IV contrast material (contradistinction to lipoma)
√ concomitant mass in retroperitoneum / thigh (in up to 10% of myxoid liposarcomas) as multicentric lesion / metastasis
√ mass of near water density / hypoechoic / hypointense on T1WI + hyperintense on T2WI in myxoid liposarcoma (high content of myxoid cells)

LYME ARTHRITIS
Agent: spirochete Borrelia burgdorferi; transmitted by tick Ixodes dammini
Histo: inflammatory synovial fluid, hypertrophic synovia with vascular proliferation + cellular infiltration
• history of erythema chronicum migrans
• endemic areas: Lyme, Connecticut first recognized location; now also throughout United States, Europe, Australia
• recurrent attacks of arthralgias within days to 2 years after tick bite (80%)
Location: mono- / oligoarthritis of large joints (especially knee)
√ erosion of cartilage / bone (4%)
Rx: antibiotics
DDx: (1) Rheumatic fever (2) Rheumatoid arthritis (3) Gonococcal arthritis (4) Reiter syndrome

LYMPHOMA OF BONE
= RETICULUM CELL SARCOMA = HISTIOCYTIC LYMPHOMA = PRIMARY LYMPHOMA OF BONE (the generalized form of reticulum cell sarcoma is lymphoma); 2 – 6% of all primary malignant bone tumors in children
Incidence of bone marrow involvement:
  5 – 15% in Hodgkin disease;
  25 – 40% in non-Hodgkin lymphoma
  Δ bone marrow involvement indicates progression of disease
  Δ bone marrow imaging-guidance for biopsy!
NUC: 40% sensitivity; 88% specificity
MR: 65% sensitivity; 90% specificity
Histo: sheets of reticulum cells, larger than those in Ewing sarcoma (DDx: myeloma, inflammation, osteosarcoma, eosinophilic granuloma)
Age: any age; peak age in 3rd – 5th decade; 50% <40 years; 35% <30 years; M:F = 2:1
• striking contrast between size of lesion + patient's well-being
Location: lower femur, upper tibia (40% about knee), humerus, pelvis, scapula, ribs, vertebra
Site: dia- / metaphysis
√ cancellous bone erosion (earliest sign)
√ mottled permeative pattern of separate coalescent areas
√ late cortical destruction
√ lamellated / sunburst periosteal response (less than in Ewing sarcoma)
√ lytic / reactive new bone formation
√ associated soft tissue mass without calcification
√ synovitis of knee joint common

Cx: pathologic fracture (most common among malignant bone tumors)
Prognosis: 50% 5-year survival
DDx: (1)   Osteosarcoma (less medullary extension, younger patients)
(2)   Ewing tumor (systemic symptoms, debility, younger patients)
(3)   Metastatic malignancy (multiple bones involved, more destructive)

MACRODYSTROPHIA LIPOMATOSA
= neural fibrolipoma with macrodactyly = increase in size of all elements + structures of a digit
Histo: infiltration of epineurium + perineurium by fibrofatty tissue
Age: growth stops at puberty
Location: 2nd or 3rd digit of hand / foot; multiple digits may be involved
√   osseous overgrowth of phalanx often with distal splaying
√   dorsal deviation
√   clinodactyly
√   overgrowth of fat
√   long, broad, splayed phalanges
DDx: Klippel-Trenaunay-Weber syndrome, neurofibromatosis, chronic vascular stimulation, Proteus syndrome

MALIGNANT FIBROUS HISTIOCYTOMA
= MFH = MALIGNANT FIBROUS XANTHOMA
= XANTHOSARCOMA = MALIGNANT HISTIOCYTOMA
= FIBROSARCOMA VARIANT
Incidence: most common primary malignant soft tissue tumor of extremities / retroperitoneum after age 45
Histo: spindle-cell neoplasm of a mixture of fibroblasts + cells resembling histiocytes with nuclear atypia and pleomorphism in pinwheel arrangement; closely resembles high-grade fibrosarcoma
Age: 1st – 8th decade; average age of 50 years; M:F = 3:2
•   painless soft tissue mass present for a few months

Location: potential to arise in any organ (ubiquitous mesenchymal tissue); meta-diaphyseal in long bones (75%): femur (45%), tibia (20%), 50% about knee; humerus (10%); ilium (10%); spine; sternum; clavicle; rarely small bones of hand + feet
@ Soft tissue
    Location: lower extremity (1/3) > upper extremity > retroperitoneum
    √   mass usually >5 cm in size
    √   poorly defined calcifications (7 – 20%)
    √   occasional secondary involvement of adjacent bone with periosteal reaction, cortical erosion, pathologic fracture
    DDx: (1)   Liposarcoma (younger patient, presence of fat, calcifications rare)
        (2)   Rhabdomyosarcoma
        (3)   Synovial sarcoma

@ Bone (130 cases only)
    Associated with   prior radiation therapy / bone infarcts / Paget disease / fibrous dysplasia
    •   painful, tender, rapidly enlarging mass
    Site: metaphysis of long bones (most common)
    √   radiolucent defect with ill-defined margins (2.5 – 10 cm in diameter)
    √   extensive mineralization / small areas of focal calcification
    √   permeation + cortical destruction
    √   expansion in smaller bones (ribs, sternum, fibula, clavicle)
    √   occasionally lamellated periosteal reaction (especially in presence of pathologic fracture)
    √   soft tissue extension
    Cx: pathologic fracture (30 – 50%)
    DDx: (1) metastasis (2) fibrosarcoma (often with sequestrum) (3) reticulum cell sarcoma (4) osteosarcoma
@ Lung (extremely rare)
    √   solitary pulmonary nodule without calcification
    √   diffuse infiltrate

NUC: √   increased uptake of Tc-99m MDP (mechanism not understood)
    √   increased uptake of Ga-67 citrate
US: √   well-defined mass with hyperechoic + hypoechoic (necrotic) areas
CT: √   mass of muscle density with hypodense areas (necrosis)
    √   invasion of abdominal musculature, but not IVC / renal veins (DDx to renal cell carcinoma)
Angio: √   hypervascularity + early venous return
Prognosis: 2-year survival rate of 60%; 5-year survival rate of 50%; local recurrence rate of 44%; metastatic rate of 42% (lung, lymph nodes, liver, bone)

MARFAN SYNDROME
= ARACHNODACTYLY = autosomal dominant familial disorder of connective tissue (abnormal cross-linking of collagen fibers) with high penetrance but extremely variable expression, new mutations in 15%
Prevalence: 5:100,000; M:F = 1:1

A.   MUSCULOSKELETAL MANIFESTATIONS
    •   tall thin stature with long limbs, arm span greater than height
    •   muscular hypoplasia + hypotonicity
    •   scarcity of subcutaneous fat (emaciated look)
    √   generalized osteopenia
    @ Skull
        •   elongated face
        √   dolichocephaly
        √   prominent jaw
        √   high arched palate
    @ Hand
        •   Steinberg sign = protrusion of thumb beyond the confines of the clenched fist (found in 1.1% of normal population)

- metacarpal index (averaging the 4 ratios of length of 2nd through 5th metacarpals divided by their respective middiaphyseal width) >8.8. (male) or 9.4 (female)
- √ arachnodactyly = elongation of phalanges + metacarpals
- √ flexion deformity of 5th finger

@ Foot
- √ pes planus
- √ club foot
- √ hallux valgus
- √ hammer toes
- √ disproportionate elongation of 1st digit of foot

@ Spine
- ratio of measurement between symphysis and floor + crown and floor >0.45
- √ pectus carinatum / excavatum (common)
- √ scoliosis / kyphoscoliosis (45 – 60%)
- √ increased incidence of Scheuermann disease and spondylosis
- √ dural ectasia
  - √ increased interpeduncular distance
  - √ posterior scalloping
  - √ presacral + lateral sacral meningoceles
  - √ expansion of sacral spinal canal
  - √ enlargement of sacral foramina
- √ winged scapulae

@ Joints
- ligamentous laxity + hypermobility + instability
- √ premature osteoarthritis
- √ patella alta
- √ genu recurvatum
- √ recurrent dislocations of patella, hip, clavicle, mandible
- √ slipped capital femoral epiphysis
- √ progressive protrusio acetabuli (50%), bilateral > unilateral, F > M

B. OCULAR MANIFESTATIONS
- bilateral ectopia lentis, usually upwards
- contracted pupils (absence of dilator muscle)
- myopia
- strabismus
- retinal detachment
- flat cornea

C. CARDIOVASCULAR MANIFESTATIONS (60%)
Δ Cause of death in 93%!
- chest pain, palpitations, shortness of breath, fatigue
- mid-to-late systolic murmur + one / more clicks

Associated with congenital heart defect (33%): incomplete coarctation, ASD

@ AORTA (cause of death in 55%)
- √ aortic root dilatation / aneurysm of ascending aorta (cystic medial necrosis) without calcifications
- √ "tulip bulb" = symmetrical dilatation of aortic sinuses of Valsalva (58%)
- √ myxomatous degeneration of aortic annulus

@ MITRAL VALVE
- √ "floppy valve syndrome" (95%) = redundant chordae tendineae with mitral valve prolapse

Cx: (1) Aortic dissection (2) Aortic regurgitation (in 81% if root diameter >5 cm; in 100% if root diameter >6 cm) (3) Mitral regurgitation (4) Cor pulmonale (secondary to chest deformity) (5) Aortic rupture

D. PULMONARY MANIFESTATIONS
- √ cystic lung disease
- √ recurrent spontaneous pneumothoraces

E. ABDOMINAL MANIFESTATION
- √ recurrent biliary obstruction

DDx: (1) Homocystinuria (osteoporosis)
(2) Ehlers-Danlos syndrome
(3) Congenital contractural arachnodactyly (ear deformities, NO ocular / cardiac abnormalities)
(4) Type III MEN (medullary thyroid carcinoma, mucosal neuromas, pheochromocytoma, marfanoid habitus)

MASSIVE OSTEOLYSIS
= GORHAM DISEASE = "VANISHING BONE" SYNDROME = PHANTOM BONE = HEMANGIOMA OF BONE
Infrequent disorder of unknown etiology with unpredictable course + progression
Histo: massive proliferation of hemangiomatous / lymphangiomatous tissue with large sinusoid spaces + fibrosis
Age: children + adults <40 years
Associated with: soft tissue hemangiomas without calcifications
- frequently history of severe trauma
- little / no pain
Location: any bone; most commonly major long bones, innominate bone, spine, thorax, short tubular bones of hand + feet (unusual)
- √ progressive relentless destruction of bone
- √ lack of reaction (no periosteal reaction, no repair)
- √ advancing edge of destruction not sharply delineated
- √ tapering margins of bone ends at sites of osteolysis with conelike spicule of bone (early changes)
- √ no respect for joints
- √ may destroy all bones in a particular area

MASTOCYTOSIS
= URTICARIA PIGMENTOSA
= mast cell accumulation in multiple organs
Age: <6 months (50%)
Associated with leukemia
- skin lesions
- hepatomegaly
- lymphadenopathy
- pancytopenia
@ Skeletal involvement (70%)
- √ osteoporosis

√ coarsened trabeculae
√ scattered well-defined sclerotic foci with focal /
diffuse involvement; often alternating with areas of
bone rarefaction
Predilected sites: skull, spine, ribs, pelvis, humerus,
femur

MELORHEOSTOSIS
Nonhereditary disease of unknown etiology;
often incidental finding
Age: slow chronic course in adults; rapid progression in
children
Associated with   osteopoikilosis, osteopathia striata,
tumors / malformations of blood vessels (hemangioma,
vascular nevi, glomus tumor, AVM, aneurysm,
lymphedema, lymphangiectasia)
• severe pain + limited joint motion (bone may encroach
on nerves, blood vessels, or joints)
• thickening + fibrosis of overlying skin (resembling
scleroderma)
• muscle atrophy (frequent)

Location:
diaphysis, usually monomelic with at least two bones
involved in dermatomal distribution (follows spinal
sensory nerve sclerotomes); entire cortex / limited
to one side of cortex; more common in lower limb; skull,
spine, ribs rarely involved
√ "candle wax dripping" = continuous / interrupted streaks
/ blotches of sclerosis along tubular bone beginning at
proximal end extending distally with slow progression
√ may cross joint with joint fusion
√ small opacities in scapula + hemipelvis (similar to
osteopoikilosis)
√ discrepant limb length
√ flexion contractures of hip + knee
√ genu valgum / varus
√ dislocated patella

DDx: (1) Osteopoikilosis (generalized)
(2) Fibrous dysplasia (normal bone structure not
lost, not as dense)
(3) Engelmann disease
(4) Hyperostosis of neurofibromatosis, tuberous
sclerosis, hemangiomas
(5) Osteoarthropathy

MENISCAL TEAR
Type of tear:
1. Horizontal cleavage tear primarily involving the central
horizontal plane of meniscus (most common): usually
degenerative
2. Parrot beak tear = fraying of free edge, usually
degenerative tear in body of lateral meniscus near the
junction of body + posterior horn
3. Bucket handle tear = longitudinal vertical tear with an
unstable displaced inner fragment usually in medial
rarely in lateral meniscus: traumatic
4. Flap tear = oblique + incomplete tear: traumatic, at
times degenerative

5. Peripheral tear = vertical tear in peripheral third of
meniscus: traumatic
6. Meniscocapsular separation = tearing of peripheral
attachments of meniscus

Associated with: ligamentous injury
• asymptomatic in up to 20% of older individuals

Site of injury: medial: lateral = 3 – 4:1; posterior horn >
midbody > anterior horn

MR:
Accuracy:
89 – 94% for medial meniscal tear;
88 – 98% for lateral meniscal tear;
91 – 96% for anterior cruciate ligament tear;
up to 99% for posterior cruciate ligament tear
√ grade 3 signal = high signal intensity extending to free
edge of meniscus (on more than one image / imaging
plane)
√ alteration of normal shape / size
√ edge irregularity
√ truncation

FALSE-POSITIVE:
A. Normal variants simulating tears:
1. Superior recess on posterior horn of medial
meniscus
2. Popliteal hiatus of lateral meniscus
3. Transverse ligament connecting anterior horns of
medial + lateral meniscus
B. Healed meniscus
√ persistent grade 3 signal at least up to 6 months
C. Degenerative changes
√ grade 1 signal = globular increase in intensity
√ grade 2 signal = linear signal not extending to
articular surface

Arthrography: 60 – 97% accuracy
Arthroscopy: 84 – 99% accuracy

MESOMELIC DWARFISM
Heritable bone dysplasia
A. **Langer type**
autosomal recessive
• mental impairment
√ mesomelic shortening of limbs
√ hypoplasia of ulna + fibula
√ hypoplasia of mandible with short condyles
B. **Nievergelt type**
autosomal dominant
√ severe mesomelic shortening of lower limbs
√ marked thickening of tibia + fibula in central portion
√ clubfoot (frequent)
C. **Lamy-Bienenfeld type**
autosomal dominant
• ligamentous laxity
√ shortening of radius + ulna + tibia
√ absent fibula
√ normal femur + humerus

√ shortening of all long bones at birth, most marked in tibia + radius
√ modelling deformity with widening of diaphysis
√ mild to moderate bowing
√ hypoplasia of fibula with absent lateral malleolus
√ short + thick ulna with hypoplastic distal end
√ Madelung deformity of wrist
√ hypoplasia of a vertebral body may be present

METAPHYSEAL CHONDRODYSPLASIA
= severe short-limbed dwarfism
√ metaphyseal flaring (Erlenmeyer flask deformity) extending into diaphysis

A. **Schmid type** (most common)
autosomal dominant
• waddling gate
Distribution: more marked in lower limbs; mild involvement of hands + wrists
√ shortened bowed long bones
√ widened epiphyseal growth plates
√ irregular widened cupped metaphyses
√ coxa vara
√ genu varum
DDx: vitamin D-refractory rickets

B. **McKusick type**
autosomal recessive (eg, in Amish)
• sparse brittle hair, deficient pigmentation
• normal intelligence
√ shortening of long bones with normal width
√ cupped + widened metaphyses with lucent defects
√ short middle phalanges + narrow distal phalanges becoming triangular and bullet-shaped (more frequent in hands than feet)
√ widened costochondral junctions + cystic lucencies

C. **Jansen type** (less common)
sporadic occurence with wide spectrum
• intelligence normal / retarded
• serum calcium levels often elevated
Distribution: symmetrical involvement of all long + short tubular bones
√ widened epiphyseal plates
√ expanded irregular + fragmented metaphyses (unossified cartilage extending into diaphyses)
DDx: rickets

D. **Pyle disease** = Metaphyseal dysplasia
• often tall
• often asymptomatic
Distribution: major long bones, tubular bones of hands, medial end of clavicle, sternal end of ribs, innominate bone
√ splaying of proximal + distal ends of long bones with thinned cortex
√ relative constriction of central portion of shafts
√ craniofacial hyperostosis
√ genu valgum

METASTASES TO BONE
15 – 100 times more common than primary skeletal neoplasms

Frequency:

if primary known		if primary unknown	
breast	35%	prostate	25%
prostate	30%	lymphoma	15%
lung	10%	breast	10%
kidney	5%	lung	10%
uterus	2%		
thyroid	2%		
stomach	2%		
colon	1%		
others	13%		

SOLITARY BONE LESION
Δ of all causes only 7% due to metastasis
Δ in patients with known malignancy due to metastasis (55%), trauma (25%), infection (10%)
Location: axial skeleton (64 – 68%), ribs (45%), extremities (24%), skull (12%)

METASTASES IN PRIMARY BONE TUMORS
1. Osteosarcoma: 2% with distant metastases, adjuvant therapy has changed the natural history of the disease in that bone metastases occur in 10% of osteosarcomas without metastases to the lung
2. Ewing sarcoma: 13% with distant metastases

mnemonic: "**S**everal **K**inds **O**f **H**orribly **N**asty **T**umors **L**eap **P**romptly **T**o **B**one"
Sarcoma, **S**quamous cell carcinoma
Kidney tumor
Ovarian cancer
Hodgkin disease
Neuroblastoma
Testicular cancer
Lung cancer
Prostate cancer
Thyroid cancer
Breast cancer

Breast cancer:	extensive osteolytic lesions; involvement of entire skeleton; pathologic fractures common
Thyroid + kidney:	often solitary; rapid progression with bone expansion (bubbly); frequently associated with soft tissue mass (distinctive)
Rectum + colon:	may resemble osteosarcoma with sunburst pattern + osteoblastic reaction
Neuroblastoma:	extensive destruction, resembles leukemia (metaphyseal band of rarefaction), mottled skull destruction + increased intracranial pressure, perpendicular spicules of bone
Hodgkin tumor:	upper lumbar + lower thoracic spine, pelvis, ribs; osteolytic / occasionally osteoblastic lesions
Ewing tumor:	extensive osteolytic / osteoblastic reaction

Mode of spread: through blood stream / lymphatics /
                    direct extension
Location: predilection for marrow-containing skeleton
            (skull, spine, ribs, pelvis, humeri, femora)
√ single / multiple lesions of variable size
√ usually nonexpansile
√ joint spaces + intervertebral spaces preserved (cartilage resistant to invasion)

(a) OSTEOLYTIC
   Most common cause: neuroblastoma (in childhood);
      lung cancer (in adult male); breast cancer (in adult
      female), thyroid cancer; kidney; colon
   √ may begin in spongy bone (associated with soft
      tissue mass in ribs)
   √ vertebral pedicles often involved (not in multiple
      myeloma)

(b) OSTEOBLASTIC
   = evidence of slow-growing neoplasm
   Primary:
      prostate, breast, lymphoma, malignant carcinoid,
      medulloblastoma, mucinous adenocarcinoma of GI
      tract, TCC of bladder, pancreas, neuroblastoma
   Most common cause: prostate cancer (in adult male);
      breast cancer (in adult female)
   mnemonic: "5 **B**ees **L**ick **P**ollen"
      Brain (medulloblastoma)
      Bronchus
      Breast
      Bowel (especially carcinoid)
      Bladder
      Lymphoma
      Prostate
   √ frequent in vertebrae + pelvis
   √ may be indistinguishable from Paget disease

(c) MIXED: breast, prostate, lymphoma
(d) EXPANSILE / BUBBLY: kidney, thyroid
(e) PERMEATIVE: Burkitt lymphoma, Mycosis fungoides
(f) "Sunburst" periosteal reaction (infrequent):
      prostatic carcinoma, retinoblastoma, neuroblastoma
      (skull), GI tract
(g) Soft tissue mass: thyroid, kidney
(h) Calcifying metastases:
      mnemonic: "BOTTOM"
      Breast
      Osteosarcoma
      Testicular
      Thyroid
      Ovary
      Mucinous adenocarcinoma of GI tract

NUC:
   Pathophysiology: accumulation of tracer at sites of
                        reactive bone formation
   False-negative scan: very aggressive metastases
   False-positive scan: degeneration, healing fractures,
                         metabolic disorders
   Baseline scan:
   (a) high sensitivity for many metastatic tumors to
      bone (particularly carcinoma of breast, lung,
      prostate); 5% of metastases have normal scan;
      5 – 40% occur in appendicular skeleton

(b) substantially less sensitive than radiographs in
   infiltrative marrow lesions (multiple myeloma,
   neuroblastoma, histiocytosis)
(c) screening of asymptomatic patients
   — useful in: prostate cancer, breast cancer
   — not useful in: non-small cell bronchogenic
      carcinoma, gynecologic malignancy, head
      and neck cancer
√ multiple asymmetric areas of increased uptake
√ axial > appendicular skeleton (dependent on
   distribution of bone marrow); vertebrae, ribs, pelvis
   involved in 80%
√ superscan in diffuse bony metastases

Follow-up scan:
√ stable scan = suggestive of relative good prognosis
√ increased activity in:
   (a) enlargement of bone lesions / appearance of
      new lesions indicate progression of the disease
   (b) "flare phenomenon" (in 20 – 61%) = transient
      increase in lesion activity secondary to healing
      under antineoplastic treatment, maximum
      between 1 and 3 months, unrelated to eventual
      therapeutic response
   (c) avascular necrosis particularly in hips, knees,
      shoulders caused steroid therapy
   (d) osteoradionecrosis / radiation-induced
      osteosarcoma
√ decreased activity in:
   (a) predominately osteolytic destruction
   (b) metastases under radiotherapy; as early as
      2 – 4 months with minimum of 2000 rads

ROLE OF BONE SCAN IN BREAST CANCER
   Routine preoperative bone scan not justified:
      Stage I : unsuspected metastases in 2%, mostly
                  single lesion
      Stage II : unsuspected metastases in 6%
      Stage III: unsuspected metastases in 14%
   Follow-up bone scan:
      At 12 months no new cases; at 28 months in 5%
      new metastases; at 30 months in 29% new
      metastases
      Conversion from normal: Stage I : in 7%
                                Stage II : in 25%
                                Stage III: in 58%
      With axillary lymph node involvement conversion
      rate 2.5 x of those without
      Serial follow-up examinations are important to
      assess therapeutic efficacy + prognosis

ROLE OF BONE SCAN IN PROSTATE CANCER
   Stage B : 5% with skeletal metastases
   Stage C : 10% with skeletal metastases
   Stage D : 20% with skeletal metastases
   Test sensitivities for detection of osseous metastases:
   (a) Scintigraphy 1.0
   (b) Radiographic survey 0.68
   (c) Alkaline phosphatase 0.5
   (d) Acid phosphatase 0.5

DDx: pulmonary metastasis (SPECT helpful in distinguishing nonosseous lung from overlying rib uptake)

MR:
ideal for bone marrow imaging due to high contrast between bone marrow fat + water-containing metastatic deposits
(1) Focal lytic lesion:
√ hypointense on T1WI + hyperintense on T2WI
(2) Focal sclerotic lesion:
√ hypointense on T1WI + T2WI
(3) Diffuse inhomogeneous lesions:
√ inhomogeneously hypointense on T1WI + hyperintense on T2WI
(4) Diffuse homogeneous lesions:
√ homogeneously hypointense on T1WI + hyperintense on T2WI

Skeletal metastases in children
1. Neuroblastoma (most often)
2. Retinoblastoma
3. Embryonal rhabdomyosarcoma
4. Hepatoma
5. Ewing tumor

Skeletal metastases in adult
mnemonic: **"Common Bone Lesions Can Kill The Patient"**

Colon
Breast
Lung
Carcinoid
Kidney
Thyroid
Prostate

METATROPHIC DYSPLASIA
= HYPERPLASTIC ACHONDROPLASIA
= METATROPHIC DWARFISM
metatrophic = "changeable" (change in proportions of trunk to limbs over time secondary to developing kyphoscoliosis in childhood)
• longitudinal double skin fold overlying coccyx

√ long bones short with dumbbell-like / trumpet-shaped configuration (exaggerated metaphyseal flaring)
√ "hourglass" phalanges (short with widened ends)
√ wide separation of major joint spaces (thick articular cartilage)
√ delayed ossification of flat irregular epiphyses

@ Chest
√ cylindrical narrowed elongated thorax
√ short + wide ribs
√ pectus carinatum
@ Vertebrae
√ odontoid hypoplasia with atlantoaxial instability
√ progressive kyphoscoliosis
√ platyspondyly + very wide intervertebral spaces
√ wedge- / keel-shaped vertebral bodies

@ Pelvis
√ coccygeal appendage similar to a tail (rare but CHARACTERISTIC)
√ short squared iliac bones + irregular acetabula
√ narrowed greater sciatic notch
Prognosis: compatible with life, increased disability from kyphoscoliosis
DDx: achondroplasia, mucopolysaccharidoses

MUCOPOLYSACCHARIDOSES
= lysosomal storage disorder from deficiency of specific lysosomal enzymes involved in degradation of mucopolysaccharides

Type I = Hurler   Type V = Scheie
Type II = Hunter   Type VI = Maroteaux-Lamy
Type III = Sanfilippo   Type VII = Sly
Type IV = Morquio

Δ all autosomal recessive except for Hunter (x-linked)
Associated with: valvular heart disease
• corneal clouding
• retardation (prominent in types I, II, III, VII)
• skeletal involvement dominates in types IV and VI
√ scaphocephaly, macrocephaly; thick calvarium; hypertelorism
√ platyspondyly with kyphosis + dwarfism
√ irregularity at anterior aspect of vertebral bodies
√ atlantoaxial subluxation (laxity of transverse ligament / hypoplasia or absence of odontoid)
√ limb contractures
√ broad hands
√ hepatosplenomegaly
@ Brain
√ brain atrophy
√ varying degree of hydrocephalus
√ multiple white matter changes within cerebral hemispheres (diffuse hypodense areas, prolongation of T1 + T2)
Cx: Cord compression at atlantoaxial joint (types IV + VI)
Dx: combination of clinical features, radiographic abnormalities correlated with genetic + biochemical studies
Prenatal Dx: occasionally successful analysis of fibroblasts cultured from amniotic fluid

Hurler Syndrome
= GARGOYLISM = PFAUNDLER-HURLER DISEASE
= MPS I-H; autosomal recessive disease
Cause: homozygous for MPS III gene with excess chondroitin sulfate B due to deficient X-L iduronidase (= Hurler corrective factor)
Incidence: 1:10,000 births
Age: usually appears >1st year
• dwarfism
• progressive mental deterioration after 1 – 3 years
• large head; sunken bridge of nose; hypertelorism
• early corneal clouding progressing to blindness
• "gargoyle" features = everted lips + protruding tongue
• teeth widely separated + poorly formed
• progressive narrowing of nasopharyngeal airway

- protuberant abdomen (secondary to dorsolumbar kyphosis + hepatosplenomegaly)
- urinary excretion of chondroitin sulfate B (dermatan sulphate) + heparan sulfate
- Reilly bodies (metachromic granules) in white blood cells or bone marrow cells

@ Skull (earliest changes >6 months of age)
  √ frontal bossing
  √ calvarial thickening
  √ premature fusion of sagittal + lambdoid sutures
  √ deepening of optic chiasm
  √ enlarged J-shaped sella (undermining of anterior clinoid process)
  √ small facial bones
  √ wide mandibular angle + underdevelopment of condyles
  √ communicating hydrocephalus

@ Extremities
  √ thick periosteal cloaking of long bone diaphyses (early changes)
  √ swelling of diaphyses + tapering of either end: distal humerus, radius, ulna, proximal ends of metacarpals, ribs
  √ enlargement of shaft due to dilatation of medullary canal with cortical thinning
  √ deossification
  √ flexion deformities of knees + hips
  √ trident hands; clawing (occasionally)
  √ delayed maturation of irregular carpal bones

@ Spine
  √ thoracolumbar kyphosis with lumbar gibbus
  √ oval centra with normal / increased height + anterior beak at T12/L1/L2

  √ long slender pedicles
  √ spatulate rib configuration
@ Pelvis
  √ widely flared iliac wings
  √ constriction of iliac bones
  √ coxa valga
Prognosis: death by age 10 – 15 years

Morquio Syndrome

= KERATOSULFATURIA = MPS IV;
  autosomal recessive; excess keratosulfate
Incidence: 1:40,000 births
Etiology: N-acetylgalactosamine-6-sulfatase deficiency resulting in defective degradation of keratin sulfate (mainly in cartilage, nucleus pulposus, cornea)
Age: normal at birth; skeletal changes manifest within first 18 months

- excessive urinary excretion of keratan sulfate
- normal intelligence
- weakness + hypotonia
- dwarfism with short trunk (<4 feet tall)
- head thrust forward + sunken between high shoulders
- normal intelligence
- corneal opacities evident around age 10
- progressive deafness
- short nose, wide mouth, spacing between teeth
- semicrouching stance + knock knees from flexion deformities of knees + hips

@ Skull
  √ mild dolichocephaly
  √ hypertelorism

Mucopolysaccharidoses

Type	Eponym	Inheritance	Enzyme deficiency	Urinary glycosaminoglycan	Neurologic signs
I-H	Hurler	autosomal recessive	alpha-L-iduronidase	dermatan sulfate	marked
II	Hunter	X-linked recessive	iduronate sulfatase	dermatan / heparan sulfate	mild to moderate
III	Sanfilippo	autosomal recessive		heparan sulfate	mental deterioration
	A		heparan sulfate sulfatase		
	B		N-acetyl-alpha-D-glucosaminidase		
	C		alpha-glucosamine-N-acetyl-transferase		
	D		N-acetylglucosamine-6-sulfate sulfatase		
IV	Morquio A–D	autosomal recessive	N-acetylgalactosamine-6-sulfate sulfatase beta-galactosidase	keratan sulfate	none
I-S(V)	Scheie	autosomal recessive	alpha-L-iduronidase	heparan sulfate	none
VI	Maroteaux-Lamy	autosomal recessive	arylsulfatase B	dermatan sulfate	none
VII	Sly	autosomal recessive	beta-glucuronidase	dermatan sulfate heparan sulfate	variable

√ poor mastoid air cell development
√ short nose + depression of bridge of nose
√ prominent maxilla
@ Chest
  √ increased A-P diameter + marked pectus carinatum
  √ slight lordosis with wide short ribs
  √ bulbous costochondral junctions
  √ failure of fusion of sternal segments
@ Spine
  √ hypoplasia / absence of odontoid process of C2
  √ C1-C2 instability with anterior subluxation
  √ thick C2-body with narrowing of vertebral canal
  √ atlas close to occiput / posterior arch of C1 within foramen magnum
  √ platyspondyly = universal vertebra plana esp. affecting lumbar spine (DDx: normal height in Hurler syndrome)
  √ ovoid vertebral bodies with central anterior beak / tongue at lower thoracic / upper lumbar vertebrae
  √ mild gibbus at thoracolumbar transition = low dorsal kyphosis
  √ exaggerated lumbar lordosis
  √ widened intervertebral disc spaces
@ Pelvis
  √ "goblet-shaped" / "wine glass" pelvis = constricted iliac bodies + elongated pelvic inlet + flared iliac wings
  √ oblique hypoplastic acetabular roofs
@ Femur
  √ initially well-formed femoral head epiphysis, involution + fragmentation by age 3 – 6 years
  √ lateral subluxation of femoral heads; later hip dislocation
  √ wide femoral neck + coxa valga deformity
@ Tibia
  √ delayed ossification of lateral proximal tibial epiphysis
  √ sloping of superior margin of tibia plateau laterally + severe genu valgum
@ Hand & Foot
  √ short bones of forearm with widening of proximal ends
  √ delayed appearance + irregularity of carpal centers
  √ small irregular carpal bones
  √ proximally pointed short metacarpals 2 – 5
  √ enlarged joints; hand + foot deformities (flat feet)
  √ ulnar deviation of hand

Cx: cervical myelopathy (traumatic quadriplegia / leg pains / subtle neurologic abnormality) most common cause of death secondary to C2 abnormality; frequent respiratory infections (from respiratory paralysis)
Rx: early fusion of C1 – C2
Prognosis: may live to adulthood
DDx:
  (1) Hurler syndrome (normal / increased vertebral height; vertebral beak inferior)
  (2) Spondyloepiphyseal dysplasia (autosomal dominant, present at birth, absent flared ilia / deficient acetabular ossification, small acetabular angle, deficient ossification of pubic bones, varus deformity of femoral neck, minimal involvement of hand + foot, myopia)

MULTIPLE EPIPHYSEAL DYSPLASIA
= FAIRBANK DISEASE = ? tarda form of chondrodystrophia calcificans congenita
√ mild limb shortening
√ irregular mottled calcifications of epiphyses (in childhood + adolescence)
√ epiphyseal irregularities + premature degenerative joint disease, especially of hips (in adulthood)
√ short phalanges
DDx: Legg-Perthes disease, hypothyroidism

MULTIPLE MYELOMA
Most common primary malignant neoplasm in adults
Histo:
  normal / pleomorphic plasma cells (not pathognomonic), may be mistaken for lymphocytes (lymphosarcoma, reticulum cell sarcoma, Ewing tumor, neuroblastoma)
  (a) diffuse infiltration: myeloma cells intimately admixed with hematopoietic cells
  (b) tumor nodules: displacement of hematopoietic cells by masses entirely composed of myeloma cells
Age: usually 5th – 8th decade; 98% >40 years; rare < age 30; M:F = 2:1
  (a) DISSEMINATED FORM: >40 years of age (98%); M:F = 3:2
  (b) SOLITARY FORM: mean age 50 years
• bone pain (68%)
• normochromic normocytic anemia (62%)
• RBC rouleau formation
• renal insufficiency (55%)
• hypercalcemia (30 – 50%)
• proteinuria (88%)
• Bence-Jones proteinuria (50%)
• increased globulin production (monoclonal gammopathy)
Location:
  A. DISSEMINATED FORM:
    scattered; axial skeleton predominant site; vertebrae (50%) > ribs > skull > pelvis > long bones (distribution correlates with normal sites of red marrow)
  B. SOLITARY FORM:
    vertebrae > pelvis > skull > sternum > ribs
  C. SPINAL PLASMA CELL MYELOMA
    √ sparing of posterior elements
    √ paraspinal soft tissue mass with extradural extension
    √ scalloping of anterior margin of vertebral bodies (osseous pressure from adjacent enlarged lymph nodes)

√ generalized osteoporosis with accentuation of trabecular pattern, especially in spine (early)

√ punched out appearance of widespread osteolytic areas (skull, long bones) with endosteal scalloping and uniform size

√ diffuse osteolysis (pelvis, sacrum)

√ expansile osteolytic lesions (ballooning) in ribs, pelvis, long bones

√ soft tissue mass adjacent to bone destruction (= extrapleural + paraspinal mass adjacent to ribs / vertebral column)

√ periosteal new-bone formation exceedingly rare

√ involvement of mandible (rarely affected by metastatic disease)

√ vertebral pedicles usually spared (no red marrow) (DDx: metastatic disease)

√ sclerosis may occur after chemotherapy, radiotherapy, fluoride administration

√ sclerotic form of multiple myeloma (1 – 3%)
  (a) solitary sclerotic lesion: frequently in spine
  (b) diffuse sclerosis
  associated with POEMS syndrome:
    Polyneuropathy
    Organomegaly
    Endocrine abnormalities
    M-protein
    Skin changes

MR (recognition dependent on knowledge of normal range of bone marrow appearance for age):
  √ hypointense focal areas on T1WI (25%)
  √ hyperintense focal areas on T2WI (53%)
  √ absence of fatty infiltration (nonspecific)

SENSITIVITY OF BONE SCANS VS. RADIOGRAPHS
  Radiographs: in 90% of patients and 80% of sites
  Bone scan :   in 75% of patients and 24 – 54% of sites
  Gallium scan : in 55% of patients and 40% of sites
  Δ 30% of lesions only detected on radiographs
  Δ 10% of lesions only detected on bone scans

Cx: (1) renal involvement frequent
       (2) predilection for recurrent pneumonias (leukopenia)
       (3) secondary amyloidosis in 6 – 15%
       (4) pathologic fractures occur often

Prognosis: 20% 5-year survival; death from renal insufficiency, bacterial infection, thromboembolism

DDx:
— with osteopenia: (1) Postmenopausal osteoporosis
                     (2) Hyperparathyroidism
— with lytic lesion: (1) Metastatic disease
                       (2) Amyloidosis
                       (3) Myeloid metaplasia
— with sclerotic lesion: (1) Osteopoikilosis
                          (2) Lymphoma
                          (3) Osteoblastic metastasis
                          (4) Mastocytosis
                          (5) Myelosclerosis
                          (6) Fluorosis
                          (7) Lymphoma
                          (8) Renal osteodystrophy

MYELOMATOSIS
  √ generalized deossification without discrete tumors
  √ vertebral flattening

MYELOPROLIFERATIVE DISORDERS

= autonomous clonal disorder initiated by an acquired pluripotential hematopoietic stem stell

Types:
  1. Polycythemia vera
  2. Chronic granulomatous leukemia = chronic myelogenous leukemia
  3. Essential idiopathic thrombocytopenia
  4. Agnogenic myeloid metaplasia (= primary myelofibrosis + extramedullary hematopoiesis in liver + spleen)

Pathophysiology:
  — self-perpetuating intra- and extramedullary hematopoietic cell proliferation without stimulus
  — trilinear panmyelosis (RBCs, WBCs, platelets)
  — myelofibrosis with progression to myelosclerosis
  — myeloid metaplasia = extramedullary hematopoiesis (normocytic anemia, leukoerythroblastic anemia, reticulocytosis, low platelet count, normal / reduced WBC count)

MYELOSCLEROSIS

= AGNOGENIC MYELOID METAPLASIA
= MYELOPROLIFERATIVE SYNDROME
= PSEUDOLEUKEMIA
= hematologic disorder of unknown etiology with gradual replacement of bone marrow elements by fibrosis

Characterized by
  (1) extramedullary hematopoiesis
  (2) progressive splenomegaly
  (3) anemia
  (4) variable changes in number of granulocytes + platelets; often predated by polycythemia vera

Age: usually >50 years
Path: fibrous / bony replacement of bone marrow; extramedullary hematopoiesis

Associated with:
  metastatic carcinoma, chemical poisoning, chronic infection (TB), acute myelogenous leukemia, polycythemia vera, McCune-Albright syndrome, histiocytosis
  • dyspnea, weakness, fatigue, weight loss, hemorrhage
  • normochromic normocytic anemia; polycythemia may precede myelosclerosis in 59%
  • dry marrow aspirate

Location: red marrow-containing bones in 40% (thoracic cage, pelvis, femora, humeral shafts, lumbar spine, skull, peripheral bones)

√ splenomegaly

√ widespread diffuse increase in density (ground glass)

√ "jail bar" ribs

√ sandwich / rugger jersey spine

√ generalized increase in bone density in skull + obliteration of diploic space; scattered small rounded radiolucent lesions; or combination of both

NUC:
  √ diffuse increased uptake of bone tracer in affected skeleton, possibly "superscan"
  √ increased uptake at ends of long bones
DDx:
  (a) with splenomegaly: chronic leukemia, lymphoma, mastocytosis
  (b) without splenomegaly: osteoblastic metastases, fluorine poisoning, osteopetrosis, chronic renal disease

MYOSITIS OSSIFICANS

Types:
  (1) Myositis ossificans progressiva
  (2) Localized myositis ossificans secondary to TRAUMA (60%)
  (3) Myositis ossificans associated with NEUROLOGIC DISORDERS = Paraosteoarthropathy
  (4) Localized myositis ossificans of UNKNOWN ORIGIN:
      ? trauma; ? healed phase of dermatomyositis
DDx:
  (1) Osteosarcoma
  (2) Synovial sarcoma
  (3) Fibrosarcoma
  (4) Parosteal sarcoma (usually metaphyseal with thick densely mineralized attachment to bone)
  (5) Posttraumatic periostitis (ossification of subperiosteal hematoma with broad-based attachment to bone)
  (6) Acute osteomyelitis (substantial soft-tissue edema + early periosteal reaction)
  (7) Tumoral calcinosis (periarticular calcific masses of lobular pattern with interspersed lucent soft-tissue septa)
  (8) Osteochondroma (stalk contiguous with normal adjacent cortex + medullary space)

Myositis Ossificans Circumscripta

  = localized noneoplastic reactive heterotopic formation of fibrous tissue, cartilage + bone within soft tissues; usually in proximity to bone
Histo: outer zone of well-formed mature trabeculated dense bone surrounding a zone of immature osteoid; innermost zone with focal hemorrhage, loose cellular fibroconnective stroma, foci of degenerated muscle
Age: adolescents, young adults; M>F
  • history of direct trauma (75%)

Site:
  (a) within muscle: anterolateral aspect of thigh + arm; temporal muscle; small muscles of hands; gluteal muscle; **"rider's bone"** (adductor longus); **"fencer's bone"** (brachialis); **"dancer's bone"** (soleus); breast, elbow, knee
  (b) periosteal at tendon insertion: **Pellegrini-Stieda disease** (medial collateral ligament of knee)
  √ well-defined partially ossified soft tissue mass (develops in 5 – 6 weeks)

√ circumferential / centrifugal calcification / ossification
  = well-defined mineralization at periphery with a less distinct + inhomogeneous lucent center
  (DDx: sarcoma with ill-defined periphery + calcified ossific center)
√ radiolucent zone toward bone (DDx: periosteal sarcoma on stalk)
√ may be attached to cortex by short sessile base
√ ± periosteal reaction
MR:
  √ isointense / slightly hyperintense core on T1WI, increasing in intensity on T2WI
  √ increased peritumoral signal intensity on T2WI (= edema of diffuse myositis)
  √ focal signal abnormality within bone marrow (= marrow edema)
Angio:
  √ numerous fine vessels + diffuse capillary stain
Prognosis: ? resorption in 1 year

Myositis Ossificans Progressiva

  = FIBRODYSPLASIA OSSIFICANS PROGRESSIVA
  = congenital / idiopathic disease with remissions + exacerbation
Age: onset within 1st decade
  • initially subcutaneous painful masses on neck, shoulders, upper extremities
  • progressive involvement of remaining musculature of back, chest, abdomen, lower extremities
  • lesions may ulcerate and bleed
  • muscles of back + proximal extremities become rigid followed by thoracic kyphosis
  • inanition secondary to jaw trismus (masseter, temporal muscle)
  • "wry neck" = torticollis
  • respiratory failure (thoracic muscles affected)
A. ECTOPIC OSSIFICATION
  √ rounded / linear calcification in neck / shoulders, hips, proximal extremity, trunk, palmar + plantar fascia
  √ ossification of voluntary muscles, complete by 20 – 25 years (sparing of sphincters + head)
B. SKELETAL ANOMALIES
  may appear before ectopic ossification
  √ microdactyly of big toes (90%) and thumbs (50%)
    = usually only one large phalanx present / synostosis of metacarpal + proximal phalanx (first sign)
  √ phalangeal shortening of hand + foot
  √ hallux valgus
  √ progressive fusion of vertebral bodies
  √ diminished growth of cervical vertebral bodies
  √ ± bony ankylosis

NAIL-PATELLA SYNDROME

  = FONG DISEASE = ILIAC HORNS = FAMILIAL ONYCHO-OSTEODYSPLASIA
  = OSTEO-ONYCHODYSOSTOSIS
  = symmetrical meso- and ectodermal anomalies
  • aplasia / hypoplasia of thumb + index fingernails

- renal failure in later life
√ hypoplasia / absence of patella
√ bilateral posterior iliac horns in 80% (independent ossification center) DIAGNOSTIC
√ flared iliac crest with prominent anterior spines
√ radial head / capitellum hypoplasia (DDx: congenital dislocation of radial head)
√ clinodactyly
√ short 5th metacarpal
√ mandibular cysts (occasionally)

NEUROPATHIC ARTHROPATHY

= CHARCOT JOINT = change in sensory nerves associated with trauma

Pathogenesis: (1) decreased pain sensation produces repetitive trauma
(2) sympathetic dysfunction results in local hyperemia + bone resorption

Causes:
A. Congenital
1. Myelomeningocele
2. Congenital indifference to pain = asymbolia
B. Acquired
(a) central neuropathy
1. Injury to brain / spinal cord
2. Syringomyelia (in 1/3 of patients): shoulder joint affected
3. Neurosyphilis = tabes dorsalis (in 15 – 20% of patients): knees, hips, tarsals, ankles affected
4. Spinal cord tumors / infection
(b) peripheral neuropathy
1. Diabetes mellitus (most common cause, although incidence low): hands + feet affected
2. Leprosy
3. Peripheral nerve injury
(c) others
1. Scleroderma, Raynaud disease, Ehlers-Danlos syndrome
2. Rheumatoid arthritis, psoriasis
3. Amyloid infiltration of nerves, adrenal hypercorticism
C. Iatrogenic
prolonged use of pain-relieving drugs
mnemonic: "DS6"
Diabetes
Syphilis
Steroids
Spinal cord injury
Spina bifida
Syringomyelia
Scleroderma

√ persistent joint effusion (first sign)
√ narrowing of joint space
√ hypertrophic spurs
√ increased density of subchondral bone
√ calcification of synovial membrane
√ fragmentation of eburnated subchondral bone

√ joint subluxation (laxity of periarticular soft tissues) + dislocations
√ progressive rapid resorption of head + neck of humerus or femur
√ "pencil point" deformity of metatarsal heads
√ NO juxtaarticular osteoporosis
√ "bag-of-bones" effect in late stage (= marked deformities around joint)
mnemonic: "5 Ds"
√ **D**ense subchondral bone
√ **D**estruction of articular cortex
√ **D**eformity (pencil point)
√ **D**ebris (loose bodies)
√ **D**islocation

NONOSSIFYING FIBROMA

= FIBROXANTHOMA = NONOSTEOGENIC FIBROMA
= XANTHOMA = XANTHOGRANULOMA OF BONE
= FIBROUS METAPHYSEAL-DIAPHYSEAL DEFECT
= FIBROUS MEDULLARY DEFECT

Incidence: up to 40% of all children >2 years of age
Etiology: lesion resulting from proliferative activity of a fibrous cortical defect that has expanded into medullary cavity
Histo: whorled bundles of spindle-shaped fibroblasts + scattered multinucleated giant cells + foamy xanthomatous cells
Age: 8 – 20 years; 75% in 2nd decade of life
- usually asymptomatic
Location: shaft of long bone; mostly in bones of lower extremity, especially about knee (distal femur + proximal tibia); distal tibia; fibula
Site: eccentric metaphyseal, several cm shaftwards from epiphysis, mostly intramedullary, rarely purely diaphyseal
<u>Multiple fibroxanthomas</u> (in 8 – 10%)
associated with neurofibromatosis, fibrous dysplasia, Jaffe-Campanacci syndrome
√ multilocular ovoid bubbly osteolytic area
√ alignment along long axis of bone, about 2 cm in length
√ dense sclerotic border toward medulla; V- or U-shaped at one end
√ endosteal scalloping + thinning ± overlying bulge
√ migrates toward center of diaphysis
√ resolves with age
√ minimal / mild uptake on bone scan
Prognosis: spontaneous healing in most cases
Cx: (1) Pathologic fracture (not uncommon)
(2) Hypophosphatemic vitamin D-resistant rickets + osteomalacia (tumor may secrete substance that increases renal tubular resorption of phosphorus)
DDx: (1) Adamantinoma (midshaft of tibia)
(2) Chondromyxoid fibroma (bulging of cortex more striking)

JAFFE-CAMPANACCI SYNDROME

= nonossifying fibroma with extraskeletal manifestations in children
- mental retardation

- hypogonadism
- ocular defect
- cardiovascular congenital defect
- café-au-lait spots

NOONAN SYNDROME
= PSEUDO-TURNER = MALE TURNER SYNDROME
= phenotype similar to Turner syndrome but with normal karyotype (occurs in both males + females)
Striking familial incidence
- short / may have normal height
- webbed neck
- agonadism / normal gonads
- delayed puberty
- mental retardation

√ osteoporosis
√ retarded bone age
√ cubitus valgus
@ Skull
  √ mandibular hypoplasia with dental malocclusion
  √ hypertelorism
  √ biparietal foramina
  √ dolichocephaly, microcephaly / cranial enlargement
  √ webbed neck
@ Chest
  √ sternal deformity: pectus excavatum / carinatum
  √ right-sided congenital heart disease (valvar pulmonic stenosis, ASD, eccentric hypertrophy of left ventricle, PDA, VSD)
  √ coronal clefts of spine
  √ may have pulmonary lymphangiectasis
@ Gastrointestinal tract
  √ intestinal lymphangiectasia
  √ eventration of diaphragm
  √ renal malrotation, renal duplication, hydronephrosis, large redundant extrarenal pelvis
DDx: Turner syndrome (mental retardation rare, renal anomalies frequent)

OCHRONOSIS
= ALKAPTONURIA = inherited absence of homogentisic acid oxidase with excessive homogentisic acid production + deposition in connective tissue including cartilage, synovium, and bone
Histo: abnormally pigmented cartilage subject to deterioration resulting in calcification + denudation of cartilaginous tissue
M:F = 2:1
- black pigment in soft tissues (in 2nd decade): yellowish skin; gray pigmentation of sclera; bluish tinge of ears + nose cartilage
- alkaptonuria with black staining of diapers
- heart failure, renal failure (pigment deposition)
@ Spine
  Age: middle age
  Site: lumbar region with progressive ascension
  √ laminated calcification of multiple intervertebral discs
  √ disc space drastically narrowed

√ multiple "vacuum" phenomena (common)
√ osteoporosis of adjoining vertebrae
√ massive osteophytosis + ankylosis of spine (in older patient)
√ spotty calcifications in tissue anterior to vertebral bodies
@ Joints
  √ hypertrophic changes in humeral head
  √ severe premature progressive osteoarthritic changes in shoulder, knee, hip, spine of young patients
  √ intraarticular osseous bodies
  √ small calcifications in paraarticular soft tissues + tendon insertions

ORODIGITO-FACIAL SYNDROME
= ORO-FACIAL-DIGITAL SYNDROME
Etiology: autosomal trisomy of chromosome No. 1 with 47 chromosomes; X-linked dominant
Sex: nuclear chromatin pattern female (lethal in male)
Associated with   renal polycystic disease
- mental retardation
- hypertelorism
- cleft lip + tongue

√ cleft in palate + jaw bone
√ hypoplasia of mandible + occiput of skull
√ abnormal dentition
√ clinodactyly, syndactyly, brachydactyly (metacarpals may be elongated)

OSGOOD-SCHLATTER DISEASE
= avascular necrosis of tibial tuberosity
- local pain + tenderness on pressure, swelling of overlying soft tissue
Age: 10 – 15 years; boys
√ fragmentation of tibial tubercle displaced away from the shaft
√ sometimes increased density
√ comparison with other side (irregular development normal)

OSSIFYING FIBROMA
Closely related to fibrous dysplasia + adamantinoma
Age: 2nd – 4th decade; M < F
Histo: maturing cellular fibrous spindle cells with osteoblastic activity producing many calcific cartilaginous + bone densities
Location: frequently in face

@ Mandible, maxilla
  - painless expansion of tooth-bearing portion of jaw
  √ 1 – 5 cm well-circumscribed round / oval tumor
  √ moderate expansion of intact cortex
  √ homogeneous tumor matrix
  √ dislodgement of teeth
@ Tibia
  √ eccentric ground-glass lesion (resembling fibrous dysplasia)
Cx: frequent recurrences

OSTEITIS CONDENSANS ILII
Incidence: 2% of population
Cause: chronic stress secondary to instability of pubic symphysis
Age: young multiparous women
- associated with low back pain when instability of pubic symphysis present

√ triangular area of sclerosis along inferior anterior aspect of ileum adjacent to SI joint (joint space uninvolved)
√ similar triangle of reparative bone on sacral side
√ usually bilateral + symmetric; occasionally unilateral
√ sclerosis dissolves in 3 – 20 years following stabilization of pubic symphysis
DDx:
  (1) Ankylosing spondylitis (affects ilium + sacrum, joint space narrowing, involvement of other bones)
  (2) Rheumatoid arthritis (asymmetric, joint destruction)
  (3) Paget disease (thickened trabecular pattern)

OSTEOARTHRITIS
= DEGENERATIVE JOINT DISEASE = decreased chondroitin sulfate with age creates unsupported collagen fibrils followed by cartilage degeneration

√ joint space narrowing
√ sclerosis / eburnation of subchondral bone in areas of stress
√ subchondral cyst formation (geodes)
√ osteophytosis at articular margin / non-stressed area
@ Hand + foot
  Target area: 1st MCP; trapezioscaphoid; DIP > PIP; 1st MTP
  √ radial subluxation of 1st metacarpal base
  √ Bouchard nodes = osteophytosis at PIP joint
  √ Heberden nodes = osteophytosis at DIP joint: M:F = 1:10
@ Hip
  √ superior migration of femoral head (less frequently medial / axial)
  √ femoral + acetabular osteophytes, sclerosis, cyst formation
  √ thickening / buttressing of medial femoral cortex
@ Knee
  √ medial femorotibial compartment usually first to be involved
  √ varus deformity
@ Spine
  √ sclerosis + narrowing of intervertebral apophyseal joints
  √ osteophytosis usually associated with discogenic disease

EROSIVE OSTEOARTHRITIS
= inflammatory form of osteoarthrosis
Predisposed: postmenopausal females
Site: DIP + PIP joints of hands; bilateral + symmetric
√ "bird-wing" / "sea-gull" joint configuration = central erosions
√ may lead to bony ankylosis

DDx: Rheumatoid arthritis, Wilson disease, chronic liver disease, hemochromatosis

EARLY OSTEOARTHRITIS
mnemonic: "**E**arly **O**steo**A**rthritis"
  Epiphyseal dysplasia, multiple
  Ochronosis
  Acromegaly

OSTEOBLASTOMA
= GIANT OSTEOID OSTEOMA = OSTEOGENIC FIBROMA OF BONE = OSSIFYING FIBROMA
= rare benign tumor with unlimited growth potential + capability of malignant transformation
Incidence: <1% of all primary bone tumors; 3% of all benign bone tumors
Age: mean age of 16 – 19 years; 6 – 30 years (90%); 2nd decade (55%); 3rd decade (20%); M:F = 2:1
Path: lesion >1.5 cm; smaller lesions are classified as osteoid osteoma
Histo: numerous multinucleated giant cells (osteoclasts), irregularly arranged osteoid + bone; very vascular connective tissue stroma; trabeculae broader + longer than in osteoid osteoma

Location: (rarely multifocal)
  (a) spine (33 – 37%): 62 – 94% in dorsal elements, secondary extension into vertebral body (28%); cervical spine (31%), dorsal spine (34%), lumbar spine (31%), sacrum (3%)
  (b) long bones (26 – 32%): femur (50%), tibia (19%), humerus (19%), radius (8%), fibula (4%); unusual in neck of femur
  (c) small bones of hand + feet (15 – 26%): dorsal talus neck (62%), calcaneus (4%), scaphoid (8%), metacarpals (8%), metatarsals (8%)
  (d) calvarium + mandible (= cementoblastoma)
Site: diaphyseal (58%), metaphyseal (42%); eccentric (46%), intracortical (42%), centric (12%), may be periosteal
- asymptomatic in <2%
- dull pain of insidious onset (84%), worse at night in 7 – 13%
- response to salicylates in 7%
- localized swelling, tenderness, decreased range of motion (29%)
- painful scoliosis in 50% (with spinal / rib location) secondary to muscle spasm
- mild muscle weakness to paraplegia due to cord compression
- occasional systemic toxicity (high WBC, fever)

√ radiolucent nidus >2 cm (range of 2 – 12 cm) in size
√ well demarcated (83%)
√ ± stippled / ringlike small flecks of matrix calcification
√ tumor matrix radiolucent (25 – 64%) / ossified (36 – 72%)
√ reactive (22 – 91%) / no reactive (9 – 56%) sclerosis
√ cortical expansion (75 – 94%) / destruction (20 – 22%)

√ progressive expansile lesion that may rapidly increase in size (25%)
√ sharply defined soft tissue component
√ thin shell of periosteal new bone (58 – 77%) / no periosteal reaction
√ scoliosis (35%)
√ osteoporosis due to disuse + hyperemia in talar location
√ rapid calcification after radiotherapy
NUC:
    √ intense focal accumulation of bone agent (100%)
Angio:
    √ tumor blush in capillary phase (50%)
MR:
    √ low to intermediate intensity on T1WI
    √ mixed to high intensity on T2WI
    √ surrounding edema

Prognosis: 10% recurrence after excision; incomplete curettage can effect cure due to cartilage production + trapping of host lamellar bone
DDx:
    (1) Osteo- / chondrosarcoma (periosteal new bone)
    (2) Osteoid osteoma (dense calcification + halo of bone sclerosis, <2 cm due to limited growth potential)
    (3) Cartlaginous tumors (lumpy matrix calcification)
    (4) Giant cell tumor (no calcification, epiphyseal involvement)
    (5) Aneurysmal bone cyst
    (6) Osteomyelitis
    (7) Hemangioma
    (8) Lipoma
    (9) Epidermoid
    (10) Fibrous dysplasia
    (11) Metastasis
    (12) Ewing sarcoma

OSTEOCHONDROSIS DISSECANS
= OSTEOCHONDRITIS DISSECANS
= OSTEOCHONDRAL FRACTURE
= fragmentation + possible separation of a portion of the articular surface
Etiology:
    (1) subchondral fatigue fracture as a result of shearing, rotatory / tangentially aligned impaction forces
    (2) ? autosomal dominant trait associated with short stature, endocrine dysfunction, Scheuermann disease, Osgood-Schlatter disease, tibia vara, carpal tunnel syndrome
Age: adolescence; M > F
• asymptomatic / vague complaints
• clicking, locking, limitation of motion
• swelling, pain aggravated by movement
Location:
    (a) knee: medial (in 10% lateral) femoral condyle close to fossa intercondylaris; bilateral in 20 – 30%
    (b) humeral head
    (c) capitellum of elbow
    (d) talus
√ purely cartilaginous fragment unrecognized on plain film

√ fracture line parallels joint surface
√ mouse = osteochondrotic fragment
    Location: posterior region of knee joint, olecranon fossa, axillary / subscapular recess of glenohumeral joint
√ mouse bed = sclerosed pit in articular surface
√ soft-tissue swelling, joint effusion

OSTEOGENESIS IMPERFECTA
= PSATHYROSIS = FRAGILITAS OSSIUM = LOBSTEIN DISEASE
= heterogeneous group of a generalized connective tissue disorder leading to micromelic dwarfism characterized by bone fragility, blue sclerae, and dentinogenesis imperfecta
Incidence: overall in 1:28,500 (20,000 – 60,000) live births; M:F = 1:1
Histo: immature collagen matrix

Clinical types:
    1. OSTEOGENESIS IMPERFECTA CONGENITA
       = disease manifest at birth (occurring in utero); autosomal dominant; corresponds to Type II; lethal variety
    2. OSTEOGENESIS IMPERFECTA TARDA
       = usually not manifest at birth; recessive / sporadic corresponds to Type I + IV; nonlethal variety

• soft skull (caput membranaceum)
• hyperlaxity of joints
• blue sclerae
• poor dentition
• otosclerosis
• thin loose skin
√ diffuse demineralization, deficient trabecular structure, cortical thinning
√ defective cortical bone: increase in diameter of proximal ends of humeri + femora; slender fragile bone; multiple cyst-like areas
√ multiple fractures + pseudarthrosis with bowing (vertebral bodies, long bones)
√ normal / exuberant callus formation
√ rib thinning / notching
√ thin calvarium
√ sinus + mastoid cell enlargement
√ thickened undermineralized otic capsule (= otosclerosis)
√ Wormian bones persisting into adulthood
√ basilar impression (= platybasia)
√ biconcave vertebral bodies + Schmorl nodes, increased height of intervertebral disc space
√ bowing deformities after child begins to walk
Cx: (1) impaired hearing / deafness from otosclerosis (20 – 60%)
        (2) death from intracranial hemorrhage (abnormal platelet function)

Osteogenesis Imperfecta Type I
Autosomal dominant; compatible with life
Age at presentation: 2 – 6 years
• blue sclerae

- presenile deafness
- normal / abnormal dentinogenesis
√ infants of normal weight + length
√ osteoporosis
√ fractures in neonate (occurring during delivery)
OB-US: √ marked bowing of long bones
         √ NO IUGR

Osteogenesis Imperfecta Type II
= CONGENITAL LETHAL OSTEOGENESIS
   IMPERFECTA
Autosomal recessive / sporadic; perinatal lethal form
Incidence: 1:54,000 births; most frequent variety
- blue sclerae
- ligamentous laxity + loose skin
√ shortened broad crumpled long bones
√ bone angulations, bowing, demineralization
√ localized bone thickening from callus formation
√ thin beaded ribs ± fractures resulting in bell-shaped /
   narrow chest
√ thin poorly ossified skull
√ spinal osteopenia
√ platyspondyly
OB-US:
   A normal sonogram after 17 weeks MA excludes the
   diagnosis!
   √ increased through-transmission of skull (extremely
      poor mineralization)
      √ unusually good visualization of brain surface
      √ unusually good visualization of orbits
      √ increased visualization of intracranial arterial
         pulsations
   √ abnormal compressibility of skull vault with
      transducer
   √ decreased visualization of skeleton
   √ <u>multiple</u> fetal fractures + deformities of long bones +
      ribs
      √ wrinkled appearance of bone (= more than one
         fracture in single bone)
      √ beaded ribs (callus formation around fractures)
   √ abnormally short limbs
   √ small thorax (collapse of thoracic cage)
   √ decreased fetal movement
   √ infants small for gestational age (frequent)
Prognosis: stillborn / death shortly after birth due to
               pulmonary hypoplasia

Osteogenesis Imperfecta Type III
Autosomal recessive / dominant; progressively
deforming disorder compatible with life
- bluish sclerae during infancy which turn pale with time
- joint hyperlaxity (50%)
√ decreased ossification of skull
√ normal vertebrae + pelvis
√ progressive deformities of limbs + spine into
   adulthood
√ shortened + bowed long bones
√ ± rib fractures
√ multiple fractures present at birth in 2/3 of cases
√ fractures heal well

OB-US:
   √ short + bowed long bones
   √ fractures
   √ humerus almost normal in shape
   √ normal thoracic circumference
Prognosis: progressive limb + spine deformities
               during childhood / adolescence

Osteogenesis Imperfecta Type IV
Autosomal dominant; mildest form with best prognosis
- normal scleral color
- little tendency to develop hearing loss
√ tubular bones of normal length; mild femoral bowing
   may occur
√ osteoporosis
OB-US: √ bowing of long bones

OSTEOID OSTEOMA
= benign skeletal neoplasm composed of osteoid + woven
   bone less than 1.5 cm in diameter per definition
Incidence: 12% of benign skeletal neoplasms
Etiology: ? inflammatory response
Histo: small highly vascularized nidus of osteoid-laden
           trabeculae surrounded by zone of reactive bone
           sclerosis; osteoblastic rimming; indistinguishable
           from osteoblastoma
Age: 10 – 20 years (51%); 2nd + 3rd decade (73%); 5 –
         25 years (90%); range of 19 months – 56 years;
         uncommon <5 and >40 years of age; M:F = 2:1;
         uncommon in Blacks
- tender to touch + pressure
- local pain (95 – 98%) weeks to years in duration, worse
   at night, decreased by activity
- salicylates give relief in 20 – 30 minutes in 75 – 90%
- prostaglandin E2 elevated 100 x normal
Location:
   (a) meta- / diaphysis of long bones (73%): upper end of
        femur (43%), hands (8%), feet (4%); frequent in
        proximal tibia + femoral neck, fibula, humerus; no
        bone exempt
   (b) spine (14%): predominantly in posterior elements
        (pedicle, lamina, spinous process) of lower thoracic
        + upper lumbar spine
   (c) vertebral body, skull, rib, ischium, mandible, patella
Classification:
Cortical osteoid osteoma (most common)
   = nidus within cortex
   √ solid / laminated periosteal reaction
   √ fusiform sclerotic cortical thickening in shaft of long
      bone
   √ radiolucent area within center of osteosclerosis
Cancellous osteoid osteoma (intermediate frequency)
   = intramedullary
   Δ Intraarticular lesion difficult to identify with delay in
      diagnosis of 4 months – 5 years!
   Site: juxta- / intraarticular at femoral neck, vertebral
           posterior elements, small bones of hands +
           feet
   √ little osteosclerosis / sclerotic cortex distant to nidus
      (functional difference of intraarticular periosteum)

√ joint space widened (effusion, synovitis)

Subperiosteal osteoid osteoma (rare)

= round soft tissue mass adjacent to bone

Site: juxta- / intraarticular at medial aspect of femoral neck, hands, feet (neck of talus)

√ juxtacortical mass excavating the cortex (bony pressure atrophy) with almost no reactive sclerosis

√ radiolucent nidus (75%) of <1.5 cm in size

√ painful scoliosis concave toward lesion / kyphoscoliosis / hyperlordosis / torticollis with spinal location (due to spasm)

√ osteoarthritis (50%) with intraarticular site 1.5 – 22 years after onset of symptomatology

√ regional osteoporosis (probably due to disuse)

∆ radiographically difficult areas: vertebral column, femoral neck, small bones of hand + feet

NUC:

√ intensely increased radiotracer uptake (increased blood flow + new bone formation)

√ double density sign = small area of focal activity (nidus) superimposed on larger area of increased tracer uptake

CT (for detection + precise localization of nidus):

√ small well-defined round / oval nidus surrounded by variable amount of dense bone

√ nidus enhances on dynamic scan

√ nidus with variable amount of mineralization (50%): punctate / amorphous / ringlike / dense

MR (diminished conspicuity of lesion compared to CT):

√ nidus isointense to muscle on T1WI

√ signal intensity increases to between that of muscle + fat / remains low on T2WI

Angio:

√ highly vascularized nidus with intense circumscribed blush appearing in early arterial phase + persisting late into venous phase

Prognosis: no growth progression, infrequent regression

Rx: complete surgical excision of nidus (reactive bone regresses subsequently)

DDx:

(1) Cortical osteoid osteoma: Brodie abscess, sclerosing osteomyelitis, syphilis, bone island, stress fracture, osteosarcoma, Ewing sarcoma, metastasis, subperiosteal aneurysmal bone cyst, osteoblastoma (progressive growth)

(2) Intraarticular osteoid osteoma: inflammatory / septic / tuberculous / rheumatoid arthritis, nonspecific synovitis, Legg-Calvé-Perthes disease

OSTEOFIBROUS DYSPLASIA

= entity previously mistaken for fibrous dysplasia

Age: newborn up to 5 years

Histo: fibrous tissue surrounding trabeculae in a whorled storiform pattern

Location: normally confined to tibia (mid-diaphysis in 50%), lesion begins in anterior cortex; ipsilateral fibula affected in 20%

√ enlargement of tibia with anterior bowing

√ cortex thin / invisible

√ periosteal expansion

√ sclerotic margin (DDx: nonosteogenic fibroma, chondromyxoid fibroma)

√ spontaneous regression in 1/3

Cx: pathologic fracture in 25%, fractures will heal with immobilization; infrequently complicated by pseudarthrosis

DDx: fibrous dysplasia, Paget disease

OSTEOMA

= benign tumor of membranous bone (hamartoma)

Age: adult life

Associated with: Gardner syndrome (multiple osteomas + colonic polyposis)

Location: inner / outer table of calvarium (usually from external table), paranasal sinuses (frontal / ethmoid sinuses), mandible, nasal bones

√ well-circumscribed round extremely dense structureless lesion usually <2 cm in size

FIBROUS OSTEOMA

Probably a form of fibrous dysplasia

Age: childhood

√ less dense than osteoma / radiolucent

√ expanding external table without affecting internal table

DDx: enostoma, bone island, bone infarct (located in medulla)

OSTEOMYELITIS

Acute Osteomyelitis

Age: most commonly affects children

Organisms:

(a) newborns: S. aureus, group B streptococcus, Escherichia coli

(b) children: S. aureus (blood cultures in 50% positive)

(c) adults: S. aureus (60%), enteric species (29%), Streptococcus (8%)

(d) drug addicts: Pseudomonas (86%), Klebsiella, Enterobacteriae; (57 days average delay in diagnosis)

(e) sickle cell disease: Salmonella

Cause:

(a) genitourinary tract infection (72%) (b) lung infection (14%) (c) dermal infection (14%)

Sites:

@ Lower extremity (75%)

@ Vertebrae (53%): lumbar (75%) > thoracic > cervical

@ Radial styloid (24%)

@ Sacroiliac joint (18%)

• leukocytosis + fever (66%)

A. ACUTE NEONATAL OSTEOMYELITIS

Age: onset <30 days of age

• little / no systemic disturbance

√ multicentric involvement more common; often joint involvement

√ bone scan falsely negative / equivocal in 70%

B. ACUTE OSTEOMYELITIS IN INFANCY
    Age: <18 months of age
    Pathomechanism:
        spread to epiphysis because transphyseal
        vessels cross growth plate into epiphysis
    √ striking soft tissue component
    √ subperiosteal abscess with extensive periosteal
       new bone
    Cx: frequent joint involvement
    Prognosis: rapid healing

C. ACUTE OSTEOMYELITIS IN CHILDHOOD
    Age: 2 – 16 years of age
    Pathomechanism:
        transphyseal vessels closed; metaphyseal
        vessels adjacent to growth plate loop back
        toward metaphysis locating the primary focus of
        infection into metaphysis; abscess formation in
        medulla with cortical spread
    √ sequestration frequent
    √ periosteal elevation (with disruption of periosteal
       blood supply)
    √ small single / multiple osteolytic areas in
       metaphysis
    √ extensive periosteal reaction parallel to shaft
       (after 3 – 6 weeks); may be "lamellar nodular"
       (DDx: osteoblastoma, eosinophilic granuloma)
    √ shortening of bone with destruction of epiphyseal
       cartilage
    √ growth stimulation by hyperemia + premature
       maturation of adjacent epiphysis
    √ midshaft osteomyelitis less frequent site
    √ serpiginous tract with small sclerotic rim
       (PATHOGNOMONIC)

D. ACUTE OSTEOMYELITIS IN ADULTHOOD
    √ delicate periosteal new bone
    √ joint involvement common
Radiographs:
    √ initial radiographs often normal (notoriously poor in
       early phase of infection)
    √ localized soft tissue swelling adjacent to
       metaphysis with obliteration of usual fat planes
       (after 3 – 10 days)
    √ area of bone destruction (lags 7 – 14 days behind
       pathologic changes)
    √ involucrum = cloak of laminated / spiculated
       periosteal reaction (develops after 20 days)
    √ sequestrum = detached necrotic cortical bone
       (develops after 30 days)
    √ cloaca formation = space in which dead bone
       resides
MR:
    √ bone marrow hypointense on T1WI + hyperintense
       on T2WI (= water-rich inflammatory tissue)
    √ focal / linear cortical involvement hyperintense on
       T2WI
    √ hyperintense halo surrounding cortex on T2WI =
       subperiosteal infection
    √ abscess = hyperintense fluid collection surrounded
       by hypointense pseudocapsule on T2WI + Gd-
       DTPA enhancement of granulation tissue

√ hyperintense adjacent soft tissues on T2WI
NUC (accuracy approx. 90%):
    (1) Ga-67 scans: 100% sensitivity; increased
         uptake 1 day earlier than for Tc-99m MDP
         Δ Gallium helpful for chronic osteomyelitis!
    (2) Static Tc-99m diphosphonate: 83% sensitivity
         5 – 60% false-negative rate in neonates +
         children because of (a) masking effect of
         epiphyseal plates (b) early diminished blood flow
         with infection (c) spectrum of uptake pattern from
         hot to cold
    (3) Three-phase skeletal scintigraphy:
         92% sensitivity, 87% specificity
         Phase 1 : Radionuclide angiography = perfusion
                    phase of regional blood flow
         Phase 2: "blood pool" images
         Phase 3: "bone uptake"
         DDx: Cellulitis (decrease in activity over time)
    (4) WBC-scan:
         (a) In-111-labeled leukocytes: best agent for
              acute infections
         (b) Tc-99m labeled leukocytes: preferred over
              In-111-leukocyte imaging especially in
              extremities
         Δ WBC scans have largely replaced gallium
           imaging for acute osteomyelitis due to
           improved photon flux + improved dosimetry
           (higher dose allowed relative to In-111)
           allowing faster imaging + greater resolution
    √ local increase in radiopharmaceutical uptake
       (positive within 24 – 72 hours)
    √ "cold" area in early osteomyelitis subsequently
       becoming "hot" if localized to long bones / pelvis
       (not seen in vertebral bodies)
Cx:
    (1) Soft tissue abscess (2) Fistula formation
    (3) Pathologic fracture (4) Extension into joint
    (5) Growth disturbance due to epiphyseal involvement
    (6) Neoplasm (7) Amyloidosis (8) Severe deformity
    with delayed treatment

Chronic Osteomyelitis
    √ thick irregular sclerotic bone with radiolucencies,
       elevated periosteum, chronic draining sinus

Sclerosing Osteomyelitis of Garré
    = low grade infection, no purulent exudate
    Location: mandible (most commonly)
    √ focal bulge of thickened cortex (sclerosing
       periosteal reaction)
    DDx: Osteoid osteoma, stress fracture

Chronic Recurrent Multifocal Osteomyelitis
    = benign self-limited disease of unknown etiology
    Age: children + adolescents; M:F = 1:2
    Histo: nonspecific subacute / chronic osteomyelitis
    • pain, soft tissue swelling, limited motion
    Location: tibia > femur > clavicle > fibula
    Site: metaphyses of long bones; often symmetric
    √ small areas of bone lysis, often confluent

Brodie Abscess

= subacute pyogenic osteomyelitis (smoldering indolent infection)

Organism: S. aureus (most common)

Histo: granulation tissue + eburnation

Age: more common in children; M > F

Location: tibial metaphysis (most common)

√ central area of lucency surrounded by dense reactive sclerosis

√ channel-like configuration toward growth plate

√ may persist for many months

MR:

√ "double line" effect = high signal intensity of granulation tissue surrounded by low signal intensity of bone sclerosis

DDx: Osteoid osteoma

Epidermoid Carcinoma

Etiology: complication of chronic osteomyelitis (0.5 – 1.6%)

Histo: squamous cell carcinoma (90%); occasionally: basal cell carcinoma, adenocarcinoma, fibrosarcoma, angiosarcoma, reticulum cell sarcoma, spindle cell sarcoma, rhabdomyosarcoma, parosteal osteosarcoma, plasmacytoma

Age: 30 – 80 (mean 55) years; M >> F; after 20 years of osteomyelitis

• exacerbation of symptoms with increasing pain, enlarging mass

• change in character / amount of sinus drainage

Location: at site of chronically / intermittently draining sinus; tibia (50%), femur (20%)

√ lytic lesion superimposed on changes of chronic osteomyelitis

√ soft tissue mass

√ pathologic fracture

Prognosis: (1) early metastases in 20% (within 18 months)

(2) no recurrence in 80%

OSTEOPATHIA STRIATA

= VOORHOEVE DISEASE

• usually asymptomatic (similar to osteopoikilosis)

Location: all long bones affected; the only bone sclerosis primarily involving metaphysis (with extension into epi- and diaphysis)

√ longitudinal striations of dense bone in metaphysis

√ radiating densities of "sunburst" appearance from acetabulum into ileum

OSTEOPETROSIS

= ALBERS-SCHÖNBERG DISEASE = MARBLE BONE DISEASE = rare hereditary disorder

Path:

defective osteoclast function with failure of proper reabsorption + remodeling of primary spongiosum; bone sclerotic + thick but structurally weak + brittle

A. INFANTILE AUTOSOMAL RECESSIVE TYPE

• failure to thrive

• premature senile appearance of facies

• severe dental caries

• anemia, leukocytopenia, thrombocytopenia (severe marrow depression)

• cranial nerve compression (optic atrophy, deafness)

• hepatosplenomegaly (extramedullary hematopoiesis)

• lymphadenopathy

• subarachnoid hemorrhage (due to thrombocytopenia)

May be associated with

renal tubular acidosis + cerebral calcification

Prognosis:

survival beyond middle life uncommon (death due to recurrent infection, massive hemorrhage, terminal leukemia)

B. BENIGN ADULT AUTOSOMAL DOMINANT TYPE

• 50% asymptomatic

• recurrent fractures, mild anemia

• occasionally cranial nerve palsy

Prognosis: normal life expectancy

√ diffuse osteosclerosis = generalized dense amorphous structureless bones with obliteration of normal trabecular pattern; mandible least commonly involved

√ cortical thickening with medullary encroachment

√ Erlenmeyer flask deformity = clublike long bones due to lack of tubulization + flaring of ends

√ bone-within-bone appearance

√ "sandwich" vertebrae

√ alternating sclerotic + radiolucent transverse metaphyseal lines (phalanges, iliac bones) as indicators of fluctuating course of disease

√ longitudinal metaphyseal striations

√ obliteration of mastoid cells, paranasal sinuses, basal foramina by osteosclerosis

√ sclerosis predominantly involving base of skull; calvaria often spared

Cx: (1) usually transverse fractures (common because of brittle bones) with abundant callus + normal healing

(2) crowding of marrow (myelophthisic anemia + extramedullary hematopoiesis)

(3) frequently terminates in acute leukemia

Rx: bone marrow transplant

DDx: (1) Heavy metal poisoning

(2) Melorheostosis (limited to one extremity)

(3) Hypervitaminosis D

(4) Pyknodysostosis

(5) Fibrous dysplasia of skull / face

OSTEOPOIKILOSIS

= OSTEOPATHIA CONDENSANS DISSEMINATA

Often autosomal dominant; M > F

• asymptomatic

Histo: compact bone islands

Location: in most metaphyses + epiphyses (rarely extending into midshaft); concentrated at glenoid + acetabulum, wrist, ankle, pelvis; rare in skull, ribs, vertebral centra, mandible

√ small foci of ovoid / lenticular opacification (2 – 10 mm) in cancellous bone
√ long axis of lesions parallel to long axis of bone
Prognosis: not progressive, no change after cessation of growth
DDx: (1) Epiphyseal dysplasia (metaphyses normal)
            (2) Melorheostosis (diaphyseal involvement)

OSTEOSARCOMA
Prevalence: 4 – 5:1,000,000
TYPES & FREQUENCY
    A. Conventional osteosarcoma   72%
        osteoblastic / chondroblastic / fibroblastic
    B. Variants
        (a) Clinical variants
            1. Osteosarcoma of jaw   6%
            2. Postradiation osteosarcoma   4%
            3. Osteosarcoma in Paget disease   3%
            4. Multifocal osteosarcoma   <1%
            5. Osteosarcoma in benign condition   <1%
                (fibrous dysplasia, osteoblastoma)
        (b) Surface variants
            1. Parosteal osteosarcoma   4%
            2. Dedifferentiated parosteal osteosa. <1%
            3. Periosteal osteosarcoma   <1%
            4. High-grade surface osteosarcoma   <1%
        (c) Morphological variants
            1. Telangiectatic osteosarcoma   3%
            2. Dedifferentiated chondrosarcoma   3%

Prognosis:
    dependent on age, sex, tumor size, site, classification; best predictor is degree of tissue necrosis in postresection specimen following chemotherapy (91% survival with tumor necrosis >90%, 14% survival with <90% tumor necrosis)

Osteosarcomatosis
    = SCLEROSING OSTEOGENIC SARCOMA
    = OSTEOBLASTIC OSTEOGENIC SARCOMA
    = SCLEROSING OSTEOGENIC SARCOMATOSIS
Etiology: (a) multicentric type of osteosarcoma
               (b) multiple metastatic bone lesions
Classification (Amstutz):
    Type I   multiple synchronous bone lesions occurring within 5 months + patient ≤ 18 years of age
    Type II   multiple synchronous bone lesions occurring within 5 months + patient >18 years of age
    Type IIIa early metachronous metastatic osteosarcoma occurring 5 to 24 months after diagnosis
    Type IIIb late metachronous metastatic osteosarcoma occurring >24 months after diagnosis
Age: Amstutz type I = 4 – 18 (mean 11) years
          Amstutz type II = 19 – 63 (mean 30) years
Site: metaphysis of long bones; may extend into epiphyseal plate / begin in epiphysis

√ multicentric simultaneously appearing lesions
√ densely opaque (osteoblastic)
√ lesions bilateral + symmetrical
√ early: bone islands
√ late: entire metaphysis fills with sclerotic lesions breaking through cortex
√ lesions are of same size
√ lung metastases (62%)
Prognosis: uniformly poor with early death
DDx: heavy metal poisoning, sclerosing osteitis, progressive diaphyseal dysplasia, melorheostosis, osteopoikilosis, bone infarction, osteopetrosis

Central Osteosarcoma
Most common malignant primary bone tumor in young adults + children; 2nd most common primary malignant bone tumor after multiple myeloma
Histo: arising from undifferentiated mesenchymal tissue; forming fibrous / cartilaginous / osseous matrix (mostly mixed) that produces osteoid / immature bone
Age: bimodal distribution 10 – 25 years and >60 years; 21% <10 years; 68% <15 years; 70% between 10 and 30 years;   M:F = 3:2;
          >35 years: related to preexisting conditions (Paget disease, previously irradiated bone)
• painful swelling (1 – 2 months duration)
• fever (frequent)
• slight elevation of alkaline phosphatase
• diabetes mellitus (paraneoplastic syndrome) in 25%

Location: long bones, femur (40%), tibia (16%); 50 – 75% at knee; proximal humerus (15%); cylindrical bone <30 years; flat bone (ilium) >50 years
Site: meta- / diaphysis
√ usually large bone lesion >5 cm when first detected
√ osteolytic / almost normal density / extremely dense (50%) lesion
√ sunburst / onion-peel periosteal reaction + Codman triangle
√ moth-eaten bone destruction + cortical disruption
√ soft tissue mass with tumor new bone (osseous / cartilaginous type)
√ transepiphyseal spread before plate closure (75 – 88%); physis does NOT act as a barrier to tumor spread
√ spontaneous pneumothorax (due to subpleural metastases)
NUC:
    √ intensely increased activity on bone scan (hypervascularity, new bone formation)
    √ soft tissue extension demonstrated, especially with SPECT
    √ bone scan establishes local extent (extent of involvement easily overestimated due to intensity of uptake), skip lesions, metastases to bone + soft tissues

MR (preferred modality):
√ clearly defines marrow extent (best on T1WI), vascular involvement, soft-tissue component (best on T2WI)

Metastases (in 2% at presentation):
(a) hematogenous lung metastases (15%): calcifying; spontaneous pneumothorax secondary to subpleural cavitating nodules rupturing into pleural space
(b) lymph nodes, liver, brain (may be calcified)
(c) skeletal metastases uncommon (unlike Ewing sarcoma); discontinuous tumor foci in marrow cavity in up to 10%

Cx:
(1) pathologic fracture (significant number)
(2) radiation-induced osteosarcoma (30 years delay)

Prognosis:
(1) amputation: 20% 5-year survival; 15% develop skeletal metastases; 75% dead within <2 years
(2) multidrug chemotherapy: 55% 4-year survival more proximal lesions carry higher mortality (0% 2-year survival for axial primary)

DDx: Osteoid osteoma, sclerosing osteomyelitis, Charcot joint

Periosteal Osteosarcoma

1% of all osteosarcomas
Histo: centrally malignant osteoid with peripheral lobules of cartilage extending perpendicular from cortical surface
Age: peak 10 – 20 years (range of 13 – 70 years)

Location: proximal tibia, distal femur at the medial / anterior aspects, humerus, fibula, ilium
Site: metaphysis / diaphysis of long bone; limited to periphery of cortex with normal endosteal margin + medullary canal (resembles parosteal sarcoma)
√ sessile elliptical growth at periosteum
√ short spicules of bone at right angles to shaft
√ tumor 7 – 12 cm in length, 2 – 4 cm in width
√ small uncalcified soft tissue component beyond calcified margins
√ tumor base closely attached to cortex over entire extent of tumor
√ NO cortical destruction / medullary cavity invasion
√ may lie in apparent depression on bone surface
Prognosis: 80 – 90% cure rate (better prognosis than central osteosarcoma with 50% 5-year survival)
DDx: juxtacortical chondrosarcoma

Parosteal Osteosarcoma

= JUXTACORTICAL OSTEOSARCOMA;
4% of osteosarcomas; slowly growing lesion with fulminating course if tumor reaches medullary canal
Histo: often cartilaginous cap (as in benign osteo- / chondrosarcoma)
Age: peak age 38 years (range of 12 – 58 years); 50% > age 30 (for central osteosarcoma 75% < age 30); M:F = 2:3

Location: posterior aspect of distal femur (50%), either end of tibia, proximal humerus, rare in other long bones
Site: adjacent to metaphyseal cortex in close relationship to periosteum
√ dense masses of homogeneous new bone extending away from cortex
√ lobulated round tumor periphery
√ small trabeculae may be present
√ initially fine radiolucent line separating tumor mass from cortex (30 – 40%)
√ tumor stalk grows with tumor obliterating radiolucent line
√ tumor periphery less dense than center (DDx: myositis ossificans with periphery more dense)
√ large soft tissue component with osseous + cartilaginous elements
Prognosis: 80 – 90% treated successfully (best prognosis of all osteosarcomas)
DDx: osteochondroma, myositis ossificans, juxtacortical hematoma, extraosseous osteosarcoma

Extraosseous Osteosarcoma

Infrequent
Histo: same as in osseous osteosarcoma
Mean age: 45 years
Location: thigh, retroperitoneum, buttock, back, orbit, submental, upper + lower extremities, axilla, abdomen, neck, kidney, breast
√ large soft tissue tumor
√ >50% calcified

OXALOSIS

Rare inborn error of metabolism
Etiology: excessive amounts of oxalic acid combine with calcium and deposit throughout body (kidneys, soft tissue, bone)
• hyperoxaluria = urinary excretion of oxalic acid >50 mg/day
• progressive renal failure

√ osteoporosis = cystic rarefaction + sclerotic margins in tubular bones on metaphyseal side, may extend throughout diaphysis
√ erosions on concave side of metaphysis near epiphysis (DDx: hyperparathyroidism)
√ bone-within-bone appearance of spine
√ nephrocalcinosis (2° HPT: subperiosteal resorption, rugger jersey spine, sclerotic metaphyseal bands)
Cx: pathologic fractures

PACHYDERMOPERIOSTOSIS

= OSTEODERMOPATHIA HYPERTROPHICANS (TOURAINE-SOLENTE-GOLE) = PRIMARY HYPERTROPHIC OSTEOARTHROPATHY
Autosomal dominant
Age: 3 – 38 years with progression into late 20s / 30s; M >> F
• large skin folds of face + scalp

Location: epiphyses + diametaphyseal region of tubular
             bones; distal third of bones of legs + forearms
             (early); distal phalanges rarely involved
√ enlargement of paranasal sinuses
√ irregular periosteal proliferation of phalanges + distal
  long bones (hand + feet) beginning in epiphyseal region
  at tendon / ligament insertions
√ thick cortex, BUT NO narrowing of medulla
√ clubbing
√ may have acro-osteolysis
Prognosis: progression ceases after several years
DDx: pulmonary osteoarthropathy, thyroid acropachy

PAGET DISEASE

= OSTEITIS DEFORMANS = multifocal chronic skeletal
  disease of probable viral etiology
Incidence: 3% of individuals >40 years; higher
                incidence in northern latitudes
Age: >55 years (in 3%); >85 years (in 10%);
          unusual <40 years; M:F = 2:1
Histo: increased resorption + increased bone formation;
            newly formed bone is abnormally soft with
            disorganized trabecular pattern ("mosaic pattern")
            causing deformity
(a)   ACTIVE PHASE = OSTEOLYTIC PHASE
       = aggressive bone resorption with lytic lesions,
       replacement of hematopoietic bone marrow by fibrous
       connective tissue with numerous large vascular
       channels
(b)   INACTIVE PHASE = QUIESCENT PHASE
       = decreased bone turnover with skeletal sclerosis +
       cortical accretion + loss of excessive vascularity
(c)   MIXED PATTERN (common) = lytic + sclerotic
       phases usually coexist
•   asymptomatic (1/5)
•   fatigue
•   enlarged hat size
•   peripheral nerve compression
•   neurologic disorders from compression of brainstem
    (basilar invagination)
•   hearing loss, blindness, facial palsy (narrowing of neural
    foramina) — rare
•   pain (a) from primary disease process — rare
    (b) pathologic fracture (c) malignant transformation
    (d) degenerative joint disease / rheumatic disorder
    aggravated by skeletal deformity
•   local hyperthermia of overlying skin
•   high-output congestive heart failure from markedly
    increased perfusion (rare)
•   increased alkaline phosphatase (increased bone
    formation)
•   hydroxyproline increased (increased bone resorption)
•   normal serum calcium + phosphorus
Sites: usually polyostotic + asymmetric; pelvis (75%) >
          lumbar spine > thoracic spine > proximal femur >
          calvarium > scapula > distal femur > proximal tibia
          > proximal humerus
Sensitivity: scintigraphy + radiography (60%)
                scintigraphy only (27%)
                radiography only (13%)

√ thick coarse trabeculae + cortical thickening
√ cyst-like areas (fat-filled marrow cavity / blood-filled
  sinusoids / liquefactive degeneration + necrosis of
  proliferating fibrous tissue)
@ Skull (involvement in 29 – 65%)
   √   inner + outer table involved
   √   diploic widening
   √   osteoporosis circumscripta = well-defined lysis,
       most commonly in calvarium anteriorly, occasionally
       in long bones (destructive active stage)
   √   "cotton wool" appearance = mixed lytic + blastic
       pattern of thickened calvarium (late stage)
   √   basilar invagination with encroachment on foramen
       magnum
   √   deossification + sclerosis in maxilla
   √   sclerosis of base of skull
@ Long bones (almost invariable at end of bone; rarely in
   diaphysis)
   √   "candle flame" / "blade of grass" lysis = advancing
       tip of V-shaped lytic defect in diaphysis of long
       bone originating in subarticular site
       (CHARACTERISTIC)
   √   lateral curvature of femur, anterior curvature of tibia
       (commonly resulting in fracture)
@ Small / flat bones
   √   bubbly destruction + periosteal successive layering
@ Pelvis
   √   thickened trabeculae in sacrum, ilium; rarefaction in
       central portion of ilium
   √   thickening of ileopectineal line
   √   acetabular protrusion (DDx: metastatic disease not
       deforming) + secondary degenerative joint disease
@ Spine (upper cervical, low dorsal, midlumbar)
   √   lytic / coarse trabeculations at periphery of bone
   √   "picture frame vertebra" = bone-within-bone
       appearance = enlarged square vertebral body with
       reinforced peripheral trabeculae + radiolucent inner
       aspect, typically in lumbar spine
   √   "ivory vertebra" = blastic vertebra with increased
       density
   √   ossification of spinal ligaments, paravertebral soft
       tissue, disc spaces
Bone scan:
   √   usually markedly increased uptake (symptomatic
       lesions strikingly positive)
   √   normal scan in some sclerotic burned-out lesions
   √   marginal uptake in lytic lesions
   √   enlargement + deformity of bones
Bone marrow scan:
   √   sulfur colloid bone marrow uptake is decreased
       (marrow replacement by cellular fibrovascular tissue)
MR:
   √   hypointense area / area of signal void on T1WI +
       T2WI (cortical thickening, coarse trabeculation)
   √   widening of bone
   √   reduction in size + signal intensity of medullary cavity
       (replacement of high signal-intensity fatty marrow by
       increased medullary bone formation)
   √   focal areas of higher signal intensity than fatty marrow
       (= cyst-like fat-filled marrow spaces)

√ areas of decreased signal intensity within marrow on T1WI + increased intensity on T2WI (= fibrovascular tissue resembling granulation tissue)

Cx:
(1) Sarcomatous transformation into chondro- / osteo- / fibrosarcoma in <5%
(2) Fracture: "banana fracture" = tiny horizontal cortical infractions on convex surfaces of lower extremity long bones (lateral bowing of femur, anterior bowing of tibia); compression fractures of vertebrae (soft bone despite increased density)
(3) Extradural spinal block (bone-forming phase / compression fractures) with neurologic deficits
(4) Giant cell tumor, especially in skull + facial bones

Rx: calcitonin, diphosphonate, mithramycin
Detection of recurrence:
(a) in 1/3 detected by bone scan
(b) in 1/3 detected by biomarkers (alkaline phosphatase, urine hydroxyproline)
(c) in 1/3 by scan + biomarkers simultaneously
√ diffuse (most common) / focal increase in tracer uptake
√ extension of uptake beyond boundaries of initial lesion
DDx: Osteosclerotic metastases, Hodgkin disease, vertebral hemangioma

PANNER DISEASE
= osteonecrosis of capitellum

PARAOSTEOARTHROPATHY
= HETEROTOPIC BONE FORMATION = ECTOPIC OSSIFICATION = MYOSITIS OSSIFICANS
Common complication following surgical manipulation, total hip replacement (62%) and chronic immobilization (spinal cord injury / neuromuscular disorders)
Mechanism: pluripotent mesenchymal cell lays down matrix for formation of heterotopic bone similar to endosteal bone
Causes: Para- / quadriplegia (40 – 50%), myelomeningocele, poliomyelitis, severe head injury, cerebrovascular disease, CNS infections (tetanus, rabies), surgery (commonly following total hip replacement)
Evolution: calcifications seen 4 – 10 weeks following insult; progression for 6 – 14 months; trabeculations by 2 – 3 months; stable lamellar bone ankylosis in 5% by 12 – 18 months
√ largest quantity of calcifications around joints, especially hip, along fascial planes
√ disuse osteoporosis of lower extremities
√ renal calculi (elevation of serum calcium levels)
Radiographic grading system (Brooker):
0   no soft-tissue ossification
I   separate small foci of ossification
II   >1 cm gap between opposing bone surfaces of heterotopic ossifications
III   <1 cm gap between opposing bone surfaces
IV   bridging ossification

Bone scan:
√ tracer accumulation in ectopic bone
√ assessment of maturity for optimal time of surgical resection (indicated by same amount of uptake as normal bone)
Cx: Ankylosis in 5%
Rx: 1000 – 2000 rad within 4 days following surgical removal

PHENYLKETONURIA
High incidence of X-ray changes in phenylalanine-restricted infants:
√ metaphyseal cupping of long bones (30 – 50%), especially wrist
√ calcific spicules extending vertically from metaphysis into epiphyseal cartilage (DDx to rickets)
√ sclerotic metaphyseal margins
√ osteoporosis
√ delayed skeletal maturation
DDx: Homocystinuria

PHOSPHORUS POISONING
Etiology: (1) ingestion of metallic phosphorus (yellow phosphorus)
(2) treatment of rachitis or TB with phosphorized cod liver oil
Location: long tubular bones, ilium
√ multiple transverse lines (intermittent treatment with phosphorus)
√ lines disappear after some years

PIERRE ROBIN SYNDROME
May be associated with: CHD, defects of eye and ear, hydrocephalus, microcephaly
• glossoptosis
√ micrognathia = hypoplastic receding mandible
√ arched ± cleft palate
√ rib pseudarthrosis
Cx: airway obstruction (relatively large tongue), aspiration

PIGMENTED VILLONODULAR SYNOVITIS
= PVNS
Histo: (1) hyperplasia of undifferentiated connective tissue with large cells ingesting hemosiderin / lipoid (foam / giant cells)
(2) villonodular appearance of synovial membrane ± fibrosis
(3) pressure erosion / invasion of adjoining bone
Age: mainly 2nd – 4th decade (range 12 – 68 years); 50% <40 years
• hemorrhagic "chocolate" effusion without trauma
• pain of long duration, decreased range of motion, joint locking
Location: knee, ankle, hip, elbow, shoulder, tarsal + carpal joints; predominantly monarticular (DDx: degenerative arthritis)
√ soft tissue swelling around joint (effusion + synovial proliferation)
√ dense soft tissues (hemosiderin deposits)

√ subchondral pressure erosion at margins of joint
√ multiple sites of deossification appearing as cysts
√ NO calcifications, osteoporosis, joint space narrowing (until late)
DDx: Synovial sarcoma (solitary calcified mass outside joint)

INTRAARTICULAR LOCALIZED NODULAR SYNOVITIS
= synovial lining without hemosiderin

POLAND SYNDROME
May be associated with aplasia of mamilla / breast; Autosomal recessive
√ unilateral absence of the sternocostal head of the pectoralis major muscle
√ ipsilateral syndactyly + brachydactyly
√ rib anomalies

POLIOMYELITIS
√ osteoporosis
√ soft tissue calcification / ossification
√ intervertebral disc calcification
√ rib erosion commonly on superior margin of 3rd + 4th rib (secondary to pressure from scapula)
√ "bamboo" spine (resembling ankylosing spondylitis)
√ sacroiliac joint narrowing

POPLITEAL CYST
= BAKER CYST = synovial cyst in the posterior aspect of knee joint
Pathophysiology:
formed by escape of synovial effusion into one of the bursae; fluid trapped by one-way valvular mechanism
(a) Bunsen-type valve = expanding cyst compresses the communicating channel
(b) ball-type valve = ball composed of fibrin + cellular debris plugs the communication channel
Etiology: (1) arthritis (rheumatoid arthritis most common)
(2) internal derangement
(3) pigmented villonodular synovitis
• pseudophlebitis syndrome (= pain + swelling in calf)

Location:
(a) gastrocnemio-semimembranous bursa = posterior to gastrocnemius muscle at level of medial condyle
(b) supralateral bursa = between lateral head of gastrocnemius muscle + distal end of biceps muscle superior to lateral condyle (uncommon)
(c) popliteal bursa = beneath lateral meniscus + anterior to popliteal muscle (uncommon)
√ communication with bursa (documented on arthrogram)
√ hypointense collection on T1WI + hyperintense on T2WI
√ cyst may dissect down calf between gastrocnemius + soleus
Cx: may rupture (sudden severe pain)
DDx: other synovial cysts about the knee:
(1) Meniscal cyst (at lateral / medial side of joint line; associated with horizontal cleavage tears)
(2) Tibiofibular cyst (at proximal tibiofibular joint which communicates with knee joint in 10%)

(3) Cruciate cyst (surrounding anterior / posterior cruciate ligaments following ligamentous injury)

PROGERIA
= HUTCHINSON-GILFORD SYNDROME
= autosomal recessive inheritance; most commonly in populations with consanguineous marriages (Japanese, Jewish)
Age: shortly after adolesence; M:F = 1:1

Characteristic habitus + stature:
• symmetric retardation of growth
• absent adolescent growth spurt
• dwarf with short stature + light body weight
• spindly extremities with stocky trunk
• beak-shaped nose + shallow orbits
Premature senescence:
• birdlike appearance
• graying of hair + premature baldness
• hyperpigmentation
• voice alteration
• diffuse arteriosclerosis
• bilateral cataracts
• osteoporosis
Scleroderma-like skin changes:
• atrophic skin + muscles
• circumscribed hyperkeratosis
• telangiectasia
• tight skin
• cutaneous ulcerations
• localized soft-tissue calcifications
Endocrine abnormalities:
• diabetes
• hypogonadism

√ generalized osteoporosis
@ Skull
  √ thin cranial vault
  √ delayed sutural closure + Wormian bones
  √ hypoplastic facial bones (maxilla + mandible)
@ Chest
  √ narrow thorax + slender ribs
  √ progressive resorption with fibrous replacement of outer portions of thinned clavicles (HALLMARK)
  √ coronary artery + heart valve calcifications with cardiac enlargement
@ Extremities & Joints
  √ short + slender long bones
  √ coxa valga
  √ valgus of humeral head
  √ acro-osteolysis of terminal phalanges (occasionally)
  √ flexion + extension deformities of toes (hallux valgus, pes planus)
  √ excessive degenerative joint disease of major + peripheral joints
  √ neurotrophic joint lesions (feet)
  √ widespread osteomyelitis + septic arthritis (hands, feet, limbs)
@ Soft tissue
  √ soft-tissue atrophy of extremities

√ soft tissue calcifications around bony prominences (ankle, wrist, elbow, knee)

√ peripheral vascular calcifications = premature atherosclerosis

Prognosis:
most patients die in their 30's / 40's from complications of arteriosclerosis (myocardial infarction, stroke) or neoplasm (sarcoma, meningioma, thyroid carcinoma)

DDx: Cockayne syndrome (mental retardation, retinal atrophy, deafness, family history)

PSEUDOACHONDROPLASIA

- normal face + head

√ limb shortening

√ irregular epiphyses

√ scoliosis

√ coxa vara

√ marked shortening of bones in hands + feet

PSEUDOFRACTURES

= LOOSER LINES = LOOSER ZONES = OSTEOID SEAMS = MILKMAN SYNDROME = insufficiency stress fractures + nonunion (incomplete healing due to mineral deficiency)

Associated with:
(1) Osteomalacia / rickets (2) Paget disease ("banana fracture") (3) Osteogenesis imperfecta tarda (4) Fibrous dysplasia (5) Organic renal disease (6) Renal tubular dysfunction (7) Congenital hypophosphatasia (8) Congenital hyperphosphatasia ("juvenile Paget disease") (9) Vitamin D malabsorption / deficiency (10) Neurofibromatosis

mnemonic: "POOF"
Paget disease
Osteomalacia
Osteogenesis imperfecta
Fibrous dysplasia

Common sites:
scapulae (axillary margin, lateral + superior margin), femoral neck + shaft, pubic + ischial rami, ribs, proximal 1/3 of ulna, distal 1/3 of radius, phalanges, metatarsals, metacarpals, clavicle

√ typically bilateral + symmetric at right angles to bone margin

√ 2 – 3 mm stripe of lucency at right angle to cortex (= osteoid seams formed within stress-induced infractions (PATHOGNOMONIC) + nonunion (= incomplete healing due to mineral deficiency)

√ paralleled by marginal sclerosis in later stages

PSEUDOHYPOPARATHYROIDISM

= PHypoPT = congenital X-linked dominant abnormality with renal + skeletal resistance to PTH due to (1) end organ resistance (2) presence of antienzymes (3) defective hormone

May be associated with hyperparathyroidism due to hypocalcemia; F > M

- short obese stature
- mental retardation
- corneal + lenticular opacity
- abnormal dentition (hypoplasia, delayed eruption, excessive caries)
- hypocalcemia + hyperphosphatemia (resistant to PTH injection)
- normal levels of PTH

√ brachydactyly in bones in which epiphysis appears latest (metacarpal, metatarsal bones I, IV, V) (75%)

√ accelerated epiphyseal maturation resulting in dwarfism + coxa vara / valga

√ multiple diaphyseal exostoses (occasionally)

√ calcification of basal ganglia + dentate nucleus

√ calcification / ossification of skin + subcutaneous tissue

PSEUDOPSEUDOHYPOPARATHYROIDISM

= PPHypoPT = different expression of same familial disturbance with identical clinical + radiographic features as Pseudohypoparathyroidism

- short stature, round facies
- NO blood chemical changes (normal calcium + phosphorus)
- normal response to injection of PTH

√ brachydactyly

PSORIATIC ARTHRITIS

Types:
(1) true psoriatic arthritis (31%)
(2) psoriatic arthritis resembling rheumatoid arthritis (38%)
(3) concomitant rheumatoid + psoriatic arthritis (31%)

- pitting, discoloration, hyperkeratosis, subungual separation, ridging of nails (in 80%)
- positive HLA-B27 in 80%; negative rheumatoid factor

Location: widely variable distribution + asymmetry

√ NO juxta-articular osteoporosis (DDx: rheumatoid arthritis)

√ periosteal reaction frequent

	PHypoPT	PPHypoPT
√ calcification of basal ganglia	44%	8%
√ soft tissue calcifications	55%	40%
√ metacarpal shortening (4 + 5 always involved)	75%	90%
√ metatarsal shortening (3 + 4 involved)	70%	99%

@ Hands + feet
Target area: DIP, PIP, MCP
√ asymmetrical destruction of distal interphalangeal joints + ankylosis
√ resorption of terminal tufts with "pencil-in-cup" deformity (hands + feet)
√ ivory phalanx
√ destruction of interphalangeal joint of 1st toe with exuberant periosteal reaction + bony proliferation at distal phalangeal base (PATHOGNOMONIC)
@ Axial skeleton
√ asymmetrical + incomplete nonmarginal syndesmophyte formation (thoracic area, lower cervical and upper lumbar regions)
√ squaring of vertebrae in lumbar region
√ paravertebral soft tissue calcifications, separate from edges of vertebrae
√ bilateral sacroiliac joint widening, increased density, fusion

PYKNODYSOSTOSIS

= autosomal recessive disease;
  probably variant of cleidocranial dysostosis
Age: children;   M:F = 2:1

• dwarfism (resembling osteopetrosis)
• mental retardation (10%)
• widened hands + feet
• dystrophic nails
• yellowish discoloration of teeth
• characteristic facies (beaked nose, receding jaw)

√ brachycephaly + platybasia
√ wide cranial sutures, Wormian bones
√ thick skull base
√ hypoplasia of mandible + obtuse mandibular angle
√ hypoplasia + nonpneumatization of paranasal sinuses
√ nonsegmentation of C1/2 and L5/S1
√ generalized increased density of long bones with thickened cortices
√ clavicular dysplasia
√ hypoplastic tapered terminal tufts
√ multiple spontaneous fractures
DDx:
(1) Osteopetrosis (no mandibular / skull abnormality, no phalangeal hypoplasia, no transverse metaphyseal bands, anemia, Erlenmeyer flask deformity; "bone-within-bone" appearance)
(2) Cleidocranial dysostosis (no dense bones / terminal phalangeal hypoplasia, short stature)

RADIATION INJURY TO BONE

Pathogenesis: vascular compromise with obliterative endarteritis + periarteritis followed by damage to osteoblasts with decreased matrix production (growing bone + periosteal new bone most sensitive)
A. RADIATION OSTEITIS
   Dose: (a)   600 – 1200 rad: histological recovery retained

        (b)   >1200 rad   :   pronounced cellular damage
√ temporary growth cessation with recovery
√ periostitis
√ increased fragility with sclerosis
√ aseptic necrosis
√ osteoradionecrosis
MR:
   √ increased intensity of spinal bone marrow on T1WI + T2WI corresponding to radiation port (fatty infiltration)
B. BENIGN NEOPLASM
   Most likely in patients <2 years of age at treatment; with doses of 1600 – 6425 rads; latent period of 9 – 14 years
   1. Exostosis = Osteochondroma
   2. Osteoblastoma
C. MALIGNANT NEOPLASM
   1. Sarcoma (5.5% of all osteogenic sarcomas)
      Criteria: (a) microscopic evidence of altered histology of the original lesion
              (b) malignancy occuring within radiated field
              (c) latency period of >5 years
              (d) histologic proof of sarcoma
   • pain, soft tissue mass, rapid progression of lesion

REITER SYNDROME

= triad of (1) arthritis (2) uveitis (3) urethritis; 98% male
Types:
   (1) endemic type (venereal)
   (2) epidemic (postdysenteric)
• Hx of sexual exposure / diarrhea 3 – 11 days before onset of urethritis
• mucocutaneous lesions (keratosis blennorrhagia, balanitis circinata sicca)
• uveitis, conjunctivitis
• positive HLA-B27 in 76%
Location: asymmetric mono- / pauciarticular
√ polyarthritis
√ articular soft tissue swelling + joint space narrowing in 50% (particularly knees, ankles, feet)
√ widening + inflammation of Achilles + patella tendons
√ "fluffy" periosteal reaction (DISTINCTIVE) at metatarsal necks, proximal phalanges, calcaneal spur, tibia + fibula at ankle and knee
√ juxtaarticular osteoporosis (rare in acute stage)

CHRONIC CHANGES
• recurrent joint attacks in a few cases
√ calcaneal spur at insertion of plantar fascia + Achilles tendon
√ periarticular deossification
√ marginal erosions, loss of joint space
√ bilateral sacroiliac changes indistinguishable from ankylosing / psoriatic spondylitis
√ isolated osteophyte usually in thoracolumbar area, separated from vertebral body
Cx: gastric ulcer + hemorrhage; aortic incompetence; heart block; amyloidosis

RELAPSING POLYCHONDRITIS

= generalized recurring inflammation + destruction of cartilage in joints, ears, nose, larynx, airways

Etiology: acquired metabolic disorder (? abnormal acid mucopolysaccharide metabolism / hypersensitivity / altered immunity

Histo: loss of cytoplasm in chondrocytes; plasma cell + lymphocyte infiltration

- saddle-nose deformity
- swollen + tender ears, cauliflower ears
- hearing loss (obstruction of external auditory meatus)
- cough, hoarseness, dyspnea (collapse of trachea)
- arthralgia

@ Head
- √ calcification of pinna of ear

@ Chest
- √ ectasia + collapsibility with narrowing of trachea and mainstem bronchi
- √ generalized + localized emphysema
- √ aortic aneurysm (10%), mostly in ascending aorta, may be multiple / dissecting
- √ costochondritis

@ Bone
- √ periarticular osteoporosis
- √ erosive changes in carpal bones resembling rheumatoid arthritis
- √ soft tissue swelling around joints + styloid process of ulna
- √ erosive irregularities in sacroiliac joints
- √ disc space erosion + increased density of articular plates

Rx: corticosteroids

RENAL OSTEODYSTROPHY

= combination of (a) osteomalacia (adults) / rickets (children) (b) 2° HPT with osteitis cystica fibrosa + soft tissue calcifications (c) osteosclerosis

Classification:
- (1) Glomerular form = acquired renal disease: chronic glomerulonephritis (common)
- (2) Tubular form = congenital renal osteodystrophy:
    1. Vitamin D-resistent rickets = Hypophosphatemic rickets
    2. Fanconi syndrome = impaired resorption of glucose, phosphate, amino acids, bicarbonate, uric acid, sodium, water
    3. Renal tubular acidosis

Pathogenesis:
- (a) Renal insufficiency causes a decrease in vitamin D conversion + vitamin D deficiency which slows intestinal calcium absorption; *vitamin D resistance predominates* and calcium levels stay low (Ca x P product remains almost normal secondary to hyperphosphatemia); low calcium levels lead to OSTEOMALACIA
- (b) Renal insufficiency with diminished filtration results in phosphate retention; maintenance of Ca x P product lowers serum calcium directly, which in turn increases PTH production (2° HPT); *2° HPT predominates* associated with mild vitamin D resistance and leads to an increase in Ca x P product with SOFT TISSUE CALCIFICATION in kidney, lung, joints, bursae, blood vessels, heart as well as OSTEITIS FIBROSA
- (c) Mixture of (a) and (b): increased serum phosphate inhibits vitamin D activation via feedback regulation
- phosphate retention
- hypocalcemia

A. OSTEOMALACIA (adult)
Due to acquired insensitivity to vitamin D / antivitamin D factor
(a) diffuse form:
- √ osteopenia = diminution in number of trabeculae + thickening of stressed trabeculae = increased trabecular pattern

(b) focal form:
- √ Milkman fracture / Looser zones = incomplete compression fractures with little or no callus response; bilateral symmetric

B. RICKETS (children)
Most apparent in areas of rapid growth such as knee joints
- √ diffuse bone demineralization
- √ widened growth plate
- √ irregular zone of provisional calcification
- √ metaphyseal cupping + fraying
- √ bowing of long bones
- √ slipped capital femoral epiphysis

C. OSTEITIS FIBROSA
Secondary to hypocalcemia + hyperphosphatemia followed by increased parathormone production
- √ subperiosteal bone resorption (most constant + specific): radial aspect of phalanges, distal end of clavicles, medial tibia plateau, medial humerus neck, distal ulna, phalangeal tufts, lamina dura of teeth
- √ subchondral + subligamentous bone resorption = widening of symphysis, sacroiliac joints, resorption of ischial tuberosity
- √ spotty deossification of skull (wooly / granular salt and pepper skull)
- √ metaphyseal fractures, slipped epiphyses
- √ brown tumor + chondrocalcinosis (more common in 1° HPT)

D. OSTEOSCLEROSIS
One of the most common radiologic manifestations; most commonly with chronic glomerulonephritis
- √ diffuse chalky density: thoracolumbar spine in 60% (rugger jersey spine); also in pelvis, ribs, long bones, facial bones, base of skull (children)

E. SOFT TISSUE CALCIFICATIONS
(a) metastatic secondary to hyperphosphatemia (elevated Ca x P product)
(b) dystrophic secondary to tissue injury
Location: (a) arterial (b) periarticular = tumoral
(c) visceral, cutaneous + subcutaneous
- √ fluffy amorphous "tumoral" calcification

Rx:
1. Decrease of phosphorus absorption in bowel (in hyperphosphatemia)
2. Vitamin D$_3$ administration (if vitamin D resistance predominates)
3. Parathyroidectomy for 3° HPT (= autonomous HPT)

Congenital Renal Osteodystrophy
Vitamin D-resistant Rickets
= PHOSPHATE DIABETES = PRIMARY HYPOPHOSPHATEMIA = FAMILIAL HYPOPHOSPHATEMIC RICKETS

X-linked dominant renal tubular abnormality characterized by
(1) impaired resorption of phosphate in proximal renal tubule (2) decreased intestinal resorption of calcium + phosphate
Age: <1 year

- hypophosphatemia + hyperphosphaturia
- increased alkaline phosphatase
- hypocalcemia (secondary to intestinal malabsorption)
√ classic rachitic changes, occasionally dwarfism
Rx: phosphate infusion + large doses of vitamin D

Fanconi Syndrome
Triad of
(1) hyperphosphaturia
(2) amino aciduria
(3) renal glucosuria (normal blood glucose)
Etiology: renal tubular defect
√ rickets, osteomalacia, osteitis fibrosa, osteosclerosis
Prognosis: functional renal impairment likely when bone changes occur
Rx: large doses of vitamin D + alkalinization

Renal Tubular Acidosis
- systemic acidosis, bone lesions
√ rickets, osteomalacia, pseudofractures, nephrocalcinosis, osteitis fibrosa (rare)

(a) Lightwood syndrome = salt-losing nephritis (self-limited form)
   - NO nephrocalcinosis
(b) Butler-Albright syndrome (severe form)
   - nephrocalcinosis

RHEUMATOID ARTHRITIS
= generalized connective tissue disease
Age: highest incidence 40 – 50 years;
M:F = 1:3 if <40 years; M:F = 1:1 if >40 years
Pathogenesis: synovitis with synovial hypertrophy leads to impaired nutrition with chondronecrosis, joint narrowing, subluxation, and ankylosis
Diagnostic criteria of American Rheumatism Association (at least 4 criteria should be present):

(1) morning stiffness (2) swelling of ≥3 joints particularly wrist, metatarsophalangeal or proximal interphalangeal joints for >6 weeks (3) symmetric swelling (4) typical radiographic changes (5) rheumatoid nodules (6) positive rheumatoid factor
- morning stiffness
- fatigue, weight loss
- carpal tunnel syndrome
- positive rheumatoid factor (94%)
- positive latex flocculation test
Location: symmetric involvement of diarthrodial joints
Target areas:
all five MCP, PIP, interphalangeal joint of thumb, all wrist compartments (especially radiocarpal, inferior radioulnar, pisiform-triquetral joints); medial aspect of MTP + interphalangeal joints of foot (esp. great toe); earliest changes seen in 2nd + 3rd MCP, 3rd PIP

EARLY SIGNS:
√ fusiform periarticular soft tissue swelling (result of effusion)
√ regional osteoporosis (disuse + local hyperthermia)
√ widened joint space
√ marginal + central bone erosions (less common in large joints); site of first erosion is classically base of proximal phalanx of 4th finger
√ changes in the ulnar styloid + distal radioulnar joint
√ atlantoaxial dislocation >2.5 mm
√ giant synovial cyst
LATE SIGNS:
√ diffuse loss of interosseous space
√ flexion + extension contractures with ulnar subluxation + dislocation
√ marked destruction + fractures of joint space
√ extensive destruction of bone ends
√ bony fusion
√ elevation of humeral heads (tear / atrophy of rotator cuff)
√ resorption of distal clavicle
√ erosion of superior margins of posterior portions of ribs 3 – 5
√ destruction + narrowing of disc spaces + irregular vertebral body outlines + absence of osteophytosis
√ destruction of zygapophyseal joints without osteophyte formation
√ resorption of spinous processes
√ "stepladder appearance" of cervical spine due to subaxial subluxations
√ protrusio acetabuli (from osteoporosis)
√ synovial herniation + cysts (eg, popliteal cyst)
√ calcaneal plantar spur

Cystic rheumatoid arthritis
= intraosseous cystic lesions as dominant feature
Pathogenesis: increased pressure in synovial space from joint effusion decompresses through microfractures of weakened marginal cortex into subarticular bone
∆ increase in size + extent of cysts correlates with increased level of activity + absence of synovial cysts

Age: as above; M:F = 1:1
- seronegative in 50%

√ juxtaarticular subcortical lytic lesions with well-defined sclerotic margins

√ relative lack of cartilage loss, osteoporosis, joint disruption

DDx: gout (presence of urate crystals), pigmented villonodular synovitis (monarticular)

EXTRAARTICULAR MANIFESTATIONS (76%)

A. **Felty Syndrome** (<1%)
   = rheumatoid arthritis (present for >10 years) + splenomegaly + neutropenia
   Age: 40 – 70 years; F > M; rare in blacks
   - rapid weight loss
   - therapy refractory leg ulcers
   - brown pigmentation over exposed surfaces of extremities

B. SJÖGREN SYNDROME (15%)
   = keratoconjunctivitis + xerostomia + rheumatoid arthritis

C. PULMONARY MANIFESTATIONS
   √ pleural effusion, mostly unilateral, without change for months, usually not associated with parenchymal disease
   √ interstitial fibrosis with lower lobe predominance
   √ rheumatoid nodules (30%): well-circumscribed, peripheral, with frequent cavitation
   √ Caplan syndrome (= hyperimmune reactivity to silica inhalation with rapidly developing multiple pulmonary nodules)
   √ pulmonary hypertension secondary to arteritis

D. SUBCUTANEOUS NODULES
   (in 5 – 35% with active arthritis) over extensor surfaces of forearm + other pressure points (eg, olecranon) without calcifications (DDx to gout)

E. CARDIOVASCULAR INVOLVEMENT
   1. Pericarditis (20 – 50%)
   2. Myocarditis (arrhythmia, heart block)
   3. Aortitis (5%) of ascending aorta ± aortic valve insufficiency

F. RHEUMATOID VASCULITIS
   Mimicks periarteritis nodosa;
   - polyneuropathy, cutaneous ulceration, gangrene, polymyopathy, myocardial / visceral infarction

G. NEUROLOGIC SEQUELAE
   1. Distal neuropathy (related to vasculitis)
   2. Nerve entrapment (atlantoaxial subluxation, carpal tunnel syndrome, Baker cyst)

H. LYMPHADENOPATHY (up to 25%)
   √ splenomegaly (1 – 5%)

Juvenile Rheumatoid Arthritis

= rheumatoid arthritis in patients <16 years of age; M < F

Classification:
(1) Juvenile-onset adult type (10%)
   - IgM RA factor positive; age 8 – 9; poor prognosis

√ erosive changes; perfuse periosteal reaction; hip disease with protrusio

(2) Polyarthritis of the ankylosing spondylitic type
   - iridocyclitis; boys age 9 – 11 years
   √ peripheral arthritis; fusion of greater trochanter; complete fusion of both hips; heel spur

(3) **Still disease**
   (a) systemic (b) polyarticular (c) pauciarticular + iridocyclitis (30%)
   - fever, rash, lymphadenopathy, hepatosplenomegaly; pericarditis, dwarfism
   - fatal kidney disease in 20%
   Age: 2 – 4 and 8 – 11 years of age; M < F
   Location: involvement of carpometacarpal joints ("squashed carpi" in adulthood), hind foot, hip (40 – 50%)
   √ periosteal reaction of phalanges; broadening of bones; accelerated bone maturation + early fusion (stunting of growth)

- morning stiffness, arthralgia
- subcutaneous nodules (10%)
- skin rash (50%)
- fever, lymphadenopathy

Location: early involvement of large joints (hips, knees, ankles, wrists, elbows); later of hands + feet

√ radiologic signs similar to rheumatoid arthritis (except for involvement of large joints first, late onset of bony changes, more ankylosis, wide metaphyses)

√ periarticular soft tissue swelling

√ thinning of joint cartilage

√ large cyst-like lesions removed from articular surface (invasion of bone by inflammatory pannus); rare in children

√ articular erosions at ligamentous + tendinous insertion sites

√ joint destruction may resemble neuropathic joints

√ juxtaarticular osteoporosis

√ "balloon epiphyses" + "gracile bones" (epiphyseal overgrowth + early fusion with bone shortening secondary to hyperemia)

@ Hand / foot
   √ "rectangular" phalanges (periostitis + cortical thickening)
   √ ankylosis in carpal joints

@ Axial skeleton
   √ ankylosis of cervical spine (apophyseal joints), sacroiliac joints
   √ subluxation of atlantoaxial joint (66%)
   √ thoracic spinal compression fractures

@ Chest
   √ ribbon ribs
   √ pleural + pericardial effusions
   √ interstitial pulmonary lesions (simulating scleroderma, dermatomyositis)
   √ solitary pulmonary nodules, may cavitate

Prognosis: complete recovery (30%); secondary amyloidosis

RICKETS

= osteomalacia during enchondral bone growth

Age: 4 – 18 months

Histo: zone of preparatory calcification does not form, heap up of maturing cartilage cells; failure of osteoid mineralization also in shafts so that osteoid production elevates periosteum

- irritability, bone pain, tenderness
- craniotabes
- rachitic rosary
- bowed legs
- delayed dentition
- swelling of wrists + ankles

Location: metaphyses of long bones subjected to stress are particularly involved (wrists, ankles, knees)

√ poorly mineralized epiphyseal centers with delayed appearance

√ irregular widened epiphyseal plates (increased osteoid)

√ increase in distance between end of shaft and epiphyseal center

√ cupping + fraying of metaphysis with thread-like shadows into epiphyseal cartilage (weight-bearing bones)

√ cortical spurs projecting at right angles to metaphysis

√ coarse trabeculation (NO ground glass pattern as in scurvy)

√ periosteal reaction may be present

√ deformities common (bowing of soft diaphysis, molding of epiphysis, fractures)

√ bowing of long bones

√ frontal bossing

Causes & Classification of Rickets

I.   *ABNORMALITY IN VITAMIN D METABOLISM*
Associated with reactive hyperparathyroidism
  A. Vitamin D deficiency
       (a) Dietary lack of vitamin D
            = famine osteomalacia
       (b) Lack of sunshine exposure
       (c) Malabsorption of vitamin D
            = gastroenterogenous rickets
            1. pancreatitis + biliary tract disease
            2. steatorrhea, celiac disease, postgastrectomy
            3. inflammatory bowel disease
  B. Defective conversion of vitamin D to 25-OH-cholecalciferol in liver
       1. Liver disease
       2. Anticonvulsant drug therapy (= induction of hepatic enzymes that accelerate degradation of biologically active vitamin D metabolites)
  C. Defective conversion of 25-OH-D3 to 1,25-OH-D3 in kidney
       1. Chronic renal failure = renal osteodystrophy
       2. Vitamin D-dependent rickets = autosomal recessive enzyme defect of 1-OHase

II. *ABNORMALITY IN PHOSPHATE METABOLISM*
not associated with hyperparathyroidism secondary to normal serum calcium

  A. Phosphate deficiency
       1. Intestinal malabsorption of phosphates
       2. Ingestion of aluminum salts [$Al(OH)_2$] forming insoluble complexes with phosphate
       3. Low phosphate feeding in prematurely born infants
       4. Severe malabsorption state
       5. Parenteral hyperalimentation
  B. Disorders of renal tubular reabsorption of phosphate
       1. Renal tubular acidosis (renal loss of alkali)
       2. deToni-Debré-Fanconi syndrome
            = hypophosphatemia, glucosuria, aminoaciduria
       3. Vitamin D-resistant rickets
       4. Cystinosis
       5. Tyrosinosis
       6. Lowe syndrome
  C. Hypophosphatemia with nonendocrine tumors
       = Oncogenic rickets = elaboration of humeral substance which inhibits tubular reabsorption of phosphates
       1. Sclerosing hemangioma
       2. Hemangiopericytoma
       3. Ossifying mesenchymal tumor
       4. Nonossifying fibroma
  D. Hypophosphatasia

III. *CALCIUM DEFICIENCY*
       1. Dietary rickets = milk-free diet (extremely rare)
       2. Malabsorption
       3. Consumption of substances forming chelates with calcium

CLASSIFICATION OF RICKETS

I.   Primary vitamin D deficiency rickets
II.   Gastrointestinal malabsorption
       A. Partial gastrectomy
       B. Small intestinal disease: gluten-sensitive enteropathy / regional enteritis
       C. Hepatobiliary disease: chronic biliary obstruction / biliary cirrhosis
       D. Pancreatic disease: chronic pancreatitis
III.   Primary hypophosphatemia; vitamin D deficiency rickets
IV.   Renal disease
       A. Chronic renal failure
       B. Renal tubular disorders: renal tubular acidosis
       C. Multiple renal defects
V.   Hypophosphatasia + pseudohypophosphatasia
VI.   Fibrogenesis imperfecta osseum
VII.   Axial osteomalacia
VIII. Miscellaneous
       Hypoparathyroidism, hyperparathyroidism, thyrotoxicosis, osteoporosis, Paget disease, fluoride ingestion, ureterosigmoidostomy, neurofibromatosis, osteopetrosis, macroglobulinemia, malignancy

ROTATOR CUFF LESIONS
Rotator Cuff Tear
Etiology:
  (1) Attritional change + tendon degeneration due to aging, repeated microtrauma as a result of impingement between humeral head + coracoacromial arch, overuse of shoulder from professional / athletic activities
  (2) Acute trauma (rare)
Age: most commonly >50 years

Location: "critical zone" of supraspinatus tendon 1 cm medial to tendon attachment (area of relative hypovascularity)
Classification:
  (a) complete rupture = full-thickness tear bridging the subacromial bursa to glenohumeral joint
      — pure transverse tear
      — pure vertical / longitudinal tear
      — tear with retraction of tendon edges
      — global tear = massive avulsion of cuff
  (b) incomplete rupture = partial tear involving bursal / synovial surface or remain intratendinous
MR:
  √ focal / generalized intense / markedly increased signal intensity on T2WI (= fluid within cuff defect) in <50%
  √ low / moderate signal intensity on T2WI (= severely degenerated tendon, intact bursal / synovial surface, granulation / scar tissue filling the region of torn tendinous fibers)
  √ cuff defect with contour irregularity
  √ adjunct criteria:
      √ fluid within subacromial-subdeltoid bursa
      √ retraction of musculotendinous junction
      √ abrupt change in the signal character at boundary of the lesion
      √ supraspinatus muscle atrophy
US (scans in hyperextended position, 75 – 100% sensitive, 43 – 97% specific, 65 – 95% negative predictive value, 55 – 75% positive predictive value):
  √ nonvisualization of rotator cuff (large tear), most reliable sign
  √ unilateral discontinuity manifested as hypoechoic focus without apposition of deltoid muscle to humeral head (defect filled with fluid / reactive tissue), reliable sign
  √ abrupt + sharply demarcated focal thinning
  √ abnormal unilateral area of hyperechogenicity (small tear filled with granulation tissue / hypertrophied synovium)
  False-negatives: longitudinal tear, partial tear
  False-positives: intraarticular biceps tendon, soft-tissue calcification, small scar / fibrous tissue

Subacromial-Subdeltoid Bursitis
  common finding in rotator cuff tears
  √ peribursal fat totally / partially obliterated + replaced by low-signal intensity tissue on all pulse sequences
  √ fluid accumulation within bursa

Supraspinatus Tendinitis / Tendon Degeneration
Cause: impingement, acute / chronic stress
  √ increase in signal intensity in tendon on proton-density images without disruption of tendon
  √ tendinous enlargement + inhomogeneous signal pattern

Impingement Syndrome
  = lateral shoulder pain with abduction; common cause of rotator cuff tears
Cause:
  (1) Acromioclavicular joint arthritis
  (2) Subacromial spur
  (3) Fibrous thickening of subacromial bursa

RUBELLA
Age: infants
• neonatal dwarfism (growth retardation)
• failure to thrive
• cataracts, deafness
• mental deficiency
• thrombocytopenic purpura

  √ "celery-stalk" sign (50%) = metaphyseal irregular margins + coarsened trabeculae extending longitudinally from epiphysis; distal end of femur > proximal end of tibia, humerus
  √ no periosteal reaction
  √ congenital heart disease (PDA)
  √ peripheral pulmonary artery stenosis
  √ hepatosplenomegaly
  √ pneumonia
  √ necrosis of myocardium

Prognosis: osseous manifestations disappear in 1 – 3 months
DDx: (1) CMV (brain calcifications, not seen in rubella)
       (2) Congenital syphilis (diaphysitis + epiphysitis)
       (3) Toxoplasmosis

SARCOIDOSIS
Osseous involvement in 15 – 20%
• unimpaired joint function, joints are rarely involved

Location: small bones of hands + feet (middle + distal phalanges)
  √ reticulated "lace-like" trabecular pattern in metaphyseal ends of middle + distal phalanges, metacarpals, metatarsals
  √ well-defined cystlike lesions of varying size
  √ neuropathic-like destruction of terminal phalanges (DDx: scleroderma)
  √ endosteal sclerosis + periosteal new bone (infrequent)
  √ vertebral involvement unusual: destructive lesions with sclerotic margin
  √ diffuse sclerosis of multiple vertebral bodies
  √ paravertebral soft tissue mass (DDx: indistinguishable from tuberculosis)
  √ osteolytic changes in skull

SCLERODERMA

= PROGRESSIVE SYSTEMIC SCLEROSIS (PPS)
= multisystem connective tissue disorder of unknown etiology characterized by progressive interstitial fibrosis + chronic inflammation of the microvasculature (initially hypertrophy and finally atrophy of collagen fibers)

Age: 4th – 5th decade; F > M
- atrophy + thickening of skin and musculature
- weakness, generalized debility
- renal failure (from nephrosclerosis)
- pericarditis

@ Hands
  - Raynaud phenomenon
  - thickened skin + edema
  - arthralgia (rheumatoid factor in 30%)
  - √ "tapered fingers" = atrophy + resorption of soft tissues of fingertips
  - √ calcinosis = punctate soft tissue calcifications (fingertips, axilla, ischial tuberosity, forearms, lower legs, face)
  - √ osteolysis
    - √ "penciling" / "autoamputation" of terminal tufts beginning at volar aspect with proximal progression
    - √ bony erosions of carpal bones, distal radius + ulna, mandible, ribs, clavicle, humerus, acromion, cervical spine
    - √ bilateral resorption of trapezium + radial subluxation of associated metacarpal base
  - √ NO significant osteoporosis
  - √ ± flexion contractures of fingers (from tendon sheath inflammation + fibrosis)
  - √ arthritis
    Location: DIP, PIP, 1st CMC, MCP
    - √ soft-tissue swelling + periarticular osteoporosis
    - √ central / marginal erosions
    - √ joint space narrowing (late)
  - *DDx:*   rheumatoid, psoriatic, erosive arthritis

@ Chest
  - cough, dyspnea, hematemesis
  - √ pulmonary fibrosis with diffuse reticulate infiltrate predominantly in lower lungs

@ GI tract
  - difficulty in swallowing
  - √ atony of esophagus, duodenum
  - √ segmentation, dilatation, delay in transit of small bowel
  - √ sacculations + pseudosacculations in colon; wide-mouthed small bowel diverticula / pseudodiverticula on mesenteric side
  - √ hepatomegaly

SCURVY

= BARLOW DISEASE = vitamin C deficiency with defective osteogenesis from abnormal osteoblast function

Age: 6 – 9 months (maternal vitamin C protects for first 6 months)
- irritability
- tenderness + weakness of lower limbs

- scorbutic rosary of ribs
- bleeding of gums (teething)
- legs drawn up + widely spread = pseudoparalysis

Location: distal femur (esp. medial side), proximal and distal tibia + fibula, distal radius + ulna, proximal humerus, sternal end of ribs

- √ Wimberger ring = sclerotic ring around epiphysis
- √ white line of Fränkel = metaphyseal zone of preparatory calcification (DDx: lead / phosphorus poisoning, bismuth treatment, healing rickets)
- √ Trümmerfeld zone = radiolucent zone on shaft side of Fränkel's white line (site of subepiphyseal infraction)
- √ Parke corner sign = subepiphyseal infraction / comminution resulting in mushrooming / cupping of epiphysis (DDx: syphilis, rickets)
- √ Pelkan spurs = metaphyseal spurs projecting at right angles to shaft axis
- √ "ground glass" osteoporosis (CHARACTERISTIC)
- √ cortical thinning
- √ subperiosteal hematoma with calcification of elevated periosteum (sure radiographic sign of healing)
- √ soft tissue edema (rare)

SEPTIC ARTHRITIS

Organism:
  most often due to S. aureus; Gonorrhea (indistinguishable from tuberculous arthritis, but more rapid); Brucellar arthritis (indistinguishable from tuberculosis, slow infection); Salmonella (commonly associated with sickle cell disease / Gaucher disease)
  (a) <4 years of age: Streptococcus pyogenes, S. aureus, Haemophilus influenzae
  (b) >4 years of age: S. aureus
  (c) >10 years of age: S. aureus, Neisseria gonorrhoeae

Location: lower extremity (75%) with hip + knee in 90%
- pain, limp, pseudoparalysis
- warmth, swelling
- septic clinical picture
- bacteremia, leukocytosis

ACUTE SIGNS:
- √ initial radiographs frequently normal
- √ soft tissue swelling (first sign secondary to local hyperemia + edema)
- √ joint distension (effusion) ± subluxation of hip and humerus in children
- √ joint space narrowing = rapid development of destruction of articular cartilage (not in tuberculous arthritis)

SUBACUTE SIGNS after 8 – 10 days:
- √ small erosions in articular cortex / loss of entire cortical outline (marginal erosions in tuberculosis)
- √ reactive bone sclerosis in underlying bone
- √ subchondral bone destruction (by synovial proliferation)
- √ defective reparation / ankylosis (if entire cartilage is destroyed)
- √ local bone atrophy (immobility)
- √ metaphyseal bone destruction (if osteomyelitis is source of septic joint)

Dx: prompt arthrocentesis + blood culture
Cx: (1) bone growth disturbance (lengthening,
          shortening, angulation)
       (2) chronic degenerative arthritis
       (3) ankylosis
       (4) osteonecrosis

SHORT–RIB POLYDACTYLY SYNDROME
= group of autosomal recessive disorders characterized
  by short limb dysplasia, constricted thorax, postaxial
  polydactyly (on ulnar / fibular side)
TYPE I = SALDINO-NOONAN SYNDROME
TYPE II = MAJEWSKI TYPE
TYPE III = NAUMOFF TYPE
√ severe micromelia
√ pointed femurs at both ends (Type I); widened
  metaphyses (Type III)
√ narrow thorax
√ extremely short horizontally oriented ribs
√ distorted underossified vertebral bodies + incomplete
  coronal clefts
√ polydactyly
√ cleft lip / palate
Prognosis: uniformly lethal

SICKLE CELL ANEMIA
Abnormal Hemoglobins:
  Hb S = DNA mutation substituting glutamic acid in
          position 6 on beta-chain with valine
  Hb C = DNA mutation substituting glutamic acid in
          position 6 on beta-chain with lysine
  (a) homozygous   = Hb SS with sickle cell anemia
  (b) heterozygous = Hb SA with sickling trait but no
                       anemia
                     = Hb SC with sickle cell S-C
                       disease (less severe form)
                     = Hb S-thalassemia, seen
                       occasionally
Incidence: 8 – 13% of American blacks carry sickling
             factor (Hb S); 1:40 with sickle cell trait will
             manifest sickle cell anemia (Hb SS); 1:120
             with sickle cell trait will manifest Hb SC
             disease
Pathogenesis:
  altered shape + plasticity of RBCs under lowered
  oxygen tension lead to increased blood viscosity, stasis,
  "log jam" occlusion of small blood vessels, infarction,
  necrosis, superinfection; sickling occurs in areas of
  (a) slow flow (spleen, liver, renal medulla)
  (b) rapid metabolism (brain, muscle, fetal placenta)

• hemolytic anemia (altered RBCs rapidly destroyed by
  RES), jaundice
• chronic leg ulcers, priapism
• abdominal crisis
• rheumatic-like joint pain
• skeletal pain (osteomyelitis, cellulitis, bone marrow
  infarction)
• splenomegaly (in children + infants), later organ atrophy
Cx: high incidence of infections (lung, bone, brain)

Prognosis: death <40 years
(1) DEOSSIFICATION DUE TO MARROW
     HYPERPLASIA
     √ porous decrease in bone density of skull (25%)
     √ widening of diploe with decrease in width of outer
       table (22%)
     √ vertical hair-on-end striations (5%)
     √ osteoporosis with thinning of trabeculae
     √ biconcave "fish" vertebrae (bone softening) in 70%
     √ widening of medullary space + thinning of cortices
     √ coarsening of trabecular pattern in long + flat bones
     √ rib notching
     √ pathologic fractures
(2) THROMBOSIS AND INFARCTION
     Location: in diaphysis of small tubular bones
                (children); in metaphysis + subchondrium
                of long bones (adults)
     √ osteolysis (in ACUTE infarction)
     √ dystrophic medullary calcification
     √ periosteal reaction (bone-within-bone appearance)
     √ juxtacortical sclerosis
     √ Lincoln log = Reynold sign = H-vertebrae = step-like
       endplate depression
     √ articular disintegration
     √ collapse of femoral head (DDx: Perthes with
       involvement of metaphysis)
     MR:
       √ diffusely decreased signal of marrow on short +
         long TR/TE images (= hematopoietic marrow
         replacing fatty marrow)
       √ focal areas of decreased signal intensity on short
         TR/TE + increased intensity on long TR/TE
         (= acute marrow infarction)
       √ focal areas of decreased signal intensity on short
         TR/TE + long TR/TE images (= old infarction /
         fibrosis)
(3) SECONDARY OSTEOMYELITIS
     Organism: Salmonella in unusual frequency, also
                 Staphylococcus
     √ periostitis (DDx: indistinguishable from bone
       infarction)
     √ dactylitis = hand-foot syndrome
(4) GROWTH EFFECTS (secondary to diminished blood
     supply)
     Location: particularly in metacarpal / phalanx
     √ bone shortening = premature epiphyseal fusion
     √ epiphyseal deformity with cupped metaphysis
     √ cup / peg-in-hole defect of distal femur
     √ diminution in vertebral height (shortening of stature
       + kyphoscoliosis)
@ Abdomen
     √ splenomegaly < age 10
     √ small fibrotic spleen
     √ autoinfarction of spleen (function lost by age 5)
     √ cholelithiasis
Acute splenic sequestration crisis
     = venous drainage obstruction of small intrasplenic
       veins / within sinusoids
     • sudden splenic enlargement
     • rapid fall in hematocrit + rise in reticulocytes

√ enlarged spleen
√ multiple lesions at periphery of spleen:
  hypoechoic by US, of low attenuation by CT,
  hyperintense on T1WI + T2WI (due to
  heorrhage)
Prognosis: in 50% death <2 years of age
@ Kidney
• hematuria
• hyposthenuria
• nephrotic syndrome
• renal tubular acidosis (distal)
• hyperuricemia
• progressive renal insufficiency
√ normal urogram (70%)
√ papillary necrosis (20%)
√ focal renal scarring (20%)
√ smooth large kidney (4%)
MR:
  √ decreased cortical signal on T2-weighted
    images
@ Chest
√ cardiomegaly + congestive heart failure

Bone marrow scintigraphy:
√ usually symmetric marked expansion of hematopoietic
  marrow beyond age 20 involving entire femur,
  calvarium, small bones of hand + feet (normally only
  in axial skeleton + proximal femur and humerus)
√ bone marrow defects indicative of acute / old
  infarction
Tc-99m diphosphonate scan:
√ increased overall skeletal uptake (high bone-to-soft
  tissue ratio)
√ prominent activities at knees, ankles, proximal
  humerus (delayed epiphyseal closure / increased
  blood flow to bone marrow)
√ bone marrow expansion (calvarial thickening with
  relative decrease in activity along falx insertion)
√ decreased / normal uptake on bone scan within 24
  hours in acute infarction / posthealing phase
  following infarction (cyst formation)
√ increased uptake on bone scan after 2 – 10 days
  persistent for several weeks in healing infarction
√ increased uptake on bone scan within 24 – 48 hours
  in osteomyelitis
√ increased blood-pool activity + normal delayed image
  on bone scan in cellulitis
√ renal enlargement with marked retention of tracer in
  renal parenchyma (medullary ischemia + failure of
  countercurrent system) in 50%
√ persistent splenic uptake (secondary to
  degeneration, atrophy, fibrosis, calcifications)
Tc-99m sulfur colloid scan:
√ functional asplenia

SICKLE CELL TRAIT
Hb SA carrier; mild disease with few episodes of crisis +
  infection; sickling provoked only under extreme stress
  (unpressurized aircraft, anoxia with CHD, prolonged
  anesthesia, marathon running)

Incidence: in 8 – 10% of American blacks
• may have normal blood count
• recurrent gross hematuria
√ splenic infarction

SC DISEASE
Hb SC carrier
Incidence: 3% of American blacks
• retinal hemorrhages
• hematuria due to multiple infarctions
√ aseptic necrosis of hip

SICKLE-THAL DISEASE
Resembling clinically Hb SS patients
• anemia (no normal adult hemoglobin)
√ persistent splenomegaly

SJÖGREN SYNDROME
= multisystem disorder associated with collagen-vascular
  disease affecting (1) salivary + lacrimal glands
  (2) mucosa + submucosa of pharynx
  (3) tracheobronchial tree (4) reticuloendothelial system
  (5) joints
TRIAD: keratoconjunctivitis sicca, xerostomia, rheumatoid
         arthritis
Age: 35 – 70; female predominance
• dry eyes
• dry mouth
• decreased sweating
• decreased vaginal secretions

√ sialectasis
√ rheumatoid arthritis
√ interstitial lymphocytic pneumonitis + fibrosis
√ pseudolymphoma (disorder between lymph node
  hyperplasia and neoplasm)
√ bilateral lower lobe bronchiectasis
√ acute focal / lipoid pneumonia (oils taken to combat dry
  mouth)
Cx: Lymphoma (occurs in significant number of
        patients)

SMALLPOX
5% of infants
Location: elbow bilateral; metaphysis of long bones

√ rapid bone destruction spreading along shaft
√ periosteal reaction
√ endosteal + cortical sclerosis frequent
√ premature epiphyseal fusion with severe deformity
√ ankylosis is frequent

SOFT TISSUE CHONDROMA
Age: 3rd – 4th decade; M > F
Histo: adult-type hyaline cartilage
Location: hand + feet

√ slow-growing lobular well-demarcated mass
√ may contain calcifications / ossifications
√ scalloping of adjacent bone with sclerotic reaction

SOLITARY OSTEOCHONDROMA

= OSTEOCARTILAGINOUS EXOSTOSIS = hyperplastic / dysplastic bone disturbance originating from displaced or aberrant cartilage of the growth plate; growth ends when nearest epiphyseal plate fuses; most common benign growth of the skeleton

Age: 1st – 3rd decade; M:F = 1:1
Histo: cartilage cap containing a basal surface with enchondral ossification

• usually painless mass; painful with impingement of nerves / blood vessels

Location: long bone metaphysis of femur, humerus, proximal radius, tibia (50% about knee); scapula; rib; pelvis; spine (1 – 5%, commonly thoracic); in any bone that develops by enchondromal calcification

Type: (a) pedunculated form (b) broad-based form (c) calcific form

√ cortical bone with cartilaginous cap
√ grows at right angles + towards diaphysis (tendon pull)
√ continuity of bone cortex to host bone
√ continuity of medullary marrow space to host bone
√ metaphyseal widening

Cx: (1) Impingement on nerves / blood vessels
(2) Malignant transformation into chondro- / osteosarcoma (<1%)
√ enlargement after epiphyseal fusion (usually starts in cartilaginous cap)

SOLITARY BONE CYST

= UNICAMERAL / SIMPLE BONE CYST
Etiology: ? trauma (synovial entrapment at capsular reflection), ? vascular anomaly (blockage of interstitial drainage)
Histo: cyst filled with clear yellowish fluid often under pressure, wall lined with fibrous tissue + hemosiderin, giant cells may be present
Age: 3 – 19 years (80%); occurs during active phase of bone growth; M:F = 3:1

• asymptomatic, unless fractured

Location: proximal femur + proximal humerus (60 - 75%), fibula, at base of calcaneal neck (4%, >12 years of age), talus; rare in ribs, ilium, small bones of hand + feet (rare), NOT in spine / calvarium

Sites: centric metaphyseal, adjacent to epiphyseal cartilage (during active phase) / migrating into diaphysis with growth (during latent phase), does not cross epiphyseal plate

√ 2 – 3 cm oval radiolucency with long axis parallel to long axis of host bone
√ fine sclerotic boundary
√ scalloping + erosion of internal aspect of underlying cortex
√ photopenic area on bone scan (if not fractured)
√ "fallen fragment" sign if fractured

Prognosis: mostly spontaneous regression
DDx: (1) Enchondroma (calcific stipplings) (2) Fibrous dysplasia (more irregular lucency) (3) Eosinophilic granuloma (4) Chondroblastoma (epiphyseal)
(5) Chondromyxoid fibroma (more eccentric + expansile) (6) Giant cell tumor (7) Aneurysmal bone cyst (eccentric) (8) Hemorrhagic cyst (9) Brown tumor

SOLITARY PLASMACYTOMA

= represents early stage of multiple myeloma, precedes multiple myeloma by 1 – 20 years
Age: 5th – 7th decade

• negative marrow aspiration; no IgG spike in serum / urine

A. SOLITARY MYELOMA OF BONE

Sites: thoracic / lumbar spine (most common) > pelvis > ribs > sternum, femora, humeri (common)

√ solitary "bubbly" osteolytic grossly expansile lesion
√ poorly defined margins, Swiss-cheese pattern
√ frequently pathologic fracture (collapse of vertebra)

DDx: Giant cell tumor, aneurysmal bone cyst, osteoblastoma, solitary metastasis from renal cell / thyroid carcinoma

B. EXTRAMEDULLARY PLASMACYTOMA

Location: majority in head + neck; 80% in nasal cavity, paranasal sinuses, upper airways of trachea, lung parenchyma

SPONDYLOEPIPHYSEAL DYSPLASIA

Spondyloepiphyseal Dysplasia Congenita

Autosomal dominant / sporadic (most)

• disproportionate dwarfism with spine + hips more involved than extremities
• waddling gait + muscular weakness
• flat facies
• short neck
• deafness
√ cleft palate
@ Axial skeleton
√ hypoplasia of odontoid process (Cx: cervical myelopathy)
√ ovoid vertebral bodies + severe platyspondyly (incomplete fusion of ossification centers + flattening of vertebral bodies)
√ progressive kyphoscoliosis (short trunk) involving thoracic + lumbar spine
√ narrowing of disc spaces (resulting in short trunk)
√ broad iliac bases + deficient ossification of pubis
√ flat acetabular roof
@ Chest
√ bell-shaped thorax
√ pectus carinatum
@ Extremities
√ normal / slightly shortened limbs
√ severe coxa vara + genu valgum
√ multiple accessory epiphyses in hands + feet
√ talipes equinovarus
Cx: (1) Retinal detachment, myopia (50%)
(2) Secondary arthritis in weight-bearing joints

Spondyloepiphyseal Dysplasia Tarda

Sex-linked recessive form with milder manifestation + later clinical onset

Age: apparent by 10 years; exclusive to males
√ hyperostotic new bone along posterior 2/3 of vertebral end-plate (PATHOGNOMONIC)
√ platyspondyly with depression of anterior 1/3 of vertebral body
√ narrowing with calcification of disc spaces + spondylitic bridging
√ short trunk
√ dysplastic joints (eg, flattened femoral heads)
√ premature osteoarthritis
DDx: Ochronosis

SPONTANEOUS OSTEONECROSIS OF KNEE
= SONK
Causes: ? meniscal tear (78%), trauma with resultant microfractures, vascular insufficiency, degenerative joint disease, severe chondromalacia, gout, rheumatoid arthritis, joint bodies, intraarticular steroid injection (45 – 85%)
Age: 7th decade (range 13 – 83 years)
• acute onset of pain
Location: weight-bearing medial condyle more toward epicondylus (95%), lateral condyle (5%), may involve tibial plateau

√ radiographs usually normal (within 3 months after onset)
√ positive bone scan within 5 weeks (most sensitive)
√ flattening of weight-bearing segment of medial femoral epicondyle
√ radiolucent focus in subchondral bone + peripheral zone of osteosclerosis
√ horizontal subchondral fracture (within 6 – 9 months) + osteochondral fragment
√ periosteal reaction along medial side of femoral shaft (30 – 50%)
Cx: osteoarthritis

SPRENGEL DEFORMITY
= failure of descent of scapula secondary to fibrous / osseous omovertebral connection
Associated with: Klippel-Feil syndrome, renal anomalies
• webbed neck
• shoulder immobility
√ elevation of scapula

SUDECK DYSTROPHY
= REFLEX SYMPATHETIC DYSTROPHY = CAUSALGIA
= SHOULDER-HAND SYNDROME = POST-TRAUMATIC OSTEOPOROSIS
Etiology: (1) Injury (fracture, frostbite; may be trivial) (2) Immobilization (3) Infection (4) Myocardial infarction
• pain, tenderness, soft tissue swelling out of proportion to degree of injury
• atrophic skin changes
• vasomotor instability (Raynaud phenomenon, local vasoconstriction /-dilatation, hyperhydrosis)
• end-stage (after 6 – 12 months): contractures, atrophy of skin + soft tissues
Location: hands and feet distal to injury

√ periarticular soft tissue swelling
√ patchy demineralization = ground glass appearance (endosteal + intracortical excavation; subperiosteal bone resorption; lysis of juxtaarticular + subchondral bone)
Bone scan:
√ increased uptake particularly in periarticular bone (radiocarpal, intercarpal, carpometacarpal, metacarpophalangeal, interphalangeal joints) on delayed images
√ perfusion + blood pool phase not sensitive

SYNOVIAL CHONDROMATOSIS
= OSTEOCHONDROMATOSIS = JOINT CHONDROMA
Histo: cartilage / osteochondroma formed by synovial membrane / joint capsule; hyperplastic synovia with cartilage metaplasia (foci <2 – 3 cm)
Age: presents in 4th decade; M > F
• progressive joint pain
Sites: knee (most often involved), hip, elbow, ankle, shoulder, wrist; usually monarticular, occasionally bilateral
√ multiple calcified / ossified loose bodies in a single joint
√ varying degrees of bone mineralization (1/3 of chondromas show no radiopacity)
√ pressure erosion of adjacent bone
√ widening of joint space
√ long-standing disease may lead to degenerative joint disease
DDx:
(1) Synovial sarcoma
(2) Osteochondral fracture (Hx of trauma)
(3) Joint surface disintegration (rheumatoid arthritis, neurotrophic arthropathy, tuberculous arthritis, degenerative joint disease)

SYNOVIOMA
= SYNOVIAL SARCOMA
= slow-growing expansile malignant tumor originating in the synovial lining / bursa / tendon sheath; uncommonly intraarticular
Incidence: 10% of soft-tissue sarcomas
Histo: fibrosarcomatous + synovial component
Age: 3rd – 5th decade; M:F = 2:3
• painful soft tissue mass
Location: knee (most common), hip, ankle, elbow, wrist, hands, feet; usually solitary
√ lesion about 1 cm removed from joint cartilage
√ invasion of cortex (1/3) with wide zone of transition
√ amorphous calcifications (1/3)
√ juxtaarticular osteoporosis
√ large spheroid well-defined soft tissue mass
MR:
√ low signal intensity on T1WI
√ inhomogeneously increased signal intensity on T2WI
Rx: local excision / amputation + radiation / chemotherapy

SYPHILIS OF BONE
Congenital Syphilis
Transplacental transmission cannot occur <16 weeks gestational age

- positive rapid plasma reagin (measures quantity of antibodies to assess new infection / efficacy of Rx)
- positive microhemagglutination test for Treponema pallidum (remains reactive for life)
√ pneumonia alba
√ hepatomegaly
Location: symmetrical bilateral osteomyelitis involving multiple bones (HALLMARK)

A. Early phase
   Δ Skeletal radiography abnormal in 19% of infected newborns without overt disease!
   1. Metaphysitis
      √ lucent metaphyseal band adjacent to thin / widened zone of provisional calcification (disturbance in enchondral bone growth)
      √ frayed edge of metaphyseal-physeal junction (osteochondritis) = erosions + lytic defects
   2. Diaphyseal periostitis = "luetic diaphysitis"
      √ solid / lamellated periosteal new bone growth = bone-within-bone appearance
   3. Spontaneous epiphyseal fractures causing Parrot pseudopalsy (DDx: battered child syndrome)
   4. Bone destruction
      √ marginal destruction of spongiosa + cortex along side of shaft with widening of medullary canal (in short tubular bones)
      √ patchy rarefaction in diaphysis
   5. Wimberger sign
      √ symmetrical focal bone destruction of medial portion of proximal tibial metaphysis (ALMOST PATHOGNOMONIC)

B. Late phase
   - Hutchinson triad = dental abnormality, interstitial keratitis, 8th nerve deafness
   √ frontal bossing of Parrot = diffuse thickening of outer table
   √ saddle nose + high palate (syphilitic chondritis + rhinitis)
   √ short maxilla (maxillary osteitis)
   √ thickening at sternal end of clavicle
   √ "saber-shin" deformity = anteriorly convex bowing in upper 2/3 of tibia with bone thickening

Acquired Syphilis
= TERTIARY SYPHILIS resembles chronic osteomyelitis
√ dense bone sclerosis of long bones
√ irregular periosteal proliferation + endosteal thickening with narrow medulla
√ extensive calvarial bone proliferation with mottled pattern (anterior half + lateral skull) in outer table (DDx: fibrous dysplasia, Paget disease)
√ ill-defined lytic destruction in skull, spine, long bones (gumma formation)
√ enlargement of clavicle (cortical + endosteal new bone)
√ Charcot arthropathy = neuropathic joints (lower extremities + spine)

TARSAL COALITION
Most important congenital problem of calcaneus clinically
- asymptomatic / painful pes planus with peroneal spasm
Age: fibrous coalition at birth, ossification during 2nd decade of life
√ bone bars on lateral radiographs between calcaneus, talus, navicular
√ both feet affected in 20%
Types:
   (1) calcaneoclavicular (50%)
      √ hypoplastic talar head
      √ narrowed calcaneonavicular joint with indistinct articular margins
   (2) talocalcaneal (35%)
      √ prominent dorsal beak (66%)
      √ ball-and-socket ankle joint
      √ asymmetric anterior talocalcaneal joint
DDx: acquired intertarsal ankylosis (infection, trauma, arthritis, surgery)

THALASSEMIA SYNDROMES
PHYSIOLOGIC HEMOGLOBINS
   (a) in adulthood:
      Hb A (98% = 2 α- and 2 β-chains);
      Hb A$_2$ (2% = 2 α- and 2 δ-chains)
   (b) in fetal life, rapidly decreasing up to 3 months of newborn period:
      Hb F (= 2 α- and 2 γ-chains)

A. ALPHA-THALASSEMIA
   = decreased synthesis of α-chains leading to excess of β-chains + γ-chains (Hb H = 4 β-chains; Hb Bart = 4 γ-chains)
   - disease begins in intrauterine life as no fetal hemoglobin is produced
   - homozygosity is lethal (lack of oxygen transport)

B. BETA-THALASSEMIA
   = decreased synthesis of β-chains leading to excess of α-chains + γ-chains (= fetal hemoglobin)
   - disease manifest in early infancy
   (a) homozygous defect = thalassemia major = Cooley anemia
   (b) heterozygous defect = thalassemia minor

Thalassemia major
= COOLEY ANEMIA = MEDITERRANEAN ANEMIA
= HEREDITARY LEPTOCYTOSIS = beta-thalassemia trait inherited from both parents (= homozygous)
Incidence: 1% for American blacks; 7.4% for Greek population; 10% for certain Italian populations
Age: develops after newborn period
- retarded growth
- elevated serum bilirubin
- hyperpigmentation of skin
- hyperuricemia
- secondary sexual characteristics retarded, normal menstruation rare (primary gonadotropin insufficiency from iron overload in pituitary gland)

- hypochromic microcytic anemia (Hb 2 – 3 g/dl), nucleated RBC, target cells, reticulocytosis, decrease in RBC survival, leukocytosis
- susceptible to infection (leukopenia secondary to splenomegaly)
- bleeding diathesis (secondary to thrombocytopenia)

@   Skull:
  √   widening of diploic space with coarsened trabeculations and displacement + thinning of outer table (from marrow hyperplasia)
  √   severe hair-on-end appearance (frontal bone, NOT inferior to internal occipital protuberance)
  √   impediment of pneumatization of maxillary antra + mastoid sinuses
  √   lateral displacement of orbits
  √   rodent facies = ventral displacement of incisors (marrow overgrowth in maxillary bone) with dental malocclusion
@   Peripheral skeleton:
  √   earliest changes in small bones of hands + feet (>6 months of age)
  √   widened medullary spaces with thinning of cortices
  √   osteoporosis = atrophy + coarsening of trabeculae (marrow hyperplasia)
  √   Erlenmeyer flask deformity = bulging of normally concave outline of metaphyses
  √   premature fusion of epiphyses (10%), usually at proximal humerus + distal femur
  √   arthropathy (secondary to hemochromatosis + CPPD + acute gouty arthritis)
  √   regression of peripheral skeletal changes (as red marrow becomes yellow)
@   Chest:
  √   cardiac enlargement + congestive heart failure (secondary to anemia)
  √   paravertebral masses (= extramedullary hematopoiesis)
  √   costal osteomas = expanded posterior aspect of ribs with thinned cortices
@   Abdomen:
  √   hepatosplenomegaly
  √   gallstones

Cx:
(1) Pathologic fractures
(2) Sequelae of iron overload from transfusion therapy (absent puberty, diabetes mellitus, adrenal insufficiency, myocardial insufficiency)
Prognosis: usually death within 1st decade

Thalassemia minor

= beta-thalassemia trait inherited from one parent (= heterozygous)

- usually asymptomatic except for periods of stress (pregnancy, infection)
- microcytic hypochromic anemia (Hb 9 – 11 g/dl)
- occasionally jaundice + splenomegaly

THANATOPHORIC DYSPLASIA

= sporadic lethal skeletal dysplasia characterized by severe rhizomelia (micromelic dwarfism)
Incidence: 6.9:100,000 births; 1:6,400 – 16,700 births; most common lethal bone dysplasia

- hypotonic infants
- protuberant abdomen
- extended arms + abducted externally rotated thighs

@   Head
  √   large head with short base of skull + prominent frontal bone
  √   occasionally trilobed cloverleaf skull = "Kleeblattschädel" (huge coronal + lambdoid sutures)
@   Chest
  √   narrow chest
  √   short horizontal ribs with cupped anterior ends
  √   small scapula + normal clavicles
@   Spine
  √   normal length of trunk
  √   reduction of interpediculate space of last few lumbar vertebrae
  √   extreme generalized platyspondyly = severe H-shaped vertebra plana
  √   excessive intervertebral space height
@   Pelvis
  √   iliac wings small + square (vertical shortening but wide horizontally)
  √   flat acetabulum
  √   narrow sacrosciatic notch
  √   short pubic bones
@   Extremities
  √   severe micromelia + bowing of extremities
  √   metaphyseal flaring = "telephone handle" appearance of long bones
  √   thorn-like projections in metaphyseal area
OB-US (findings may be seen very early in pregnancy):
  √   polyhydramnios (71%)
  √   short-limbed dwarfism with extremely short + bowed "telephone receiver"-like femurs
  √   extremely small hypoplastic thorax narrowed in anteroposterior dimension
  √   protuberant abdomen
  √   short ribs
  √   macrocrania with frontal bossing ± hydrocephalus (increased HC:AC ratio)
  √   "cloverleaf skull" (in 14%) (DDx: encephalocele)
  √   diffuse platyspondyly
  √   redundant soft tissues
Prognosis: often stillborn; uniformly fatal within a few hours / days after birth (respiratory failure)
DDx:
(1) Ellis-van Creveld syndrome (extra digit, acromesomelic short limbs)
(2) Asphyxiating thoracic dysplasia (less marked bone shortening, vertebrae spared)
(3) Short-rib polydactyly syndrome
(4) Homozygous achondroplasia (both parents affected)

THROMBOCYTOPENIA-ABSENT RADIUS SYNDROME

= TAR SYNDROME = rare autosomal recessive disorder
Age: presentation at birth
May be associated with CHD (33%): ASD, tetralogy
- platelet count <100,000/mm³ (decreased production by bone marrow)
√ usually bilateral radial aplasia / hypoplasia
√ uni- / bilaterally hypoplastic / absent ulna / humerus
√ defects of hands, feet, legs
Prognosis: death in 50% in early infancy (hemorrhage)

THYROID ACROPACHY

Onset: after 18 months following thyroidectomy for hyperthyroidism (does not occur with antithyroid medication)
Incidence: 1 – 10%
- clubbing, soft tissue swelling
- eu- / hypo- / hyperthyroid state
Location: diaphyses of phalanges + metacarpals of hand; less commonly feet, lower legs, forearms
√ thick spiculated lacy periosteal reaction
DDx: (1) Pulmonary osteoarthropathy (painful)
(2) Pachydermoperiostosis
(3) Fluorosis (ligamentous calcifications)

TRANSIENT REGIONAL OSTEOPOROSIS

Cause: unknown; ? overactivity of sympathetic nervous system + local hyperemia similar to reflex sympathetic dystrophy syndrome

Regional Migratory Osteoporosis

= rapid onset of self-limiting episodes of severe localized osteoporosis and pain but repetitive occurrence of same symptoms in other regions of the same or opposite lower extremity
Etiology: unknown
- rapid onset of local pain
- diffuse erythema, swelling, increased heat
- significant disability due to severe pain on weight-bearing
Age: middle-aged males
Location: usually lower extremity (ie, ankle, knee, hip, foot)

√ rapid localized osteoporosis within 4 – 8 weeks after onset migrating from one joint to another; may affect trabecular / cortical bone
√ linear / wavy periosteal reaction
√ preservation of subchondral cortical bone
√ no joint space narrowing, bone erosion
MR:
  √ affected area has low signal intensity on T1WI, high signal intensity on T2WI (= bone marrow edema)
NUC:
  √ increased activity
Prognosis: persists for 6 – 9 months in one area; cycle of symptoms may last for several years
Rx: variable response to analgesics / corticosteroids

PARTIAL TRANSIENT OSTEOPOROSIS
= variant of regional migratory osteoporosis with more focal pattern of osteoporosis, which may eventually become more generalized
(a) Zonal form = portion of bone involved, ie, one femoral condyle / one quadrant of femoral head
(b) Radial form = only one / two rays of hand / foot involved

Transient Osteoporosis of Hip

= self-limiting disease of unknown etiology
Age: typically in middle-aged males / in 3rd trimester of pregnancy in females; M>F
- spontaneous onset of hip and groin pain
- painful swelling of joint followed by progressive demineralization
- rapid development of disability, limp, decreased range of motion
Site: hip most commonly affected; generally only one joint at a time
√ progressive marked osteoporosis of femoral head, neck, acetabulum (3 – 6 weeks after onset of illness)
√ NO joint space narrowing / subchondral bone collapse
√ diffuse increased uptake on bone scan without cold spots / inhomogeneities
Cx: pathologic fracture common
Prognosis: spontaneous recovery within 2 – 6 months; recurrence in another joint within 2 years possible
DDx:
(1) AVN (cystic + sclerotic changes, early subchondral undermining)
(2) Septic / tuberculous arthritis (joint aspiration)
(3) Monoarticular rheumatoid arthritis
(4) Metastasis
(5) Reflex sympathetic dystrophy
(6) Disuse atrophy
(7) Synovial chondromatosis
(8) Villonodular synovitis

TRANSIENT SYNOVITIS OF HIP

= OBSERVATION HIP = TRANSITORY SYNOVITIS
= TOXIC SYNOVITIS = COXITIS FUGAX
= nonspecific inflammatory reaction; most common nontraumatic cause of acute limp in a child
Etiology: unknown
Age: 5 – 10 (average 6) years; M:F = 2:1
- developing limp over 1 – 2 days
- pain in hip, thigh, knee
- Hx of recent viral illness (65%)
- mild fever (25%)
√ radiographs usually normal
√ joint effusion
  √ displacement of femur from acetabulum
  √ displacement of psoas line
  √ lateral displacement of gluteal line (least sensitive + least reliable)
√ regional osteoporosis (? hyperemia, disuse)
Prognosis: complete recovery within a few weeks
Dx: per exclusion

Rx: non-weight-bearing treatment
DDx: trauma, Legg-Perthes disease, acute rheumatoid
         arthritis, acute rheumatic fever, septic arthritis,
         tuberculosis, malignancy

TREACHER COLLINS SYNDROME

= MANDIBULOFACIAL DYSOSTOSIS
autosomal dominant
- antimongoloid eye slant, deficient lashes in lower eye
  lids, coloboma
- dysplastic ears; deafness
√ craniosynostosis
√ egg-shaped orbits = drooping of outer inferior orbital rim
√ marked hypoplasia of zygomatic arches, maxilla,
  paranasal sinuses
√ mandibular hypoplasia with broad concave curve on
  lower border of body

TRISOMY D SYNDROME

= Trisomy 13 – 15 group syndrome
Etiology: additional chromosome in D group; high
              maternal age
- severe mental retardation
- hypertonic infant
- cleft lip + palate
Associated with: capillary hemangioma of face +
                      upper trunk
- hypotelorism
- coloboma, cataract, microphthalmia
- malformed ear with hypoplastic external auditory canal
- hyperconvex nails
√ post-axial polydactyly
@ Skull
   √ deficient ossification of skull
   √ cleft / absent midline structures of facial bones
   √ poorly formed orbits
   √ slanting of frontal bones
   √ microcephaly
   √ arhinencephaly
   √ holoprosencephaly
@ Chest
   √ thin malformed ribs
   √ diaphragmatic hernia (frequent)
   √ congenital heart disease
Prognosis: death within 6 months of age

TRISOMY E SYNDROME

= Trisomy 16 – 18 group syndrome
Etiology: additional chromosome at 18 or E group
              location
Sex: usually female
- hypertonic infants
- mental + psychomotor retardation
- typical facies: micrognathia, high narrow palate with
  small buccal cavity, low-set deformed ears
- flexed ulnar-deviated fingers + short adducted thumb
- 2nd finger overlapping of 3rd (CHARACTERISTIC)
Associated with: congenital heart disease in 100%
                     (PDA, VSD); hernias; renal anomalies;
                     eventration of diaphragm

√ stippled epiphyses
@ Skull
   √ thin calvarium
   √ persistent metopic suture
   √ prominent occiput
   √ hypoplastic mandible (most constant feature) +
     maxilla
@ Chest
   √ increase in AP diameter of thorax
   √ hypoplastic sternum
   √ hypoplastic clavicles (DDx: cleidocranial dysostosis)
   √ slender + tapered ribs
   √ diaphragmatic eventration (common)
@ Pelvis
   √ small pelvis with forward rotation of iliac wings
   √ increased obliquity of acetabulum
@ Hand & Foot
   √ adducted thumb = short 1st metacarpal +
     phalanges (DIAGNOSTIC)
   √ overlap of 2nd on 3rd finger (DIAGNOSTIC)
   √ flexed ulnar-deviated fingers
   √ short 1st toe
   √ varus deformities of forefoot + dorsiflexion of toes
   √ rocker bottom foot / extreme pes planus (frequent)
OB-US:
   √ hydrocephalus
   √ cystic hygroma
   √ diaphragmatic hernia
   √ clubfoot
   √ overlapping index finger
   √ choroid plexus cyst (30%)
Prognosis: child rarely survives beyond 6 months of age

TUBERCULOSIS OF BONE

Incidence: 3 – 5% of tuberculous patients, 30% in
               patients with extrapulmonary tuberculosis
Age: any, rare in 1st year of life, M:F = 1:1
- negative skin test excludes diagnosis
- history of active pulmonary disease (in 50%)
Location: vertebral column, hip, knee, wrist, elbow
Pathogenesis:
   1. Hematogenous spread from
      (a) primary infection of lung (particularly in children)
      (b) quiescent primary pulmonary site / extraosseous
           focus
   2. Reactivation: especially in hip

Tuberculous Arthritis

= joint involvement usually secondary to adjacent
  osteomyelitis
Incidence: 84% of skeletal tuberculosis
Pathophysiology: synovitis with pannus formation
                      leads to chondronecrosis
Age: middle-aged / elderly
- chronic pain, weakness, muscle wasting
- soft-tissue swelling, draining sinus
- joint fluid: high WBC count, low glucose level, poor
  mucin clot formation (similar to rheumatoid arthritis)
Location: hip, knee > elbow, wrist, sacroiliac joint,
            glenohumeral, articulation of hand + foot

√ Phemister triad:
1. gradual narrowing of joint space (from slow cartilage destruction)
2. peripherally located (= marginal) bone erosions
3. juxtaarticular osteoporosis
√ early: extensive deossification adjacent to joint, soft tissues normal
√ late: small cyst-like erosions along joint margins in non-weight-bearing line opposing one another (DDx: pyogenic arthritis erodes articular cartilage)
√ no joint space narrowing for months
√ articular cortical bone destruction earlier in joints with little unopposed surfaces (hip, shoulder)
√ infection of subchondral bone forming "kissing sequestra"
√ increased density with extensive soft tissue calcifications in healing phase
Cx: fibrous ankylosis
Dx: synovial biopsy (in 90% positive), culture of synovial fluid (in 80% positive)

Tuberculous Osteomyelitis
Incidence: 16% of skeletal tuberculosis
Location: any bone
Site:
(a) epiphysis with spread to joint (most common)
(b) metaphysis with transphyseal spread (in child)
  DDx: pyogenic infections usually do not extend across physis
(c) diaphysis (<1%)

√ initially destructive lesion with minimal / no surrounding sclerosis
√ varying amounts of eburnation + periostitis
√ cystic tuberculosis = well-marginated osseous lesions
(a) in children (frequent): in peripheral skeleton, ± symmetric distribution, no sclerosis
(b) in adults: in skull / shoulder / pelvis / spine, with sclerosis
√ spina ventosa = tuberculous dactylitis = digit with exuberant periosteal new bone formation of fusiform appearance secondary to erosion of endosteal cortex with lamellated / solid periosteal thickening in hands + feet
Age: children <5 years (0.5 – 14%), rare in adults
• painless swelling of hand / foot

Tuberculous Spondylitis
= POTT DISEASE
= destruction of vertebral body + intervertebral disc by tuberculous mycobacterium
Incidence: 25 – 60% of skeletal tuberculosis
Age: children / adults; M>F
• insidious onset of back pain, stiffness
• local tenderness

Location: thoracolumbar area (L1 most common), frequent involvement of multiple contiguous segments
Site: vertebral body (82%) > posterior elements (18%)

Spread:
(a) hematogenous spread via paravertebral venous plexus of Batson: separate foci in 1 – 4%
(b) contiguous into disc by penetrating subchondral bone plate + cartilaginous endplate
(c) subligamentous beneath anterior / posterior longitudinal ligament into adjacent disc

√ narrowed vertebral interspaces (first change), vertebral disc space maintained longer than in pyogenic arthritis
√ erosion of vertebral endplates, destruction of centra
√ vertebra plana (in children)
√ vertebra within a vertebra (= growth recovery lines)
√ ivory vertebra (= reossification as healing response to osteonecrosis)
√ large cold fusiform abscess in paravertebral gutters / psoas, commonly bilateral, ± anterolateral scalloping of vertebral bodies
√ amorphous / teardrop-shaped calcification in paraspinal area between L1 + L5 (DDx: nontuberculous abscess rarely calcifies)
√ "gouge defect" = mild contour irregularity of anterior and lateral aspect of vertebral body (= erosion from subligamentous extension of tuberculous abscess)

Cx: angular kyphosis (= gibbus deformity), scoliosis, ankylosis, osteonecrosis, paralysis (spinal cord compression from abscess, granulation tissue, bone fragments, arachnoiditis)

Prognosis: 26 – 30% mortality rate

TUMORAL CALCINOSIS
= LIPOCALCINOGRANULOMATOSIS = progressive large nodular juxtaarticular calcified soft tissue masses in patients with normal serum calcium + phosphorus and no evidence of renal, metabolic, or collagen-vascular disease
Etiology:
autosomal dominant with variable clinical expressivity; unknown biochemical defect of phosphorus metabolism responsible for abnormal phosphate reabsorption + 1,25-dihydroxy-vitamin D formation
Path:
multilocular cystic lesions with creamy white fluid (hydroxyapatite) + many giant cells (granulomatous foreign body reaction) surrounded by fibrous capsule

Age: 1 – 79 years (onset mostly within 1st / 2nd decade); M:F = 1:1; predominantly in blacks

• progressive painful / painless soft-tissue mass with overlying skin ulceration + sinus tract draining chalky milk-like fluid
• swelling
• limitation of motion
• hyperphosphatemia + hypervitaminosis D
• normal serum calcium, alkaline phosphatase, renal function, parathyroid hormone

@ Soft tissue
  Location:
    paraarticular in hips > elbows > shoulders > feet, ribs, ischial spines; single / multiple joints; ALMOST NEVER knees; usually along extensor surface of joints (? initially a calcific bursitis)
  √ dense loculated multiglobular homogeneously calcified soft-tissue mass of 1 – 20 cm in size
  √ radiolucent septa (= connective tissue)
  √ fluid-fluid levels with milk-of-calcium consistency
  √ underlying bones NORMAL
  √ increased tracer uptake of soft tissue masses on bone scan
@ Bone
  √ diaphyseal periosteal reaction (diaphysitis)
  √ patchy areas of calcification in medullary cavity (calcific myelitis)
@ Teeth
  √ bulbous root enlargement
  √ pulp stones = intrapulp calcifications
@ Pseudoxanthoma elasticum-like features
  √ calcinosis cutis = skin calcifications
  √ vascular calcifications
  √ angioid streaks of retina
Prognosis: tendency for recurrence after incomplete excision
Rx: phosphate depletion
DDx: Chronic renal failure on hemodialysis, CPPD, paraosteoarthropathy, hyperparathyroidism

TURNER SYNDROME
= due to nondysjunction of sex chromosomes as
    (1) complete monosomy (45,XO) (2) partial monosomy (structurally altered second X-chromosome)
    (3) mosaicism (XO + another sex karyotype)
Incidence: 1:3,000 – 5,000 live births
Associated with: coarctation, aortic stenosis, horseshoe kidney (most common)
• sexual infantilism: primary amenorrhea, absent secondary sex characteristics
• short stature; absence of prepubertal growth spurt
• webbed neck; low irregular nuchal hair line
• shield-shaped chest + widely spaced nipples
• mental deficiency (occasionally)
• high palate; thyromegaly
• multiple pigmented nevi; keloid formation
• idiopathic hypertension; elevated urinary gonadotropins
@ General
  √ normal skeletal maturation with growth arrest at skeletal age of 15 years
  √ delayed fusion of epiphyses > age 20 years
  √ osteoporosis during / after 2nd decade (gonadal hormone deficiency)
  √ coarctation of aorta (10%); aortic stenosis
  √ renal ectopia / horseshoe kidney
  √ lymphedema
@ Skull
  √ basilar impression; basal angle >140°
  √ parietal thinning
  √ small bridged sella

√ hypertelorism
@ Axial skeleton
  √ hypoplasia of odontoid process + C1
  √ osteochondrosis of vertebral plates
  √ squared lumbar vertebrae; kyphoscoliosis
  √ deossification of vertebrae
  √ small iliac wings; late fusion of iliac crests
  √ android pelvic inlet with narrowed pubic arch + small sacrosciatal notches
@ Chest
  √ thinning of lateral aspects of clavicles
  √ thinned + narrowed ribs with pseudonotching
@ Hand + arm
  √ positive metacarpal sign = relative shortening of 4th metacarpal = tangential line along heads of 5th + 4th metacarpals intersects 3rd metacarpal
  √ positive carpal sign = narrowing of scaphoid-lunate-triquetrum angle <117°
  √ phalangeal preponderance = length of proximal + distal phalanx exceeds length of 4th metacarpal by >3 mm
  √ shortening of 2nd + 5th middle phalanx (also in Down syndrome)
  √ "drumstick" distal phalanges = slender shaft + large distal head
  √ "insetting" of epiphyses into bases of adjacent metaphyses (phalanges + metacarpals)
  √ Madelung deformity = shortening of ulna / absence of ulnar styloid process
  √ cubitus valgus = bilateral radial tilt of articular surface of trochlea
  √ deossification of carpal bones
@ Knee
  √ tibia vara = enlarged medial femoral condyle + depression of medial tibial plateau (DDx: Blount disease)
  √ small exostosis-like projection from medial border of proximal tibial metaphysis
@ Foot
  √ deossification of tarsal bones
  √ shortening of 1st, 4th + 5th metatarsals
  √ pes cavus
OB-US:
  √ large nuchal cystic hygroma
  √ lymphangiectasia with generalized hydrops
  √ symmetrical edema of dorsum of feet
  √ CHD (20%): coarctation of aorta (70%), left heart lesions
  √ horseshoe kidney

BONNEVIE-ULLRICH SYNDROME
= infantile form of Turner syndrome
    (1) congenital webbed neck
    (2) widely separated nipples
    (3) lymphedema of hands + feet

VAN BUCHEM DISEASE
= GENERALIZED CORTICAL HYPEROSTOSIS
  may be related to hyperphosphatasemia
• paralysis of facial nerve

- auditory + ocular disturbances (in late teens secondary to foraminal encroachment)
- increased alkaline phosphatase

Location: skull, mandible, clavicles, ribs, long bone diaphyses

√ symmetrical generalized sclerosis + thickening of endosteal cortex

√ obliteration of diploe

√ spinous processes thickened + sclerotic

DDx:

(1) Osteopetrosis (sclerosis of all bones, not confined to diaphyses)
(2) Generalized hyperostosis with pachydermia (involves entire long bones, considerable pain, skin changes)
(3) Hyperphosphatasia (infancy, widened bones but decreased cortical density)
(4) Engelmann disease (rarely generalized, involves lower limbs)
(5) Pyle disease (does not involve middiaphyses)
(6) Polyostotic fibrous dysplasia (rarely symmetrically generalized, paranasal sinuses abnormal, skull involvement)

WILLIAMS SYNDROME

= IDIOPATHIC HYPERCALCEMIA OF INFANCY

- elfin facies, dysplastic dentition
- neonatal hypercalcemia
- mental retardation

@ Skeletal manifestations

√ osteosclerosis (secondary to trabecular thickening)

√ dense broad zone of provisional calcification

√ radiolucent metaphyseal bands

√ dense vertebral endplates + acetabular roofs

√ bone islands in spongiosa

√ metastatic calcification

√ craniostenosis

@ Cardiovascular manifestations

√ supravalvular aortic stenosis, aortic hypoplasia

√ pulmonic stenosis

√ stenoses of major vessels (innominate, carotids, renal arteries)

@ GI and GU tract:

√ colonic diverticula

√ bladder diverticula

Prognosis: spontaneous resolution after 1 year in most

Rx: withhold vitamin D + calcium

DDx: Hypervitaminosis D

WILSON DISEASE

= HEPATOLENTICULAR DEGENERATION

= autosomal recessive disease with excessive copper retention due to decreased ceruloplasmin in liver

Incidence: 1:200,000

Age of onset: 7 – 50 years

- tremor, rigidity, dysarthria, dysphagia (excessive copper deposition in lenticular region of brain)
- intellectual impairment, emotional disturbance
- Kayser-Fleischer ring (= green pigmentation surrounding limbus corneae)
- jaundice / portal hypertension (liver cirrhosis)

Skeletal manifestations (in 2/3):

√ generalized deossification may produce pathologic fractures

@ Joints: shoulder (frequent), knee, hip, wrist, 2nd – 4th MCP joints

- articular symptoms in 75%: pain, stiffness, gelling of joints

√ subarticular cysts

√ premature osteoarthritis (narrowing of joint space + osteophyte formation)

√ osteochondritis dissecans

√ chondrocalcinosis

√ premature osteoarthrosis of spine, prominent Schmorl nodes, wedging of vertebrae, irregularities of vertebral plates

@ Brain

Location: basal ganglia, rarely thalamus

√ cerebral white matter atrophy

√ hypodensities, prolongation of T1 + T2

Cx: rickets + osteomalacia (secondary to renal tubular dysfunction) in minority of patients

DIFFERENTIAL DIAGNOSIS OF SKULL AND SPINE DISORDERS

SKULL
Basilar invagination
= bulging of C-spine and foramen magnum into cranial cavity

A. Primary form: associated with narrow foramen magnum + occipitalization of atlas

B. Secondary form: osteogenesis imperfecta, Paget disease

mnemonic: "COOP"

  Congenital
  Osteogenesis imperfecta
  Osteomalacia
  Paget disease

√ abnormal craniometry:
  — Lateral view:
    Chamberlain line: line between roof of hard palate to posterior lip of foramen magnum (= opisthion)
      √ tip of odontoid above this line
    McGregor line: line between hard palate to most caudal portion of occipital bone
      √ tip of odontoid >5 mm above this line
    McRae line: line between anterior lip (= basion) to posterior lip (= opisthion) of foramen magnum
      √ tip of odontoid above this line
  — Anteroposterior view:
    Digastric line: line between incisurae mastoideae (origin of digastric muscles)
      √ tip of odontoid above this line
    Bimastoid line: line connecting the tips of both mastoid processes
      √ tip of odontoid >10 mm above this line
√ C-spine + foramen magnum bulge into cranial cavity
√ elevation of posterior arch of C1

Platybasia
= flattened skull base

Cause: osteomalacia, rickets, hyperparathyroidism, fibrous dysplasia, Paget disease, Arnold-Chiari malformation

• cord symptoms
√ sphenoid angle (= angle between roof of sphenoid and clivus) >150°

Sutural abnormalities
Wide sutures
= >10 mm at birth, >3 mm at 2 years, >2 mm at 3 years of age; (sutures are splittable up to age 12 – 15; complete closure by age 30)

A. NORMAL VARIANT
    in neonate + prematurity; growth spurt occurs at 2 – 3 years and 5 – 7 years

B. CONGENITAL UNDEROSSIFICATION
    Osteogenesis imperfecta, hypophosphatasia, rickets, hypothyroidism, pyknodysostosis, cleidocranial dysplasia

C. METABOLIC DISEASE
    Hypoparathyroidism; lead intoxication; hypo- / hypervitaminosis A

D. RAISED INTRACRANIAL PRESSURE
    Cause: (1) intracerebral tumor (2) subdural hematoma (3) hydrocephalus
    Age: seen only if <10 years of age
    Location: coronal > sagittal > lambdoid > squamosal suture

E. INFILTRATION OF SUTURES
    Cause: metastases to meninges from (1) neuroblastoma (2) leukemia (3) lymphoma
    √ poorly defined margins

F. RECOVERY
    from (1) deprivational dwarfism (2) chronic illness (3) prematurity (4) hypothyroidism

Craniosynostosis
= CRANIOSTENOSIS = premature closure of sutures (normally at about 30 years of age)

Age: often present at birth; M:F = 4:1
Etiology:

A. Primary craniosynostosis
B. Secondary craniosynostosis
    (a) hematologic: sickle cell anemia, thalassemia
    (b) metabolic: rickets, hypercalcemia, hyperthyroidism, hypervitaminosis D
    (c) bone dysplasia: hypophosphatasia, achondroplasia, metaphyseal dysplasia, mongolism, Hurler disease, skull hyperostosis, Rubinstein-Taybi syndrome
    (d) syndromes: Crouzon, Apert, Carpenter, Treacher-Collins, cloverleaf skull, craniotelencephalic dysplasia, arrhinencephaly
    (e) microcephaly: brain atrophy / dysgenesis
    (f) after shunting procedures

TYPES:
Sagittal suture most commonly affected followed by coronal suture

1. **Scaphocephaly = Dolichocephaly (55%)**
   premature closure of sagittal suture (long skull)
2. **Brachycephaly = Turricephaly (10%)**
   premature closure of coronal / lambdoid sutures (short tall skull)
3. **Plagiocephaly (7%)**
   unilateral early fusion of coronal + lambdoidal suture (lopsided skull)
4. **Trigonocephaly**: premature closure of metopic suture (forward pointing skull)
5. **Oxycephaly**: premature closure of coronal, sagittal, lambdoid sutures
6. **Cloverleaf skull** = Kleeblattschädel:
   intrauterine premature closure of sagittal, coronal, lambdoid sutures

√ sharply defined thickened sclerotic suture margins

√ delayed growth of BPD in early pregnancy

Wormian bones
= intrasutural ossicles in lambdoid, posterior sagittal, temperosquamosal sutures; normal up to 6 months of age (most frequently)

mnemonic: "PORK CHOPS I"
Pyknodysostosis
Osteogenesis imperfecta
Rickets in healing phase
Kinky hair syndrome
Cleidocranial dysostosis
Hypothyroidism / **H**ypophosphatasia
Otopalatodigital syndrome
Primary acro-osteolysis (Hajdu-Cheney) /
    Pachydermoperiostosis / **P**rogeria
Syndrome of Down
Idiopathic

Increased skull thickness
A. Generalized
1. Chronic severe anemia (eg, thalassemia, sickle cell disease)
2. Cerebral atrophy following shunting of hydrocephalus
3. Engelmann disease: mainly skull base
4. Hyperparathyroidism
5. Acromegaly
6. Osteopetrosis
B. Focal
1. Meningioma
2. Fibrous dysplasia
3. Paget disease
4. Dyke-Davidoff-Mason syndrome
5. Hyperostosis frontalis interna
= dense hyperostosis of inner table of frontal bone;
M < F

mnemonic: "HIPFAM"
Hyperostosis frontalis interna
Idiopathic
Paget disease
Fibrous dysplasia
Anemia (sickle cell, iron deficiency, thalassemia, spherocytosis)
Metastases

Hair-on-end skull
mnemonic: "SHITE"
Sickle cell disease
Hereditary spherocytosis
Iron deficiency anemia
Thalassemia major
Enzyme deficiency (glucose-6-phosphate dehydrogenase deficiency causes hemolytic anemia)

Leontiasis ossea
= overgrowth of facial bones causing leonine (lion-like) facies
1. Fibrous dysplasia
2. Paget disease
3. Craniometaphyseal dysplasia

4. Hyperphosphatasia

Abnormally thin skull
A. Generalized
1. Obstructive hydrocephalus
2. Cleidocranial dysostosis
3. Progeria
4. Rickets
5. Osteogenesis imperfecta
6. Craniolacuna
B. Focal
1. Neurofibromatosis
2. Chronic subdural hematoma
3. Arachnoid cyst

Inadequate calvarial calcification
1. Achondroplasia
2. Osteogenesis imperfecta
3. Hypophosphatasia

Osteolytic lesion of skull
A. Normal variant
1. Emissary vein
connecting venous systems inside + outside skull
√ bony channel <2 mm in width
2. Venous lake
= outpouching of diploic vein
√ extremely variable in size, shape, and number
√ irregular well-demarcated contour
3. Pacchionian granulations
√ usually multiple lesions with irregular contour in parasagittal location (within 3 cm of superior sagittal sinus) primarily involving the inner table;
Associated with   impressions by arachnoid granulations
4. Parietal foraminae
nonossification of embryonal rests in parietal fissure; bilateral at superior posterior angles of parietal bone; hereditary transmission
B. Trauma
1. Surgical burr hole
2. Leptomeningeal cyst
C. Infection
1. Osteomyelitis
2. Hydatid disease
3. Syphilis
4. Tuberculosis
D. Congenital
1. Epidermoid / dermoid
2. Neurofibromatosis (asterion defect)
3. Meningoencephalocele
4. Fibrous dysplasia
5. Osteoporosis circumscripta of Paget disease
E. Benign tumor
1. Hemangioma
2. Brown tumor
3. Eosinophilic granuloma
F. Malignant tumor
1. Solitary / multiple metastases
2. Multiple myeloma

3. Leukemia
4. Neuroblastoma

SOLITARY LYTIC LESION IN SKULL
   mnemonic: "MFT HOLE"
     Metastasis, **M**yeloma
     Fibrous dysplasia
     Tuberculosis, **T**rauma
     Histiocytosis X
     Osteomyelitis
     Leptomeningeal cyst
     Epidermoid / dermoid

MULTIPLE LYTIC LESIONS IN SKULL
   mnemonic: "BAMMAH"
     Brown tumor
     AVM
     Myeloma
     Metastases
     Amyloidosis
     Histiocytosis

Lytic area in bone flap
   mnemonic: "RATI"
     Radiation necrosis
     Avascular necrosis
     Tumor
     Infection

Button sequestrum
   mnemonic: "TORE ME"
     Tuberculosis
     Osteomyelitis
     Radiation
     Eosinophilic granuloma
     Metastasis
     Epidermoid

Absent greater sphenoid wing
   mnemonic: "M FOR MARINE"
     Meningioma
     Fibrous dysplasia
     Optic glioma
     Relapsing hematoma
     Metastasis
     Aneurysm
     Retinoblastoma
     Idiopathic
     Neurofibromatosis
     Eosinophilic granuloma

Tumors of the central skull base
  A. DEVELOPMENTAL
    1. Encephalocele
  B. INFECTION / INFLAMMATION
    1. Extension from paranasal sinus / mastoid infection
    2. Complication of trauma
    3. Fungal disease: mucormycosis in diabetics, aspergillosis in immunosuppressed patients

    4. Sinus + nasopharyngeal sarcoidosis
    5. Radiation necrosis
  C. BENIGN
    1. Juvenile angiofibroma
    2. Meningioma
    3. Chordoma
    4. Pituitary tumor
    5. Paget disease
    6. Fibrous dysplasia
  D. MALIGNANT
    1. Metastasis: prostate, lung, breast
    2. Chondrosarcoma
    3. Nasopharyngeal carcinoma
    4. Rhabdomyosarcoma
    5. Perineural tumor spread: head + neck neoplasm

J-shaped sella
   mnemonic: "NO NOAH"
     Normal variant
     Osteogenesis imperfecta
     Neurofibromatosis
     Optic glioma
     Achondroplasia
     Hurler syndrome

MANDIBLE & MAXILLA

Mandibular hypoplasia
  1. Pierre-Robin syndrome
  2. Treacher-Collins syndrome
  3. Chromosomal abnormalities
  4. Pyknodysostosis

Destruction of temperomandibular joint
   mnemonic: "HIRT"
     Hyperparathyroidism
     Infection
     Rheumatoid arthritis
     Trauma

Radiolucent lesion of mandible
  A. SHARPLY MARGINATED LESION
    (a) around apex of tooth
      1. Radicular cyst
      2. Cementinoma
    (b) around unerupted tooth
      1. Dentigerous cyst
      2. Ameloblastoma
    (c) unrelated to tooth
      1. Simple bone cyst
      2. Fong disease
      3. Basal cell nevus syndrome: multiple basal cell epitheliomas, mandibular cysts, extensive calcification of falx + tentorium, brachydactyly, bifid ribs, scoliosis
  B. POORLY MARGINATED LESIONS
    √ "floating teeth": suggestive of primary / secondary malignancy
    √ resorption of tooth root: hallmark of benign process

(a) Infection
   1. Osteomyelitis: actinomycosis
(b) Radiotherapy
   1. Osteoradionecrosis
(c) Malignant neoplasm
   1. Osteosarcoma (1/3 lytic, 1/3 sclerotic, 1/3 mixed)
   2. Local invasion from gingival / buccal neoplasms (more common)
   3. Metastasis from breast, lung, kidney in 1% (in 70% adenocarcinoma)
(d) Other
   1. Eosinophilic granuloma: "floating tooth"
   2. Fibrous dysplasia
   3. Osteocementoma
   4. Ossifying fibroma (very common)

Tooth mass

A. CYSTIC LESION
1. **Radicular cyst** (commonest)
   Cause: deep carious lesion / deep filling / trauma
   Site: intimately associated with apex of nonvital tooth
   √ apical lucency
2. **Ameloblastoma = adamantinoma of jaw**
   locally aggressive lesion from enamel-type epithelial tissue elements around tooth; 1/3 arise from dentigerous cyst
   Age: 4 – 5th decade; M:F = 1:1
   Location: mandible (75%), maxilla (25%), in region of bicuspids + molars (angle of mandible commonly affected)
   √ uni- / multilocular lytic lesion with scalloped margin + cortical expansion
   √ may be associated with impacted tooth / resorption of the root of a tooth
   Prognosis: frequently local recurrence even more aggressive after excision

3. **Primordial cyst**
   arising from follicle of tooth that never developed
   √ absent tooth
4. **Giant cell reparative granuloma**
   unrelated to tooth (nonodontogenic)
   √ lucent smooth multiloculated lesion
5. **Traumatic bone cyst**
   in association with vital tooth
   √ sharply marginated lucent lesion with finger-like projections between roots
6. **Dentigerous cyst**
   = epithelial-lined cyst from odontogenic epithelium developing around unerupted tooth
   Location: maxilla (may expand into maxillary sinus), posterior mandible
   √ cystic expansile lesion containing tooth
   Cx: may degenerate into ameloblastoma (rare)

B. SCLEROTIC LESION
1. **Cementinoma** = fibro-osteoma = periapical cemental dysplasia

Histo: spindle-cell fibroblastic proliferation + cementum
Age: 30 – 40 years of age; most common in women
Location: in anterior portion of mandible, at apex of vital tooth
√ often multicentric
√ mixed lucent + sclerotic lesion with little expansion, calcifies with time
DDx: ossifying fibroma, fibrous dysplasia, Paget disease

2. True cementoma = benign cementoblastoma
3. Gigantiform cementoma
4. **Hypercementosis**
   = bulbous enlargement of a root
   (a) idiopathic (b) associated with Paget disease
5. Benign fibro-osseous lesions
   (a) ossifying fibroma: young adults; mandible > maxilla
   (b) monostotic fibrous dysplasia: M < F, younger patients
   (c) condensing osteitis = focal chronic sclerosing osteitis
   √ near apex of nonvital tooth
6. Paget disease
   involvement of jaw in 20%; maxilla > mandible
   Location: bilateral, symmetric involvement
   √ widened alveolar ridges
   √ flat palate
   √ loosening of teeth
   √ hypercementosis
   √ may cause destruction of lamina dura
7. **Torus mandibularis** = exostosis
   Site: midline of hard palate; lingual surface of mandible in region of bicuspids

SPINE

Small vertebral body
1. Radiation therapy
   during early childhood in excess of 1000 rads
2. Juvenile rheumatoid arthritis
   Location: cervical spine
   √ atlantoaxial subluxation may be present
   √ vertebral fusion may occur
3. Eosinophilic granuloma
   Location: lumbar / lower thoracic spine
   √ compression deformity / vertebra plana
4. Gaucher disease
   = deposits of glucocerebrosides within RES
   √ compression deformity
5. Platyspondyly generalisata
   = flattened vertebral bodies associated with many hereditary systemic disorders (achondroplasia, spondyloepiphyseal dysplasia tarda, mucopolysaccharidosis, osteopetrosis, neurofibromatosis, osteogenesis imperfecta, thanatophoric dwarfism)
   √ disc spaces of normal height

VERTEBRA PLANA
   mnemonic: " FETISH"
   Fracture
   Eosinophilic granuloma
   Tumor (metastasis, myeloma)
   Infection
   Steroids (avascular necrosis)
   Hemangioma

Enlarged vertebral body
1. Paget disease
   √ "picture framing"; bone sclerosis
2. Gigantism
   √ increase in height of body + disc
3. Myositis ossificans progressiva
   √ bodies greater in height than width
   √ osteoporosis
   √ ossification of ligamentum nuchae

Enlarged vertebral foramen
1. Neurofibroma
2. Congenital absence / hypoplasia of pedicle
3. Dural ectasia (Marfan syndrome, Ehlers-Danlos syndrome)
4. Intraspinal neoplasm
5. Metastatic destruction of pedicle

Vertebral border abnormality
Straightening of anterior border
1. Ankylosing spondylitis
2. Paget disease
3. Psoriatic arthritis
4. Reiter disease
5. Rheumatoid arthritis
6. Normal variant

Anterior scalloping of vertebrae
1. Aortic aneurysm
2. Lymphadenopathy
3. Tuberculosis
4. Multiple myeloma (paravertebral soft tissue mass)

Posterior scalloping of vertebrae
in conditions associated with dural ectasia
A.   Increased intraspinal pressure
   1. Communicating hydrocephalus
   2. Ependymoma
B.   Mesenchymal tissue laxity
   1. Neurofibromatosis (secondary to dural ectasia / spinal tumor)
   2. Marfan syndrome
   3. Ehlers-Danlos syndrome
   4. Posterior meningocele
C.   Bone softening
   1. Mucopolysaccharidoses: Hurler, Morquio, Sanfilippo
   2. Acromegaly (lumbar vertebrae)
   3. Ankylosing spondylitis (lax dura acting on osteoporotic vertebrae)

4. Achondroplasia

mnemonic: "DAMN MALE SHAME"
   Dermoid
   Ankylosing spondylitis
   Meningioma
   Neurofibromatosis

   Marfan syndrome
   Acromegaly
   Lipoma
   Ependymoma

   Syringohydromyelia
   Hydrocephalus
   Achondroplasia
   Mucopolysaccharidoses
   Ehlers-Danlos syndrome

Bony projections from vertebra
1. Hurler syndrome = gargoylism
   √ rounded appearance of vertebral bodies
   √ mild kyphotic curve with smaller vertebral body at apex of kyphosis displaying tongue-like beak at anterior half (usually at T12 / L1)
   √ "step-off" deformities along anterior margins
2. Hunter syndrome
   less severe changes than in Hurler syndrome
3. Morquio disease
   √ flattened + widened vertebral bodies
   √ anterior "tongue-like" elongation of central portion of vertebral bodies
4. Hypothyroidism = cretinism
   √ small flat vertebral bodies
   √ anterior "tongue-like" deformity (in children only)
   √ widened disc spaces + irregular endplates
5. Spondylosis deformans
   √ osteophytosis along anterior + lateral aspects of endplates with horizontal + vertical course as a result of shearing of the outer annular fibers (Sharpey fibers connecting the annulus fibrosus to adjacent vertebral body)
6. Diffuse idiopathic skeletal hyperostosis (DISH) = Forrestier disease
   √ flowing calcifications + ossifications along anterolateral aspect of >4 contiguous thoracic vertebral bodies ± osteophytosis
7. Ankylosing spondylitis
   √ bilateral symmetric syndesmophytes (ossification of annulus fibrosus)
   √ "bamboo spine"
   √ "discal ballooning" = biconvex intervertebral discs secondary to osteoporotic deformity of endplates
   √ straightening of anterior margins of vertebral bodies (erosion)
   √ ossification of paraspinal ligaments
8. Fluorosis
   √ vertebral osteophytosis + hyperostosis
   √ sclerotic vertebral bodies + kyphoscoliosis
   √ calcification of paraspinal ligaments

Spine ossification
A. Syndesmophyte = ossification of annulus fibrosus
    associated with: ankylosing spondylitis, ochronosis
B. Osteophyte
    = ossification of anterior longitudinal ligament
    associated with: osteoarthritis
C. Flowing anterior ossification
    = ossification of disc, anterior longitudinal ligament, paravertebral soft tissues
    associated with: diffuse idiopathic skeletal hyperostosis
D. Paravertebral ossification
    associated with: psoriatic arthritis, Reiter syndrome

Vertebral endplate abnormality
1. Osteoporosis (senile / steroid-induced)
   √ "fish vertebrae" (DDx: osteomalacia, Paget disease, hyperparathyroidism)
   √ bone sclerosis along endplates
2. Sickle cell disease
   √ "H-vertebrae" = compression of central portions from subchondral infarcts (DDx: other anemias, Gaucher disease)
3. Schmorl node
   = intraosseous herniation of nucleus pulposus at center of weakened endplate in disc herniation / Scheuermann disease
4. Limbus vertebrae
   = intraosseous herniation of disc material at junction of vertebral bony rim of centra + endplate (anterosuperior corner)
5. "Ring" epiphysis
   = normal aspect of developing vertebra (between 6 and 12 years of age)
   √ small step-like recess at corner of anterior edge of vertebral body
6. Renal osteodystrophy
   √ "rugger-jersey spine" = horizontal bands of increased opacity subjacent to vertebral endplates
7. Myelofibrosis
   √ "rugger-jersey spine"
8. Osteopetrosis
   √ "sandwich" / "hamburger" vertebrae = sclerotic endplates alternate with radiolucent midportions of vertebral bodies

Schmorl node
= chondrification defects where periosteal vessels penetrate cartilage plates of disc
√ concave defects at upper and lower vertebral endplates with sharp margins produced by superior / inferior herniation of disc material
MR: √ node of similar signal intensity as disc
      √ low signal intensity of rim
      √ associated with narrowed disc space
DDx: mnemonic: "SHOOT"
    Scheuermann disease
    Hyperparathyroidism
    Osteoporosis
    Osteomalacia
    Trauma

Vacuum phenomenon in intervertebral disc space
= liberation of nitrogen gas from surrounding tissues into clefts with an abnormal nucleus or annulus attachment
Incidence: in up to 20% of plain radiographs / in up to 50% of spinal CT in patients > age 40
Cause:
   1. Primary / secondary degeneration of nucleus pulposus
   2. Intraosseous herniation of disc (= Schmorl node)
   3. Spondylosis deformans
   4. Adjacent vertebral metastatic disease with vertebral collapse
   5. Infection (extremely rare)

Bone-within-bone vertebra
= "ghost vertebra" following stressful event during vertebral growth phase in childhood
   1. Stress line of unknown cause
   2. Leukemia
   3. Heavy metal poisoning
   4. Thorotrast injection, TB
   5. Rickets
   6. Scurvy
   7. Hypothyroidism
   8. Hypoparathyroidism

Ivory vertebra
mnemonic: "**M**y **O**nly **S**ister **L**eft **H**ome **O**n **F**riday **P**ast"
    Myelosclerosis
    Osteoblastic metastasis
    Sickle cell disease
    Lymphoma
    Hemangioma
    Osteopetrosis
    Fluorosis
    Paget disease

Expansile lesion of vertebrae
A. INVOLVEMENT OF MULTIPLE VERTEBRAE
    Metastases, multiple myeloma / plasmacytoma, lymphoma, hemangioma, Paget disease, angiosarcoma, eosinophilic granuloma
B. INVOLVEMENT OF TWO / MORE CONTIGUOUS VERTEBRAE
    Osteochondroma, chordoma, aneurysmal bone cyst, myeloma
C. BENIGN LESION
    1. Osteochondroma (1 – 5% in spine)
       commonly thoracic, posterior elements, large dense calcified mass with ill-defined borders
    2. Osteoblastoma (40% in spine)
       M:F = 2:1; commonly cervical, posterior elements, may involve body if large, well-defined borders, calcified tumor matrix in 50%, rarely malignant degeneration

3. Giant cell tumor (5% in spine)
   commonly sacrum, expansile lytic lesion of
   vertebral body with well-defined borders;
   secondary invasion of posterior elements;
   malignant degeneration in 15 – 20%
4. Osteoid osteoma (25% in spine)
   commonly lower thoracic / upper lumbar spine,
   posterior elements (pedicle, lamina, spinous
   process), painful scoliosis with concavity toward
   lesion
5. Aneurysmal bone cyst (20% in spine)
   commonly cervical / thoracic spine, posterior
   elements, well-defined margins, arising from
   primary bone lesion (giant cell tumor, fibrous
   dysplasia) in 50%, may involve two contiguous
   vertebrae
6. Hemangioma (30% in spine)
   10% incidence in general population; commonly
   lower thoracic / upper lumbar spine, vertebral
   body, "accordion" / "corduroy" appearance
7. Hydatid cyst (1% in spine)
   slow-growing destructive lesion, well-defined
   sclerotic borders, endemic areas
8. Paget disease
   vertebral body ± posterior elements, enlargement
   of bone, "picture framing"; bone sclerosis
9. Eosinophilic granuloma (6% in spine)
   most often cervical / lumbar spine, vertebral
   body, "vertebra plana"; multiple involvement
   common
10. Fibrous dysplasia (1% in spine)
    vertebral body, nonhomogeneous trabecular
    "ground glass" appearance
D. MALIGNANT
   1. Chordoma (15% in spine)
      particularly 2nd cervical vertebra, within vertebral
      body
      √ total destruction + collapse + anterior soft
        tissue mass
      √ sclerosis adjacent to bone
      √ violates disc space
   2. Metastases (especially from lung, breast)
      Age: >50 years of age;
      Clue: pedicles often destroyed
   3. Multiple myeloma / plasmacytoma
      Clue: vertebral pedicles usually spared
   4. Angiosarcoma
      10% involve spine, most commonly lumbar
   5. Osteosarcoma, chondrosarcoma, lymphoma

Bone tumors favoring vertebral bodies
mnemonic: "CALL HOME"
   Chordoma
   Aneurysmal bone cyst
   Leukemia
   Lymphoma
   Hemangioma
   Osteoid osteoma, **O**steoblastoma
   Myeloma, **M**etastasis
   Eosinophilic granuloma

Primary vertebral tumors in children
in order of frequency
1. Osteoid osteoma
2. Benign osteoblastoma
3. Aneurysmal bone cyst
4. Ewing sarcoma

Blowout lesion of posterior elements
mnemonic: "GO APE"
   Giant cell tumor
   Osteoblastoma
   Aneurysmal bone cyst
   Plasmacytoma
   Eosinophilic granuloma

Primary tumor of posterior elements
mnemonic: "A HOG"
   Aneurysmal bone cyst
   Hydatid cyst, **H**emangioma
   Osteoblastoma, **O**steoid osteoma
   Giant cell tumor

Segmentation anomalies of vertebral bodies
during 9 – 12th week of gestation two ossification centers
form for the ventral + dorsal half of vertebral body

1. **Asomia** = agenesis of vertebral body
   √ complete absence of vertebral body
   √ hypoplastic posterior elements may be present
2. **Hemivertebra**
   (a) Unilateral wedge vertebra
       √ right / left hemivertebra
       √ scoliosis at birth
   (b) Dorsal hemivertebra
       √ rapidly progressive kyphoscoliosis
   (c) Ventral hemivertebra (extremely rare)
3. **Coronal cleft**
   = failure of fusion of anterior + posterior ossification
     centers
   May be associated with: premature male infant,
       chondrodystrophia calcificans congenita
   Location: usually in lower thoracic + lumbar spine
   √ vertical radiolucent band just behind midportion of
     vertebral body; disappears mostly by 6 months of life
4. **Butterfly vertebra**
   = failure of fusion of lateral halves secondary to
     persistence of notochordal tissue
   may be associated with: anterior spina bifida ±
       anterior meningocele
   √ widened vertebral body with butterfly configuration
     (AP view)
   √ adaptation of vertebral endplates of adjacent vertebral
     bodies
5. **Block vertebra**
   = congenital vertebral fusion
   Location: lumbar / cervical
   √ height of fused vertebral bodies equals the sum of
     heights of involved bodies + intervertebral disc
   √ "waist" at level of intervertebral disc space

6. Hypoplastic vertebra
7. Klippel-Feil syndrome

Cervical spine fusion
mnemonic: "SPAR BIT"
Senile hypertrophic ankylosis (DISH)
Psoriasis
Ankylosing spondylitis
Reiter disease
Block vertebra (Klippel-Feil)
Infection
Trauma

SPINAL DYSRAPHISM
= abnormal / incomplete fusion of midline embryologic mesenchymal, neurologic, bony structures

External signs (in 50%)
- subcutaneous lipoma
- hypertrichosis
- pigmented nevi
- skin dimple
- bladder + bowel dysfunction
- pathologic plantar response
- spastic gait disturbance
- foot deformities
- absent tendon reflexes
- sinus tract

Spina bifida
= incomplete closure of bony elements of the spine (lamina + spinous processes) posteriorly

Spina bifida occulta
= OCCULT SPINAL DYSRAPHISM
= skin covered defect; 15% of spinal dysraphism
- rarely leads to neurologic deficit in itself
Associated with:
vertebral defect (85 – 90%), lumbosacral dermal lesion (80%), ie, hairy tuft, dimple, sinus, nevus, hyperpigmentation, hemangioma, subcutaneous mass
1. Diastematomyelia
2. Lipomeningocele
3. Tethered cord syndrome
4. Filum terminale lipoma
5. Intraspinal dermoid
6. Epidermoid cyst
7. Myelocystocele
8. Split notochord syndrome
9. Meningocele
10. Dorsal dermal sinus
11. Tight filum terminale syndrome

Spina bifida aperta
= SPINA BIFIDA CYSTICA
= posterior protrusion of all / parts of the contents of the spinal canal through a bony spina bifida; 85% of spinal dysraphism
- associated with neurologic deficit in >90%

1. Simple meningocele
= herniation of CSF-filled sac without neural elements

2. Myelocele
= midline plaque of neural tissue lying exposed at the skin surface
3. Myelomeningocele
= a myelocele elevated above skin surface by expansion of subarachnoid space ventral to neural plaque
4. Myeloschisis
= surface presentation of neural elements completely uncovered by meninges

Atlantoaxial subluxation
= displacement of atlas with respect to axis
(1) Posterior atlantoaxial subluxation (rare)
(2) Anterior atlantoaxial subluxation (common)
= distance between dens + anterior arch of C1 (measurement along midplane of atlas on lateral view):
(a) predental space: >2.5 mm; >4.5 mm (in children)
(b) retrodental space: <18 mm

Causes of subluxation:
(a) Congenital
1. Occipitalization of atlas
0.75% of population; fusion of basion + anterior arch of atlas
2. Congenital insufficiency of transverse ligament
3. Os odontoideum / aplasia of dens
4. Down syndrome (20%)
5. Morquio syndrome
6. Bone dysplasia
(b) Arthritis
due to laxity of transverse ligament or erosion of dens
1. Rheumatoid arthritis
2. Psoriatic arthritis
3. Reiter syndrome
4. Ankylosing spondylitis
5. SLE
rare: in gout + CPPD
(c) Inflammatory process
Pharyngeal infection in childhood, retropharyngeal abscess, coryza, otitis media, mastoiditis, cervical adenitis, parotitis, alveolar abscess
√ dislocation 8 – 10 days after onset of symptoms
(d) Trauma (very rare without odontoid fracture)
(e) Marfan disease

mnemonic: "J-TRAP"
Juvenile rheumatoid arthritis
Trauma
Retropharyngeal spondylitis
Ankylosing spondylitis
Psoriasis

PSEUDOSUBLUXATION
= ligamentous laxity in infants allows for movement of the vertebral bodies on each other, esp. C2 on C3

Intramedullary lesion

15% of spinal canal tumors in adults; 6% of spinal cord tumors in children (1/3 of spinal neoplasms in childhood)
A. Tumor
(a) primary:
1. Ependymoma
2. Astrocytoma
3. Oligodendroglioma (3%)
4. Lipoma
Location: — cervical region: astrocytoma
— thoracic region: teratoma-dermoid
— lumbar region: ependymoma, astrocytoma, dermoid
(b) metastatic: eg, malignant melanoma, breast, lung
B. Cystic lesion
may show delayed filling of cystic space on CT-myelography
1. Syringomyelia
2. Hydromyelia
3. Reactive cyst
4. Hemangioblastoma
C. Vascular
1. Cord concussion = reversible local edema
2. Hemorrhagic contusion
3. Cord transection
4. AVM
D. Chronic infection
1. Sarcoid
2. Transverse myelitis
3. Multiple sclerosis

mnemonic: "EAGLE MASH"
Ependymoma
Astrocytoma
Glioma
Lipoma, **L**ymphoma
Epidermoid
Metastasis
Abscess
Syringomyelia
Hydromyelia, **H**ematoma

Intradural extramedullary mass

1. Neurofibroma (25 – 35%)
2. Meningioma (25 – 45% of all spinal tumors)
3. Lipoma
4. Dermoid
commonly conus / cauda equina; associated with spinal dysraphism (1/3)
5. Ependymoma
commonly filum terminale; NO spinal dysraphism
6. "Drop metastases" from CNS tumors
7. Metastases from outside CNS
with subarachnoid hemorrhage: malignant melanoma, choriocarcinoma, hypernephroma, bronchogenic carcinoma
others: breast, lymphoma,
√ predominantly dorsal location
√ single / multiple nodules
√ thickening of meninges

√ matted nerve roots
8. Arachnoid cyst
9. Neurenteric cyst
10. Hemangioblastoma

mnemonic: "MAMA N"
Metastasis
Arachnoiditis
Meningioma
AVM, **A**rachnoid cyst
Neurofibroma

Epidural extramedullary lesion

Epidural space = space between dura mater + bone containing epidural venous plexus, lymphatic channels, connective tissue, fat
Incidence: 30% of all spinal tumors

A. Tumor
(a) benign
1. Dermoid, epidermoid
2. Lipoma: over several segments
3. Fibroma
4. Neurinoma (with intradural component)
5. Meningioma (with intradural component)
6. Ganglioneuroblastoma, ganglioneuroma
(b) malignant
1. Hodgkin disease
2. Lymphoma: most commonly in dorsal space
3. Metastasis: breast, lung — most commonly from involved vertebrae without extension through dura
4. Paravertebral neuroblastoma
B. Disc disease
1. Bulging disc
2. Herniated nucleus pulposus
3. Sequestered nucleus pulposus
C. Osseous spinal stenosis, spondylosis
D. Inflammation: epidural abscess
E. Hematoma

mnemonic: "MANDELIN"
Metastasis, **M**eningioma
Arachnoiditis, **A**rachnoid cyst
Neurofibroma
Dermoid / epidermoid
Ependymoma
Lipoma
Infection (TB, cysticercosis)
Normal but tortuous roots

CSF seeding of intracranial neoplasms

occurs more frequently in pediatric age group than in adults
1. Medulloblastoma: up to 33%
2. Ependymoma: after local recurrence, more common in infra- than supratentorial ependymomas
3. Anaplastic glioma
4. Germinoma
5. Pineoblastoma, pineocytoma

Less common: malignant choroid plexus papilloma,
                angioblastic meningioma
Location: lumbosacral + dorsal thoracic spine

√   thickened + nodular nerve roots
√   nodular + irregularly narrowed thecal sac
√   enlarged cord (from coating of outer wall of spinal
    cord)
√   Gd-DTPA enhancement

Tumors of nerve roots and nerve sheaths
= NEURINOMA

A. arising from nerve sheath
   1. **Schwannoma**
      Schwann cell = cell that surrounds peripheral
      nerves providing mechanical protection, producing
      myelin sheath, serving as a tract for nerve
      regeneration
      Histo: cellular component (Antoni type A tissue)
               + myxoid component (Antoni type B tissue)
      Location: (most commonly) cervical spine roots,
                vagus nerve, sympathetic plexus
      √ solitary fusiform well-encapsulated lesion

   2. Neurilemoma
      = nerve fibers diverge and course over the surface
      of the tumor mass

B. originating from nerve
   1. Neuroma

   2. **Neurofibroma**
      = tumor of nerve sheath composed of Schwann
      cells + fibroblasts with involvement of nerve,
      nerve fibers run through mass
      Histo: swirls of neuronal elements
      Associated with   neurofibromatosis type 1;
      M:F = 1:1
      Δ Only 10% of patients with neurofibromas have
      von Recklinghausen disease!
      Location: any level, but particularly cervical
      (a)   peripheral nerves
            √ non-encapsulated well-circumscribed
              fusiform mass of peripheral nerves
      (b)   intradural extramedullary mass
            √ well-defined mass with dumbbell
              configuration (= extradural component
              extends through neural foramen)
            √ widening of intervertebral foramen + erosion
              of pedicles
            √ scalloping of vertebral bodies
      √ hypo- (CHARACTERISTIC) / isodense to
        skeletal muscle
      √ usually NO contrast enhancement
      MR:
        √ isointense to cord on T1W images
        √ hyperintense tumor on T2W images compared
          with surrounding fat
      DDx: Conjoined nerve root sleeve

Cord atrophy
1. Multiple sclerosis
2. Amyotrophic lateral sclerosis
3. Cervical spondylosis
4. Sequelae of trauma
5. Ischemia
6. Radiation therapy
7. AVM of cord

Delayed uptake of water-soluble contrast in cord lesion
1. Syringohydromyelia
2. Cystic tumor of cord
3. Osteomalacia

exceedingly rare: 4. Demyelinating disease
                    5. Infection
                    6. Infarction

Extraarachnoid myelography
A. SUBDURAL INJECTION
   √   spinal cord, nerve roots, blood vessels not outlined
   √   irregular filling defects
   √   slow flow of contrast material
   √   CSF pulsations diminished
   √   contrast material pools at injection site within anterior
       / posterior compartments

B. EPIDURAL INJECTION
   √   contrast extravasation along nerve roots
   √   contrast material lies near periphery of spinal canal
   √   intraspinal structures are not well outlined

Lumbosacral postsurgical syndrome
= signs of dysfunction and disability + pain and
  paresthesia following surgery

Cause:
A. Biomechanical failure
   1. Primary disc herniation
   2. Recurrent disc herniation
      (onset 1 week – 1 month)

B. Failure of surgical treatment
   1. Residual disc herniation
      (onset <1 week)
   2. Perioperative intraspinal hemorrhage
      (onset <1week)
   3. Spinal / meningeal / neural inflammation
      (onset 1 week – 1 month)
   4. Intraspinal scar formation (onset >1 month)
      (a)   Epidural fibrosis
            √ enhancing epidural plaque / mass
      (b)   Fibrosing arachnoiditis
            √ clumping of nerve roots
            √ adhesion of roots to wall of thecal sac
            √ abnormal enhancement of thickened
              meninges + matted nerve roots
   5. Remote phenomena unrelated to spine

Failed back surgery syndrome
= failure of improvement following back surgery in 5 –
   15%
Δ Interpretation in immediate postoperative period
   difficult, stabilization of findings occurs in 2 – 6 months

A. OSSEOUS CAUSES
   1. Spondylolisthesis
   2. Central stenosis
   3. Foraminal stenosis
   4. Pseudarthrosis
B. SOFT-TISSUE CAUSES
   1. Adhesive arachnoiditis
      √ thickened irregular clumped nerve roots
   2. Infection
   3. Hemorrhage
   4. Epidural fibrosis (scarring)
      √ heterogeneous enhancement on early T1WI
         (maximum at about 5 minutes post injection)
   5. Recurrent disc herniation
      √ no enhancement on early T1WI
         (appears enhanced ≥ 30 minutes post injection)

C. SURGICAL ERRORS
   1. Wrong level / side of surgery
   2. Direct nerve injury

Cauda equina syndrome
= constellation of signs + symptoms resulting from
   compressive lesion in lower lumbar spinal canal
Cause:
   (1) Displaced disc fragment
   (2) Intra- / extramedullary tumor
   (3) Osseous: Paget disease, osteomyelitis,
       osteoarthrosis of facet joints, complication of
       ankylosing spondylitis

- diminished sensation in lower lumbar + sacral
  dermatomes
- wasting + weakness of muscles
- decreased ankle reflexes
- impotence
- disturbed sphincter function + overflow incontinence
- decreased sphincter tone

ANATOMY OF SKULL AND SPINE

FORAMINA OF BASE OF SKULL
on inner aspect of middle cranial fossa 3 foramina are
oriented along an oblique line in the greater sphenoidal
wing from anteromedial behind the superior orbital fissure
to posterolateral
  mnemonic: "rotos"
    foramen **rot**undum
    foramen **o**vale
    foramen **s**pinosum

Foramen rotundum
  = canal within greater sphenoid wing connecting middle
    cranial fossa + pterygopalatine fossa
  Location: inferior and lateral to superior orbital fissure
  Course: extends obliquely forward + slightly inferiorly
              in a sagittal direction parallel to superior
              orbital fissure
  Contents:
    (a) nerves: V_2 (maxillary nerve)
    (b) vessels: (1) artery of foramen rotundum
                     (2) emissary vv.
  √ best visualized by coronal CT

Foramen ovale
  = canal connecting middle cranial fossa + infratemporal
    fossa
  Location: medial aspect of sphenoid body, situated
              posterolateral to foramen rotundum
              (endocranial aspect) + at base of lateral
              pterygoid plate (exocranial aspect)
  Contents:
    (a) nerves: (1) V_3 (mandibular nerve)
                     (2) lesser petrosal nerve (occasionally)
    (b) vessels: (1) accessory meningeal artery
                     (2) emissary vv.

Foramen spinosum
  Location: on greater sphenoid wing posterolateral to
              foramen ovale (endocranial aspect) + lateral
              to eustacian tube (exocranial aspect)
  Contents:
    (a) nerves: (1) recurrent meningeal branch of
                          mandibular nerve
                     (2) lesser superficial petrosal nerve
    (b) vessels: (1) middle meningeal a.
                     (2) middle meningeal v.

Foramen lacerum
  Fibrocartilage cover (occasionally), carotid artery rests
    on endocranial aspect of fibrocartilage
  Location: at base of medial pterygoid plate
  Contents: (inconstant)
    (a) nerve: nerve of pterygoid canal (actually
                    pierces cartilage)
    (b) vessel: meningeal branch of ascending
                    pharyngeal a.

Foramen magnum
  Contents:
    (a) nerves: (1) medulla oblongata
                     (2) spinal accessory n.
    (b) vessels: (1) vertebral a.
                     (2) anterior spinal a.
                     (3) posterior spinal a.

Pterygoid canal
  = VIDIAN CANAL
  = within sphenoid body connecting pterygopalatine fossa
    anteriorly to foramen lacerum posteriorly
  Location: at base of pterygoid plate below foramen
              rotundum
  Contents:
    (a) nerves: Vidian nerve = nerve of pterygoid canal
                    = continuation of greater superficial petrosal nerve
                    (from cranial nerve VII) after its union with deep
                    petrosal nerve
    (b) vessel: Vidian artery = artery of pterygoid canal
                    = branch of terminal portion of internal maxillary a.
                    arises in pterygopalatine fossa + passes through
                    foramen lacerum posterior to Vidian n.

Hypoglossal canal
  = ANTERIOR CONDYLAR CANAL
  Location: in posterior cranial fossa anteriorly above
              condyle starting above anterolateral part of
              foramen magnum, continuing in an
              anterolateral direction + exiting medial to
              jugular foramen
  Contents:
    (a) nerves: cranial nerve 12 (hypoglossal nerve)
    (b) vessels: (1) pharyngeal artery
                     (2) branches of meningeal artery

Jugular foramen
  Location: at the posterior end of petro-occipital suture
              directly posterior to carotid orifice
  A. anterior part:
      (1) inferior petrosal sinus
      (2) meningeal branches of pharyngeal artery +
             occipital artery
  B. intermediate part:
      (1) cranial nerve 9 (glossopharyngeal nerve)
      (2) cranial nerve 10 (vagus nerve)
      (3) cranial nerve 11 (accessory nerve)
  C. posterior part: internal jugular vein

MENINGES OF SPINAL CORD
  A. Periosteum
      = continuation of outer layer of cerebral dura mater
  B. Epidural space
      consists of loose areolar tissue + rich plexus of veins
      (a) cervical + thoracic spine: spacious posteriorly,
             potential space anteriorly

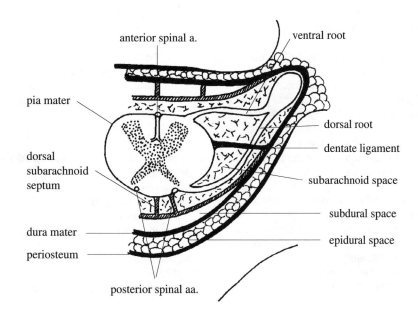

anterior spinal a.

ventral root

pia mater

dorsal root

dentate ligament

dorsal subarachnoid septum

subarachnoid space

subdural space

dura mater

epidural space

periosteum

posterior spinal aa.

Menges of Spinal Cord

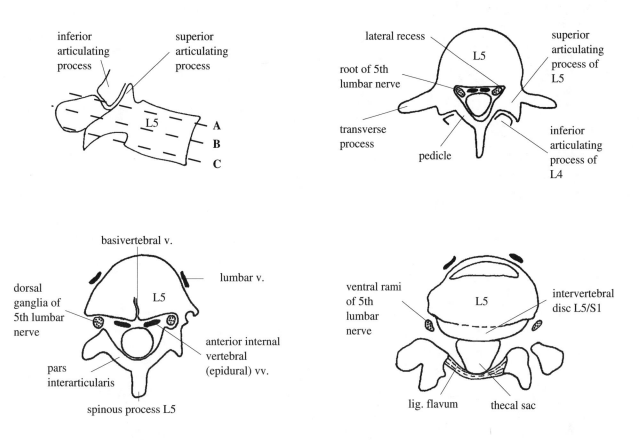

inferior articulating process

superior articulating process

L5

A

B

C

lateral recess

superior articulating process of L5

root of 5th lumbar nerve

L5

transverse process

pedicle

inferior articulating process of L4

basivertebral v.

lumbar v.

dorsal ganglia of 5th lumbar nerve

L5

anterior internal vertebral (epidural) vv.

pars interarticularis

spinous process L5

ventral rami of 5th lumbar nerve

intervertebral disc L5/S1

L5

lig. flavum

thecal sac

Cross-sections through 5th lumbar vertebra

 (b) lower lumbar + sacral spine: may occupy more than half of cross-sectional area

C. Dura
 = continuation of meningeal / inner layer of cerebral dura mater; ends at 2nd sacral vertebra + forms coccygeal ligament around filum terminale; sends tubular extensions around spinal nerves; is continuous with epineurium of peripheral nerves
 Attachment: at circumference of foramen magnum, bodies of 2nd + 3rd cervical vertebrae, posterior longitudinal ligament (by connective tissue strands)

D. Subarachnoid space
 = space between arachnoid and pia mater containing CSF, reaching as far lateral as spinal ganglia
 <u>dentate ligament</u> partially divides CSF space into an anterior + posterior compartment extending from foramen magnum to 1st lumbar vertebra, is continuous with pia mater of cord medially + dura mater laterally (between exiting nerves)

 <u>dorsal subarachnoid septum</u> connects the arachnoid to the pia mater (cribriform septum)

E. Pia mater
 = firm vascular membrane intimately adherent to spinal cord, blends with dura mater in intervertebral foramina around spinal ganglia, forms filum terminale, fuses with periosteum of 1st coccygeal segment

Normal position of conus medullaris
 Δ Vertebral bodies grow more quickly than spinal cord!
Inferior-most aspect of conus:
 L2-3 level in 97.8%
 L3 level in 1.8%
 usually at L1-2 level at 3 months of age

NOTA BENE:
 If conus is at / below L3 level, a search should be made for tethering mass, bony spur, thick filum!

SKULL AND SPINE DISORDERS

ARACHNOIDITIS
Etiology: Pantopaque (inflammatory effect potentiated by blood), back surgery, hemorrhage, trauma, idiopathic
Associated with syrinx

Myelo: √ blunting of nerve root sleeves
√ blocked nerve roots without cord displacement (2/3)
√ streaking + clumping of contrast
CT: √ fusion / clumping of nerve roots
√ featureless empty-looking sac with roots adherent to wall (final stage)

ARACHNOID CYST OF SPINE
Location: dorsal to cord in thoracic region
Site:
(a) extradural cyst secondary to congenital / acquired dural defect
(b) intradural secondary to congenital deficiency within arachnoid (= true arachnoid cyst) / adhesion from prior infection or trauma (= arachnoid loculation)

√ oval sharply demarcated extramedullary mass
√ immediate / delayed contrast filling depending upon size of opening between cyst + subarachnoid space
√ local displacement + compression of spinal cord
√ higher signal intensity than CSF (from relative lack of CSF pulsations)

ARACHNOID DIVERTICULUM
= widening of root sheath with arachnoid space occupying >50% of total transverse diameter of root + sheath together
Cause: ? congenital / traumatic, arachnoiditis, infection
Pathogenesis: hydrostatic pressure of CSF

√ scalloping of posterior margins of vertebral bodies
√ myelographic contrast material fills diverticula

ARTERIOVENOUS MALFORMATION OF SPINAL CORD
Classification:
1. True intramedullary AVM
= nidus of abnormal intermediary arteriovenous structure with multiple shunts
Age: 2nd – 3rd decade
Cx: subarachnoid hemorrhage, paraplegia
Prognosis: poor (especially in midthoracic location)
2. Intradural arteriovenous fistula
= single shunt between one / several medullary arteries + single perimedullary vein
3. Dural arteriovenous fistula
= single shunt between meningeal arteries + intradural vein
4. Metameric angiomatosis

BRACHIAL PLEXUS INJURY
1. Erb-Duchenne: adduction injury affecting C5/6 (downward displacement of shoulder)
2. Klumpke: abduction injury at C7, C8, T1 (arm stretched over head)

√ pouch-like root sleeve at site of avulsion
√ asymmetrical nerve roots
√ contrast extravasation collecting in axilla
√ metrizamide in neural foraminae (CT myelography)

CAUDAL REGRESSION SYNDROME
= spectrum of anomalies including sirenomelia (= fusion of lower extremities), lumbosacral agenesis, anal atresia, malformed external genitalia, bilateral renal aplasia, pulmonary hypoplasia, Potter facies
Incidence: 1:7,500 births; infants have diabetic mothers in 17%
Etiology: disturbance of caudal mesoderm <4th week of gestation from toxic / infectious / ischemic insult
• symptoms range from isolated deformities of feet / minor muscle weakness to complete sensorimotor paralysis of both lower extremities
• anal atresia
• genitourinary anomalies, neurogenic bladder

√ total / partial unilateral sacral agenesis
√ total / partial agenesis of lumbar + sacral spine
√ fusion of caudal-most 2 or 3 vertebrae
√ narrowing of spinal canal rostral to last intact vertebra
√ characteristic wedge-shaped cord terminus (hypoplasia of distal spinal cord)
√ spinal cord may be tethered ± associated lipoma

CHORDOMA
1 – 4% of all primary malignant neoplasms of bone;
1% of all intracranial tumors
Incidence: 1:2,000,000
Etiology: originates from embryonic notocordal remnants / ectopic cordal foci (notocord appears between 4th and 7th week of embryonic development and forms nucleus pulposus)
Age: 30 – 70 years (peak age in 5th – 7th decade); M:F = 2:1; highly malignant in children
Histo: cords + clusters of large vacuolated (physaliphorous) cells containing intracytoplasmic mucous droplets; abundant extracellular mucus deposition + areas of hemorrhage
Location: (a) 50% in sacrum (b) 35% in skull base (c) 15% spinal axis (d) other sites (5%) in mandible, maxilla, scapula
Metastases (in 10 – 30%) to: lung, lymph nodes, bone, liver, skin (late)
Prognosis: almost 100% recurrence rate despite radical surgery

SACROCOCCYGEAL CHORDOMA (50 – 70%)
40% of all sacral tumors
Peak age: 40 – 60 years; M:F = 2:1
• low back pain (70%)
• constipation / fecal incontinence
• rectal bleeding (42%)
• sciatica
• frequency, urgency, straining on micturition
• sacral mass (17%)
√ presacral mass with average size of 10 cm extending superiorly + inferiorly; rarely posterior location
√ displacement of rectum + bladder
√ solid tumor with cystic areas (in 50%)
√ osteolytic midline mass in sacrum + coccyx
√ amorphous peripheral calcifications (15 – 89%)
√ secondary bone sclerosis in tumor periphery (50%)
√ honeycomb pattern with trabeculations (10 – 15%)
Prognosis: 66% 5-year survival rate (adulthood)
DDx: Giant cell tumor, plasmacytoma, metastatic adenocarcinoma, aneurysmal bone cyst, chondrosarcoma, osteomyelitis, ependymoma

SPHENO-OCCIPITAL CHORDOMA (15 – 25%)
Age: younger patient (peak age of 20 – 40 years); M:F - 1:1
• orbitofrontal headache
• visual disturbances
• ptosis
• 6th nerve palsy / paraplegia
Location: clivus, spheno-occipital synchondrosis
√ bone destruction (in 90%): clivus > sella > petrous bone > orbit > floor of middle cranial fossa > jugular fossa > atlas > foramen magnum
√ reactive bone sclerosis (rare)
√ calcifications / bone fragments (20 – 70%)
√ soft tissue extension into nasopharynx (common), into sphenoid + ethmoid sinuses (occasionally), may reach nasal cavity + maxillary antrum
√ variable degree of enhancement
MR:
   √ large intraosseous mass extending into prepontine cistern, sphenoid sinus, middle cranial fossa, nasopharynx
   √ posterior displacement of brainstem
   √ usually isointense to brain / occasionally inhomogeneously hyperintense on T1WI
   √ hyperintense on T2WI
DDx: meningioma, metastasis, plasmacytoma, giant cell tumor, sphenoid sinus cyst, nasopharyngeal carcinoma, chondrosarcoma

VERTEBRAL CHORDOMA (15 – 20%)
more aggressive than sacral / cranial chordomas
Age: younger patient; M:F = 2:1
• low back pain + radiculopathy
Location: cervical (particularly C2) > lumbar > thoracic spine
√ total destruction of vertebra, initially unaccompanied by collapse
√ variable extension into spinal canal

√ violates disc space to involve adjacent bodies (common)
√ anterior soft tissue mass
Cx: complete spinal block
DDx: Metastasis, primary bone tumor, primary soft tissue tumor, neuroma, meningioma

CSF FISTULA
Cause:
   (1) Trauma to skull base (most commonly)
       Δ 2% of all head injuries develop CSF fistula
   (2) Tumor: especially those arising from pituitary gland
   (3) Congenital anomalies: encephalocele
• traumatic leak: usually unilateral; onset within 48 hours after trauma, usually scanty; resolve in 1 week
• nontraumatic leak: profuse flow; may persist for years
• anosmia (in 78% of trauma cases)

Location: fractures through frontoethmoidal complex + middle cranial fossa (most commonly)
√ high-resolution thin-section CT in coronal plane followed by rescanning after low-dose intrathecal contrast material instilled into lumbar subarachnoid space
Cx: Infection (in 25 – 50% of untreated cases)

DEGENERATIVE DISC DISEASE
Pathophysiology:
   loss of disc height leads to malalignment (= rostrocaudal subluxation) of facet joints causing spine instability with arthritis, capsular hypertrophy, hypertrophy of posterior ligaments, facet fracture
Plain film:
   √ narrowing of disc space
   √ disc calcification
   √ vacuum disc phenomenon = radiolucent interspace accumulation of nitrogen gas at sites of negative pressure
   √ intervertebral osteochondrosis = loss of disc space height + bone sclerosis of adjacent vertebral bodies
   √ cartilaginous nodes = intraosseous disc herniation
   √ spondylosis deformans = endplate osteophytosis secondary to anterolateral disc displacement resulting in traction osteophytes at site of osseous attachment of annulus fibrosus fibers of Sharpey
Myelography:
   √ delineation of thecal sac, spinal cord, exiting nerve roots
CT (accuracy >90%):
   √ facet joint disease (marginal sclerosis, joint narrowing, cyst formation, bony overgrowth)
MR:
   √ endplate changes (Modic & DeRoos):
   (a) Type I   (4%) with decreased signal on T1WI + increased signal on T2WI (= vascularized fibrous tissue)
   (b) Type II   (16%) with increased signal on T1WI + isointensity on T2WI (= local fatty replacement of marrow)
   (c) Type III   with decreased signal on T1WI + T2WI (= advanced sclerosis)

NUC:
  SPECT imaging of vertebrae can aid in localizing increased uptake to vertebral bodies, posterior elements, etc.
  √ eccentrically placed increased uptake on either side of an intervertebral space (osteophytes, discogenic sclerosis)
Sequelae: (1) disc bulging (2) disc herniation (3) spinal stenosis (4) facet joint disease
TERMINOLOGY:
  1. Bulge
    = concentric smooth circumferential expansion of softened disc material beyond the confines of end-plates
  2. Protrusion
    = focal protrusion of disc material maintaining broad base with parent disc due to focally weakened / ruptured annulus
  3. Extrusion
    = prominent focal extrusion of disc material with only an isthmus of connection to parent disc
  4. Free fragment
    = frank separation of disc material from parent disc
  5. Free fragment migration
    = separated disc material travels above / below intervertebral disc space

Bulging Disc

= broad-based disc extension outward in all directions with intact but weakened annulus fibrosus + posterior longitudinal ligament
Age: common finding in individuals >40 years of age
Location: lumbar, cervical spine
√ rounded symmetric defect localized to disc space level
√ concave anterior margin of thecal sac
MR: √ nucleus pulposus hypointense on T1WI + hyperintense on T2WI (water loss through degeneration)

Herniation of Nucleus Pulposus

= HNP = focal protrusion of disc material beyond margins of adjacent vertebral endplates secondary to rupture of annulus fibrosus confined within posterior longitudinal ligament
Δ 21% of asymptomatic population has disc herniation!
• local somatic spinal pain = sharp / aching, deep, localized
• centrifugal radiating pain = sharp, well-circumscribed, superficial, "electric", confined to dermatome
• centrifugal referred pain = dull, ill-defined, deep or superficial, aching or boring, confined to somatome (= dermatome + myotome + sclerotome)
Location: L4/5 (35%) > L5/S1 (27%) > L3/4 (19%) > L2/3 (14%) > L1/2 (5%); thoracic spine affected in 3:1,000 disc operations
  (a) posterolateral (49%) = weakest point along posterolateral margin of disc at lateral recess of spinal canal (posterior longitudinal ligament tightly adherent to posterior margins of disc)

  (b) posterocentral (8%)
  (c) bilateral (on both sides of posterior ligament)
  (d) lateral / foraminal (<10%)
  (e) intraosseous / vertical = Schmorl node (14%)
  (f) extraforaminal = anterior (commonly overlooked) (29%)

Myelography:
  √ sharply angular indentation on lateral aspect of thecal sac with extension above or below level of disc space (ipsilateral oblique projection best view)
  √ asymmetry of posterior disc margin
  √ double contour secondary to superimposed normal + abnormal side (horizontal beam lateral view)
  √ narrowing of intervertebral disc space (most commonly a sign of disc degeneration)
  √ deviation of nerve root / root sleeve
  √ enlargement of nerve root secondary to edema ("trumpet sign")
  √ amputated / truncated nerve root (nonfilling of root sleeve)
MR:
  √ herniated disc material of low-signal intensity displaces the posterior longitudinal ligament and epidural fat of relative high signal intensity on T1WI
Cx: spinal stenosis

Free Fragment Herniation

= DISC SEQUESTRATION
= complete separation of disc material with rupture through posterior longitudinal ligament into epidural space

√ migration superiorly / inferiorly away from disc space with compression of nerve root above / below level of disc herniation
√ disc material noted >9 mm away from intervertebral disc space

DDx: (1) Postoperative scarring (retraction of thecal sac to side of surgery)
        (2) Epidural abscess
        (3) Epidural tumor
        (4) Conjoined nerve root (2 nerve roots arising from thecal sac simultaneously representing mass in ventrolateral aspect of spinal canal; normal variant in 1 – 3% of population)

Cervical Disc Herniation

Peak age: 3rd – 4th decade
• neck stiffness, muscle splinting
• dermatomic sensory loss
• weakness + muscle atrophy
• reflex loss
Sites: C6-7 (69%); C5-6 (19%); C7-T1 (10%); C4-5 (2%)
Sequelae:
  (1) compression of exiting nerve roots
  (2) cord compression (spinal stenosis + massive disc rupture)

DERMOID OF SPINE

= uni- / multilocular cystic tumor lined by squamous
epithelium containing skin appendages (hair follicles,
sweat glands, sebaceous glands)

Cause:
- (a) congenital dermal rest / focal expansion of dermal
   sinus
- (b) acquired from implantation of viable dermal tissue
   (by spinal needle without trocar)

Incidence: 1% of spinal cord tumors
Age at presentation: <20 years; M:F = 1:1
May be associated with   dermal sinus (in 20%)
- slowly progressive myelopathy
- acute onset of chemical meningitis (secondary to
  rupture of inflammatory cholesterol crystals from cyst
  into CSF)

Location: lumbosacral (60%), cauda equina (20%)
Site: extramedullary (60%), intramedullary (40%)
√ almost always complete spinal block on myelography
√ intensity of fat
√ occasionally hypointense on T1WI + hypodense on CT
   (secretions from sweat glands within tumor)
√ NO contrast enhancement
√ CT myelography facilitates detection

DIASTEMATOMYELIA

= SPLIT CORD = MYELOSCHISIS
= sagittal division of spinal cord into two hemicords, each
  of which contains a central canal, one dorsal horn + one
  ventral horn

Etiology: congenital malformation as a result of split
         notochord; M:F = 1:3

Path:
- (a) 2 hemicords each covered by layer of pia within
   single subarachnoid space + dural sac (60%); not
   accompanied by bony spur / fibrous band
- (b) 2 hemicords each with its own pial, subarachnoidal
   + dural sheath (40%); accompanied by fibrous band
   (in 25%), cartilaginous / bony spurs (in 75%)

Associated with: myelomeningocele
- hypertrichosis, nevus, lipoma, dimple, hemangioma
  overlying the spine (26 – 81%)
- clubfoot (50%)
- muscle wasting, ankle weakness in one leg

Location: lower thoracic / upper lumbar > upper thoracic
         > cervical spine
√ congenital scoliosis (50 – 75%)
   Δ 5% of patients with congenital scoliosis have
      diastematomyelia
√ spina bifida over multiple levels
√ anteroposterior narrowing of vertebral bodies
√ widening of interpediculate distance
√ narrowed disc space with hemivertebra, butterfly
   vertebra, block vertebra
√ fusion + thickening of adjacent laminae (90%)
- (a) fusion to ipsilateral lamina at adjacent levels
- (b) diagonal fusion to contralateral adjacent lamina
   = intersegmental laminar fusion
√ bony spur through center of spinal canal arising from
   posterior aspect of centra (<50%)

√ thickened filum terminale >2 mm (>50%)
√ tethered cord (>50%)
√ low conus medullaris below L2 level (>75%)
√ the 2 hemicords usually reunite caudal to cleft
√ defect in thecal sac on myelogram
Cx: progressive spinal cord dysfunction

DISCITIS

most common pediatric spine problem
Etiology: blood-borne bacterial invasion of vertebrae
         infecting disc via communicating vessels
         through endplate
Agents:
- (a) Pyogenic: Staphylococcus aureus (most frequent),
   Gram-negative rods (in IV drug abusers /
   immunocompromised patients)
- (b) Nonpyogenic: tuberculosis, coccidioidomycosis
Pathogenesis:
   infection starts in disc (still vascularized in children) / in
   anterior inferior corner of vertebral body (in adults) with
   spread across disc to adjacent vertebral endplate
Age peak: 6 months – 4 years and 10 – 14 years;
         average age of 6 years at presentation
- fever, irritability, malaise
- back / referred hip pain, limp
- failure to bear weight

Location: L3/4, L4/5, unusual above T9
Plain film (positive 2 – 4 weeks after onset of symptoms):
√ disc space narrowing (earliest sign) = intraosseous
   herniation of nucleus pulposus into vertebral body
   through weakened endplate
√ indistinctness of adjacent endplates with destruction
√ endplate sclerosis (during healing)
CT:
√ paravertebral inflammatory mass
√ epidural soft tissue extension with deformity of thecal
   sac
MR (preferred modality):
√ decreased marrow intensity on T1WI in two
   contiguous vertebrae
√ in early stage preserved disc height with variable
   intensity on T2WI (often increased)
√ in later stages loss of disc height with increased
   intensity on T2WI
NUC (90% sensitivity on Tc-99m MDP + Tc-99m WBC
scans):
√ positive before radiographs
√ bone scan usually positive in adjacent vertebrae (until
   age 20) secondary to vascular supply via endplates;
   may be negative after age 20
Cx: kyphosis

DORSAL DERMAL SINUS

= epithelium-lined dural tube extending from skin surface
  to intracanalicular space + frequently communicating
  with CNS / its coverings
Cause: focal area of incomplete separation of
         cutaneous ectoderm from neural ectoderm
         during neurulation

Age: encountered in early childhood – 3rd decade;
M:F = 1:1
- midline dimple / pinpoint ostium
- hyperpigmented patch / hairy nevus / capillary angioma
Location: lumbosacral (60%), occipital (25%), thoracic (10%), cervical (2%), sacrococcygeal (1%), ventral (8%)
CT myelography (best modality to define intraspinal anatomy):
√ groove in upper surface of spinous process + lamina of vertebra
√ hypoplastic spinous process
√ single bifid spinous process
√ focal multilevel spina bifida
√ laminar defect
√ dorsal tenting of dura + arachnoid
√ sinus may terminate in conus medullaris / filum terminale / nerve root / fibrous nodule on dorsal aspect of cord / dermoid / epidermoid
√ nerve roots bound down to capsule of dermoid / epidermoid cyst
√ displacement / compression of cord by extramedullary dermoids / epidermoids
√ expansion of cord by intramedullary dermoids / epidermoids
√ clumping of nerve roots from adhesive arachnoiditis

Δ 50% of dorsal dermal sinuses end in dermoid / epidermoid cysts!
Δ 20 – 30% of dermoid cysts / dermoid tumors are associated with dermal sinus tracts!
Cx:
(1) meningitis (bacterial / chemical)
(2) subcutaneous / epidural / subdural / subarachnoid / subpial abscess (bacterial ascent)
Δ dermal sinus accounts for up to 3% of spinal cord abscesses!
(3) compression of neural structures

EPIDERMOID OF SPINE
= cystic tumor lined by a membrane composed of epidermal elements of skin
Cause:
(a) congenital dermal rest / focal expansion of dermal sinus
(b) acquired from implantation of viable epidermal tissue (by spinal needle without trocar)
Incidence: 1% of spinal cord tumors
Age at presentation: 3rd – 5th decade; M>F
May be associated with dermal sinus
- slowly progressive myelopathy
- acute onset of chemical meningitis (secondary to rupture of inflammatory cholesterol crystals from cyst into CSF)
Location: upper thoracic (17%), lower thoracic (26%), lumbosacral (22%), cauda equina (35%)
Site: extramedullary (60%), intramedullary (40%)
√ almost always complete spinal block on myelography
√ displacement of spinal cord / nerve roots
√ small tumors isointense to CSF

√ NO contrast enhancement
√ CT myelography facilitates detection

EPIDURAL HEMATOMA OF SPINE
Etiology: (1) vertebral fracture / dislocation (2) traumatic lumbar puncture (3) hypertension (4) AVM (5) vertebral hemangioma (6) bleeding diathesis / anticoagulation / hemophilia (7) idiopathic (45%)
Peak age: 40 – 50 years
- acute radicular pain
- paraplegia
Location: thoracic spine (most common)
√ compression of posterior aspect of cord
√ high attenuation lesion on CT
√ iso- / slightly hypointense lesion on T1WI with marked increase in intensity on T2WI

FRACTURES OF SKULL
1. Linear fracture (most common type) (DDx: vascular groove, suture)
2. Depressed fracture surgery indicated if depression >5 mm
3. Skull-base fracture

LeFort Fracture
= all LeFort fractures involve pterygoid process
A. LeFort I = Transverse maxillary fracture caused by blow to premaxilla
Fracture line: (a) alveolar ridge (b) lateral aperture of nose (c) inferior wall of maxillary sinus
√ detachment of alveolar process of maxilla
B. LeFort II = "Pyramidal fracture"
Fracture line: arch through (a) posterior alveolar ridge (b) medial orbital rim (c) across nasal bones
√ separation of midportion of face
C. LeFort III = "craniofacial dysjunction"
Fracture line: horizontal course through (a) naso-frontal suture (b) maxillo-frontal suture (c) orbital wall (d) zygomatic arch
√ separation of entire face from base of skull

Sphenoid Bone Fracture
Incidence: involved in 15% of skull-base fractures
- CSF rhinorrhea / otorrhea
- hematotympanum
- battle sign = mastoid region ecchymosis
- racoon eyes = periorbital ecchymosis
- 7th / 8th nerve palsy
- muscular dysfunction: problems with ocular motility, mastication, speech, swallowing, eustachian tube function
√ air-fluid level in sinuses + mastoid
√ axial thin-slice high-resolution CT for best delineation of fractures
√ water-soluble intrathecal contrast material for CSF fistula

Zygomaticomaxillary Fracture

= "TRIPOD" FRACTURE = MALAR / ZYGOMATIC
COMPLEX FRACTURE

Cause: direct blow to malar eminence
- loss of sensibility of face below orbit
- deficient mastication
- double vision / ophthalmoplegia
- facial deformity

Fracture line:
   (a) lateral wall of maxillary sinus (b) orbital rim close
   to infraorbital foramen (c) floor of orbit (d) zygomatico-
   frontal suture / zygomatic arch

Blow-out Fracture

= isolated fracture of orbital floor

Cause: sudden direct blow to globe with increase in
   intraorbital pressure transmitted to the weak
   orbital floor, often associated with fracture of
   the thin lamina papyracea
- diplopia on upward gaze (entrapment of inferior
  rectus + inferior oblique muscles)
- enophthalmus
- facial anesthesia

√ soft tissue mass extending into maxillary sinus
√ complete opacification of maxillary sinus (edema +
  hemorrhage)
√ depression of orbital floor
√ posttraumatic atrophy of orbital fat leads to
  enophthalmus

FRACTURES OF CERVICAL SPINE

Frequency: C2, C6 > C5, C7 > C3, C4 > C1
Location:
   (a) upper cervical spine = C1/2 (19 – 25%):
       atlas (4%), odontoid (6%)
   (b) lower cervical spine = C3 – 7 (75 – 81%)
Site: vertebral arch (50%), vertebral body (30%),
      intervertebral disc (25%), posterior ligaments
      (16%), dens (14%), locked facets (12%), anterior
      ligament (2%)
Associated with
      thoracic / lumbar spine fracture in 5 – 15%

A. HYPERFLEXION INJURY (46 – 79%)
   1. Odontoid fracture
   2. Simple wedge fracture (stable)
   3. Teardrop fracture: most severe + unstable injury of
      C-spine
   4. Anterior subluxation
   5. Bilateral locked facets (unstable)
   6. Anterior disc space narrowing
   7. Widened interspinous distance
   8. Spinous process fracture = clay shoveler's fracture
      = sudden load on flexed spine with avulsion
      fracture of C6 / C7 / T1 (stable)

B. HYPEREXTENSION INJURY (20 – 38%)
   1. Anteriorly widened disc space
   2. Prevertebral swelling

   3. **Teardrop fracture** = avulsion of anteroinferior
      corner by anterior ligament (unstable) typically at C2
   4. Neural arch fracture of C1 (stable = anterior ring +
      transverse ligament intact)
   5. Subluxation (anterior / posterior)
   6. **Hangman's fracture** = bilateral neural arch fracture
      of C2 (unstable)
      √ prevertebral soft tissue swelling
      √ anterior subluxation of C2 on C3
      √ avulsion of anteroinferior corner of C2 (rupture of
        anterior longitudinal ligament)

C. FLEXION-ROTATION INJURY (12%)
   1. Unilateral locked facets (oblique views!, stable)

D. VERTICAL COMPRESSION (4%)
   1. **Jefferson fracture** = comminuted fracture of ring of
      C1 (unstable)
      √ lateral displacement of lateral massa (self-
        decompressing)
      (DDx: Pseudo-Jefferson fracture = lateral offset of
      lateral masses of atlas without fracture in fusion
      anomalies of anterior / posterior arches of C1, in
      children as lateral masses of atlas ossify earlier than
      C2)
   2. Burst fracture = intervertebral disc driven into
      vertebral body below (stable)
      √ several fragments, fragment from posterior
        superior margin often in spinal canal

E. LATERAL FLEXION / SHEARING (4 – 6%)
   1. Uncinate fracture
   2. Isolated pillar fracture
   3. Transverse process fracture
   4. Lateral vertebral compression

Atlas fracture

Incidence: 4% of cervical spine injuries
Site: posterior arch, anterior arch, massa lateralis,
      Jefferson fracture
Associated with:
   fractures of C7 (25%), C2 pedicle (15%), extraspinal
   fractures (58%)

Axis fracture

Incidence: 6% of cervical spine injuries
associated with fractures of C1 in 8%
   Type I = avulsion of tip of ondontoid (5 – 8%)
            √ difficult to detect
   Type II = fracture through base of dens (54 – 67%)
            Cx: nonunion
   Type III = subdental fracture (30 – 33%)
            Prognosis: good
DDx: os ondontoideum, ossiculum terminale,
       hypoplasia of dens, aplasia of dens

FRACTURES OF THORACOLUMBAR SPINE

40% of all vertebral fractures that cause neurologic deficit,
mostly complex (body + posterior elements involved)
√ diastasis of apophyseal joints

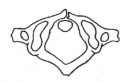
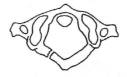
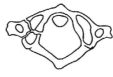
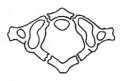

Anterior arch fracture **Posterior arch fracture** **Lateral mass fracture** **Jefferson fracture**

Atlas Fracture

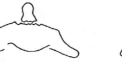

Type I **Type II** **Type III**

Axis Fracture

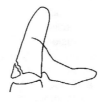
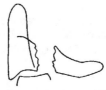

Teardrop fracture **Hangman's fracture**

Dens Fractures

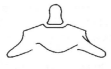
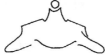

Os odontoideum **Ossiculum terminale** **Hypoplasia of dens** **Aplasia of dens**

√ disruption of interspinal ligament
√ retropulsion of body fragments into spinal canal
√ "burst" fragments at superior surface of body

Chance Fracture

= SEATBELT FRACTURE
Mechanism: shearing flexion injury (lap-type seatbelt
       injury in back-seat passengers)
• neurologic deficit infrequent
Location: L-2 or L-3
√ horizontal splitting of spinous process, neural arch +
  superior portion of vertebral body

Often associated with
(1) bone injury
    rib fractures along the course of diagonal strap;
    sternal fractures; clavicular fractures

(2) soft tissue injury
    transverse tear of rectus abdominis muscle;
    anterior peritoneal tear; diaphragmatic rupture

(3) vascular injury
    mesenteric vascular tear; transection of common
    carotid artery; injury to internal carotid artery,
    subclavian artery, superior vena cava; thoracic
    aortic tear; abdominal aortic transection

(4) visceral injury
    perforation of jejunum + ileum > large intestine >
    duodenum (free intraperitoneal fluid in 100%,
    mesenteric infiltration in 88%, thickened bowel
    wall in 75%, extraluminal air in 56%); laceration /
    rupture of liver, spleen, kidneys, pancreas,
    distended urinary bladder; uterine injury

CHANCE EQUIVALENT
= purely ligamentous disruption leading to lumbar
subluxation / dislocation
√ mild widening of posterior aspect of affected disc
space
√ widened facet joints
√ splaying of spinous processes = "empty hole sign"
on AP view

GLIOMA OF SPINAL CORD

Often associated with: syrinx

1. Ependymoma (60 – 70%)
   Location: lower spinal cord, conus medullaris, filum
   terminale; extends over several vertebral
   segments
   √ well-demarcated / diffusely infiltrating tumor
   √ occupies whole width of spinal cord
   √ focal mass with areas of extensive cystic
   degeneration, hemorrhage, and calcification
   √ erosion of vertebral body (uncommon)
   MR:
   √ intense homogeneous sharply marginated focal
   enhancement on Gd-enhanced MR
   √ hypointense tumor margin on T1WI + T2WI

2. Astrocytoma (30%)
   Histo: Low grade astrocytoma I and II (75%), high
   grade astrocytoma III and IV (8%)
   Location: thoracic + cervical spine; often extending
   into lower brainstem
   √ usually homogeneous extensive cord tumor with
   widening of spinal cord
   √ eccentric location within spinal cord
   √ dilated veins on surface of cord
   √ mass may be cystic with water-soluble
   myelographic contrast entering cystic space on
   delayed CT images
   √ patchy irregular Gd enhancement on MR

HEMANGIOBLASTOMA OF SPINE

= ANGIOBLASTOMA = ANGIORETICULOMA
Incidence: 2% of all spinal cord tumors; mostly
sporadic
Associated with: von Hippel-Lindau disease (in 1/3)
Age: middle age; M:F = 1:1
Location: intramedullary (75%), radicular (20%),
intradural extramedullary (5%); solitary in
>90%; mostly in cervicothoracic spine
√ increased interpediculate distance (mass effect)
√ expanded cord
√ intratumoral cystic component (50 – 60%)
√ large draining veins form sinuous mass along posterior
aspect of cord
√ densely staining tumor nodule
√ frequently accompanies syrinx
MR:
√ well-demarcated Gd-enhancing mass
√ curvilinear area of signal void
Cx: intramedullary hemorrhage

KLIPPEL-FEIL SYNDROME

= BREVICOLLIS = synostosis of two / more cervical
segments
May be associated with:
platybasia, syringomyelia, encephalocele, facial +
cranial asymmetry, Sprengel deformity (25 – 40%),
syndactyly, clubbed foot, hypoplastic lumbar vertebrae;
renal anomalies in 50% (agenesis, dysgenesis,
malrotation, duplication, renal ectopia); congenital heart
disease in 5% (atrial septal defect, coarctation)
• clinical triad of
  (1)   short neck
  (2)   restriction of cervical motion
  (3)   low posterior hairline
• deafness (30%)
• webbed neck
Location: cervical spine
√ fusion of vertebral bodies and posterior elements
√ ± hemivertebrae
√ may have cervicothoracic / cervical / atlanto-occipital
fusion
√ torticollis
√ scoliosis
√ rib fusion
√ Sprengel deformity (25 – 40%) = elevation + medial
rotation of scapula (may be related to presence of
anomalous omovertebral bone)
√ ear anomalies: absent auditory canal, microtia,
deformed ossicles, underdevelopment of bony labyrinth

KÜMMELL DISEASE

= intravertebral vacuum phenomenon
Cause: 1. Osteonecrosis
                2. Weeks to months following acute fracture
Pathophysiology: likely to represent gaseous release
into bony clefts within a nonhealed
fracture underneath endplate
Age: >50 years
Location: most commonly at thoracolumbar junction
√ gas collection increasing with extension + traction,
decreasing with flexion

LEPTOMENINGEAL CYST

= "Growing" fracture
Incidence: 1% of all pediatric skull fractures
Pathogenesis:
skull fracture with dural tear leads to arachnoid
herniation into dural defect; CSF pulsations produce
fracture diastasis + erosion of bone margins (apparent
2 – 3 months after injury)
Age: usually <3 years
√ skull defect with indistinct scalloped margins
√ CSF-density cyst adjacent to / in skull, may contain
cerebral tissue
MR:
√ cyst isointense with CSF + communicating with
subarachnoid space
√ area of encephalomalacia underlying fracture
(frequent)
√ intracranial tissue extending between edges of bone

LIPOMA OF SPINE
= partially encapsulated mass of fat + connective tissue with connection to leptomeninges / spinal cord
Types:
  (a) intradural lipoma (4%)
  (b) lipomyelomeningocele (84%)
  (c) fibrolipoma of filum terminale (12%)
Δ Intradural lipomas + lipomyelomeningoceles represent 35% of skin-covered lumbosacral masses + 20 – 50% of occult spinal dysraphism!

Intradural Lipoma
= subpial juxtamedullary mass totally enclosed in intact dural sac
Incidence: <1% of primary intraspinal tumors
Age peaks: first 5 years of life (24%), 2nd + 3rd decade (55%), 5th decade (16%)
• slow ascending mono- / paraparesis, spasticity, cutaneous sensory loss, defective deep sensation (with cervical + thoracic intradural lipoma)
• flaccid paralysis of legs, sphincter dysfunction (with lumbosacral intradural lipoma)
• overlying skin most often normal
• elevation of protein in CSF (30%)
Location: cervical (12%) / cervicothoracic (24%) / thoracic (30%); dorsal aspect of cord (75%), lateral / anterolateral (25%)
√ spinal cord open in midline dorsally
√ lipoma in opening between lips of placode
√ exophytic component at upper / lower pole of lipoma
√ syringohydromyelia (2%)
√ focal enlargement of spinal canal ± adjacent neural foramina
√ narrow localized spina bifida

Lipomyelomeningocele
= lipoma tightly attached to exposed dorsal surface of neural placode blending with subcutaneous fat
Incidence: 20% of skin-covered lumbosacral masses; up to 50% of occult spinal dysraphism
Age: typically <6 months of age; M<F
• semifluctuant lumbosacral mass with overlying skin intact
• sensory loss in sacral dermatomes, motor loss, bladder dysfunction
• foot deformities, leg pain
Location: lumbosacral; longitudinal extension over entire length of spinal canal (in 7%)
√ lipoma may enter central canal and extend rostrally (= "intradural intramedullary lipoma")
√ lipoma may extend upward within spinal canal external to dura (= "epidural lipoma")
√ tethered cord
√ large spinal canal
√ erosion of vertebral body + pedicles
√ posterior scalloping (50%)
√ focal spina bifida
√ segmental anomalies / butterfly vertebra (up to 43%)
√ confluent sacral foramina / partial sacral agenesis (up to 50%)

Fibrolipoma of Filum Terminale
Incidence: 6% of autopsies
• asymptomatic
Location: intradural filum, extradural filum, involvement of both portions
Prognosis: potential for development of symptoms of tethered cord

LÜCKENSCHÄDEL
= CRANIOLACUNIA = LACUNAR SKULL = mesenchymal dysplasia of calvarial ossification (developmental disturbance)
Age: present at birth
Associated with: (1) meningocele / myelomeningocele (2) encephalocele (3) spina bifida (4) cleft palate (5) Arnold-Chiari II malformation
• normal intracranial pressure
Location: particularly upper parietal area
√ honeycombed appearance about 2 cm in diameter (thinning of diploic space)
√ premature closure of sutures (turricephaly / scaphocephaly)
Prognosis: spontaneous regression within first 6 months of life
DDx:
  (1) Convolutional impressions = "digital" markings (visible at 2 years, maximally apparent at 4 years, disappear by 8 years of age)
  (2) "Beaten brass" = "hammered silver" appearance of increased intracranial pressure

MENINGIOMA OF SPINE
Incidence: 25 – 45% of all spine tumors; 2 – 3% of pediatric spinal tumors; 12% of all meningiomas
Age: >40 years + female (80%)
Location: thoracic region (82%); cervical spine on anterior cord surface near foramen magnum (2nd most common location); 90% on lateral aspect
Site: intradural extramedullary (50%); entirely epidural; intradural + epidural
• spinal cord / nerve root compression
√ bone erosion in <10%
√ scalloping of posterior aspect of vertebral body
√ widening of interpedicular distance
√ enlargement of intervertebral foramen
√ may calcify (not as readily as intracranial meningioma)
CT:
  √ solid smoothly marginated mass isodense to skeletal muscle
  √ marked enhancement
MR:
  √ isointense to grey matter on T1WI + T2WI
  √ rapid + dense enhancement after Gd-DTPA

METASTASES TO SPINE
Source:
  (a) Metastatic tumors: breast, prostate, lung, kidney, lymphoma, malignant melanoma

(b) Primary tumor: multiple myeloma
Pathogenesis: hematogenous spread to vertebral bodies
(bones with greatest vascularity)
MR:
√ patchy multifocal relatively well-defined lesions
√ diminished signal on T1WI + increased signal on
T2WI (except for blastic metastases with diminished
T1 + T2 signals)
DDx:
(1) Infection (centered around disc space)
(2) Primary vertebral tumor (rare in older patients,
almost always benign in patients <21 years of age)

MYELOCYSTOCELE

= SYRINGOCELE
= hydromyelic spinal cord + arachnoid herniated through
posterior spina bifida; least common form of spinal
dysraphism
May be associated with: GI tract anomalies, GU tract
anomalies
• cystic skin-covered mass over spine
• cloacal exstrophy (frequent)
Location: lower spine > cervical > thoracic spine
√ direct continuity of meningocele with subarachnoid
space
√ cyst communicating with widenend central canal of
spinal cord typically posteriorly + inferiorly to
meningocele
√ lordosis, scoliosis, partial sacral agenesis (common)

MYELOMENINGOCELE

= sac covered by leptomeninges containing CSF +
variable amount of neural tissue; herniated through a
defect in the posterior / anterior elements of spine
Incidence: 1:1,000 – 2,000 births (in Great Britain 1:200
births); twice as common in infants of
mothers >35 years of age; Caucasians >
Blacks > Orientals; most common congenital
anomaly of CNS
Etiology: localized defect of closure of caudal neuropore
(usually closed by 28 days)
• positive family history in 10%
• neural placode = reddish neural tissue in the middle of
back made up of open spinal cord
• normal skin / cutaneous abnormality: pigmented nevus,
abnormal distribution of hair, skin dimple, angioma,
lipoma
• MS-AFP (≥ 2.5 S.D. over mean) permits detection in
80% (positive predictive value of 2 – 5%) if defect not
covered by full skin thickness
Recurrence rate: 3 – 7% chance of NTD with previously
affected sibling / in fetus of affected parent

Associated with:
(1) Hydrocephalus (70 – 90%): requiring ventriculo-
peritoneal shunt in 90%
Δ 25% of patients with hydrocephalus have spina
bifida!
(2) Chiari II malformation (100%)
(3) Congenital / acquired kyphoscoliosis (90%)

(4) Vertebral anomalies (vertebral body fusion,
hemivertebrae, cleft vertebrae, butterfly vertebrae)
(5) Diastematomyelia (31 – 46%): spinal cord split
above (31%), below (25%), at the same level (22%)
as the myelomeningocele
(6) Duplication of central canal (5%) cephalic to + at
level of placode
(7) **Hemimyelocele** (10%) = two hemicords in
separate dural tubes separated by fibrous / bony
spur: one hemicord with myelomeningocele on one
side of midline, one hemicord normal / with smaller
myelomeningocele at a lower level
• impaired neurological function on side of
hemimyelocele
(8) Hydromyelia (29 – 77%) depending on efficacy of
hydrocephalus treatment
(9) Chromosomal anomalies

Location:
(a) **dorsal meningocele:**   lumbosacral (70% below
L2), suboccipital
(b) **anterior sacral meningocele** = prolapse through
anterior sacral bony defect; occasionally
associated with neurofibromatosis type 1, Marfan
syndrome, partial sacral agenesis, imperforate
anus, anal stenosis, tethered spinal cord, GU tract /
colonic anomalies; M:F = 1:4
(c) **lateral thoracic meningocele** through enlarged
intervertebral foramen into extrapleural aspect of
thorax; right > left side, in 10% bilateral; often
associated with neurofibromatosis (85%) + sharply
angled scoliosis convex to meningocele
√ expanded spinal canal
√ erosion of posterior surface of vertebral body
√ thinning of neural arch
√ enlarged neural foramen
(d) **lateral lumbar meningocele** through enlarged
neural foramina into subcutaneous tissue /
retroperitoneum; often associated with
neurofibromatosis / Marfan syndrome
√ expanded spinal canal
√ erosion of posterior surface of vertebral body
√ thinning of neural arch
√ enlarged neural foramen
(e) **traumatic meningocele** = avulsion of spinal nerve
roots secondary to tear in meningeal root sheath; in
C-spine after brachial plexus injury (most
commonly)
√ small irregular arachnoid diverticulum with
extension outside the spinal canal
(f) **cranial meningocele** = encephalocele

OB-US: detection rate of 85 – 90%; sensitivity dependent
on GA (fetal spine may be adequately visualized
after 16 – 20 weeks GA); false-negative rate of
24%
√ may have clubfoot / rocker-bottom foot
√ polyhydramnios
@ Spine:
√ loss of epidermal integrity

√ soft tissue mass protruding posteriorly + visualization of sac

√ widening of lumbar spine with fusiform enlargement of spinal canal

√ splaying (= divergent position) of ossification centers of laminae with cup- / wedge-shaped pattern (in transverse plane = most important section for diagnosis)

√ absence of posterior line = posterior vertebral elements (in sagittal plane)

√ gross irregularity in parallelism of lines representing laminae of vertebrae (in coronal plane)

√ anomalies of segmentation / hemivertebrae (33%) with short-radius kyphoscoliosis

√ tethered cord (with lumbar / lumbosacral myelomeningocele)

@ Head:

√ "lemon sign" = concave / linear frontal contour abnormality located at coronal suture (in 98% of fetuses ≤24 weeks + 13% of fetuses >24 weeks; positive predictive value 81 – 84%, false-positive rate of 1%)

√ "banana sign" = obliteration of cisterna magna with cerebellum wrapped around posterior brainstem secondary to downward traction of spinal cord in Arnold-Chiari malformation type II (in 96% of fetuses ≤24 weeks + in 91% of fetuses >24 weeks)

√ nonvisualization of cerebellum

√ obliterated cisterna magna (100% sensitivity)

√ absence of normal cisterna magna

√ BPD <5th percentile (65 – 79% sensitivity)

√ HC <5th percentile (35% sensitivity)

√ ventricular dilatation (40 – 90%) with choroid incompletely filling the ventricles (54 – 63% sensitivity)

Plain films:

√ bony defect in neural arch

√ deformity + failure of fusion of lamina

√ absent spinous process

√ widened interpedicular distance

√ widened spinal canal

Rx: (1) Possibly elective cesarean section at 36 – 38 weeks GA (may decrease risk of contaminating / rupturing the meningomyelocele sac)

(2) Repair within 48 hours

Postoperative complications:

(1) Postoperative tethering of spinal cord by placode / scar

(2) Constricting dural ring

(3) Cord compression by lipoma / dermoid / epidermoid cyst

(4) Ischemia from vascular compromise

(5) Syringohydromyelia

Prognosis:

(1) Mortality 15% by age 10 years

(2) Intelligence: IQ <80 (27%); IQ >100 (27%); learning disability (50%)

(3) Urinary incontinence: 85% achieve social continence (scheduled intermittent catheterization)

(4) Motor function: some deficit (100%); improvement after repair (37%)

(5) Hindbrain dysfunction associated with Chiari II malformation (32%)

(6) Ventriculitis: 7% in initial repair within 48 hours, more common in delayed repair >48 hours

NEURENTERIC CYST

= persistence of canal of Kovalevski between yolk sac + notochord

Associated with:

neurofibromatosis; meningocele; spinal malformation (stalk connects cyst and neural canal; usually no stalk between cyst and esophagus)

Location: anterior to spinal canal on mesenteric side of gut

√ midline cleft in centra (accommodates stalk)

√ anterior / posterior spina bifida

√ incomplete vertebral elements

√ diastematomyelia

√ posterior mediastinal mass

OSSIFYING FIBROMA

Peak incidence: first 2 decades of life

Histo: areas of osseous tissue intermixed with a highly cellular fibrous tissue

Sites: maxilla > frontal > ethmoid bone > mandible (rarely seen elsewhere)

√ areas of increased + decreased attenuation

√ intact inner + outer table

√ slow-growing expansile lesion

√ usually unilateral + monostotic

DDx: may be impossible to differentiate from fibrous dysplasia

OSTEOMYELITIS OF VERTEBRA

Incidence: 2 – 10% of all cases of osteomyelitis

Causes:

(1) direct penetrating trauma (most common); following surgical removal of nucleus pulposus

(2) hematogenous: associated with urinary tract infections / following GU surgery / instrumentation; diabetes mellitus; drug abuse

Pathophysiology:

infection begins in low-flow end-vascular arcades adjacent to subchondral plate

Organism: Staphylococcus aureus, Streptococcus

Peak age: 5 – 7th decade

• back pain, neurologic deficit

• fever, leukocytosis

• increased erythrocyte sedimentation rate

• positive blood / urine culture

√ disc space narrowing (earliest radiographic sign)

√ tracer uptake in adjacent portions of two vertebral bodies

Cx: secondary infection of intervertebral disc is frequent

PERINEURAL SACRAL CYST

= TARLOV CYST = cyst arising from posterior rootlets (S2 + S3 most common)

√ sacral erosion
√ may communicate with thecal sac

SACRAL AGENESIS

= CAUDAL REGRESSION SYNDROME = midline closure
defect of neural tube
Incidence: 0.005 – 0.01%
Predisposed: infants of diabetic mothers (16%)
Associated with:
(1) musculoskeletal anomalies: hip dislocation, foot
deformities, hypoplasia of extremities
(2) lack of bladder / bowel control
(3) spina bifida (myelomeningocele often not in
combination with hydrocephalus)
NOT associated with VATER syndrome
√ sacral agenesis
√ ± dural sac stenosis with high termination
√ ± tethered cord with associated lipoma, teratoma, cauda
equina cyst
Cx: neurogenic bladder (if >2 segments are missing)

SACROCOCCYGEAL TERATOMA

= rare congenital tumor arising from pluripotential cells
that are derived from the primitive knot (Henson node)
with its final resting place in the sacrococcygeal area
Incidence: 1:40,000 live births; Type I + II (80%); most
common congenital solid tumor in the
newborn; M:F = 1:4
Histo:
(1) mature benign teratoma (55 – 75%) with elements
from glia, bowel, pancreas, bronchial mucosa, skin
appendages, striated + smooth muscle, bowel
loops, bone components (metacarpal bones +
digits), well-formed teeth, choroid plexus structures
(production of CSF)
(2) immature teratoma (11 – 28%): neuroepithelial /
renal origin
(3) malignant teratoma (7 – 17%): yolk sac /
endodermal sinus tumor / embryonal carcinoma;
more common in males; metastasizes to lung,
spine, lymph nodes, liver
Age: 50 – 70% during first few days; 80% by 6 months
of age; <10% >2 years of age; M:F = 1:4
Classification:
Type I   predominantly external lesion covered by
skin with a minimal presacral component
(47%)
Type II   predominantly external tumor with significant
presacral component (35%)
Type III predominantly sacral component + external
extension (8%)
Type IV   presacral tumor with no external component
(10%)

Associated with other congenital anomalies (in 18%):
(1) vertebral (5 – 16%)
(2) musculoskeletal
(3) renal anomalies
(4) placentomegaly
(5) nonimmune hydrops

(6) curvilinear sacrococcygeal defect (rare autosomal
dominant inheritance with equal sex incidence,
low malignant potential, absence of calcifications) +
anorectal stenosis / atresia, vesicoureteral reflux
• AFP only elevated with malignant degeneration
• premature labor
• uterus large for dates
• radicular pain, constipation, urinary frequency /
incontinence

Plain film:
√ amorphous, punctate, spiculated calcifications,
possibly resembling bone (36 – 50%); suggestive of
benign tumor
√ soft tissue mass in pelvis protruding anteriorly +
inferiorly
BE:
√ anterosuperior displacement of rectum
√ luminal constriction
IVP:
√ displacement of bladder anterosuperiorly
√ development of bladder neck obstruction
Myelography:
√ intraspinal component may be present
Angio:
√ neovascularity (arterial supply by middle sacral,
internal iliac, gluteal arteries)
√ enlargement of feeding vessels
√ arterial encasement
√ arteriovenous shunting
√ early venous filling with serpiginous dilated tumor
veins
US / CT:
√ solid (25%) / mixed (60%) / cystic (15%) sacral mass
√ average size of 8 cm in diameter
√ polyhydramnios (2/3)
√ oligohydramnios, hydronephrosis, urinary ascites,
hydrops are poor prognostic factors
MR:
√ lobulated + sharply demarcated tumor extremely
heterogeneous on T1WI as a result of high signal
from fat, intermediate signal from soft tissue, low
signal from calcium
Prognosis: prevalence of malignant germ cell tumors
increases with patient's age
Δ predominantly fatty tissue tumors are usually benign
Δ hemorrhage / necrosis is suggestive of malignancy
Δ cystic lesions are less likely malignant
Cx: (1) dystocia in 6 – 13%
(2) massive intratumoral hemorrhage
(3) fetal death in utero / stillbirth
DDx: myelomeningocele, lipomeningocele, lipoma,
hemangioma, epidermal cyst, rectal duplication,
lymphangioma, chordoma, sarcoma, ependymoma

SCHEUERMANN DISEASE

= SPINAL OSTEOCHONDROSIS = KYPHOSIS
DORSALIS JUVENILIS = VERTEBRAL EPIPHYSITIS
= disorder consisting of vertebral wedging + endplate
irregularity + narrowing of intervertebral disc space

Incidence: in 31% of male + 21% of female patients with back pain

Age: onset at puberty

Location: lower thoracic / upper lumbar vertebrae; in mild cases limited to 3 – 4 vertebral bodies

√ anterior wedging of vertebral body with increased anteroposterior diameter

√ irregular-shaped + narrowed disc spaces

√ kyphosis / loss of lordosis; scoliosis

√ Schmorl nodes (intravertebral herniation of nucleus pulposus into vertebral body) = depression in contour of endplate in posterior half of vertebral body; found in up to 30% of adolescents + young adults

√ flattened area in superior surface of epiphyseal ring anteriorly = avulsion fracture of ring apophysis due to migration of nucleus pulposus through weak point between ring apophysis + vertebral endplate (fusion of ring apophysis usually occurs at about 18 years of age)

√ detached epiphyseal ring anteriorly

DDx: (1) Developmental notching of anterior vertebrae (NO wedging or Schmorl nodes)

  (2) Osteochondrodystrophy (earlier in life, extremities show same changes)

SPINAL STENOSIS
= abnormal narrowing of spinal canal, lateral recess, or neural foramen

Causes:
  A. Congenitally short pedicles (idiopathic / achondroplasia)
  B. Acquired:
      1. Hypertrophy of ligamentum flavum (most common)
      2. Superior facet joint hypertrophy
      3. Degenerative bulging disc
      4. Spondylosis, spondylolisthesis
      5. Surgical fusion
      6. Fracture
      7. Calcification of posterior longitudinal ligament
      8. Paget disease

Age: middle-aged / elderly; M>F

Location: generally involves lumbar spinal canal; cervical spinal canal may be similarly affected

√ narrowing of cervical canal <13 mm, of lumbar canal <16 mm (AP diameter)

√ interpedicular distance <25 mm

√ distorted shape of thecal sac

√ obliteration of epidural fat

Lumbar Spinal Stenosis
Causes:
  1. Achondroplasia:
      √ narrowed interpediculate distance progressive toward lumbar spine
  2. Paget disease: bony overgrowth
  3. Spondylolisthesis
  4. Operative posterior spinal fusion
  5. Herniated disc
  6. Metastasis to vertebrae
  7. Developmental / congenital

Age: presentation between 30 – 50 years of age
• low back pain
• cauda equina syndrome: paraparesis, incontinence, sensory findings in saddle-like pattern, areflexia

√ unusual small quantity of contrast material to fill thecal sac

√ anteroposterior + interpediculate diameter constricted

√ may appear as spinal block in hyperextended neck on AP views

√ thickened articular process, pedicles, laminae, ligaments

√ trefoil / cloverleaf configuration of spinal canal

√ bulging discs

SPLIT NOTOCHORD SYNDROME
= spectrum of anomalies with persistent connection between gut + dorsal ectoderm

Etiology:
failure of complete separation of ectoderm from endoderm with subsequent splitting of notochord and mesoderm around the adhesion about 3rd week of gestation

√ fistula / isolated diverticula / duplication / cyst / fibrous cord / sinus along the tract

Types:
1. **Dorsal enteric fistula**
   = fistula between intestinal cavity + dorsal midline skin traversing prevertebral soft tissue, vertebral body, spinal canal, posterior elements of spine
   • bowel ostium / exposed pad of mucous membrane in dorsal midline in newborn
   • opening passes meconium + feces
   √ dorsal bowel hernia into a skin- / membrane-covered dorsal sac after passing through a combined anterior + posterior spina bifida

2. **Dorsal enteric sinus**
   = blind remnant of posterior part of tract with midline opening to dorsal external skin surface

3. **Dorsal enteric enterogenous cyst**
   = prevertebral / postvertebral / intraspinal enteric-lined cyst derived from intermediate part of tract
   Intraspinal enteric cyst
      Age at presentation: 20 – 40 years
      • intermittent local / radicular pain worsened by elevation of intraspinal pressure
      Location: intraspinal in lower cervical / upper thoracic region
      √ enlarged spinal canal at site of cyst
      √ hemivertebrae, segmentation defect, partial fusion, scoliosis in region of cyst

4. **Dorsal enteric diverticulum**
   = tubular / spherical diverticulum arising from dorsal mesenteric border of bowel as a persistent portion of tract between gut + vertebral column

5. **Dorsal enteric cyst**
   = involution of portion of diverticulum near gut
   • mass in abdomen / mediastinum (due to bowel rotation)

SPONDYLOLISTHESIS

Cause: (a) usually bilateral spondylolysis
       (b) pseudospondylolisthesis = degenerative /
           inflammatory joint disease (eg, rheumatoid
           arthritis)

Grades I – IV (Meyerding method):
   each grade equals 1/4 anterior subluxation of superior
   on inferior vertebral body
• symptoms not related to grade

SPONDYLOLYSIS

= pars interarticularis defect between superior + inferior
   articulating processes
Incidence: 4 – 7% of population; increases with age; in
              30 – 70% other family members afflicted
Age: uncommon in infants; whites:blacks = 3:1
Cause:

   (a) congenital malformation: frequently associated with
        spina bifida occulta of S1, dorsally wedge-shaped
        body of L5, hypoplasia of L5
   (b) hereditary hypoplasia of pars leads to insufficiency
        fracture; eg, pars defect in 34% of Eskimos
   (c) pseudarthrosis following stress fracture of pars (in
        most); common in gymnastics (30%), diving,
        contact sports (football, soccer, hockey, lacrosse)
   (d) secondary spondylolysis: neoplasm, osteomyelitis,
        Paget disease, osteomalacia, osteogenesis
        imperfecta
• mostly asymptomatic

Location: L5; L4; C6 (rare); in 75% bilateral
Plain film:
   √ fracture line resembles collar of "Scottie dog"
CT:
   √ inner contour of spinal canal interrupted

SPONDYLOSIS OF CERVICAL SPINE

= progressive degeneration of intervertebral discs
   leading to proliferative changes of bone + meninges;
   more common than disc herniation as a cause for
   cervical radiculopathy
Incidence: 5 – 10% at age 20 – 30; >50% at age 45;
              >90% by age 60
• spastic gait disorder
• neck pain
Location: C4-5, C5-6, C6-7 (greater normal cervical
             motion at these levels)

Sequelae: (a) direct compression of spinal cord
           (b) neural foraminal stenosis
           (c) ischemia due to vascular compromise
           (d) repeated trauma from normal flexion /
                extension
DDx of myelopathy:
   rheumatoid arthritis, congenital anomalies of
   craniocervical junction, intradural extramedullary
   tumor, spine metastases, cervical spinal cord tumor,
   arteriovenous malformation, amyotrophic lateral
   sclerosis, multiple sclerosis, neurosyphilis

SYRINGOHYDROMYELIA

= SYRINGOMYELIA = SYRINX (used in a general
   manner reflecting difficulty in classification)
= longitudinally oriented CSF-filled cavities + gliosis within
   spinal cord frequently involving both parenchyma +
   central canal
Age: primarily childhood / early adult life
• loss of sensation to pain + temperature (interruption of
   spinothalamic tracts)
• trophic changes [skin lesions; Charcot joints in 25%
   (shoulder, elbow, wrist)]
• muscle weakness (anterior horn cell involvement)
• spasticity, hyperreflexia (upper motor neuron
   involvement)
• abnormal plantar reflexes (pyramidal tract involvement)
Location: predominantly lower end of cervical cord;
             extension into brain stem (= syringobulbia)
CT:
   √ distinct area of decreased attenuation within spinal
     cord (100%)
   √ swollen / normal-sized / atrophic cord
   √ no contrast enhancement
   √ flattened vertebral border (rare) with increased
     transverse diameter of cord
   √ change in shape + size of cord with change in position
     (rare)
   √ filling of syringohydromyelia with intrathecal contrast
     (a) early filling via direct communication with
        subarachnoid space
     (b) late filling after 4 – 8 hours (80 – 90%) secondary
        to permeation of contrast material
Myelography:
   √ enlarged cord (DDx: intramedullary tumor)
   √ "collapsing cord sign" = collapsing of cord with gas
     myelography as fluid content moves caudad in the
     erect position (rare)
MR:
   √ cystic area of low signal intensity on T1WI, increased
     intensity on T2WI
   √ presence of CSF flow-void (= low signal on T2WI)
     within cavity from pulsations
   √ beaded cavity from multiple incomplete septations
   √ cord enlargement

Hydromyelia

= PRIMARY SYRINGOHYDROMYELIA
= CONGENITAL SYRINGOHYDROMYELIA
= dilatation of persistent central canal of spinal cord (in
   70 – 80% obliterated) which communicates with 4th
   ventricle (= communicating syringomyelia)
Histo: lined by ependymal tissue
Associated with:
   (1) Chiari malformation in 20 – 70%
   (2) Spinal dysraphism
   (3) Myelocele
   (4) Dandy-Walker syndrome
   (5) Diastematomyelia
   (6) Scoliosis in 48 – 87%
   (7) Klippel-Feil syndrome
   (8) Spinal segmentation defects

(9) Tethered cord (in up to 25%)

Syringomyelia
= ACQUIRED SYRINGOHYDROMYELIA
= SECONDARY SYRINGOHYDROMYELIA
= any cavity within substance of spinal cord which may communicate with the central canal, usually extending over several vertebral segments
Histo: not lined by ependymal tissue
Pathophysiology: interrupted flow of CSF through the perivascular spaces of cord between subarachnoid space + central canal
Causes:
1. Posttraumatic syringomyelia
   Incidence: in 3.2% after spinal cord injury
   √ 0.5 – 40 cm (average 6 cm) in length
2. Postinflammatory syringomyelia
   infection, subarachnoid hemorrhage, arachnoid adhesions, S/P surgery
3. Tumor-associated syringomyelia
   spinal cord tumors, herniated disc;
   secondary to circulatory disturbance + thoracic spinal cord atrophy
4. Vascular insufficiency

Reactive Cyst
= POSTTRAUMATIC SPINAL CORD CYST
= CSF-filled cyst adjacent to level of trauma; usually single (75%)
• late deterioration in patients with spinal cord injury (not related to severity of original injury)
Rx: shunting leads to clinical improvement

TETHERED CORD
= TIGHT FILUM TERMINALE SYNDROME = LOW CONUS MEDULLARIS
= abnormally short + thickened filum terminale with low position of conus medullaris
Etiology: failure of ascent of conus (normal location of tip of conus medullaris: L 4/5 at 16 weeks of gestation, L 2/3 at birth, L1/2 >3 months of age)
Age at presentation: 5 – 15 years (in years of growth spurt); M:F = 2:3

Associated with: lipoma in 29 – 78%
• dorsal nevus, dermal sinus, hair patch (50%)
• bowel, bladder, limb dysfunction in childhood
• gait abnormalities with muscle stiffness + muscle weakness
• clubfoot
• paraplegia, paraparesis
• radiculopathy (adults)
• abnormal lower extremity reflexes
• anal / perineal pain (in adults)
• back pain (particularly with exertion)
√ lumbar spina bifida occulta with interpedicular widening
√ scoliosis (20%)
√ diameter of filum terminale >2 mm at L5-S1 level (55%), small fibrolipoma within thickened filum (23%), small filar cyst (3%), spinal cord ending in a small lipoma (13%)
√ posteriorly located tethered conus medullaris + filum terminale (supine views)
√ conus medullaris below level of L2 by age 12 (86%)
√ abnormal lateral course of nerve roots (>15° angle relative to spinal cord)
√ widened triangular thecal sac tented posteriorly (thecal sac pulled posteriorly by filum)
MR:
   √ prolonged T1 relaxation in center of spinal cord on T1WI in 25% (? myelomalacia / mild hydromyelia)
Sequelae: chronic repetitive cord ischemia with stretching of cord
Rx: decompressive laminectomy / partial removal of lipoma ± freeing of cord

TERATOMA OF SPINE
= neoplasm containing tissue belonging to all 3 germinal layers at sites where these tissues do not normally occur
Incidence: 0.15% (excluding sacrococcygeal teratoma)
Age: all ages; M:F = 1:1
Path: solid, thin- / thick-walled partially / wholly cystic with clear / milky / dark cyst fluid, uni- / multilocular, presence of bone / cartilage
Location: intra- / extramedullary
√ complete block at myelography
√ syringomyelia above level of tumor
√ spinal canal may be focally widened

DIFFERENTIAL DIAGNOSIS OF BRAIN DISORDERS

Intracranial pneumocephalus

Causes:
A. Trauma (74%):
in 3% of all skull fractures; in 8% of fractures involving paranasal sinuses (frontal > ethmoid > sphenoid > mastoid)
B. Neoplasm invading sinus (13%):
1. Osteoma of frontal / ethmoid sinus
2. Pituitary adenoma
3. Mucocele, epidermoid
4. Malignancy of paranasal sinuses
C. Infection with gas-forming organism (9%):
in mastoiditis, sinusitis
D. Surgery (4%):
hypophysectomy, paranasal sinus surgery
Mechanism (dural laceration):
(1) ball-valve mechanism during straining, coughing, sneezing
(2) vacuum phenomenon secondary to loss of CSF
Time of onset: on initial presentation (25%), usually seen within 4 – 5 days, delay up to 6 months (33%)
Mortality: 15%
Cx:
1. CSF rhinorrhea (50%)
2. Meningitis / epidural / brain abscess (25%)
3. Extracranial pneumocephalus = air collection in subaponeurotic space

Cerebral atrophy

= irreversible loss of brain substance + subsequent enlargement of intra- and extracerebral CSF-containing spaces (hydrocephalus ex vacuo = ventriculomegaly)

A. DIFFUSE BRAIN ATROPHY
Cause:
(a) Trauma, radiation therapy
(b) Drugs (dilantin, steroids, methotrexate, marijuana, hard drugs, chemotherapy), alcoholism, hypoxia
(c) Demyelinating disease (multiple sclerosis, encephalitis)
(d) Degenerative disease
eg, Alzheimer disease, Pick disease, Jakob-Creutzfeldt disease
(e) Cerebrovascular disease + multiple infarcts
(f) Advancing age, anorexia, renal failure
√ enlarged ventricles + sulci

B. FOCAL BRAIN ATROPHY
Cause: Vascular / chemical / metabolic / traumatic / idiopathic (Dyke-Davidoff-Mason syndrome)

C. REVERSIBLE PROCESS SIMULATING ATROPHY (in younger people)
Cause: Anorexia nervosa, alcoholism, catabolic steroid treatment, pediatric malignancy

Cerebellar atrophy

A. Cerebellar atrophy with cerebral atrophy
= generalized senile brain atrophy
B. Cerebellar atrophy without cerebral atrophy
1. Olivopontocerebellar degeneration / Marie ataxia / Friedreich ataxia
• onset of ataxia in young adulthood
2. Ataxia-telangiectasia
3. Ethanol- / phenytoin-toxicity
4. Idiopathic degeneration secondary to carcinoma (= paraneoplastic), usually oat cell carcinoma of lung
5. Radiotherapy
6. Focal cerebellar atrophy: (a) infarction (b) traumatic injury

HYPERDENSE INTRACRANIAL LESIONS

Increased density of falx

1. Subarachnoid hemorrhage
2. Interhemispheric subdural hematoma
3. Diffuse cerebral edema (= increased density relative to low density brain)
4. Dural calcifications (hypercalcemia from chronic renal failure, basal cell nevus syndrome, hyperparathyroidism)
5. Normal falx (can be normal in pediatric population)

Intracranial calcifications

mnemonic: "PINEEAL"
Physiologic
Infection
Neoplasm
Endocrine
Embryologic
Arteriovenous
Leftover Ls

A. Physiologic intracranial calcifications
B. Infection:
TORCH (toxoplasmosis, rubella, CMV, herpes), healed abscess, hydatid cyst, tuberculoma, cysticercosis
mnemonic:
CMV calcifications are **c**ircum**v**entricular
Toxoplasma calcifications are in**t**raparenchymal
C. Neoplasm:
Craniopharyngioma (40 – 80%), oligodendroglioma (50 – 70%), chordoma (25 – 40%), choroid plexus papilloma (10%), meningioma (20%), pituitary adenoma (3 – 5%), pinealoma (10 – 20%), dermoid (20%), lipoma of corpus callosum, ependymoma (50%), astrocytoma (15%), radiotherapy
D. Endocrine:
Hyperparathyroidism, hypervitaminosis D, hypoparathyroidism, pseudohypoparathyroidism, CO poisoning, lead poisoning

E. Embryologic:
    Neurocutaneous syndromes (tuberous sclerosis, Sturge-Weber, neurofibromatosis), Fahr disease, Cockayne syndrome, basal cell nevus syndrome
F. Arteriovenous:
    Atherosclerosis, aneurysm, AVM, hemangioma, subdural hematoma
G. Leftover Ls:
    Lipoma, lipoid proteinosis, lissencephaly

Physiologic intracranial calcification
1. Pineal calcification
    Incidence: 2/3 of adult population
    - may be physiologic >10 years of age
    - rare <6 years of age
    √ amorphous / ring-like calcification <3 mm from midline usually <10 mm in diameter
    √ approximately 30 mm above highest posterior elevation of pyramids
    CAVE: pineal calcification >10 mm suggests pineal neoplasm (teratoma / pinealoma)
2. Habenula
    Incidence: approximately in 1/3 of population
    - >10 years of age
    √ posteriorly open C-shaped calcification 4 – 6 mm anterior to pineal gland
3. Choroid plexus
    may calcify in all ventricles, most commonly in atrium of lateral ventricles
    - >3 years of age
    √ 20 – 30 mm behind + slightly below pineal on lateral projection, symmetrical on AP projection
    DDx: neurofibromatosis
4. Dura, falx, tentorium
    Incidence: 10%
    - >3 years of age
    DDx: basal cell nevus syndrome (Gorlin), pseudoxanthoma elasticum
5. Petroclinoid ligament
    between tip of dorsum sellae and apex of petrous bone
    - >5 years of age
6. Interclinoid ligament
    = interclinoid bridging
7. Arteriosclerosis of ICA
8. Basal ganglia

Basal ganglia calcification
A. Physiologic with aging
B. Metabolic
    1. Hypoparathyroidism + pseudohypoparathyroidism (60%)
    2. Wilson disease
    3. Fahr disease
    4. Cockayne syndrome
    5. Down syndrome
    6. Tuberous sclerosis
C. Trauma
    1. Childhood leukemia following methotrexate therapy

2. S/P radiation therapy
3. Birth anoxia
D. Drugs
    1. Carbon monoxide poisoning
    2. Lead intoxication
E. Infection
    1. Toxoplasmosis
    2. AIDS

Periventricular calcifications in a child
1. Tuberous sclerosis
2. Congenital infection: CMV, toxoplasmosis

Linear echogenic foci in thalamus + basal ganglia
A. In utero infection:
    = destruction of vessel wall + replacement by deposits of amorphous granular material
    1. Cytomegalovirus
    2. Rubella
    3. Toxoplasmosis
B. Chromosomal abnormality
    1. Down syndrome
    2. Trisomy 13
C. Others
    1. Perinatal asphyxia
    2. Fetal alcohol syndrome
    3. Nonimmune hydrops

Bilateral basal ganglia lesions
A. Metabolic disease
    1. Leigh disease
    2. Wilson disease
    3. Mitochondrial encephalomyopathies
    4. Hallervorden-Spatz disease
B. Poisoning
    1. Carbon monoxide poisoning
    2. Hydrogen sulfide poisoning
    3. Barbiturate intoxication
C. Others
    1. Striato-nigral degeneration
    2. Cytoplasmatically inherited striatal degeneration
    3. Hypoglycemia

Dense cerebral mass
Substrate: calcification / hemorrhage / dense protein

A. VESSEL
    1. Aneurysm
    2. Arteriovenous malformation
    3. Hematoma (acute / subacute)
B. TUMOR
    1. Lymphoma
    2. Medulloblastoma
    3. Meningioma
    4. Metastasis
        (a) from mucinous-producing adenocarcinoma
        (b) hemorrhagic metastases: melanoma, choriocarcinoma, hypernephroma, bronchogenic carcinoma, breast carcinoma (rarely)

Dense lesion near foramen of Monro
A. <u>Intraventricular lesion</u>
1. Colloid cyst
2. Meningioma
3. Choroid plexus tumor / granuloma
4. AVM of septal, thalamostriate, internal cerebral veins
B. <u>Periventricular mass</u>
1. Primary CNS lymphoma
2. Tuberous sclerosis
   (a) subependymal tuber
   (b) giant cell astrocytoma
3. Metastasis from mucin-producing adenocarcinoma / hemorrhagic metastasis (melanoma, choriocarcinoma, hypernephroma, bronchogenic carcinoma, breast carcinoma)
4. Glioblastoma of septum pellucidum
C. <u>Masses projecting superiorly from base of skull</u>
1. Pituitary adenoma
2. Craniopharyngioma
3. Aneurysm
4. Dolichoectatic basilar artery

ENHANCING BRAIN LESIONS
Sulcal enhancement
A. <u>Meningeal tumor</u>
(a) Meningeal carcinomatosis from systemic tumor: eg, breast carcinoma, small cell carcinoma of lung, malignant melanoma, lymphoma / leukemia
(b) Seeding primary CNS tumor:
   1. Medulloblastoma
   2. Pineoblastoma
   3. Ependymoma
B. <u>Meningitis</u>
pyogenic, tuberculous, fungal, cysticercosis, sarcoidosis
C. <u>Sequelae of subarachnoid hemorrhage</u>
(from fibroblastic proliferation)
D. <u>Subacute brain infarct</u>

Enhancing ventricular margins
A. <u>Subependymal spread of metastatic tumor</u>
1. Bronchogenic carcinoma (especially small cell carcinoma)
2. Melanoma
3. Breast carcinoma
B. <u>Subependymal seeding of CNS primary</u>
1. Glioma
2. Ependymoma
C. <u>Ependymal seeding of CNS primary</u>
1. Medulloblastoma
2. Germinoma
D. <u>Primary CNS lymphoma / systemic lymphoma</u>
E. <u>Inflammatory ventriculitis</u>

Dense and enhancing lesions
1. Aneurysm
2. Meningioma
3. CNS lymphoma
4. Medulloblastoma

5. Metastasis

Multifocal enhancing lesions
1. Multiple infarctions
2. Arteriovenous malformations
3. Multifocal primary / secondary neoplasms
4. Multifocal infectious processes
5. Demyelinating diseases: eg, multiple sclerosis

Innumerable small enhancing cerebral nodules
A. METASTASES
B. PRIMARY CNS LYMPHOMA
C. DISSEMINATED INFECTION
1. Cysticercosis
2. Histoplasmosis
3. Tuberculosis
D. INFLAMMATION
1. Sarcoidosis
2. Multiple sclerosis
E. SUBACUTE MULTIFOCAL INFARCTION
from hypoperfusion, multiple emboli, cerebral vasculitis (SLE), meningitis, cortical vein thrombosis

HYPERINTENSE BRAIN LESIONS

Periventricular T2WI-hyperintense lesions
A. YOUNG PATIENTS
1. <u>Multiple sclerosis</u>
2. <u>Migraine:</u> in 41% with classic migraine, in 57% with complicated migraine; presumed to represent small infarcts
3. <u>Vasculitic disorder:</u> SLE, Behçet disease, sickle cell disease
   √ triad of deep white matter lesions + cortical infarcts + hemorrhage
4. <u>Postviral leukoencephalopathy</u>
   = Acute disseminated encephalomyelitis
   = autoimmune process
   • several weeks following an exanthematous viral infection
   √ diffuse white matter abnormalities, occasionally deep grey matter involvement
   √ sparing of cortical grey matter
5. <u>Virchow-Robin space</u>
   = small subarachnoid space following pia mater along perforating nutrient end vessels into brain substance
   √ 1 – 2 mm round lesions on heavily T2WI (seen on sections through centrum semiovale + on low sections at level of anterior commissure)
6. <u>Leukodystrophy:</u> in children
   √ symmetric diffuse confluent involvement
B. ELDERLY
1. <u>État criblé</u> (sieve-like) / gliosis
   = perivascular fluid spaces predominantly at arteriolar level
   Cause: chronic ischemia due to arteriosclerosis of long penetrating arteries arising from circle of Willis (lenticulostriate + thalamoperforators)

Histo: lipohyaline deposits within vessel walls followed by partial demyelination, gliosis, interstitial edema

Incidence: in 10% without risk factors, in 84% with risk factors and symptoms

Age: >60 years (in 30 – 60%)

Location: periventricular white matter > optic radiation > basal ganglia > centrum semiovale > brainstem (usually spares corpus callosum + subcortical U-fibers)

C. PATIENTS WITH AIDS
1. HIV encephalitis:
   √ well-defined "patchy" / ill-defined "dirty white matter"
2. Toxoplasmosis
3. Lymphoma
4. Progressive multifocal leukoencephalopathy (PML)

D. PATIENTS WITH TRAUMA
1. Diffuse axonal / shearing injury
   Location: grey-white matter junction, extension along white matter tracts to corpus callosum / along corona radiata to posterior limb of internal capsule + posterolateral aspect of brainstem
2. Diffuse necrotizing leukoencephalopathy
   Cause: intrathecal methotrexate ± whole brain irradiation
   √ confluent pattern with scalloped margins within periventricular white matter extending out to subcortical U-fibers

E. PATIENTS WITH HYDROCEPHALUS
1. Transependymal CSF flow
   √ smooth halo of even thickness

HYPODENSE BRAIN LESIONS

Diffusely swollen hemispheres
A. Metabolic
1. Metabolic encephalopathy: eg, uremia, Reye syndrome, ketoacidosis
2. Anoxia: cardiopulmonary arrest, near-drowning, smoke inhalation, ARDS

B. Neurovascular
1. Hypertensive encephalopathy
2. Superior sagittal sinus thrombosis
3. Head trauma
4. Pseudotumor cerebri

C. Inflammation
eg, herpes encephalitis, CMV, toxoplasmosis

Edema of brain
Etiology:
1. Vasogenic edema (most common form)
   secondary to breakdown of blood-brain barrier with plasma extravasation;
   associated with primary brain neoplasm, metastases, hemorrhage, infarction, inflammation
2. Cytotoxic edema
   reversible increase in intracellular water content secondary to ischemia / anoxia

3. Interstitial edema
   increase in periventricular interstitial spaces secondary to transependymal flow of CSF with elevated intraventricular pressure
   √ decreased distinction between gray + white matter
   √ compressed slit-like lateral ventricles
   √ compression of cerebral sulci + perimesencephalic cisterns

CT:
√ areas of hypodensity ± mass effect
√ return to normal from nonhemorrhagic edema / brain atrophy from white matter shearing injury

MR:
√ decreased intensity on T1WI, increased intensity on T2WI

US:
√ generalized / focal increase of parenchymal echogenicity with featureless appearance
√ decreased resistive indices

Midline cystic structures
1. **Cavum septi pellucidi** = "5th ventricle"
   = thin triangular membrane consisting of two glial layers covered laterally with ependyma separating the frontal horns of lateral ventricles
   Incidence: in 80% of term infants; in 15% of adults
   Location: posterior to genu of corpus callosum, inferior to body of corpus callosum, anterosuperior to anterior pillar of fornix
   √ extends to foramen of Monro
   √ may dilate + cause obstructive hydrocephalus (rare)
2. **Cavum vergae** = "6th ventricle"
   = cavity posterior to columns of fornix; contracts after about 6th gestational month
   Incidence: in 30% of term infants; in 15% of adults
   Location: posterior to fornix, anterior to splenium of corpus callosum, inferior to body of corpus callosum, superior to transverse fornix
   √ posterior midline continuation of cavum septi pellucidi beyond foramen of Monro
3. **Cavum veli interpositi**
   = extension of quadrigeminal plate cistern above 3rd ventricle to foramen of Monro, laterally bounded by columns of fornix + thalamus
4. Colloid cyst: anterior + superior to cavum septi pellucidi
5. Arachnoid cyst: in region of quadrigeminal plate cistern
   √ curvilinear margins

Periventricular hypodensity
1. Encephalomalacia
   √ slightly denser than CSF
2. Porencephaly
   = cavity communicating with ventricle / cistern from intracerebral hemorrhage
   associated with: dilated ventricle, sulci, and fissures
   √ CSF density
3. Resolving hematoma
   • Hx of previously demonstrated hematoma
   √ may show ring enhancement + compression of adjacent structures

4. Cystic tumor
   √ mass effect + contrast enhancement

Suprasellar low-density lesion with hydrocephalus
A. CYST
   1. Arachnoid cyst
   2. Ependymal cyst of 3rd vertricle
   3. Parasitic cyst of 3rd ventricle (cysticercosis)
   4. Dilated 3rd ventricle (in aqueductal stenosis)
B. CYSTIC MASS
   1. Epidermoid
   2. Hypothalamic pilocytic astrocytoma
   3. Cystic craniopharyngioma

Nota bene: Cystic lesion may be inapparent within
             surrounding CSF; metrizamide
             cisternography is helpful in detection + to
             exclude aqueduct stenosis

Low-attenuation lesion in basal ganglia
1. Poisoning: carbon monoxide, barbiturate intoxication,
   hydrogen sulfide poisoning, cyanide poisoning,
   methanol intoxication
2. Hypoxia
3. Hypoglycemia
4. Hypotension (lacunar infarcts)
5. Wilson disease

Mesencephalic low-density lesion
1. Normal: decussation of superior cerebellar peduncles
   at level of inferior colliculi
2. Syringobulbia
   found in conjunction with syringomyelia, Arnold-Chiari
   malformation, trauma
   √ CSF density centrally
   √ intrathecal contrast enters central cavity
3. Brainstem infarction
   √ abnormal contrast enhancement after 1 week
   √ well-defined low attenuation region without
     enhancement after 2 – 4 weeks
4. Central pontine myelinolysis
   comatose patient receiving rapid correction /
   overcorrection of severe hyponatremia (following
   prolonged IV fluid administration / alcoholism)
   √ central region of diminished attenuation
5. Brainstem glioma
   √ mass with indistinct margins + vague enhancement
6. Metastasis
   √ well-defined contrast enhancement
7. Granuloma in TB / sarcoidosis (rare)

BRAIN MASSES
Classification of primary CNS tumors
A. TUMORS OF BRAIN AND MENINGES
   (a) GLIOMAS
       Astrocytoma
           1. Astrocytoma (astrocytoma grades I – II)
           2. Glioblastoma (astrocytoma grades III – IV)
       Oligodendroglioma

       Paraglioma
           1. Ependymoma
           2. Choroid plexus papilloma
       Ganglioglioma
       Medulloblastoma
   (b) PINEAL TUMOR
       1. Germinoma
       2. Teratoma
       3. Pineocytoma
       4. Pineoblastoma
   (c) PITUITARY TUMOR
       1. Pituitary adenoma
       2. Pituitary carcinoma
   (d) MENINGIOMA
   (e) NERVE SHEATH TUMOR
       1. Schwannoma
       2. Neurofibroma
   (f) MISCELLANEOUS
       1. Sarcoma
       2. Lipoma
       3. Hemangioblastoma
B. TUMORS OF EMBRYONAL REMNANTS
   (a) Craniopharyngioma
   (b) Colloid cyst
   (c) Teratoid tumor
       1. Epidermoid
       2. Dermoid
       3. Teratoma

Incidence of brain tumors
= 9% of all primary neoplasms; account for 1.2% of
  autopsied deaths

IN ALL AGE GROUPS:		IN PEDIATRIC AGE GROUP:	
Glioma	34%	Astrocytoma	50%
Meningioma	17%	Medulloblastoma	15%
Metastasis	12%	Ependymoma	10%
Pituitary adenoma	6%	Craniopharyngioma	6%
Neurinoma	4%	Choroid plexus papilloma	2%
Sarcoma	3%		
Granuloma	3%		
Craniopharyngioma	2%		
Hemangioblastoma	2%		

CNS tumors presenting at birth
1. Hypothalamic astrocytoma
2. Choroid plexus papilloma / carcinoma
3. Teratoma
4. Primitive neuroectodermal tumor
5. Medulloblastoma
6. Ependymoma
7. Craniopharyngioma

CNS tumors in pediatric age group
Incidence:
    2.4:100,000 (<15 years of age); 2nd most common
    pediatric tumor (after leukemia); 15% of all pediatric
    neoplasms; 15 – 20% of all primary brain tumors; M>F
• increased intracranial pressure
• increasing head size

A. SUPRATENTORIAL (50%)
  Age: first 2 – 3 years of life
  Covering of brain : dural sarcoma, schwannoma, meningioma (3%)
  Cerebral hemisphere : astrocytoma (37%), oligodendroglioma
  Corpus callosum : astrocytoma
  3rd ventricle : colloid cyst, ependymoma
  Lateral ventricle : ependymoma (5%), choroid plexus papilloma (12%)
  Optic chiasm : craniopharyngioma (12%), optic nerve glioma (13%), teratoma, pituitary adenoma
  Hypothalamus : glioma (8%), hamartoma
  Pineal region : germinoma, pinealoma, teratoma (8%)

B. INFRATENTORIAL (50%)
  Age: 4 – 11 years
  Cerebellum : astrocytoma (31 – 33%), medulloblastoma (26 – 31%)
  Brainstem : glioma (16 – 21%)
  4th ventricle : ependymoma (6 – 14%), choroid plexus papilloma
  mnemonic: "BE MACHO"
    Brainstem glioma
    Ependymoma
    Medulloblastoma
    AVM
    Cystic astrocytoma
    Hemangioblastoma
    Other

SUPRATENTORIAL MIDLINE TUMORS
  1. Optic + hypothalamic glioma (39%)
  2. Craniopharyngioma (20%)
  3. Astrocytoma (9%)
  4. Pineoblastoma (9%)
  5. Germinoma (6%)
  6. Lipoma (6%)
  7. Teratoma (3.5%)
  8. Pituitary adenoma (3.5%)
  9. Meningioma (2%)
  10. Choroid plexus papilloma (2%)

SUPRATENTORIAL INTRAVENTRICULAR TUMORS
  (a) Lateral ventricle (3/4)
    1. Choroid plexus tumor (44%)
    2. Giant cell astrocytoma in tuberous sclerosis (19%)
    3. Hemangioma in Sturge-Weber syndrome (12%)
  (b) Third ventricle (1/4)
    1. Astrocytoma (13%)
    2. Choroid plexus tumor (6%)
    3. Meningioma (6%)

CLASSIFICATION BY HISTOLOGY
  1. Astrocytic tumors (33.5%)
  2. "Primitive" neuroectodermal tumor = PNET (21%) highly malignant neoplasms originating from germinal matrix + containing glial + neural elements
    — Medulloblastoma (16%)
    — Ependymoblastoma (2.5%)
    — PNET of cerebral hemisphere (2.5%)
  3. Mixed gliomas (16%)
  4. Malformative tumors (11.5%)
    — Craniopharyngioma (5.5%)
    — Lipoma (4.5%)
    — Dermoid cyst (1%)
    — Epidermal cyst (0.5%)
  5. Choroid plexus tumors (4%)
  6. Ependymal tumors (4%)
  7. Tumors of meningeal tissues (3.5%)
    — Meningioma (3%)
    — Meningeal sarcoma (0.5%)
  8. Germ cell tumors (2.5%)
    — Germinoma (1.5%)
    — Teratomatous tumor (1%)
  9. Neuronal tumors
    — Gangliocytoma (1.5%)
  10. Tumors of neuroendocrine origin
    — Pituitary adenoma (1%)
  11. Oligodendroglial tumors (0.5%)
  12. Tumors of blood vessels
    — Hemangioma (1%)

Multifocal CNS tumors
  A. METASTASES FROM PRIMARY CNS TUMOR
    (a) via commissural pathways: corpus callosum, internal capsule, massa intermedia
    (b) via CSF: ventricles / subarachnoid cisterns
    (c) satellite metastases
  B. MULTICENTRIC CNS TUMOR
    (a) true multicentric gliomas (4%)
    (b) concurrent tumors of different histology (coincidental)
  C. MULTICENTRIC MENINGIOMAS (3%) without neurofibromatosis
  D. MULTICENTRIC PRIMARY CNS LYMPHOMA
  E. PHAKOMATOSES
    1. Generalized neurofibromatosis: meningiomatosis, bilateral acoustic neuromas, bilateral optic nerve gliomas, cerebral gliomas, choroid plexus papillomas, multiple spine tumors, AVMs
    2. Tuberous sclerosis: subependymal tubers, intraventricular gliomas (giant cell astrocytoma), ependymomas
    3. von Hippel-Lindau disease: retinal angiomatosis, hemangioblastomas, congenital cysts of pancreas + liver, benign renal tumors, cardiac rhabdomyomas

Calcified intracranial mass
  mnemonic: "Ca^{2+} COME"
    Craniopharyngioma
    Astrocytoma, **A**neurysm
    Choroid plexus papilloma
    Oligodendroglioma
    Meningioma
    Ependymoma

Intra- versus extra-axial mass		
	intraaxial	extraaxial
Relationship to dura / bone	no attachment until advanced	contiguous
Local bony changes	uncommon	common
Displacement of cortex	toward dura / bone	away from bone
Subarachnoid cistern	effaced	widened
Feeding arteries	pial feeding arteries	dural feeding arteries

Avascular mass of brain
mnemonic: "TEACH"
Tumor: astrocytoma, metastasis, oligodendroglioma
Edema
Abscess
Cyst, **C**ontusion
Hematoma, **H**erpes

Ring-enhancing lesion of brain
Cause:
A. NEOPLASM
    1. Primary neoplasm: high grade glioma,
       meningioma, lymphoma, leukemia, pituitary
       macroadenoma, acoustic neuroma,
       craniopharyngioma
    2. Metastatic carcinoma + sarcoma
B. ABSCESS
    1. Abscess: bacterial, fungal, parasitic
    2. Empyema of epidural / subdural / intraventricular
       spaces
C. HEMORRHAGIC-ISCHEMIC LESION
    1. Resolving infarction
    2. Aging hematoma
    3. Operative bed following resection
    4. Thrombosed aneurysm
D. DEMYELINATING DISORDER
    1. Radiation necrosis
    2. Necrotizing leukoencephalopathy after
       methotrexate

Pathogenesis:
(1) hypervascular margin of lesion = granulation tissue
    / peripheral vascular channels / hypervascular
    tumor capsule
(2) breakdown of blood-brain barrier = leakage of
    contrast out of abnormally permeable vessels into
    extracellular fluid space
(3) hypodense center = avascular / hypovascular
    (requires time to fill) / cystic degeneration

√ ring-blush
  Incidence of ring blush:
    abscess (in 73%); glioblastoma (in 48%);
    metastasis (in 33%); grade II astrocytoma (in 26%)
    [NOT in grade I astrocytoma]

Intraventricular tumor
1.	Ependymoma	20%
2.	Astrocytoma	18%
3.	Colloid cyst	12%
4.	Meningioma	11%
5.	Choroid plexus papilloma	7%
6.	Epidermoid / dermoid	6%
7.	Craniopharyngioma	6%
8.	Medulloblastoma	5%
9.	Cysticercosis	5%
10.	Arachnoid cyst	4%
11.	Subependymoma	2%
12.	AVM	2%
13.	Teratoma	1%
14.	Metastasis	

IN 4TH VENTRICLE
    1. Choroid plexus papilloma
    2. Ependymoma / glioma
    3. Hemangioblastoma
    4. Vermian metastasis
    5. AVM
    6. Epidermoid tumor (rare)
    7. Inflammatory mass
    8. Cyst
IN 3RD VENTRICLE
    1. Colloid cyst
    2. Glioma
    3. Aneurysm
    4. Craniopharyngioma
    5. Ependymoma
    6. Meningioma
    7. Choroid plexus papilloma
    8. Intraventricular neurocytoma

Jugular foramen mass
1. Glomus tumor
2. Meningioma
3. Neuroma
4. Metastasis

Dumbbell mass spanning petrous apex
1. Large trigeminal schwannoma
2. Meningioma
3. Epidermoid cyst

Posterior fossa tumor in adult

A. Extraaxial:
1. Acoustic neuroma
2. Meningioma
3. Chordoma
4. Choroid plexus papilloma
5. Epidermoid

B. Intraaxial:
1. Metastasis (lung, breast)
2. Hemangioblastoma
3. Lymphoma
4. Lipoma

CYSTIC MASS IN CEREBELLAR HEMISPHERE IN ADULT
1. Hemangioblastoma
2. Cerebellar astrocytoma
3. Metastasis
4. Lateral medulloblastoma (= "cerebellar sarcoma")
5. Choroid plexus papilloma with lateral extension

Cerebellopontine angle tumor

= extraaxial tumor arising between bone / dura and brain

√ may widen CSF space (cistern) in 25%
√ bone erosion / hyperostosis
√ sharp margination with brain

Types:
1. Acoustic neuroma = schwannoma (80%): from intracanalicular portion of 8th cranial nerve
2. Meningioma (13 – 18%)
   2nd most common extraaxial mass in posterior fossa; <5% of all intracranial meningiomas; larger + more hemispheric in shape + more homogeneously enhancing than acoustic neuroma
3. Epidermoid tumor (5%): cholesterol contents
4. Trigeminal neuroma
   from Gasserian ganglion within Meckel cave in the most anteromedial portion of petrous pyramid / trigeminal nerve root
5. Glomus jugulare tumor
   within adventitia of bulb of jugular vein at base of petrous bone with invasion of posterior fossa
6. Chordoma
7. Arachnoid cyst
8. Aneurysm of basilar / vertebral artery
9. Exophytic glioma

mnemonic: "**E**ver **G**rave **C**erebello**P**ontine **A**ngle **M**asses"
Epidermoid
Glomus jugulare tumor
Chondroma, **C**hordoma, **C**holesteatoma
Pituitary tumor, **P**ontine glioma (exophytic)
Acoustic + trigeminal neuroma, **A**neurysm of basilar / vertebral artery, **A**rachnoid cyst
Meningioma, **M**etastasis

LOW-ATTENUATION EXTRAAXIAL LESION:
1. Acoustic schwannoma (occasionally low density mass)
2. Epidermoid tumor
3. Arachnoid cyst

Lesion expanding cavernous sinus

A. TUMOR
1. Trigeminal schwannoma
2. Pituitary adenoma
3. Parasellar meningioma
4. Parasellar metastasis
5. Invasion by tumor of skull base

B. VESSEL
1. Internal carotid artery aneurysm
2. Carotid-cavernous fistula
3. Cavernous sinus thrombosis

C. Tolosa-Hunt syndrome = granulomatous invasion of cavernous sinus

Phakomatoses

= NEUROCUTANEOUS SYNDROMES
= NEUROECTODERMAL DYSPLASIAS = development of benign tumors / malformations especially in organs of ectodermal origin
1. Neurofibromatosis
2. Tuberous sclerosis
3. von Hippel-Lindau disease
4. Sturge-Weber-Dimitri syndrome
5. Ataxia-telangiectasia

CLASSIFICATION OF CNS ANOMALIES

A. DORSAL INDUCTION ANOMALY
= defects of neural tube closure
1. Chiari malformation: at 4 weeks
2. Encephalocele: at 4 weeks
3. Anencephaly
4. Spinal dysraphism
5. Hydromyelia

B. VENTRAL INDUCTION ANOMALY
1. Holoprosencephaly: 5 – 6 weeks
2. Septo-optic dysplasia: 6 – 7 weeks
3. Dandy-Walker malformation: 7 – 10 weeks
4. Agenesis of septum pellucidum

C. NEURONAL PROLIFERATION & HISTOGENESIS
1. Neurofibromatosis: 5 weeks – 6 months
2. Tuberous sclerosis: 5 weeks – 6 months
3. Primary hydranencephaly: >3 months
4. Neoplasia
5. Vascular malformation (vein of Galen, AVM, hemangioma)

D. NEURONAL MIGRATION ANOMALY
1. Schizencephaly: 2 months
2. Agyria + pachygyria: 3 months
3. Gray matter heterotopia: 5 months
4. Dysgenesis of corpus callosum: 2 - 5 months
5. Lissencephaly
6. Polymicrogyria
7. Unilateral megalencephaly

E. DESTRUCTIVE LESIONS
1. Hydranencephaly
2. Porencephaly
3. Hypoxia
4. Toxicoses

5. Inflammatory disease (TORCH)
   (a) Toxoplasmosis
   (b) Herpes simplex
   (c) Rubella
       √ punctate / nodular calcifications
       √ porencephalic cysts
       √ occasionally microcephaly
   (d) Cytomegalic inclusion disease
       √ typically punctate / stippled / curvilinear periventricular calcifications
       √ often hydrocephalus

Classification of vascular CNS anomalies
A. VASCULAR MALFORMATION
   (a) arterial
       1. Facial / brain arteriovenous malformation
   (b) capillary
       1. Facial port wine stain
   (c) venous = tangle of varices
       • soft + compressible without thrills / pulsations
       • distension with Valsalva maneuver
       √ normal angiogram
   (d) lymphatic
       1. Cystic hygroma
   (e) combinations
       1. Sturge-Weber disease
       2. Rendu-Osler-Weber disease
B. VASCULAR TUMOR
   1. Hemangioma
       (a) capillary hemangioma: seen in children, involution by 7 years of age in 95%
       (b) cavernous hemangioma: seen in adults, no involution
           √ thrombosed blood + hemosiderin
           √ normal angiogram
   2. Hemangiopericytoma
   3. Hemangioendothelioma
   4. Angiosarcoma

Absence of septum pellucidum
1. Holoprosencephaly
2. Callosal agenesis
3. Septo-optic dysplasia
4. Schizencephaly
5. Severe chronic hydrocephalus
6. Destructive porencephaly

Colpocephaly
= dilatation of trigones + occipital horns + posterior temporal horns of lateral ventricles
1. Agenesis of corpus callosum
2. Arnold-Chiari malformation
3. Holoprosencephaly

SELLA
Destruction of sella
1. Pituitary adenoma
2. Suprasellar tumor
3. Carcinoma of sphenoid + posterior ethmoid sinus
   √ opacification of sinus + destruction of walls

√ associated with nasopharyngeal mass (common)
4. Nasopharyngeal carcinoma
   (a) squamous cell carcinoma
   (b) lymphoepithelioma = Schmincke tumor = non-keratinizing form of squamous cell carcinoma
       √ sclerosis of adjacent bone
5. Metastasis to sphenoid
   from breast, kidney, thyroid, colon, prostate, lung, esophagus
6. Primary tumor of sphenoid bone (rare)
   osteogenic sarcoma, giant cell tumor, plasmacytoma
7. Chordoma
8. Mucocele of spenoid sinus (uncommon)
9. Enlarged 3rd ventricle
   aqueductal stenosis from infratentorial mass, maldevelopment

Enlarged sella
A. TUMOR
   1. Pituitary adenoma
   2. Craniopharyngioma
   3. Meningioma: hyperostosis
   4. Optic glioma: J-shaped sella
B. PITUITARY HYPERPLASIA
   1. Hypothyroidism
   2. Hypogonadism
   3. Nelson syndrome (occurring in 7% of patients subsequent to adrenalectomy)
C. CSF-SPACE
   1. Enlarged 3rd ventricle
   2. Hydrocephalus
   3. Empty sella
D. VESSEL
   1. Arterial aneurysm
   2. Ectatic internal carotid artery

mnemonic: "CHAMPS"
   Craniopharyngioma
   Hydrocephalus (empty sella)
   AVM, **A**neurysm
   Meningioma
   Pituitary adenoma
   Sarcoidosis, TB

Parasellar mass
1. Meningioma: tentorium cerebelli
2. Neurinoma (III, IV, V_1, V_2, VI)
3. Metastasis: lung, breast, kidney, GI tract, spread from nasopharynx
4. Epidermoid
5. Aneurysm
6. Carotid-cavernous fistula

mnemonic: "SATCHMO"
   Sella neoplasm with superior extension, **S**arcoidosis
   Aneurysm, ectatic carotid, carotid-cavernous sinus fistula, **A**rachnoid cyst
   Teratoma: dysgerminoma (usually), dermoid, epidermoid
   Craniopharyngioma, **C**hordoma

Hypothalamic glioma, **H**istiocytoma, **H**amartoma
Metastatic disease, **M**eningioma, **M**ucocele
Optic nerve glioma, neuroma

Intrasellar mass

1. Pituitary adenoma / carcinoma (most common cause)
2. Craniopharyngioma (2nd most common cause)
3. Meningioma: from surface of diaphragm / tuberculum sellae
4. Chordoma
5. Metastasis: lung, breast, prostate, kidney, GI tract, spread from nasopharynx
6. Intracavernous ICA aneurysm: bilateral in 25%
7. Pituitary abscess: rapidly expanding mass associated with meningitis
8. Empty sella
9. Rathke cleft cyst: commonly at junction of anterior + posterior pituitary gland
10. Granular cell tumor = myeloblastoma: benign neoplasm of posterior pituitary gland
11. Granuloma: sarcoidosis, giant cell granuloma, TB, syphilis, eosinophilic granuloma
12. Lymphoid adenohypophysitis
13. Pituitary hyperplasia, eg, in Nelson syndrome

Suprasellar mass

1. Meningioma
2. Craniopharyngioma: in 80% suprasellar
3. Chiasmal + optic nerve glioma
   in 38% of neurofibromatosis; adolescent girls;
   DDx: chiasmal neuritis
4. Hypothalamic glioma
5. Hamartoma of tuber cinereum
6. Infundibular tumor
   metastasis (esp. breast); glioma; lymphoma / leukemia; histiocytosis X; sarcoidosis, tuberculosis
   √ diameter of infundibulum >4.5 mm immediately above level of dorsum; cone-shaped (on coronal scan)
7. Germinoma
   malignant tumor similar to seminoma (= "ectopic pinealoma")
   √ frequently calcified (teratoma)
   √ CSF spread (germinoma + teratocarcinoma)
   √ enhancement on CECT (common)
8. Epidermoid / dermoid
   √ cystic lesion containing calcifications + fat
   √ minimal / no contrast enhancement
9. Arachnoid cyst
   • hydrocephalus (common), visual impairment,
   • endocrine dysfunction
   Age: most common in infancy
10. Enlarged 3rd ventricle extending into pituitary fossa
11. Suprasellar aneurysm
    √ rim calcification + eccentric position

Suprasellar mass with low attenuation

1. Craniopharyngioma
2. Dermoid / epidermoid
3. Arachnoid cyst
4. Lipoma
5. Simple pituitary cyst
6. Glioma of hypothalamus

Suprasellar mass with mixed attenuation

A. IN CHILDREN
1. Hypothalamic-chiasmatic glioma
2. Craniopharyngioma
3. Hamartoma of tuber cinereum
4. Histiocytosis
B. IN ADULTS
1. Suprasellar extension of pituitary adenoma
2. Craniopharyngioma
3. Epidermoid cyst
4. Thrombosed aneurysm
5. Low-grade hypothalamic / optic glioma
6. Inflammatory lesion: sarcoidosis, TB, sphenoid mucocele

Suprasellar mass with calcification

A. Curvilinear:
1. Giant carotid aneurysm
2. Craniopharyngioma
B. Granular:
1. Craniopharyngioma
2. Meningioma
3. Granuloma
4. Dermoid cyst / teratoma
5. Optic / hypothalamic glioma (rare)

Enhancing mass with supra- and intrasellar component

1. Pituitary adenoma
2. Meningioma
3. Germinoma
4. Hypothalamic glioma
5. Craniopharyngioma

Perisellar vascular lesion

1. ICA aneurysm
   Giant aneurysms are >2.5 cm in diameter
   √ destruction of bony sella / superior orbital fissure
   √ calcified wall / thrombus
   √ CECT enhancement, nonuniform with thrombosis
2. Ectatic carotid artery
   √ curvilinear calcifications
   √ encroachment upon sella turcica
3. Carotid-cavernous sinus fistula

PINEAL GLAND

Classification of pineal gland tumors

Incidence of pineal mass:
   <1% of all intracranial tumors, 4% of all childhood intracranial masses, 9% of all intracranial masses in Asia
Δ "pinealoma" = misnomer referring to any pineal mass

A. PRIMARY TUMOR
  (a) Germ cell origin (2/3)
      — forming embryonic tissue
        1. Germinoma (40 – 50%)
        2. Embryonal cell carcinoma
        3. Teratoma (15%): benign mature teratoma, benign immature teratoma, malignant teratoma
      — forming extraembryonic tissue
        4. Choriocarcinoma (<5%)
        5. Endodermal sinus tumor = yolk sac tumor
  (b) Pineal parenchymal cell origin (<15%)
      1. Pineocytoma
      2. Pineoblastoma
  (c) Other cell origin
      1. Retinoblastoma (trilateral retinoblastoma = left eye + right eye + pineal gland
      2. Astrocytoma
      3. Ependymoma
      4. Meningioma
      5. Hemangiopericytoma
  (d) Cysts
      1. Pineal cyst
      2. Malignant teratoma
      3. AVM, vein of Galen aneurysm
      4. Arachnoid cyst
      5. Inclusion cyst (dermoid / epidermoid)
B. SECONDARY TUMOR
  Metastasis: eg, lung carcinoma

DDx considerations:
  — female: likely NOT germ cell tumor
  — hypodense matrix: likely NOT pineal cell tumor
  — distinct tumor margins: probably pineocytoma / teratoma / germinoma
  — calcification: likely NOT teratocarcinoma, metastasis, germinoma
  — CSF seeding: NOT teratoma
  — intense enhancement: likely NOT teratoma

Intensely enhancing mass in pineal region
1. Germinoma
2. Pineocytoma / -blastoma
3. Pineal teratocarcinoma
4. Glioma of brainstem / thalamus
5. Subsplenial meningioma
6. Vein of Galen aneurysm

DEGENERATIVE DISEASES OF CEREBRAL HEMISPHERES
= progressive fatal disease characterized by destruction / alteration of gray and white matter
Etiology: genetic; viral infection; nutritional disorders (eg, anorexia nervosa, Cushing syndrome); immune system disorders (eg, AIDS); exposure to toxins (eg, CO); exposure to drugs (eg, alcohol, methotrexate + radiation)
Leukodystrophy
  = degenerative diffuse sclerosis with symmetrical bilateral white matter lesions

Leukoencephalopathy
  = disease of white matter

A. DEMYELINATING DISEASE
  = normal myelin destroyed by disease process
    1. Multiple sclerosis (most frequent primary demyelinating disease)
    2. Alzheimer disease (most common of diffuse gray matter degenerative diseases)
    3. Parkinson disease (most common subcortical degenerative disease)
    4. Creutzfeldt-Jakob disease
    5. Menkes disease (sex-linked recessive disorder of copper metabolism)
    6. Progressive multifocal leukoencephalopathy
    7. Disseminated necrotizing leukoencephalopathy
    8. Globoid cell leukodystrophy
    9. Spongiform degeneration
    10. Cockayne syndrome
    11. Spongiform leukoencephalopathy

B. DYSMYELINATING DISEASE
  = metabolic disorder (= enzyme deficiency) resulting in deficient / absent myelin sheaths
  (a) macrencephalic:
      1. Alexander disease (frontal areas affected first)
      2. Canavan disease (white matter diffusely affected)
  (b) hyperdense thalami, caudate nuclei, corona radiata
      1. Krabbe disease
  (c) family history (X-linked recessive)
      1. X-linked adrenoleukodystrophy
      2. Pelizaeus-Merzbacher disease
  (d) others
      1. Metachromatic leukodystrophy (most common hereditary leukodystrophy)
      2. Binswanger disease (SAE)
      3. Multi-infarct dementia (MID)
      4. Pick disease
      5. Huntington disease
      6. Wilson disease
      7. Reye syndrome
      8. Mineralizing microangiopathy
      9. Diffuse sclerosis

Infection in immunocompromised patients
Cause: underlying malignancy, collagen disease, cancer therapy, AIDS, immunosuppressive therapy in organ transplants
Organism: Toxoplasma, Nocardia, Aspergillus, Candida, Cryptococcus

√ ring / nodular enhancement (sufficient immune defenses): Toxoplasma, Nocardia
√ enhancement may be blunted by steroid Rx
√ poorly defined hypodense zones with rapid enlargement in size + number, particularly affecting basal ganglia + centrum semiovale (poorly localized + encapsulated infection with poor prognosis)

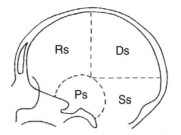

Rs = round shift Ds = distal shift Ps = Proximal shift Ss = square shift

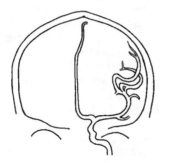

Round shift

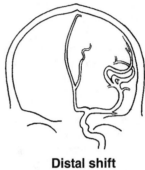

Distal shift

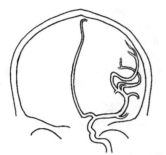

Square shift

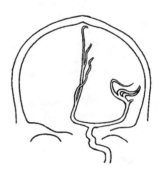

Proximal shift

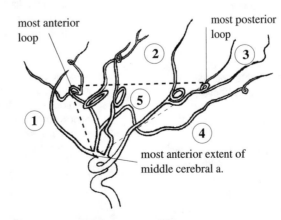

Sylvian Triangle
reference to numbers in text

AIDS may be associated with:
thrombocytopenia, lymphoma, plasmacytoma, Kaposi sarcoma, progressive multifocal leukoencephalopathy

Displacement of vessels
A. Arterial shift
(a) Pericallosal arteries
1. Round shift = frontal lesion anterior to coronal suture
2. Square shift = lesion behind foramen of Monro in lower half of hemisphere
3. Distal shift = posterior to coronal suture in upper half of hemisphere
4. Proximal shift = basifrontal lesion / anterior middle cranial fossa including anterior temporal lobe
(b) Sylvian triangle
= branches of MCA within sylvian fissure on outer surface of insula form a loop upon reaching the upper margin of the insula; serves as angiographic landmark for localizing supratentorial masses
Location of lesion:
1. anterior sylvian ... frontal region
2. suprasylvian ... posterior frontal + parietal
3. retrosylvian ... occipital, parieto-occipital
4. infrasylvian ... temporal lobe + extracerebral region
5. intrasylvian ... usually due to meningioma
6. lateral sylvian ... frontal, frontotemporal, parietotemporal
7. central sylvian ... deep posterior frontal, basal ganglia
B. Cerebral veins
= indicate the midline of the posterior part of the forebrain showing the exact location of the roof of the 3rd ventricle

Occlusive vascular disease
(a) Embolic state: √ single vascular territory
(b) Hypoperfusive state: √ multiple vascular territories
Causes:
1. Vasospasm from subarachnoid hemorrhage
2. Embolic infarction (50%)
(a) thrombus (atrial fibrillation, valvular disease, atheromatous plaques of extracerebral arteries, fibromuscular dysplasia, intracranial aneurysm, surgery, paradoxic emboli, sickle cell disease, atherosclerosis, thrombotic thrombocytopenic purpura)
• fluctuating blood pressures
• hypercoagulability
√ cerebral petechial hemorrhage within cortical / basal gray matter during 2nd week (from fragments of embolus) in up to 40%; initial ischemia is followed by reperfusion (= HALLMARK of embolic infarction)
√ "supernormal artery" on NECT = high-density material lodged in cerebral vessel near major bifurcations

√ atheromatous narrowing of vessels

(b) fat
(c) nitrogen

3. Watershed infarct
involving deep white matter between two adjacent vascular beds in global hypoperfusion secondary to poor cardiac output / cervical carotid artery occlusion
Δ 6% of cerebral infarcts have hemorrhage (red infarct)
• stroke (3rd most common cause of death in USA) (5% of stroke syndromes are caused by underlying tumor)
• TIA = transitory ischemic attack: clears within 24 hours
• RIND = reversible ischemic neurologic deficit: still evident >24 hours with eventual total recovery
• amaurosis fugax = transient monocular blindness
• weakness / numbness in an extremity
• aphasia
• dizziness, diplopia, dysarthria (vertebrobasilar ischemia)

4. Hypertension
(a) Hypertensive encephalopathy
√ diffuse white matter hypodensity (edema secondary to arterial spasm)
(b) Hypertensive hemorrhage
Location: basal ganglia (putamen, external capsule), thalamus, pons, cerebellum
(c) Lacunar infarct
secondary to occlusion of small penetrating endarteries at base of brain
Incidence: 20% of cerebral infarctions
Histo: hyalinization + arteriolar sclerosis resulting in thickening of vessel wall + luminal narrowing
Location: basal ganglia, thalamus, pons (territory of lenticulostriate, thalamoperforating, pontine perforating arteries)
√ small discrete foci of hypodensity <1 cm in diameter
(d) Subcortical arteriosclerotic encephalopathy (SAE)

5. Amyloidosis
involvement of small + medium-sized arteries of meninges + cortex
• normotensive patient >65 years of age
√ multiple simultaneous / recurrent cortical hemorrhages

6. Vasculitis
(a) Bacterial meningitis, TB, syphilis, fungus, virus, rickettsia
(b) Collagen-vascular disease: Wegener granulomatosis, polyarteritis nodosa, SLE, scleroderma, dermatomyositis

(c) Granulomatous angitis: giant cell arteritis, sarcoidosis, Takayasu disease, temporal arteritis

(d) Inflammatory arteritis: rheumatoid arteritis, hypersensitivity arteritis, Behçet disease, lymphomatoid granulomatosis

(e) Drug-induced: IV amphetamine, ergot preparations, oral contraceptives

(f) Radiation arteritis = mineralizing microangiopathy

(g) Moyamoya disease

7. Anoxic encephalopathy
cardiorespiratory arrest, near-drowning, drug overdose, CO poisoning

8. Venous thrombosis

MULTIPLE INFARCTIONS
typical in extracranial occlusive disease, cardiac output problems, small vessel disease; in 6% from a shower of emboli
Location: usually bilateral + supratentorial (3/4); supra- and infratentorial (1/4)

Cerebrovascular malformations
1. Arteriovenous malformation
2. Vein of Galen aneurysm
3. Sinus pericranii
4. Venous angioma

Occult vascular malformation
1. Cavernous angioma
2. Capillary teleangiectasia

Birth Trauma
1. **Caput succedaneum**
   $\doteq$ localized edema in presenting portion of scalp, frequently associated with microscopic hemorrhage + subcutaneous hyperemia
   Cause: commonly after vaginal delivery
   • soft superficial pitting edema
   √ crosses suture lines
2. **Subgaleal hemorrhage**
   = hemorrhage subjacent to aponeurosis covering scalp beneath the occipito-frontalis muscle
   • may become symptomatic secondary to blood loss
   • firm fluctuant mass increasing in size after birth
   • may dissect into subcutaneous tissue of neck
   • usually resolves over 2 – 3 weeks
3. **Cephalohematoma**
   = hematoma beneath outer layer of periosteum
   Cause: incorrect application of obstetric forceps / skull fracture during birth
   Incidence: 1 – 2% of all deliveries
   Location: most commonly parietal
   • firm tense mass
   • usually increase in size after birth
   • resolution in few weeks to months
   √ confined by cranial sutures
   √ crescent-shaped lesion adjacent to outer table of skull
   √ may calcify / ossify causing thickening of diploe

4. Skull fracture
   Incidence: 1% of all deliveries
   √ CT shows associated intracranial hemorrhage
5. Subdural hemorrhage
   (a) convexity hematoma (b) interhemispheric hematoma (c) posterior fossa hematoma
6. **Benign subdural effusion**
   = benign condition that resolves spontaneously
   • clear / xanthochromic fluid with elevated protein level
   √ extracerebral fluid collection accompanied by ventricular dilatation (= communicating hydrocephalus caused by impaired CSF absorption of these subdural fluid collections)

Increased intracranial pressure
1. Intracranial mass
2. Hydrocephalus
3. Malignant hypertension
4. Diffuse cerebral edema
5. Increased venous pressure
6. Elevated CSF protein
7. Pseudotumor cerebri
• papilledema
√ enlargement of perioptic nerve subarachnoid space

Prolactin elevation
Causes:
1. Interference with hypothalamic-pituitary axis:
   (a) hypothalamic tumor
   (b) parasellar tumor
   (c) sarcoidosis
   (d) histiocytosis
   (e) traumatic infundibular transection
2. Pharmacologic agents
   alpha-methyldopa, reserpine, phenothiazine, butyrophenone, tricyclic antidepressants, oral contraceptives
3. Hypothyroidism
4. Renal failure
5. Cirrhosis
6. Stress / recent surgery
7. Breast examination
8. Pregnancy
9. Lactation

Stroke
Incidence:
   3rd leading cause of death in United States (after heart disease + cancer); 2nd leading cause of death due to cardiovascular disease in U.S.; 2nd leading cause of death in patients >75 years of age; 450,000 new cases / year; 160 new strokes per 100,000 population per year; leading cause of death in Orient
Age: >55 years; M:F = 2:1
Risk factors:
   heredity, hypertension (50%), smoking, diabetes (15%), obesity, familial hypercholesterolemia, myocardial infarction, atrial fibrillation, congestive heart failure, alcoholic excess, oral contraceptives, high anxiety + stress

Etiology:
A. NONVASCULAR (5%): eg, tumor
B. VASCULAR (95%)
  1. Hemorrhagic brain infarction (12%)
    intracerebral hemorrhage (12%)
  2. Ischemic brain infarction (78%)
    (a) Occlusive disease of extracranial (35%) /
        intracranial (10%) arteries = large vessel
        disease between aorta + penetrating arterioles
        <u>Atherosclerosis</u>
        — critical stenosis, thrombosis,
        — plaque hemorrhage / ulceration / embolism
        <u>Non-atherosclerotic disease</u>
        — elongation, coil, kinks (up to 20%)
        — fibromuscular dysplasia (typically spares
           origin + proximal segment of ICA)
        — aneurysm (rare) may occur in cervical /
           petrous portion / intracranially
        — dissection (traumatic / spontaneous)
        — arteritis (Takayasu, giant cell)
    (b) Small vessel disease of penetrating arteries
        = recipients of emboli
    (c) Cardiogenic emboli (6 – 23%)
        <u>Ischemic heart disease with mural thrombus</u>
        — acute myocardial infarction (3% risk/year)
        — cardiac arrhythmia
        <u>Valvular heart disease</u>
        — post-inflammatory (rheumatic) valvulitis
        — infective endocarditis (20% risk/year)
        — nonbacterial thrombotic endocarditis (30%
           risk/year)
        — mitral valve prolapse (low risk)
        — mitral stenosis (20% risk/year)
        — prosthetic valves (1 – 4% risk/year)
        <u>Nonvalvular atrial fibrillation</u> (6% risk/year)
        <u>Left atrial myxoma</u> (27 – 55% risk/year)
    (d) Vasospasm due to subarachnoid hemorrhage
        (10%)
    (e) Veno-occlusive disease (2%)
    (f) others (4%)
        — Cerebral arteritis (collagen disease,
           lymphoid granulomatosis, temporal
           arteritis, Behçet disease)
        — Post-endarterectomy thrombosis /
           embolism / restenosis
May be preceded by   TIA
  Δ 10 – 14% of all strokes are preceded by TIA!
  Δ 60% of all strokes ascribed to carotid disease are
    preceded by TIA!
Prognosis:
  (1) death during hospitalization (25%): alteration in
      consciousness, gaze preference, dense hemiplegia
      have a 40% mortality rate
  (2) survival with varying degrees of neurologic deficit
      (75%)
  (3) good functional recovery (40%)
Indications for cerebrovascular testing:
  1. TIA = transient ischemic attack
  2. Progression of carotid disease to 95 – 98% stenosis
  3. Cardiogenic cerebral emboli

Temporal classification:
  1. **TIA** = transient ischemic attack
  2. **RIND** = reversible ischemic neurologic deficit
    = fully reversible prolonged ischemic event resulting
    in minor neurologic dysfunction for >24 hours
    Incidence: 16 per 100,000 population per year
  3. **Progressing stroke** = stepwise / gradually
    progressing accumulative neurologic deficit evolving
    over hours / days
  4. **Slow stroke** = rare clinical syndrome presenting as
    developing neuronal fatigue with weakness in lower /
    proximal upper extremity after exercise; occurs in
    patients with occluded internal carotid artery
  5. **Completed stroke** = severe + persistent stable
    neurologic deficit = cerebral infarction (death of
    neuronal tissue) as endstage of prolonged ischemia
    • level of consciousness correlates well with size of
      infarction
    Prognosis: 6 – 11% recurrent stroke rate

Transient ischemic attack

= brief episode of transient focal neurological deficit owing
  to ischemia of <24 hours duration with return to pre-
  attack status

Incidence: 31 per 100,000 population per year;
             increasing with age up to 300; 105,000 new
             cases per year in United States; M>F
Cause: (1) embolic: usually from ulcerative plaque at
             carotid bifurcation
      (2) hemodynamic: fall in perfusion pressure
             distal to a high-grade stenosis / occlusion

Risk factors:
  (1) Hypertension (linear increase in probability of stroke
      with increase in diastolic blood pressure)
  (2) Cardiac disorders (prior myocardial infarction,
      angina pectoris, valvular heart disease,
      dysrhythmia, congestive heart failure)
  (3) Diabetes mellitus
  (4) Cigarette smoking (weak)

Prognosis: 5.3% stroke rate per year for 5 years after
             first TIA; per year 12% increase of stroke /
             myocardial infarction / death; complete
             stroke in 33% within 5 years; complete
             stroke in 5% in 1 month

A. CAROTID TIA (2/3)
  • carotid attacks <6 hours in 90%
  • transient weakness / sensory dysfunction
    CLASSICALLY in
    (a) hand / face with embolic event
    (b) proximal arm + lower extremity with
        hemodynamic event (watershed area)
  — motor dysfunction = weakness, paralysis,
      clumsiness of one / both limbs on same side
  — sensory alteration = numbness, loss of sensation,
      paresthesia of one / both limbs on same side

— speech / language disturbance = difficulty in speaking (dys- / aphasia) / writing, in comprehension of language / reading / performing calculations

— visual disturbance = loss of vision in one eye, homonymous hemianopia, amaurosis fugax

• paresis (mono-, hemiparesis) in 61%
• paresthesia (mono-, hemiparesthesia) in 57%
• amaurosis fugax (= transient premonitory attack of impaired vision due to retinal ischemia) in 12% caused by transient hypotension or emboli of platelets / cholesterol crystals which may be revealed by funduscopy
• facial paresthesia in 30%

B. VERTEBROBASILAR TIA (1/3)
• vertebrobasilar events <2 hours in 90%
— motor dysfunction = as with carotid TIA but sometimes changing from side to side including quadriplegia, diplopia, dysarthria, dysphagia
— sensory alteration = as with carotid TIA usually involving one / both sides of face / mouth / tongue
— visual loss = as with carotid TIA including uni- / bilateral homonymous hemianopsia
— disequilibrium of gait / postural disturbance, ataxia, imbalance / unsteadiness
— drop attack = sudden fall to the ground without loss of consciousness
• binocular visual disturbance in 57%
• vertigo in 50%
• paresthesia in 40%
• diplopia in 38%
• ataxia in 33%
• paresis in 33%
• headaches in 25%
• seizures in 1.5%

ACCELERATING / CRESCENDO TIA
= repeated periodic events of neurologic dysfunction with complete recovery to normal in interphase

Rx: 1. Carotid endarterectomy (1% mortality, 5% stroke)
2. Anticoagulation
3. Antiplatelet agent: aspirin, ticlopedine
— in patients with recently symptomatic TIA / minor stroke + >70% carotid artery stenosis: prophylactic carotid endarterectomy + chronic low-dose aspirin therapy

Pulsatile tinnitus ± vascular tympanic membrane
= perception of a rhythmic cardiac synchronous sound

A. No abnormality (20%)
B. Normal vascular variants (21%)
  1. Aberrant ICA
    = result of anastomosis of enlarged inferior tympanic artery with enlarged caroticotympanic artery when cervical ICA is underdeveloped
  2. Dehiscent jugular bulb
    √ absence of bony plate separating jugular bulb from middle ear cavity
    √ jugular bulb bulges into middle ear cavity
  3. High-riding non-dehiscent jugular bulb (= jugular megabulb)
    √ high jugular bulb with diverticulum projecting cephalad into petrous temporal bone
C. Acquired vascular lesions (25%)
  1. Dural AVM
  2. Extracranial arteriovenous fistula
  3. Stenotic vascular lesion: carotid artery atherosclerosis, fibromuscular dysplasia, carotid artery dissection
  4. Aneurysm involving horizontal segment of petrous ICA
D. Temporal bone tumors (31%)
  1. Paraganglioma (27%): glomus tympanicum, glomus jugulare
  2. Meningioma
  3. Hemangioma
E. Miscellaneous
  1. Cholesterol granuloma

ANATOMY OF BRAIN

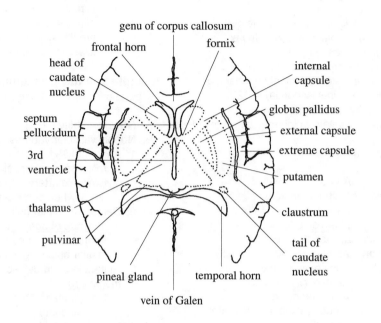

Axial section through level of 3rd ventricle

genu of corpus callosum
frontal horn
fornix
head of caudate nucleus
internal capsule
septum pellucidum
globus pallidus
external capsule
extreme capsule
3rd ventricle
putamen
thalamus
claustrum
pulvinar
tail of caudate nucleus
pineal gland
temporal horn
vein of Galen

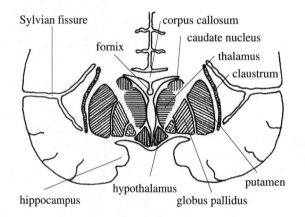

Coronal section through level of basal ganglia

Sylvian fissure
corpus callosum
caudate nucleus
fornix
thalamus
claustrum
hippocampus
hypothalamus
globus pallidus
putamen

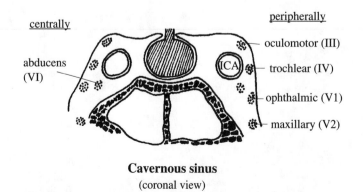

Cavernous sinus
(coronal view)

centrally
peripherally
abducens (VI)
oculomotor (III)
ICA
trochlear (IV)
ophthalmic (V1)
maxillary (V2)

Classification of brain anatomy
A. **Prosencephalon** = forebrain
   1. **Telencephalon** = cerebrum
      = cerebral hemispheres, putamen, caudate nucleus
   2. **Diencephalon**
      = thalamus, hypothalamus, epithalamus (= pineal gland + habenula), globus pallidus

B. **Mesencephalon** = midbrain
   = short segment of brainstem above pons; traverses the hiatus in tentorium cerebelli; contains cerebral peduncles, tectum, colliculi (corpora quadrigemina)

C. **Rhombencephalon** = hindbrain
   1. **Metencephalon** = cerebellar hemispheres, vermis
   2. **Myelencephalon** = medulla oblongata, pons

Basal nuclei
= BASAL GANGLIA (earlier incorrect designation)
A. Amygdaloid body
B. Claustrum
C. Corpus striatum
   (1) Caudate
   (2) Lentiform nucleus
      (a) pallidum = globus pallidus
      (b) putamen

Pituitary gland
= HYPOPHYSIS CEREBRI within hypophyseal fossa of sphenoid, covered superiorly by sellar diaphragm (= dura mater) which has an aperture for the infundibulum centrally
Size:
   adult size is achieved at puberty
   Height in adult females = 7 (range 4 – 10) mm
   Height in adult males   = 5 (range 3 – 7) mm
Shape:
   √ flat / downwardly convex superior border

A. ANTERIOR LOBE
   = larger anterior portion of adenohypophysis
   Origin: ectodermal derivative of stomatodeum
   Function:
      (a) chromophil cells
         1. acidophil cells = α cells
            somatotropin (STH), lactogenic hormone (LTH)
         2. basophil cells = β cells
            adrenocorticotropin (ACTH), thyrotropin (TSH), follicle-stimulating hormone (FSH), interstitial-cell-stimulating hormone (ICSH), luteinizing hormone (LH), melanocyte-stimulating hormone (MSH)
      (b) chromophobe cells = 50% of epithelial cell population, of unknown significance
   MRI:
      √ larger homogeneous component isointense to white matter on T1WI + T2WI
      √ prominent contrast enhancement (during first 3 minutes)

B. PARS INTERMEDIA
   = posterior portion of adenohypophysis; separated from anterior lobe by hypophyseal cleft in fetal life
   Origin: pouch of Rathke
   √ not visible with imaging techniques

C. POSTERIOR LOBE
   = major portion of neurohypophysis
   Origin: diencephalic outgrowth (termination point of axons from supraoptic + paraventricular nuclei of hypothalamus)
   Function: vasopressin = antidiuretic hormone (ADH), oxytocin transported along neurosecretory hypothalamohypophyseal tract
   MRI:
      √ hyperintense on T1WI + isointense on T2WI in comparison to anterior lobe (? due to relaxing agent of phospholipid / neurosecretory granules / vasopressin)

D. PITUITARY STALK = INFUNDIBULUM
   arises from anterior aspect of floor of 3rd ventricle (infundibular recess)
   √ joins posterior lobe at junction of anterior + posterior lobes
   √ up to 3 mm thick superiorly, up to 2 mm thick inferiorly
   √ usually in midline, may be slightly tilted to one side
   MRI:
      √ prominent contrast enhancement

Pineal gland
Development:
   from area of ependymal thickening at the most caudal portion of roof of 3rd ventricle that evaginates into a pine cone-shaped mass during 7th week of gestation; initially contains ependyma lining in central cavity that connects with 3rd ventricle
Function:
   1. regulation of long-term biologic rhythm (eg, onset of puberty)
   2. regulation of short-term biologic rhythm (eg, diurnal / circadian) due to photoperiodic clues via accessory optic pathway

Histo:
   (a) pinealocytes with dendritic processes (= neuronal cells) make up 95% of population
   (b) neuroglial supporting cells make up 5% of population

Location: attached to upper aspect of posterior border of 3rd ventricle, lies within CSF of quadrigeminal cistern, anterior to pineal gland is cistern of velum interpositum (= cistern of transverse fissure)

Size: 8 mm long, 4 mm wide
√ pineal calcifications: none <5 years of age, in 8 – 10% at 8 – 14 years of age, in 40% by 20 years of age

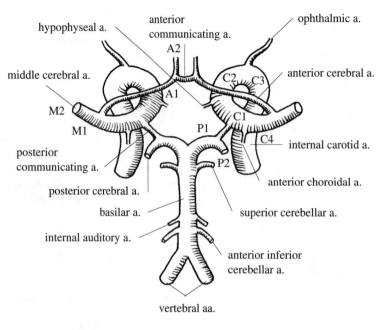

hypophyseal a.
anterior communicating a.
A2
ophthalmic a.
middle cerebral a.
C2 C3
anterior cerebral a.
M2
A1
M1
P1
C1
C4
internal carotid a.
posterior communicating a.
P2
posterior cerebral a.
anterior choroidal a.
basilar a.
superior cerebellar a.
internal auditory a.
anterior inferior cerebellar a.
vertebral aa.

Circle of Willis

CEREBRAL VESSELS

External carotid artery branches
mnemonic: "**A**ll **S**ummer **L**ong **E**mily **O**gled **P**eter's **S**porty **I**suzu"
Ascending pharyngeal artery
Superior thyroid artery
Lingual artery
External maxillary = facial artery
Occipital artery
Posterior auricular artery
Superficial temporal artery
Internal maxillary artery

Internal carotid artery
A.   CERVICAL SEGMENT
ascends posterior and medial to ECA; enters carotid canal of petrous bone; NO branches

B.   PETROUS SEGMENT
ascends briefly, in carotid canal bends anteromedially in a horizontal course (anterior to tympanic cavity + cochlea); exits near petrous apex through posterior portion of foramen lacerum; ascends to juxtasellar location where it pierces dural layer of cavernous sinus
Branches:
1. **Caroticotympanic a.:** to tympanic cavity, anastomoses with anterior tympanic branch of maxillary a. + stylomastoid a.
2. **Pterygoid (vidian) a.:** through pterygoid canal; anastomoses with recurrent branch of greater palatine a.

C.   CAVERNOUS SEGMENT
ascends to posterior clinoid process, then turns anteriorly + superomedially through cavernous sinus; exits medial to anterior clinoid process piercing dura
Branches:
1. **Meningohyphyseal trunk**
   (a) tentorial branch
   (b) dorsal meningeal branch
   (c) inferior hypophyseal branch
2. **Anterior meningeal a.:** supplies dura of anterior fossa; anastomoses with meningeal branch of posterior ethmoidal a.
3. Cavernous rami supply trigeminal ganglion, walls of cavernous + inferior petrosal sinuses

D.   SUPRACLINOID SEGMENT
ascends posterior + lateral between oculomotor + optic nerve
Branches:
   mnemonic: "OPA"
   Ophthalmic a.
   Posterior communicating a.
   Anterior choroidal a.
1. **Ophthalmic a.** exits from ICA medial to anterior clinoid process, travels through optic canal inferolateral to optic nerve
   (a) recurrent meningeal branch: dura of anterior middle cranial fossa
   (b) posterior ethmoidal a.: supplies dura of planum sphenoidale
   (c) anterior ethmoidal a.
2. **Superior hypophyseal a.:** optic chiasm, anterior lobe of pituitary
3. **Posterior communicating a.** (PCom)

4. **Anterior choroidal a.**
5. **Middle + anterior cerebral arteries**
(MCA, ACA)

CAROTID SIPHON
flow direction: C4 — C1
(a) C4 segment = before origin of ophthalmic a.
(b) C3 segment = genu of ICA
(c) C2 segment = supraclinoid segment after origin of ophthalmic a.
(d) C1 segment = terminal segment of ICA between pCom + ACA

Vertebral artery
originates from subclavian a. proximal to thyrocervical trunk; left vertebral a. usually greater than right cerebral a.; left vertebral a. may originate directly from aorta (5%)

A. PREVERTEBRAL SEGMENT
ascends posterosuperiorly between longus colli + anterior scalene muscle; enters transverse foramina at C6
Branches: muscular branches
B. CERVICAL SEGMENT
ascends through transverse foramina in close proximity to uncinate processes
Branches:
1. **Anterior meningeal a.**
C. ATLANTIC SEGMENT
exits transverse foramen of atlas; passes posteriorly in a groove on superior surface of posterior arch of atlas; pierces atlanto-occipital membrane + dura mater to enter cranial cavity
Branches:
1. **Posterior meningeal branch** to posterior falx + tentorium
D. INTRACRANIAL SEGMENT
ascends anteriorly + laterally around medulla to reach midline at pontomedullary junction; anastomoses with contralateral side to form basilar artery at clivus

Branches:
1. **Anterior + posterior spinal a.**
2. **Posterior inferior cerebellar a.** (PICA)
3. **Anterior inferior cerebellar a.** (AICA)
4. **Internal auditory a.**
5. **Superior cerebellar a.**
6. **Posterior cerebral a.** (PCA)
7. Medullary + pontine perforating branches

Anterior cerebral artery (ACA)
A. HORIZONTAL PORTION = A 1 SEGMENT = segment between origin and anterior communicating a. (ACom)
(a) Inferior branches
supply superior surface of optic nerve + chiasm
(b) superior branches
penetrate brain to supply anterior hypothalamus, septum pellucidum, anterior commissure, fornix columns, anterior inferior portion of corpus striatum (largest striatal artery = medial lenticulostriate artery = recurrent **artery of Heubner** for anteroinferior portion of head of caudate, putamen, anterior limb of internal capsule)

B. INTERHEMISPHERIC PORTION = A 2 SEGMENT = segment after origin of anterior communicating a. (ACom); ascends in cistern of lamina terminalis
Branches:
1. **Medial orbitofrontal a.:** along gyrus rectus
2. **Frontopolar a.**
3. **Callosomarginal a.:** within cingulus gyrus
4. **Pericallosal a.:** over corpus callosum within callosal cistern
(a) Superior internal parietal a.: anterior portion of precuneus + convexity of superior parietal lobule
(b) Inferior internal parietal a.
(c) Posterior pericallosal a.
from callosomarginal / pericallosal artery:
— Anterior + middle + posterior internal frontal aa.

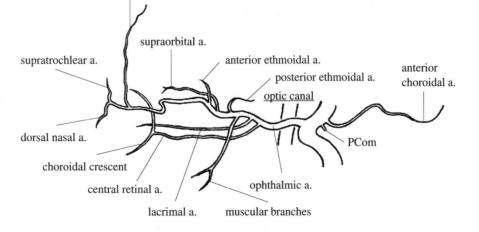

Ophthalmic artery

— Paracentral a.: supplies precentral +
postcentral gyri

Middle cerebral artery

= largest branch of ICA arising lateral to optic chiasm;
passes horizontal in lateral direction just ventral to
anterior perforated substance to enter sylvian fissure
where it divides into 2 / 3 / 4 branches

Branches: 1. **Anterior temporal a.**

2. **Ascending frontal a.** (candelabra) /
prefrontal a.
3. **Precentral a.** = Pre-Rolandic a.
4. **Central a.** = Rolandic a.
5. **Anterior parietal a.** = Post-Rolandic a.
6. **Posterior parietal a.**
7. **Angular a.**
8. **Middle temporal a.**
9. **Posterior temporal a.**
10. **Temporooccipital a.**

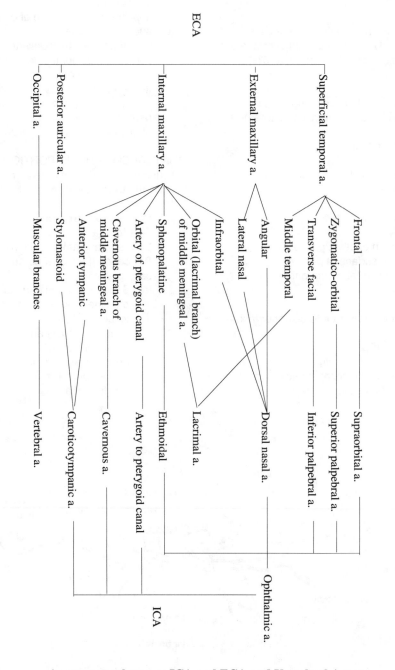

Anastomoses between ICA and ECA and Vertebral Artery

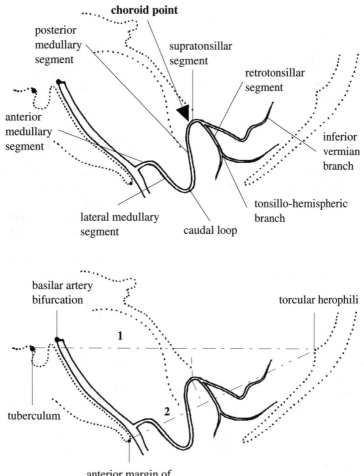

Posterior inferior cerebellar artery

Posterior cerebral artery

originates from bifurcation of basilar artery within interpeduncular cistern (in 15% as a direct continuation of posterior communicating artery); lies above oculomotor nerve and circles midbrain above the tentorium cerebelli
Branches:
1. Mesencephalic perforating branches: tectum + cerebral peduncles
2. Posterior thalamoperforating aa.: midline of thalamus + hypothalamus
3. Thalamogeniculate aa.: geniculate bodies + pulvinar
4. Posterior medial choroidal a.: circles midbrain parallel to PCA; enters lateral aspect of quadrigeminal cistern; passes lateral and above pineal gland and enters roof of 3rd ventricle; supplies quadrigeminal plate + pineal gland
5. Posterior lateral choroidal a.: courses lateral and enters choroidal fissure; anterior branch to temporal horn + posterior branch to choroid plexus of trigone and lateral ventricle + lateral geniculate body

6. Cortical branches:
   (a) Anterior inferior temporal a.
   (b) Posterior inferior temporal a.
   (c) Parietooccipital a.
   (d) Calcarine a.
   (e) Posterior pericallosal a.

Posterior inferior cerebellar artery

= PICA = last and largest branch of vertebral artery
Parts:
1. Premedullar segment = caudal loop around medulla, may descend below level of foramen magnum
2. Retromedullar segment = ascending portion up to the level of 4th ventricle and tonsils
3. Supratonsillar segment = the most cranial point is the choroidal point

P1 segment = horizontal segment between origin of PICA + pCom
P2 segment = segment downstream from pCom take-off

Variations: commonly asymmetric; hypoplastic / absent in 20% [vascular supply then provided by anterior inferior cerebellar artery (AICA)]

Orthotopic **choroid point** established by:

1. perpendicular line from choroid point onto Twining's line = TTT-line (Twining's Tuberculum-Torcula line) bisects TTT-line (length of anterior portion 52 – 60%)
2. perpendicular line from choroid point cuts CT-line (Clivus-Torcular line) <1 mm anterior / <3 mm posterior to junction of anterior and middle thirds of CT-line

Arterial anastomoses of the brain

Anastomoses via the arteries at the base of the brain

A.   Circle of Willis
   1. right ICA — right ACA — aCom — left ACA — left ICA
   2. ICA — pCom — basilar a.
   3. ICA — anterior choroidal a. — posterior choroidal a. — PCA — basilar a.
B.   Persistent anastomotic remnants
   transient carotid-basilar anastomoses appearing consecutively in embryonic life (normally involute by 35th day):
   1. **Persistent trigeminal artery**
      Incidence: 0.03 – 0.6% of angiograms
      Frequently associated with
      (a) ipsilateral hypoplastic PCA
      (b) aneurysm at origin
      √ 12 – 24 mm short wide connection between the cavernous portion of ICA and upper third of basilar artery (beneath posterior communicating artery)

2. **Persistent hypoglossal artery**
   Incidence: 30 cases in literature
   Associated with
   (a) hypoplasia / absence of vertebral arteries
   (b) origin of PICA from this vessel
   √ arterial connection between ICA (several cm above carotid sinus) and proximal portion of basilar artery (just above vertebrobasilar junction); enters cranium through hypoglossal canal

3. **Persistent proatlantal artery**
   = most caudal anastomotic channel between anterior + posterior circulation without clinical significance
   Incidence: 4 cases described
   √ arises from ICA at C2, travels through foramen magnum, connects to vertebral artery

4. **Persistent acoustic (otic) artery**
   Incidence: 8 cases
   • may compress cranial nerves VII + VIII
   √ arterial connection between cervical portion of ICA + vertebral artery in region of 12th nerve

Anastomoses via surface vessels

A.   Leptomeningeal anastomoses of the cerebrum: ACA — MCA — PCA
B.   Leptomeningeal anastomoses of the cerebellum: Superior cerebellar a. — AICA — PICA

Rete mirabile

ECA — middle meningeal a. / superficial temporal a. — leptomeningeal aa. — ACA / MCA

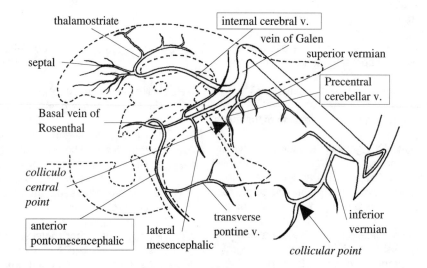

Cerebral Veins

Cerebral veins

Important vascular markers:

1. Pontomesencephalic v. = anterior border of brainstem
2. Precentral cerebellar v. = position of tectum
   △ colliculocentral point = midpoint of Twining's line at knee of precentral cerebellar vein
3. Venous angle = acute angle at junction of thalamostriate with internal cerebral v. = posterior aspect of foramen of Monro
4. Internal cerebral vv. = demarcate caudad border of splenium of corpus callosum superiorly + pineal gland inferiorly
5. Copular point = junction of inferior + superior retrotonsillar tributaries draining cerebellar tonsils in region of copular pyramids of vermis

Cerebrospinal fluid

Total volume:
50 ml in newborn, 150 ml in adult

Composition:
inorganic salts like those in plasma, traces of protein + glucose

Production:
0.3 – 0.4 ml/min resulting in 500 ml/day; secreted into ventricles by choroid plexuses (80 – 90%), 10 – 20% formed by parenchyma of the cerebrum + spinal cord

Circulation:
from ventricles through foramina of Magendie + Luschka of 4th ventricle into cisterna magna + basilar cisterns; 80% of CSF flows initially into suprasellar cistern + cistern of lamina terminalis, the ambient / superior cerebellar cisterns, eventually ascending over supero-lateral aspects of each hemisphere; 20% initially enters spinal subarachnoid space + eventually recirculates into cerebral subarachnoid space

Cerebral aqueduct:
pulsatile flow (due to brain motion during cardiac cycle) + net outflow into 4th ventricle; diameter of 2.6 – 4.2 mm; peak outflow velocity of 6 – 51 mm/sec; inflow velocity of 3 – 28 mm/sec

Absorption:
into venous system by

(a) arachnoid villi of superior sagittal sinus (villi behave as one-way valves with an opening pressure between 20 – 50 mm of CSF)
(b) cranial + spinal nerves with eventual absorption by lymphatics (50%)
(c) prelymphatic channels of capillaries within brain parenchyma
(d) vertebral venous plexuses, intervertebral veins, posterior intercostal + upper lumbar veins into azygos + hemiazygos veins

BRAIN DISORDERS

ABSCESS OF BRAIN
Pyogenic Abscess
= focal area of necrosis with formation of surrounding membrane beginning in area of cerebritis

Cause:
1. Extension from paranasal sinus infection (41%) / mastoiditis / otitis media (5%) / facial soft tissue infection / dental abscess
2. Generalized septicemia (32%):
   (a) Lung (most common): bronchiectasis, empyema, lung abscess, bronchopleural fistula, pneumonia
   (b) Heart (less common): CHD with R-L shunt, AVM, bacterial endocarditis
   (c) Osteomyelitis
3. Penetrating trauma or surgery
4. Cryptogenic (25%)

Predisposed: diabetes mellitus, patients on steroids / immunosuppressive drugs, congenital / acquired immunologic deficiency

Organism: Anaerobic streptococcus (most common), Bacteroides, Staphylococcus; in 20% multiple organisms; in 25% sterile contents

Pathophysiology:
Stage I: vascular congestion, petechial hemorrhage, edema
Stage II: cerebral softening + necrosis
Stage III: (after 2 – 3 weeks) liquefaction, cavitation + capsule consisting of inner layer of granulation tissue, a middle collagenous layer and an outer astroglial layer; edema outside abscess capsule

Location: typically at corticomedullary junction; frontal + temporal lobes; supratentorial : infratentorial = 2:1

NCCT:
√ zone of low density with mass effect (92%)
√ slightly increased rim density (4%), development of collagen layer takes 10 – 14 days
√ gas within lesion (4%) is diagnostic of gas-forming organism

CECT:
√ ring enhancement (90%) with peripheral zone of edema
√ homogeneous enhancement in lesions <0.5 cm
√ edema + contrast enhancement suppressed by steroids
√ smooth regular 1 – 3 mm thick wall with relative thinning of medial wall (secondary to poorer blood supply of white matter)
√ multiloculation + subjacent daughter abscess in white matter

MR: (most sensitive modality)
√ centrally increased / variable intensity with hypointense rim on T2WI
√ outside border of increased signal intensity on T2WI (edema)

Cx:
(1) Development of daughter abscesses toward white matter
(2) Rupture into ventricular system / subarachnoid space (thinner abscess capsule formation on medial wall of abscess related to fewer blood vessels) producing ventriculitis ± meningitis

DDx: primary / metastatic neoplasm, subacute infarction, resolving hematoma

Granulomatous Abscess
1. Tuberculoma
2. Sarcoid abscess
3. Fungal abscess
commonly in immunocompromised patients

ACRANIA
= EXENCEPHALY
= very rare developmental anomaly characterized by partial / complete absence of calvarium + complete but abnormal development of brain tissue
√ absence of calvarium
√ hemispheres surrounded by thin membrane
Prognosis: uniformly lethal

ADRENOLEUKODYSTROPHY
= inherited metabolic disorder characterized by progressive demyelination of cerebral white matter + adrenal insufficiency

Etiology:
defective peroxisomal fatty acid oxidation with accumulation of very long chain fatty acids (cholesterol esters) in gray and white matter + adrenal cortex

Dx: assay of plasma, red cells, cultured skin fibroblasts for the presence of increased amounts of very long chain fatty acids

Mode of inheritance:
(a) X-linked recessive in boys (common)
(b) autosomal recessive in neonates (uncommon)

Histo: PAS cytoplasmic inclusions in brain, adrenals, other tissues

Age: 3 – 10 years (X-linked recessive)

• deteriorating vision (27%), loss of hearing (50%)
• ataxia
• optic disk pallor
• adrenal gland insufficiency (abnormal increased pigmentation, elevated ACTH levels)
• altered behavior, mental deterioration, death

Location:
disease process usually starts in central occipital white matter, advances anteriorly through internal + external capsules + centrum semiovale, centripetal progression to involve subcortical white matter, interhemispheric spread via corpus callosum particularly splenium, involvement of optic radiation ± auditory system ± pyramidal tract

CT:
- √ large symmetric low-density lesions in occipitoparietotemporal white matter (80%) advancing toward frontal lobes + cerebellum
- √ thin curvilinear / serrated enhancing rims near edges of lesion
- √ initial frontal lobe involvement (12%)
- √ calcifications within hypodense areas (7%)
- √ cerebral atrophy in late stage (progressive loss of cortical neurons)

MR:
- √ hypointensity on T1WI in affected areas (hypointense atrophic splenium of corpus callosum)
- √ hyperintense bilateral confluent areas on T2WI

Prognosis:
usually fatal within several years after onset of symptoms

ADRENOMYELONEUROPATHY
= clinically milder form with later age of onset
- • symptoms of spinal cord demyelination + peripheral neuropathy

AGENESIS OF CORPUS CALLOSUM
= COMPLETE DYSGENESIS OF CORPUS CALLOSUM
= failure of formation of corpus callosum originating from the lamina terminalis at 7 – 13 weeks from where a phalanx of callosal tissue extends backwards arching over the diencephalon; usually developed by 20 weeks

Incidence: 0.7 – 5.3%

Histo:
axons from cerebral hemispheres that would normally cross continue along medial walls of lateral ventricles as longitudinal callosal bundles of Probst that terminate randomly in occipital + temporal lobes

Associated with:
- (a) CNS anomalies (85%):
  1. Dandy-Walker cyst (11%)
  2. Interhemispheric arachnoid cyst may be continuous with 3rd and lateral ventricles
  3. Hydrocephalus (30%)
  4. Midline intracerebral lipoma of corpus callosum often surrounded with ring of calcium (10%)
  5. Arnold-Chiari II malformation (7%)
  6. Midline encephalocele
  7. Porencephaly
  8. Holoprosencephaly
  9. Hypertelorism median cleft syndrome
- (b) Cardiovascular, gastrointestinal, genitourinary anomalies (62%)
- • normal brain function unusual but possible; neurologic abnormalities
- • intellectual impairment; seizures
- √ absence of septum pellucidum + corpus callosum
- √ concave medial wall of frontal horns (bundles of Probst)
- √ laterally convex frontal horns in case of absent genu of corpus callosum
- √ "high-riding third ventricle" = upward displacement of widened 3rd ventricle often to level of bodies of lateral ventricle

- √ anterior interhemispheric fissure adjoins elevated 3rd ventricle ± communication (PATHOGNOMONIC)
- √ "interhemispheric cyst" = interhemispheric CSF collection as an upward extension of 3rd ventricle
- √ enlarged foramina of Monro
- √ radial arrangement of sulci of medial hemisphere terminating at the roof of the 3rd ventricle (on sagittal images)
- √ colpocephaly (= dilatation of trigones + occipital horns + posterior temporal horns in the absence of splenium due to disorganization of dorsal white matter)
- √ "bat-wing" appearance of lateral ventricles (= wide separation of lateral ventricles with straight parallel parasagittal orientation with absent callosal body)
- √ failure of normal convergence of calcarine + parietooccipital sulci
- √ persistent eversion of cingulate gyrus (rotated inferiorly + laterally) with absence on midsagittal images
- √ incomplete formation of Ammon's horn in the hippocampus

Angio:
- √ wandering straight posterior course of pericallosal arteries (lateral view)
- √ wide separation of pericallosal arteries secondary to intervening 3rd ventricle (anterior view)
- √ separation of internal cerebral veins
- √ loss of U-shape in vein of Galen

DDx:
- (1) Prominent cavum septi pellucidi + cavum vergae (should not be mistaken for 3rd ventricle)
- (2) Arachnoid cyst in midline (suprasellar, collicular plate) raising and deforming the 3rd ventricle and causing hydrocephalus

PARTIAL AGENESIS OF CORPUS CALLOSUM
= milder form of callosal dysgensis (best seen by MR)
- (a) genu only
- (b) genu + part of the body
- (c) genu + entire body
- (d) genu + body + splenium (without rostrum)

AIDS
= DNA retrovirus infection attacking monocytes + macrophages which leads to deficient cell-mediated immunity

Incidence: 1% of population in United States is HIV-seropositive; 187,000 new cases in 1991

Histo: formation of microglial nodules instead of granulomas in 75 – 80% of autopsied brains

- • neurological symptoms as initial complaint in 10%, ultimately afflict up to 60%: headache, memory loss, confusion, dementia, focal deficit from mass lesion

- Δ any male with neurologic symptoms between age 20 and 50 has AIDS until proven otherwise
- Δ unusual presentations are clues to HIV infection: pan-sinusitis, mastoiditis, parotid cysts, cervical adenopathy, hypointense spine

DIFFUSE CHANGES:
(1) HIV / CMV encephalopathy (most common complication)
both viruses occur always in combination
- dementia in up to 60% during course of disease
- cognitive dysfunction in up to 90%
- √ patchy white matter lesions (= subacute leukoencephalitis) in 31%

FOCAL CHANGES:
(1) Primary CNS lymphoma
(2) Toxoplasmosis
(3) Progressive multifocal leukoencephalopathy
(4) Cryptococcosis
Location: extension along Virchow-Robin spaces
√ hydrocephalus + cortical / central atrophy (with inadequate immune response)
√ enhancing granulomatous meningitis (with sufficient immune response)
√ bilateral nonenhancing hyperintense abnormalities in lenticulostriate region (= gelatinous pseudocyst) on T2WI
(5) Other opportunistic CNS infections: tuberculosis, neurosyphilis

Rx: azidothymidine (AZT)

ALEXANDER DISEASE

= FIBRINOID LEUKODYSTROPHY
Age: as early as first few weeks of life
- macrocephaly
- failure to attain developmental milestones
- progressive spastic quadriparesis
- intellectual failure

Location: frontal white matter gradually extending posteriorly into parietal region + internal capsule
CT:
√ low density white matter lesion
√ contrast enhancement near tip of frontal horn
MR:
√ prolonged T1 + T2 relaxation times
Prognosis: death in infancy / early childhood

ALZHEIMER DISEASE

most common of diffuse gray matter diseases with large loss of cells from cerebral cortex + other areas
- slowly progressing memory loss, dementia
- √ "cracked walnut" appearance = symmetrically enlarged sulci in high convexity area

ANENCEPHALY

= failure of closure of the rostral end of the neural tube between 4 – 5th week MA
Incidence: 1:1,000 births (3.5:1,000 in South Wales); M:F = 1:4; most common congenital defect involving CNS
Recurrence rate: 3 – 4%
Etiology: multifactorial (genetic + environmental)

Path: absence of cerebral hemispheres + cranial vault; partial / complete absence of diencephalic + mesencephalic structures; hypophysis + rhombencephalic structures usually preserved
Risk factors: family history of neural tube defect; twin pregnancy
Associated anomalies:
spinal dysraphism (17 – 50%), cleft lip / palate (2%), clubfoot (2%), umbilical hernia, amniotic band syndrome

√ absence of cranium cephalad to orbits
√ bulging eyes (frog-like appearance)
√ short neck
√ polyhydramnios (40 – 50%) after 26 weeks GA (due to failure of normal fetal swallowing) / oligohydramnios

Prognosis: uniformly fatal within hours to days of life; in 53% premature birth; in 68% stillbirth
DDx: microcephaly, acrania, encephalocele, amniotic band syndrome

ANEURYSM OF CNS

Etiology:
(a) congenital (97%) = "berry aneurysm" in 2% of population (in 20% multiple); associated with aortic coarctation + adult polycystic kidney disease
(b) infectious (3%) = mycotic aneurysm
(c) arteriosclerotic: fusiform shape
(d) traumatic
(e) neoplastic
(f) fibromuscular disease
(g) collagen vascular disease

Location of aneurysm:
(a) by autopsy:
(a) Circle of Willis (80%):
MCA bifurcation > ICA at origin of PCom > ACom > ICA at bifurcation into ACA + MCA
(b) Posterior fossa (20%)
(b) by angiography (= symptomatic aneurysms):
PCom (38%) > ACom (36%) > MCA bifurcation (21%) > ICA bifurcation > tip of basilar artery (2.8%)
(c) by risk of bleeding: 1 – 2% per year ACom (70% bleed), PCom (2nd highest risk)

LOCATION OF BLOOD SUGGESTING SITE OF ANEURYSM:
(a) according to location of subarachnoid hemorrhage:
1. Anterior chiasmatic cistern   : ACom
2. Septum pellucidum   : ACom
3. Intraventricular   : ACom, ICA, MCA
4. Sylvian fissure   : MCA, ICA, PCom
5. Anterior pericallosal cistern   : ACA, ACom
6. Symmetric distribution in subarachnoid space: ACA + basilar artery
(b) according to location of cerebral hematoma:
1. inferomedial frontal lobe   : ACom
2. temporal lobe   : MCA
3. corpus callosum   : pericallosal artery

(c) intraventricular hemorrhage
   from aneurysms at ACom, MCA, pericallosal artery
   (CAVE: blood may have entered in retrograde
   manner from subarachnoid location)

Rupture size: 5 – 15 mm
Clues for bleeding aneurysm:
   (a) the largest aneurysm (87%)
   (b) anterior communicating artery (70%)
   (c) contralateral side of all visualized aneurysms
       (60%), non-visualization due to spasm

MULTIPLE ANEURYSMS
   Cause: congenital aneurysms in 20%, mycotic
       aneurysms in 22%
   mirror image aneurysms = 35% of patients with one
       MCA aneurysm have one on the contralateral side
   CECT: detection rate of aneurysms at PCom (40%),
       ACom / MCA, basilar artery (80%)

Prognosis:
   (1) Death in 10% within 24 hours from concomitant
       intracerebral hemorrhage, extensive brain
       herniation, massive infarcts + hemorrhage within
       brainstem
   (2) Survivors frequently recover completely within a few
       days
   (3) Cerebral ischemia + infarction
   (4) Recurrence within 2 weeks (increased mortality)
   Cx: subdural hematoma

Giant Aneurysm
   = aneurysm larger than 2.5 cm in diameter, usually
     presenting with intracranial mass effect
   Incidence: 25% of all aneurysms
   Age: no age predilection; M:F= 2:1
   Location: (arise from arteries at the base of the brain)
   (a) middle fossa: cavernous segment of ICA
       (43%), supraclinoid segment of ICA, terminal
       bifurcation of ICA, middle cerebral artery
   (b) posterior fossa: at tip of basilar artery, AICA,
       vertebral artery
   Skull film:
       √ predominantly peripheral curvilinear calcification
         (22%)
       √ bone erosion (44%)
       √ pressure changes on sella turcica (18%)
   CECT:
       √ "target sign" = centrally opacified vessel lumen +
         ring of thrombus + enhanced fibrous outer wall
       √ simple ring-blush (75%) of fibrous outer wall with
         total thrombosis
       √ little / no surrounding edema
   MR:
       √ mixed signal intensity (combination of subacute +
         chronic hemorrhage, calcification)
   Cx: subarachnoid hemorrhage in <30%

Mycotic Aneurysm
   = 3% of all intracranial aneurysms, multiple in 20%

Source: subacute bacterial endocarditis (65%),
   acute bacterial endocarditis (9%), meningitis
   (9%), septic thrombophlebitis (9%), myxoma
Location: peripheral to first bifurcation of major vessel
   (64%); often located near surface of brain
   especially over convexities
   (a) suprasellar cistern = circle of Willis
   (b) inferolateral sylvian fissure = middle
       cerebral artery trifurcation
   (c) genu of corpus callosum = origin of
       callosomarginal artery
   (d) bottom of 3rd ventricle = pericallosal
       artery
NCCT:
   √ aneurysm rarely visualized; indirect evidence from
     focal hematoma secondary to rupture
   √ zone of increased density / calcification
   √ increased density in subarachnoid, intraventricular,
     intracerebral spaces (extravasated blood)
   √ focal / diffuse lucency of brain (edema / infarction /
     vasospasm)
CECT:
   √ intense homogeneous enhancement within round /
     oval mass contiguous to vessels
   √ incomplete opacification with mural thrombus
Cx: develop recurrent bleeding more frequently than
   congenital aneurysms

Supraclinoid Carotid Aneurysm
   = 38% of intracranial aneurysms
   Sites: (a) at origin of posterior communicating artery
       (65%)
   (b) at bifurcation of internal carotid artery (23%)
   (c) at origin of ophthalmic artery (12%) medial
       to anterior clinoid process; most likely to
       become giant aneurysm
Presentation: • bitemporal hemianopsia (extrinsic
       compression on chiasm)

   √ calcification is rare (frequent in atherosclerotic
     cavernous sinus aneurysm)

Cavernous Sinus Aneurysm
   Age: 20 – 70 years, peak 5 – 6th decade; F >> M
   Cause: sinus thrombophlebitis
   • progressive visual impairment
   • cavernous sinus syndrome: trigeminal nerve pain,
     oculomotor nerve paralysis
   Site: extradural portion of cavernous sinus ICA

   √ undercutting of anterior clinoid process
   √ erosion of lateral half of sella
   √ erosion of posterior clinoid process
   √ invasion of middle cranial fossa
   √ enlargement of superior orbital fissure
   √ erosion of tip of petrous pyramid
   √ rim-like calcification (33%)
   √ displacement of thin bony margins without sclerosis
   Rx often inoperable; balloon embolization ± parent
       artery occlusion

AQUEDUCTAL STENOSIS

= focal reduction in size of aqueduct at level of superior colliculi / intercollicular sulcus (normal range of 0.2 – 1.8 mm^2)

Embryology:
aqueduct develops about the 6th week of gestation + decreases in size until birth due to growth pressure from adjacent mesencephalic structures

Incidence: 0.5 – 1:1,000 births; most frequent cause of congenital hydrocephalus (20 – 43%); recurrence rate in siblings of 1 – 4.5%; M:F = 2:1

Etiology:
(a) postinflammatory (50%): secondary to perinatal infection (toxoplasmosis, CMV, syphilis, mumps, influenza virus) or intracranial hemorrhage = destruction of ependymal lining of aqueduct with adjacent marked fibrillary gliosis

(b) developmental: aqueductal forking (= marked branching of aqueduct into channels) / narrowing / transverse septum (X-linked recessive inheritance in 25% of males)

(c) neoplastic (extremely rare): pinealoma, meningioma, tectal astrocytoma (may be missed on routine CT scans, easily differentiated by MR)

May be associated with other congenital anomalies (16%): thumb deformities

√ enlargement of lateral + 3rd ventricles with normal-sized 4th ventricle (4th ventricle may be normal with communicating hydrocephalus)

Prognosis: 11 – 30% mortality

ARACHNOID CYST

= CSF-containing intraarachnoid cyst without ventricular communication / brain maldevelopment

Incidence: 1% of all intracranial masses

Origin:
(1) congenital: arising from clefts / duplication of arachnoid membrane with expansion by secretory activity of arachnoid cells = **true arachnoid cyst**

(2) acquired: following hemorrhage / infection in neonatal period = loculation of CSF surrounded by arachnoidal scarring with expansion by osmotic filtration / ball-valve mechanism = **leptomeningeal cyst = secondary arachnoid cyst = acquired arachnoid cyst**

Histo: cyst filled with clear fluid, thin wall composed of cleaved arachnoid membrane lined by ependymal / meningothelial cells

Age: presentation at any time during life
• often asymptomatic
• symptomatic due to mass effect, hydrocephalus, seizures, headaches, hemiparesis, intracranial hypertension, craniomegaly, developmental delay, visual loss, precocious puberty, bobble-head doll syndrome

Location: (arise in CSF cisterns between brain + dura)
(a) floor of middle fossa near tip of temporal lobe (sylvian fissure) in 50%
(b) suprasellar / chiasmatic cistern (may produce endocrinopathy) in 10%
(c) posterior fossa (1/3): cerebellopontine angle (11%), quadrigeminal plate cistern (10%), in relationship to vermis (9%), prepontine / interpeduncular cistern (3%)
(d) interhemispheric fissure, cerebral convexity, anterior infratentorial midline

√ forward bowing of anterior wall of cranial fossa + elevation of sphenoid ridge
√ extraaxial unilocular thin-walled CSF-density cyst with well-defined smooth angular margins
√ compression of subarachnoid space + subjacent brain (minimal mass effect)
√ may erode inner table of calvarium
√ NO enhancement (intrathecal contrast penetrates into cyst on delayed scans)

MR (best modality):
√ well-circumscribed lesion with same signal intensity as CSF ± mass effect on surrounding structures

Cx: (1) hydrocephalus (30 – 60%)
          (2) concurrent subdural / intracystic hemorrhage

Prognosis: favorable if removed before onset of irreversible brain damage

Rx: fenestration / cyst-peritoneal shunting

CT-DDx:
epidermoid, dermoid, subdural hygroma, infarction, porencephaly

US-DDx:
choroid plexus cyst, porencephalic cyst (communicates with ventricle), cystic tumor (solid components), midline cyst associated with agenesis of corpus callosum, dorsal cyst associated with holoprosencephaly, Dandy-Walker cyst (extension of 4th ventricle, developmental delay), vein of Galen aneurysm

ARTERIOVENOUS FISTULA

= abnormal communication between artery + vein resulting in tremendous amount of flow due to high pressure gradient; leading to enlargement + elongation of draining veins

Cause:
(1) Vessel laceration (delay between trauma + clinical manifestation due to delayed lysis of hematoma surrounding arterial laceration)
(2) Angiodysplasia: fibromuscular disease, neurofibromatosis, Ehlers-Danlos syndrome
(3) Congenital fistula

• pulsatile mass + thrill / bruit
• ± neurologic symptoms / deficit (due to arterial steal)

Location:
(a) carotid-cavernous sinus fistula (most common)
(b) vertebral artery fistula
(c) external carotid fistula (rare)

ARTERIOVENOUS MALFORMATION

= congenital abnormality consisting of dilated tortuous arteries + veins with racemose tangle of closely packed pathologic vessels resulting in shunting of blood from arterial to venous side without intermediary capillary network; most common vascular lesion

Age: 80% by end of 4th decade; 20% <20 years of age
- headaches, seizures (nonfocal in 40%), mental deterioration
- progressive hemispheric neurologic deficit (50%)
- ictus from acute intracranial hemorrhage (50%)

Location:
  (a) supratentorial (90%): parietal > frontal > temporal lobe > paraventricular > intraventricular region > occipital lobe
  (b) infratentorial (10%)

Vascular supply:
  (a) pial branches of ICA in 73% of supratentorial location, in 50% of posterior fossa location
  (b) dural branches of ECA in 27% with infratentorial lesions

Skull film:
  √ speckled / ring-like calcifications (15 – 30%)
  √ thinning / thickening of skull at contact area with AVM
  √ prominent vascular grooves on inner table of skull (dilated feeding arteries + draining veins) in 27%
NCCT:
  √ irregular mass with large feeding arteries + draining veins
  √ mixed density (60%): dense large vessels + hemorrhage + calcifications
  √ isodense lesion (15%): may be recognizable by mass effect
  √ low density (15%): brain atrophy due to ischemia
  √ not visualized (10%)
CECT:
  √ serpiginous dense enhancement in 80% (tortuous dilated vessels)
  √ No enhancement in thrombosed AVM
  √ No avascular spaces within AVM
  √ lack of mass effect / edema (unless thrombosed / bleeding)
  √ rapid shunting
  √ thickened arachnoid covering
  √ adjacent atrophic brain
MR:
  √ flow void (imaging with GRASS gradient echo + long TR sequences)
Angio:
  √ grossly dilated efferent + afferent vessels with a racemose tangle ("bag of worms"), arteriovenous shunting
  √ negative angiogram (compression by hematoma / thrombosis)
Prognosis: 10% mortality; 30% morbidity; 2% risk per year of recurrent bleeding

Wyburn-Mason syndrome
  = telangiectasias of skin + retinal cirsoid aneurysm + AVM involving entire optic tract (optic nerve, thalamus, geniculate bodies, calcarine cortex);
  May be associated with AVMs of posterior fossa, neck, mandible / maxilla presenting in childhood

ASTROCYTOMA
Incidence:
  70 – 75% of all primary intracranial tumors; most common brain tumor in children (40 – 50% of all primary pediatric intracranial neoplasms)
Location:
  cerebral hemisphere (lobar), thalamus, pons, midbrain, may spread across corpus callosum (incidence of occurrence proportional to amount of white matter); no particular lobar distribution;
  in children: supratentorial (30%), cerebellum (40%), brainstem (20%)

Classification:
  1. Well-differentiated astrocytoma
  2. Anaplastic astrocytoma
  3. Malignant glioblastoma

Well-differentiated = Low Grade Astrocytoma
Incidence: 9% of all primary intracranial tumors
Age: 20 – 40 years; M > F
Histo:
  homogeneous relatively uniform appearance with proliferation of well-differentiated multipolar fibrillary / protoplasmic astrocytes; mild nuclear pleomorphism + mild hypercellularity; poorly defined borders with infiltration of white matter + basal ganglia + cortex; mitoses rare; no significant tumor vascularity / necrosis / hemorrhage
Location: posterior fossa in children, supratentorial in adults (typically lobar)

√ may develop a cyst with high protein content (rare)
CT:
  √ usually hypodense lesion with minimal mass effect + NO peritumoral edema
  √ well-defined tumor margins
  √ central calcifications (frequent)
  √ minimal / no contrast enhancement (normal capillary endothelial cells)
MR:
  √ well-defined hypointense lesion with little mass effect / vasogenic edema / heterogeneity on T1WI
  √ hyperintense on T2WI
  √ little / no enhancement on Gd-DTPA
  √ cyst with content hyperintense to CSF (protein content)
  √ hyperintense area within tumor mass (paramagnetic effect of methemoglobin)
  √ inhomogeneous gadolinium-DTPA enhancement of tumor nodule
Angio: √ majority avascular

Prognosis:
  3 – 10 years postoperative survival; occasionally converting into more malignant form several years after presentation

Anaplastic Astrocytoma
Incidence: 11% of all primary intracranial neoplasms

Histo:
multipolar fibrillary / protoplasmic astrocytes; mitoses + vascular endothelial proliferation common; frequently vasogenic edema; no necrosis / hemorrhage
Location: typically lobar
MR:
√ well-defined slightly heterogeneous hypointense lesion on T1WI with prevalent edema
√ hyperintense on T2WI
√ ± enhancement on Gd-DTPA

Pilocytic Astrocytoma
= JUVENILE PILOCYTIC ASTROCYTOMA
= most benign histologic subtype of astrocytoma
Histo: alternating pattern of compact bipolar pilocytic (hairlike) astrocytes arranged mostly around vessels + loosely aggregated protoplasmic astrocytes undergoing microcystic degeneration
Age: predominantly in children + young adults; peak age between birth and 9 years of age; M:F = 1:1
Associated with   neurofibromatosis
Location: cerebellum, optic nerve / chiasm, around 3rd ventricle

√ mural tumor nodule located in wall of cerebellar cyst
√ multilobulated / dumbbell appearance along optic pathway
√ rarely calcifies
√ micro- / macrocysts in cerebellar location
√ increased heterogeneous signal intensity on early Gd-DTPA enhanced T1WI; homogeneous enhancement on delayed images
Prognosis: relatively benign clinical course, almost never recurs after surgical excision; NO malignant transformation to anaplastic form

ATAXIA-TELEANGIECTASIA
= autosomal recessive disorder characterized by telangiectasias of skin + eye, cerebellar ataxia, sinus + pulmonary infections, immunodeficiencies, propensity to develop malignancies
Incidence: 1:40,000 livebirths
Path: neuronal degradation + atrophy of cerebellar cortex (? from vascular anomalies)
• cerebellar ataxia at beginning of walking age
• progressive neurologic deterioration
• oculomotor abnormalities, dysarthric speech, choreoathetosis, myoclonic jerks
• mucocutaneous telangiectasias: bulbar conjunctiva, ears, face, neck, palate, dorsum of hands, antecubital + popliteal fossa
• recurrent bacterial + viral sinopulmonary infections
√ cerebellar cortical atrophy: diminished cerebellar size, dilatation of 4th ventricle, increased cerebellar sulcal prominence
√ cerebral hemorrhage (rupture of telangiectatic vessels)

√ cerebral infarct (emboli shunted through vascular malformations in lung)
Cx:
1. Bronchiectasis + pulmonary failure (most common cause of death)
2. Malignancies (10 – 15%): lymphoma, leukemia, epithelial malignancies

BASAL GANGLIA HEMATOMA
= rupture of small distal microaneurysms in the lenticulo-striate arteries in patients with poorly controlled systemic arterial hypertension
Cx: (1) Dissection into adjacent ventricles (2/3)
   (2) Porencephaly
   (3) Atrophy with ipsilateral ventricular dilatation

BASAL GANGLIA INFARCT
= occlusion of small penetrating arteries at base of brain (lenticulostriate / thalamoperforating arteries) = lacunar infarct (infarcts <1 cm in size)
Cause:
(1) Embolism (2) Hypoperfusion (3) Carbon monoxide poisoning (4) Drowning (5) Vasculopathy (hypertension, microvasculopathy, aging)
√ dense homogeneous enhancement outlining caudate nucleus, putamen, globus pallidus, thalamus
√ dense round nodular enhancement / peripheral ring enhancement

BINSWANGER DISEASE
= ENCEPHALOPATHIA SUBCORTICALIS PROGRESSIVA = SUBCORTICAL ARTERIOSCLEROTIC ENCEPHALOPATHY (SAE)
Path: atherosclerosis in small arteries of subcortical white matter
Age: middle age
• psychiatric changes, intellectual impairment, slowly progressive dementia, transient neurologic deficits, seizures, spasticity, syncope
√ multifocal hypodense lesions (periventricular, centrum semiovale) with sparing of U fibers
√ lacunar infarcts in basal ganglia
√ sulcal enlargement + dilated lateral ventricles (brain atrophy)
DDx: leukodystrophy, progressive multifocal leukoencephalopathy, multiple sclerosis

CANAVAN DISEASE
= SPONGIFORM LEUKODYSTROPHY
= spongy degeneration of brain in infancy; autosomal recessive, most common in Ashkenazi Jews
Cause: unknown
Age: 3 – 6 months
• marked hypotonia
• macrocephaly
• seizures
• failure to attain motor milestones
• spasticity
• intellectual failure
• optic atrophy

√ diffuse symmetric white matter abnormality
√ cortical atrophy
CT:
  √ low density white matter
MR:
  √ white matter hypointense on T1WI + hyperintense on T2WI
Prognosis: death in 2nd year of life

CAPILLARY TELANGIECTASIA
= abnormal dilated capillaries separated by normal neural tissue; commonly "cryptic"
May be associated with: hereditary Rendu-Osler-Weber syndrome, ataxia-telangiectasia syndrome
• usually asymptomatic (incidental finding at necropsy)
Location: mostly in pons; usually multiple / may be solitary
√ poorly defined area of dilated vessels (resembling petechiae)
Prognosis: bleeding uncommon; bleeding in pons usually fatal

CAVERNOUS HEMANGIOMA OF BRAIN
= CAVERNOUS ANGIOMA = CAVERNOMA = well-circumscribed nodule of honeycomb-like large sinusoidal vascular spaces separated by fibrous collagenous bands without intervening neural tissue
Age: 3rd – 6th decade; M > F
• seizures
Location: cerebrum (mainly subcortical) > pons > cerebellum; solitary > multiple
NCCT: √ extensive calcifications = hemangioma calcificans (20%)
  √ small round hyperdense region (CLUE)
  √ minimal surrounding edema
CECT: √ minimal / intense enhancement
  √ low attenuation areas due to thrombosed portions
Angio: √ negative ("cryptic / occult vascular malformation" = OCVM)

CEPHALOCELE
= defect in skull + dura with extracranial extension of intracranial structures
ENCEPHALOCELE = herniation of brain tissue + meninges + CSF
CRANIAL MENINGOCELE = herniation of meninges + CSF only
Incidence:
  1 – 4 per 10,000 livebirths; 5 – 20% of all craniospinal malformations; predominant neural axis anomaly in fetuses spontaneously aborted <20 weeks GA
Cause:
  failure of surface ectoderm to separate from neuroectoderm early in embryonic development
  @ Skull base
    (1) faulty closure of neural tube
    (2) failure of basilar ossification centers to unite
  @ Calvarium
    (1) defective induction of bone

  (2) pressure erosion of bone by intracranial mass / cyst
In 60% associated with:
  (1) Spina bifida (7 – 30%)
  (2) Corpus callosum dysgenesis
  (3) Chiari malformation
  (4) Dandy-Walker malformation
  (5) Meckel-Gruber syndrome (= encephalocele + microcephaly + cystic dysplastic kidneys + polydactyly)
  (6) Amniotic band syndrome: multiple irregular asymmetric off-midline encephaloceles
  (7) Chromosomal anomalies in 44% (trisomy 18)
• alpha-fetoprotein in amniotic fluid may be elevated
• CSF rhinorrhea
• meningitis

Occipital Encephalocele (75%)
Most common encephalocele in western hemisphere
Associated with Dandy-Walker malformation, Chiari malformation
• external occipital mass
√ supra- and infratentorial structures involved with equal frequency
√ skull defect (visualized in 80%)
√ flattening of basiocciput
√ ventriculomegaly
√ lemon sign = inward depression of frontal bones (33%)
√ cyst-within-a-cyst (ventriculocele = herniation of 4th ventricle into cephalocele)
√ acute angle between mass + skin line of neck and occiput
Prognosis: 50% survival in liveborns, 74% retarded
DDx: cystic hygroma

Frontoethmoidal Encephalocele (15%)
= sincipital cephalocele
Most common variety in Southeast Asia
Types: naso-ethmoidal, nasofrontal, naso-orbital, interfrontal
Associated with midline craniofacial dysraphism (dysgenesis of corpus callosum, interhemispheric lipoma, anomalies of neural migration)
• external mass near dorsum of nose, orbits, forehead
• hypertelorism

Sphenoidal Encephalocele (10%)
= basal encephalocele
Age: present at end of first decade of life
• clinically occult
• mass in nasal cavity, nasopharynx, mouth, posterior portion of orbit
• mouth breathing due to nasopharyngeal obstruction
• nasopharyngeal mass increasing with Valsalva
• diminished visual acuity with hypoplasia of optic discs
• hypothalamic-pituitary dysfunction
Associated with agenesis of corpus callosum (80%)
Types:
  (a) sphenopharyngeal = through sphenoid body

(b)   sphenoorbital = through superior orbital fissure
(c)   sphenoethmoidal = through sphenoid + ethmoid
(d)   transethmoidal = through cribriform plate
(e)   sphenomaxillary = through maxillary sinus

Parietal Encephalocele   (uncommon)
Associated with   dysgenesis of corpus callosum, large interhemispheric cyst

√ cranium bifidum = cranioschisis = "split cranium" (= skull defect) = smooth opening with well-defined sclerotic rim of cortical bone
√ hole in sphenoid bone (seen on submentovertex film)
√ hydrocephalus in 15 – 80% (from associated aqueductal stenosis, Arnold-Chiari malformation, Dandy-Walker cyst)
√ nonenhancing expansile homogeneous paracranial mass
√ mantle of cerebral tissue often difficult to image in encephalocele (except with MR)
√ intracranial communication often not visualized
√ metrizamide / radionuclide ventriculography diagnostic
√ microcephaly (20%)
√ polyhydramnios
DDx: sonographic refraction artifact at skull edge; may be impossible to differentiate from mucocele

CEREBELLAR ASTROCYTOMA
2nd most frequent tumor of posterior fossa in children
Incidence: 10 – 20% of pediatric brain tumors
Histo: mostly grade I
Age: children > adults; no specific age peak; M:F = 1:1
Path:
(1)   cystic lesion with tumor nodule ("mural nodule") in cyst wall (50%); (midline astrocytomas cystic in 50%, hemispheric astrocytomas cystic in 80%)
(2)   solid mass with cystic (= necrotic) center (40 – 45%)
(3)   solid tumor without necrosis (<10%)
• cerebellar signs: truncal ataxia, dysdiadochokinesia
Location: originating in midline with extension into cerebellar hemisphere (30%) > vermis > tonsils > brainstem
√ calcifications (20%): dense / faint / reticular / punctate / globular; mostly in solid variety
√ may develop extreme hydrocephalus (quite large when finally symptomatic)
CT:
√ round / oval cyst with density of cyst fluid > CSF
√ round / oval / plaque-like mural nodule with intense homogeneous enhancement
√ cyst wall slightly hyperdense + nonenhancing (= compressed cerebellar tissue)
√ uni- / multilocular cyst (= necrosis) with irregular enhancement of solid tumor portions
√ round / oval lobulated fairly well-defined iso- / hypodense solid tumor with hetero- / homogeneous enhancement

MR:
√ hypointense on T1WI + hyperintense on T2WI
√ enhancement of solid tumor portion
Angio:
√ avascular
Prognosis:
malignant transformation exceedingly rare
—   40% 25-year survival rate for solid cerebellar astrocytoma
—   90% 25-year survival rate for cystic juvenile pilocytic astrocytoma

DDx of solid astrocytoma:
(1)   medulloblastoma (hyperdense mass, noncalcified)
(2)   ependymoma (fourth ventricle, 50% calcify)
DDx of cystic astrocytoma:
(1)   Hemangioblastoma (lesion <5 cm)
(2)   Arachnoid cyst
(3)   Trapped 4th ventricle
(4)   Megacisterna magna
(5)   Dandy-Walker cyst

CEREBRITIS
= focal area of inflammation within brain substance
CT: √ area of decreased density ± mass effect
√ no contrast enhancement (initially) / central or patchy enhancement (later)
MR: √ focal area of increased intensity on T2WI
Cx: brain abscess

CHIARI MALFORMATION
A.   CHIARI I MALFORMATION (adulthood)
= herniation of cerebellar tonsils below foramen magnum
frequent isolated hindbrain abnormality of little consequence without supratentorial anomalies
Associated with:
(1)   syringohydromyelia (20 – 30%)
(2)   hydrocephalus (25 – 44%)
(3)   basilar impression (25%)
(4)   occipitalization of C1 (10%)
(5)   Klippel-Feil anomaly (10%)
(6)   incomplete ossification of C1-ring (5%)
NOT associated with myelomeningocele!

• benign cerebellar ectopia <3 mm of no clinical consequence; 3 – 5 mm of uncertain significance; >5 mm clinical symptoms likely
• no symptoms in childhood (unless associated with hydrocephalus / syringomyelia)
• may have cranial nerve dysfunction / dissociated anesthesia of lower extremities in adulthood
√ downward displacement of cerebellar tonsils + medial part of the inferior lobes of the cerebellum 5 mm below the level of the foramen magnum
√ pointed / triangular tonsils
√ obliteration of cisterna magna
√ elongation of 4th ventricle which remains in normal position
√ slight anterior angulation of lower brainstem

B. CHIARI II MALFORMATION (childhood)
= ARNOLD-CHIARI MALFORMATION
= most common and serious complex of anomalies secondary to a too small posterior fossa involving hindbrain, spine, mesoderm

HALLMARK is dysgenesis of hindbrain with
(1) caudally displaced 4th ventricle
(2) caudally displaced brainstem
(3) tonsillar + vermian herniation through foramen magnum

Associated with:
(1) lumbar myelomeningocele (almost all patients)
(2) dysgenesis of corpus callosum (80 – 85%)
(3) obstructive hydrocephalus (50 – 98%) following closure of myelomeningocele
(4) absence of septum pellucidum (40%)
(5) syringohydromyelia
(6) excessive cortical gyration (stenogyria = histologically normal cortex; polymicrogyria = histologically abnormal cortex)

NOT associated with basilar impression / C1-assimilation / Klippel-Feil deformity!

- newborn: respiratory distress, apneic spells, bradycardia, impaired swallowing, poor gag reflex, retrocollis, spasticity of upper extremities
- teenager: gradual loss of function + spasticity of lower extremiites

Skull film:
√ Lückenschädel (most prominent near torcular herophili / vertex) in 85% = dysplasia of membranous skull disappearing by 6 months of age
√ scalloping of clivus + posterior aspect of petrous pyramids (from pressure of cerebellum) in 70 – 90% leading to shortening of IAC
√ small posterior fossa
√ enlarged foramen magnum + enlarged upper spinal canal secondary to molding in 75%
√ absent / hypoplastic posterior arch of C1 (70%)

@ Supratentorial
√ hydrocephalus (duct of Sylvius dysfunctional but probe patent); may not become evident until after repair of myelomeningocele (90%)
√ colpocephaly (= enlargement of occipital horns + atria) due to maldeveloped occipital lobes
√ hypoplasia / absence of splenium + rostrum of corpus callosum (80 – 90%)
√ "bat-wing" configuration of frontal horns on coronal views = frontal horns pointing inferiorly with blunt superolateral angle secondary to prominent impressions by enlarged caudate nucleus
√ "hourglass ventricle" = small biconcave 3rd ventricle secondary to large massa intermedia
√ interdigitation of medial cortical gyri (hypoplasia + fenestration of falx in up to 100%)
√ wide prepontine + supracerebellar cisterns
√ nonvisualization of aqueduct (in up to 70%)

√ stenogyria = multiple small closely spaced gyri at medial aspect of occipital lobe secondary to dysplasia (in up to 50%)
@ Cerebellum
√ "cerebellar peg" = protrusion of vermis + hemispheres through foramen magnum (90%) resulting in craniocaudal elongation of cerebellum
√ hypoplastic poorly differentiated cerebellum (poor visualization of folia on sagittal images) secondary to severe degeneration
√ elongated / obliterated vertically oriented thin-tubed 4th ventricle with narrowed AP diameter exiting below foramen magnum (40%)
√ obliteration of CPA cistern + cisterna magna by cerebellum growing around brainstem
√ dysplastic tentorium with wide U-shaped incisura inserting close to foramen magnum (95%)
√ "tectal beaking" = fusion of midbrain colliculi into a single beak pointing posteriorly and invaginating into cerebellum
√ V-shaped widened quadrigeminal plate cistern (due to hypoplasia of cingulate gyri)
√ "towering cerebellum" = "pseudomass" = cerebellar extension above incisura of tentorium
√ triple peak configuration = corners of cerebellum wrapped around brainstem pointing anteriorly + laterally (on axial images)
√ flattened superior portion of cerebellum secondary to temporoparietal herniation
√ vertical orientation of shortened straight sinus
@ Spinal cord
√ medulla + pons displaced into cervical canal
√ "cervicomedullary kink" = herniation of medulla posterior to spinal cord (up to 70%) at level of dentate ligaments
√ widened anterior subarachnoid space at level of brainstem + upper cervical spine (40%)
√ AP diameter of pons narrowed
√ upper cervical nerve roots ascend toward their exit foramina
√ syringohydromyelia
√ low-lying often tethered conus medullaris below L2

C. CHIARI III MALFORMATION
most severe rare abnormality; probably unrelated to type I and II Chiari malformation
√ occipitocervical / high cervical meningomyeloencephalocele
Prognosis: survival usually not beyond infancy

D. CHIARI IV MALFORMATION
extremely rare anomaly probably erroneously included as type of Chiari malformation
√ agenesis of cerebellum
√ hypoplasia of pons
√ small + funnel-shaped posterior fossa

CHOROID PLEXUS CYST
= cyst arising from neuroepithelial folds within choroid plexus

Incidence: 0.9 – 3.6% in sonographic population;
50% of autopsied brains; 71% of autopsied
fetuses with trisomy 18 have choroid plexus
cysts bilaterally >10 mm in diameter
Histo: no epithelial lining, filled with clear fluid
May be associated with   aneuploidy (trisomy 18 + 21)
• usually asymptomatic
√ round anechoic cyst, frequently at level of atrium
√ usually 2 – 8 mm in size (average 4.5 mm)
Cx: hydrocephalus (if large)
Prognosis:
usually disappears by 28th week; may persist; in 95% of
no significance; risk of trisomy 18 is lower than risk of
fetal loss due to amniocentesis (approximately 1:200)

CHOROID PLEXUS PAPILLOMA

Incidence: 0.5 – 0.6% of all intracranial tumors;
2 – 5% of brain tumors in childhood
Age: 20 – 40% <1 year of age; 86% <5 years of age;
middle age; in 75% <2 years of age; M >> F
Path: large aggregation of choroidal fronds producing
great quantities of CSF; occasionally found
incidentally on postmortem examination
• signs of increased intracranial pressure
Location:
    (a)   glomus of choroid plexus in trigone of lateral
ventricles, L > R (in children)
    (b)   4th ventricle + cerebellopontine angle (in adults)
    (c)   3rd ventricle (unusual)
    (d)   multiple in 7%
√ large mass with smooth lobulated border
√ small foci of calcifications (common)
√ engulfment of glomus of choroid plexus (distinctive
feature)
√ asymmetric diffuse ventricular dilatation (CSF
overproduction / decreased absorption secondary to
obstruction of arachnoid granulations from repeated
occult hemorrhage)
√ dilatation of temporal horn in atrial location (obstruction)
√ growth into surrounding white matter (occasionally,
more common a feature of choroid plexus carcinoma)
CT:
    √ iso- / mildly hyperdense with intense homogeneous
enhancement on CECT
MR:
    √ isointense / slightly hyperintense lesion on T1WI +
slightly hypointense on T2WI relative to white matter
    √ surrounded by hypointense signal on T1WI +
hyperintense signal on T2WI (CSF)
    √ intraventricular enhancing island of tumor on Gd-
DTPA
US:
    √ echogenic mass adjacent to normal choroid plexus
Angio:
    √ supplied by anterior + posterior choroidal arteries
Cx: (1)   transformation into malignant choroid plexus
papilloma = choroid plexus carcinoma
    (2)   hydrocephalus (in children) secondary to
increased intracranial pressure from CSF-
overproduction

Rx: surgical removal (24% operative mortality) cures
hydrocephalus
DDx: intraventricular meningioma, ependymoma,
metastasis, cavernous angioma, xanthogranuloma,
astrocytoma

COCKAYNE SYNDROME

= autosomal recessive diffuse demyelinating disease
Age: beginning at age 1
• dwarfism
• progressive physical + mental deterioration
• retinal atrophy + deafness
√ brain atrophy / microcephaly
√ calcifications in basal ganglia + cerebellum
√ skeletal changes superficially similar to progeria
DDx: Progeria

COLLOID CYST

Incidence: 2% of glial tumors of ependymal origin;
0.5 – 1% of CNS tumors
Histo: ciliated + columnar epithelium; mucin-secreting;
squamous cells of ependymal origin; tough
fibrous capsule
Age: young adults; M > F
Location: exclusively arising from inferior aspect of
septum pellucidum protruding into anterior
portion of 3rd ventricle between columns of
fornix
• positional headaches (transient obstruction secondary
to ball valve mechanism at foramen of Monro)
• gait apraxia
• change in mental status ± dementia (related to
increased intracranial pressure)
• papilledema (may become medical emergency with
acute herniation)

√ ± sellar erosion
√ spherical iso- / hyperdense lesion on NCCT with smooth
surface
√ fluid contents:
    (a)   in 20% similar to CSF (= isodense)
    (b)   in 80% mucinous fluid, proteinaceous debris,
hemosiderin, desquamated cells (= hyperdense)
√ may show enhancement of border (draped choroid
plexus / capsule)
√ 3rd ventricular enlargement (to accommodate cyst
anteriorly)
√ asymmetric lateral ventricular enlargement (invariably)
√ occasionally widens septum pellucidum
MR:
    √ lesion hyperintense on T1WI + hyperintense on T2WI
in 60% (related to large protein molecules /
paramagnetic effect of magnesium, copper, iron in
cyst)
DDx: meningioma, ependymoma of 3rd ventricle (rare)
with enhancement

CONTUSION OF BRAIN

Incidence: in 21% of head trauma patients;
children:adults = 2:1

Path: tissue necrosis, capillary disruption, petechial hemorrhage followed by liquefaction + edema after 4 – 7 days

Mechanism: acceleration-deceleration forces

1. **Coup** = impact on stationary brain
   Location: frontal + temporal regions (often bilateral), beneath an acute subdural hematoma
2. **Contrecoup** = impact of moving brain on stationary calvarium
   Location: common in frontal, particularly supraorbital, temporal, occipital region at apices of cerebral gyri with variable extension into white matter
3. **White matter shearing injury** = diffuse impact injury with rotational forces = cortex and deep structures move at different speed resulting in shearing stress along the course of white matter tracts especially at gray-white matter junction with axonal tears followed by wallerian degeneration
   Location: corpus callosum, internal capsule, basal ganglia, thalamus, upper brainstem, cerebellar peduncles, corticomedullary junction

- confusion
- focal cerebral dysfunction
- seizures, personality changes
- focal neurologic deficits (late changes)

CT (sensitive to hemorrhage in acute phase):
- √ focal / multiple (29%) poorly defined areas of irregular contour + inhomogeneous increased density (hemorrhage) + surrounding edema
- √ isodense hemorrhage after 2 – 3 weeks
- √ some degree of contrast enhancement (leaking new capillaries)
- √ area of slightly low attenuation + mass effect (diffuse petechial hemorrhage); associated with delayed hematoma formation
- √ diffuse cerebral swelling without hemorrhage in immediate posttraumatic period (common in children) due to hyperemia / ischemic edema

MR (best modality to demonstrate exact extent of hemorrhagic contusional involvement in subacute + chronic phase):
- √ initially decreased intensity (deoxyhemoglobin of acute hemorrhage) surrounded by hyperintense edema on T2WI
- √ hyperintense on T1WI + T2WI in subacute phase (secondary to Met-Hb)
- √ hyperintense gliosis + hypointense hemosiderin on T2WI in chronic phase

Cx: (1) Encephalomalacia (= scarred brain)
(2) Porencephaly (= formation of cystic cavity lined with gliotic brain and communicating with ventricles / subarachnoid space)
(3) Hydrocephalus as a result from adhesions caused by subarachnoid blood

Prognosis: poor

CRANIOPHARYNGIOMA

Incidence: 3 – 4% of all intracranial neoplasms; 15% of supratentorial + 50% of suprasellar tumors in children; most common suprasellar mass

Origin: from epithelial rests along vestigial craniopharyngeal duct (Rathke pouch)

Path: benign tumor originating from neuroepithelium in craniopharyngeal duct + primitive buccal epithelium

Histo: cystic (rich in liquid cholesterol) / complex / solid

Age: from birth – 7th decade; bimodal age distribution: age peaks in 1st – 2nd decade (75%) + in 5th decade (25%); M>F

- diabetes insipidus (compression of pituitary gland)
- growth retardation (compression of hypothalamus)
- bitemporal hemianopsia (compression of optic nerve chiasm)
- headaches from hydrocephalus (compression of foramen of Monro / aqueduct of Sylvius)

Location:
(a) pituitary stalk / tuber cinereum
(b) suprasellar (20%)
(c) intrasellar (10%)
(d) intra- and suprasellar (70%)

Ectopic craniopharyngioma
(e) floor of anterior 3rd ventricle (more common in adults)
(f) sphenoid bone

Skull films:
- √ normal sella (25%)
- √ enlarged J-shaped sella with truncated dorsum
- √ thickening + increased density of lamina dura in floor of sella (10%)
- √ extensive sellar destruction (75%)
- √ curvilinear / flocculent / stippled calcifications / lamellar ossification; calcifications seen in youth in 70 – 90%, in adults in 30 – 40%

CT:
- √ multilobulated inhomogeneous suprasellar mass
- √ solid (15%) / mixed (30%) / cystic lesion (54 – 75%) (cystic appearance secondary to cholesterol, keratin, necrotic debris with higher density than CSF)
- √ enhancement of solid lesion, peripheral enhancement of cystic lesion
- √ marginal hyperdense lesion (calcification / ossification) in 100%
- √ ± obstructive hydrocephalus
- √ extension into middle > anterior > posterior cranial fossa (25%)

MR (relatively ineffective in demonstrating calcifications):
- √ hyper- / iso- / hypointense on T1WI (variable secondary to hemorrhage / cholesterol-containing proteinaceous fluid)
- √ markedly hyperintense on T2WI
- √ marginal enhancement of solid components with gadopentetate dimeglumine

Angio:
- √ usually avascular
- √ lateral displacement, elevation, narrowing of supraclinoid segment of ICA
- √ posterior displacement of basilar artery

DDx: (1)   Epidermoid (no contrast enhancement)
       (2)   Rathke cleft cyst (small intrasellar lesion)

CYSTICERCOSIS OF BRAIN

larva of pork tapeworm (Taenia solium) frequently
involving CNS, muscles, heart, fat tissue

Incidence: CNS involvement in up to 90%

Location: meninges (39%) esp. in basal cisterns,
       parenchyma (20%), intraventricular (17%),
       mixed (23%), intraspinal (1%)

A. Acute phase (= focal meningoencephalitis)
   • focal seizures
   √ single / multiple small focal enhancing lesions;
     transitory with resolution in a few months
   √ diffusely edematous white matter
   √ homogeneously enhancing small nodules often with
     extensive edema (DDx: metastases without edema)

B. Chronic phase (= involution with subsequent
   calcification + cyst formation)
   √ small focal calcifications (= probably dead larvae);
     may appear within 8 months – 10 years after acute
     infection along gray-white matter junction
   √ well-defined cystic areas of CSF density (= racemose
     cysts) without associated edema (= living larvae)
   √ "rice-like" muscle calcifications rarely visible

RADIOGRAPHIC TYPES

1. Parenchymal type
   √ multiple / solitary cystic lesions up to 6 cm in size;
     many terminate as calcified granulomata (larvae not
     dead unless completely calcified)
   √ encephalitic form may occur in children

2. Meningeal / racemose type
   √ ventricular dilatation indicating diffuse meningeal
     inflammatory process
   √ lucent cystic lesions in basal cisterns (= racemose
     cysts) with variable enhancement

3. Intraventricular type
   √ obstructive hydrocephalus caused by blockage
     within various portions of ventricular system from
     solitary / multiple cysts

4. Mixed type (frequent)

DANDY-WALKER MALFORMATION

= characterized by (1) enlarged posterior fossa with high
   position of tentorium (2) dys- / agenesis of cerebellar
   vermis (3) cystic dilatation of 4th ventricle filling nearly
   entire posterior fossa

Cause: congenital atresia of foramina of **L**uschka
       (**l**ateral) + **M**agendie (**m**edian)

Incidence: 12% of all congenital hydrocephaly

Path: defect in vermis connecting an ependyma-lined
       retrocerebellar cyst with 4th ventricle
       (PATHOGNOMONIC)

Associated midline anomalies   (in >60%):
   (1)   dysgenesis of corpus callosum (20 – 25%), lipoma
         of corpus callosum
   (2)   holoprosencephaly (25%)
   (3)   malformation of cerebral gyri (dysplasia of cingulate
         gyrus) (25%)

   (4)   cerebellar heterotopia + malformation of cerebellar
         folia (25%)
   (5)   malformation of inferior olivary nucleus
   (6)   hamartoma of tuber cinereum
   (7)   syringomyelia
   (8)   cleft palate
   (9)   occipital encephalocele (<5%)

other associations:
   (1)   polymicrogyria / gray matter heterotopia (5 – 10%)
   (2)   polydactyly
   (3)   cardiac anomalies

Skull film:
   √ large skull secondary to hydrocephalus +
     dolichocephaly
   √ diastatic lambdoid suture
   √ disproportionately large expanded posterior fossa
   √ torcular herophili and lateral sinuses high above
     lambdoid angle = torcular-lambdoid inversion

CT / US / MR:
   √ hypoplasia / absence of cerebellar vermis: total
     (25%), partial (75%)
   √ superiorly displaced superior vermis cerebelli
   √ small + widely separated cerebellar hemispheres
   √ anterior + lateral displacement of ± hypoplastic
     cerebellar hemispheres
   √ large posterior fossa cyst with extension through
     foramen magnum = diverticulum of roofless 4th
     ventricle
   √ elevated insertion of tentorium cerebelli
   √ cerebellar hemispheres in apposition without
     intervening vermis following shunt procedure
   √ absence of falx cerebelli
   √ scalloping of petrous pyramids
   √ hydrocephalus (in 72% open communication with 3rd
     ventricle; in 39% patent 4th ventricle; in 28%
     aqueductal stenosis; in 11% incisural obstruction);
     unusual at birth but present by 3 months of age in
     75%
   √ anterior displacement of pons

Angio:
   √ high position of transverse sinus
   √ elevated great vein of Galen
   √ elevated posterior cerebral vessels
   √ anterosuperiorly displaced superior cerebellar arteries
     above the posterior cerebral arteries
   √ small / absent PICA with high tonsillar loop

Cx: trapping of cyst above tentorium = "keyhole
       configuration"

Prognosis: 22 – 50% mortality

DDx: posterior fossa extraaxial cyst, arachnoid cyst,
       isolated 4th ventricle, giant cisterna magna,
       porencephaly

DANDY-WALKER VARIANT

= dysgenetic cerebellar vermis + cystic dilatation of 4th
   ventricle <u>without</u> enlargement of posterior fossa;
   More common than Dandy-Walker malformation
   √ 4th ventricle smaller + better formed
   √ retrocerebellar cyst smaller

√ communication between retrocerebellar cyst and subarachnoid space through a patent foramen of Magendie may be present

√ posterior fossa smaller than in usual Dandy-Walker syndrome

DERMOID OF CNS

= pilosebaceous mass lined with skin appendages originating from the inclusion of epithelial cells + skin appendages during closure of neural tube

Incidence: 1% of all intracranial tumors

Path: ectodermal + mesodermal lesion = squamous epithelium, mesodermal cells (hair follicles, sweat + sebaceous glands)

Age: <30 years (appears in adulthood secondary to slow growth); M < F

Location:

(a) spinal canal (most common): extra- / intramedullary in lumbosacral region

(b) posterior fossa within vermis / 4th ventricle (predilection for midline)

(c) posterior to superior orbital fissure, may be associated with bone defect

• bouts of chemical / bacterial meningitis possible

√ thick-walled inhomogeneous mass with focal areas of fat

√ mural / central calcifications / bone (possible)

√ may have sinus tract to skin surface (dermal sinus) if located in midline at occipital / nasofrontal region

√ fat-fluid level if cyst ruptures into ventricles, fat droplets in subarachnoid space

√ NO contrast enhancement

MR:

√ variointense on T1WI (hyperintense with contents of liquified cholesterol products)

√ shortened T1 + T2 relaxation times (= fat)

DIFFUSE SCLEROSIS

sporadic, young adults, fulminant course

• dementia, deafness

√ low attenuation regions in both hemispheres without symmetry

DYKE-DAVIDOFF-MASON SYNDROME

= unilateral cerebral atrophy with ipsilateral small skull

• seizures

• hemiparesis

• mental retardation

Age: presents in adolescence

√ unilateral thickening of skull

√ unilateral decrease in size of cranial fossa

√ unilateral overdevelopment of sinuses

√ contraction of a hemisphere / lobe

√ compensatory enlargement of adjacent ventricle + sulci with midline shift

EMPTY SELLA SYNDROME

= extension of subarachnoid space into sella turcica, which becomes exposed to CSF pulsations secondary to defect in diaphragma sellae; characterized by normal

/ molded pituitary gland + normal or enlarged sella (empty sella = misnomer)

Incidence: 24% in autopsy study

A. PRIMARY EMPTY SELLA (anatomic spectrum)

Incidence: 10% of adult population; M:F = 1:4

Probable causes:

(1) pituitary enlargement followed by regression during pregnancy

(2) involution of a pituitary tumor

(3) congenital weakness of diaphragma sellae occurs more frequently in patients with increased intracranial pressure

• usually asymptomatic

• increased risk for CSF rhinorrhea

• NO endocrine abnormalities

B. SECONDARY EMPTY SELLA

= postsurgical when diaphragma sellae has been disrupted

• visual disturbance

• headaches

√ slowly progressive symmetrical / asymmetrical (double floor) enlargement of sella

√ remodeled lamina dura remains mineralized

√ small rim of pituitary tissue displaced posteriorly + inferiorly

√ infundibulum sign = infundibulum extends to floor of sella

DDx: cystic tumor, large herniated 3rd ventricle (displaced infundibulum)

EMPYEMA OF BRAIN

A. SUBDURAL EMPYEMA

20% of all intracranial bacterial infections

Cause: paranasal sinusitis, otitis media, calvarial osteomyelitis, infection after craniotomy or ventricular shunt placement, penetrating wound, contamination of meningitis-induced subdural effusion

Location: frontal + inferior cranial space in close proximity to paranasal sinuses; 80% over convexity extending into interhemispheric fissure or posterior fossa

√ hypo- / isodense crescentic / lentiform zone adjacent to inner table

√ may show mass effect (sulcal effacement, ventricular compression, shift)

√ thin curvilinear rim of enhancement (7 – 10 days later) adjacent to brain

√ severe sinusitis / mastoiditis (may be most significant indicator)

Mortality: 30% (neurosurgical emergency)

Cx: venous thrombosis, infarction, seizures, hemiparesis, hemianopsia, aphasia, brain abscess

DDx: subacute / chronic subdural hematoma

B. EPIDURAL EMPYEMA

same causes as above

No neurologic deficits (dura minimizes pressure exerted on brain)

√ thick enhancing rim

ENCEPHALITIS

= term generally reserved for diffuse inflammatory process of viral etiology (herpes simplex, California encephalitis, Eastern equine encephalitis, St. Louis encephalitis, Western equine encephalitis)
√ diffuse mild cerebral edema
√ small infarctions / hemorrhage (less frequent)

Herpes Simplex Encephalitis (HSE)

= most common cause of nonepidemic necrotizing meningoencephalitis in USA
Organism: HSV type I (in adults); HSV type II (in neonates from transplacental infection)
• confusion, disorientation
• preceding viral syndrome, fever, headache, seizures
Location: temporal > frontal > parietal lobes; propensity for limbic system (olfactory tract, temporal lobes, cingulate gyrus, insular cortex); predominantly unilateral
CT (principal role is to identify biopsy site):
√ may be negative in first 3 days
√ poorly defined bilateral areas of decreased attenuation
√ spared putamen forms sharply defined concave / straight border (DDx: infarction, glioma)
√ compression of lateral ventricles, sylvian fissure (brain edema)
√ patchy peripheral / gyral / cisternal enhancement (50%), may persist for several months
√ tendency for hemorrhage + rapid dissemination in brain
MR:
√ increased signal intensity on T2WI
NUC:
Agents: standard brain imaging (eg, Tc-99m DTPA), newer brain agents (eg, I-123 iodoamphetamine / Tc-99m HMPAO)
SPECT imaging improves sensitivity
√ characteristic focal increase in activity in temporal lobes on brain scintigraphy (blood-brain barrier breakdown)
Dx: fluorescein antibody staining / viral culture from brain biopsy
Mortality: 70%
Rx: adenine arabinoside
DDx: low-grade glioma, infarct, abscess

Postinfectious Encephalitis

following viral illness / vaccination
Acute disseminated encephalomyelitis (ADEM)
= autoimmune disorder following measles, mumps, varicella, pertussis, rubella infection / vaccination
• seizures + focal neurologic signs 7 – 14 days after clinical onset of viral infection
Histo: diffuse perivenous inflammatory process resulting in areas of demyelination
Location: subcortical white matter of both hemispheres asymmetrically
CT: √ hypodense white matter
MR: √ focal areas of prolonged T1 + T2

Rx: corticosteroids result in dramatic improvement
Prognosis: complete recovery / some permanent neurologic damage (10 – 20%)
DDx: simulating multiple sclerosis (rarely recurrent episodes as in multiple sclerosis)

Human Immunodeficiency Virus Encephalitis

often in combination with CMV encephalitis
Histo: microglial nodules + perivascular multinucleated giant cells accompanying gliosis of deep white + gray matter
√ predominantly central CNS atrophy
√ symmetric periventricular / diffuse white matter disease without mass effect (hypodense on CT, high-intensity on T2WI)

EPENDYMOMA

= in majority benign slow-growing neoplasm of mature well-differentiated ependymal cells lining the ventricles
Incidence: most commonly in children; 5 – 9% of all primary CNS neoplasms; 15% of posterior fossa tumors in children; 63% of spinal intramedullary gliomas
Histo: benign aggregates of ependymocytes in form of perivascular pseudorosettes; may have papillary pattern (difficult DDx from choroid plexus papilloma)
Age: (a) supratentorial: at any age (atrium / foramen of Monro)
(b) posterior fossa: <10 years; age peaks at 5 and 34 years; M:F = 0.8:1
Associated with: neurofibromatosis
• increased intracranial pressure (90%)
Location:
(a) infratentorial: floor of 4th ventricle (70% of all intracranial ependymomas)
(b) supratentorial: frontal > parietal > temperoparietal juxtaventricular region (uncommonly intra-ventricular), lateral ventricle, 3rd ventricle
(c) conus (40 – 65% of all spinal intramedullary gliomas)
in children: infratentorial in 70%, supratentorial in 30%
√ small cystic areas in 15 – 50% (central necrosis)
√ fine punctate multifocal calcifications (25 – 50%)
√ intratumoral hemorrhage (10%)
√ frequently grows into brain parenchyma extending to cortical surface (particularly in frontal + parietal lobes)
√ may invaginate into ventricles
√ expansion frequently through foramen of Luschka into cerebellopontine angle (15%) or through foramen of Magendie caudad into cisterna magna (up to 60%) (CHARACTERISTIC)
√ direct invasion of brainstem / cerebellum (30 – 40%)
√ insinuation around blood vessels + cranial nerves
√ communicating hydrocephalus (100%) secondary to protein exudate elaborated by tumor clogging resorption pathways
CT:
√ sharply marginated multilobulated iso- / slightly hyperdense 4th ventricular mass

√ thin well-defined low-attenuation halo (distended effaced 4th ventricle)

√ heterogeneous / moderately uniform enhancement of solid portions (80%)

MR:

√ low to intermediate heterogeneous signal intensity on T1WI

√ hypointense tumor margins on T1WI + T2WI in 64% (hemosiderin deposits)

√ foci of high signal intensity on T2WI (= necrotic areas / cysts) + low signal intensity (= calcification / hemorrhage)

√ fluid-fluid level within cysts

√ homogeneous Gd-DTPA enhancement of tumor

Cx: subarachnoid dissemination via CSF (rare) (DDx: malignant ependymoma, ependymoblastoma)

Rx: surgery (difficult to resect due to adherence to surrounding brain) + radiation (partially radiosensitive) + chemotherapy

DDx of cerebellar ependymoma:

(1) Astrocytoma (hypodense, displaces 4th ventricle from midline, cystic lucency, intramedullary)

(2) Medulloblastoma (hyperdense, calcifications in only 10%)

(3) Trapped 4th ventricle (no contrast enhancement)

EPIDERMOID OF CNS

Incidence: 0.2 – 1.8% of all primary intracranial neoplasms; most common congenital intracranial tumor which typically enlarges with somatic growth becoming symptomatic in adulthood

Etiology: ectodermal lesion = inclusion of epithelial elements during closure of neural tube in 5th week of fetal life (early inclusion results in midline lesion, later inclusion results in more lateral location)

Path: "pearly tumor" = well-defined solid lesion with glistening irregular nodular surface lined by stratified squamous epithelium becoming cystic by progressive desquamation of keratinized debris + formation of cholesterol crystals = PRIMARY / CONGENITAL CHOLESTEATOMA

Age: 10 – 60 years, peak age in 4th – 5th decade; M:F = 1:1

• cranial neuropathy from cerebellopontine epidermoids

• hydrocephalus in suprasellar epidermoids

• chemical meningitis (secondary to leakage of tumor contents into subarachnoid space) in middle cranial fossa epidermoids

Location: may be intra- / extradural

(a) cerebellopontine angle (most common)

(b) suprasellar region (common)

(c) perimesencephalic cisterns

(d) within ventricles

(e) skull vault

√ signal intensity similar to CSF

√ soft infiltrating lesion surrounding vessels + cranial nerves

√ little mass effect, no edema / hydrocephalus

√ NO contrast enhancement

√ may be associated with dermal sinus tract at occipital / nasofrontal region if midline in location

CT:

√ typically lobulated round low density mass

√ bony erosion with sharply defined well-corticated margins

√ calcification (1%)

MR:

√ heterogeneous hypointense lesion on T1WI + hyperintense on T2WI

√ angiographically avascular

√ papillary / frondlike surface on cisternography

EPIDURAL HEMATOMA OF BRAIN

= EXTRADURAL HEMATOMA = within potential space between naked inner table + calvarial periosteum (dura layer), which is bound down at suture margins

Incidence: 2% of all serious head injuries; in <1% of all children with cranial trauma; uncommon in infants

Associated with: skull fracture in 40 – 85% (best demonstrated on skull radiographs)

Mechanism of injury:

(a) laceration of meningeal artery / vein adjacent to inner table from fracture of calvarium (91%)

(b) avulsion of venous vessels from points of calvarial perforations

(c) disruption of dural venous sinuses (major cause in younger children)

• transient loss of consciousness

• lucent interval

• 3rd nerve palsy (sign of cerebral herniation)

• somnolence (24 – 96 hours after accident): medical emergency!

Δ DANGEROUS because of focal mass effect + rapid onset!

Types:

I acute epidural hematoma (58%) from arterial bleeding

II subacute hematoma (31%)

III chronic hematoma (11%) from venous bleeding

Location:

(a) in 66% temporoparietal (most often from laceration of middle meningeal artery)

(b) in 29% at frontal pole, parieto-occipital region, between occipital lobes, posterior fossa (most often from laceration of venous sinuses)

CT:

√ fracture line in area of epidural hematoma

√ expanding biconvex elliptical extraaxial fluid collection (most frequent) = under high pressure

√ high density in acute stage (60 – 90 HU)

√ mass effect ("compression cone effect") with effacement of gyri + sulci from:

— epidural hematoma (57%)

— hemorrhagic contusion (29%)

— cerebral edematous swelling (14%)

√ separation of venous sinuses / falx from inner table of skull

Δ The ONLY hemorrhage displacing falx / venous sinuses away from inner table!

√ marked stretching of vessels

√ signs of arterial injury (rare): contrast extravasation, arteriovenous fistula, middle meningeal artery occlusion, formation of false aneurysm

Angio:
√ meningeal arteries displaced away from inner table of skull

Rx: after surgical evacuation return of ventricular system to midline

DDx: Chronic subdural hematoma (may have similar shape as acute epidural hematoma)

FIBROMUSLAR DYSPLASIA

= nonatherosclrotic angiopathy of unknown pathogenesis

Incidence: <1% of cerebral angiographies

Age: 2/3 >50 years; M:F = 1:9

Associated with: brain ischemia (up to 50%), intracranial aneurysms (up to 30%), intracranial tumors (30%), bruits, trauma

Location:
cervical + intracranial ICA (85%), vertebral artery (7%); both anterior + posterior circulation (8%); bilateral (60 – 65%)

Δ simultaneous involvement of renal / muscular arteries in 3%

Angiography:
√ length of affected vessel from 0.5 cm to several cm

Types:
1. Medial fibroplasia = fibromuscular hyperplasia (80%)
   √ string of beads = alternating zones of widening + narrowing
   √ tubular narrowing
2. Intimal fibroplasia
   √ smooth concentric tubular narrowing (DDx: Takayasu arteritis, sclerosing arteritis, vessel spasm, arterial hypoplasia)
3. Subadventitial hyperplasia
4. Atypical fibromuscular dysplasia
   (= ? variant of intimal fibroplasia)
   √ web = smooth / corrugated mass involving only one wall of vessel + projecting into lumen (DDx: atherosclerotic disease, posttraumatic aneurysm)

Cx: dissection (in 3%), macroaneurysm

Prognosis: tends to remain stable / minimal progression

Rx: only when symptoms progress

GLIOBLASTOMA MULTIFORME

most malignant form of astrocytoma (Grade IV); results from severe anaplasia of preexisting Grade I / II astrocytoma

Incidence: most common primary brain tumor; 50% of all intracranial tumors

Age: all ages; peak incidence at 5 – 55 years; M:F = 3:2

Path:
multilobulated appearance; frequently quite extensive vasogenic edema intermixed with infiltrating neoplasm; necrosis is essential for pathologic diagnosis

Histo:
highly cellular, often bizarrely pleomorphic / undifferentiated multipolar astrocytes; common mitoses + vascular endothelial proliferation; frequently hemorrhagic + necrotic with cyst formation (tumor outgrows blood supply); no capsule; deeply invasive

Location:
white matter of frontal > temporal lobes; relative sparing of basal ganglia + gray matter; common in corpus callosum ("butterfly glioma"), thalamus, quadrigeminal region, pons, rarely in cerebellum; multifocal in 2 – 5%

Spread:
follows white matter tracts into corpus callosum (36%); readily crosses midline = "butterfly" glioma (clue: invasion of septum pellucidum); frontal + temporal gliomas tend to invade basal ganglia; may invade pia, arachnoid and dura (mimicking meningioma); may reach subependymal surface of ventricles (subependymal carpet)

NECT:
√ inhomogeneous low-density mass with irregular shape + poorly defined margins (hypodense solid tumor / cavitary necrosis / tumor cyst / peritumoral edema)
√ compression + displacement of ventricles, cisterns, brain parenchyma
√ iso- / hyperdense portions (hemorrhage) in 5%
√ rarely calcifies (if coexistent with lower grade glioma / after radio- or chemotherapy)

CECT:
Enhancement pattern: contrast enhancement due to breakdown of blood-brain barrier / neovascularity / areas of necrosis
  (a) diffuse homogeneous enhancement
  (b) nonhomogeneous enhancement
  (c) ring pattern (occasionally enhancing mass within the ring)
  (d) low-density lesion with contrast fluid level (leakage of contrast)
√ almost always ring blush of variable thickness: multiscalloped ("garland"), round / ovoid; may be seen surrounding ventricles (subependymal spread); tumor usually extends beyond enhancement margins
√ sedimentation level secondary to cellular debris / hemorrhage / accumulated contrast material in tumoral cyst

MR:
√ poorly defined lesion with some mass effect / vasogenic edema / heterogeneity
√ hemosiderin deposits (gradient echo images)
√ hemorrhage (hypointensity on T2- and T2*-weighted images)
√ T1WI + gadolinium-DTPA enhancement separate tumor nodules from surrounding edema, central necrosis and cyst formation

Angio:
√ neovascularity + early draining veins
√ avascular lesion

PET:
√ increase in glucose utilization rate

Prognosis: 1 – 2 years postoperative survival

GANGLION CELL TUMOR
Gangliocytoma
rare benign tumor
Incidence: 0.1%
Histo: purely neuronal tumor (no glial components); ganglion cells without stain for glial fibrillary acetic protein

Ganglioglioma
glial component that may show neoplastic differentiation
√ cyst foration + calcifications
√ contrast enhancement

GLIOMA
growth along white matter tracts, tendency to increase in grade with time; may be multifocal
CELL OF ORIGIN
1. Astrocyte ...Astrocytoma
2. Oligodendrocyte ...Oligodendroglioma
3. Ependym ...Ependymoma
4. Medulloblast ...Medulloblastoma
(PNET = primitive neuroectodermal tumor)
5. Choroid plexus ...Choroid plexus papilloma

FREQUENCY OF INTRACRANIAL GLIOMAS
Glioblastoma multiforme	51%
Astrocytoma	25%
Ependymoma	6%
Oligodendroglioma	6%
Spongioblastoma polare	3%
Mixed gliomas	3%
Astroblastoma	2%

Location: (a) central white matter of cerebrum (adults); 15 – 30% of all gliomas
(b) cerebellar hemisphere + brainstem (children)
Contrast enhancement:
Δ increases in proportion to degree of anaplasia
Δ diminished intensity of enhancement with steroid therapy
A. LOW-GRADE GLIOMAS (Grade I / II) = LOW-GRADE ASTROCYTOMA
Histo: diffuse growth pattern with proliferation of well-differentiated fibrillary astrocytes, mild nuclear pleomorphism, mild hypercellularity, rarely mitotic figures
benign non-metastasizing; blood-brain barrier may remain intact
Distribution: proportional to amount of white matter
Prognosis: 3 – 10 years postoperative survival
B. ANAPLASTIC ASTROCYTOMA = GRADE III GLIOMA
Histo: less well differentiated with greater degree of hypercellularity + pleomorphism, mitoses + vascular endothelial proliferation common, NO necrosis

Distribution: proportional to amount of white matter
Prognosis: 2 years postoperative survival
C. GLIOBLASTOMA MULTIFORME = GRADE IV GLIOMA
most common of all gliomas
Peak age: 5 – 6th decades
Histo: highly cellular, bizarrely pleomorphic / undifferentiated cells, prominent endothelial proliferation, tumor necrosis (HALLMARK); histologically malignant
Prognosis: 1 year postoperative survival

Brainstem Glioma
Incidence: 1%; 12 – 15% of all pediatric brain tumors; 20 – 30% of infratentorial brain tumors
Histo: usually anaplastic astrocytoma / glioblastoma multiforme with infiltration along fiber tracts
Age: in children + young adults; peak age 3 – 13 years; M:F = 1:1
• become clinically apparent early before ventricular obstruction occurs
• ipsilateral progressive multiple cranial nerve palsies
• contralateral hemiparesis
• cerebellar dysfunction: ataxia, nystagmus
• eventually respiratory insufficiency
Location: pons > midbrain > medulla; often unilateral at medullopontine junction
Δ medullary + mesencephalic gliomas are more benign than pontine gliomas!
Growth pattern:
(a) diffuse infiltration of brainstem with symmetric expansion + rostrocaudal spread into medulla / thalamus + spread to cerebellum
(b) focally exophytic growth into adjacent cisterns (cerebellopontine, prepontine, cisterna magna)
√ asymmetrically expanded brainstem
√ flattening + posterior displacement of 4th ventricle + aqueduct of Sylvius
√ compression of prepontine + interpeduncular cistern (in upward transtentorial herniation)
√ paradoxical widening of CP angle cistern with tumor extension into CP angle
√ paradoxical anterior displacement of 4th ventricle with tumor extension into cisterna magna
CT:
√ isodense / hypodense mass with indistinct margins
√ hyperdense foci (= hemorrhage) uncommon
√ absent / minimal / patchy contrast enhancement (50%)
√ ring enhancement in necrotic / cystic tumors (most aggressive)
√ prominent enhancement in exophytic lesion
√ hydrocephalus uncommon (because of early symptomatology)
MR: (better evaluation in subtle cases)
√ hypointense on T1WI + hyperintense on T2WI
√ ± engulfment of basilar artery
Angio:
√ anterior displacement of basilar artery + anterior pontomesencephalic vein

√ posterior displacement of precentral cerebellar vein
√ posterior displacement of posterior medullary + supratonsillar segments of PICA
√ lateral displacement of lateral medullary segment of PICA
Prognosis: 10 – 30% 5-year survival rate
Rx: radiation therapy
DDx: focal encephalitis, resolving hematoma, vascular malformation, tuberculoma, infarct, multiple sclerosis, metastasi, lymphoma

Hypothalamic / Chiasmatic Glioma
Point of origin often undeterminable: hypothalamic gliomas invade chiasm, chiasmatic gliomas invade hypothalamus
Incidence: 10 – 15% of supratentorial tumors in children
Age: 2 – 4 years; M:F = 1:1
Associated with von Recklinghausen disease (20 – 50%)
• diminished visual acuity (50%) with optic atrophy
• diencephalic syndrome (in up to 20%): marked emaciation, pallor, unusual alertness, hyperactivity, euphoria
• obese child
• sexual precocity
• diabetes insipidus
√ obstructive hydrocephalus
√ suprasellar hypodense lobulated mass with dense inhomogeneous enhancement
√ hypointense on T1WI + hyperintense on T2WI

GLOBOID CELL LEUKODYSTROPHY
= KRABBE DISEASE
Cause: deficiency of galactosylceramide beta-galactosidase resulting in cerebroside accumulation + destruction of oligodendrocytes
Dx: biochemical assay from white blood cells / skin fibroblasts
Age: 3 – 6 months
• restlessness + irritability
• marked spasticity
• optic atrophy
• hyperacusis
√ symmetric hyperdense lesions in thalami, caudate nuclei, corona radiata
√ decreased attenuation of white matter
√ brain atrophy with enlargement of ventricles
Prognosis: death within first few years of life

HALLERVORDEN-SPATZ DISEASE
rare metabolic disorder with abnormal iron retention in basal ganglia
Age: 2nd decade of life
Histo: hyperpigmentation + symmetrical destruction of globus pallidus + substantia nigra
• progressive gait impairment + rigidity of limbs
• slowing of voluntary movements, dysarthria
• choreoathetotic movement disorder
• mental deterioration

CT:
√ low (= tissue destruction) / high density foci (= dystrophic calcification) in globus pallidus
MR:
√ initially hypointense globus pallidus on T2WI (= iron deposition)
√ later hyperintense foci on T2WI (= tissue destruction + gliosis)

HAMARTOMA OF CNS
Rare tumor
(a) sporadic
(b) associated with tuberous sclerosis; may degenerate into giant cell astrocytoma
Age: 0 – 30 years
Location: temporal lobe, hamartoma of tuber cinereum, subependymal in tuberous sclerosis
√ cyst with little mass effect, possibly with focal calcifications
√ usually no enhancement

HEAD TRAUMA
Indications for radiographic skull series:
Only in conjunction with positive CT scan findings!
1. Evaluation of depressed skull fracture / fracture of base of the skull
Indications for CT:
1. Loss of consciousness (more than transient)
2. Altered mental status during observation
3. Focal neurologic signs
4. Clinically suspected basilar fracture
5. Depressed skull fracture
6. Penetrating wound
Indications for MR:
1. Postconcussive symptomatology
2. Diagnosis of small sub- / epidural hematoma
3. Suspected shear injury
4. Vascular damage (eg, pseudoaneurysm formation due to basilar skull fracture)
A. INTRACEREBRAL HEMORRHAGE
1. Hematoma
2. Contusion
B. EXTRACEREBRAL HEMORRHAGE
1. Subdural hematoma
in adults: dura inseparable from skull
2. Epidural hematoma
in children: dura easily stripped away from skull
3. Subarachnoid hemorrhage
common accompaniment to severe cerebral trauma
C. OTHER POSTTRAUMATIC LESIONS
1. Pneumocephalus
2. Penetrating foreign body

HEMANGIOBLASTOMA OF CNS
= benign autosomal dominant tumor of vascular origin
Incidence: 1 – 2.5% of all intracranial neoplasms
Age: (a) adulthood (>80%): 20 – 50 years, average age of 33 years; M > F
(b) childhood (<20%): in von Hippel-Lindau disease (10 – 20%); girls

Associated with:
  (a) von Hipel-Lindau disease, may have multiple hemangioblastomas (only 20% of patients show other stigmata)
  (b) pheochromocytoma (often familial)
  (c) syringomyelia
  (d) spinal cord hemangioblastomas
- erythrocytemia in 20% (tumor elaborates stimulant)
Location: paravermian cerebellar hemisphere > spinal cord > cerebral hemisphere / brainstem; multiple lesions in 10%
√ solid (1/3) / cystic / cystic + mural nodule
√ solid portion often intensely hemorrhagic
√ almost never calcifies
CT:
  √ cystic sharply marginated mass of CSF-density (2/3)
  √ peripheral mural nodule with homogeneous enhancement (50%
  √ occasionally solid with intense homogeneous enhancement
MR:
  √ well-demarcated tumor mass moderately hypointense on T1WI + T2WI
  √ hyperintense areas on T1WI (= hemorrhage)
  √ hypointense areas on T1WI + hyperintense areas on T2WI (= cyst formation)
  √ intralesional vermiform areas of signal dropout (= high velocity blood flow)
  √ heterogeous enhancement on Gd-DTPA with
nonenhancing foci of cyst formation + calcification + rapidly flowing blood
  √ perilesional Gd-DTPA enhancing areas of slow-flowing blood vessels feeding + draining the tumor
  √ peripheral hyperintense rim on T2WI (= edema)
Angio:
  √ densely stained tumor nidus within cyst ("contrast loading")
  √ staining of entire rim of cyst
  √ draining vein
DDx: (1) astrocytoma (>5 cm, calcifications, no angiographic contrast blush of mural nodule, no erythrocytemia)
  (2) Arachnoid cyst (if mural nodule not visualized)
  (3) Metastasis

HEMATOMA OF BRAIN
Etiology:
  1. Aneurysm (36%)
  2. Hypertension (36%)
     Age: >60 years; often large hemorrhage located in basal ganglia (putamen in 50%) / thalamus (25%), pons + brainstem (10%), cerebellum (10%), cerebral hemisphere (5%)
  3. AVM (11%)
  4. Trauma
     (a) blunt / penetrating trauma (bullet, ice pick, skull fragment)
     (b) brain contusion: coup and contrecoup lesions; white matter shearing injury
  5. Bleeding into tumor (eg, metastasis, glioma)

6. Hypocoagulable state
7. Hemorrhagic infarction

Sequelae of trauma:
  1. Posttraumatic hydrocephalus (1/3)
     = obstruction of CSF pathways secondary to intracranial hemorrhage; develops within 3 months
  2. Generalized cerebral atrophy (1/3)
     = result of ischemia + hypoxia
  3. Encephalomalacia
     √ focal areas of decreased density, but usually higher density than CSF
  4. Pseudoporencephaly
     = CSF-filled space communicating with ventricle / subarachnoid space from cystic degeneration
  5. Subdural hygroma
     = localized collection of CSF in subdural space secondary to (a) result of chronic subdural hematoma (b) arachnoidal tear acting as a ball valve
     Age: most often in elderly + young children
     √ may resolve spontaneously
  6. Leptomeningeal cyst
     = progressive protrusion of leptomeninges through traumatic calvarial defect
  7. Cerebrospinal fluid leak
     - rhinorrhea, otorrhea (indicating basilar fracture with meningeal tear)
  8. Carotid-cavernous fistula
  9. Traumatic pseudoaneurysm
     = excavated encapsulated hematoma communicating with arterial lumen
     Location: branches of ACA + MCA, intracavernous portion of ICA, PCom
  10. Posttraumatic abscess
     secondary to (a) penetrating injury (b) basilar skull fracture (c) infection of traumatic hematoma
  11. Vascular compression
     compression of PCA against tentorial margin secondary to uncal herniation leads to infarction of PCA territory

Stages of cerebral hematomas
  Resolution: resorption from outside toward the center; rate depends on size of hematoma (usually 1 – 6 weeks)
  FALSE-NEGATIVE CT:
  1. impaired clotting
  2. anemia
  √ iso- / hypodense stage

Acute hemorrhage
  Time period: <24 hours
  NCCT:
  √ homogeneous consolidated high-density lesion with irregular well-defined margins increasing in density during day 1 – 3 (hematoma attenuation dependent on hemoglobin concentration + rate of clot retraction)

√ usually surrounded by low attenuation (edema, contusion) appearing within 24 – 48 hours
   (a) irregular shape in trauma
   (b) spherical + solitary in spontaneous hemorrhage
√ less mass effect compared with neoplasms

MR:
√ center of hematoma isointense on T1WI + markedly hypointense on T2WI (= deoxygenation of blood clot forms paramagnetic deoxy-hemoglobin in intact hypoxic RBCs, dependent on degree of surrounding oxygen tension)
√ surrounding tissue isointense on T1WI / hyperintense on T2WI (edema)

Subacute hemorrhage
Time period: days – 1 month
NCCT:
√ increase in size of hemorrhagic area over days / weeks
√ high density lesion within 1st week; often with layering
√ gradual decrease in density from periphery inwards (1 – 2 HU per day) during 2nd + 3rd week
√ isodense hematoma from 3rd – 10th week with perilesional ring of lucency
CECT:
√ peripheral rim enhancement at inner border of perilesional lucency (1 – 6 weeks after injury) in 80% (secondary to blood-brain barrier breakdown / luxury perfusion / formation of hypervascular granulation tissue)
√ ring blush may be diminished by administration of corticosteroids

MR:
√ center of hematoma isointense on T1WI, moderately hypointense onT2WI
√ periphery hyperintense on T1WI, hyperintense on T2WI (= progressive conversion of deoxy-hemoglobin to methemoglobin after 3 – 4 days)

√ rim isointense on T1WI, markedly hypointense on T2WI (= paramagnetic hemosiderin phagocytized by macrophages appearing during 2nd week; present for years)
√ surrounding edema isointense on T1WI + hyperintense on T2WI

Chronic hemorrhage
Time period: 1 month – years
CT:
√ hypodense phase (4 – 6 weeks) secondary to fluid uptake by osmosis
√ decreased density (3 – 6 months) / invisible
√ after 10 weeks lucent hematoma with ring blush (DDx: tumor)
MR:
√ center hyperintense on T1WI + T2WI (= extracellular methemoglobin of lysed RBCs, present for months to 1 year)
√ periphery hyperintense on T1WI + T2WI
√ rim isointense on T1WI + hypointense on T2WI; rim gradually increases over weeks in thickness, eventually fills in entire hematoma (= hemosiderin laden macrophages) = HALLMARK

HETEROTOPIC GRAY MATTER
= collection of cortical neurons in an abnormal location secondary to arrest of migrating neuroblasts from ventricular walls to brain surface between 7 – 24 weeks of GA
Frequency: 3% of healthy population
May be associated with: agenesis of corpus callosum, aqueductal stenosis, microcephaly, schizencephaly
• seizures
Location:
   (1) nodular form: usually symmetric bilateral in subependymal region / periventricular white matter with predilection for posterior + anterior horns
   (2) laminar form: deep / subcortical regions within white matter (less common)
√ single / multiple bilateral subependymal nodules along lateral ventricles

MR appearance of hemorrhage

Phase	Composition	T1	T2	Comments
hyperacute	Oxyhemoglobin	high	high	hyperacute bleed in < 1 hr.
	Deoxyhemoglobin			deoxygenation
acute	intracellular	**iso**	**low**	within intact hypoxic RBCs
	extracellular	iso	iso	after lysis of RBCs
	Methemoglobin			oxidation
	intracellular	**high**	**low**	after 3 - 4 days in intact RBCs
subacute	extracellular	**high**	**high**	may be present for months to years
chronic	Hemosiderin	low	low	within macrophages present for years
	Fibrous tissue	low	low	
	Serous fluid	iso	high	
	Edema	iso	high	

√ NO surrounding edema, isointense with gray matter on all sequences, no intensity change following contrast

DDx: subependymal spread of neoplasm, subependymal hemorrhage, vascular malformation, tuberous sclerosis, intraventricular meningioma, neurofibromatosis

HOLOPROSENCEPHALY

= lack of cleavage / diverticulation of the forebrain (= prosencephalon) laterally (cerebral hemispheres), transversely (telencephalon, diencephalon), horizontally (optic + olfactory structures) as a consequence of arrested lateral ventricular growth in 6-week embryo; cortical brain tissue develops to cover the monoventricle and fuses in the midline; posterior part of the monoventricle becomes enlarged and saclike

Incidence: 1:16,000;   M:F = 1:1

A. ALOBAR   = no hemispheric development
B. SEMILOBAR = some hemispheric development
C. LOBAR   = frontal and temporal lobation + small monoventricle

Associated with: polyhydramnios (60%), renal + cardiac anomalies; chromosomal anomalies (predominantly trisomy 13 + 18)

Associated borderline syndromes secondary to diencephalic malformation:
1. Anophthalmia
2. Microphthalmia
3. Aplasia of pituitary gland
4. Olfactogenital dysplasia
5. Septo-optic dysplasia

DDx:
1. Severe hydrocephalus (roughly symmetrically thinned cortex)
2. Dandy-Walker cyst (normal supratentorial ventricular system)
3. Hydranencephaly (frontal + parietal cortex most severely affected)
4. Agenesis of corpus callosum with midline cyst (lateral ventricles widely separated with pointed superolateral margins)

Alobar Holoprosencephaly

= extreme form in which the prosencephalon does not divide
- minimal motor activity, little sensory response (ineffective brain function); seizures
- severe facial anomalies ("the face predicts the brain"):
  1. Normal face in 17%
  2. Cyclopia (= midline single orbit); may have proboscis (= fleshy supraorbital prominence) + absent nose
  3. Ethmocephaly = 2 hypoteloric orbits + proboscis between eyes and absence of nasal structures
  4. Cebocephaly = 2 hypoteloric orbits + single nostril with small flattened nose + absent nasal septum
  5. Median cleft lip + cleft palate + hypotelorism
  6. Others: micrognathia, trigonocephaly (early closure of metopic suture), microphthalmia, microcephaly

√ thalami fused
√ absence of septum pellucidum, falx cerebri, interhemispheric fissure, corpus callosum, fornix, optic tracts, olfactory bulb (= arrhinencephaly), internal cerebral veins, superior + inferior straight sagittal sinus, vein of Galen, 3rd ventricle, tentorium, sylvian fissure, opercular cortex
√ "horseshoe" / "boomerang" configuration of brain = peripheral rim of cerebral cortex displaced rostrally (coronal plane)
  (a) pancake configuration = cortex covers monoventricle to edge of dorsal cyst
  (b) cup configuration = more cortex visible posteriorly
  (c) ball configuration = complete covering of monoventricle without dorsal cyst
√ crescent-shaped monoventricle = single large ventricle without occipital or temporal horns
√ dorsal cyst occupying most of calvarium + widely communicating with single ventricle; posterior fossa contents may be hypoplastic
√ protrusion of anteriorly placed fused thalami + basal ganglia into monoventricle
√ midbrain, brainstem, cerebellum structurally normal
√ cerebral mantle pachygyric
√ midline clefts in maxilla + palate

Prognosis: death within 1st year of life / stillborn
DDx: massive hydrocephalus, hydranencephaly

Semilobar Holoprosencephaly

= intermediate form with incomplete cleavage of prosencephalon (more midline differentiation + beginning of sagittal separation)
- mild facial anomalies: midline cleft lip + palate
- hypotelorism
- mental retardation
√ single ventricular chamber with partially formed occipital horns + rudimentary temporal horns
√ peripheral rim of brain tissue is several cm thick
√ thalami anteriorly situated, abnormally rotated and partially fused resulting in small 3rd ventricle
√ absence of septum pellucidum + corpus callosum + olfactory bulb
√ rudimentary falx cerebri + interhemispheric fissure form caudally with partial separation of occipital lobes
√ incomplete hippocampal formation

Prognosis: infants survive frequently into adulthood

Lobar Holoprosencephaly

= mildest form with two cerebral hemispheres + two distinct lateral ventricles
- usually not associated with facial anomalies except for hypotelorism
- mild to severe mental retardation, spasticity, athetoid movements
√ closely apposed bodies of lateral ventricles with occipital + frontal horns
√ mild dilatation of lateral ventricles
√ colpocephaly
√ unseparated frontal horns of angular squared shape + flat roof (on coronal images)

√ falx cerebri + interhemispheric fissure extend into frontal area
√ corpus callosum usually present
√ septum pellucidum + sylvian fissures are usually absen
√ hippocampal formation nearly normal
√ basal ganglia + thalami may be fused / separated
√ pachygyria (= abnormaly wide + plump gyri), lissencephaly (= o gyri)
Prognosis: survival into adulthood

HYDATID DISEASE OF BRAIN

= canine tapeworm (Echinococcus granulosus) in sheep- and cattle-grazing areas
Location: liver (60%), lung (25%), CNS (2%)
               subcortical

√ usually single, large round, sharply marginated smooth-walled hypodense cyst
√ no significant surrounding edema; no rim enhancement
√ development of daughter cysts (after rupture / following diagnostic puncture)

HYDRANENCEPHALY

= liquefaction necrosis of cerebral hemispheres replaced by a thin membranous sac of leptomeninges in outer layer + remnants of cortex and white matter in inner layer, filled with CSF + necrotic debris

Incidence: 0.2% of infant autopsies
Etiology:
absence of supaclinoid ICA system (? vascular occlusion / infection with toxoplasmosis or CMV) = ultimate form of porencephaly
• seizures; respiratory failure; generalized flaccidity
• decerebrate state with vegetative existence

√ normal skull size / macrocrania / microcrania
√ complete filling of hemicranium with membranous sac
√ absence of cortical mantle (inferomedial aspect of temporal lobe, inferior aspect of frontal lobe, occipital lobe may be identified in some patients)
√ brainstem usually atrophic
√ cerebellum almost always intact
√ thalamic, hypothalamic, mesencephalic structures usually preserved + project into cystic cavity
√ central brain tissue can be asymmetric
√ choroid plexus present
√ falx cerebri + tentorium cerebelli usually intact, may be deviated in aymmetric involvement, may be incomplete / absent

Prognosis:
not compatible with prolonged extrauterine life (no intellectual improvement from shunting)
DDx: (1)   Severe hydrocephalus (some identifiable cortex present)
       (2)   Alobar holoprosencephaly (facial midline anomalies)
       (3)   Schizencephaly (some spared cortical mantle)

HYDROCEPHALUS

= excessof CSF due to imbalance of CSF formation + absorption resulting in increased intraventricular pressure

Pathophysiology:
A. Overproduction (rare)
B. Impaired absorption
   1. Blockage of CSF flow within ventricular system, cisterna magna, basilar cisterns, cerebral convexities
   2. Blockage of arachnoid villi / lymphatic channels of cranial nerves, spinal nerves, adventitia of cerebral vessels

Compensated hydrocephalus = new equilibrium established at higher intracranial pressure due to opening of alternate pathways (arachnoid membrane / stroma of choroid plexus / extracellular space of cortical mantle = transependymal flow of CSF)

Skull film: Signs of raised intracranial pressure
A. YOUNG INFANT / NEWBORN
   √   increase in craniofacial ratio
   √   bulging of anterior fontanelle
   √   sutural diastasis
   √   macrocephaly + frontal bossing
   √   "hammered silver" appearance = prominent digital impressions (wide range of normals in 4 – 10 years of age)
B. ADOLESCENT / ADULT (changes in sella turcica)
   √   atrophy of anterior wall of dorsum sellae
   √   shortening of the dorsum sellae producing pointed appearance
   √   erosion / thinning / discontinuity of floor of sella
   √   depression of floor of sella with bulging into sphenoid sinus
   √   enlargement of sella turcica
   DDx: osteoporotic sella (aging, excessive steroid hormone)

Signs favoring hydrocephalus over white matter atrophy:
√   commensurate dilatation of temporal horn with lateral ventricles (most reliable sign)
√   narrowing of ventricular angle (= angle between anterior / superior margins of frontal horns at level of foramen of Monro) due to concentric enlargement
   √   Mickey Mouse ears on axial scans
√   enlargement of frontal horn radius (= widest diameter of frontal horns taken at 90° angle to long axis of frontal horn)
   √   rounding of frontal horn shape
√   enlargement of ventricular system disproportionate to enlargement of cortical sulci (due to compression of brain tissue against skull + consequent sulcal narrowing)
√   interstitial edema from transependymal flow of CSF
   √   periventricular hypodensity
   √   rim of prolonged T1 + T2 relaxation times surrounding lateral ventricles

Hydrocephalic distortion of ventricles + brain:
- √ atrial diverticulum = herniation of ventricular wall through choroidal fissure of ventricular trigone into supracerebellar + quadrigeminal cisterns
- √ dilatation of suprapineal recess expanding into posterior incisural space resulting in inferior displacement of pineal gland / shortening of tectum in rostral-caudal direction / elevation of vein of Galen
- √ enlargement of anterior recess of 3rd ventricle extending into suprasellar cistern

Obstructive Hydrocephalus
= obstruction to normal CSF flow + absorption

Communicating Hydrocephalus
= EXTRAVENTRICULAR HYDROCEPHALUS
= elevated intraventricular pressure secondary to blockade beyond the outlet of 4th ventricle within the subarachnoid pathways
Incidence: 38% of congenital hydrocephaly
Pathophysiology:
unimpeded CSF flow through ventricles, impeded CSF flow over convexities / impeded reabsorption by arachnoid villi
Cause:
Subarachnoid hemorrhage (most common cause), meningeal carcinomatosis (medulloblastoma, germinoma, leukemia, lymphoma, adenocarcinoma), purulent / tuberculous meningitis, subdural hematoma, craniosynostosis, achondroplasia, Hurler syndrome, venous obstruction (obliteration of superior sagittal sinus), absence of Pacchioni granulations
- √ symmetric enlargement of lateral, 3rd, and often 4th ventricles
- √ dilatation of subarachnoid cisterns
- √ normal / effaced cerebral sulci
- √ symmetric low attenuation of periventricular white matter (transependymal migration of CSF)
- √ delayed ascent of radionuclide tracer over convexities
- √ persistence of radionuclide tracer in lateral ventricles for up to 48 hours

Changes after successful shunting:
- √ diminished size of ventricles + increased prominence of sulci
- √ cranial vault may thicken
- *Cx:* subdural hematoma (result from precipitous decompression)

Noncommunicating Hydrocephalus
= INTRAVENTRICULAR HYDROCEPHALUS = blockade of CNS flow within the ventricular system with dilatation of ventricles proximal to obstruction
Pathogenesis:
increased CSF pressure causes ependymal flattening with breakdown of CSF-brain barrier leading to myelin destruction + compression of cerebral mantle (brain damage)

Location:
- (a) Lateral ventricular obstruction
  Cause: ependymoma, intraventricular glioma, meningioma
- (b) Foramen of Monro obstruction
  Cause: 3rd ventricular colloid cyst, tuber, papilloma, meningioma, septum pellucidum cyst / glioma, fibrous membrane (post infection), giant cell astrocytoma
- (c) Third ventricular obstruction
  Cause: large pituitary adenoma, teratoma, craniopharyngioma, glioma of 3rd ventricle, hypothalamic glioma
- (d) Aqueductal obstruction
  Cause: Congenital web / atresia (often associated with Chiari malformation), fenestrated aqueduct, tumor of mesencephalon / pineal gland, tentorial meningioma, S/P intraventricular hemorrhage or infection
- (e) Fourth ventricular obstruction
  Cause: Congenital obstruction, Dandy-Walker syndrome, inflammation (TB), tumor within 4th ventricle (ependymoma), extrinsic compression of 4th ventricle (astrocytoma, medulloblastoma, large CPA tumors, posterior fossa mass), isolated / trapped 4th ventricle
- √ enlarged lateral ventricles (enlargement of occipital horns precedes enlargement of frontal horns)
- √ effaced cerebral sulci
- √ periventricular edema with indistinct margins (especially frontal horns)
- √ radioisotope cisternography: no obstruction if tracer reaches ventricle

Nonobstructive Hydrocephalus
= secondary to rapid CSF production
Cause: Choroid plexus papilloma
- √ ventricle near papilloma enlarges
- √ intense radionuclide uptake in papilloma
- √ enlarged anterior / posterior choroidal artery and blush

Congenital Hydrocephalus
= multifactorial CNS malformation during the 3rd / 4th week after conception
Etiology:
(1) aqueductal stenosis (43%)
(2) communicating hydrocephalus (38%)
(3) Dandy-Walker syndrome (13%)
(4) other anatomic lesions (6%)
- (a) Genetic factors: spina bifida, aqueductal stenosis (X-linked recessive trait with a 50% recurrence rate for male fetuses), congenital atresia of foramina of Luschka and Magendie (Dandy-Walker syndrome; autosomal recessive trait with 25% recurrence rate), cerebellar agenesis, cloverleaf skull, trisomy 13 – 18

(b) Nongenetic etiology: tumor compressing 3rd / 4th ventricle, obliteration of subarachnoid pathway due to infection (syphilis, CMV, rubella, toxoplasmosis), proliferation of fibrous tissue (Hurler syndrome), Chiari malformations, vein of Galen aneurysm, choroid plexus papilloma, vitamin A intoxication

Incidence: 0.3 – 1.8 : 1,000 pregnancies
Associated with:
(a) Intracranial anomalies (37%): hypoplasia of corpus callosum, encephalocele, arachnoid cyst, arteriovenous malformation
(b) extracranial anomalies (63%): spina bifida in 25 – 30% (with spina bifida hydrocephalus is present in 80%), renal agenesis, multicystic dysplastic kidney, VSD, tetralogy of Fallot, anal agenesis, malrotation of bowel, cleft lip / palate, Meckel syndrome, gonadal dysgenesis, arthrogryposis, sirenomelia
(c) chromosomal anomalies (11%): trisomy 18 + 21, mosaicism, balanced translocation
• elevated amniotic alpha-fetoprotein level
OB-US: (assessment difficult prior to 20 weeks GA as ventricles ordinarily constitute a large portion of cranial vault)
√ polyhydramnios (in 30%)
√ lateral width of ventricular atrium ≥10 mm (size usually constant between 16 weeks MA and term)
√ BPD >95th percentile (usually not before third trimester)
Recurrence rate: <4%
Mortality: (1) fetal death in 24%
           (2) neonatal death in 17%
Prognosis: poor with
           (1) associated anomalies
           (2) shift of midline (porencephaly)
           (3) head circumference >50 cm
           (4) absence of cortex (hydranencephaly)
           (5) cortical thickness <10 mm

Infantile Hydrocephalus
• ocular disturbances: paralysis of upward gaze, abducens nerve paresis, nystagmus, ptosis, diminished pupillary light response
• spasticity of lower extremities (from disproportionate stretching of paracentral corticospinal fibers)
Etiology:
1. Communicating hydrocephalus
2. Aqueductal stenosis
3. Chiari II malformation
4. Dandy-Walker malformation

mnemonic: "**A VP-S**hunt **C**an **D**ecompress **T**he **H**ydrocephalic **C**hild"
Aqueductal stenosis
Vein of Galen aneurysm
Postinfectious
Superior vena cava obstruction
Chiari malformation
Dandy-Walker syndrome

Tumor
Hemorrhage
Choroid plexus papilloma

Normal Pressure Hydrocephalus
= NPH = ADAM SYNDROME
= pressure gradient between ventricle + brain parenchyma inspite of normal CSF pressure
Cause: communicating hydrocephalus with incomplete arachnoidal obstruction from neonatal intraventricular hemorrhage, spontaneous subarachnoid hemorrhage, intracranial trauma, infection, surgery
Age: 50 – 70 years
• dementia, gait apraxia, incontinence
    mnemonic: wacky, wobbly and wet
√ communicating hydrocephalus with prominent temporal horns
√ ventricles dilated out of proportion to any sulcal enlargement
√ upward bowing of corpus callosum
√ flattening of cortical gyri against inner table of calvarium (DDx: rounded gyri in generalized atrophy)

NORMAL PRESSURE HYDROCEPHALUS
    mnemonic: "PAM the HAM"
    Paget disease
    Aneurysm
    Meningitis
    Hemorrhage (from trauma)
    Achondroplasia
    Mucopolysaccharidosis

HYGROMA
= CSF-fluid collection within subdural space following tear of leptomeninges after 6 – 30 days following trauma; common in children
Cause: (1) previous subdural hematoma
         (2) tear in arachnoid with secondary ball valve mechanism
√ radiolucent crescentic-shaped collection (as in acute subdural hematoma)
MR:
    √ isointense to CSF / hyperintense to CSF on T1WI (increased protein content)
Prognosis: often spontaneous resorption

HYPOTHALAMIC HAMARTOMA
= HAMARTOMA OF TUBER CINEREUM
= rare congenital malformation composed of normal neuronal tissue
Age: <2 years of age; M>F
Histo: heterotopic collection of neurons, astrocytes, oligodendroglial cells (closely resembling histologic pattern of tuber cinereum)
• isosexual precocious puberty
• gelastic seizures, hyperactivity
• neurodevelopmental delay
Location: mamillary bodies / tuber cinereum of thalamus, rarely within hypothalamus itself

√ well-defined round / oval mass projecting from base of brain into suprasellar / interpeduncular cistern
√ attached to tuber cinereum / mamillary bodies by thin stalk (pedunculated)
CT:
  √ round homogeneous mass isodense with brain tissue
  √ NO enhancement
MR:
  √ well-defined round pedunculated mass suspended from tuber cinereum / mamillary bodies
  √ isointense on T1WI + iso- / slightly hyperintense on T2WI

IDIOPATHIC INTRACRANIAL HYPERTENSION

= PSEUDOTUMOR CEREBRI = BENIGN INTRACRANIAL HYPERTENSION (BIH) secondary to (a) elevation in blood volume (85%) (b) decrease in regional cerebral blood flow with delayed CSF absorption (10%)
Etiology:
1. Sinovenous occlusive disease, SVC occlusion, obstruction of dural sinus, obstruction of both internal jugular veins
2. Dural AVM
3. S/P brain biopsy with edema
4. Endocrinopathies
5. Hypervitaminosis A
6. Hypocalcemia
7. Menstrual dysfunction, pregnancy, menarche, birth control pills
8. Drug therapy

Predilection for   obese young to middle-aged women
• headache
• papilledema
• elevated opening pressures on lumbar puncture
√ normal ventricular size / pinched ventricles
√ increased volume of subarachnoid space

INFARCTION OF BRAIN

= brain cell death
Pathophysiology:
  Distal microstasis occurs within 2 minutes after occlusion of cerebral artery; regional cerebral blood flow is acutely decreased in area of infarction + remains depressed for several days at center of infarct; arterial circulation time may be prolonged in entire hemisphere; rapid development of vasodilatation due to hypoxia, hypercapnia, tissue acidosis; delayed filling + emptying of arterial channels in area of infarction (= arteriolar-capillary block) well into venous phase; by end of 1st week regional blood flow commonly increases to rates even above those required for metabolic needs (= hyperemic phase = luxury perfusion)

Detection rate by CT:
  80% for cortex + mantle, 55% for basal ganglia, 54% for posterior fossa
  Δ positive correlation between degree of clinical deficit and CT sensitivity

CT sensitivity:
    on day of ictus: 48%
    1 – 2 days later: 59%
    7 – 10 days later: 66%
    10 – 11 days later: 74%
Location: cerebrum:cerebellum = 19:1;
  (a) supratentorial
    — cerebral mantle (70%) in territory of MCA (50%), PCA (10%), watershed between MCA + ACA (7%), ACA (4%)
    — basal ganglia + internal capsule (20%),
  (b) infratentorial (10%)
    upper cerebellum (5%), lower cerebellum (3%), pons + medulla (2%)

TIA and RIND
√ hypodense small lesions located peripherally near / within cortex without enhancement
√ lesions detected in only 14%, contralateral lesion present in 14% (CT of marginal value)

Acute Ischemic Infarction
(a) Substage I (ictus – 24 hours)
  NCCT:
    √ initially normal finding within first 24 – 48 hours (secondary to delayed onset of cerebral edema)
    √ focal decrease in attenuation with effacement of sulci (8%)
  CECT:
    √ no iodine accumulation in affected cortical region
  MR: (positive as early as 1 – 6 hours)
    √ contrast-enhanced cortical arterial vessels in area of brain injury (collateral circulation via leptomeningeal anastomoses with slow blood flow)
    √ subtle low signal intensity on T1WI, high signal intensity on T2WI (masking of gyral infarcts on heavily T2WI due to sulcal CSF intensity)
(b) Substage II (24 hours – 7 days)
  NCCT:
    √ hypodense wedge-shaped lesion with base at cortex in a vascular distribution (in 70%) due to vasogenic + cytotoxic edema
    √ mass effect (23 – 75%): sulcal effacement, transtentorial herniation, displaced subarachnoid cisterns + ventricles
  CECT:
    √ gyral enhancement along cortex
  MR:
    √ intravascular enhancement sign (77%) = Gd-pentetate enhancement of vessels supplying infarct after 1 – 3 days
    √ meningeal enhancement sign = Gd-pentetate enhancement of meninges adjacent to infarct after 2 – 6 days
  Angio:
    √ narrowed / occluded vessels supplying the area of infarction

√ delayed filling + emptying of involved vessels
√ early draining vein
√ luxury perfusion of infarcted area (rare) = loss of small vessel autoregulation due to local increase in pH

NUC:
   Δ Newer imaging agents (eg, Tc-99m HM-PAO) may be positive within minutes of the event, while both CT and MRI are normal
   √ hemispheric hypoperfusion throughout all phases
   √ defect corresponding to non-perfused vascular territory
   √ "flip-flop sign" in radionuclide angiogram (15%) = decreased uptake during arterial + capillary phase followed by increased uptake during venous phase
   √ "luxury perfusion syndrome" (14%) = increased perfusion

Subacute Ischemic Infarction
Time period: 7 – 21 days = paradoxical phase with resolution of edema + onset of coagulation necrosis
NCCT:
   √ "fogging phenomenon" = low density area less apparent
   √ decrease of mass effect + ex vacuo dilatation of ventricles (in 57%)
CECT:
   √ gyral blush + ring enhancement (breakdown of blood brain barrier + luxury perfusion) for 2 – 8 weeks (in 65 – 80% within first 4 weeks)
   √ no enhancement in 1/5 of patients
MR:
   √ parenchymal Gd-pentetate enhancement

Chronic Ischemic Infarction
= demyelination + gliosis complete (focal brain atrophy after 8 weeks)
NCCT:
   √ loss of volume + enlargement of subarachnoid space
   √ ipsilateral dilatation of basal cisterns + ventricles
   √ prominent sulci + thinning of gyri in vicinity of infarction
   √ cyst development in vascular distribution
MR:
   √ patchy region with increased intensity on T2WI

Hemorrhagic Infarction
Incidence: 6% of clinically diagnosed brain infarcts
Path: petechial hemorrhages in various degrees of coalescence

√ hyperdensity localized to cortex + adjacent white matter hypodensity appearing within a previously imaged hypodense infarct

INIENCEPHALY
= complex developmental anomaly characterized by (1) exaggerated lordosis (2) rachischisis (3) imperfect formation of skull base at foramen magnum
M:F = 1:4
Associated with other anomalies (in 84%): anencephaly, encephalocele, hydrocephalus, cyclopia, absence of mandible, cleft lip / palate, diaphragmatic hernia, omphalocele, gastroschisis, single umbilical artery, CHD, polycystic kidney disease, arthrogryposis, clubfoot
√ dorsal flexion of head
√ abnormally short + deformed spine
Prognosis: almost uniformly fatal
DDx: (1) Anencephaly (2) Klippel-Feil syndrome
      (3) Cervical myelomeningocele

INTRAVENTRICULAR NEUROCYTOMA
= INTRAVENTRICULAR NEUROBLASTOMA
= benign primary neoplasm of lateral + 3rd ventricles
Incidence: unknown; tumor frequently mistaken for intraventricular oligodendroglioma
Age: young adult
Histo: uniform round cells with central round nucleus + fine chromatine stippling ± perivascular pseudorosettes, focal microcalcifications (closely resembling oligodendroglioma but with neuronal differentiation into synapselike junctions)

Location: body ± frontal horn of lateral ventricle, may extend into 3rd ventricle
√ coarsely calcified entirely intraventricular well-circumscribed tumor
√ mild to moderate contrast enhancement
√ attachment to septum pellucidum CHARACTERISTIC
√ ± hemorrhage into tumor / ventricle
√ hydrocephalus
√ peritumoral edema extremely uncommon
MR:
   √ isointense relative to cortical gray matter on T1WI + T2WI with heterogeneous areas due to calcifications, cystic spaces, vascular flow voids
DDx:
   (1) Intraventricular oligodendroglioma (no hemorrhage)
   (2) Astrocytoma (peritumoral edema in 20%)
   (3) Meningioma (almost exclusively in trigone)
   (4) Ependymoma (in + around 4th ventricle / trigone, in childhood)
   (5) Subependymoma (in + around 4th ventricle, young adults)
   (6) Choroid plexus papilloma (body + temporal horn of lateral ventricle, intense enhancement)
   (7) Colloid cyst (anterior 3rd ventricle / foramen of Monroe, calcifications uncommon)
   (8) Craniopharyngioma (extraventricular origin)
   (9) Teratoma + dermoid cyst (fat attenuation)

JAKOB-CREUTZFELDT DISEASE
= transmissible slow virus infection developing over weeks
• rapidly progressive dementia in middle age

JOUBERT SYNDROME
- episodic hyperpnea
- abnormal eye movement
- ataxia, mental retardation

Path:
- (1) nearly total aplasia of cerebellar vermis
- (2) dysplasia + heterotopia of cerebellar nuclei
- (3) near total absence of pyramidal decussation
- (4) anomalies in structure of inferior olivary nuclei, descending trigeminal tract, solitary fascicle, dorsal column nuclei

√ 4th ventricle triangular-shaped at mid-level + bat-wing-shaped superiorly
√ cerebellar hemispheres appose one another in midline
√ superior cerebellar peduncles surrounded by CSF

LIPOMA
= congenital tumor developing within subarachnoid space as a result of abnormal differentiation of the meninx primitiva (which differentiates into pia mater, arachnoid, inner meningeal layer of dura mater)

Incidence: <1% of brain tumors
Age: presentation in childhood / adulthood
Associated with congenital anomalies
- (a) in anterior location: various degrees of agenesis of corpus callosum (in 50 – 80%)
- (b) in posterior location (in <33%)
- asymptomatic in 50%

Location:
quadrigeminal region, midline lesion at genu of corpus callosum (25 – 50%), tuber cinereum, chiasmatic / interpeduncular / sylvian / CP angle / cerebellomedullary cistern
CT:
√ well-circumscribed mass with CT density of -100 HU
√ occasionally calcified rim (esp. in corpus callosum)
√ no enhancement
MR:
√ hyperintense mass on T1WI + less hyperintense on T2WI (CHARACTERISTIC)

Lipoma of Corpus Callosum
= congenital pericallosal tumor not actually involving the corpus callosum as a result of faulty disjunction of neuroectoderm from cutaneous ectoderm during process of neurulation
Incidence: approx. 30% of intracranial lipomas
Associated with:
- (1) anomalies of corpus callosum (almost always)
- (2) frontal bone defect (frequent) = encephalocele
- (3) cutaneous frontal lipoma
- in 50% symptomatic:
  - seizure disorders, mental retardation, dementia
  - emotional lability, headaches
  - hemiplegia

Plain film:
√ midline calcification with associated lucency of fat density

CT:
√ area of marked hypodensity immediately superior to lateral ventricles with possible extension inferiorly between ventricles / anteriorly into interhemispheric fissure
√ curvilinear peripheral / nodular central calcification within fibrous capsule (frequent)
MR:
√ hyperintense midline mass superior + posterior to corpus callosum on T1WI
√ no callosal fibers dorsal to lipoma
√ branches of pericallosal artery frequently course through lipoma
DDx: dermoid (denser, extraaxial), teratoma

LISSENCEPHALY
= "smooth brain" = AGYRIA-PACHYGYRIA COMPLEX
= most severe of neuronal migration anomalies; autosomal recessive disease with abnormal cortical stratification

agyria = absence of gyri on brain surface
pachygyria = focal / diffuse area of few broad flat gyri

A. COMPLETE LISSENCEPHALY = AGYRIA
most frequently parieto-occipital in location
B. INCOMPLETE LISSENCEPHALY
= areas of both agyria + pachygyria, pachygyric areas most frequently in frontal + temporal regions
Histo: thick gray + thin white matter with only four cortical layers I, III, V, VI (instead of six layers)

Often associated with
- (1) CNS anomalies: microcephaly, hydrocephalus, agenesis of corpus callosum, hypoplastic thalami
- (2) micromelia, clubfoot, polydactyly, camptodactyly, syndactyly, duodenal atresia, micrognathia, omphalocele, hepatosplenomegaly, cardiac + renal anomalies
- micrencephaly
- severe mental retardation
- hypotonia + occasional myoclonic spasm
- early seizures refractory to medication

√ smooth thickened cortex with diminished white matter
√ figure-eight appearance of cerebrum on axial images due to shallow widened vertically oriented sylvian fissures
√ absent sulci and gyri (brain looks similar to that in fetuses <23 weeks GA)
√ middle cerebral arteries close to inner table of calvarium (absence of sulci to course within)
√ small splenium + absent rostrum of corpus callosum
√ hypoplastic brainstem (lack of formation of corticospinal + corticobulbar tracts)
√ ventriculomegaly (atrium + occipital horns)
√ midline round calcification in area of septum pellucidum (CHARACTERISTIC)
√ polyhydramnios (50%)
Prognosis: death by age 2

DDx: Polymicrogyria (= formation of multiple small gyri mimicking pachgyria on CT + MR, broad thickened gyri with frequent gliosis subjacent to polymicrogyric cortex as the most important differentiating feature)

LYMPHOID HYPOPHYSITIS
= autoimmune disorder with lymphocytic infiltration of pituitary gland
Associated with: thyrotoxicosis + hypopituitarism
Age: predilection for postpartum women
√ enlarged homogeneously enhancing pituitary gland; spontaneous regression

LYMPHOMA
A.   PRIMARY LYMPHOMA = RETICULUM CELL SARCOMA = HISTIOCYTIC LYMPHOMA = MICROGLIOMA
Increased incidence in immunosuppressed patients (transplant, AIDS)
B.   SECONDARY = SYSTEMIC LYMPHOMA

Δ Primary lymphoma more common than secondary!
Δ Primary lymphoma indistinguishable from secondary!

Clues: (1) multicentric involvement of deep hemispheres
         (2) association with immunosuppression
         (3) steroid response
Incidence: 0.8 – 2% of all intracranial tumors; M>F
Peak age: 40 – 60 years
Location:
   paramedian structures preferentially affected; basal ganglia (50%), leptomeninges (30%), posterior fossa / brainstem (10 – 20%), thalamus, corpus callosum, periventricular white matter, vermis cerebelli, parenchymal mass (<5%); multicentricity not uncommon
Spread:
   typically infiltrating; may cross anatomic boundaries + midline, diffuse leptomeningeal spread; subependymal spread + ventricular encasement

√ commonly large discrete solitary lesion (57%)
   Δ large lesion suggests lymphoma!
√ small + symmetric multiple nodular lesions (43 - 81%)
√ diffusely infiltrating lesion with blurred margins
√ usually mildly hyperdense (33%) / occasionally isodense / low-density area (least common)
√ little mass effect with significant peritumoral edema
√ homogeneously dense + well-defined / irregular + patchy periventricular contrast enhancement
√ commonly thick-walled ring enhancement
√ spontaneous regression (unique feature)
MR:
   √ isointense / slightly hypointense on T1WI
   √ slightly hyperintense / occasionally isointense or slightly hypointense on T2WI
   √ homogeneous Gd-DTPA enhancement if perivascular infiltration present
Angio:
   √ avascular

DDx: (1) Glioma (may be bilateral with involvement of basal ganglia + corpus callosum, may show dense homogeneous enhancement with vascularity)
       (2) Meningioma
       (3) Metastases (known primary, at gray-white matter junction)
       (4) Abscess
       (5) Progressive multifocal leukencephalopathy
       (6) Multiple sclerosis
       (7) Subacute infarction
       (8) Toxoplasmosis (often multiple lesions)

SPINAL EPIDURAL LYMPHOMA
   (a)   invasion of epidural space through intervertebral foramen from paravertebral lymph nodes
   (b)   destruction of bone with vertebral collapse (less common)
   (c)   direct involvement of CNS (rare)

LEUKEMIA
   CNS affected in 10% of patients with acute leukemia
   √ enlargement of ventricles + sulci due to atrophy (31%)
   √ sulcal / fissural / cisternal enhancement (meningeal infiltration) in 5%
Prognosis: 3 – 5 months survival if untreated

MEDULLOBLASTOMA
most malignant infratentorial neoplasm; most common neoplasm of posterior fossa in childhood (followed by cerebellar astrocytoma)
Incidence:
   15 – 20% of all pediatric intracranial tumors; 30 – 40% of all posterior fossa neoplasms in children; 2 – 10% of all intracranial gliomas
Origin: from external granular layer of inferior medullary velum (= roof of 4th ventricle)
Histo: completely undifferentiated cells (50%), desmoplastic variety (25%), glial / neuronal differentiation (25%)
Age: 40% within first 5 years of life; 75% in first decade; between ages 5 – 14 (2/3); between ages 15 – 35 (1/3); M:F = 2 – 4:1
• duration of symptoms <1 month prior to diagnosis: nausea, vomiting, headaches, increasing head size, ataxia
Site: (a)   vermis cerebelli + roof of 4th ventricle (younger age group) in 91%
        (b)   cerebellar hemisphere (older age group)
Size: usually >2 cm in diameter
√ well-defined vermian mass with widening of space between cerebellar tonsils
√ encroachment on 4th ventricle / aqueduct with hydrocephalus (85 – 95%)
√ shift / invagination of 4th ventricle
√ rapid growth with extension into cerebellar hemisphere / brainstem (more often in adults)
√ extension into cisterna magna + upper cervical cord, occasionally through foramina of Luschka into cerebellopontine angle cistern

√ mild / moderate surrounding edema (90%)
CT:
  Classic features in 53%:
    √ slightly hyperdense (70%) / isodense (20%) / mixed (10%) lesion
    √ rapid intense homogeneous enhancement (97%) due to usually solid tumor
  Atypical features:
    √ cystic / necrotic areas (10 – 16%) with lack of enhancement
    √ calcifications in 13%
    √ hemorrhage in 3%
    √ supratentorial extension
MR:
  √ mixed / hypointense on T1WI
  √ hypo- / iso- / hyperintense on T2WI
  √ usually homogeneous Gd-DTPA enhancement with hypointense rim
  √ cerebellar folia blurred

Cx: (1) Subarachnoid metastatic spread (30 – 100%) via CSF pathway to spinal cord + cauda equina ("drop metastases" in 40%), cerebral convexities, sylvian fissure, suprasellar cistern, retrograde into lateral + 3rd ventricle
        √ continuous "frosting" of tumor on pia
      (2) Metastases outside CNS (axial skeleton, lymph nodes, lung) after surgery
Rx: surgery + radiation therapy (extremely radiosensitive)
DDx of midline medulloblastoma:
  ependymoma, astrocytoma (hypodense)
DDx of eccentric medulloblastoma:
  astrocytoma, meningioma, acoustic neuroma

MENINGIOMA
Incidence:
  most common extraaxial tumor; 15 – 18% of intracranial tumors in adults; 1 – 2% of primary brain tumors in children; 33% of all incidental intracranial neoplasms
Origin: derived from meningothelial cells concentrated in arachnoid villi which penetrate the dura (sagittal sinus, exit of cranial nerves, choroid plexus)
Histologic classification:
  (a) meningothelial = syncytial type composed of large cells thought to be of arachnoidal origin (= arachnoid "cap" cells)
  (b) fibroblastic type interlacing strands of fibrous tissue composed of collagen + reticulin fibers
  (c) transitional type features of meningothelial + fibroblastic forms
  (d) angioblastic / malignant type probably hemangiopericytoma / hemangioblastoma arising from vascular pericytes
Age: peak incidence 45 years (range 35 – 70 years); rare <20 years (in children >50% malignant, M>F); M:F = 1:2
Associated with: neurofibromatosis (multiple, occurrence in childhood)

TYPES:
  (a) Globular meningioma (most common): compact rounded mass with invagination of brain; flat at base; contact to falx / tentorium / basal dura / convexity dura
  (b) Meningioma en plaque: pronounced hyperostosis of adjacent bone particularly along base of skull; difficult to distinguish hyperostosis from tumor cloaking the inner table (DDx: Paget disease, chronic osteomyelitis, fibrous dysplasia, metastasis)
  (c) Multicentric meningioma (2 – 9%) 16% in autopsy series; tendency to localize to a single hemicranium; present clinically at earlier age; global / mixed; CSF seeding is exceptional; in 50% associated with neurofibromatosis type 2
Location:
  (a) convexity = lateral hemisphere (20 – 34%)
  (b) parasagittal = medial hemisphere (18 – 22%)
    — falcine meningioma (5%) below superior sagittal sinus, usually extending to both sides
  (c) sphenoid ridge + middle cranial fossa (17 – 25%)
  (d) frontobasal (10%)
  (e) posterior fossa (9 – 15%)
    — cerebellar convexity (5%)
    — tentorium cerebelli (2 – 4%)
    — cerebellopontine angle (2 – 4%)
    — clivus (<1%)
  (f) spine (12%)
Atypical location:
  (a) cerebellopontine angle (<5%)
  (b) optic nerve sheath (<2%)
  (c) intraventricular (2 – 5%): 80% in lateral, 15% in 3rd, 5% in 4th ventricle; from infolding of meningeal tissue during formation of choroid plexus
    Δ most common trigonal intraventricular mass in adult!
  (d) ectopic = extradural (<1%): intradiploic space, outer table of skull, scalp, paranasal sinus, parotid gland, parapharyngeal space, mediastinum, lung, adrenal gland
Plain film:
  √ hyperostosis at site close to / within bone (exostosis, enostosis, sclerosis)
  √ blistering at paranasal sinuses (ethmoid, sphenoid) ± sclerosis (= pneumosinus dilatans)
  √ enlarged meningeal grooves (if location in vault), enlarged foramen spinosum
  √ calcification (= psammoma bodies)
CT:
  √ well-defined mass with smooth sharp margins
  √ abutting meningeal surface
  √ "cortical buckling" of underlying brain
  √ isodense / hyperdense lesion (psammomatous calcifications) on NECT
  √ calcifications in circular / radial pattern (20%) (DDx: osteoma)
  √ "intraosseous meningioma" = permeation of bone with intra- and extracerebral soft tissue component (DDx: fibrous dysplasia)

√ hyperostosis of adjacent bone (18%)
√ intense uniform enhancement on CECT (absence of blood-brain barrier)
√ minimal peritumoral edema (in up to 75%): NO correlation between tumor size + amount of edema (DDx: intraaxial lesion)
√ cystic component: major in 2%, minor in 15%
MR (100% detection rate with gadolinium DTPA):
√ hypo- to isointense on T1WI + iso- to hyperintense on T2WI (intensity depends on amount of cellularity versus collagen elements)
√ homogeneous / heterogeneous texture (tumor vascularity, cystic changes, calcifications)
√ arcuate bowing of white matter + cortical effacement
√ tumor-brain interface of low intensity vessels + high intensity cerebrospinal cleft on T2WI
√ contrast enhancement for 3 – 60 minutes on T1WI
√ linear "tail" extending from tumor mass along dural surface on Gd-DTPA enhanced scans in 60% (= meningothelial tumor nodules)
Angio:
√ "mother-in-law" phenomenon (contrast material shows up early and stays late into venous phase)
√ "sunburst" / "spoke-wheel" pattern of tumor vascularity with hypervascular cloudlike stain
√ early draining vein (rare: perhaps in angioblastic meningioma)
√ en plaque meningioma is poorly vascularized
Vascular supply:
1. vault: middle meningeal artery
2. sphenoid plane + tuberculum: recurrent meningeal branch of ophthalmic a.
3. tentorium: meningeal branch of meningohypophyseal trunk of ICA
4. intraventricular: choroidal vessels
5. clivus + posterior fossa: vertebral artery / ascending pharyngeal artery
6. falx: partly middle meningeal artery + others

Cx: local invasion of venous sinuses

ATYPICAL MENINGIOMA (15%)
1. Low attenuation area of necrosis, old hemorrhage, cyst formation, fat (DDx: malignant glioma, metastasis)
   (a) **Cystic meningioma** (14%)
       intratumoral central / eccentric cyst (necrosis, cystic degeneration), extratumoral cyst (reactive arachnoid cyst) (DDx: cystic / necrotic glioma)
   (b) **Lipoblastic meningioma** (5%)
       metaplastic change of meningothelial cells into adipocytes
2. Heterogeneous / ring enhancement (secondary to bland tumor infarction / necrosis in aggressive histologic variants / true cyst formation from benign fluid accumulation)
3. "En plaque" morphology
4. "Comma shape" = combination of semilunar component bounded by dural interface + spherical component growing beyond dural margin

5. Sarcomatous transformation with spread over hemisphere + invasion of cerebral parenchyma (leptomeningeal supply)
6. **Meningeal hemangiopericytoma**
   √ multilobulated contour
   √ narrow dural base / "mushroom" shape
   √ large intratumoral vascular signals
   √ bone erosion
   √ prominent peritumoral edema
   √ mutliple irregular feeding vessels on angiogram

Sphenoid Wing Meningioma
1. Hyperostotic meningioma en plaque
   • slowly progressive unilateral painless exophthalmos
   • numbness in distribution of cranial nerve V_1 + V_2
   • headaches, seizures
2. Meningioma arising from middle third of sphenoid ridge
   • headaches, seizures
   √ compression of regional frontal + temporal lobes
3. Meningioma arising from clinoid process
   √ encasement of carotid + middle cerebral arteries
   √ compression of optic nerve + chiasm
4. Meningioma of planum sphenoidale
   √ subfrontal growth + posterior growth into sella turcica and clivus
   √ hyperostotic blistering of planum sphenoidale

Suprasellar Meningioma
Origin: from arachnoid + dura along tuberculum sellae / diaphragma sellae; NOT from within pituitary fossa
• hypothalamic / pituitary dysfunction (rare)
√ irregular hyperostosis = blistering adjacent to sinus (HALLMARK of meningiomas at planum sphenoidale / tuberculum sellae)
√ pneumatosis sphenoidale = increased pneumatization of sphenoid in area of anterior clinoids + dorsum sellae (DDx: normal variant)
√ broad base of attachment
√ intense homogeneous enhancement (may be impossible to differentiate from supraclinoid carotid aneurysm on CT)
√ blood supply: posterior ethmoidal branches of ophthalmic artery, branches of meningohypophyseal trunk
DDx: metastasis, glioma, lymphoma

MENINGTIS
1. Pachymeningitis: affecting dura mater
2. Leptomeningitis: affecting pia mater / arachnoid (most common)
• headaches, stiff neck
• confusion, disorientation
• positive CSF lab analysis
ROLE of CT and MR:
(1) to exclude parenchymal abscess, ventriculitis, localized empyema
(2) to evaluate paranasal sinuses / temporal bone as source of infection

(3) to monitor complications: hydrocephalus, subdural effusion, infarction

Purulent Meningitis
Cause: otitis media / sinusitis
Organism:
  (a) adults: Meningococcus, Streptococcus pneumoniae, Staphylococcus aureus, beta-hemolytic Streptococcus
  (b) children: Haemophilus influenzae, Escherichia coli, Neisseria meningitidis
NECT:
  √ often normal
  √ increased density in subarachnoid space (increased vascularity), esp. in children
  √ small ventricles secondary to diffuse cerebral edema
CECT:
  √ marked curvilinear meningeal enhancement over cerebrum (frontal + parietal lobes) and interhemispheric + sylvian fissures
  √ obliteration of basal cisterns with enhancement (common)
MR (most sensitive modality):
  √ hyperintense plaques on T2WI
  √ enhancement with Gd-DTPA
Cx:
  (1) Cerebritis
  (2) Ventriculitis = ependymitis (secondary to retrograde spread)
  (3) Brain atrophy
  (4) Brain infarction (arteritis, venous thrombosis)
  (5) Subdural effusion [sterile subdural effusion secondary to H. influenzae meningitis (in children) may turn into empyema]
  (6) Hydrocephalus (cellular debris blocking foramen of Monro, aqueduct, 4th ventricular outlet / intraventricular septa / arachnoid adhesions)
  (7) Cranial nerve dysfunction
Prognosis:
  Δ Cerebral infarction + edema are predictive of poor outcome
  Δ Enlargement of ventricles + subarachnoid spaces + subdural effusions have no predictive value
Mortality: 10% (5th common cause of death in children between 1 and 4 years of age)
DDx: meningeal carcinomatosis

Granulomatous Meningitis
Histo: thick exudate, perivascular inflammation, granulation tissue + reactive fibrosis
(1) Tuberculous meningitis = basilar meningitis: part of generalized miliary tuberculosis / primary tuberculous infection; in infants + small children
(2) Sarcoidosis
  may be associated with single / multiple intracerebral masses
(3) Fungal meningitis: cryptococcosis, candidiasis, coccidioidomycosis (endemic), blastomycosis, mucormycosis (diabetics), nocardiosis, actinomycosis, aspergillosis (under chronic corticosteroid therapy)

• acute life-threatening process / chronic indolent disease
May be associated with cerebritis, abscess formation

√ hydrocephalus
CT:
  √ obliteration of basal cisterns, sylvian fissure, suprasellar cistern (isodense cisterns secondary to filling with debris)
  √ intense contrast enhancement of gyri + involved subarachnoid spaces
  √ calcification of meninges
  √ decreased attenuation of white matter
MR:
  √ high signal intensity of basilar cisterns on T2WI
  √ enhancement with gadopentetate dimeglumine

Cx: (1) hydrocephalus (obliteration of basal cisterns; blocking of CSF flow + CSF absorption)
     (2) infarction (due to arteritis)

METACHROMATIC LEUKODYSTROPHY
= MLD = most common hereditary (autosomal recessive) leukodystrophy
Cause: deficiency of arylsulfatase A resulting in severe deficiency of myelin lipid sulfatide within macrophages + Schwann cells
Age of presentation: before age 3 (2/3), in adolescence (1/3)

A. LATE INFANTILE FORM
  Age: 2nd year of life
  • gait disorder + strabismus
  • impairment of speech
  • spasticity
  • intellectual deterioration
  Prognosis: death within 4 years of onset
B. JUVENILE FORM
  Age: 5 – 7 years
C. ADULT FORM
  • organic mental syndrome
  • progressive corticospinal, corticobulbar, cerebellar, extrapyramidal signs

√ progressive loss of hemispheric brain tissue
CT:
  √ symmetric low density of white matter adjacent to ventricles (esp. centrum ovale and frontal horns)
  √ progressive atrophy
  √ no contrast enhancement
MR:
  √ progressive symmetrical areas of hypointensity on T1WI
  √ hyperintensity on T2WI (increased water)
Prognosis: death within several years

METASTASES TO BRAIN
Incidence: 14 – 37% of all intracranial tumors

Metastatic primary:
Six tumors account for 95% of all brain metastases:
1. Bronchial carcinoma (47%): RARELY squamous cell carcinoma
2. Breast carcinoma (17%)
3. GI-tract tumors (15%): colon, rectum
4. Hypernephroma (10%)
5. Melanoma (8%)
6. Choriocarcinoma

In childhood:
1. Leukemia / lymphoma
2. Neuroblastoma

Δ Brain metastases from sarcomas are exceptionally rare!
Location: (a) corticomedullary junction of brain (most characteristic)
(b) subarachnoid space = carcinomatous meningitis (15%)
(c) subependymal spread (frequent in breast carcinoma)
(d) skull (5%)

HEMORRHAGIC METASTASES (in 3 – 4%):
1. Malignant melanoma
2. Choriocarcinoma
3. Oat cell carcinoma of lung
4. Renal cell carcinoma
5. Thyroid carcinoma

CYSTIC METASTASES:
1. Squamous cell carcinoma of lung
2. Adenocarcinoma of lung

CALCIFIED METASTASES:
1. Mucin-producing neoplasm
2. Cartilage- / bone-forming sarcoma
3. Effective radiochemotherapy

Presentation:
— multiple lesions (2/3), single lesion (1/3)
— cerebral hemispheres (57%), cerebellum (29%), brainstem (32%)
— nodular deposits to dura are common
√ multiple lesions of different sizes + locations
√ surrounding edema usually exceeds tumor volume
CT:
√ solid enhancement in small tumors / ring-like enhancement in large tumors
MR: A combination of T2WI + contrast-enhanced T1WI offer greatest sensitivity
√ hypointense mass relative to edema on T2WI
√ hypointensity more pronounced in melanoma + mucinous adenocarcinoma (paramagnetic effect)
√ homogeneous / ring / nodular mixed enhancement after Gd-DTPA; often more than one metastatic focus identified in region of colliding edema
√ asymmetric enhancement of dura with dural spread
√ leptomeningeal enhancement (eg, in metastatic ependymoma)

MICROCEPHALY
= clinical syndrome characterized by a head circumference below the normal range

Incidence: 1.6:1,000 or 1:6,200 – 1:8,500 births
Etiology:
(1) Undiagnosed intrauterine infection (toxoplasmosis, rubella, CMV, herpes, syphilis), toxic agents, hypoxia, radiation
(2) Premature craniosynostosis
(3) Chromosomal abnormalities (trisomies)
(4) Meckel-Gruber syndrome
Often associated with:
microencephaly, macrogyria, pachygyria, atrophy of basal ganglia, decrease in dendritic arborization
√ AC:HC discrepancy
√ head circumference <3 S.D. below the mean
√ ape-like sloping of forehead
√ dilatation of lateral ventricles
√ poor growth of fetal cranium
√ intracranial contents may not be visible (rare)
Prognosis: normal to severe mental retardation (depending on degree of microcephaly)

MINERALIZING MICROANGIOPATHY
= RADIATION-INDUCED LEUKOENCEPHALOPATHY
= sequelae of radiotherapy combined with methotrexate therapy for leukemia
• 85% without neurologic deficits
CT:
√ thin reticular / serrated linear calcifications near corticomedullary junction, especially in frontal + posterior parietal lobes and in basal ganglia
√ symmetric low attenuation process in white matter near corticomedullary area
MR:
√ confluent diffuse periventricular distribution spreading peripherally with an irregular scalloped edge

MOYAMOYA DISEASE
= progressive obstructive / occlusive cerebral arteritis affecting distal ICA at bifurcation into its branches (anterior 2/3 of circle of Willis), usually involving both hemispheres
Etiology: unknown
Age: predominantly in children + young adults
• headaches
• behavorial disturbances
• recurrent hemiparetic attacks
√ stenosis of distal internal carotid + proximal middle + anterior cerebral arteries
√ large network of vessels in basal ganglia ("puff of smoke") + upper brainstem fed by basilar artery, anterior + middle cerebral arteries (dilatation of lenticulostriate + anterior choroidal arteries)
√ anastomoses between dural meningeal + leptomeningeal arteries
Cx: subarachnoid hemorrhage (occasionally)

MULTIPLE SCLEROSIS
= most frequent form of chronic inflammatory demyelinating disease of unknown etiology, which reduces the lipid content and brain volume; characterized by a relapsing + remitting course

Histo: myelin degeneration at junctions of pial veins resulting in scar (= plaque)

Age: young adults; M:F = 1:1

- headaches, dizziness, nausea, recurrent sensory changes
- Schumacher criteria:
  (1) CNS dysfunction (2) involvement of two / more parts of CNS (3) predominant white matter involvement (4) two / more episodes lasting >24 hours less than 1 month apart (5) slow stepwise progression of signs + symptoms (6) at onset 10 – 50 years of age
- Rudick red flags (suggests diagnosis other than MS):
  (1) no eye findings (2) no clinical remission (3) totally local disease (4) no sensory findings (5) no bladder involvement (6) no CSF abnormality

@ Brain
  Location:
  subependymal periventricular location (along lateral aspects of atria + occipital horns), corpus callosum, internal capsule, centrum semiovale, corona radiata, optic nerves, chiasm, optic tract, brainstem (ventrolateral aspect of pons at 5th nerve root entry), cerebellar peduncles, cerebellum; rather symmetric involvement of cerebral hemispheres
  CT:
  √ normal CT scan (18%)
  √ nonspecific atrophy of brain (45%): enlarged ventricles, prominent sulci
  √ periventricular (near atria) multifocal nonconfluent lesions with distinct margins + without mass effect on ventricles (location not always correlating well with symptoms)
    (a) NECT: isodense / lucent
    (b) CECT: transient enhancement during acute stage (active demyelination) for about 2 weeks; may require double dose of contrast; ultimately disappearance / permanent scar
  MR (modality of choice):
    (a) for optic nerve lesions: short T1 inversion recovery pulse sequence
    (b) for cortical lesions: long TR pulse sequences
    √ well-marginated discrete foci of varying size with high signal intensity on T2WI + proton density images (= loss of hydrophobic myelin produces increase in water content); hypointense on T1WI
    √ Gd-DTPA enhancement of lesions on T1WI (up to 8 weeks following acute demyelination)

@ Spine
  most common demyelinating process of spinal cord
  Location: predilection for cervical region
  Site: eccentric involvement of dorsal + lateral elements abutting subarachnoid space
  √ acute tumefactive MS = cord swelling + enhancement
    DDx: (1) cord tumor (follow-up after 6 weeks without decrease in size of lesion)
            (2) transverse myelitis

NEONATAL INTRACRANIAL HEMORRHAGE
Germinal Matrix Bleed
= GERMINAL MATRIX RELATED HEMORRHAGE
Germinal matrix
  = highly vascular subependymal tissue adjacent to lateral ventricles in which the cells that compose the brain are generated; has its largest volume around 26 weeks GA; decreases in size with increasing fetal maturity; usually involutes by 32 – 34 weeks of gestation

Cause: (1) prematurity (2) hypoxia (3) birth trauma (4) coagulopathy

Pathogenesis: friable vascular bed ruptures under hypertension, hypoxia, acidosis

Incidence: in premature neonates <32 weeks of age; in 43% of infants <1,500 gms; up to 50% without prenatal care, in 5 – 10% with prenatal care

Location:
  subependymal; region of the caudate nucleus and caudothalamic notch / groove remains metabolically active the longest (most frequently involved); parenchymal damage manifests as periventricular leukomalacia in more premature infants

GRADES
  I : subependymal hemorrhage confined to germinal matrix
  II : subependymal / choroid plexus hemorrhage ruptured into nondilated ventricle
  III : intraventricular hemorrhage with ventricular enlargement
  IV : massive intraventricular + intraparenchymal hemorrhage with ventricular dilatation

Time of onset: within first 3 days of life (86%); within first week of life (91%)

Optimum for screening: 7 – 14 days of life

US (100% sensitivity + 91% specificity for lesions >5 mm; 27% sensitivity + 88% specificity for lesions ≤5 mm):
  √ region of increased echogenicity inferior to floor of frontal horn + anterior to foramen of Monro (= caudothalamic notch bleed)
  √ highly echogenic mass, commonly lateral to frontal horns / in parietal lobe, rare in occipital lobe + thalamus
  √ echogenic material in ventricles (acute phase) becoming sonolucent in a few weeks (= intraventricular hemorrhage)
  √ irregular bulky choroid plexus
  √ echogenic ventricular surfaces
  √ ventricular dilatation
    (a) temporary blockage of arachnoid villi by hemorrhagic particulate matter; often resolves
    (b) obliterative arachnoiditis in cisterna magna from severe hemorrhage with permanent progressive hydrocephalus

Cx:
  (1) Cavitation of hemorrhage
  (2) Unilocular subependymal cyst
  (3) Unilocular porencephalic cyst

(4) Ventriculomegaly (scarring of pacchionian granulations, septation of ventricles)
(5) Mental retardation, cerebral palsy
(6) Death in 25% (IVH most common cause of neonatal death)
Prognosis:
(1) Grade I + II: good with normal developmental scores (12 – 18% risk of handicap)
(2) Grade III + IV: 54% mortality; motor disabilities, cognitive defects

Intraventricular Hemorrhage
Etiology: (a) germinal matrix hemorrhage (b) bleeding from choroid plexus
• seizures, dystonia, obtundation, intractable acidosis
• bulging anterior fontanelle, drop in hematocrit, bloody / proteinaceous CSF
√ IVH usually cleared within 7 – 14 days

Periventricular Leukoencephalopathy
Periventricular Leukomalacia
= PVL = focal necrosis of deep white matter as a result of ischemic infarction involving the watershed zones between central and peripheral vascularity; nonhemorrhagic (more often) / hemorrhagic
Incidence:
5% of premature infants; 7 – 22% at autopsy (85% of infants between 900 and 2,200 g surviving beyond 6 days); in 34% of infants <1500 g; in 59% of infants surviving longer than 1 week on assisted ventilation; only 28% detected by cranial sonography
Histo: edema, white matter necrosis, evolution of cysts / diminished myelin
Pathogenesis:
immature autoregulation of periventricular vessels secondary to deficient muscularis of arterioles limits vasodilation in response to hypoxemia + hypercapnia + hypotension of perinatal asphyxia

• spastic diplegia / quadriparesis (affecting descending fibers from motor cortex)
• mental retardation
• severe hearing / visual impairments
• convulsive disorders
Location:
bilateral paralleling both lateral ventricles, dorsal + lateral to external angle of lateral ventricular trigones, frontal cerebral white matter near foramen of Monro
MR:
√ hyperintense periventricular signals on T2WI in peritrigonal region
√ thinning of posterior body + splenium of corpus callosum (= degeneration of transcallosal fibers)
US (50% sensitivity + 87% specificity):
√ increased periventricular echogenicity (PVE) (appearing 2 days – 2 weeks after insult)
√ bilateral often asymmetric zones, occasionally extending to cortex
√ infrequently accompanied by IVH

Late changes:
√ periventricular cystic PVL = cystic degeneration of ischemic areas (= multiple small never septated periventricular cysts in relationship to lateral ventricles appear 2 – 3 weeks after development of echodensities + disappear after 1 – 3 months)
√ brain atrophy secondary to thinning of periventricular white matter always at trigones, occasionally involving centra semiovale
√ ventriculomegaly (after disappearance of cysts) with irregular outline of body + trigone of lateral ventricles
√ deep prominent sulci abutting the ventricles with little / no interposed white matter (DDx: schizencephaly)
√ enlarged interhemispheric fissure

Prognosis: very poor
DDx: tissue damage from ventriculitis (sequelae of meningitis), metabolic disorders, in utero ischemia (eg, maternal cocaine abuse)

Periventricular Hemorrhagic Infarction
= hemorrhagic necrosis of periventricular white matter, usually large + asymmetric
Associated with   IVH in 80%
Incidence: 15% of infants with IVH have periventricular hemorrhagic infarction
Pathogenesis:
intraventricular / germinal matrix blood clot leads to obstruction of terminal veins
Histo: perivascular hemorrhage of medullary veins near ventricular angle
Age: peak occurrence at 4th postnatal day

• spastic hemiparesis (affects lower + upper extremities equally)
Location: dorsal + lateral to external angle of lateral ventricle; 67% unilateral; 33% bilateral but asymmetric

√ unilateral / asymmetric bilateral triangular "fan-shaped" echodensities
√ extension from frontal to parietooccipital regions / localized
Late changes:
√ single large cyst = porencephaly
√ bumpy ventricle / false accessory ventricle
Prognosis:
59% overall mortality with echodensities >1 cm

Encephalomalacia
= more extensive brain damage than PVL; may include all of white matter in subcortex + cortex
Associated with:
(1) Neonatal asphyxia
(2) Vasospasm
(3) Inflammation of CNS
√ cysts often not communicating

NEUROBLASTOMA

Age at presentation: <2 years (50%); <4 years (75%);
 <8 years (90%); peak age <3 years
- abdominal mass (45%)
- neurologic signs (20%)
- bone pain / limp (20%)
- orbital ecchymosis / proptosis (12%)
- catecholamine production (95%) with paroxysmal
 episodes of flushing, tachycardia, hypertension,
 headaches, sweating, intractable diarrhea, acute
 cerebellar encephalopathy
- positive bone marrow aspiration (70%)

Location: adrenal gland (67%), chest (13%), neck
 (5%), intracranial (2%); commonly involvement
 of multiple skeletal sites
NUC (overall sensitivity of detection better than
 radiography):
 CAVE: symmetric lytic neuroblastoma metastases
 occur frequently in metaphyseal areas where
 normal epiphyseal activity obscures lesions
 √ purely lytic lesions may present as photopenic areas
 √ soft tissue uptake of Tc-99m phosphate in 60%
 √ frequently GA-67 uptake in primary site of
 neuroblastoma
Prognosis: 2-year survival (a) in 60% for age <1 year
 (b) in 20% for ages 1 – 2 years (c) in 10% for
 ages >2 years

A.   PRIMARY CEREBRAL NEUROBLASTOMA (rare)
 Age: childhood / early adolescence
 √ large hypodense / mixed-density mass with well-
 defined margins
 √ intratumoral coarse dense calcifications
 √ central cystic / necrotic zones with hemorrhage
 Cx: metastasizes via subarachnoid space to dura +
 calvarium
B.   SECONDARY NEUROBLASTOMA (common)
 metastatic to:
 @ liver
 @ skeleton
 √ osteolysis with periosteal new bone formation
 √ sutural diastasis
 √ hair-on-end appearance of skull
 @ orbit: √ unilateral proptosis
 Δ Neuroblastoma usually not metastatic to brain!

Olfactory Neuroblastoma
 = very malignant tumor arising from olfactory mucosa
 Types:
 1. Esthesioneuroepithelioma
 2. Esthesioneurocytoma
 3. Esthesioneuroblastoma
 √ mass in superior nasal cavity with extension into
 ethmoid + maxillary sinuses
 Cx: distant metastases in 20%

NEUROFIBROMATOSIS
Peripheral Neurofibromatosis   (90%)
 = VON RECKLINGHAUSEN DISEASE
 = NEUROFIBROMATOSIS 1

= dysplasia of mesodermal + neuroectodermal tissue with
 potential for diffuse systemic involvement; autosomal
 dominant with abnormalities of long arm of chromosome
 17; 50% spontaneous mutants; variable expressivity
Incidence: 1:3,000;   M:F = 1:1;   most common of
 phakomatoses
Diagnostic criteria (at least two must be present):
 (1) >6 café-a-lait spots >5 mm in greatest diameter
 (>15 mm in postpubertal individuals)
 (2) ≥2 neurofibromas of any type / one plexiform
 neurofibroma
 (3) freckling in axilla / inguinal region
 (4) optic glioma
 (5) ≥2 Lisch nodules (= pigmented hamartomas of iris)
 (6) distinctive osseous lesion (eg, sphenoid dysplasia /
 thinning of long bone cortex)
 (7) first-degree relative with peripheral
 neurofibromatosis
Path:
 pure neurofibromas (= tumor of nerve sheath with
 involvement of nerve, nerve fibers run through mass)
 + neurilemomas (nerve fibers diverge and course over
 the surface of the tumor mass); frequently combined
 (1) discrete round mass
 (2) plexiform = tortuous tangles / fusiform
 enlargement of peripheral nerves
 (PATHOGNOMONIC)
May be associated with:
 (1) MEA IIb (pheochromocytoma + medullary
 carcinoma of thyroid + multiple neuromas)
 (2) CHD (10 fold increase):   pulmonary valve stenosis,
 ASD, VSD, IHSS

A. CNS MANIFESTATIONS
 @ Intracranial
 1. Optic pathway glioma
 isolated to single optic nerve ± extension to other
 optic nerve, chiasm, optic tracts
 Histo: pilocytic astrocytoma with perineural /
 subarachnoid spread (optic nerve is
 embryologically part of hypothalamus
 and develops gliomas instead of
 schwannomas)
 Δ in up to 30% of all neurofibromatosis patients
 Δ 10% of all optic nerve gliomas are associated
 with neurofibromatosis
 2. Cerebral gliomas
 astrocytomas of tectum, brainstem, gliomatosis
 cerebri (= unusual confluence of astrocytomas)
 3. Hydrocephalus
 obstruction usually at aqueduct of Sylvius
 Cause: benign aqueductal stenosis, glioma of
 tectum / tegmentum of mesencephalon
 4. Vascular dysplasia
 = occlusion / stenosis of distal internal carotid
 artery, proximal middle / anterior cerebral
 artery
 √ moyamoya phenomenon (60 – 70%)
 5. Schwannomas of cranial nerves 3 – 12 (most
 commonly 5 + 8)

6. Craniofacial plexiform neurofibromas
   = locally aggressive congenital lesion composed
   of tortuous cords of Schwann cells, neurons +
   collagen with progression along nerve of origin
   (usually small unidentified nerves)
   Location: commonly orbital apex, superior
                orbital fissure
7. CNS hamartomas (75 – 90%)
   Location: pons, globus pallidus, cerebellar
                white matter
   √ multiple foci of isointensity on T1WI +
     hyperintensity on T2WI without mass effect

@ Spine
   1. Paraspinal neurofibromas
      √ tumors of varying sizes at nearly every level
        throughout the spinal canal
      √ enlargement of neural foramina
      √ spinal cord displaced to contralateral side
      √ hypodense to muscle on CT
      √ slightly hyperintense to muscle on T1WI,
        hyperintense periphery + hypointense core on
        T2WI
   2. Lateral meningocele
      = diverticula of thecal sac extending through
        widened neural foramina
      Cause: dysplasia of meninges focally
                  stretched by CSF pulsations
      Location: thoracic level (most common)
      √ erosion of bony elements with marked posterior
        scalloping + widening of neural foramina

B. SKELETAL MANIFESTATIONS (in 30 – 80%)
   • dwarfism caused by scoliosis
   @ Orbit:
      • pulsatile exophthalmus / unilateral proptosis
        (herniation of subarachnoid space + temporal
        lobe into orbit)
      √ Harlequin appearance to orbit = partial absence
        of greater and lesser wing of sphenoid bone +
        orbital plate of frontal bone (failure of
        development of membranous bone)
      √ hypoplasia + elevation of lesser wing of sphenoid
      √ defect in sphenoid bone ± extension of middle
        cranial fossa structures into orbit
      √ concentric enlargement of optic foramen (optic
        glioma)
      √ enlargement of orbital margins + superior orbital
        fissure (plexiform neurofibroma of peripheral and
        sympathetic nerves within orbit / optic nerve
        glioma)
      √ sclerosis in the vicinity of optic foramen (optic
        nerve sheath meningioma)
      √ deformity + decreased size of ipsilateral ethmoid
        + maxillary sinus

   @ Skull:
      √ macrocranium + macroencephaly
      √ calvarial defect adjacent to left lambdoid suture
        = parietal mastoid (rare)

@ Spine:
   √ sharply angled kyphoscoliosis (50%) in lower
     thoracic + lumbar spine; kyphosis predominates
     over scoliosis; incidence increases with age
     Cause: abnormal development of vertebral bodies
   √ hypoplasia of pedicles, transverse + spinous
     processes
   √ posterior scalloping of vertebral bodies with dural
     ectasia (secondary to weakened meninges
     allowing transmission of normal CSF pulsations)
   √ enlarged intervertebral foramina
     (a) intrathoracic / lateral meningocele (protrusion
         of spinal meninges through intervertebral
         foramina)
     (b) "dumbbell" neurofibroma of spinal nerves
     CT: √ fusiform / spherical low-attenuation mass
         (20 – 30 HU)
     US: √ hypoechoic well-circumscribed cylindrical
         lesion
@ Chest:
   √ twisted "ribbon-like" ribs in upper thoracic
     segments accompanying kyphoscoliosis
   √ localized cortical notches / depression of inferior
     margins of ribs (DDx: aortic coarctation)
   √ intrathoracic meningoceles
   √ lung + mediastinal neurofibromas
   √ progressive pulmonary interstitial fibrosis
@ Appendicular skeleton:
   √ anterolateral bowing of lower half of tibia (most
     common) / fibula (frequent) / upper extremity
     (uncommon) ± pseudarthrosis secondary to
     deossification with bowing-fracture in 1st year of
     life
   √ atrophic thinned / absent fibulas
   √ periosteal dysplasia = traumatic subperiosteal
     hemorrhage with abnormally easy detachment of
     periosteum from bone
   √ subendosteal sclerosis
   √ bone erosion from periosteal / soft tissue
     neurofibromas
   √ intramedullary longitudinal streaks of increased
     density
   √ single / multiple cystic lesions within bone
     (? deossification / non-ossifying fibroma)
   √ focal gigantism = unilateral overgrowth of a limb
     bone; marked enlargement of a digit in a hand /
     foot (overgrowth of ossification center)

C. NEURAL CREST TUMORS
   1. Pheochromocytoma: • hypertension in adults
   2. Parathyroid adenomas: • hyperparathyroidism

D. VASCULAR LESIONS
   Schwann cell proliferation within vessel wall
   1. Cranial artery stenosis
   2. Renal artery stenosis: very proximal, funnel-
      shaped (one of the most common causes of
      hypertension in childhood)
   3. Renal artery aneurysm
   4. Thoracic / abdominal aortic coarctation

E. GI TRACT MANIFESTATIONS (25%)
- pain, intestinal bleeding, obstruction

Location: jejunum > stomach > ileum > duodenum
- (a) solitary pattern = single neurofibroma, neuroma, ganglioneuroma
  - √ subserosal / -mucosal filling defect
- (b) plexiform pattern = regional enlargement of nerve root trunks
  - √ multiple polypoid filling defects
- √ multiple leiomyomas ± ulcer

F. OCULAR MANIFESTATIONS (6%)
- buphthalmos = congenital glaucoma
1. Pigmented iris hamartomas <2 mm (Lisch nodules) in >90%, mostly bilateral; appear in childhood
2. Plexiform neurofibroma (most common)
3. Optic glioma: in 12% of patients, in 4% bilateral; 75% in 1st decade
   - √ extension into optic chiasm (up to 25%), optic tracts + optic radiation
   - √ increased intensity on T2WI if chiasm + visual pathways involved
4. Perioptic meningioma
5. Choroidal hamartoma: in 50% of patients

G. SKIN MANIFESTATIONS
1. Café-au-lait spots
   of "coast of California" type (= smooth outline): ≥6 in number >5 mm in greatest diameter usually develop within 1st year of life / >15 mm in size in postpubertal individuals
2. Axillary freckling (in 66%)
3. Cutaneous neurofibroma
   begin to appear around puberty
   - (a) localized = fibroma molluscum = string of pearls along peripheral nerve
   - (b) plexiform neurofibroma = elephantiasis neuromatosa

Cx: malignant transformation to malignant neurofibromas + malignant schwannomas (3 – 13%), glioma, xanthomatous leukemia

Neurofibromatosis with Bilateral Acoustic Neuromas

= CENTRAL NEUROFIBROMATOSIS
= NEUROFIBROMATOSIS 2
= autosomal dominant, abnormality of chromosome 22
Incidence: 1:50,000

Diagnostic criteria:
- (a) bilateral 8th nerve masses
- (b) first degree relative with unilateral 8th nerve mass / neurofibroma, meningioma, glioma, schwannoma, juvenile subcapsular lenticular opacity

- NO Lisch nodules, skeletal dysplasia, optic pathway glioma, vascular dysplasia, learning disability
- café-au-lait spots (<50%): pale, <5 in number
- cutaneous neurofibroma: minimal in size + number / absent

@ Intracranial
1. Bilateral acoustic schwannomas
2. Schwannoma of other cranial nerves
3. Multiple meningiomas: intraventricular in choroid plexus of trigone, parasagittal, sphenoid ridge, olfactory groove, along intracranial nerves
4. Meningiomatosis = dura studded with innumerable small meningiomas

@ Spinal
- symptoms of cord compression
1. Multiple paraspinal neurofibromas
2. Spinal cord ependymomas
3. Meningioma of spinal cord (thoracic region)

NEUROMA

Incidence: 8% of all intracranial tumors
Age: 20 – 50 years
- slow growth; not painful

Acoustic Neuroma

= 5 – 7% of all intracranial tumors; 85% of all intracranial neuromas; 80% of cerebellopontine angle tumors
Age: usually 35 – 60 years; M:F = 1:2
Associated with
1. Central neurofibromatosis (95%)
2. Contralateral acoustic neuroma (25%)
3. Peripheral neurofibromatosis (5%)
- unilateral sensorineural hearing loss (acoustic neuromas account for 10%)
- tinnitus
- diminished corneal reflex
- unsteadiness, vertigo, ataxia, dizziness
- pain

Doubling time: 2 years
Location:
- (a) arises from within internal auditory canal (IAC) at the glial-Schwann cell junction of the vestibular division of 8th nerve (95%)
- (b) may arise in cerebellopontine angle cistern outside IAC with intracanalicular extension (5%)

Plain film:
- √ erosion of IAC: a difference in canal height of >2 mm is abnormal

CT:
- √ round mass based at the IAC with adjacent IAC canal widening (rarely within cerebellopontine angle cistern without bone widening)
- √ usually solid tumor with uniformly dense tumor enhancement
- √ hypodense / isodense (50% may be missed without CECT)
- √ may have cyst formation in / adjacent to tumor (15%)
- √ ring enhancement may be seen
- √ NO calcification
- √ widening / obliteration of ipsilateral cerebellopontine angle cistern
- √ shift / asymmetry of 4th ventricle with hydrocephalus

√ intrathecal contrast / carbon dioxide insufflation (for tumors <5 mm)

MR (most sensitive test with Gd-DTPA enhancement):
  √ moderately hypointense on T1WI + hyperintense on T2WI if solid
  √ very hyperintense on T2WI if cystic
  √ intensely enhancing homogeneous mass / ringlike enhancement (if cystic) after Gd-DTPA

Angio:
  √ elevation + posterior displacement of anterior inferior cerebellar artery (AICA) on basal view
  √ elevation of the superior cerebellar artery (large tumors)
  √ displacement of basilar artery anteriorly / posteriorly + contralateral side
  √ compression / posterior + lateral displacement of petrosal vein
  √ posterior displacement of choroid point of PICA
  √ vascular supply frequently from external carotid artery branches
  √ rarely hypervascular tumor with tumor blush

Trigeminal Neuroma

3 – 5% of intracranial neuromas, 0.26% of all brain tumors

Origin: arising from Gasserian ganglion within Meckel cave at the most anteromedial portion of the petrous pyramid / trigeminal nerve root

Age: 35 – 60 years; M:F = 1:2

Symptoms of location in middle cranial fossa:
  • facial paresthesia / hypesthesia
  • exophthalmus, ophthalmoplegia

Symptoms of location in posterior cranial fossa:
  • facial nerve palsy
  • hearing impairment, tinnitus
  • ataxia, nystagmus

Location: (a) middle cranial fossa (46%) (b) posterior cranial fossa (29%) (c) in both fossae (25%)
  √ erosion of petrous tip
  √ enlargement of contiguous fissures, foramina, canals
  √ dumbbell / saddle-shaped mass (extension into middle cranial fossa + through tentorial incisura into posterior fossa)
  √ isodense mass with dense inhomogeneous enhancement (tumor necrosis + cyst formation)
  √ distortion of ipsilateral quadrigeminal cistern
  √ displacement + cutoff of posterior 3rd ventricle
  √ anterior displacement of temporal horn
  √ angiographically avascular / hypervascular mass

OLIGODENDROGLIOMA

= uncommon form of slowly growing glioma; presenting with large size at time of diagnosis

Incidence: 2 – 10% of intracranial gliomas; 5 – 7% of all primary intracranial neoplasms

Histo: mixed glial cells (50%), astrocytic components (30%); hemorrhage + cyst formation infrequent

Age: 30 – 50 years
  • seizures

Location:
  most commonly in cerebral hemispheres (propensity for periphery of frontal lobes) involving cortex + white matter, thalamus, corpus callosum; occasionally around / in ventricles ("subependymal oligodendroglioma") rare in cerebellum + spinal cord
  √ large nodular clumps of calcifications (in 45% on plain film; in 90% on CT)

CT:
  √ round / oval hypodense lesion with mass effect (75%)
  √ commonly no / minimal tumor enhancement (75%), pronounced in high grade tumors
  √ may be adherent to dura (mimicking meningiomas)
  √ ± erosion of inner table of skull
  √ cystic changes (uncommon)
  √ edema (in 50% of low-grade, in 80% of high-grade tumors)

MR:
  √ well-circumscribed heterogeneous hypointense lesion on T1WI + hyperintense on T2WI
  √ little edema / mass effect
  √ solid / peripheral / mixed enhancement
  √ calcification may not be detected

Cx: malignant metaplasia + CSF seeding

DDx:
  (1) Astrocytoma (no large calcifications)
  (2) Ganglioglioma (in temporal lobes + deep cerebral tissues
  (3) Ependymoma (enhancing tumor, often with internal bleeding producing fluid levels)
  (4) Glioblastoma (infiltrating, enhancing, edema, no calcifications)

PARAGONIOMIASIS OF BRAIN

Oriental lung fluke (Paragonimus westermani) producing arachnoiditis, parenchymal granulomas, encapsulated abscesses
  √ isodense / inhomogeneous masses surrounded by edema
  √ ring enhancement

PELIZAEUS-MERZBACHER DISEASE

= rare X-linked sudanophilic leukodystrophy (5 types with different times of onset, rate of progression, genetic transmission)

Age: neonatal period
  • bizarre pendular nystagmus + head shaking
  • cerbellar ataxia
  • slow psychomotor development

CT:
  √ hypodense white matter
  √ progressive white matter atrophy

MR:
  √ lack of myelination (appearance of newborn retained)
  √ hyperintense internal capsule, optic radiations, proximal corona radiata on T1WI
  √ near complete absence of hypointensity in supratentorial region on T2WI
  √ mild / moderate prominence of cortical sulci

Prognosis: death in adolescence / early adulthood

PICK DISEASE
= rare form of presenile dementia similar to Alzheimer disease; may be inherited with autosomal dominant mode; M < F
√ focal cortical atrophy of anterior frontal + temporal lobes
√ dilatation of frontal + temporal horns of lateral ventricle

PINEAL CYST
= small nonneoplastic cyst of pineal gland
Incidence: 25 – 40% on autopsy, 4% on MRI
Types:
   (a) developmental = persistence of ependymal-lined pineal diverticulum
   (b) degenerative = glial-lined secondary cavitation within area of gliosis
• never associated with Parinaud syndrome
• never cause of hydrocephalus
• may be symptomatic when large
CT:
   √ normal-sized gland (80%), slightly >1 cm in 20%
   √ isodense to CSF in surrounding cistern (infrequently noted)
MR:
   √ sharply marginated ovoid mass in pineal region
   √ slight impression on superior colliculi (sagittal image)
   √ isointense to CSF on T1WI + slightly hyperintense to CSF on T2WI (due to phase coherence in cysts but not in moving CSF)
   √ may have higher signal intensity than CSF due to high protein content
   √ contrast may diffuse from enhanced rim of residual pineal tissue into fluid center (no blood-brain barrier) on delayed sequence images

PINEAL GERMINOMA
= DYSGERMINOMA = PINEALOMA = ATYPICAL TERATOMA (former inaccurate names)
= malignant primitive germ cell neoplasm
Incidence: most common pineal tumor (>50% of all pineal tumors)
Histo: identical to testicular seminoma + ovarian dysgerminoma, NO capsule facilitates invasion
Age: 10 – 25 years; M:F = 10:1
May be associated with   ectopic pinealoma = secondary focus in inferior portion of 3rd ventricle
• precocious puberty frequent in children <10 years of age
• Parinaud syndrome = paralysis of upward gaze (compression of mesencephalic tectum)
Location of germinomas: pineal gland (80%), suprasellar region (20%), basal ganglia, thalamus
√ displacement of calcified pineal gland
√ hydrocephalus (compression of aqueduct of Sylvius)
√ well-defined lesion restricted to pineal gland
√ may infiltrate quadrigeminal plate / thalamus
CT:
   √ infiltrating variodense homogeneous mass (attenuation usually similar to grey matter)

√ rarely psammomatous calcifications within tumor, but pineal calcifications in 100% (40% in normal population)
√ moderate / marked uniform contrast enhancement
MR:
   √ round / lobular well-circumscribed relatively homogeneous mass isointense to gray matter
   √ hypointense mass on T2WI (occasionally)
   √ strong Gd-DTPA enhancement
Cx: metastatic spread via CSF (frequent)
Rx: combination of irradiation (very radiosensitive) + chemotherapy (adriamycin, cisplatin, cyclophosphamide)
Prognosis: 75% survival after radiation therapy alone

PINEAL TERATOCARCINOMA
= highly malignant variant of germ cell tumors
Types:
   1. Choriocarcinoma
   2. Embryonal cell carcinoma
   3. Endodermal sinus tumor
Histo: arising from primitive germ cells, frequently containing more than one cell type
Age: <20 years; males
• Parinaud syndrome
• tumor markers elevated in serum + CSF
√ intratumoral hemorrhage (esp. choriocarcinoma)
√ invasion of adjacent structures
√ intense homogeneous contrast enhancement
Cx: seeding via CSF

PINEAL TERATOMA
= benign tumor containing one / all three germ cell layers (pineal region most common site of teratomas)
Incidence: 15% of all pineal masses (2nd most common tumor in pineal region)
Age: <20 years; M:F = 2 – 8:1
• Parinaud syndrome = paralysis of upward gaze (compression / infiltration of superior colliculi)
• hypothalamic symptoms
• headache
• somnolence (related to hydrocephalus)

Location: pineal, parapineal, suprasellar, 3rd ventricle
√ well-defined rounded / irregular lobulated extremely heterogenous mass of fat, cartilage, hair, linear / nodular calcifications + cysts
   ∆ Fat is absent in all other pineal tumors!
√ may show heterogeneous / rim-like contrast enhancement (limited to solid-tissue areas)
Angio:
   √ elevation of internal cerebral vein
   √ posterior displacement of precentral vein
CT:
   √ heterogeneous mass with fat, calcification, cystic + solid areas
MR:
   √ variegated appearance on all pulse sequences with hyperintense areas of fat on T1WI
Cx: chemical meningitis with spontaneous rupture

PINEOBLASTOMA

= highly malignant tumor derived from primitive pineal parenchymal cells

Histo:

unencapsulated highly cellular primitive small round cell tumor (similar to medulloblastoma, neuroblastoma, retinoblastoma)

Age: any age, more common in children; M < F

CT:

√ poorly marginated iso- / slightly hyperdense mass

√ may contain dense tumor calcifications

√ peripherally displaced preexisting normal pineal calcification (= "exploded pineal pattern")

√ intense homogeneous contrast enhancement

MR:

√ iso- / moderately hypointense on T1WI + iso- / hyperintense on T2WI

√ dense homogeneous Gd-DTPA enhancement

Spread:

(1) direct extension posteriorly with invasion of cerebellar vermis + anteriorly into 3rd ventricle

(2) throughout CSF (frequent) along meninges / via ventricles

PINEOCYTOMA

= rare slow-growing unencapsulated tumor composed of mature pineal parenchymal cells

Age: any age; M:F = 1:1

√ well-marginated slightly hyperdense / isodense mass

√ dense focal tumor calcifications possible

√ peripherally displaced preexisting normal pineal calcification (= "exploded pineal pattern")

√ well-defined homogeneous enhancement

MR:

√ intermediate intensity on T1WI + T2WI

√ may be isointense to CSF but containing trabeculations (DDx to pineal cyst)

√ mild to moderate Gd-DTPA enhancement

Cx: some metastasize via CSF

PITUITARY ADENOMA

= benign slow-growing neoplasms arising from adenohypophysis (= anterior lobe); account for 5 – 18% of all intracranial neoplasms

FORMER CLASSIFICATION:

A. Chromophobe adenoma (80%)

associated with hypopituitarism;

elevation of prolactin, TSH, GH serum levels

√ greatest sella enlargement; calcified in 5%

however: functioning microadenomas are part of chromophobe adenomas

B. Acidophilic / eosinophilic adenoma (15%)

increased GH secretion (acromegaly), prolactin, TSH

√ tumor of intermediate size

C. Basophilic adenoma (5%)

associated with ACTH secretion (Cushing syndrome), LH, FSH

√ small tumor

Plain film: (UNRELIABLE !)

√ enlargement of sella + sloping of sella floor

√ erosion of anterior + posterior clinoid processes

√ erosion of dorsum sellae

√ calcification in <10%

√ may present with mass in nasopharynx

Functioning Pituitary Adenoma

Adenoma may secrete multiple hormones!

1. PROLACTINOMA (most frequent)

• prolactin levels do not closely correlate with tumor size

Female:

• women during childbearing age

• amenorrhea

• galactorrhea

• elevated prolactin levels (usually >100 ng/ml)

Male:

• headache

• impotence

• visual disturbance

√ characteristic lateral location, anteriorly / inferiorly; variable in size

Rx: bromocriptine

2. CORTICOTROPHIC ADENOMA

ACTH-secreting tumor

√ central location; posterior lobe; usually <5 mm in size

• Cushing disease (truncal obesity, abdominal striae, glycosuria, osteoporosis, proximal muscle weakness, hirsutism, amenorrhea, hypertension, elevated cortisol levels in plasma and urine)

Rx: suppression by high doses of dexamethasone of 8 mg/day

3. SOMATOTROPHIC ADENOMA

• gigantism, acromegaly, elevated GH >10 ng/ml, no rise in GH after administration of glucose / TRH

√ hypodense region, may be less well-defined, variable size

4. Thyroid-stimulating hormone, follicle-stimulating hormon / luteinizing hormone

CECT (dynamic bolus injection):

√ upward convexity of gland

√ increased height >10 mm

√ deviation of pituitary stalk

√ floor erosion of sella

√ gland asymmetry

√ focal hypodensity (most specific for adenoma)

√ shift of pituitary tuft / density change in region of adenoma

MR:

Highest sensitivity on coronal non-enhanced T1WI (70%) + 3 D FLASH sequence (69%) + combination of both (90%)

Δ 1/3 of lesions are missed with enhancement

Δ 1/3 of lesions are missed without enhancement

√ focus of low / high signal intensity

DDx: simple pituitary cyst

Pituitary Macroadenoma

= tumor usually >10 mm in size, usually nonfunctioning (70 – 80% of pituitary adenomas)

Incidence: 10%; M:F = 1:1

Age: 25 – 60 years

- hypopituitarism, bitemporal hemianopia (with superior extension), pituitary apoplexy, hydrocephalus, cranial nerve involvement (III, IV, VI)

Extension into: suprasellar cistern / cavernous sinus / sphenoid sinus + nasopharynx

√ occasionally tumor hemorrhage

CT: √ tumor isodense to brain tissue
   √ roughly homogeneous enhancement
   √ calcifications infrequent

MR: allows differentiation from aneurysm

Cx: (1) Obstructive hydrocephalus (at foramen of Monro)
   (2) Encasement of carotid artery
   (3) Pituitary apoplexy (rare)

Pituitary Microadenoma

= very small adenomas <10 mm

- usually become clinically apparent by hormone production (20 – 30% of all pituitary adenomas)

∆ prolactin elevation (>25 ng/ml in females)
   4 – 8 x normal : adenoma demonstrated in 71%
   >8 x normal : adenoma demonstrated in 100%

- **incidentaloma** = nonfunctioning microadenoma / pituitary cyst

√ NO imaging features to distinguish between different types of adenomas

MRI:
   √ small mass of lower signal intensity on pre- and postcontrast T1WI
   √ occasionally isointense on precontrast images + hyperintense on postcontrast images
   √ focal bulge on surface of gland
   √ focal depression of sellar floor
   √ deviation of pituitary stalk

PITUITARY APOPLEXY

= massive hemorrhage into pituitary adenoma / dramatic necrosis / sudden infarction of pituitary gland; area of destruction must be >70% to produce pituitary insufficiency

Sheehan Syndrome = postpartum infarction of anterior pituitary gland

- severe headache, nausea, vomiting
- stiff neck
- sudden visual loss / diplopia
- obtundation (frequent)
- secondary hypothyroidism

NCCT: √ increased density

PORENCEPHALY

= focal cavity as a result of localized brain destruction

A. AGENETIC PORENCEPHALY
   = Schizencephaly (= true porencephaly)

B. ENCEPHALOCLASTIC PORENCEPHALY
   Time of injury: during first half of gestation
   Histo: necrotic tissue completely reabsorbed without surrounding glial reaction (= liquefaction necrosis)
   MR:
     √ smooth-walled cavity filled with CSF on all pulse sequences (= porencephalic cyst)
     √ lined by white matter

C. ENCEPHALOMALACIA
   = Pseudoporencephaly = Acquired porencephaly
   Cause: infectious, vascular
   Time of injury: after end of 2nd trimester (brain has developed capacity for glial response)
   Location: parasagittal watershed areas with sparing of periventricular region + ventricular wall
   CT:
     √ hypodense regions
   MR:
     √ hypointense on T1WI + hyperintense on T2WI
     √ surrounding hyperintense rim on T2WI (= gliosis)
     √ glial septae coursing through cavity identified on T1WI + proton density images
   US:
     √ septations in cavity well visualized

PRIMITIVE NEUROECTODERMAL TUMOR

= PNET = group of very undifferentiated tumors arising from germinal matrix cells of primitive neural tube

Incidence: <5% of supratentorial neoplasms in children

Age: mainly in children <5 years of age; M:F = 1:1

Histo: highly cellular tumors composed of >90 – 95% of undifferentiated cells (histologically similar to medulloblastoma, pineoblastoma, peripheral neuroblastoma)

- signs of increased intracranial pressure / seizures

Location:
   (a) supratentorial: deep cerebral white matter (most commonly in frontal lobe), pineal gland, in thalamic + suprasellar territories (least frequently)
   (b) posterior fossa (= medulloblastoma)

√ large cellular lesion with tendency for necrosis (65%), cyst formation, calcifications (71%), hemorrhage (10%)

√ thin rim of edema

√ contrast enhancement of solid tumor portion

CT:
   √ solid tumor portions hyperdense (due to high nuclear to cytoplasmic ratio)

MR:
   √ mildly hypointense on T1WI + hyperintense on T2WI
   √ remarkably inhomogeneous due to cyst formation + necrosis
   √ areas of signal dropout due to calcifications
   √ hyperintense areas on T1WI + variable intensity on T2WI due to hemorrhage
   √ inhomogeneously enhancing mass with tumor nodules + ring-like areas surrounding central necrosis after Gd-DTPA

PROGRESSIVE MULTIFOCAL LEUKOENCEPHALOPATHY

= PML = progressive fatal demyelinating disease in patients with impaired immune system (leukemia, lymphoma, carcinomatosis, AIDS, tuberculosis, sarcoidosis, organ transplant)

Etiology: virus infection (probably latent papovavirus)

Pathophysiology: destruction of oligodendrogliocytes leading to areas of demyelination + edema

Histo: intranuclear inclusion bodies within swollen oligodendrocytes (viral particles in nuclei), absence of significant perivenous inflammation

• progressive neurologic deficits, visual disturbances, dementia, ataxia, spasticity
• normal CSF fluid

Location: predilection for parietooccipital white matter

CT:
  √ multicentric confluent white matter lesions of low attenuation with scalloped borders
  √ NO contrast enhancement
  √ NO mass effect

MR:
  √ patchy high-intensity lesions of white matter away from ependyma in asymmetric distribution on T2WI

Prognosis: death usually within 6 months

DDx in early stages: primary CNS lymphoma

REYE SYNDROME

= hepatitis + encephalitis following viral upper respiratory tract infection with Hx of large doses of aspirin ingestion

Age: in children + young adults

• obtundation rapidly progressing to coma
√ initially (within 2 – 3 days) small ventricles
√ later progressive enlargement of lateral ventricles + sulci
√ markedly diminished attenuation of white matter

Mortality: 15 – 85% (from white matter edema + demyelination)

Dx: liver biopsy

SARCOIDOSIS OF CNS

Incidence: CNS involvement in 3 – 8%

• cranial neuropathy (facial > acoustic > optic > trigeminal nerves) secondary to granulomatous infiltration + leptomeningeal fibrosis
• peripheral neuropathy + myopathy
• aseptic meningitis
• diffuse encephalopathy
• hypothalamic dysfunction
• seizures
• improvement following therapy with steroids

Location: affects meninges + cranial nerves more often than brain

√ diffuse meningeal enhancement (most common) / meningeal nodules (less common) from leptomeningeal invasion
  Site: particularly in basal cisterns (suprasellar, sellar, subfrontal regions) with extension to optic chiasm, hypothalamus, pituitary gland
√ dense enhancement of falx + tentorium (granulomatous invasion of dura)

√ isodense / hyperdense homogeneously enhancing small single / multiple nodules (invasion of brain parenchyma via perivascular spaces of Virchow-Robin)
  Site: periphery of parenchyma, intraspinal
√ hydrocephalus most common finding (from arachnoiditis / adhesions)

SCHIZENCEPHALY

= AGENETIC PORENCEPHALY = TRUE PORENCEPHALY

= gray-matter lined parenchymal clefts extending from subarachnoid space to subependyma of lateral ventricles

Cause: segmental developmental failure of cell migration to form cerebral cortex / destruction of portion of germinal matrix

Time of injury: before formation of hemispheres

Often associated with   polymicrogyria, microcephaly, gray matter heterotopia

Types:
  (a) clefts with fused lips
      (may be missed in imaging planes parallel to the plane of cleft)
      √ walls appose one another obliterating CSF space
  (b) clefts with separated lips
      √ CSF fills cleft from lateral ventricle to subarachnoid space

• seizure disorder
• mild / moderate developmental delay
• mental retardation possible
• blindness possible (optic nerve hypoplasia in 33%)

Location: most commonly near pre- and postcentral gyri; uni- / bilateral

√ full-thickness cleft through hemisphere with irregular margins
√ gray-matter lining of cleft (PATHOGNOMONIC) extending through entire hemisphere
√ polymicrogyria / pachygyria of cortex adjacent to cleft
√ bilateral often symmetric intracranial cysts, usually around sylvian fissure
√ asymmetrical dilatation of lateral ventricles with midline shift
√ wide separation of lateral ventricles + squaring of frontal lobes
√ absence of cavum septi pellucidi (80 - 90%) + corpus callosum

Prognosis: severe intellectual impairment, spastic tetraplegia, blindness

DDx:
  (1) Pseudoporencephaly = Acquired porencephaly
      = local parenchymal destruction secondary to vascular / infectious / traumatic insult (almost always unilateral)
  (2) Arachnoid cyst
  (3) Cystic tumor

SEPTO-OPTIC DYSPLASIA

= DeMORSIER SYNDROME

= rare anterior midline anomaly with (1) hypoplasia of optic nerves (2) hypoplasia / absence of septum pellucidum;
often considered a mild form of lobar holoprosencephaly
M:F = 1:3
Associated with schizencephaly (50%)

- diminished visual acuity (hypoplasia of optic discs), nystagmus, occasionally hypotelorism
- hypothalamic hypopituitarism (66%):
diabetes insipidus (in 50%), growth retardation (deficient secretion of growth hormone + tyroid stimulating horone)
- seizures, hypotonia
√ small optic canals
√ hypoplasia of optic nerves + chiasm + infundibulum
√ bulbous dilatation of anterior recess of 3rd ventricle
√ absent septum pellucidum
√ thin corpus callosum
√ dilatation of chiasmatic + suprasellar cisterns
√ fused dilated box-like frontal horns squared off dorsally + pointing inferiorly

SINUS PERICRANII
= subperiosteal venous angiomas adherent to skull and connected by anomalous diploic veins to a sinus / cortical vein
- soft painless scalp mass that reduces under compression
Location: frontal bone
√ calvarial thinning + defect
CT:
  √ sessile sharply marginated homogeneous densely enhancing mass adjacent to outer table of skull, perforating it and connecting it with another similar structure beneath the inner table
Angio:
  √ extracalvarial sinus may not opacify secondary to slow flow

SPONGIFORM LEUKOENCEPHALOPATHY
rare, hereditary, > age 40
- deteriorating mental function
√ confluent areas of diminished attenuation

STURGE-WEBER-DIMITRI SYNDROME
= ENCEPHALOTRIGEMINAL ANGIOMATOSIS
= MENINGOFACIAL ANGIOMATOSIS
= vascular malformation with capillary venous angiomas involving face, choroid of eye, leptomeninges
Cause: persistence of transitory primordial sinusoidal plexus stage of vessel development; usually sporadic
- seizures (90%) in 1st year of life
- mental deficiency (>50%)
- increasing crossed hemiparesis (35 – 65%)
- hemiatrophy of body contralateral to facial nevus (secondary to hemiparesis)
- ipsilateral glaucoma (often)
- homonomous hemianopsia

A. FACIAL MANIFESTATION
- congenital facial port wine stain (nevus flammeus) = telangiectasia of trigeminal region; usually 1st ± 2nd division of 5th nerve; usually unilateral
  — V_1 associated with occipital lobe angiomatosis
  — V_2 associated with parietal lobe angiomatosis
  — V_3 associated with frontal lobe angiomatosis

B. CNS MANIFESTATION
√ leptomeningeal venous angiomas confined to pia mater
Location: parietal > occipital > frontal lobes
Angio:
  √ capillary blush
  √ abnormally large veins in subependymal + periventricular regions
  √ abnormal deep medullary veins draining into internal cerebral vein (= venous shunt)
  √ failure to opacify superficial cortical veins in calcified region (markedly slow blood flow / thrombosis of dysgenetic superficial veins)
√ cortical hemiatrophy beneath meningeal angioma due to anoxia (steal)
√ "tram track" gyriform cortical calcifications >2 years of age; in layers 2-3(-4-5) of opposing gyri underlying pial angiomatosis; bilateral in up to 20%
Location: temporo-parieto-occipital area, occasionally frontal, rare in posterior fossa
√ subjacent white matter hypodense on CT with slight prolongation of T1 + T2 relaxation times (gliosis)
√ choroid plexus enlargement ipsilateral to angiomatosis
√ ipsilateral thickening of skull + orbit (bone apposition as result of subdural hematoma secondary to brain atrophy)
√ elevation of sphenoid wing + petrous ridge
√ enlarged ipsilateral paranasal sinuses + mastoid air cells
√ thickened calvarium (= widening of diploic space)
C. ORBITAL MANIFESTATION (30%)
Path: angiomatous malformation of choroid
√ buphthalmos = enlarged + elongated globe as result of increased intraocular pressure
Cx: glaucoma, retinal detachment
D. VISCERAL MANIFESTATION
localized / diffuse angiomatous malformation located in intestine, kidneys, spleen, ovaries, thyroid, pancreas, lungs

SUBARACHNOID HEMORRHAGE
Cause:
A. Spontaneous
(1) ruptured aneurysm (72%) (2) AV malformation (10%) (3) hypertensive hemorrhage (4) hemorrhage from tumor (5) embolic hemorrhagic infarction (6) blood dyscrasia, anticoagulation therapy (7) eclampsia (8) intracranial infection (9) spinal vascular malformation (10) cryptogenic in 6% (negative 4-vessel angiography; seldom recurrent)

B. Trauma
concomitanto cerebral contusion
(a) injury to leptomeningeal vessels at vertex
(b) rupture of major intracerebral vessels (less common)
Location: (a) focal, overlying site of contusion
(b) interhemispheric fissure, paralleling falx cerebri
(c) spread diffusely throughout subarachnoid space (rare in trauma)

NCCT (accuracy of detection 60 – 90% depending on time of scan; high within 4 – 5 days of onset):
√ increased density in basal cisterns, superior cerebellar cistern, sylvian fissure, cortical sulci, intraventricular, intracerebral
√ along interhemispheric fissure = on lateral aspect irregular dentate pattern due to extension into paramedian sulci with rapid clearing after several days
MR (relatively insensitive):
√ deoxyhemoglobin effects not appreciable in acute phase (secondary to higher oxygen tension in CSF, counterbalancing effects of very long T2 of CSF, pulsatile flow effects of CSF)
√ low signal intensity on brain surfaces in recurrent subarachnoid hemorrhages (hemosiderin deposition)

Prognosis: clinical course depends on amount of subarachnoid blood
Cx:
(1) Acute obstructive hydrocephalus (in <1 week) secondary to intraventricular hemorrhage / ependymitis obstructing aqueduct of Sylvius or outlet of 4th ventricle
(2) Delayed communicating hydrocephalus (after 1 week) secondary to fibroblastic proliferation in subarachnoid space and arachnoid villi
(3) Cerebral vasospasm + infarction (develops after 72 hours, at maximum between 5 – 17 days, amount of blood is prognostic parameter)
(4) Transtentorial herniation (cerebral hematoma, hydrocephalus, infarction, brain edema)

SUBDURAL HEMATOMA OF BRAIN
Incidence: in 5% of head trauma patients
Age: predominantly in infants + elderly (large subarachnoid space with freedom to move in cerebral atrophy)
Pathogenesis:
most often due to venous bleeding from "bridging veins" (= subdural veins), which connect cerebral cortex to dural sinuses and travel through the subarachnoid space and potential space between dura and arachnoid membranes, veins tear at portion attached to sinus
Location: potential space between dura + leptomeninges
DDx: (1) Arachnoid cyst (extension into sylvian fissure)
(2) Subarachnoid hemorrhage (extension into sulci)

Acute Subdural Hematoma
Usually follows severe trauma, manifest within hours after injury
Associated with: underlying brain injury (50%) with worse long-term prognosis than epidural hematoma, skull fracture (1%)
Location: along cerebral convexity, frequent extension into interhemispheric fissure, along tentorial margins, beneath temporal + occipital lobes; bilateral in 15 – 25% of adults (common in elderly) and in 80 – 85% in infants
√ extraaxial peripheral crescentic fluid collection between skull and cerebral hemisphere usually with
√ concave inner margin (hematoma minimally pressing into brain substance)
√ convex outer margin following normal contour of cranial vault
√ hyperdense (<1 week) / isodense (1 – 3 weeks) / hypodense (3 – 4 weeks)
√ occasionally with blood-fluid level
False-negative CT scan:
high-convexity location, beam-hardening artifact, volume averaging with high density of calvarium obscuring flat "en plaque" hematoma, isodense hematoma during 10 – 20 days post injury
Δ 38% of small subdural hematomas are missed!
√ after surgical evacuation: underlying parenchymal injury becomes more obvious
√ after healing: ventricular + sulcal enlargement

Cx: Arteriovenous fistula (meningeal artery + vein caught in fracture line)
Prognosis: may progress to subacute + chronic stage / may disappear spontaneously

INTERHEMISPHERIC SUBDURAL HEMATOMA
Most common acute finding in child abuse (whiplash forces on large head with weak neck muscles)
√ predominance for posterior portion of interhemispheric fissure
√ crescentic shape with flat medial border
√ unilateral increased attenuation with extension along course of tentorium
√ anterior extension to level of genu of corpus callosum

SUBDURAL HEMORRHAGE IN NEWBORN
Cause: mechanical trauma during delivery (excessive vertical molding of head)
1. Posterior fossa hemorrhage
(a) tentorial laceration with rupture of vein of Galen / straight sinus / transverse sinus
(b) occipital osteodiastasis = separation of squamous portion from exoccipital portion of occipital bone
√ high-density thickening of affected tentorial leaf extending down posterior to cerebellar hemisphere (better seen on coronal views)
√ mildly echogenic subtentorial collection
Cx: death from compression of brainstem, acute hydrocephalus

2. Supratentorial hemorrhage
   (a) laceration of falx near junction with tentorium with rupture of inferior sagittal sinus (less common than tentorial laceration)
   √ hematoma over corpus callosum in inferior aspect of interhemispheric fissure
   (b) convexity hematoma from rupture of superficial cortical veins
   √ usually unilateral subdural convexity hematoma accompanied by subarachnoid blood
   √ underlying cerebral contusion
   √ sonographic visualization of convexities difficult

Subacute Subdural Hematoma
CT:
   √ isodense hematoma (1 – 3 weeks) may be recognizable by mass effect with effacement of cortical sulci, deviation of lateral ventricle, midline shift, white matter buckling, displacement of gray-white matter junction
   √ contrast enhancement of inner membrane
   AID in Dx: contrast enhancement defines cortical-subdural interface
MR:
   √ modality of choice in subacute stage because of high sensitivity for Met-Hb on T1WI (esp. superior to CT during isodense phase)
   √ allows differentiation of subdural from epidural blood secondary to low signal of dura

Chronic Subdural Hematoma
Following minor injury some time ago; rarely associated with parenchymal injury
Histo: hematoma enclosed by thick + vascular membrane which forms after 3 – 6 weeks
Pathogenesis:
   vessel fragility accounts for repeated episodes of rebleeding following minor injuries that tear fragile capillary bed within neomembrane surrounding subdural hematoma
• history of trauma often absent
• ill-defined neurological signs + symptoms

   √ crescentic-shaped hematoma conforming to configuration of brain (early)
   √ usually biconvex lenticular configuration (late), esp. after compartmentalization secondary to formation of fibrous septa
   √ low density lesion, sometimes as low as CSF
   √ high density components of collection (after common rebleeding)
   √ fluid-fluid level
   √ displacement / absence of sulci, displacement of ventricles + parenchyma
   √ No midline shift if bilateral (25%)
   √ CECT demonstrates medially displaced cortical vein or membrane around hematoma (1 – 4 weeks after injury)
DDx: Acute epidural hematoma (similar biconvex shape)

TERATOMA OF CNS
Incidence: 0.5% of primary intracranial neoplasms; 2% of intracranial tumors before age 15
Histo: mostly benign, occasionally containing primitive elements + highly malignant

Location: pineal + parapineal region > floor of 3rd ventricle > posterior fossa > spine (associated with spina bifida)
   √ heterogeneous midline lesion, occasionally homogeneous soft tissue mass (DDx: astrocytoma)
   √ contains fat + calcium
   √ hydrocephalus (common)

TOXOPLASMOSIS OF BRAIN
Organism: obligate intracellular protozoan parasite Toxoplasma gondii, can live in any cell except for nonnucleated RBCs
Infection: ingestion of cysts / transplacental transmission of trophozoites; acquired through blood transfusion + organ transplantation
Histo: inflammatory solid / cystic granulomas as a result of glial mesenchymal reaction surrounded by edema + microinfarcts due to vasculitis
• asymptomatic
• lymphadenopathy
• malaise, fever

A. AIDS INFECTION
   • meningoencephalitic symptoms
   • seizures
   • pseudotumor cerebri syndrome
   Location: basal ganglia (75%), scattered throughout brain parenchyma
   √ solitary (up to 39%) / multiple lesions with nodular / thin-walled (common) ring enhancement + surrounding white matter edema
   √ double-dose delayed CT scans with higher detection rate for multiple lesions (64 – 72%)
   Dx: improvement on antitoxotherapy within 1 – 2 weeks / biopsy
   DDx: CNS lymphoma (particularly with single lesion)
      Δ Multiple lesions suggest toxoplasmosis!

B. INTRAUTERINE INFECTION
   • Toxoplasma gondii found in ventricular fluid
   • chorioretinitis
   • mental retardation
   √ multiple irregular, nodular / cyst-like / curvilinear calcifications in periventricular area + choroid plexus (= necrotic foci); bilateral; 1 – 20 mm in size; increasing in number + size (usually not developed at time of birth)
   √ microcephaly with little postnatal growth
   √ hydrocephalus with return to normal / persistence of large head size
   √ thickened vault, sutures apposed / overlapping
   Dx: demonstration of elongated teardrop-shaped trophozoites in histologic sections of tissue

TUBERCULOMA OF BRAIN

= result of granuloma formation within cerebral substance

Incidence: 0.15% of intracranial masses in Western countries, 30% in underdeveloped countries

Age: infant, small child, young adult

Associated with: tuberculous meningitis in 50%

• history of previous extracranial TB (in 60%)

Location: more common in posterior fossa (62%), cerebellar hemispheres; may be associated with tuberculous meningitis

√ solitary (70%) / multiple (30 – 60%) lesions; may be multiloculated

NCCT:
√ isodense (72%) / hyperdense lesion of 0.5 – 4 cm in diameter with mass effect (93%)
√ surrounding edema (72%) less marked than in pyogenic abscess
√ central calcification (29%)

CECT:
√ homogeneous enhancement
√ ring blush (nearly all) with smooth / slightly shaggy margins + thick wall around an isodense center (DDx: in pyogenic abscess less thick + more regular)
√ "target sign" = central calcification in isodense lesion + ring-blush (DDx: giant aneurysm)
√ homogeneous blush in tuberculoma en plaque along dural plane (6%) (DDx: meningioma en plaque)

TUBEROUS SCLEROSIS

= BOURNEVILLE DISEASE = EPIPLOIA

= autosomal dominant neuroectodermal disorder with low penetrance (frequent skips in generations); sporadic in 50 – 80%; characterized by TRIAD consisting of
(1) Adenoma sebaceum (30%)
(2) Seizures (80%)
(3) Mental retardation (70%)
mnemonic: zits, fits, nitwits

Frequency: 1:150,000 livebirths

Prognosis: 30% dead by age 5; 75% dead by age 20

@ CNS INVOLVEMENT

• myoclonic seizures (80 – 90%): often first + most common sign of tuberous sclerosis with onset at 1st – 2nd year, decreasing in frequency with age

• mental retardation (50 – 82%): mild to moderate (1/3) moderate to severe (2/3); progressive; observed in adulthood; common if onset of seizures before age 5 years

1. **Subependymal hamartomas**
   Location:
   along ventricular surface of caudate nucleus, on lamina of sulcus thalamo-striatus immediately posterior to foramen of Monro (most often), along frontal + temporal horns or 3rd + 4th ventricle (less commonly)
   √ multiple subependymal nodules with "candle drippings" appearance at lining of lateral ventricles
   √ calcification with increasing age (in up to 88%)
   MR:
   √ subependymal nodules protruding into adjacent ventricle isointense with white matter

√ minimal / no contrast enhancement

2. **Giant cell astrocytoma**
   = large subependymal nodule located near foramen of Monro with tendency for enlargement + growth into ventricle
   Incidence: 5 – 15%; M:F = 1:1
   √ hydrocephalus (obstruction at foramen of Monro)
   √ hypo- / isodense well-demarcated rounded lesion in the region of foramen of Monro
   √ hypo- / isointense on T1WI + hyperintense on T2WI
   √ uniformly enhancing mass
   √ frequent extension into frontal horn / body of lateral ventricle
   Cx: degeneration into higher grade astrocytoma

3. **Tubers** (in 56%)
   = CORTICAL HAMARTOMAS
   Histo: clusters of atypical glial cells surrounded by giant cells with frequent calcifications (if >2 years of age) = hamartomas
   Frequency: multiple (75%); bilateral (30%)
   √ noncalcified hypodense brain lesions of abnormal myelination within broadened cortical gyri
   √ cortical tubers calcified (in 15% <1 year of age, in 50% by age 10)
   MR:
   √ relaxation time similar to white matter (if uncalcified)
   √ multiple nodules of high signal intensity on T2WI, iso- / hypointense on T1WI (fibrillary gliosis / demyelination)

4. **Heterotopic islands in white matter**
   Histo: grouping of bizarre and gigantic neuronal cells associated with gliosis + areas of demyelination
   CT:
   √ hypodense well-defined regions within cerebral white matter without contrast enhancement
   √ calcification of all / part of nodule
   MR:
   √ subtle hypointense region on T1WI + well-defined hyperintense area on T2WI

DDx of CNS lesions:
(1) Intrauterine CMV / toxoplasma infection (smaller lesions, brain atrophy, microcephaly)
(2) Basal ganglia calcification in hypoparathyroidism / Fahr disease (location)
(3) Sturge-Weber, calcified AVM (diffuse atrophy, not focal)
(4) Heterotopic grey matter (along medial ventricular wall, isodense, associated with agenesis of corpus callosum, Chiari malformation)

@ SKIN INVOLVEMENT

• Adenoma sebaceum (80 – 90%) = wart-like nodules of brownish red color averaging 4 mm in size with bimalar distribution ("butterfly rash")
   Age: first discovered at age 1 – 5 years; family history in 30%
   Path: small hamartomas from neural elements with blood vessel hyperplasia = angiofibromas

Location: nasolabial folds, eventually covers nose + middle of cheeks
- Shagreen rough skin patches(80%) = "pigskin" = "peau d'orange" = patches of fibrous hyperplasia; in intertriginous + lumbar location
- Ash leaf patches = hypopigmented macules shaped like ash / spearmint leaf on trunk + extremities (earliest manifestation in infancy)
- Ungual fibromas (15 – 50%): sub- / periungual with erosion of distal tuft
- Café-au-lait spots: incidence similar to that in general population

@ OCULAR INVOLVEMENT
- Phakoma (>50%) = whitish disc-shaped retinal hamartoma = astrocytic proliferation in / near optic disc, often multiple + usually in both eyes
- √ small calcifications in region of optic nerve head
- √ optic nerve glioma

@ RENAL INVOLVEMENT
- renal failure in severe cases (5%)
- hypertension
1. Angiomyolipoma (40 – 80%): usually multiple + bilateral; risk of spontaneous hemorrhage (subcapsular / perinephric)
2. Multiple cysts of varying size in cortex + medulla mimicking adult polycystic kidney disease
   Path: cysts lined by columnar epithelium with foci of hyperplasia projecting into cyst lumen

@ LUNG INVOLVEMENT (1%)
- √ interstitial fibrosis in lower lung fields + miliary nodular pattern may progress to honeycomb lung (lymphangioleiomyomatosis = smooth muscle proliferation around blood vessels)
- √ cystic changes of lung parenchyma
- √ spontaneous pneumothorax (50%)
- √ chylothorax
- √ cor pulmonale

@ HEART INVOLVEMENT
- congenital cardiomyopathy
- √ circumscribed / diffuse subendocardial rhabdomyoma (in 5%)

@ BONE INVOLVEMENT
- √ sclerotic calvarial patches (45%) = "bone islands" involving diploe + internal table; frontal + parietal location
- √ thickening of diploe (long-term phenytoin therapy)
- √ bone islands in pelvic brim, vertebrae, long bones
- √ periosteal thickening of long bones
- √ bone cysts with undulating periosteal reaction in distal phalanges (most common), metacarpals, metatarsals (DDx: sarcoid, neurofibromatosis)

@ OTHER VISCERAL INVOLVEMENT
1. Adenomas + lipomyomas of liver
2. Adenomas of pancreas
3. Tumors of spleen

@ VASCULAR INVOLVEMENT (rare)
- √ thoracic + abdominal arterial aneurysms
Path: vascular dysplasia with intimal + medial abnormalities of large muscular + musculoelastic arteries

UNILATERAL MEGALENCEPHALY
= hamartomatous overgrowth of all / part of a cerebral hemisphere with migration defects
- intractable seizure disorder at early age

- √ moderately / marked enlargement of hemisphere
- √ pachygyria + heterotopia of gray matter
- √ gliosis (low density in white matter on CT, prolonged T1 + T2 relaxation times on MR)
- √ lateral ventricle enlarged in proportion to enlargement of affected hemisphere
- √ frontal horn of ipsilateral ventricle straight + pointing anterolaterally

Rx: partial / complete hemispheric resection

VEIN OF GALEN ANEURYSM
= central AVM directly draining into secondarily enlarged vein of Galen (aneurysm is misnomer), fed by anterior cerebral artery, anterior + posterior choroidal arteries, lenticulostriate + thalamic perforating arteries
Age at presentation: neonatal period; detectable in utero >30 weeks GA; M:F = 2:1
- cardiac failure (36%)
- cranial bruit
- headache
- seizures, focal neurologic signs (5%)
- macrocrania from obstructive hydrocephalus

May be associated with porencephaly, nonimmune hydrops

- √ smoothly marginated midline mass posterior to indented 3rd ventricle
- √ prominent serpiginous thalamic network
- √ dilated straight + transverse sinus + torcular herophili
- √ dilatation of lateral + 3rd ventricle (37%)
NCCT:
- √ homogeneous slightly hyperdense mass
- √ hyperdense intracerebral hematoma (ruptured AVM)
- √ focal hypodense zones (ischemic changes)
CECT:
- √ marked homogeneous enhancement of serpentine structures + vein of Galen + straight sinus
OB-US:
- √ median tubular cystic space with high-velocity turbulent flow demonstrated by pulsed / color Doppler
- √ brain infarction / leukomalacia (steal phenomenon with hypoperfusion)
- √ cardiac enlargement (high-output heart failure)
- √ dilated veins of head + neck
- √ hydrocephalus (aqueductal obstruction / posthemorrhagic impairment of CSF absorption)

Cx: subarachnoid hemorrhage
Rx: ligation, excision, embolization of vessels from transtorcular / transarterial approach
Prognosis: high morbidity + mortality (94%)
DDx: pineal tumor, arachnoid / colloid / porencephalic cyst

VENOUS ANGIOMA

= cluster of dilated medullary veins, which drain into an enlarged vein; bleed rarely

Histo: venous channels without internal elastic lamina, separated by gliotic neural tissue that may calcify; probably representing persistent fetal venous system

√ no arterial vessels
√ radially oriented veins at periphery of lesion converging to one vein

DDx: Sturge-Weber disease (diffuse pial angiomatosis with venous-type capillaries)

VENOUS SINUS THROMBOSIS

Septic causes (esp. in childhood):
Mastoiditis, sub- / epidural empyema, meningitis, encephalitis, brain abscess, face + scalp cellulitis, septicemia

Aseptic causes:
(a) Tumor compressing sinuses: meningioma, leukemia
(b) Trauma: fracture through sinus wall, cranial surgery
(c) Low-flow state: CHF, CHD, dehydration, shock
(d) Hypercoagulability: polycythemia vera, idiopathic thrombocytosis, thrombocytopenia, sickle cell disease, cryofibrinogenemia, pregnancy, contraceptive steroids, disseminated intravascular coagulopathy
(e) Chemotherapy: eg, ARA-C
• headaches, seizures
• stroke symptomatology

NCCT:
√ high attenuation material (clotted blood) in sagittal sinus / straight sinus / cerebral cortical vein = "cord sign" (rare)
√ compression of lateral ventricles in 32% (infarction / edema)
√ unilateral (2/3) / bilateral (1/3) parenchymal hemorrhage involving gray + white matter (20%)
CECT:
√ "delta sign" / "empty triangle" = filling defect in straight sinus / superior sagittal sinus (in 70%)
√ gyral enhancement in periphery of infarction (30 – 40%)
√ intense tentorial enhancement secondary to collaterals (rare)
√ dense transcortical medullary vein
Angio:
√ nonfilling of thrombosed sinus
√ filling of cortical veins, deep venous system, cavernous sinus
√ parasagittal hemorrhages (highly specific for superior sagittal sinus thrombosis) secondary to cortical venous infarction
MR:
√ high signal within sinus on T1WI + T2WI
Prognosis: high mortality

VENTRICULITIS

= EPENDYMITIS = inflammation of ependymal lining of one / more ventricles

Cause: (1)   rupture of periventricular abscess (thinner capsule wall medially)
(2)   retrograde spread of infection from basal cisterns

CECT (necessary for diagnosis):
√ thin uniform enhancement of involved ependymal lining
√ often associated with intraventricular inflammatory exudate + septations

Cx: Obstructive hydrocephalus (occlusion at foramen of Monro / aqueduct)
DDx: Ependymal metastases, lymphoma, infiltrating glioma

VENTRICULOPERITONEAL SHUNT COMPLICATION

A. SHUNT MALFUNCTION
   Cause: occlusion of catheter by choroid plexus / glial tissue, disconnection of tubes
   • symptoms of increased intracranial pressure
   • persistent bulging of anterior fontanelle
   • excessive rate of head growth
   √ increasing ventricular size
   √ shuntogram (by scintigram / contrast radiography) determines site of obstruction
   √ brain edema tracking along shunt + within interstices of centrum semiovale (with partial obstruction)
   √ formation of white matter cyst surrounding ventricular catheter

B. SHUNT INFECTION
   Incidence: 1 – 5%
   • intermittent low-grade fever
   • anemia, dehydration, hepatosplenomegaly
   • stiff neck
   • swelling + redness over shunting tract
   • peritonitis
   √ ventriculitis (= enlarged ventricles with irregular enhancing ventricular wall ± septations)

C. ABDOMINAL COMPLICATIONS
   1. Ascites
   2. Pseudocyst formation
   3. Perforation of viscus / abdominal wall
   4. Intestinal obstruction

D. SUBDURAL HEMATOMA
   Cause: precipitous drainage of markedly enlarged ventricles
   Age: usually seen in children >3 years of age
   Prognosis: small hematomas are insignificant

E. GRANULOMATOUS LESION
   = rare granulomatous reaction adjacent to shunt tube within / near ventricle
   √ irregular contrast-enhancing mass along course of shunt tube

F. SLIT VENTRICLE SYNDROME
    = symptoms from shunt failure in absence of
       ventricular enlargement (poorly defined syndrome)
    √ normal imaging studies

VISCERAL LARVA MIGRANS OF BRAIN
roundworm nematode (Toxocara canis)
√ small calcific nodules, especially in basal ganglia +
   periventricular
DDx: tuberous sclerosis

VON HIPPEL-LINDAU DISEASE
= vHL= RETINOCEREBELLAR ANGIOMATOSIS
= uncommon autosomal dominant disease with variable
   penetrance; 20% familial; M:F = 1:1
Dx:
   (a) >1 hemangioblastoma of CNS
   (b) 1 hemangioblastoma + visceral manifestation
   (c) 1 manifestation + known family history

@ CNS MANIFESTATION
   Age at presentation: 25 – 35 years
   • cerebellar symptoms: vertigo, dysdiadochokinesia,
      dysmetria, Romberg sign
   • signs of increased intracranial pressure: headache,
      vomiting
   • vision changes: reactive retinal inflammation with
      exudate + hemorrhage, retinal detachment,
      glaucoma, cataract, uveitis, decreasing visual acuity,
      eye pain
   • spinal cord symptoms (uncommon): loss of
      sensation, impaired proprioception

   1. Retinal angiomatosis = **von Hippel tumor** (>50%)
       earliest manifestation of disease; multiple in up to
       66%, bilateral in up to 50%
       Dx: indirect ophthalmoscopy + fluorescein
              angiography
       √ small tumors rarely detected by imaging studies
       √ retinal detachment
       √ thick calcified retinal density (calcified angioma-
         induced hematoma)

   2. Hemangioblastomas of CNS = **Lindau tumor**
       = most commonly recognized manifestation of vHL
         disease; multifocal in 10%

   Δ 4 – 20% of single hemangioblastomas occur in
      von Hippel-Lindau disease
   Age: 15 – 40 years
   Site: posterior fossa (88%) mostly in cerebellar
          hemisphere (90%), some in vermis, a few
          close to 4th ventricle, medulla, spinal cord
   CT:
      √ cystic mass in 75%, solid (iso- / hyperdense /
        mixed) in 25%
      √ intense tumor blush / blushing mural nodule
      √ NO calcifications (DDx: cystic astrocytoma
        calcifies in 25%)
   MR:
      √ small tubular areas of flow void within solid
        nodule (= enlarged feeding + draining vessels)
      √ prolongation of T1 + T2 relaxation times with
        contrast enhancement in solid tumor
   Angio: to identify small tumor nodule + other small
           hemangioblastomas
   Prognosis: frequent recurrence after resection

@ ADRENAL pheochromocytoma (in up to 10 – 15%)

@ RENAL
   • elevated erythropoeitin with polycythemia (10 – 20%)
   1. Multiple cortical cysts (75%)
   2. Angiomas
   3. Renal cell carcinoma (in up to 40%): age of 20 – 50
       years, in 10% bilateral, frequently multicentric

MULTIPLE ORGAN NEOPLASMS
   @ Kidney   : renal cell carcinoma (up to 40%)
                      renal angioma (up to 45%)
   @ Liver   : adenoma, angioma
   @ Pancreas   : cystadenoma / adenocarcinoma
   @ Epididymis   : adenoma
   @ Adrenal gland: pheochromocytoma

MULTIPLE ORGAN CYSTS
   (1) Kidney (usually multiple cortical cysts in 75 – 100%
        at early age, most common abdominal
        manifestation)
   (2) Pancreas (in 9 – 72% often numerous cysts;
        second most common affected abdominal organ)
   (3) Others: liver, spleen, omentum, mesentery,
        epididymis, adrenals, lung, bone

DIFFERENTIAL DIAGNOSIS OF ORBITAL DISORDERS

Intraconal lesion
mnemonic: "**M**el **M**et **R**ita **M**ending **H**ems **O**n **P**oor
Charlie's **G**rave"

Melanoma
Metastasis
Retinoblastoma
Meningioma
Hemangioma
Optic glioma
Pseudotumor
Cellulitis
Grave disease

Intraconal lesion with optic nerve involvement
1. Optic nerve glioma
2. Optic nerve sheath meningioma (10% of orbital neoplasm)
3. Optic neuritis
4. Inflammatory pseudotumor (may surround optic nerve)
5. Intraorbital lymphoma (may surround optic nerve, older patient)
6. Elevated intracranial pressure
   = distension of optic sheath
   √ bilateral tortuous enlarged optic nerve-sheath complex

Intraconal lesion without optic nerve involvement
1. Cavernous hemangioma
2. Orbital varix
3. Carotid-cavernous fistula
4. Arteriovenous malformation
   least common of orbital vascular malformations (congenital, idiopathic, traumatic)
   √ irregularly shaped intensely enhancing mass of enlarged vessels
   √ associated with dilated superior / inferior ophthalmic vein
5. Hematoma
6. Lymphangioma
7. Neurilemoma
   √ commonly adjacent to superior orbital fissure, inferior to optic nerve
   √ local bone erosion

Extraconal lesion
Extraconal-intraorbital lesion
A. BENIGN TUMOR
   1. Dermoid cyst
   2. **Teratoma**
      <1% of all pediatric orbital tumors
      √ ± areas of fat, cartilage, bone
      √ expansion of bony orbit ± bone defect

3. Capillary hemangioma
4. Lymphangioma
5. Plexiform neurofibroma
6. Inflammatory orbital pseudotumor
7. Histiocytosis X
   lesion usually arises from bone
B. MALIGNANT TUMOR
   1. Lymphoma / Leukemia
   2. Metastasis
   3. Rhabdomyosarcoma

Extraconal-extraorbital lesion
A. FROM SINUS
   maxillary / sphenoid sinuses are rare locations of origin
   1. Tumor: squamous cell carcinoma (80%), adenocarcinoma, adenoid cystic carcinoma, lymphoma
   2. Paranasal sinusitis:
      most common cause of orbital infection; originating from ethmoid sinuses (in children), from frontal sinus (in adolescence)
      Organism: Staphylococcus, Streptococcus, Pneumococcus
      √ preseptal / orbital edema / cellulitis
      √ subperiosteal / orbital abscess
      √ mucormycosis (in diabetics) destroys bone + extends into cavernous sinus
      Cx: (1) epidural abscess (2) subdural empyema (3) cavernous sinus thrombosis (4) meningitis (5) cerebritis (6) brain abscess
   3. Mucocele
B. FROM SKIN
   1. Orbital cellulitis
C. FROM LACRIMAL GLAND
   √ mass arising from superolateral aspect of orbit

mnemonic: "MOLD"
   Metastasis
   Others (rhabdomyosarcoma, lymphangioma, sinus lesion)
   Lymphoma, **L**acrimal gland tumor
   Dermoid

Orbital mass in childhood
1. Dermoid cyst   46%
2. Inflammatory lesion   16%
3. Dermolipoma   7%
4. Capillary hemangioma   4%
5. Rhabdomyosarcoma   4%
6. Leukemia / lymphoma   2%
7. Optic nerve glioma   2%
8. Lymphangioma   2%
9. Cavernous hemangioma   1%

PRIMARY MALIGNANT ORBITAL TUMORS
1. Retinoblastoma   86.0%
2. Rhabdomyosarcoma   8.1%
3. Uveal melanoma   2.3%
4. Sarcoma   1.7%

SECONDARY MALIGNANT ORBITAL TUMORS
1. Leukemia   36.7%
2. Sarcoma   14.3%
3. Hodgkin lymphoma   11.0%
4. Neuroblastoma   9.2%
5. Wilms tumor   6.7%
6. Non-Hodgkin lymphoma   5.6%
7. Histiocytosis   3.9%
8. Medulloblastoma   3.5%

ORBITAL VASCULAR TUMORS
1. Orbital varix
2. Arteriovenous malformation
3. Carotid-cavernous fistula
4. Hemangioma: capillary / cavernous
5. Blood cyst
6. Arterial malformation
7. Glomus tumor
8. Hemangiopericytoma

mnemonic: "LO VISHON"
Leukemia, **L**ymphoma
Optic nerve glioma
Vascular malformation: hemangioma, lymphangioma
Inflammation
Sarcoma: ie, rhabdomyosarcoma
Histiocytosis
Orbital pseudotumor, **O**steoma
Neuroblastoma

Mass in superolateral quadrant of orbit
1. Lacrimal gland tumor
2. Dermoid cyst
3. Metastasis (breast, prostate, lung)
4. Lymphoma
5. Leukemic infiltration of lacrimal gland
6. Sarcoidosis
7. Wegener granulomatosis
8. Pseudotumor
9. Frontal sinus mucocele

Extraocular muscle enlargement
A. Endocrine
   1. Grave disease (50%)
   2. Acromegaly
B. Inflammation
   1. **Myositis**
      • rapid onset of proptosis, erythema of lids, conjunctival injection
      Location: single muscle (in adults);
                  multiple muscles (in children)
      √ enlarged extraocular muscle
      √ positive response to steroids
   2. Orbital cellulitis

3. Sjögren disease, Wegener granulomatosis, lethal midline granuloma, SLE
   4. Sarcoidosis
   5. Foreign body reaction
C. Tumor
   1. Pseudotumor
   2. Rhabdomyosarcoma
   3. Metastasis, lymphoma, leukemia
D. Vascular
   1. Spontaneous / traumatic hematoma
   2. Arteriovenous malformation
   3. Carotid-cavernous sinus fistula

GLOBE
Ocular lesion
Intraocular calcifications
1. Retinoblastoma
2. **Astrocytic hamartoma**
   associated with tuberous sclerosis
   + neurofibromatosis
   Location: retina / near optic disc
   √ typically unilateral (DDx to drusen)
3. **Choroidal osteoma**
   young woman; mature bone
   √ very dense curvilinear mass aligned with choroidal margin of globe
4. **Optic drusen**
   = accretions of hyaline material on / near surface of optic disc; often familial
   • headache, visual field defects
   • pseudopapilledema
   √ small flat / round calcification at junction of retina + optic nerve
   √ bilateral in 75%
5. Scleral calcifications
   (a) in systemic hypercalcemic states (HPT, hypervitaminosis D, sarcoidosis, secondary to chronic renal disease)
   (b) in elderly: at insertion of extraocular muscles
6. Retrolental fibroplasia
7. **Phthisis bulbi**
   secondary to trauma or infection
   √ small contracted calcified disorganized nonfunctioning globe

Noncalcified ocular process
1. Uveal melanoma
2. Metastasis
   86% of ocular lesions within globe; usually in vascular choroid
   Origin: breast, lung, GI tract, GU tract, cutaneous melanoma, neuroblastoma
   √ bilateral in 30%
3. **Choroidal hemangioma**
   most common benign tumor in adults
   may be associated with: Sturge-Weber syndrome
   √ focal thickening of posterior wall of globe
   √ enhancement similar to choroid
4. **Vitreous lymphoma**
   √ diffuse ill-defined soft tissue density

5. Developmental anomalies
    (a) **Primary glaucoma** = enlargement of eye secondary to narrowing of Schlemm canal
    (b) **Coloboma** = congenital incomplete closure of embryonic choroidal fissure affecting eyelid / iris / retina / macula; autosomal dominant trait; bilateral in 60%
        √ small globe with cystic outpouching of vitreous at site of optic nerve attachment
        DDx: duplication cyst, axial (high) myopia
    (c) **Staphyloma** = berry-like protrusion of cornea / pear-shaped sacculation of posterior pole secondary to high myopia, glaucoma, trauma

Microphthalmia

= congenital underdevelopment / acquired diminution of globe
A. BILATERAL with cataract
    1. Congenital rubella
    2. Persistent hyperplastic vitreous
    3. Retinopathy of prematurity
    4. Retinal folds
    5. Lowe syndrome
    √ small globe + small orbit
B. UNILATERAL
    1. Trauma / surgery
    2. Inflammation with disorganization of eye (phthisis bulbi)
    √ shrunken calcified globe + normal orbit

Macrophthalmia

= enlargement of globe
1. Myopia
2. Juvenile glaucoma
3. Buphthalmos = severe form of juvenile glaucoma

Dense vitreous in pediatric age group

1. Retinoblastoma
2. Persistent hyperplastic primary vitreous
3. Coats disease
4. Norrie disease
5. Retrolental fibroplasia
6. Sclerosing endophthalmitis

Leukokoria

= abnormal white / pinkish / yellowish pupillary light reflex
A. TUMOR
    1. Retinoblastoma (most common cause)
    2. Medulloepithelioma (rare)
B. DEVELOPMENTAL
    1. Persistent hyperplastic primary vitreous (2nd most common cause)
    2. Coats disease
    3. Retrolental fibroplasia
    4. Coloboma of choroid / optic disk
C. INFECTION
    1. Uveitis
    2. Larval granulomatosis

D. DEGENERATIVE
    1. Posterior cataract
E. TRAUMA
    1. Organized vitreous hemorrhage
    2. Long-standing retinal detachment

Optic nerve enlargement

A. TUMOR:
    1. Optic nerve glioma
    2. Optic nerve sheath meningioma
    3. Infiltration by leukemia / lymphoma
B. FLUID:
    4. Perineural hematoma
    5. Papilledema of intracranial hypertension
    6. Patulous subarachnoid space
C. INFLAMMATION:
    7. Optic neuritis
    8. Sarcoidosis

√ fusiform thickening
    = lens-shaped thickening of nerve-sheath complex
    (a) with central lucency: meningioma
    (b) without central lucency: optic nerve glioma
√ excrescentic thickening
    = single / multiple nodules along nerve-sheath complex usually due to tumor
√ tubular enlargement
    = uniform enlargement of nerve-sheath complex
    (a) with central lucency: subarachnoid process (metastases, perineuritis, meningioma, perineural hemorrhage)
    (b) without central lucency: papilledema, leukemia, lymphoma, sarcoid, optic nerve glioma

LACRIMAL GLAND

Lacrimal gland lesion

A. INFLAMMATION
    1. **Dacryoadenitis**
    2. **Mikulicz syndrome**
        = nonspecific enlargement of lacrimal + salivary glands
        Associated with   sarcoidosis, lymphoma, leukemia
    3. **Sjögren syndrome**
        = lymphocytic infiltration of lacrimal + salivary glands
        • decreased lacrimation, xerostomia
        Often associated with   rheumatoid arthritis, systemic lupus erythematosus, scleroderma, polymyositis
    4. Sarcoidosis
B. TUMOR
    (a) benign: granuloma, cyst, benign mixed tumor (= pleomorphic adenoma)
    (b) malignant: malignant mixed tumor (= pleomorphic adenocarcinoma), adenoid cystic carcinoma, lymphoma, metastasis (rare)

Ophthalmoplegia

Lesions of
1. Oculomotor nerve (III)
   innervates medial rectus, superior rectus, inferior rectus, inferior oblique muscle, pupilloconstrictor, levator palpebrae
2. Trochlear nerve (IV)
   innervates superior oblique muscle
3. Abducens nerve (VI)
   innervates lateral rectus muscle

Anopia

A. Monocular defects
   1 = monocular blindness (optic nerve lesion in fracture of optic canal, amaurosis fugax)
B. Bilateral heteronymous defects
   2 = bitemporal hemianopia (chiasmatic lesion)
C. Bilateral homonymous defects
   3   = homonymous hemianopia
   4   = upper right-sided quadrantanopia
   5   = central hemianoptic scotoma

3,4,5 = most common type of hemianopia (CVA, brain tumor)

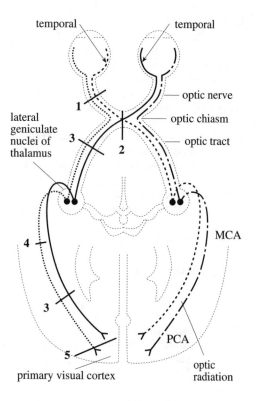

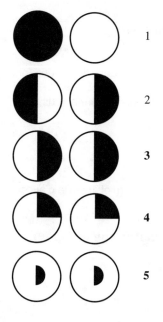

Types of Anopia

ANATOMY OF ORBIT

Orbital connections

Superior orbital fissure

Boundaries:
— medial : body of sphenoid
— above : lesser wing of sphenoid = optic strut
— below : greater wing of sphenoid
— lateral : frontal bone

Contents:
(a) nerves: III oculomotor n.
IV trochlear n.
V_1 ophthalmic branch of trigeminal n.:
  (a) lacrimal nerve
  (b) frontal nerve
VI abducens n.
sympathetic filaments of internal carotid plexus
(b) veins: superior + inferior ophthalmic vein
(c) arteries: 1. meningeal branch of lacrimal artery
2. orbital branch of middle meningeal artery

Inferior orbital fissure

Location: between floor + lateral wall of orbit; connects with pterygopalatine + infratemporal fossa

Contents:
(a) nerves: infraorbital + zygomatic nn.
branches from pterygopalatine ganglion
(b) veins: connection between inferior orbital v. + pterygoid plexus

Optic canal

completely formed by lesser wing of sphenoid
Contents:
(a) nerve: optic nerve (I)
(b) vessel: ophthalmic a.

Normal orbit measurements

Muscles
medial rectus muscle ....4.1 ± 0.5 mm
inferior rectus muscle................4.9 ± 0.8 mm
superior rectus muscle..............3.8 ± 0.7 mm
lateral rectus muscle ....2.9 ± 0.6 mm
superior oblique muscle ....2.4 ± 0.4 mm
Superior ophthalmic vein
axial CT....................................1.8 ± 0.5 mm
coronal CT ....2.7 ± 1.0 mm
Optic nerve sheath
retrobulbar ....5.5 ± 0.8 mm
waist.......................................4.2 ± 0.6 mm
Globe position
behind interzygomatic line ....9.9 ± 1.7 mm

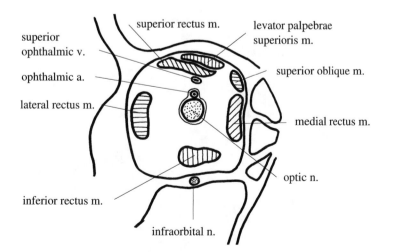

Coronal orbital tomogram through mid-orbit

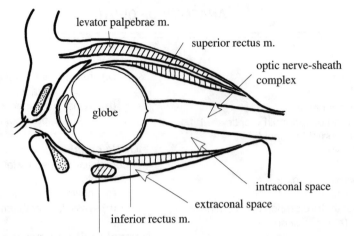

Orbital spaces

globe:	subdivided into anterior + posterior segments by lens
optic nerve-sheath complex:	optic nerve surrounded by meningeal sheath as extension from cerebral meninges
intraconal space:	orbital fat, ophthalmic a., superior ophthalmic v., nerves I, III, IV, V_1, VI
conus:	incomplete fenestrated musculofascial system extending from bony orbit to anterior third of globe, consists of extraocular muscles + interconnecting fascia
extraconal space:	between muscle cone + bony orbit containing fat, lacrimal gland, lacrimal sac, portion of superior ophthalmic v.

ORBITAL DISORDERS

CAROTID-CAVERNOUS SINUS FISTULA
Etiology:
- (1) Trauma: laceration of ICA within cavernous sinus
  - (a) usually secondary to basal skull fracture (cavernous ICA + small cavernous branches fixed to dura)
  - (b) penetrating trauma
- (2) Spontaneous: rupture of an intracavernous ICA aneurysm

Route of drainage:
- (a) superior ophthalmic vein (common)
- (b) contralateral cavernous sinus
- (c) petrosal sinus
- (d) cortical veins (rare)
- pulsating exophthalmus, chemosis, conjunctival edema, persistent bruit
- restricted extraocular movement
- decrease in vision due to increase in intraocular pressure (50%) = indication for emergent treatment

√ enlarged edematous extraocular muscles
√ dilatation of superior ophthalmic vein / facial veins / internal jugular vein
√ focal / diffuse enlargement of cavernous sinus
√ occasionally sellar erosion / enlargement
√ enlargement of superior orbital fissure (in chronic phase)
US + MR:
  √ arterial flow in cavernous sinus + superior ophthalmic vein
Angio:
  √ ipsilateral ICA contrast injection shows wall of ICA to be incomplete
  √ contralateral ICA contrast injection + compression of involved ICA
Rx: latex / silicone balloon detached inside cavernous sinus to plug laceration (ocular signs resolve within 7 – 10 days)

COATS DISEASE
= Pseudoglioma = congenital vascular malformation of the retina characterized by multiple telangiectasis + detachment of retina secondary to leakage of lipoproteinaceous exudate from these vessels with accumulation in retina + subretinal space
Age: 6 – 8 years; M:F = 2:1
- may present with unilateral leukokoria (if retina massively detached)
√ unilateral dense vitreous in normal sized globe
√ NO focal mass / calcification
DDx: persistent hyperplastic vitreous, retinopathy of prematurity

DACRYOADENITIS
= infection of lacrimal gland
Organism: staphylococci (most common), mumps, infectious mononucleosis, influenza

√ homogeneous enlargement of lacrimal gland
√ ± compression of globe

DERMOID CYST OF ORBIT
Most common benign orbital tumor in childhood (45% of all masses)
Age: 1st decade
Histo: contains keratin, hair, stratified epithelium + dermal appendages within thick capsule; usually arises in fetal cleavage planes (sutures)
Location: in anterior extraconal orbit, upper temporal quadrant (60%), upper nasal quadrant (25%)
√ well-defined cystic mass ± negative HU numbers
√ thick surrounding capsule
√ ± expansion / erosion of bony orbit
MR:
  √ high signal intensity on T1WI + T2WI

ENDOPHTHALMITIS
- A. INFECTIOUS ENDOPHTHALMITIS
  most commonly related to eye injury / surgery
  √ increased attenuation of vitreous
  √ uveal-scleral thickening
  √ decreased attenuation of lens
- B. SCLEROSING ENDOPHTHALMITIS
  = TOXOCARA CANIS ENDOPHTHALMITIS
  = granulomatous uveitis resulting in subretinal exudate, retinal detachment, organized vitreous; chorioretinitis in 80%, bilateral in 85%
  Age: 2 – 8 years
  Mode of infection: playing in soil contaminated by dog excrement
  - convulsions
  √ obliteration of vitreous cavity with increase in density
  √ contrast enhancement of sclera
  √ intracranial calcifications
  Dx: enzyme-linked immunosorbent assay

GRAVES DISEASE OF ORBIT
= THYROID OPHTHALMOPATHY
= ENDOCRINE EXOPHTHALMUS
Δ Most common cause of uni- / bilateral proptosis in adult!
= increase in orbital pressure produces ischemia, edema, fibrosis of muscles
Etiology: produced by long-acting thyroid stimulating factor (LATS)
Age: adulthood; 5% younger than 15 years; M:F = 1:4
Histo: deposition of hygroscopic mucopolysaccharides + glycoprotein (early) + collagen (late); infiltration by mast cells and lymphocytes, edema, muscle fiber necrosis, lipomatosis, fatty degeneration
Time of onset: signs + symptoms usually develop within one year of the onset of hyperthyroidism
- proptosis
- lid lag = upper eyelid retraction

- periorbital swelling
- conjunctival injection
- restricted ocular motility (correlates with increase in mean muscle diameters)
- optic neuropathy (associated with apical crowding)
- hyperthyroidism; euthyroidism (in 10 – 15%); severity of orbital involvement unrelated to degree of thyroid dysfunction

STAGING (Werner's modified classification):
Stage I: eyelid retraction without symptoms
Stage II: eyelid retraction with symptoms
Stage III: proptosis >22 mm without diplopia
Stage IV: proptosis >22 mm with diplopia
Stage V: corneal ulceration
Stage VI: loss of sight

Location:
all muscles equally affected with similar proportional enlargements; superior muscle group most commonly when only single muscle involved [former notion: inferior > medial > superior rectus muscle + levator palpebrae > lateral rectus muscle]; bilateral in 70 – 85%; single muscle in 10%; asymmetrical involvement in 10 – 30%
√ proptosis = globe protrusion >21 mm anterior to interzygomatic line on axial scans at level of lens
√ swelling of muscles maximally in midportion (relative sparing of tendinous insertion at globe) = "Coke-bottle" sign
√ slight uveal-scleral thickening
√ apical crowding = orbital apex involved late (pressure on optic nerve)
√ dilatation of superior ophthalmic vein (compromised orbital venous drainage at orbital apex due to enlarged extraocular muscles)
√ increase in diameter of retrobulbar optic nerve sheath (dural distension due to accumulation of CSF in subarachnoid space with optic neuropathy)
√ increased density of orbital fat (late)
MR:
   √ high signal intensity in enlarged eye muscles on T2WI (edema in acute inflammation)
Prognosis: in 90% spontaneous resolution within 3 – 36 months; in 10% decrease in visual acuity (corneal ulceration / optic neuropathy)
Rx: short- and long-term steroid therapy, radiation, surgical decompression, correction of eyelid position
DDx: pseudotumor (usually includes tendon of eye muscles)

HEMANGIOMA OF ORBIT
Most common benign orbital tumor
(a) CAPILLARY HEMANGIOMA
      most common vascular tumor of orbit in children; 5 – 15% of all pediatric orbital masses
      Age: first 2 weeks of life; 95% in <6 months of age; M < F
      Histo: proliferation of endothelial cells with multiple capillaries

- proptosis, chemosis (= edema) of eyelid + conjunctiva exaggerated by crying
- associated with skin angioma (90%)
√ mass with enhancement equal to / greater than orbital muscle
√ poorly marginated (suggesting malignant cause)
√ activity in radionuclide flow studies
Prognosis: often increase in size for 6 – 10 months followed by spontaneous involution within 1 – 2 years
(b) CAVERNOUS HEMANGIOMA
      usually tumor of adulthood;
      1 – 2% of childhood orbital masses
      Age: 20 – 40 years; F > M
      Histo: large dilated venous channels with flattened endothelial cells surrounded by fibrous pseudocapsule
- slowly progressive unilateral proptosis, diplopia, diminished visual acuity (optic nerve compression)

Location: 83 – 94% retrobulbar (intraconal)
√ sharply demarcated oval mass in superior-temporal portion of conus (2/3) often sparing orbital apex
√ displacement (not involvement) of optic nerve
√ expansion of bony orbit
√ uniform / inhomogeneous (when thrombosed) enhancement
√ small calcifications (phleboliths)
√ puddling of contrast material on angiography

INFECTION OF ORBIT
Cause: bacterial infection extending from paranasal sinuses (especially ethmoid + frontal sinuses), face, eyelid, nose, teeth, lacrimal sac through thin lamina papyracea + valveless facial veins into orbit
Organism: staphylococci, streptococci, pneumococci
- lid edema, ocular pain, ophthalmoplegia
- fever, elevated WBC
Location: preseptal = periorbital soft tissue; subperiosteal; peripheral = extraconal fat; extraocular muscles; central = intraconal fat; optic nerve complex; globe; lacrimal gland
Cx: epidural abscess, subdural empyema, cavernous sinus thrombosis, cerebral abscess, osteomyelitis

Abscess of Orbit
Location: most commonly in subperiosteal space on medial wall
√ subperiosteal fluid collection
√ displacement of thickened periosteal membrane + increased enhancement
√ displacement of adjacent fat + extraocular muscles
MR:
   √ hyperintensity on T1WI + T2WI

Cellulitis of Orbit
√ thickening of eyelids + septum
√ proptosis
√ scleral thickening

√ enlargement + displacement of extraocular muscles (frequently medial rectus muscle)

√ increased attenuation of orbital fat + obliteration of fat planes

√ opacification of ethmoid + maxillary sinuses

DDx: cannot be differentiated from edema, chloroma, leukemic infiltrate

Edema of Orbit

Location: usually confined to preseptal structures (eyelid, face); involvement of orbital structures (rare)

√ swelling of eyelids / face

√ increased attenuation of orbital fat + obliteration of fat planes

√ displacement + enlargement of extraocular muscles

MR:

√ hyperintensity on T2WI

LYMPHANGIOMA OF ORBIT

Incidence: 3.5:100,000; 1 – 2% of orbital childhood masses; 8% of expanding orbital lesions

Histo:

dilated lymphatics, dysplastic venous vessels, smooth muscle, areas of hemorrhage

(a) simple / capillary lymphangioma
= lymphatic channels of capillary size

(b) cavernous lymphangioma
= dilated microscopic channels

(c) cystic hygroma
= macroscopic multilocular cystic mass

Age: 1st decade or later

• proptosis (sudden proptosis from spontaneous intratumoral hemorrhage = CARDINAL FEATURE; exacerbated during upper respiratory infections [rare])

• associated with lesions on lid, conjunctiva, cheek

• coincident lymphangiomatous cysts in oral mucosa

Location: usually medial to optic nerve with intra- and extraconal component, crossing anatomic boundaries (conal fascia / orbital septum)

√ poorly defined multilobulated inhomogeneous lesion

√ single / multiple cystlike areas with rim enhancement (after hemorrhage) = blood cyst = "chocolate cyst"

√ areas of enhancement (= venous channels) / ring enhancement (after hemorrhage)

√ rarely contains phleboliths (DDx: hemangioma, orbital varix)

√ mild to moderate enlargement of orbit

MR:

√ may show hematoma of various duration within lesion

Prognosis: no involution, progression slows with termination of body growth

DDx: orbital varix

LYMPHOMA OF ORBIT

Usually presents without evidence of systemic disease; subsequent development of systemic disease frequent

Incidence: 3rd most common cause of proptosis after orbital pseudotumor + cavernous hemangioma

Age: 50 years on average

Type: usually non-Hodgkin B-cell lymphoma; Hodgkin disease rare

• painless swelling of eyelid

• exophthalmos (late in course of disease)

Location: extraconal (especially lacrimal gland, anterior extraconal space, retrobulbar) > intraconal > optic nerve-sheath complex; may be bilateral

Δ Lacrimal gland is a common site for leukemic infiltration!

Growth types:

(a) well-defined high-density mass (most commonly about lacrimal gland)

(b) diffuse infiltration (tends to involve entire intraconal region)

√ slight to moderate enhancement

METASTASIS TO ORBIT

Origin: only in 50% known; carcinoma of breast + lung (adults); neuroblastoma, Ewing sarcoma, leukemia, Wilms tumor (children)

Location: 12% intraorbital, 86% intraocular especially in posterior temporal portion of uvea (vascular layer between retina + sclera) near macula; may be bilateral

CT:

√ small areas of thickening + increased density

√ subretinal fluid

NORRIE DISEASE

= RETINAL DYSPLASIA

= X-linked recessive disease; ? inherited form of persistent hyperplastic primary vitreous

• seizures, mental deficiency (50%)

• hearing loss, deafness by age 4 (30%)

• leukokoria, cataract, blindness

√ microphthalmia

√ dense vitreous with blood-fluid level

√ cone-shaped central retinal detachment

√ calcifications

OPTIC NERVE GLIOMA

= JUVENILE PILOCYTIC ASTROCYTOMA

= most common cause of optic nerve enlargement

Incidence: 1% of all intracranial tumors, 2% of childhood orbital masses; 80% of primary tumors of optic nerve

Histo: proliferation of well-differentiated astrocytes = low-grade glial neoplasm; most commonly pilocytic astrocytoma (in children) + glioblastoma (in adults)

Age: 1st decade (80%); peak age around 5 years; M < F

Associated with neurofibromatosis in 10 – 50% (± bilateral optic gliomas)

Δ 15% of patients with neurofibromatosis have optic nerve gliomas!

• decreased visual acuity, minimal axial proptosis

√ tubular / fusiform / excrescentic well-circumscribed enlargement of optic nerve
√ posterior extension along optic tracts in 60 – 70% (indicates nonresectability)
√ calcifications (rare)
√ same attenuation as normal optic nerve; slight contrast enhancement
√ ipsilateral optic canal enlargement (90%) >3 mm / 1 mm difference compared with contralateral side
MR: more sensitive than CT in detecting intracanalicular + intracranial extent
√ isointense to muscle on T1WI
√ hyperintense on T2WI
DDx: optic nerve sheath meningioma (no intracranial extension along optic pathway)

OPTIC NERVE SHEATH MENINGIOMA
= PERIOPTIC MENINGIOMA
Incidence: 10% of all intraorbital neoplasms; <2% of intracranial meningiomas
Age: middle-aged + elderly females; slightly more aggressive in children
Occasionally associated with
     neurofibromatosis (usually in teenagers)

Primary origin:
     arising from arachnoid rests in the meningeal investiture of optic nerves in orbit / middle fossa
• progressive loss of visual acuity over months (optic atrophy), proptosis

√ tubular (most commonly) / fusiform / excrescentic thickening of optic nerve
√ sphenoid bone hyperostosis
√ frequently calcified (HIGHLY SUGGESTIVE)
CECT: enhancement is the rule
     √ dense linear bands (axial view) as "tram tracks" / ring-like (coronal view) due to tumor enhancement around non-enhancing optic nerve
     √ minimal extension into optic canal (not uncommon)
MR:
     √ extrinsic soft tissue mass surrounding optic nerve
     √ hypointense to fat on T1WI

OPTIC NEURITIS
= nerve involvement by inflammation, degeneration, demyelination
Etiology: (1) multiple sclerosis (involves optic nerve in 1/3) (2) inflammation secondary to ocular infection (3) degeneration (toxic, metabolic, nutritional) (4) ischemia (5) meningitis / encephalitis
• sudden onset of central vision defect
• orbital pain
CT:
     √ normal / mildly enlarged optic nerve + chiasm
     √ may show enhancement
MR:
     √ mild enlargement + enhancement of optic nerve well demonstrated on axial T1WI

PERSISTENT HYPERPLASTIC PRIMARY VITREOUS
= rare condition with persistence + hyperplasia of embryonic hyaloid vascular system of primary vitreous (= hyaloid canal of Cloquet); friable vessels may lead to intravitreal hemorrhage
May be associated with   any severe ocular malformation / optic dysplasia (eg, Norrie disease)

— Primary vitreous
     = fibrillar ectodermal + mesodermal tissue consisting primarily of embryonic hyaloid vascular system
     Occupies space between lens + retina, involutes by 6th month of gestation
— Hyaloid artery
     = important source of intraocular nutrition until 8th month of gestation
     Arises from dorsal opthalmic artery at 3rd week of gestation; grows anteriorly with branches supplying vitreous + posterior aspect of lens
— Secondary / adult vitreous
     Begins to form during 3rd gestational month; gradually replaces primary vitreous, which is reduced to a small S-shaped remnant (hyaloid canal = Cloquet canal) and serves as lymph channel

• unilateral leukokoria
• seizures, mental deficiency, hearing loss
• cataract
CT:
     √ microphthalmia = small hypoplastic globe
     √ small optic nerve
     √ deformity of globe + lens
     √ dense vitreous
     √ vitreous fluid-fluid levels (from breakdown of recurrent hemorrhage in subhyaloid / subretinal space)
     √ enhancing cone-shaped central retrolental density extending from lens through vitreous body to back of orbit, just lateral to optic nerve
     √ NO calcifications
MR:
     √ hyperintense vitreous body on T1WI + T2WI from vitreous hemorrhage / proteinaceous fluid
     √ hypointense thin triangular band with base near optic disk and apex at posterior surface of lens
Cx:
     (1) Glaucoma, cataract from recurrent spontaneous intraocular hemorrhage
     (2) Proliferation of embryonic tissue
     (3) Retinal detachment from organizing hemorrhage / traction
     (4) Hydrops / atrophy of globe + resorption of lens

PSEUDOTUMOR OF ORBIT
= IDIOPATHIC INFLAMMATORY PSEUDOTUMOR
= nongranulomatous inflammatory process affecting all intraorbital soft tissues
Etiology:
     (a) cause not apparent at time of study: bacterial, viral, foreign body

(b) systemic disease presently not apparent: sarcoidosis, collagen, endocrine

(c) idiopathic: probably abnormal immune response

Incidence: 25% of all cases of unilateral exophthalmos; most common cause of an intraorbital mass lesion in adult

Age: young female

Histo: lymphocytic infiltrate

May be associated with: Wegener granulomatosis, sarcoidosis, fibrosing mediastinitis, retroperitoneal fibrosis, thyroiditis, cholangitis, vasculitis, lymphoma

• unilateral painful ophthalmoplegia
• proptosis, chemosis, lid injection
• limitation of ocular movement

Location: retrobulbar fat (76%), extraocular muscle (57%), optic nerve (38%), uveal-scleral area (33%), lacrimal gland (5%)

(a) Tumefactive type (common)
  √ discrete / poorly defined intra- / extraconal mass = "pseudotumor" close to surface margin of globe

(b) Myositic type (unusual)
  √ enlargement of one / more extraocular muscles close to insertion in globe with ill-defined margins
  √ typically involves muscles + tendon insertions (DDx to Graves disease with muscle involvement only)

√ increased density of retro-orbital fat (may involve anterior compartment)
√ thickening and enhancement of sclera near Tenon capsule
√ enlarged lacrimal gland
√ proptosis

MR:
  √ lesion isointense to fat on T2WI

Prognosis:
(1) remitting / chronic + progressive course
(2) rapid dramatic + lasting response to steroid therapy

DDx:
lymphoma (may be confused with lymphoma clinically, radiographically, pathologically), thyroid ophthalmopathy (tapering of distal muscles, painless proptosis), radiation therapy

RETINOBLASTOMA

= primary intraocular malignant tumor of childhood arising from photoreceptor cells (neuroectoderm) of retina

(a) sporadic
(b) autosomal dominant (10 – 40%): bilateral (25 – 31%), multicentric within same eye (25 – 33%), often accompanied by small cell tumor in pineal region

Incidence: 1:15,000 – 30,000 live births; most common intraocular malignancy in childhood

Age: 18 months at presentation; 98% in children <2 years of age

Histo: Flexner-Wintersteiner rosettes

May be associated with:
(1) Pinealoblastoma = **Trilateral retinoblastoma** (rare variant) = bilateral retinoblastomas + neuroectodermal pineal tumor
(2) Osteosarcoma + other CNS neoplasms

• "cat's eye" = leukokoria (whitish mass behind lens)
• decreased visual acuity, eye pain
• strabismus, proptosis (less common)

Location: posterolateral wall of globe (most commonly); 60% unilateral, 40% bilateral

CT:
  √ solid smoothly marginated lobulated retrolental hyperdense mass in endophytic type (rarer exophytic type grows subretinally causing retinal detachment)
  √ partial punctate / complete calcification (50 – 95%)
  √ dense vitreous (common)
  √ extraocular extension (in 25%): optic nerve enlargement, abnormal soft tissue in orbit, intracranial extension
  √ contrast enhancement usual

Cx:
(1) Metastases to: meninges (via subarachnoid space), bone marrow, liver, lymph nodes
(2) radiation-induced sarcomas develop in 15 – 20%

Prognosis: spontaneous regression in 1%; calcifications = favorable prognostic sign; contrast enhancement = poor prognostic sign

DDx:
(1) Retinoma = Retinocytoma (benign variant)
(2) Toxocara canis infection (no calcification)
(3) Retrolental fibroplasia
(4) Coats disease (subretinal exudation, no calcification)
(5) Norrie disease (retinal dysplasia)
(6) Persistent hyperplastic primary vitreous (hypoplastic globe, no calcification)

RETROLENTAL FIBROPLASIA

= RETINOPATHY OF PREMATURITY

Predisposed: premature infants with respiratory distress syndrome requiring prolonged oxygen therapy

Severity directly related to:
(1) degree of prematurity
(2) birth weight
(3) amount of oxygen used in therapy

• leukokoria in severe cases (traction retinal detachment, usually bilateral + temporal)
√ dense vitreous bilaterally
√ calcifications in choroid + lens

RHABDOMYOSARCOMA

Most common primary malignant orbital tumor in childhood

Δ 10% occur primarily in orbit
Δ 10% metastasize to / invade orbit

Incidence: 3 – 4% of all pediatric orbital masses

Histo:
arising from undifferentiated mesenchyma of orbital soft tissues (not from striated muscle)
(1) embryonal type (75%)
(2) alveolar type (15%)
(3) pleomorphic type (10%)

Age at presentation: average 7 years; 90% by 16 years;
                          M > F
Rarely associated with   neurofibromatosis
• rapidly progressive exophthalmos + proptosis of upper
  lid
Location: superior orbit / retrobulbar (71%), lid (22%),
             conjunctiva (7%)
√ large soft tissue density mass with ill-defined margins
  (extraocular muscles not involved)
√ ± extension into preseptal space, adjacent sinus, nasal
  cavity, intracranial cavity with bony erosion
√ may show significant enhancement
Metastases: lung, bone marrow, cervical lymph nodes
             (rare)
Prognosis:
  (1) 40% survival after exenteration
  (2) 80 – 90% survival after radiation therapy
       (4,000 – 5,000 rad) + chemotherapy (vincristine,
       cyclophosphamide, adriamycin)

UVEAL MELANOMA

Most common primary intraocular neoplasm in adult
Caucasian
Age: 50 – 70 years
Location: choroid (85 – 93%) > ciliary body (4 – 9%) >
             iris (3 – 6%); almost always unilateral

• retinal detachment, vitreous hemorrhage
• astigmatism, glaucoma
√ ill-defined hyperdense thickening of wall of globe with
  inward bulge
MR:
  √ sharply circumscribed hyperdense lesion on T1WI
    (paramagnetic properties of melanin)
Metastases to: globe, optic nerve; liver, lung, subcutis

VARIX OF ORBIT

Etiology:
  (a) Congenital: venous malformation / venous wall
       weakness
  (b) Acquired: intraorbital / intracranial AVM
• intermittent exophthalmus associated with straining
• frequent blindness
√ involvement of superior / inferior orbital vein; phleboliths
  rare
√ may produce bony erosion without sclerotic reaction
√ enlargement of mass during Valsalva maneuver /
  jugular vein compression
√ well-defined markedly enhancing mass
√ spontaneous thrombosis (common)
MR:
  √ flow void (rapid flow) / flow-related enhancement
    (slow flow)

DIFFERENTIAL DIAGNOSIS OF EAR, NOSE AND THROAT DISORDERS

EAR
Temporal bone sclerosis
1. Otosclerosis
2. **Paget disease** = osteoporosis circumscripta
   - sensorineural / mixed hearing loss (cochlear involvement / stapes fixation in oval window)
   - √ usually lytic changes beginning in petrous pyramid + progressing laterally; otic capsule last to be affected
   - √ calvarial changes ± basilar impression
3. **Fibrous dysplasia**
   monostotic with temporal bone involvement
   - painless mastoid swelling
   - conductive hearing loss (from narrowing of EAC / middle ear)
   - √ homogeneously dense thickened bone (fibro-osseous tissue less dense than calvarial bone)
   - √ expanded bone with preserved cortex
   - √ lytic lesions (less frequent)
   - √ sparing of membranous labyrinth, facial nerve canal, IAC is the rule
4. Osteogenesis imperfecta
   - √ changes similar to otosclerosis
   van der Hoeve syndrome = osteogenesis imperfecta + otosclerosis + blue sclera
5. Meningioma
5. Metastasis
6. Ossifying fibroma
7. Osteosarcoma
8. Osteopetrosis

External ear masses
A. CONGENITAL
   1. Atresia
B. INFLAMMATORY
   1. Malignant external otitis
   2. **Keratosis obturans**
      bilateral process in association with chronic sinusitis + bronchiectasis
      Age: <40 years
   3. Cholesteatoma
C. BENIGN TUMOR
   1. **Exostosis** = surfer's ear
      Cause: irritation by cold water
      √ projecting into EAC; often multiple + bilateral
   2. **Osteoma**
      √ may invade adjacent bone; single in EAC / mastoid
   3. **Ceruminoma**
      from apocrine + sebaceous glands; bone erosion mimics malignancy
D. MALIGNANT TUMOR
   1. Squamous cell carcinoma
      - often long history of chronic suppurative otitis media = "malignant otitis"

2. Basal cell carcinoma
3. Melanoma, adenocarcinoma, adenoid cystic carcinoma
4. Metastases
   (a) hematogeneous: breast, prostate, lung, kidney, thyroid
   (b) direct spread: skin, parotid, nasopharynx, brain, meninges
   (c) systemic: leukemia, lymphoma, myeloma
5. Histiocytosis X: in 15% of patients

Middle ear masses
A. CONGENITAL
   1. **Aberrant internal carotid artery**
      - vascular tympanic membrane
      - pulsatile tinnitus
      - √ tubular soft tissue density entering middle ear cavity posterolateral to cochlea, crossing mesotympanum along cochlear promontory, exiting anteromedial to become horizontal portion of carotid canal
      - √ protrusion into middle ear without bony margin
   2. **Dehiscent jugular bulb**
      - pulsatile tinnitus
      - vascular tympanic membrane
      - √ middle ear soft tissue mass contiguous with jugular foramen
      - √ absence of bony plate separating jugular bulb from posteroinferior middle ear
      DDx: Jugular megabulb (rises above floor of EAC but with preservation of bony plate)
B. INFLAMMATORY
   1. Cholesteatoma
   2. Cholesterol granuloma
   3. Granulation tissue
      - √ linear strands partially opacifying middle ear cavity without bony erosion
C. BENIGN TUMOR
   1. Glomus tumor (multiple in 10%; 8% malignant)
      (a) Glomus tympanicum: at cochlear promontory
         - √ seldom erodes bone
      (b) Glomus jugulare: at jugular foramen
         - √ invasion of middle ear from below
         - √ destruction of bony roof of jugular fossa + bony spur separating vein from carotid artery
   2. Facial neuroma
      - persistent Bell palsy (in 5% caused by neurinoma)
      Location: intracanalicular > IAC
      - √ tubular mass in enlarged / scalloped facial canal
   3. Ossifying hemangioma
   4. Choristoma = ectopic mature salivary tissue
   5. Meningioma
D. MALIGNANT TUMOR
   1. Squamous cell carcinoma

2   Metastasis
3. Rhabdomyosarcoma
    Location: orbit > nasopharynx > ear
4. Adenocarcinoma (rare), adenoid cystic carcinoma

Inner ear masses
A. CONGENITAL
   1. Congenital / primary cholesteatoma = epidermoid tumor (3rd most common CPA tumor)
B. INFLAMMATION
   1. Cholesterol granuloma
   2. Petrous apex mucocele
C. TUMOR
   1. Glomus jugulare tumor
   2. Hemangioma, fibro-osseous lesion
   3. Metastasis
   4. Facial nerve neurinoma
   5. Large CPA tumors: acoustic neuroma, meningioma (2nd most common CPA tumor)

Lesion causing pulsatile tinnitus
A. CONGENITAL VASCULAR PSEUDOTUMOR
   1. Aberrant internal carotid artery
   2. Dehiscent / high jugular bulb
B. VASCULAR
   1. Aneurysm / AVM / fistula of temporal bone region
   2. High-grade arterial stenosis
C. TUMOR
   1. Paraganglioma: glomus tympanicum / jugulare

SINUSES
Opacification of maxillary sinus
A. WITHOUT BONE DESTRUCTION
   1. Sinus aplasia / hypoplasia
      Age: NOT routinely visualized at birth, by age 6 antral floor at level of middle turbinate, by age 15 of adult size
      Location: uni- / bilateral
      √ depression of orbital floor with enlargement of orbit
      √ lateral displacement of lateral wall of nasal fossa with large turbinate
   2. Maxillary dentigerous cyst
      usually containing a tooth / crown; without tooth = primordial dentigerous cyst
   3. Ameloblastoma
   4. Acute sinusitis
      √ air-fluid level
B. WITH BONE DESTRUCTION
   1. Maxillary sinus tumor
   2. Infection: aspergillosis, mucormycosis, TB, syphilis
   3. Wegener granulomatosis; lethal midline granuloma
   4. Blow-out fracture

Paranasal sinus masses
1. Mucocele
2. Mucus retention cyst
   = blockage of secretion in ducts secondary to allergy / inflammation

3. Polyp
    secondary to atopic hypersensitivity (adult) / cystic fibrosis (child)
4. Antrochoanal polyp
5. Inverting papilloma
6. Sinusitis
7. Carcinoma

Granulomatous lesions of sinuses
A. Chronic irritants
    1. beryllium
    2. chromate salts
B. Infection
    1. Tuberculosis
    2. Actinomycosis
    3. Rhinoscleroma
    4. Yaws
    5. Blastomycosis
    6. Leprosy
    7. Rhinosporidiosis
    8. Syphilis
    9. Leishmaniosis
    10. Glanders
C. Autoimmune disease
    1. Wegener granulomatosis
D. Lymphoma-like lesions
    1. Midline granuloma
E. Unclassified
    1. Sarcoidosis

Opacified sinus + expansion / destruction
mnemonic: "PLUMP FACIES"
Plasmacytoma
Lymphoma
Unknown etiology: Wegener granulomatosis
Mucocele
Polyp
Fibrous dysplasia, **F**ibroma (ossifying)
Aneurysmal bone cyst, **A**ngiofibroma
Cancer
Inverting papilloma
Esthesioneuroblastoma
Sarcoma: ie, rhabdomyosarcoma

NOSE
Nasal vault masses
A. BENIGN
   1. Sinonasal polyp
   2. Inverted papilloma
   3. Hemangioma
      • history of epistaxis
   4. Pyogenic granuloma
      √ pedunculated lobular mass
   5. Granuloma gravidarum
      = nasal hemangioma of pregnancy
   6. Hemangiopericytoma
   7. Juvenile nasopharyngeal angiofibroma
      √ arises in superior nasopharynx with extension into nose via posterior choana

B. MALIGNANT
1. Lymphoma
2. Melanoma
3. Vascular metastasis

PHARYNX
Parapharyngeal space mass
1. Asymmetric pterygoid venous plexus
   - √ racemose enhancing area along medial border of lateral pterygoid muscle
2. Atypical second branchial cleft cyst
   Age: child / young adult
   - protruding parotid gland
   - bulging posterolateral pharyngeal wall
   - √ cystic mass projecting from deep margin of faucial tonsil toward skull base
3. Abscess
   Origin: pharyngitis (most common), dental infection, parotid calculus disease, penetrating trauma
4. Pleomorphic adenoma of ectopic salivary tissue

Pharyngeal mucosal space mass
1. Asymmetric fossa of Rosenmüller
   - = lateral pharyngeal recess = asymmetry in amount of lymphoid tissue
2. Tonsillar abscess
   - sore throat, fever, painful swallowing
3. Postinflammatory retention cyst
   - √ 1 – 2 cm well-circumscribed cystic mass
4. Postinflammatory calcification
   - remote history of severe pharyngitis
   - √ multiple clumps of calcification
5. Benign mixed tumor
   - pedunculated mass arising from minor salivary glands
   - √ oval / round well-circumscribed mass protruding into airway
6. Squamous cell carcinoma
   - √ infiltrating mass with epicenter medial to + invading parpharyngeal space
   - √ middle ear fluid (eustachian tube malfunction)
   - √ cervical adenopathy
7. Non-Hodgkin lymphoma
8. Minor salivary gland malignancy
9. Thornwaldt cyst

Masticator space mass
1. Asymmetric accessory parotid gland
   Incidence: 21% of general population
   Location: usually on surface of masseter muscle
   - √ prominent salivary gland tissue
2. Benign masseteric hypertrophy
   Cause: bruxism (= nocturnal gnashing of teeth)
   - √ homogeneous enlargement of one / both masseters
3. Odontogenic abscess
   - bad dentition + trismus
4. Sarcoma (chondro-, osteo-, soft tissue sarcoma)
   - √ infiltrating mass with mandibular destruction
5. Malignant schwannoma
   - √ tubular mass along cranial nerve V$_3$

6. Non-Hodgkin lymphoma
7. Infiltrating squamous cell carcinoma

Carotid space mass
A. Vascular lesion
1. Ectatic common / internal carotid artery
2. Carotid artery aneurysm / pseudoaneurysm
3. Asymmetric internal jugular vein
4. Jugular vein thrombosis
B. Benign tumor
1. Paraganglioma (carotid body tumor + glomus vagale)
2. Schwannoma
3. Neurofibroma
C. Malignant tumor
1. Nodal metastasis from squamous cell carcinoma
2. Non-Hodgkin lymphoma

Retropharyngeal space mass
A. Infection
1. Reactive lymph adenopathy
   - √ nodes >10 mm in diameter
2. Abscess
   - √ bow-tie shape
B. Benign tumor
1. Hemangioma
2. Lipoma
C. Malignant tumor
1. Metastasis from squamous cell carcinoma, melanoma, thyroid carcinoma
2. Non-Hodgkin lymphoma
3. Direct invasion by squamous cell carcinoma

Prevertebral space mass
A. Pseudotumor
1. Anterior disc herniation
2. Vertebral body osteophyte
B. Inflammation
1. Vertebral body osteomyelitis
2. Abscess
C. Tumor
1. Chordoma
2. Vertebral body metastasis: lung, breast, prostate, non-Hodgkin lymphoma

PAROTID GLAND
Parotid gland enlargement
A. Localized inflammatory disease
1. Chronic recurrent sialadenitis
2. Sialosis
3. Sarcoidosis
4. Tuberculosis
5. Cat-scratch fever
6. Syphilis
7. Abscess
8. Reactive adenopathy
B. Systemic autoimmune related disease
1. Sjögren disease (= myoepithelial sialadenitis)
2. Mikulicz disease

C. Neoplasm
  (a) benign tumor
    1. Pleomorphic / monomorphic adenoma
    2. Cystadenolymphoma (= Warthin tumor)
    3. Benign lymphoepithelial cysts (AIDS)
    4. Lipoma
    5. Facial neuroma
    6. Oncocytoma
  (b) primary malignant tumor
    1. Mucoepidermoid carcinoma
    2. Adenoid cystic carcinoma (= cylindroma)
    3. Malignant mixed tumor
    4. Adenocarcinoma
    5. Acinus cell carcinoma
  (c) metastatic tumor
    Δ Parotid gland undergoes late encapsulation, which leads to incorporation of lymph nodes!
    1. Squamous cell carcinoma
    2. Melanoma
    3. Non-Hodgkin lymphoma
D. Lymphoproliferative disorders
  1. Lymphoma
  2. Primary Non-Hodgkin lymphoma
E. Congenital
  1. First branchial cleft cyst

Multiple lesions of parotid gland
  1. Warthin tumor
  2. Metastases to lymph nodes: squamous cell carcinoma of skin, malignant melanoma, Non-Hodgkin lymphoma
  3. Benign lymphoepithelial cysts (AIDS)

Facial nerve paralysis
  A. INTRACRANIAL SEGMENT
    (a) intraaxial
      brainstem glioma, metastasis, multiple sclerosis, cerebrovascular accident, hemorrhage
      • cranial nerve VI also involved
    (b) extraaxial
      CPA tumor (acoustic neuroma, meningioma, epidermoid), CPA inflammation (sarcoidosis, basilar meningitis), vertebrobasilar dolichoectasia, AVM, aneurysm
      • cranial nerve VIII also involved
  B. INTRATEMPORAL SEGMENT
    fracture, cholesteatoma, paraganglioma, hemangioma, facial nerve schwannoma, metastasis, Bell palsy, otitis media
      • loss of lacrimation, hyperacusis, loss of taste
  C. EXTRACRANIAL PAROTID SEGMENT
    forceps delivery, penetrating facial trauma, parotid surgery, parotid malignancy, malignant otitis externa
      • preservation of lacrimation, stapedius reflex, taste

AIRWAYS
Airway obstruction in children
Nasopharyngeal narrowing
  (a) Congenital: Choanal atresia, choanal stenosis, encephalocele

  (b) Inflammatory: Adenoidal enlargement, polyps
  (c) Neoplastic: Juvenile angiofibroma, rhabdomyosarcoma, teratoma, neuroblastoma, lymphoepithelioma
  (d) Traumatic: Foreign body, hematoma, rhinolith

Oropharyngeal narrowing
  (a) Congenital: Glossoptosis + micrognathia (Pierre Robin, Goldenhar, Treacher Collins syndrome), macroglossia (cretinism, Beckwith-Wiedemann syndrome)
  (b) Inflammatory: Abscess, tonsillar hypertrophy
  (c) Neoplastic: Lingular tumor / cyst
  (d) Traumatic: Hematoma, foreign body

Retropharyngeal narrowing
  = potential space (normally <3/4 of AP diameter of adjacent cervical spine in infants / <3 mm in older children)
  (a) Congenital: Branchial cleft cyst, ectopic thyroid
  (b) Inflammatory: Retropharyngeal abscess
  (c) Neoplastic: Cystic hygroma (originating in posterior cervical triangle with extension toward midline + into mediastinum), neuroblastoma, neurofibromatosis, hemangioma
  (d) Traumatic: Hematoma, foreign body
  (e) Metabolic: Hypothyroidism

Vallecular narrowing
  = valleys on each side of glossoepiglottic folds between base of tongue + epiglottis
  (a) Congenital: Congenital cyst, ectopic thyroid, thyroglossal cyst
  (b) Inflammatory: Abscess
  (c) Neoplastic: Teratoma
  (d) Traumatic: Foreign body, hematoma

Supraglottic narrowing
  = area between epiglottis and true vocal cords
  (a) Congenital: Aryepiglottic fold cyst
  (b) Inflammatory: Acute bacterial epiglottitis, angioneurotic edema
  (c) Neoplastic: Retention cyst, cystic hygroma, neurofibroma
  (d) Traumatic: Foreign body, hematoma, radiation, caustic ingestion
  (e) Idiopathic: Laryngomalacia

Glottic narrowing
  = area of true vocal cords
  (a) Congenital: Laryngeal atresia, laryngeal stenosis, laryngeal web (anterior commissure)
  (b) Neoplastic: Laryngeal papillomatosis
  (c) Neurogenic: Vocal cord paralysis (most common)
  (d) Traumatic: Foreign body, hematoma

Subglottic narrowing
= short segment between undersurface of true vocal cords + inferior margin of cricoid cartilage is the narrowest portion of child's airway
(a) Congenital: Congenital subglottic stenosis
(b) Inflammatory: Croup
(c) Neoplastic: Hemangioma, papillomatosis
(d) Traumatic: Acquired stenosis (result of prolonged endotracheal intubation in 5%), granuloma
(e) Idiopathic: Mucocele = mucous retention cyst (rare complication of prolonged endotracheal intubation)

Tracheal narrowing
A. ANTERIOR COMPRESSION
  (a) Congenital
    1. Congenital goiter
    2. Innominate artery syndrome
      √ pulsatile indentation
      Rx: surgical attachment of innominate artery to manubrium
  (b) Inflammatory
    1. Cervical / mediastinal abscess
  (c) Neoplastic
    1. Cervical / intrathoracic teratoma:
      √ amorphous calcifications + ossifications
    2. Thymoma
    3. Thyroid tumors
    4. Lymphoma
  (d) Traumatic: Hematoma
B. POSTERIOR TRACHEAL COMPRESSION
  (a) Congenital
    1. Vascular ring
      — complete: double aortic arch, right aortic arch
      — incomplete: anomalous right subclavian artery
      √ posterior indentation of esophagus + trachea
    2. Pulmonary sling
      = anomalous left pulmonary artery arising from right pulmonary artery, passing between trachea + esophagus enroute to left lung
    3. Bronchogenic cyst
      most common between esophagus + trachea at level of carina
  (b) inflammatory: abscess
  (c) neoplastic: neurofibroma
  (d) traumatic: esophageal foreign body, esophageal stricture, hematoma
C. INTRINSIC TRACHEAL CAUSES
  (a) Congenital:
    1. Congenital tracheal stenosis: generalized /segmental
      = complete cartilaginous ring (instead of horseshoe shape)
    2. Congenital tracheomalacia = immaturity of tracheal cartilage

• expiratory stridor
  √ tracheal collapse on expiration
(b) Neoplastic: papilloma, fibroma, hemangioma
(c) Traumatic: acquired stenosis (endotracheal + tracheostomy tubes), granuloma, acquired tracheomalacia (cartilage degeneration after inflammation, extrinsic pressure, bronchial neoplasia, TE fistula, foreign body)

Inspiratory stridor in children
1. Croup
2. Congenital subglottic stenosis
3. Subglottic hemangioma
4. Airway foreign body
5. Esophageal foreign body
6. Epiglottitis

LARYNX
Epiglottic enlargement
A. Normal variant
  1. Prominent normal epiglottis
  2. Omega epiglottis
B. Inflammation
  1. Acute / chronic epiglottitis
  2. Angioneurotic edema
  3. Stevens-Johnson syndrome
  4. Caustic ingestion
  5. Radiation therapy
C. Masses
  1. Epiglottic cyst
  2. Aryepiglottic cyst
  3. Foreign body

Aryepiglottic cyst
1. Retention cyst
2. Lymphangioma
3. Cystic hygroma
4. Thyroglossal cyst
• may be symptomatic at birth
√ well-defined mass in aryepiglottic fold

Vocal cord paralysis
1. Birth injury
2. Arnold-Chiari malformation
3. Intracranial tumor
4. Mediastinal mass / cyst
5. Vascular ring
6. Thyroidectomy
7. Malignancy
√ fixed vocal cords (fluoroscopy)

Congenital cystic lesions of neck
Δ 95% of all branchial cleft anomalies arise from 2nd branchial apparatus!
1. **Second branchial cleft cyst**
   = incomplete obliteration of 2nd branchial cleft tract (cervical sinus) resulting in sinus tract / fistula / cyst
   Age: young to middle-aged adult

Location: parotid space near mandibular angle,
             parapharyngeal space
- history of multiple parotid abscesses unresponsive
  to drainage + antibiotics
- otorrhea (if connected to external auditory canal)
√ cystic oval / round mass near mandibular angle
√ displacement of sternocleidomastoid muscle
  posteriorly, carotid artery + jugular vein
  posteromedially, submandibular gland anteriorly
√ may insinuate between internal + external carotid
  artery (PATHOGNOMONIC)
√ cyst may enlarge after upper respiratory tract
  infection / injury
DDx: necrotic neural tumor, cervical abscess,
          submandibular gland cyst, cystic
          lymphangioma, necrotic metastatic /
          inflammatory lymphadenopathy

2. **First branchial cleft cyst**
   Residual embryonic tract begins near submandibular
   triangle + ascends through the parotid gland,
   terminates at junction of cartilaginous + bony external
   auditory canal
   Incidence: 8% of all branchial cleft anomalies
   Age: middle-aged women
   - enlarging mass near lower pole of parotid gland
   DDx: inflammatory parotid cyst, benign cystic parotid
             tumor, necrotic metastatic lymphadenopathy

3. **Cervical thymic cyst**
   forms along migratory tract of thymic tissue into
   mediastinum
   Age: <5 years of age; M>F
   No association with myasthenia gravis!
   Location: from angle of mandible to anterior mid-neck
   √ uni- / multilocular mostly unilateral cyst

4. **Parathyroid cyst**
   Age: 30 – 50 years
   - hormonally inactive
   √ non-colloidal cyst near lower pole of thyroid gland

5. Thyroglossal duct cyst

6. **Lymphangioma**
   Histo:
   (a) capillary lymphangioma
       = capillary-sized lymphatic channels
   (b) cavernous lymphangioma
       = moderately dilated lymphatic spaces
   (c) cystic lymphangioma = cystic hygroma
       = enormously dilated lymphatic channels
   Age: present at birth (65%), clinically apparent by
             end of 2nd year (90%)
   - may cause dyspnea / dysphagia
   Location: neck (posterior triangle), superior
                mediastinum, axilla, chest wall, groin
   Prognosis: spontaneous regression (10 – 15%)

7. **Dermoid cyst**
   (1) Cystic teratoma
   (a) epidermoid cyst = lined by simple squamous
       epithelium without adnexal structures
   (b) dermal cyst = epithelial-lined cyst containing
       hair + sebaceous glands

   (c) teratoid cyst = lined with squamous /
       respiratory epithelium containing derivatives of
       skin appendages + endoderm + mesoderm
   (2) Non-teratomatous epithelial-lined cyst
   Location:
   — dorsum of nose in infants (most common)
   — midline anterior floor of mouth:
   (a) sublingual between mylohyoid muscle +
       tongue (DDx: inclusion cyst, ranula)
   (b) submental between platysma + mylohyoid
       muscle

Air-containing masses of neck
1. Laryngocele
2. Tracheal diverticulum
   arising from anterior wall of trachea close to thyroid
3. Zenker diverticulum
4. Lateral pharyngeal diverticulum
   located in tonsillar fossa / vallecula / pyriform fossa

THYROID
Congenital Dyshormonogenesis
1. TRAPPING DEFECT
   = defective cellular uptake of iodine into thyroid,
     salivary glands, gastric mucosa;
   Δ high doses of inorganic iodine facilitate diffusion
     into thyroid permitting a normal rate of thyroid
     hormone synthesis
   Δ normal ratio of iodine concentrations for gastric
     juice:plasma = 20:1
   √ nearly entire dose of administered radioiodine is
     excreted within 24 hours
2. ORGANIFICATION DEFECT
   = deficient peroxidase activity, which catalyzes the
     oxidation of iodide by H_2O_2 to form
     monoiodotyrosine (MIT) / diiodotyrosine (DIT)
   - high serum TSH
   - low serum T_4
   - diffuse symmetric thyromegaly
   √ high thyroidal uptake of radioiodine / pertechnetate
   √ rapid I-131 turnover
   √ positive perchlorate washout test
   Pendred syndrome = autosomal recessive trait of
     deficient peroxidase regeneration characterized by
     hypothyroidism + goiter + nerve deafness
3. DEIODINASE (DEHALOGENASE) DEFECT
   = deficient deiodination of MIT / DIT to release iodide
     which is reutilized to synthesize thyroid hormone
     production
   - hypothyroidism
   - identification of MIT + DIT in serum + urine
     following administration of I-131
   - "intrinsic" iodine deficiency goiter
   √ high thyroidal I-131 uptake
   √ rapid intrathyroidal turnover of I-131
4. THYROXIN-BINDING GLOBULIN (TBG) DEFICIENCY
   - abnormal T_4 transport
   - low bound serum T_4 concentration
   - euthyroid

5. END-ORGAN RESISTANCE TO THYROID
   HORMONE
   • high serum T_4
   • euthyroid / hypothyroid
   • growth retardation
   √ goiter
   √ stippled epiphyses

Hyperthyroidism
1. Graves disease (most common)
2. Toxic nodular goiter
3. Iodine-induced hyperthyroidism = Jod-Basedow
4. Thyroiditis
   (a) Hashimoto thyroiditis = chronic lymphocytic
       thyroiditis
   (b) Subacute thyroiditis = de Quervain thyroiditis
   (c) Painless thyroiditis
   US: √ decrease in overall echogenicity
          √ discrete nodules (50%)
5. Thyrotoxicosis medicamentosa / factitia
   surreptitious self-administration of thyroid hormones
6. Struma ovarii
   = ovarian teratoma containing thyroid tissue
7. Hydatidiform mole / choriocarcinoma / testicular
   trophoblastic carcinoma
   = stimulation of thyroid by HCG
8. Pituitary hyperthyroidism = pituitary neoplasm
   • ± acromegaly
   • ± hyperprolactinemia
9. Thyroid carcinoma / hyperfunctioning metastases
   very rare (25 cases)

Hypothyroidism
A. PRIMARY HYPOTHYROIDISM (most common)
   = thyroid's inability to produce sufficient thyroid
     hormone
   1. Agenesis of thyroid
   2. Congenital dyshormonogenesis
   3. Chronic thyroiditis
   4. Previous radioiodine therapy
   5. Ectopic thyroid (1:4,000)
B. SECONDARY HYPOTHYROIDISM
   = failure of anterior pituitary to release sufficient
     quantities of TSH
   1. Sheehan syndrome
   2. Head trauma
   3. Pituitary tumor (primary / secondary)
   4. Aneurysm
   5. Surgery
C. TERTIARY / HYPOTHALAMIC HYPOTHYROIDISM
   = failure of hypothalamus to produce sufficient
     amounts of TRH

Decreased / no uptake of radiotracer
A. BLOCKED TRAPPING FUNCTION
   1. Iodine load (most common)
      = dilution of tracer within flooded iodine pool (from
        administration of radiographic contrast / iodine-
        containing medication)
      Δ Suppression usually lasts for 4 weeks!

2. Exogenous thyroid hormone (replacement therapy)
   suppresses TSH release
B. BLOCKED ORGANIFICATION
   1. Antithyroid medication (propylthiouracil (PTU) /
      methimazole) / goitrogenic substances
   √ Tc-99m uptake not inhibited
C. DIFFUSE PARENCHYMAL DESTRUCTION
   1. Subacute / chronic thyroiditis
D. HYPOTHYROIDISM
   1. Congenital hypothyroidism
   2. Surgical / radioiodine ablation
   3. Thyroid ectopia (struma ovarii, intrathoracic goiter)

Prominent pyramidal lobe
= distal remnant of thyroid descent tract
1. Normal variant: present in 10%
2. Hyperthyroidism
3. Thyroiditis
4. S/P thyroid surgery
DDx: Esophageal activity from salivary excretion
       (disappears after glass of water)

Thyroid calcifications
= benign calcifications = stromal calcifications in adenoma
  √ coarse calcifications with rough outline
  √ alignment along periphery of lesion
  √ irregular distribution

Psammoma bodies
= microcalcifications (<1 mm) occur in 54% of thyroid
  neoplasms
√ seen on xeroradiography in 94%
1. Papillary carcinoma   61%
2. Follicular carcinoma   26%
3. Undifferentiated carcinoma   13%

Cystic areas in thyroid
A. Anechoic fluid + smooth regular wall:
   1. Colloid accumulation in goiter = colloid-filled dilated
      macrofollicle
   2. Simple cyst (extremely uncommon)
B. Solid particles + irregular outline:
   1. Intranodular hemorrhage in goiter
   2. Liquefaction necrosis in adenoma / goiter
   3. Abscess

Thyroid nodule
Incidence: (increasing with age)
   (a) 4 – 8% by palpation (>2 cm in 2%, 1 – 2 cm in 5%,
       <1 cm in 1%); M:F = 1:4
   (b) 50% by autopsy / thyroid US if clinically normal:
       multiple in 38%, solitary in 12% (occult small
       cancers found in 4%)
A. BENIGN
   1. Adenomatous hyperplasia / degenerative involuted
      nodule (50%)
   2. Follicular adenoma (20%)
   3. Ectopic parathyroid adenoma
   4. Inflammatory lymph node in subacute + chronic
      thyroiditis

5. Hemorrhage / hematoma: frequently associated with adenomas
6. Abscess

B. MALIGNANT
1. Thyroid carcinoma
2. Nonthyroidal neoplasm
  metastasis from breast, lung, kidney, malignant melanoma, Hodgkin disease

C. Hürthle cell carcinoma
√ very thin hypoechoic halo

D. Carcinoma in situ
√ echogenic area inside a goiter nodule

PROBABILITY OF A COLD NODULE FOR THYROID CANCER:
Δ Solitary cold nodules by scintigraphy are multinodular by US in 20 – 25%!
(a) 15 – 25% for solitary cold nodule
(b) 1 – 6% for multiple nodules (DDx: multinodular goiter)
(c) with history of neck irradiation in childhood
  — solitary nodule found in 70% (cancerous in 31%)
  — multiple nodules found in 25% (cancerous in 37%)
  — normal thyroid scan found in 5% (cancer detected in 20%)

Discordant thyroid nodule

= nodule hyperfunctioning on Tc-99m pertechnetate scan + hypofunctioning on I-131 scan, which indicates reduced organification capacity

Causes:
1. Malignancy : follicular / papillary carcinoma
2. Benign lesion: follicular adenoma / adenomatous hyperplasia
  (autonomous nontoxic nodules have accelerated iodine turnover and discharge radioiodine as hormone within 24 hours)

Hot thyroid nodule

Incidence: 8% of Tc-99m pertechnetate scans

1. Adenoma
  (a) Autonomous adenoma = TSH-independent
    • hyper- / euthyroid
    √ partial / total suppression of remainder of gland
  (b) Adenomatous hyperplasia = TSH-dependent
    secondary to defective thyroid hormone production
2. Thyroid carcinoma (extremely rare)
  √ discordant uptake
N.B.: any hot nodule on Tc-99m scan must be imaged with I-123 to differentiate between autonomous or cancerous lesion

Cold thyroid nodule

A. Benign tumor
1. Nonfunctioning adenoma
2. Cyst (11 – 20%)
3. Involutional nodule
4. Parathyroid tumor

B. Inflammatory mass
1. Focal thyroiditis
2. Granuloma
3. Abscess

C. Malignant tumor
1. Carcinoma
2. Lymphoma
3. Metastasis

US features of cold nodule:
√ hypoechoic (71%)
√ isoechoic (22%)
√ mixed echogenicity (4%)
√ hyperechoic (3%)
√ cystic (rarely malignant)

mnemonic: "CATCH LAMP"
Cyst
Adenoma (most common)
Thyroiditis
Carcinoma
Hemorrhage
Lymphoma
Abscess
Metastasis
Parathyroid

ANATOMY AND FUNCTION OF NECK ORGANS

Paranasal sinuses
Mucus production of 1 l/day; irritants are propelled toward nasopharynx at a rate of 1 cm/minute

A. Maxillary sinus
Size: 6 – 8 cm at birth
Extension: 4 – 5 mm below level of nasal cavity by age 12
Walls: roof = floor of orbit; posterior wall abuts pterygopalatine fossa
Plain film: visible at 4 – 5 months
Ostium: maxillary ostium + infundibulum enter middle meatus within posterior aspect of hiatus semilunaris; additional ostia may be present

B. Ethmoid sinuses
Size: adult size by age 12; 3 – 18 air cells per side
Walls: roof = floor of anterior cranial fossa; lateral wall = lamina papyracea

Plain film: visible at 1 year of age
(a) anteromedial group
2 – 8 cells with a total area of 24 x 23 x 11 mm
Ostia: opening into anterior aspect of hiatus semilunaris of middle meatus (anterior group), opening into ethmoid bulla (middle group)
(b) posterior group
1 – 8 cells, larger cells, total area smaller than that of anteromedial group
Ostium: into superior meatus

C. Frontal sinus
Size: 28 x 24 x 20 mm in adults, rapid growth until the late teens
Walls: posterior wall = anterior cranial fossa; inferior wall = anterior portion of roof of orbit
Plain film: visible at age 6 years
Ostium: into frontal recess of middle meatus via nasofrontal duct

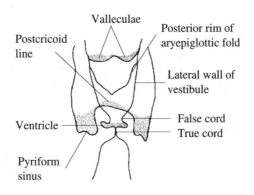

Frontal laryngopharyngogram during phonation

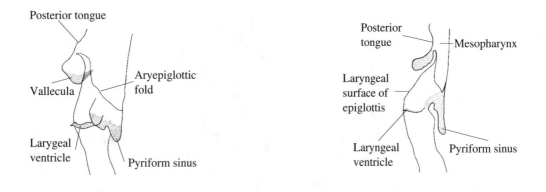

Lateral laryngogram

during phonation   **during quiet breathing**

D. **Sphenoid sinus**
Size: 20 x 23 x 17 mm in adults, small evagination of
sphenoethmoidal recess at birth, invasion of
sphenoid bone begins at age 5 years
Walls: roof = floor of sella turcica; anterior wall shared
with ethmoid sinuses; posterior wall = clivus;
inferior wall = roof of nasopharynx
Ostium: 10 mm above sinus floor into sphenoethmoidal
recess posterior to superior meatus

Ostiomeatal unit

= area of superomedial maxillary sinus + middle meatus
that conveys mucociliary drainage of frontal sinus,
anterior + middle ethmoid sinuses, and maxillary sinus
into nose
Components:
1. Infundibulum
= flattened cone-like passage between inferomedial
border of orbit / ethmoid bulla (laterally) + uncinate
process (medially)
2. Uncinate process
= lateral wall of nose below hiatus semilunaris in
middle meatus
3. Ethmoid bulla
√ located in cephalad recess of middle meatus
4. Hiatus semilunaris
located just inferior to ethmoid bulla in middle meatus
Ostia:
(1) multiple ostia from anterior ethmoid air cells (at
its anterior aspect)
(2) maxillary ostium infundibulum (at its posterior
aspect)

Anatomic variations predisposing to ostiomeatal
narrowing:
1. Concha bullosa = aerated middle turbinate
2. Oversized ethmoid bulla

3. Haller cells = inferiorly extending ethmoid cells
below ethmoid bulla adhering to roof of maxillary
sinus
4. Uncinate process bulla
5. Bowed nasal septum
6. Paradoxical middle turbinate = convexity of
turbinate directed toward lateral nasal wall
7. Deviation of uncinate process

Branchial cleft development

— 6 paired branchial arches are responsible for
formation of lower face + neck
— each branchial cleft arch contains a central core of
cartilage + muscle, a blood vessel and a nerve
— arches form 5 ectodermal "clefts" / grooves on outer
aspect of neck + 5 endodermal pharyngeal pouches
separated by a membrane
Formation: during 4th – 7th week of embryonic
development

1st branchial arch = maxillo-mandibular arch
(a) ventral / mandibular prominence
(b) dorsal / maxillary prominence
nerve: mandibular division of trigeminal nerve
pouch forms: mastoid air cells + eustachian tube
cleft forms: external auditory canal + tympanic cavity

2nd branchial arch = hyoid arch
nerve: facial nerve
arch forms: thyroid gland
pouch forms: palatine tonsil + tonsillar fossa
cleft involutes completely by 9th fetal week;
2nd arch overgrows 2nd + 3rd + 4th clefts to form
cervical sinus which creates a tract that runs from
supraclavicular area just lateral to carotid sheath, turns
medially at mandibular angle between external +
internal carotid artery, terminates in tonsillar fossa

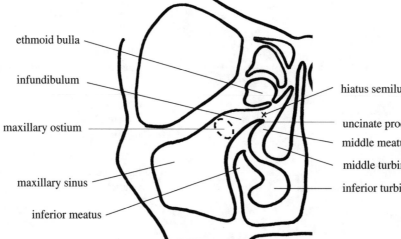

ethmoid bulla

infundibulum

maxillary ostium

maxillary sinus

inferior meatus

hiatus semilunaris

uncinate process
middle meatus
middle turbinate
inferior turbinate

Coronal scan of ostiomeatal unit

<u>3rd branchial arch</u>
sunk into retrohyoid depression
nerve: glossopharyngeal nerve
arch forms: glossoepiglottic fold
pouch forms:
(a) thymus gland, which descends into mediastinum by 9th fetal week
(b) inferior parathyroid glands passing down with the thymus

<u>4th branchial arch</u>
sunk into retrohyoid depression
nerve: superior laryngeal branch of vagus nerve
arch forms: epiglottis + aryepiglottic folds
pouch forms: superior parathyroid glands
cleft forms: ultimobranchial body, which provides parafollicular = "C" cells of thyroid

<u>5th + 6th branchial arches</u>
cannot be recognized externally
nerve: recurrent laryngeal branch of vagus nerve

Deep Spaces of Suprahyoid Head & Neck
Pharyngeal mucosal space
adenoids, faucial + lingual tonsils
superior + middle constrictor muscles
salpingopharyngeal muscle
levator palatini muscle
torus tubarius

Parapharyngeal space
fat
internal maxillary artery
ascending pharyngeal artery
pharyngeal venous plexus
branches of cranial nerve V_3

Retropharyngeal space
fat
medial + lateral retropharyngeal nodes

Prevertebral space
prevertebral muscles
scalene muscles
vertebral artery + vein
brachial plexus
phrenic nerve

Carotid space
internal carotid artery
internal jugular vein
cranial nerves IX — XII

Parotid space
parotid gland
intraparotid lymph nodes
external carotid + internal maxillary arteries
retromandibular vein
facial nerve

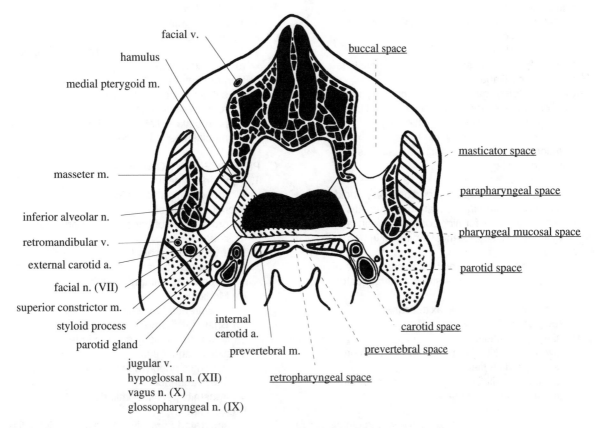

facial v.
hamulus
medial pterygoid m.
masseter m.
inferior alveolar n.
retromandibular v.
external carotid a.
facial n. (VII)
superior constrictor m.
styloid process
parotid gland
jugular v.
hypoglossal n. (XII)
vagus n. (X)
glossopharyngeal n. (IX)
internal carotid a.
prevertebral m.
buccal space
masticator space
parapharyngeal space
pharyngeal mucosal space
parotid space
carotid space
prevertebral space
retropharyngeal space

Transaxial scan through level of lower nasopharynx

Hypopharynx
= compartment of aerodigestive tract betwen oropharynx above + larynx below

1. Pyriform sinus
   = two symmetric stalactites of air hanging from hypopharynx behind larynx
   — inferior wall: level of cricoarytenoid joint
   — anteromedial wall: lateral wall of aryepiglottic fold
   — lateral wall: abuts posterior ala of thyroid cartilage
   — posterior wall: most lateral aspect of posterior hypopharyngeal wall

2. Postcricoid area = pharyngoesophageal junction
   extends from level of arytenoid cartilages to inferior border of cricoid cartilage

3. Posterior hypopharyngeal wall
   extends from level of valleculae to cricoarytenoid joints

Larynx
Vertical length: 44 mm (males), 36 mm (females), at 4th – 6th cervical vertebrae

A. SUPRAGLOTTIS
   extends from tip of epiglottis to laryngeal ventricles
   1. Vestibule
      = air-space within supraglottic larynx
   2. Epiglottis
      = leaf-shaped cartilage that functions as a lid to endolarynx
      (a) petiole = stem of epiglottis
      (b) thyroepiglottic ligament = connects petiole to thyroid cartilage
      (c) hyoepiglottic ligament = connects epiglottis to hyoid bone, covered by a mucosal fold between the valleculae (glossoepiglottic fold)
   3. False vocal cords = ventricular folds
      = mucosal surface of ventricular ligaments
   4. Arytenoid cartilages
   5. Aryepiglottic folds
      = tissue between cephalad portion of arytenoid cartilage + inferolateral margin of epiglottis
      √ soft-tissue folds forming border between lateral pyriform sinuses + central laryngeal lumen
   6. Ventricle
      = fusiform fossa bounded by crescentic edge of false cords superiorly + straight margin of true cords inferiorly
      √ generally not visible on axial scans
   7. Pre-epiglottic space
   8. Paralaryngeal space
      √ low-density tissue between true + false cords and thyroid cartilage
      √ continuous with preepiglottic space anteriorly + aryepiglottic folds superiorly
   9. Preepiglottic space
      √ low-density tissue between anterior margin of epiglottis + thyroid cartilage

B. GLOTTIS
   1. True vocal cords
      = extend from vocal process of arytenoid cartilage to anterior commissure
      √ vocal cords adduct during phonation of "E" / breath holding
   2. Anterior commissure
      √ <1 mm soft tissue behind thyroid cartilage (during abduction of vocal cords with quiet breathing)
   3. Posterior commissure
      = mucosal surface lining anterior portion of cricoid cartilage between arytenoid cartilages

C. SUBGLOTTIS
   extends from undersurface of true cords to inferior surface of cricoid cartilage
   1. Conus elasticus
      = fibroelastic membrane extending from cricoid cartilage to medial margin of true vocal cords + forming lateral wall of subglottis

Temporal bone

A. SQUAMOUS PORTION
   = lateral wall of middle cranial fossa + floor of temporal fossa

B. MASTOID PORTION
   1. Mastoid antrum
   2. Aditus ad antrum
      connects epitympanum (= attic) of middle ear cavity to mastoid antrum
   3. Körner septum
      = small bony projection extending inferiorly from roof of mastoid antrum as part of petrosquamosal suture between lateral + medial mastoid air cells

C. PETROUS PORTION = inner ear
   1. Tegmen tympani
      = roof of tympanic cavity
   2. Arcuate eminence
      = prominence of bone over superior semicircular canal
   3. Internal auditory canal (IAC)
      (a) Porus acusticus internus
         = opening of internal auditory canal
      (b) Modiolus
         = entrance to cochlea
      (c) Crista falciformis
         = horizontal bony septum in IAC
   4. Vestibular aqueduct
      = transmits endolymphatic duct
   5. Cochlear aqueduct
      = transmits perilymphatic duct
   6. Petrous apex
      = separated from clivus by petro-occipital fissure + foramen lacerum

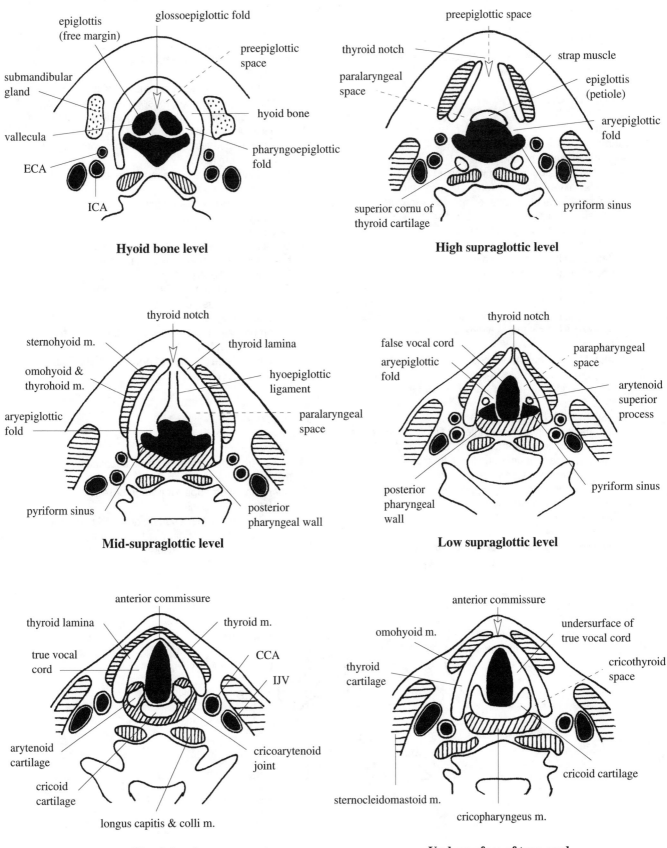

Hyoid bone level

High supraglottic level

Mid-supraglottic level

Low supraglottic level

Glottic level

Undersurface of true cord

D. TYMPANIC PORTION
1. External auditory canal (EAC)
   medial border formed by tympanic membrane, which attaches superiorly at scutum + inferiorly at tympanic annulus

E. STYLOID PORTION

Middle ear

Borders:
— anterior wall = carotid wall
— posterior wall = mastoid wall including
  (a) facial nerve recess for descending facial nerve
  (b) pyramidal eminence for stapedius muscle
  (c) sinus tympani (clinically blind spot)
— superior wall = tegmen tympani
— inferior wall = jugular wall
— lateral wall   = tympanic membrane
— medial wall   = labyrinthine wall

A. EPITYMPANUM
= tympanic cavity above the line drawn between the inferior tip of scutum + tympanic portion of facial nerve
Contents: malleus head, body + short process of incus, Prussak space (= area between incus + lateral wall of epitympanum)

B. MESOTYMPANUM
= tympanic cavity between inferior tip of scutum + line drawn parallel to inferior aspect of bony EAC
Contents: manubrium of malleus, long process of incus, stapes, tensor tympani muscle (innervated by V_3), stapedius muscle (innervated by VII)

C. HYPOTYMPANUM
= shallow trough in floor of miidle ear

Inner ear

1. Cochlea
   2 1/2 turns, basal first turn opens into round window posteriorly, encircles central bony axis of modiolus
2. Vestibule
   = largest part of membranous labyrinth with subunits of utricle + saccule (not separately visualized); separated from middle ear by oval window
3. Semicircular canals
   — superior semicircular canal forms convexity of arcuate eminence
   — posterior semicircular canal points posteriorly along line of petrous ridge
   — lateral / horizontal semicircular canal juts into epitympanum
4. Cochlear aqueduct
   contains 8 mm long perilymphatic duct, extends from basal turn of cochlea to lateral border of jugular foramen paralleling IAC
   Function: regulates CSF + perilymphatic fluid pressure
5. Vestibular aqueduct
   encompasses endolymphatic duct, extends from vestibule to endolymphatic sac
   Function: equilibration of endolymphatic fluid pressure

Facial nerve

Segments:
(a) intracranial segment
    = from brainstem to porus acusticus internus
(b) internal auditory canal
    = in anterosuperior portion of IAC
(c) labyrinthine segment
    = short segment curling anteriorly over top of cochlea; terminates in anterior genu (geniculate ganglion)

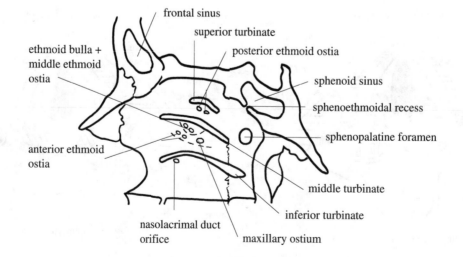

View of Lateral Nasal Wall (turbinates removed)

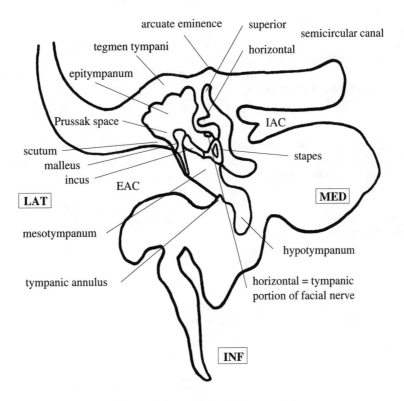

Coronal tomogram of temporal bone

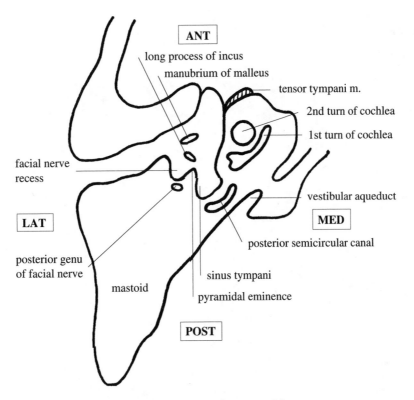

Axial tomogram of temporal bone

(d) tympanic segment
  = segment from anterior to posterior genu just underneath lateral semicircular canal
(e) mastoid segment
  = from posterior genu to stylomastoid foramen
(f) parotid segment
  = extracranial segment between superficial + deep lobes of parotid gland

Function:
1. Lacrimation (via greater superficial petrosal nerve)
2. Stapedius reflex: sound damping
3. Taste of anterior 2/3 of tongue (via chorda tympani nerve to lingual nerve)
4. Facial expression (platysma)
5. Secretion of lacrimal + submandibular + sublingual glands (via nervus intermedius)

Thyroid hormones

free hormone	:	T_4	(0.03%)
		T_3	(0.4%)
Thyroxin binding globulin (TBG)	:	binds T_4	(70%)
		and T_3	(38%)
Thyroxin binding prealbumin (TBPA)	:	binds T_4	(10%)
		and T_3	(27%)
Albumin	:	binds T_4	(20%)
		and T_3	(35%)

ELEVATION OF TBG
  (1) Pregnancy (2) Estrogen administration (3) Genetic trait
REDUCTION IN TBG
  (1) Androgens (2) Anabolic steroids (3) Glucocorticoids
  (4) Nephrotic syndrome
  (5) Chronic hepatic disease
INHIBITION OF T_4 BINDING TO TBG: salicylates

EAR, NOSE AND THROAT DISORDERS

ADENOID CYSTIC CARCINOMA
= CYLINDROMA
Incidence: 4 – 15% of all salivary gland tumors
Histo: (a) tubular (b) cribriform (c) solid
Age: 3rd – 9th decade; maximum between 40 and 70 years
Location:
@ Minor salivary glands (most common; 25 – 31% of malignant neoplasms in minor salivary glands)
• nasal obstruction + swelling
@ Submandibular gland (15% of tumors in this gland)
@ Parotid gland (2 – 6% of tumors in this gland; arises from peripheral parotid ducts with propensity for perineural spread along facial nerve)
• hard mass + facial nerve pain / paralysis
√ infiltrating parotid mass
MR:
√ hypo- to hyperintense (high signal corresponds to low cellularity) on T2WI
Metastases to: lung, cervical lymph nodes, bone, liver
Prognosis:
slow relentless malignant course with repeat recurrences; the greater the cellularity the worse the prognosis (requires entire tumor); 60 – 69% 5-year survival rate; 40% 10-year survival rate
Rx: repeat surgical excision + radiation therapy

ADENOMATOUS HYPERPLASIA OF THYROID
(1) Cystic form = colloid cyst
US: √ anechoic areas in nodule (hemorrhage / colloid degeneration)
√ calcific deposits
(2) Solid form = degenerative nodule

ANTROCHOANAL POLYP
= benign antral polyp, which widens the sinus ostium and extends into nasal cavity; 5% of all nasal polyps
Age: teenagers + young adults
√ antral clouding
√ ipsilateral nasal mass
√ NO sinus expansion

APICAL PETROSITIS
= PETROUS APICITIS
Etiology: spread from middle ear + mastoid infection; requires presence of air cells in petrous apices (which is found 30% of population)
• **Gradenigo syndrome:** otorrhea (otitis media) + retroorbital pain (trigeminal pain) + 6th nerve palsy
√ air cell opacification (fluid in ipsilateral middle ear + mastoid)
√ bone destruction (osteomyelitis)

BENIGN MIXED TUMOR OF PAROTIS
= PLEOMORPHIC ADENOMA
Incidence: 80% of all benign parotid tumors

Histo: mixture of epithelial + myoepithelial cells
Age: usually >50 years
• slow-growing lump in cheek
√ round / oval / lobulated sharply marginated mass
√ rarely dystrophic calcifications
√ variable contrast enhancement
CT:
√ low-density center if large (mucoid matrix)
MR:
√ hyperintense mass on T2WI
√ hyperintense areas in center (mucoid matrix)

CAROTID ARTERY DISSECTION
= hematoma within media splitting off the vessel wall and causing a false lumen within media
Etiology:
A. SPONTANEOUS CAROTID DISSECTION
(1) non-recalled minor / trivial trauma
(2) primary arterial disease: Marfan syndrome (fibromuscular dysplasia in 15%), cystic medial necrosis
B. TRAUMATIC CAROTID DISSECTION
blunt / penetrating trauma (automobile accident, boxing, accidental hanging, diagnostic carotid compression, manipulative therapy)

Age: 18 – 76 years (66% between 35 and 50 years)
Associated with: hypertension (36%), smoking (47%), migraine (11%), fibromuscular disease (14%)
Site:
(a) Subintimal dissection = close to intima
(b) Subadventitial dissection = close to adventitia
Location:
cervical ICA usually at level of C1-2 (60%), vertebral artery (20%), both ICA + vertebral artery (10%); multiple simultaneous dissections (33%); bilateral carotid dissections (15%), bilateral vertebral dissections (5%)
• unilateral anterior headache (86%), neck pain (25%)
• TIA / stroke (58%), amaurosis fugax (12%)
• oculosympathetic paresis (52%)
• bruit (48%)

Angiography:
√ string sign = elongated tapered irregular luminal stenosis extending to base of skull (76%)
√ abrupt luminal reconstitution at level of bony carotid canal (42%)
√ finger-like / saccular aneurysm (40%), often in upper cervical / subcranial region
√ intimal flap (29%), sometimes creating double-barrel lumen
√ slow ICA-MCA flow
√ tapered "flame-like" / "radish tail-like" occlusion (17%), often distal to carotid bulb
Prognosis: complete / excellent recovery (8%)
Rx: best therapy not clear; anticoagulants

CAROTID ARTERY STENOSIS

High-grade ICA stenosis is associated with increased risk for TIA, stroke, carotid occlusion, embolism arising from thrombi forming at site of narrowing

Increased risk for stroke:
- (a) significant ICA stenosis (compromised blood flow)
  Reduction of blood flow occurs at 50 – 60% diameter stenosis / 75% area stenosis
  Δ 2% risk of stroke with nonsignificant stenosis
  Δ 16% incidence of stroke with significant stenosis
  Δ 2% incidence of subsequent stroke following endarterectomy
- (b) intraplaque hemorrhage (embolic stroke)

Histo:
Arteriosclerosis = generic term for all structural changes resulting in hardening of the arterial wall

1. Diffuse intimal thickening
   = growth of intima through migration of medial smooth muscle cells into subendothelial space through fenestrations in internal elastic lamella associated with increasing amounts of collagen, elastic fibers, glycosaminoglycans
   Age: beginning at birth slowly progressing to adult life

2. Atherosclerosis
   = intimal pool of necrotic proteinaceous + fatty substances within hardened arterial wall
   Location: large + medium-sized elastic and muscular arteries
   - (a) fatty streak = superficial yellow-gray flat intimal lesion characterized by focal accumulation of subendothelial smooth muscle cells + lipid deposits
   - (b) fibrous plaque = whitish protruding lesion consisting of central core of lipid + cell debris surrounded by smooth muscle cells, collagen, elastic fibers, proteoglycans; a fibrous cap separates the lipid core (= atheroma) from the vessel lumen
   - (c) complicated lesion = fibrous plaque with degenerative changes such as calcification, plaque hemorrhage, intimal ulceration / rupture, mural thrombosis
     Plaque hemorrhage from thin-walled blood vessels in vascularized plaque may cause ulceration, thrombosis + embolism, and luminal narrowing
     Δ in 93% of symptomatic patients
     Δ in 27% of asymptomatic patients
     Plaque ulceration exposes thrombogenic subendothelial collagen + lipid-rich material
     Δ frequent in plaques occupying >85% of lumen
     Δ 12.5% stroke incidence per year

3. Mönckeberg sclerosis = medial calcification
4. Hypertensive arteriosclerosis

Predilection sites of arterial stenosis:

	Incidence of lesions	
	Stenosis	Occlusion
Right ICA origin	33.8%	8.6%
Left ICA origin	34.1%	8.7%
Right vertebral artery origin	18.4%	4.8%
Left vertebral artery origin	22.3%	2.2%
Right carotid siphon	6.7%	9.0%
Left carotid siphon	6.6%	9.2%
Basilar artery	7.7%	0.8%
Right MCA	3.5%	2.2%
Left MCA	4.1%	2.1%

COURSE OF CAROTID ARTERY STENOSIS
1. Stable stenosis (68%)
2. Progressive stenosis to >50% diameter reduction (25%)

Angiography:
@ Extracranial
  √ smooth asymmetrical excrescence encroaching upon vessel lumen
  √ crater / niche = ulceration
  √ mound within base of crater = mural thrombus
  √ Holman carotid slim sign = diffuse narrowing of entire ICA distal to high-grade stenosis due to decrease in perfusion pressure
  √ occlusion of ICA
@ Intracranial
  √ carotid siphon stenosis
  √ retrograde flow in ophthalmic artery filled from ECA
  √ small vessel occlusion
  √ focal areas of slow flow
  √ early draining vein = reactive hyperemia = "luxury perfusion" due to shunting between arterioles + venules surrounding an area of ischemia
  √ ICA-MCA slow flow = delayed arrival + washout of ICA-MCA distribution in comparison to ECA

Risk of carotid endarterectomy:
1% mortality; 2% risk of intraoperative neurologic deficit

Carotid Duplex Ultrasound
Indications for carotid duplex US:
- (1) Screening for suspected extracranial carotid disease
  - (a) high-grade flow-limiting stenosis
  - (b) low-grade stenosis with hemorrhage
- (2) Nonhemispheric neurologic symptomatology
- (3) History of transient ischemic attack / stroke
- (4) Asymptomatic carotid bruit
- (5) Retinal cholesterol embolus
- (6) Preoperative evaluation before major cardiovascular surgery
- (7) Intraoperative monitoring of vascular patency during endarterectomy
- (8) Sequential evaluation after endarterectomy
- (9) Monitoring of known plaque during medical treatment

Accuracy of duplex scans: (in comparison to arteriography for ICA lesions)
91 – 94% sensitivity, 85 – 99% specificity for >50% ICA diameter stenosis

DUPLEX CATEGORIES OF INTERNAL CAROTID ARTERY LESIONS
incorporating B-mode and Doppler spectrum analysis

A. <u>No lesion</u>
- √ peak systole <125 cm/s
- √ clear window under systole
- √ no evidence of plaque
- √ no spectral broadening

B. <u>Minimal Disease</u>
- = 0 – 15% diameter reduction
- √ peak systole <125 cm/s
- √ clear window under systole
- √ minimal plaque
- √ minimal spectral broadening in deceleration phase of systole

C. <u>Moderate Disease</u>
- = 16 – 49% diameter reduction
- √ peak systole <125 cm/s
- √ no window under systole
- √ moderate plaque
- √ spectral broadening throughout systole

D. <u>Severe Disease</u> = <u>Hemodynamically Significant Lesion</u>
- (a) 50 – 79% diameter reduction
  - √ peak systole >125 cm/s
  - √ increased diastolic flow
  - √ marked spectral broadening throughout cardiac cycle
  - √ velocity ratio of ICA/CCA = 2.0
- (b) 80 – 99% diameter reduction
  - √ peak systole >125 cm/s
  - √ end-diastole >135 cm/s
  - √ no window under systole
  - √ spectral broadening throughout systole
  - √ "string sign" on color Doppler with slow-flow sensitivity setting

E. <u>Occluded Vessel</u>
- √ no signal in ICA
- √ absence of diastolic flow in CCA (high impedance flow)
- √ diastolic flow reversal in CCA
- √ increased diastolic flow in ECA (if ECA assumes the role of primary supplier of blood to brain)
- √ increase in peak systolic velocities in contralateral ICA (due to collateral flow)
- √ no evidence of color Doppler flow in low-flow sensitivity setting

PLAQUE CHARACTERIZATION

A. <u>Homogeneous plaque</u> = stable plaque
- *Histo:* deposition of fatty streaks + fibrous tissue; rarely shows intraplaque hemorrhage / ulcerations
- *Prognosis:*
  - Δ neurologic deficits develop in 4%
  - Δ ipsilateral infarction on CT in 12%
  - Δ ipsilateral symptoms develop in 22%
  - Δ progressive stenosis develops in 18%
- √ homogenous uniform echo pattern with smooth surface

B. <u>Heterogeneous plaque</u>
- = unstable plaque = mixture of high, medium and low level echoes with smooth / irregular surface; may fissure / tear resulting in intraplaque hemorrhage / ulceration + thrombus formation (embolus / increasing stenosis)
- B-mode ultrasound has 90 – 94% sensitivity, 75 – 88% specificity, 90% accuracy for intraplaque hemorrhage
- *Histo:* lipid-laden macrophages, monocytes, leukocytes, necrotic debris, cholesterol crystals, calcifications
- *Prognosis:*
  - Δ neurologic deficits develop in 27%
  - Δ ipsilateral infarction on CT in 24%
  - Δ ipsilateral symptoms develop in 50%
  - Δ progressive stenosis develops in 77%

Doppler Spectrum Analysis

Diameter stenosis classification	(%)	ICA/CCA peak systolic ratio	ICA/CCA peak diastolic ratio	Peak systolic velocity (cm/sec)	kHz[†]	Peak diastolic velocity (cm/sec)	kHz[†]
normal – mild	0 – 40	<1.5 – 1.8	<2.4 – 2.6	<110 > 25	<3.5	<40	<1.5
moderate	41 – 59	<1.8	<2.4 – 2.6	>120 – 130	>3.5	<40	<1.5
severe	60 – 79	>1.8	>2.4 – 2.6	>130	>5.0	>40	>1.5
critical	80 – 99	>3.7	>5.5	>250	>8.0	>80 – 135	>4.5
† = based on 5 MHz pulsed Doppler carrier frequency at 60° flow angle (Blackshear, Bluth)							
	0 – 50	<2:1		<125		<40	
	50 – 75	>2:1		125 – 225		40 – 100	
	75 – 90	>3:1	>5:1	225 – 325		>100	
	>90	>4:1	>9:1	>325		>100	
(Gosink)	>95	resistive CCA	distortion	may be decreased		may be decreased	

√ anechoic areas within plaque (= hemorrhage)
√ heterogeneous complex echo pattern

C. Ulcerated plaque
Neither arteriography nor US has proved reliable!
√ isolated crater within surface of plaque
√ proximal + distal undercutting of plaque
√ anechoic area within plaque extending to surface
√ reversed flow vortices extending into plaque by color Doppler associated with high-grade stenosis

INDIRECT METHODS OF EVALUATION
1. Oculoplethysmography (OPG)
= measurement of opthalmic artery pressure + pulse arrival time by air calibrated system
Contraindications: glaucoma, retinal detachment, recent eye surgery / trauma, lens implants
2. Periorbital bidirectional Doppler
= insonation of frontal + supraorbital arteries to assess flow direction around orbit and to detect crossover flow through the circle of Willis (through contra- and ipsilateral compression)
3. Transcranial Doppler
= insonation to establish flow direction in basal cerebral arteries through temporal bone (MCA, ACA, PCA, terminal portion of ICA), foramen magnum (both vertebral arteries, basilar artery), orbit (carotid siphon)
Δ Nondiagnostic in up to 35%!

Errors in Duplex Ultrasound
1. Error in proper localization of stenosis (6%)
Cause: ECA stenosis placed into ICA / carotid bifurcation or vice versa
2. Mistaking patent ECA branches for carotid bifurcation (4%)
Cause: complete occlusion of ICA not recognized
√ disparity in position of bifurcation
√ no difference in pulsatility waveform
√ high resistance waveform in CCA
3. Interpreter error in estimating severity of stenosis (2.5%)
usually overestimation, rarely underestimation
√ absence of one / more components for diagnosis which are
(a) significant elevation of peak velocity
(b) poststenotic turbulence
(c) extension of high velocity into diastole
4. Superimposition of ECA + ICA (2%)
Cause: strict coronal orientation of ECA + ICA
√ superimposition can be avoided by rotation of head to opposite side
5. Severe stenosis mistaken for occlusion
minimal flow not detectable; angiogram necessary with delayed images
6. Weak signals misinterpreted as occlusion
7. Normal / weak signals in severe stenosis
Cause: severe stenosis causes a decrease in blood flow + peak velocity with return to normal velocity levels

√ high resistivity in CCA
8. Point of maximum frequency shift not identified
Cause: extremely small lumen / short segment of stenosis
√ unexplained (poststenotic) coarse turbulence
√ ipsilateral ECA collateral flow
√ abnormal CCA resistivity
9. Stenosis obscured by plaque / strong Doppler shift in overlying vessel
10. Inaccessible stenosis
√ abnormal CCA resistivity
√ abnormal oculoplethysmography
11. Unreliable velocity measurements
(a) higher velocities: hypertension, severe bradycardia, obstructive contralateral carotid disease
(b) lower velocities: arrhythmia, aortic valvular lesion, severe cardiomyopathy, proximal obstructive carotid lesion ("tandem lesion"), >95% ICA stenosis
(c) aliasing = high velocities are displayed in reversed direction below zero baseline due to Doppler frequency exceeding half the pulse repetition frequency
Remedy: shift zero baseline, increase pulse repetition frequency, increase Doppler angle, decrease transducer frequency, use continuous wave Doppler probe

CHOLESTEATOMA
= KERATOMA = epithelium-lined sac filled with keratin debris leading to bone destruction by pressure + demineralizing enzymes

Primary Cholesteatoma
= CONGENITAL CHOLESTEATOMA = EPIDERMOID CYST (2%)
= derived from aberrant embryonic ectodermal rests in temporal bone (commonly petrous apex) / epidural space / meninges
• conductive hearing loss in child with NO history of middle ear inflammatory disease
• cholesteatoma seen through intact tympanic membrane
Associated with EAC dysplasia
Location:
(a) epitympanum
(b) petrous pyramid: internal auditory canal first involved
(c) meninges: scooped out apppearance of petrous ridge
(d) cerebellopontine angle: erosion of porus, shortening of posterior canal wall
(e) jugular fossa: erosion of posteroinferior aspect of petrous pyramid

Secondary Cholesteatoma
= INFLAMMATORY CHOLESTEATOMA (98%)
Cause:
ingrowth of squamous cell epithelium of EAC through eardrum in

(a) chronic inflammation of ear with invagination of posterosuperior retraction pocket
(b) marginal perforation of eardrum
Age: usually >40 years
- whitish-pearly mass behind intact tympanic membrane (invasion of middle ear cavity and mastoid) diagnosed otoscopically in 95%
- facial paralysis (compression of nerve VII at geniculate ganglion)
- sensorineural hearing loss (compromise of nerve VIII in internal auditory canal / involvement of cochlea or labyrinth)
- severe vertigo (labyrinthine fistula)
Types:
1. **Pars flaccida cholesteatoma** = Primary acquired cholesteatoma = Attic cholesteatoma (most common)
   √ increasing width of attic
   √ initally destruction of lateral wall of attic, particularly the drum spur (scutum) with invasion of Prussak space
   √ extension posteriorly through aditus ad antrum into mastoid antrum
   √ destruction of Körner septum
2. **Pars tensa cholesteatoma** = Secondary acquired cholesteatoma (less frequent)
   √ displacement of auditory ossicles
   √ erosion of ossicular chain: first affecting long process of incus

√ nondependent homogeneous mass
√ perforation of tympanic membrane posterosuperiorly (pars flaccida = Shrapnell membrane)
√ poorly pneumatized mastoid (frequent association)
√ erosion of tegmen tympani (with more extensive cholesteatoma)
√ destruction of labyrinthine capsule (less common) involving the lateral semicircular canal first
√ erosion of facial canal
MRI:
   √ iso- / hypointense relative to cortex on T1WI
   √ no enhancement with Gd-DTPA (enhancement is related to granulation tissue)
Cx:
(1) Intratemporal: ossicular destruction, facial nerve paralysis (1%), labyrinthine fistula, automastoidectomy, complete hearing loss
(2) Intracranial: meningitis, sigmoid sinus thrombosis, temporal lobe abscess, CSF rhinorrhea
DDx: chronic otitis media, granulation tissue = cholesterol granuloma, brain herniation through tegmen defect, neoplasm (rhabdomyosarcoma, squamous cell carcinoma)

CHOLESTEROL GRANULOMA
= CHOLESTEROL CYST
Histo:
   cholesterol crystals surrounded by foreign-body giant cells; embedded in fibrous connective tissue with varying proportions of hemosiderin-laden macrophages, chronic inflammatory cells and blood vessels; brownish fluid contains cholesterol crystals + blood
- blue (vascular) tympanic membrane without pulsatile tinnitus
√ ossicles remain intact
CT: √ nonenhancing middle ear mass
MRI: √ hyperintense signal on T1WI + T2WI (DDx to cholesteatoma, which is isointense to brain on T1WI)

CHRONIC RECURRENT SIALADENITIS
- painful periodic unilateral enlargement of parotid gland
- milky discharge may be expressed
Sialography:
   √ Stenson duct irregularly enlarged / sausage-shaped
   √ pruning of distal parotid ducts
   √ ± calculi
CT: √ diffusely enlarged dense gland
   √ dilated Stenson duct ± calculi
Cx: Mucocele

CROUP
= ACUTE LARYNGOTRACHEOBRONCHITIS
= ACUTE VIRAL SPASMODIC LARYNGITIS
= lower respiratory tract infection
Organism: parainfluenza, respiratory syncitial virus
Age: >6 months of age, peak incidence 2 – 3 years
- history of viral lower respiratory infection
- hoarse cry + "brassy" cough
- inspiratory difficulty with stridor
- fever
√ thickening of vocal cords
√ NORMAL epiglottis + aryepiglottic folds
√ "steeple sign" = subglottic "inverted V" = symmetrical funnel-shaped narrowing 1 – 1.5 cm below lower margins of pyriform sinuses on AP radiograph (loss of normal "shouldering" of air column caused by mucosal edema + external restriction by cricoid), accentuated on expiration, paradoxical inspiratory collapse, less pronounced during expiration
√ narrow + indistinct subglottic trachea on lateral radiograph
√ inspiratory ballooning of hypopharynx (nonspecific sign of any acute upper airway obstruction)
√ distension of cervical trachea on expiration
Prognosis: usually self-limiting

CYSTIC HYGROMA
= CYSTIC LYMPHANGIOMA = single / multiloculated fluid-filled cavities on either side of fetal neck + head ± trunk secondary to congenital blockage of lymphatic drainage (= noncommunication of jugular lymphatic sac with jugular vein)
Incidence: 1:6,000 pregnancies
Age: 50 – 65% present at birth; up to 90% evident by age 2
Path:
(1) capillary lymphangioma
(2) cavernous lymphangioma

(3) cystic lymphangioma = hygroma
macroscopic multilocular mass with cysts of varying
size lined with single layer of endothelium
containing serous / milky fluid

Associated with:
(1) Turner syndrome (45 XO, mosaic) in 73%
(2) Trisomies 13, 18, 21, 13q, 18p, 22
(3) Noonan syndrome
(4) Fetal alcohol syndrome
(5) Distichiasis-lymphedema syndrome
(6) Familial pterygium colli
• ± dyspnea / dysphagia with encroachment upon
trachea, pharynx, esophagus
• rapid increase in size (from infection / hemorrhage)
Location:
posterior neck (75%), mediastinum (3 – 10%, in 1/2
extension from neck), axilla (20%), chest wall (14%),
face (10%), retroperitoneum, abdominal viscera, groin,
scrotum, bones
√ thin-walled fluid-filled structure with multiple septa +
solid cyst wall components
√ isolated nuchal cysts
√ webbed neck (= pterygium colli) following later
communication with jugular veins
√ nonimmune hydrops + progressive peripheral edema
√ fetal ascites
√ oligo- / polyhydramnios / normal amount of fluid
√ bradycardia
Cx: (1) compression of airways / esophagus
        (2) slow growth / sudden enlargement
             (hemorrhage, inflammation)
Prognosis:
(1) Intrauterine demise (33%)
(2) Mortality of 100% with hydrops
(3) Spontaneous regression (10 – 15%)
Rx: surgical excision (difficult since mass does not
        follow tissue planes)
DDx: twin sac of blighted ovum, cervical meningocele,
        encephalocele, cystic teratoma, nuchal edema,
        branchial cleft cyst, vascular malformation, lipoma,
        abscess

EPIGLOTTITIS
= ACUTE BACTERIAL EPIGLOTTITIS = life-threatening
infection with edema of epiglottis + aryepiglottic folds
Organism: Haemophilus influenzae type B,
              Pneumococcus, Streptococcus group A
Age: >3 years, peak incidence 6 years
• abrupt onset of respiratory distress with inspiratory
stridor
• severe dysphagia
Location: purely supraglottic lesion; associated subglottic
            edema in 25%
Lateral radiograph should be taken in erect position only!
(frontal view irrelevant)
√ enlargement of epiglottis + thickening of aryepiglottic
folds
√ circumferential narrowing of subglottic portion of
trachea during inspiration
√ ballooning of hypopharynx + pyriform sinuses

√ cervical kyphosis
Cx: Mortal danger of suffocation secondary to hazard of
        complete airway closure; patient needs to be
        accompanied by physician experienced in
        endotracheal intubation

EXTERNAL AUDITORY CANAL DYSPLASIA
Incidence: 1:10,000 births; family history in 14%
Etiology: (a) isolated (b) Trisomy 13, 18, 21 (c) Turner
              syndrome (d) Maternal rubella (e) Craniofacial
              dysostosis (f) Mandibulofacial dysostosis
SPECTRUM
1. Stenosis of EAC
2. Fibrous atresia of EAC
3. Bony atresia (in position of tympanic membrane)
4. Decreased pneumatization of mastoid (mastoid cells
    begin to form in 7th fetal month)
5. Decreased size / absence of tympanic cavity
6. Ossicular changes (rotation, fusion, absence)
7. Ectopic facial nerve = anteriorly displaced vertical
    (mastoid) portion of facial nerve canal
8. Decrease in number of cochlear turns / absence of
    cochlea
9. Dilatation of lateral semicircular canal
• bilateral in 29%; M:F = 6:4
• pinna deformity
• stenotic / absent auditory canal
Cx: congenital cholesteatoma (infrequent)

FOLLICULAR ADENOMA OF THYROID
(1) Toxic adenoma
(2) Toxic multinodular goiter = hyperfunctioning adenoma
     within multinodular goiter; usually occurs in nodule
     >2.5 cm in size
(3) Nonfunctioning adenoma
√ mass with increased / decreased echogenicity
√ "halo sign" = complete hypoechoic ring with regular
border surrounding isoechoic solid mass

FRACTURE OF TEMPORAL BONE
A. LONGITUDINAL FRACTURE (75%)
   = fracture parallel to the axis of petrous pyramid arising
   in squamosa of temporal bone through tegmen
   tympani, EAC (external auditory canal), middle ear,
   terminating in foramen lacerum
• bleeding from EAC (disruption of tympanic
membrane)
• NO neurosensory hearing loss
• otorrhea (CSF leak with ruptured tympanic
membrane; rare)
• conductive hearing loss (dislocation of auditory
ossicles — most commonly incus as the least
anchored ossicle)
• facial nerve palsy (10 – 20%) due to edema / fracture
of facial canal near geniculate ganglion; frequent
spontaneous recovery

√ pneumocephalus
√ herniation of temporal lobe
√ incudostapedial joint dislocation (weakest joint)

√ disrupted ice cream cone relationship on direct
coronal CT scan
  √ fracture of "molar tooth" on direct sagittal CT scan
√ mastoid air cells opaque / with air-fluid level
Plain film views: Stenver / Owens projection
B. TRANSVERSE FRACTURE (25%)
= fracture perpendicular to axis of petrous pyramid
originating in occipital bone extending anteriorly
across the base of skull + across the petrous pyramid
- irreversible neurosensory hearing loss (fracture
across IAC / labyrinthine capsule)
- persistent vertigo
- facial nerve palsy in 50% (injury in IAC); less frequent
spontaneous recovery because of disruption of nerve
fibers
- rhinorrhea (CSF leak with intact tympanic membrane)
- bleeding into middle ear
Plain film views: posteroanterior (transorbital) + Towne
projection

GLOMUS TUMOR
= CHEMODECTOMA = NON-CHROMAFFIN
  PARAGANGLIOMA
Origin: tumor arising from nonchromaffin paraganglion
cells of neuroectodermal origin; differs from
adrenal medulla only in its nonchromaffin feature
Path: histologically similar to pheochromocytoma,
storage of catecholamines (usually
nonfunctioning)
Age: range of 6 months – 80 years; peak age in 5 – 6th
decade; F:M = 4:1
Associated with: pheochromocytoma
Location:
anywhere in paraganglionic tissue between glomus
jugulotympanicum and base of bladder: carotid body,
skull base, temporal region, trachea, periaortic region,
mandible, ciliary ganglion of the eye, retroperitoneal
region, cervical vagus nerve, laryngeal branches of
vagus nerve
Synchronous multicentricity in 3 – 26%:
(a) autosomal dominant in 25 – 35%
(b) non-hereditary in <5%

Glomus Tympanicum
Most common tumor in middle ear
- hearing loss, pulsatile tinnitus
- reddish purple mass behind tympanic membrane
Location: on cochlear promontory of middle ear
CT:
  √ globular soft tissue mass abutting promontory
  √ intense enhancement
  √ usually small at presentation (early involvement of
ossicles)
  √ erosion + displacement of ossicles
  √ inferior wall of middle ear cavity intact
Angio: √ difficult to visualize because of small size

Glomus Jugulare
Most common tumor in jugular fossa with intracranial
extension

Origin: adventitia of jugular bulb
- tinnitus, hearing loss
- vascular tympanic membrane
Location: at dome of jugular bulb
√ soft tissue mass in jugular bulb region /
hypotympanicum / middle ear space
√ intense enhancement
√ destruction of posteroinferior petrous pyramid +
corticojugular spine of jugular foramen
√ destruction of ossicles (usually incus), otic capsule,
posteromedial surface of petrous bone
MR:
  √ "salt and pepper" appearance due to multiple small
tumor vessels
Angio: (filming of entire neck for concurrent glomus
  tumors)
  √ hypervascular mass with persistent homogeneous
reticular stain
  √ invasion / occlusion of jugular bulb by thrombus /
tumor
  √ supplied by tympanic branch of ascending
pharyngeal artery, meningeal branch of occipital
artery, posterior auricular artery via stylomastoid
branch, internal carotid artery, internal maxillary
artery
  √ arteriovenous shunting
Cx: malignant transformation with metastases to
regional lymph nodes (in 2 – 4%)

Glomus Vagale
Origin: near ganglion nodosum of vagus nerve at base
of skull close to jugular foramen
Extension: (a)   downward into parapharyngeal space
  (2/3)
(b)   intracranially (dumbbell shape)
- slow growing + asymptomatic
√ spherical / ovoid mass with sharp interfacing margins
and homogeneous enhancement
√ highly vascular mass + neovascularity + intense
tumor blush
Cx: malignant transformation with metastases in
15% to regional lymph nodes + lung (other
paragangliomas in 10%)

Carotid Body Tumor
Embryology:
derived from mesoderm of 3rd branchial arch + neural
crest ectoderm cells, which differentiate into
sympathogonia (= forerunner of paraganglionic cells);
Δ Chemodectoma is misnomer (not derived from
  chemoreceptor cells)!
Histo:
nests of epithelioid cells ("Zellballen") with granular
eosinophilic cytoplasm separated by trabeculated
vascularized connective tissue
Δ chromaffin-positive granules (= catecholamines)
  may be present
Function of carotid body:
5 x 3 x 2 mm carotid body regulates pulmonary
ventilation through afferent input by way of

glossopharyngeal nerve to the medullary reticular formation

Stimulus: hypoxia > hypercapnia > acidosis

Effect: increase in respiratory rate + tidal volume; increase in sympathetic tone (heart rate, blood pressure, vasoconstriction, elevated catecholamines)

- painless pulsatile firm neck mass below the angle of the jaw, laterally mobile but vertically fixed

Location: adventitia of carotid bifurcation; bilateral in 5% with sporadic occurrence, in 32% with autosomal dominant transmission

√ enhancing oval mass with splaying of ICA + ECA

Cx: malignant transformation in 6% with metastases to regional lymph nodes, brachial plexus, cerebellum, lung, bone, pancreas, thyroid, kidney, breast

GOITER

Adenomatous Goiter

= MULTINODULAR GOITER

US: (89% sensitivity, 84% specificity, 73% positive predictive value, 94% negative predictive value)

√ increased size + asymmetry of gland

√ multiple 1 – 4 cm solid nodules

√ areas of hemorrhage + necrosis

√ coarse calcifications may occur within adenoma (secondary to hemorrhage + necrosis)

Diffuse Goiter

US:

√ increase in glandular size, R lobe > L lobe

√ NO focal textural changes

√ calcifications not associated with nodules

Iodine-Deficiency Goiter

Not a significant problem in United States because of supplemental iodine in food

Etiology: chronic TSH stimulation

- low serum T_4

√ high I-131 uptake

JOD-BASEDOW PHENOMENON (2%)

= development of thyrotoxicosis (= excessive amounts of T_4 synthesized + released) if normal dietary intake is resumed / iodinated contrast medium administered

Incidence: most common in individuals with long standing multinodular goiter

Age: >50 years

√ multinodular goiter with in- / decreased uptake (depending on iodine pool)

Toxic Nodular Goiter

= PLUMMER DISEASE

= autonomous function of one / more thyroid adenomas

Peak age: 4 – 5th decade; M:F = 1:3

- elevated T_4
- suppressed TSH

√ nodular thyroid with hot nodule + suppression of remainder of gland

√ stimulation scan will disclose normal uptake in remainder of gland

√ increased radioiodine uptake by 24 hours of approximately 80%

Rx: I-131 treatment with empirical dose of 25 – 29 mCi

Intrathoracic Goiter

= extension of cervical thyroid tissue / ectopic thyroid tissue (rare) into mediastinum

Incidence: 5% of resected mediastinal masses; most common cause of mediastinal masses

Location: usually anterior, 25% posterior exclusively on right side

- mostly asymptomatic
- symptoms of tracheal + esophageal + recurrent laryngeal nerve compression

√ continuity with cervical thyroid / lack of continuity (with narrow fibrous / vascular pedicle)

√ mass of high HU + well-defined borders

√ frequent focal calcifications

√ inhomogeneous texture with low-density areas (= degenerative cystic areas)

√ marked + prolonged enhancement

GRAVES DISEASE

= DIFFUSE TOXIC GOITER

= autoimmune disorder with thyroid stimulating antibodies (LATS) producing hyperplasia + hypertrophy of thyroid gland

Peak age: 3rd – 4th decade; M:F = 1:7

- elevated T_3 + T_4
- depressed TSH production
- dermopathy = pretibial myxedema (5%)
- ophthalmopathy = periorbital edema, lid retraction, ophthalmoplegia, proptosis, malignant exophthalmus

√ diffuse thyroid enlargement

√ uniformly increased uptake

√ incidental nodules superimposed on preexisting adenomatous goiter (5%)

US: (identical to diffuse goiter)

√ global enlargement of 2 – 3 x the normal size

√ normal / diffusely hypoechoic pattern

Rx: I-131 treatments (for adults):

Dose: 80 – 120 μCi/g of gland with 100% uptake (taking into account estimated weight of gland + measured radioactive iodine uptake for 24 hours)

Cx: 10 – 30% develop hypothyroidism within 1st year + 3%/year rate thereafter

HYPOPHARYNGEAL CARCINOMA

Histo: squamous cell carcinoma

May be associated with   Plummer-Vinson syndrome (= atrophic mucosa, achlorhydria, sideropenic anemia) affecting women in 90%

- sore throat, intolerance to hot / cold liquids (early signs)
- dysphagia, weight loss (late signs)
- cervical adenopathy (in 50% at presentation)

Stage:
- T1   tumor limited to one subsite
- T2   tumor involves >1 subsite / adjacent site without fixation of hemilarynx
- T3   same as T2 with fixation of hemilarynx
- T4   invasion of thyroid / cricoid cartilage / soft tissue of neck

Pyriform sinus carcinoma
Incidence: 60% of hypopharyngeal carcinomas
- may escape clinical detection if located at inferior tip; often origin of "cervical adenopathy with unknown primary" (next to primaries in lingual + faucial tonsils and nasopharynx)
- √ invasion of posterior ala of thyroid cartilage, cricothyroid space, soft tissue of neck in T4 lesion

Prognosis: poor due to early soft tissue invasion

Postcricoid carcinoma
Incidence: 25% of hypopharyngeal carcinomas
- √ difficult assessment due to varying thickness of inferior constrictor + prevertebral muscles

Prognosis: 25% 5-year survival (worst prognosis)

Posterior pharyngeal wall carcinoma
Incidence: 15% of hypopharyngeal carcinomas
- √ invasion of retropharyngeal space with extension into oro- and nasopharynx
- √ retropharyngeal adenopathy

INVERTING PAPILLOMA
= most common of epithelial papillomas; commonly occurring after nasal surgery

M>F

Path: hyperplastic epithelium inverts into underlying stroma

Location: most often arising from the lateral nasal wall extending into ethmoid / maxillary sinuses, at junction of antrum + ethmoid sinuses, uniquely unilateral
- unilateral nasal obstruction, epistaxis, postnasal drip, sinus headache
- distinctive absence of allergic history
- √ commonly involves antrum + ethmoid sinus
- √ widening of infundibulum / outflow tract of antrum
- √ destruction of medial antral wall / lamina papyracea of orbit (pressure necrosis)
- √ septum may be bowed to opposite side (NO invasion)
- √ homogeneous enhancement

MR:
- √ may have intermediate to low intensity on T2WI (DDx: squamous cell carcinoma)

Cx: (1) cellular atypia / squamous cell carcinoma (10%)
(2) recurrence (25 – 50%)

JUVENILE ANGIOFIBROMA
= most common benign nasopharyngeal tumor, can grow to enormous size and locally invade vital structures

Incidence: 0.5% of all head and neck neoplasms

Age: teenagers; exclusively in males

- recurrent + severe epistaxis
- nasal speech due to nasal obstruction
- facial deformity (less common)

Location: nasopharynx / posterior nares

Extension: posterolateral wall of nasal cavity; via pterygopalatine fossa into retroantral region / orbit / middle cranial fossa; laterally into infratemporal fossa
- √ widening of pterygopalatine fossa (90%)
- √ anterior bowing of posterior antral wall
- √ invasion of sphenoid sinus (2/3) from tumor erosion through floor of sinus
- √ widening of inferior + superior orbital fissures (spread into orbit via inferior orbital fissure + into middle cranial fossa via superior orbital fissure)
- √ highly vascular nasopharyngeal mass (only enhances on CT scan immediately after bolus injection); supplied primarily by internal maxillary artery

MR:
- √ intermediate signal intensity on T1WI with discrete punctate areas of hypointensity (secondary to highly vascular stroma)

NOTE: Biopsy contraindicated!

LABYRINTHITIS
Cause: toxins, viral illness (mumps, measles), bacterial infection
- √ no abnormalities with viral causes

Labyrinthitis ossificans
Cause: suppurative infection (tympanogenic, meningogenic, hematogenic), trauma, surgery, tumor, severe otosclerosis)
- bi - / unilateral profound deafness
- √ inner ear structures filled with bone

LARYNGEAL CARCINOMA
98% of all malignant laryngeal tumors; in 2% sarcomas

Risk factors: smoking, alcohol abuse, airborne irritants

Histo: squamous cell carcinoma

Suggestive of lymph node metastasis:
- √ lymph node >1.5 cm in cross-section
- √ proximity to laryngeal mass
- √ cluster of >3 lymph nodes 6 – 15 mm in size

Supraglottic Carcinoma
Incidence: 20 – 30% of all laryngeal cancers

Metastases: early to lymph nodes of deep cervical chain, in 25 – 55% at time of presentation
- symptomatic late in course of disease (often T3 / T4)

Stage:
- T1   tumor confined to site of origin
- T2   involvement of adjacent supraglottic site / glottis without cord fixation
- T3   tumor limited to larynx with cord fixation or extension to postcricoid area / medial wall of pyriform sinus / preepiglottic space
- T4   extension beyond larynx with involvement of oropharynx (base of tongue) / soft tissue of neck / thyroid cartilage

A. ANTERIOR COMPARTMENT
  1. **Epiglottic carcinoma**
    √ circumferential relatively symmetric growth
    √ extension into preepiglottic space ± base of tongue ± paraglottic space
  Prognosis: better than for tumors of posterolateral compartment
B. POSTEROLATERAL COMPARTMENT
  1. **Aryepiglottic fold (marginal supraglottic) carcinoma**
    √ exophytic growth from medial surface of aryepiglottic fold
    √ growth into fixed portion of epiglottis + paraglottic (= paralaryngeal) space
  2. **False vocal cord / laryngeal ventricle carcinoma**
    √ submucosal spread into paraglottic space
    √ ± destruction of thyroid cartilage
    √ ± involvement of true vocal cords
  Prognosis: poorer than for cancer of the anterior compartment

Glottic Carcinoma
Incidence: 50 – 60% of all laryngeal cancers
- early detection due to hoarseness

Stage:
  T1 tumor confined to vocal cord with normal mobility
  T2 supra- / subglottic extension ± impaired mobility
  T3 fixation of true vocal cord
  T4 destruction of thyroid cartilage / extension outside larynx

Patterns of tumor invasion:
  (1) anterior extension into anterior commissure
    √ >1 mm thickness of anterior commissure
    √ invasion of contralateral vocal cord via anterior commissure
  (2) posterior extension to arytenoid cartilage, posterior commissure, cricoarytenoid joint
  (3) subglottic extension
    √ tumor >5 mm inferior to level of vocal cords
  (4) deep lateral extension into paralaryngeal space
Prognosis: T1 carcinoma rarely metastasizes (0 – 2%) due to absence of lymphatics within true vocal cords

Subglottic Carcinoma
Incidence: 5% of all laryngel cancers
- late detection due to minimal symptomatology

Stage:
  T1 confined to subglottic area
  T2 extension to vocal cords ± mobility
  T3 tumor confined to larynx + cord fixation
  T4 cartilage destruction / extension beyond larynx
Prognosis: poor due to early metastases to cervical lymph nodes (in 25% at presentation)

LARYNGEAL PAPILLOMATOSIS
Squamous papilloma is the most common benign tumor of the larynx
Etiology: human papilloma virus type 6 (Papova virus)

Histo: core of vascular connective tissue covered by stratified squamous epithelium
Age of onset: 1 – 54 years; M:F = 1:1; bimodal distribution
  (a) <10 years (diffuse involvement)
  (b) 21 – 50 years (usually single papilloma)
- progressive hoarseness / aphonia
- repeated episodes of respiratory distress
- inspiratory stridor, asthma-like symptoms
- cough
- recurrent pneumonia
- hemoptysis
Location: (a) uvula, palate (b) vocal cord (c) subglottic extension (50 – 70%) (d) pulmonary involvement (1 – 6%)
√ thickened lumpy cords
√ bronchiectasis

Cx:
  (1) Tracheobronchial papillomatosis (2 – 5%)
    √ solid pulmonary nodules in mid + posterior lung fields
    √ 2 – 3 cm large thin-walled cavity with 2 – 4 mm thick nodular wall
    √ peripheral atelectasis + obstructive pneumonitis
  (2) Pulmonary papillomatosis
    from aerial metastases (bronchoscopy, laryngoscopy, tracheal intubation) 10 years after initial diagnosis
    √ irregularities of tracheal / bronchial walls
  (3) Malignant transformation into invasive squamous cell carcinoma
Rx: CO_2 laser resection

LARYNGOCELE
= abnormally dilated appendix / sacculus of laryngeal ventricle (= anteriorly located blind pouch within laryngeal ventricle between false + true vocal cords; normal appendix relatively large in infancy, visible in 10% of adults during phonation)
Pathogenesis: chronic increase in intraglottic pressure
Cause: excessive coughing, playing wind instrument, blowing glass, obstruction of appendicular ostium (= secondary laryngocele) by chronic granulomatous disease, laryngeal neoplasm
Types:
  (a) internal = in parapharyngeal space confined within thyrohyoid membrane + supraglottis
  (b) external = protrusion above thyroid cartilage + through thyrohyoid membrane presenting as lateral neck mass near hyoid bone
  (c) mixed (44%) = internal + external component joined through connection at thyrohyoid membrane
- hoarseness / stridor (internal laryngocele)
- anterior neck mass just below angle of mandible (external laryngocele)
Site: unilateral (80%), bilateral (20%)
√ cystic mass that can be followed to level of ventricle
√ increase in size during Valsalva maneuver
√ decrease in size during compression

√ may be filled with fluid
Cx: infection (pyolaryngocele), formation of mucocele

LARYNGOMALACIA
= immaturity of cartilage; most common cause of stridor in neonate + young infant
• only cause of stridor to get worse at rest
√ hypercollapsible larynx during inspiration (supraglottic portion only)
√ backward bent of epiglottis + anterior kink of aryepiglottic folds during inspiration
Prognosis: transient (disappears by age 1 year)

LINGUAL THYROID
= solid embryonic rest of thyroid tissue, which remains ectopic along the tract of thyroglossal duct
Incidence: in 10% of autopsies (within tongue <3 mm); M << F
• may be only functioning thyroid tissue (70 – 80%)
• asymptomatic (usually)
• may enlarge causing dysphagia / dyspnea
Location: midline dorsum of tongue near foramen cecum (majority), thyroglossal duct, trachea
CT: √ small focus of intrinsic high attenuation
Cx: malignancy in 3% (papillary carcinoma)

MALIGNANT EXTERNAL OTITIS
= severe bacterial infection of the soft tissues + bones of base of skull
Organism: almost always Pseudomonas aeruginosa
Age: elderly
Predisposed: diabetes mellitus / immunocompromised
• unrelenting otalgia, headache
• purulent otorrhea unresponsive to topical antibiotics
• may cause malfunction of nerves VII, IX, X, XI
Location: at bone-cartilage junction of EAC
Spread of infection:
   (a) inferiorly into soft tissues inferior to temporal bone, parotid space, nasopharyngeal masticator space
   (b) posteriorly into mastoid
   (c) anteriorly into temporomandibular joint
   (d) medially into petrous apex
CT:
  √ soft-tissue density in external auditory canal (100%)
  √ fluid in mastoid / middle ear (89%)
  √ disease around eustachian tube (64%)
  √ obliteration of fat planes beneath temporal bone (64%)
  √ involvement of parapharyngeal space (54%)
  √ masticator space disease (27%)
  √ mass effect in nasopharynx (54%)
  √ bone erosion of clivus (9%)
  √ intracranial extension (9%)
Cx: bone destruction, osteomyelitis, abscess
Prognosis: 20% recurrence rate
DDx: malignant neoplasm

MUCOCELE
Most common lesion to cause expansion of paranasal sinus; increased incidence in cystic fibrosis

Etiology: accumulation of mucoid secretions behind an obstructed paranasal sinus ostium with expansion of sinus cavity + thinning of sinus walls
Age: usually adulthood
• history of chronic nasal polyposis + pansinusitis
• commonly present with unilateral proptosis
• palpable mass in superomedial aspect of orbit (frontal mucocele)
• pain

Sites: frontal (60%) > ethmoid (30%) > maxillary (10%) > sphenoid (rare)
√ soft tissue density mass
√ sinus cavity expansion (DDx: never in sinusitis)
√ bone erosion / remodeling at late stage (impossible DDx from neoplasm)
√ surrounding zone of bone sclerosis (from chronic infection)
√ macroscopic calcification in 5% (especially with superimposed fungal infection)
√ pyocele = superimposed infection (rare)
√ uniform lack of enhancement
Cx: may protrude into orbit displacing medial rectus muscle laterally
DDx: paranasal sinus carcinoma, Aspergillus infection (enlargement of medial rectus muscle + optic nerve, focal / diffuse areas of increased attenuation), chronic infection, inverting papilloma

MUCOEPIDERMOID CARCINOMA
= most common malignant lesion of parotid gland
Path: arises from glandular ductal epithelium
• rock-hard mass
• pain / itching over course of facial nerve
• facial nerve paralysis

√ well-circumscribed parotid mass (low-grade lesion) / infiltrating poorly marginated lesion (high-grade lesion)

OTIC CAPSULE DYSPLASIA
Mondini malformation = any dysplasia of inner ear

Cochlear Aplasia
= Michel aplasia = agenesis of cochlea
• total sensorineural hearing loss
√ region of otic capsule normally occupied by cochlea is replaced by dense labyrinthine + pneumatized bone
√ marked enlargement of vestibule into region of lateral + superior semicircular canals

Single-Cavity Cochlea
= saccular defect / cavity in otic capsule in the position normally occupied by cochlea without recognizable modiolus, osseous spiral lamina, interscalar septum
• profound hearing loss discovered in early childhood
May be associated with recurrent bacterial meningitis, perilymphatic fistula of oval window
√ cystic cochlea (= developed basal turn, middle + apical turn occupy common nondeveloped space)

Insufficient Cochlear Turns
= normal basilar turn + varying degrees of hypoplasia of middle and apical turns

Small Internal Auditory Canal
= decrease in the diameter of IAC due to hypoplasia / aplasia of cochlear nerve (portion of cranial nerve VIII)
- total sensorineural hearing loss
- √ hypoplastic anteroinferior quadrant of IAC

Large Vestibule
Associated with   underdeveloped lateral semicircular canal
- √ lateral semicircular canal smaller
- √ vestibule extends further into lateral + superior aspects of otic capsule

Large Vestibular Aqueduct
= Vestibular aqueduct syndrome
- unilateral congenital deafness (commonly missed)
- √ vestibular aqueduct >2 mm in diameter

OTOSCLEROSIS
= OTOSPONGIOSIS
= replacement of dense otic capsule by more vascular bone in active phase (misnomer) with restoration of density during reparative sclerotic phase
Etiology: unknown; frequently hereditary
Age: young adult Caucasian; M:F = 1:2

A. STAPEDIAL = FENESTRAL OTOSCLEROSIS (80 – 90%)
Location: anterior oval window margin (= fissula antefenestrum); bilateral in 85%
- tinnitus early in course (2/3)
- progressive conductive hearing loss (stapes fixation in oval window)
- √ oval window too wide (lytic phase)
- √ new bone formation on anterior oval window margin ± posterior oval window margin ± round window
- √ complete plugging of oval window = obliterative otosclerosis (in 2%)

B. COCHLEAR = RETROFENESTRAL OTOSCLEROSIS (10 – 20%)
Invariably associated with   fenestral otosclerosis
- progressive sensorineural hearing loss (involvement of otic capsule / cytotoxic enzyme diffusion into fluid of membranous labyrinth)
- √ lucent halo around cochlea (may appear as 3rd turn to cochlea) in early phase
- √ bony proliferation in reparative sclerotic phase difficult to diagnose because of same density as cochlea

DDx: Paget disease, osteogenesis imperfecta

PARANASAL SINUS CARCINOMA
Location: maxillary sinus (80%), nasal cavity (10%), ethmoid sinus (5 – 6%), frontal + sphenoid sinus (rare)

Maxillary Sinus Carcinoma
Incidence: 80% of all paranasal sinus carcinomas
Histo: squamous cell carcinoma (80%)
Age: >40 years in 95%; M:F = 2:1
- asymmetry of face, tumor in oral / nasal cavity
- √ bone destruction (in 90%) predominates over expansion
- √ nodal metastases in 10 – 18%

Nasopharyngeal Carcinoma
Incidence: 10% of paranasal sinus carcinomas; 0.25 – 0.5% of all malignant tumors in whites; M>F
Predisposed: Chinese population
Histo: squamous cell carcinoma (>85%)
Mean age: 40 years
- asymptomatic for a long time
- history of chronic sinusitis / nasal polyps (15%)
- unilateral nasal obstruction
Location: turbinates (50%) > septum > vestibule > posterior choanae > floor
Extension: skull base, intracranially (cranial nerve V most commonly affected)
- √ polypoid or papillary (2/3)
- √ bone invasion (1/3)
MR:
- √ signal intensity similar to that of adjacent mucosa

Ethmoid Sinus Carcinoma
Incidence: 5 – 6% of paranasal sinus carcinomas
Histo: squamous cell carcinoma (>90%), sarcoma, adenocarcinoma, adenoid cystic carcinoma; frequently secondarily involved from maxillary sinus carcinoma
- nasal obstruction, bloody discharge
- anosmia, broadening of nose

PHARYNGEAL ABSCESS
Etiology: spread of infection from tonsils / pharynx
Age: children > adults
- trismus (most common presenting symptom) from involvement of pterygoid muscle
- sore throat
- low-grade fever
- √ isodense / low-density mass with unsharp margins
- √ rim enhancement
Cx: Mycotic aneurysm of carotid artery (within 10 days)

RETROPHARYNGEAL ABSCESS / HEMORRHAGE
Etiology: upper respiratory tract infection, perforating injury of pharynx / esophagus, suppuration of infected lymph node
Organism: Staphylococcus, mixed flora
Age: usually <1 year
- fever, neck stiffness, dysphagia
- √ thickness of retropharyngeal space >3/4 of AP diameter of vertebral body
- √ reversal of cervical lordosis
- √ anterior displacement of airway
- √ may contain gas and gas-fluid level

RHABDOMYOSARCOMA

= most common soft-tissue tumor in children; 3rd most common primary childhood malignancy of head + neck (following brain tumors + retinoblastomas)

Incidence: 5 – 15% of all malignant tumors in children <15 years of age

Age: 2 – 5 years (peak prevalence); <10 years (70%)
• cranial nerve palsy

Location: head and neck (orbit most common), paranasal sinus, middle ear, nasopharyngeal musculature (1/3); most common primary extracranial tumor invading the cranial vault in childhood

Metastases: lymph nodes (50%), lung, bone

√ bulky nasopharyngeal mass
√ extension into cranial vault through fissures + foramina (up to 35%) usually involving cavernous sinus
√ bone destruction
√ uniform enhancement

CT:
√ isodense with brain
√ expanded foramen / fissure

MR (imaging modality of choice):
√ signal intensity intermediate between muscle and fat on T1WI + hyperintense on T2WI

Prognosis: 12.5% 5-year survival

RHINOCEREBRAL MUCORMYCOSIS

= paranasal sinus infection caused by nonseptated fungi Rhizopus arrhizus and Rhizopus oryzae

Spread: fungus first involves nasal cavity, then extends into maxillary / ethmoid sinuses / orbits / intracranially along ophthalmic artery / cribriform plate (frontal sinuses are spared)

Predisposed:
(1) poorly controlled diabetes mellitus (2) chronic renal failure (3) cirrhosis (4) malnutrition (5) cancer (6) prolonged antibiotic therapy (7) steroid therapy (8) cytotoxic drug therapy (9) AIDS (10) extensive burns
• black crusting of nasal mucosa (in diabetics)
• small ischemic areas (invasion of arterioles + small arteries)
√ nodular thickening involving nasal septum + turbinates
√ mucoperiosteal thickening + clouding of ethmoids
√ focal areas of bone destruction

Cx: (1) blindness (2) cranial nerve palsy (3) hemiparesis
Prognosis: high mortality rate

SARCOIDOSIS

blacks:whites = 10:1
Location: eye, lacrimal glands, salivary glands (40%), larynx (5%), involvement of intra- and extraparotid lymph nodes (rare)
√ granulomas may enhance
√ enlargement of optic canal (optic neuritis)
√ thickening of larynx with enhancement of granulomas
√ multiple small granulomas of septum + turbinates

Heerfordt syndrome

(1) Parotid enlargement
• diffuse bilateral painless enlargement (10 – 30%)
• xerostomia
CT: √ diffusely dense multinodular gland / enlargement of lymph nodes within gland
(2) Uveitis
(3) Facial nerve paralysis

SIALOSIS

= nontender noninflammatory recurrent enlargement of parotid gland

Cause: cirrhosis, alcoholism, diabetes, malnutrition, hormonal insufficiency (ovarian / pancreatic / thyroid), drugs (sulfisoxazole, phenylbutazone), radiation therapy

Histo: serous acinar hypertrophy + fatty replacement of gland

Sialography:
√ sparse peripheral ducts

CT:
√ enlarged / normal-sized gland
√ diffusely dense gland in end-stage

SINUSITIS

Incidence:
most common paranasal sinus problem; most common chronic disease diagnosed in United States; complicating common colds in 0.5% (3 – 4 colds/year in adults, 6 – 8 colds/year in children)

Cause:
(1) Obstruction of major ostia
(a) middle meatus draining frontal, maxillary, anterior ethmoid sinus
(b) sphenoethmoid recess draining posterior ethmoid sphenoid sinus
(2) Ineffective mucociliary clearing secondary to contact of two mucosal surfaces

Primary focus:
anterior ethmoid-middle meatal complex = area responsible for drainage of frontal + maxillary sinuses

√ air-fluid level (= retention of secretions secondary to mucosal swelling, which leads to narrowing of ostia + ostial dysfunction)
√ opacification of sinus
√ mucosa >5 mm thick on Water view

A. BACTERIAL SINUSITIS
Organism:
Streptococcus pneumoniae + Haemophilus influenzae (>50%); Branhamella catarrhalis, viruses, fungi (Aspergillus fumigatus)
√ solitary antral disease (obstruction of sinus ostium)
√ uniform enhancement

B. ALLERGIC SINUSITIS
√ involves multiple sinuses
√ bilaterally symmetric
√ uniform enhancement

Cx:
(1) **Retention cyst** (10%) = smoothly marginated soft-tissue mass from obstruction of mucous gland (commonly in floor of maxilla)
(2) Orbital extension through neurovascular foramina, dehiscences, or thin bones

(3) Septic thrombophlebitis
(4) Intracranial extension: meningitis, epidural abscess, subdural empyema, venous sinus thrombosis, cerebral abscess

SUBGLOTTIC HEMANGIOMA
Most common subglottic soft-tissue mass causing upper respiratory tract obstruction in neonates
- croup-like symptoms in neonatal period
- hemangiomas elsewhere (skin, mucosal membranes) in 50%
√ eccentric thickening of subglottic portion of trachea (AP view)
√ arises from posterior wall below true cords (lateral view)

SUBGLOTTIC STENOSIS
A. CONGENITAL SUBGLOTTIC STENOSIS
- croup-like symptoms, often self-limiting disease
Location: 1 – 2 cm below vocal cords
√ circumferential symmetrical narrowing of subglottic portion of trachea during inspiration
√ NO change in degree of narrowing with expiration
B. ACQUIRED SUBGLOTTIC STENOSIS
following prolonged endotracheal intubation (in 5%)

THORNWALDT CYST
= midline congenital pouch / cyst lined by ectoderm within nasopharyngeal mucosal space
Origin: persistent focal adhesion between notochord + ectoderm extending to the pharyngeal tubercle of the occipital bone
Incidence: 4% of autopsies
Peak age: 15 – 30 years
- asymptomatic incidental finding
- persistent nasopharyngeal drainage
- halitosis
- foul taste in mouth

Location: posterior roof of nasopharynx
√ smoothly marginated cystic mass of few mm to 3 cm in size
√ low density, not enhancing
√ NO bone erosion
Cx: infection of cyst
DDx: Rathke pouch (occurs in craniopharyngeal canal located anteriorly + cephalad to Thornwaldt cyst)

THYROGLOSSAL DUCT CYST
Embryogenesis:
thyroglossal duct = duct along which thyroid gland descends to its final position from foramen cecum at base of tongue passing anteriorly / posteriorly / through precursor of hyoid bone; duct usually involutes by 8th week of fetal life; thyroid elements remain in thyroglossal duct in 5%
Histo: cyst lined by squamous cell mucosa
Age: <10 years in 50%; 2nd peak at 20 – 30 years
- midline neck mass
- ± history of previous incision and drainage of an "abscess" in area of cyst

Location: suprahyoid (20%), hyoid (15%), infrahyoid (65%)
√ midline / paramedian cystic mass of 2 – 4 cm
√ infrahyoid strap muscles beak over edge of cyst
Cx: infection; thyroglossal duct carcinoma (<1%)
Rx: complete surgical removal

THYROID CARCINOMA
Age: <30 years; M>F
- history of neck irradiation
- rapid growth
- stone-hard nodule
√ hypoechoic mass
√ irregular ill-defined border without halo
√ NO hemorrhage / liquefaction necrosis

RADIATION-INDUCED THYROID CANCER
Incidence increases with doses of thyroidal irradiation from 6.5 – 1,500 rad (higher doses are associated with hypothyroidism)
Peak occurence: 5 – 30 (up to 50) years post irradiation
Thyroid abnormalities in 20%:
(a) in 14% adenomatous hyperplasia, follicular adenoma, colloid nodules, thyroiditis
(b) in 6% thyroid cancer
Δ Nondetectable microscopic foci of cancer in 25% of patients operated on for benign disease!
Δ In patients with multiple cold nodules frequency of cancer is 40%

WHOLE-BODY SCAN in metastatic thyroid carcinoma
Indication: to detect metastases of thyroid carcinoma after total thyroidectomy; preferred over bone scan (only detects 40%) for skeletal metastases
Δ metastases not detectable in presence of normal functioning thyroid tissue because uptake is much less in metastases
Δ Tc-99m pertechnetate is useless because of high background activity + lack of organification
Technique:
(1) T_4 replacement therapy discontinued
(2) short-acting T_3 is administered for 4 – 6 weeks
(3) T_3 replacement therapy discontinued 10 – 14 days prior to whole-body scan
(4) measurement of TSH level to confirm adequate elevation (TSH >50 mIU/ml; administration of exogenous TSH not desirable because of uneven stimulation)
(5) oral administration of 5 – 10 mCi I-131
(6) whole-body scan after 24, 48, 72 hours (low background activity)

N.B.: posttherapy scan (1 week after therapeutic dose) identifies more lesions than diagnostic scan
Normal sites of accumulation: nasopharynx, salivary glands, stomach, colon, bladder, liver (I-131-labeled thyroxine produced by carcinoma is metabolized in

liver), breasts in lactating women (breast feeding must be terminated after administration of I-131) CONTRAINDICATED during pregnancy!

TREATMENT for follicular / papillary cancer:
(1) Surgery: total thyroidectomy + modified radical neck dissection
(2) Postoperative radioiodine treatment with I-131 (multiple treatments are usually necessary)
    Δ Radioiodine therapy only appropriate for papillary / mixed / follicular thyroid carcinomas (NOT for medullary or anaplastic carcinomas)
    (a) ablative dose to destroy remaining thyroid tissue 6 weeks following surgery; no thyroid hormone replacement 3 – 4 weeks prior to therapy
        Dose = [(weight (g) x 80–120 µCi/g) ÷ % uptake of I-123 by 24 hours] x 100 approx. 100 mCi I-131 orally
    (b) treatment of metastases
        Dose: 100 – 200 mCi (dose increase with regional lymph node / lung / bone metastases to 150, 175, 200 mCi) Administration of 150 mCi of I-131 with an uptake of 0.5% per gram of tumor tissue and a biologic half-life of 4 days will produce 25,000 rads to tumor)
    Δ Rapid turnover rates may exist in some metastases (lower dose advisable)
    Δ Treatment of large tumors incomplete (range of beta radiation is a few mm)
    Cx:
        radiation thyroiditis, radiation parotitis, GI-symptoms (nausea, diarrhea), minimal bone marrow depression, leukemia (2%), anaplastic transformation (uncommon), lung fibrosis (with extensive pulmonary metastases + dose >200 mCi)
(3) Thyroid replacement therapy exogenous thyroid hormone to suppress TSH stimulation of metastases
(4) External radiation therapy for anaplastic carcinoma + metastases without iodine uptake
FOLLOW-UP: Thyroglobulin >50 ng/ml indicates functioning metastases

Papillary Carcinoma of Thyroid
60% of all thyroid carcinomas
Peak age: 5th decade; F>M
Histo: unencapsulated well-differentiated tumor
    (a) purely papillary
    (b) mixed with follicular elements (more common, especially under age 40)
Metastases:
    (1) Lymphogenic spread to regional lymph nodes (40%, in children almost 90%)
    (2) Hematogenous spread to lung (4%), bone (rare)
NUC:
√ tumor usually concentrates radioiodine (even some purely papillary tumors)

US:
    √ tumor of decreased echogenicity
    √ purely solid / complex mass with areas of necrosis, hemorrhage, cystic degeneration
X-ray:
    √ punctate / linear psammomatous calcifications at tumor periphery
Prognosis:
    90% 10-year survival for occult + intrathyroidal cancer; 60% 10-year survival for extrathyroidal cancer; worse prognosis with increasing age

Follicular Carcinoma of Thyroid
20% of all thyroid cancers; slow growing
Peak age: 5th decade; F > M
Histo: encapsulated well-differentiated tumor without papillary elements; in 25% multifocal; cytologically impossible to distinguish between well-differentiated follicular carcinoma + follicular adenoma (vascular invasion is only criteria)
Early hematogenous spread to:
    (a) lung
    (b) bone (30%): almost always osteolytic (more frequent than in papillary carcinoma)
√ psammoma bodies + stromal calcium deposits
NUC:
    √ usually concentrates pertechnetate, but fails to accumulate I-123
US:
    √ indistinguishable from benign follicular adenoma
Prognosis:
    90% 10-year survival with slight / equivocal angioinvasion; 35% 10-year survival with moderate / marked angioinvasion

Anaplastic Carcinoma of Thyroid
15% of all thyroid cancers
Age: 6 – 7th decade; M:F=1:1
NUC:
    √ NO radioiodine uptake
Prognosis: 5% 5-year survival; average survival time of 6 – 12 months

Medullary Carcinoma of Thyroid
1 – 5% of all thyroid cancers; sporadic / familial
Histo: arises from parafollicular C-cells, associated with amyloid deposition in primary + metastatic sites
Mean age: 60 years for sporadic variety; in adolescence with MEN
May be associated with:
    (1) MEN IIa = pheochromocytoma + parathyroid hyperplasia
    (2) MEN IIb = without parathyroid component

Metastases: early spread to lymph nodes (50%), lung, liver, bone
• elevated calcitonin (from tumor production) stimulated by pentagastrin + calcium infusion

NUC:
√ NO uptake by radioiodine / pertechnetate
√ frequently shows increased uptake of Tl-201
√ granular calcifications within fibrous stroma / amyloid masses (50%)
Prognosis:
90% 10-year survival without nodal metastases
42% 10-year survival with nodal metastases
Rx: total thyroidectomy + modified radical neck dissection

THYROIDITIS

Hashimoto Thyroiditis
= CHRONIC LYMPHOCYTIC THYROIDITIS
Most frequent cause of goitrous hypothyroidism in adults in the USA (iodine-deficiency is the more common cause worldwide)
Etiology: autoimmune process with marked familial predisposition; antibodies are typically present; functional organification defect
Peak age: 4 – 5th decade; M > F
• firm rubbery lobular goiter
• gradual painless enlargement
• thyrotoxicosis in early stage (4%)
• decreased thyroid reserve
• hypothyroidism at presentation (20%)
√ moderate enlargement of both lobes (18%)
NUC:
√ low tracer uptake (occasionally increased) with poor visualization (4%)
√ prominent pyramidal lobe
√ positive perchlorate washout test
√ patchy tracer distribution
√ multiple (40%) / single cold defects (28%) / normal thyroid (8%)
US:
√ initially diffusely decreased echogenicity + slight lobulation of contour
√ later densely echogenic (fibrosis) + acoustical shadows
Cx: hypothyroidism

De Quervain Thyroiditis
= SUBACUTE THYROIDITIS
Etiology: probably viral
Histo: lymphocytic infiltration + granulomas + foreign body giant cells
Peak age: 2 – 5th decade; M:F = 1:5
• upper respiratory tract infection precedes onset of symptoms by 2 – 3 weeks
• painful tender gland + fever; only mild enlargement
• hyperthyroidism (50%) secondary to severe destruction
• short-lived hypothyroidism (25%) secondary to hormone depletion of gland

NUC:
√ abnormally low radioiodine uptake with clinical and laboratory evidence of hyperthyroidism
√ poor visualization of thyroid (initially)
√ single / multiple hypofunctional areas (occasionally)
√ increased uptake during phase of hypothyroidism (late event)

Cx: permanent hypothyroidism (rare)
Prognosis: usually full recovery

Painless Thyroiditis
Histo: resembles chronic lymphocytic thyroiditis
• clinical presentation similar to subacute thyroiditis
• NOT painful / tender

Acute Suppurative Thyroiditis
US:
√ focal / diffuse enlargement; possibly abscess
√ decreased echogenicity

WARTHIN TUMOR
= PAPILLARY CYSTADENOMA LYMPHOMATOSUM
Incidence: 2nd most common benign tumor of parotid gland; bilateral in 10%
Age: about 50 years; M > F
Origin: from heterotopic salivary gland tissue within parotid lymph nodes
• slow-growing mass

√ well-circumscribed single / multiple tumors in parotid region usually 3 – 4 cm in size
MR:
√ hypointense compared to fat / surrounding parotid tissue on T2WI

WEGENER GRANULOMATOSIS
= necrotizing granulomatous vasculitis
Mean age of onset: 40 years; M:F = 2:1
Triad:
(1)   Upper respiratory tract
    (a)   nasal cavity:
        • erosion of nasal septum
        • saddle nose deformity
        √ progressive destruction of nasal cartilage + bone (DDx: relapsing polychondritis)
        √ granulomatous masses filling nasal cavities
    (b)   sinuses (maxillary antra most frequently):
        √ thickening of mucosa
(2)   Lungs
    • hemoptysis
    √ multiple pulmonary nodules
(3)   Glomerulonephritis
Rx: cyclophosphamide

DIFFERENTIAL DIAGNOSIS OF CHEST DISORDERS

ABNORMAL LUNG PATTERNS

1. Mass
   - = any localized density not completely bordered by fissures / pleura
2. Consolidative (alveolar) pattern
   commonly produced by alveolar filling,
   ALSO by alveolar collapse, airway obstruction,
   confluent interstitial thickening
3. Interstitial pattern
4. Vascular pattern
   - (a) increased vessel size: CHF, pulmonary arterial hypertension, shunt vascularity, lymphangitic carcinomatosis
   - (b) decreased vessel size: emphysema, thromboembolism
5. Bronchial pattern
   - √ wall thickening: bronchitis, asthma, bronchiectasis
   - √ density without air bronchogram (= complete airway obstruction)
   - √ lucency of air trapping (= partial airway obstruction with ball valve mechanism)

ALVEOLAR (CONSOLIDATIVE) PATTERN

= pattern of filled air spaces

Classic appearance of air space consolidation:
- √ **A**cinar rosettes: rounded poorly defined nodules in size of acini (6 – 10 mm), best seen at periphery of densities
- √ **A**ir alveologram / bronchogram
- √ **B**utterfly / bat-wing distribution: perihilar / bibasilar
- √ **C**oalescent / confluent cloud-like ill-defined opacities
- √ **C**onsolidation in diffuse, perihilar / bibasilar, segmental / lobar, multifocal / lobular distribution
- √ **C**hanges occur rapidly (labile / fleeting)

CT:
- √ poorly marginated densities within primary lobule (up to 1 cm in size)
- √ rapid coalescence with neighboring lesions in segmental distribution
- √ predominantly central location with sparing of subpleural zones
- √ air bronchograms

Diffuse air space disease

A. INFLAMMATORY EXUDATE = "PUS"
1. Lobar pneumonia
2. Bronchopneumonia: especially Gram-negative organisms
3. Unusual pneumonias
   - (a) viral: extensive hemorrhagic edema especially in immuno-compromised patients with hematologic malignancies + transplants
   - (b) pneumocystis
   - (c) fungal: Aspergillus, Candida, Cryptococcus, Phycomycetes
   - (d) tuberculosis
4. Aspiration

B. HEMORRHAGE = "BLOOD"
1. Trauma: Contusion
2. Pulmonary embolism, thromboembolism
3. Bleeding diathesis: leukemia, hemophilia, anticoagulants, DIC
4. Vasculitis: Wegener granulomatosis, Goodpasture syndrome, SLE, mucormycosis, aspergillosis, Rocky Mountain spotted fever, infectious mononucleosis
5. Idiopathic pulmonary hemosiderosis
6. Bleeding metastases: choriocarcinoma

C. TRANSUDATE = "WATER"
1. Cardiac edema
2. Neurogenic edema
3. Hypoproteinemia
4. Fluid overload
5. Renal failure
6. Radiotherapy
7. Shock
8. Toxic inhalation
9. Drug reaction
10. Adult respiratory distress syndrome

D. SECRETIONS = "PROTEIN"
1. Alveolar proteinosis
2. Mucous plugging

E. MALIGNANCY = "CELLS"
1. Bronchioloalveolar cell carcinoma
2. Lymphoma

F. INTERSTITIAL DISEASE simulating air space disease, eg, "alveolar sarcoid"

mnemonics:
"**P**lease **P**ut **A** **H**ot-**L**ight **A**t
The **S**ithouse **F**irst"   "AIRSPACED"

Pulmonary edema	**A**spiration
Pneumonia	**I**nhalation
Alveolar proteinosis, carcinoma, microlithiasis	**R**enal (uremia)
	Swimming (drowning)
Hyaline membrane disease, Hemorrhage, Heroin	**P**neumonia
	Alveolar proteinosis
Lymphoma	**C**ardiovascular
Aspiration	**E**dema
Tuberculosis	**D**rug reaction
Sarcoidosis	
Fungus	

Acute alveolar infiltrate
mnemonic: "I 2 CHANGE FAST"
Infarct
Infection

Contusion
Hemorrhage
Aspiration
Near drowning
Goodpasture syndrome
Edema
Fungus
Allergic sensitivity
Shock lung
Tuberculosis

Chronic alveolar infiltrate
mnemonics:

"PALS GET MOD"	"STALLAG"
Proteinosis	**S**arcoidosis
Alveolar cell carcinoma	**T**uberculosis
Lymphoma	**A**lveolar cell ca.
Sarcoidosis	**L**ymphoma
Granulomatosis	**L**ipoid pneumonia
Eosinophilic granuloma	**A**lveolar proteinosis
Tuberculosis	**G**oodpasture syndr.
Microlithiasis	
Oil aspiration	
DIP (not consolidative)	

Eosinophilic lung disease
= PULMONARY INFILTRATION WITH BLOOD / TISSUE EOSINOPHILIA (PIE)

Classification:
1. IDIOPATHIC EOSINOPHILIC LUNG DISEASE
   (a) Transient pulmonary eosinophilia = Löffler syndrome
       • peripheral eosinophilia
   (b) Chronic eosinophilic pneumonia
       • no peripheral eosinophilia
2. EOSINOPHILIC LUNG DISEASE OF PECIFIC ETIOLOGY
   (a) drug induced: nitrofurantoin, penicillin, sulfonamides, ASA, tricyclic antidepressants, hydrochlorothiazide, cromolyn sodium, mephenesin
   (b) parasite induced: tropical eosinophilia (ascariasis, schistosomiasis), strongyloidiasis, ancylostomiasis (hookworm), filariasis, Toxocara canis (visceral larva migrans), Dirofilaria immitis, amebiasis (occasionally — in right lower + middle lobe)
   (c) fungus induced: allergic bronchopulmonary aspergillosis, bronchocentric granulomatosis
   (d) Pulmonary eosinophilia with asthma
3. EOSINOPHILIC LUNG DISEASE ASSOCIATED WITH ANGIITIS ± GRANULOMATOSIS
   (a) Wegener granulomatosis
   (b) Polyarteritis nodosa
   (c) Allergic granulomatosis (Churg-Strauss)
       = variant of polyarteritis nodoa
       Strongly associated with history of asthma
       • peripheral eosinophilia in >30%

(d) Lymphomatoid granulomatosis
    may lead to lymphoma
    √ CXR similar to Wegener granulomatosis
(e) Bronchocentric granulomatosis
    = granulomas forming around bronchi + vasculitis
    • often associated with long history of asthma
    √ bronchial obstruction
(f) Necrotizing "sarcoidal" angiitis
(g) Rheumatoid disease
(h) Scleroderma
(i) Dermatomyositis
(j) Sjögren syndrome
(k) CREST

INTERSTITIAL LUNG DISEASE
= thickening of lung interstices (= interlobular septa)

(a) Major lymphatic trunks
    1. Lymphangitic carcinomatosis
    2. Congenital pulmonary lymphangiectasia
(b) Pulmonary veins (increased pulmonary venous pressure)
    1. Left ventricular failure
    2. Venous obstructive disease
(c) Supporting connective tissue network
    1. Interstitial edema
    2. Chronic interstitial pneumonia
    3. Pneumoconioses
    4. Collagen-vascular disease
    5. Interstitial fibrosis
    6. Amyloid
    7. Tumor infiltration within connective tissue
    8. Desmoplastic reaction to tumor

INTERSTITIAL LUNG PATTERN
1. Linear form
   (a) **reticulations**
       = network of interlacing lines in all directions
   (b) **Kerley lines** = septal lines
       = thickened connective septa
       √ Kerley A lines = relatively long fine linear shadows in upper lungs, deep within lung parenchyma
       √ Kerley B lines = short horizontally oriented lines extending to pleura, perpendicular to pleura in costophrenic angles + retrosternal clear space
       √ Kerley C lines = "spider web" appearance covering entire lung
2. Nodular form
   = small sharp numerous uniform nodules with even distribution
3. Destructive form = honeycomb lung

SIGNS OF ACUTE INTERSTITIAL DISEASE
√ thickening of interlobular fissures
√ Kerley-lines
√ peribronchial cuffing = thickened bronchial wall + peribronchial sheath (when viewed end on)

√ perihilar haze = blurring of hilar shadows
√ blurring of pulmonary vascular markings
√ increased density at lung bases
√ small pleural effusions

SIGNS OF CHRONIC INTERSTITIAL DISEASE
√ irregular visceral pleural surface

√ reticulations
  (a) fine reticulations = early potentially reversible /
      minimal irreversible alveolar septal abnormality
  (b) coarse reticulations
      in 75% related to environmental disease,
      sarcoidosis, collagen-vascular disorders, chronic
      interstitial pneumonia

√ **nodularity**
  in 90% related to infectious / noninfectious
  granulomatous process, metastatic malignancy,
  pneumoconioses, amyloidosis

√ **linearity**
  cardiogenic / noncardiogenic interstitial pulmonary
  edema, lymphangitic malignancy, diffuse bronchial
  wall disorders (cystic fibrosis, bronchiectasis,
  hypersensitivity asthma)

√ **honeycombing** = rounded radiolucencies <1 cm in
  diameter set off against a background of increased
  lung density (endstage lung)

HRCT of interstitial disease:
  √ thick irregular saw-toothed appearance of interlobar
    fissures, vascular borders, bronchial walls

√ sharply marginated noncoalescing interstitial nodules

√ interstitial reticulation:
  √ large network of polyhedral reticular elements of 15
    – 25 mm in diameter with central pulmonary artery
    (secondary lobular architecture);
    associated with   interstitial pulmonary edema,
                        lymphangitic carcinomatosis
  √ predominantly subpleural small reticular elements
    of 6 – 10 mm in diameter with small cystic changes
    ("honeycombing")
    associated with   interstitial fibrosis,
                           lymphangioleiomyomatosis, diffuse amyloidosis
  √ fine diffusely distributed network of 2 – 3 mm basic
    elements
    associated with   miliary TB, reactions to
                        methotrexate

√ ground glass opacities (diffuse interstitial thickening +
  obliteration of air space)

Generalized interstitial disease
  mnemonic: "HIDE FACTS"
    Hamman-Rich, **H**emosiderosis
    Infection, **I**rradiation, **I**diopathic
    Dust, **D**rugs
    Eosinophilic granuloma, **E**dema
    Fungal, **F**armer's lung
    Aspiration (oil), **A**rthritis (rheumatoid, ankylosing
      spondylitis)
    Collagen disease
    Tumor, **T**B, **T**uberous sclerosis
    Sarcoidosis, **S**cleroderma

Distribution of Diffuse Lung Disease

Means of distribution	Peripheral lung	Central lung
Perfusion	Hematogenous metastases Adult respiratory distress syndrome Fat embolism Usual interstitial pneumonitis Scleroderma Rheumatoid arthritis Bleomycin sulfate administration	Acute hydrostatic pulmonary edema
Ventilation	Chronic eosinophilic pneumonia Asbestosis Diffuse panbronchiolitis	Allergic bronchopulmonary aspergillosis Bronchitis Centrilobular emphysema Hypersensitivity pneumonitis
Lymph flow		Sarcoidosis Silicosis Coal worker's pneumoconiosis Eosinophilic granuloma Postprimary tuberculosis

Reticulonodular pattern
mnemonic:
"**P**lease **D**on't **E**at **S**tale **T**una **F**ish **S**andwiches **E**very
Morning"
Pneumoconiosis
Drugs
Eosinophilic granuloma
Sarcoidosis
Tuberculosis
Fungal disease
Schistosomiasis
Exanthem (measles, chickenpox)
Metastases (thyroid)

Acute diffuse fine reticulations
A. ACUTE INTERSTITIAL EDEMA
    1. Congestive heart failure
    2. Fluid overload
    3. Uremia
    4. Hypersensitivity
B. ACUTE INTERSTITIAL PNEUMONIA
    1. Viral pneumonia
    2. Mycoplasma pneumonia
    3. Pneumocystis carinii pneumonia

mnemonic: "HELP"
Hypersensitivity
Edema
Lymphoproliferative
Pneumonitis (viral)

Chronic diffuse fine reticulations
A. VENOUS OBSTRUCTION
    1. Atherosclerotic heart disease
    2. Mitral stenosis
    3. Left atrial myxoma
    4. Pulmonary veno-occlusive disease
    5. Sclerosing mediastinitis
B. LYMPHATIC OBSTRUCTION
    1. Lymphangiectasia (pediatric patient)
    2. Mediastinal mass   (lymphoma)
    3. Lymphoma / leukemia
    4. Lymphangitic carcinomatosis:
        predominantly basilar distribution
        (a) bilateral (breast, stomach, colon, pancreas)
        (b) unilateral (lung tumor)
    5. Lymphocytic interstitial pneumonitis
C. INHALATIONAL DISEASE
    1. Silicosis: small nodules + reticulations
    2. Asbestosis: basilar distribution, pleural
                    thickening + calcifications
    3. Hard metals
    4. Allergic alveolitis
D. GRANULOMATOUS DISEASE
    from a nodular to a reticular pattern if
        (a) nodules line up along bronchovascular
            bundles
        (b) interlobular septa show fibrotic changes
    1. Sarcoidosis: hilar + mediastinal adenopathy
                       (may have disappeared)

2. Eosinophilic granuloma: upper lobe distribution
E. COLLAGEN-VASCULAR DISEASE
    reticulations in late stages
    1. Rheumatoid lung
    2. Scleroderma
F. DRUG REACTIONS
G. IDIOPATHIC
    1. Usual interstitial pneumonitis (UIP)
    2. Desquamative interstitial pneumonitis (DIP)
    3. Tuberous sclerosis: smooth muscle proliferation
    4. Lymphangiomyomatosis
    5. Idiopathic pulmonary hemosiderosis
    6. Alveolar proteinosis (late complication)
    7. Amyloidosis
    8. Interstitial calcification (chronic renal failure)

mnemonic: "LIFE lines"
Lymphangitic spread
Inflammation / infection
Fibrosis
Edema

Coarse reticulations
= architectural destruction of interstitium = end-stage
  scarring of lung = **honeycomb lung**
√ coarse reticular interstitial densities with intervening
  cystic spaces
√ rounded radiolucencies <1 cm in areas of increased
  lung density
√ small lung volume (decreased compliance)
Cx: (1)   intercurrent pneumothoraces
        (2)   bronchogenic carcinoma = scar carcinoma

Cause:
A. INHALATIONAL DISEASE
    (a) Pneumoconioses
        1. Asbestosis: basilar distribution, shaggy heart,
            pleural thickening + calcifications
        2. Silicosis: upper lobe predominance, ± pleural
            thickening, ± hilar and mediastinal lymph
            adenopathy
        3. Berylliosis
    (b) Chemical inhalation (late)
        1. Silo-filler's disease (nitrogen dioxide)
        2. Sulfur dioxide, chlorine, phosgene, cadmium
    (c) Extrinsic allergic alveolitis (hypersensitivity to
        organic dusts)
    (d) Oxygen toxicity: sequelae of RDS therapy with
        oxygen
    (e) Chronic aspiration
        eg, mineral oil: localized process in medial basal
        segments / middle lobe
B. GRANULOMATOUS DISEASE
    1. Sarcoidosis
    2. Eosinophilic granuloma
C. COLLAGEN-VASCULAR DISEASE
    1. Rheumatoid lung
    2. Scleroderma
    3. Ankylosing spondylitis: upper lobes
    4. SLE: rarely produces honeycombing

D. IATROGENIC
1. Drug hypersensitivity
2. Radiotherapy
E. IDIOPATHIC
1. Usual interstitial pneumonitis (UIP)
honeycombing in 50%, severe volume loss in 45%
2. Desquamative interstitial pneumonitis (DIP)
honeycombing in 12.5%, severe volume loss in 23%
√ basilar patchy air consolidations
3. Lymphangiomyomatosis
4. Tuberous sclerosis (rare)
5. Neurofibromatosis (rare)
DDx: Bronchiectasis, cavitary metastases (rare)

Distribution of interstitial disease
mnemonics:

Basilar distribution	**Apical distribution**
"BAD LASS RF"	"CASSET"
Bronchiectasis	**C**ystic fibrosis
Aspiration	**A**nkylosing spondylitis
DIP, **D**ermatomyositis	**S**ilicosis
Lymphangitic spread	**S**arcoidosis
Asbestosis	**E**osinophilic granuloma
Sarcoidosis	**T**uberculosis, fungus
Scleroderma	
Rheumatoid arthritis	
Furadantin	

Honeycomb lung
mnemonic: "HIPS RDS"   "SHIPS BOATS"

Histiocytosis X	**S**arcoidosis
Interstitial pneumonia	**H**istiocytosis
Pneumoconiosis	**I**diopathic (UIP)
Sarcoidosis	**P**neumoconiosis
	Scleroderma
Rheumatoid lung	**B**leomycin, **B**usulfan
Dermatomyositis	**O**xygen toxicity
Scleroderma	**A**rthritis (rheumatoid),
	Amyloidosis,
	Allergic alveolitis
	Tuberous sclerosis, **TB**
	Storage disease (Gaucher)

Reticulations + pleural effusion
A. ACUTE
1. Edema
2. Infection: viral, mycoplasma (very rare)
B. CHRONIC
1. Congestive heart failure
2. Lymphangitic carcinomatosis
3. Lymphoma / leukemia
4. SLE
5. Rheumatoid disease
6. Lymphangiectasia
7. Lymphangiomyomatosis
8. Asbestosis

Reticulations + hilar adenopathy
1. Sarcoidosis
2. Silicosis
3. Lymphoma / leukemia
4. Lung primary: particularly oat cell carcinoma
5. Metastases: lymphatic obstruction / spread
6. Fungal disease
7. Tuberculosis
8. Viral pneumonia (rare combination)

Diffuse fine nodular disease + miliary nodules
√ very small (1 – 4 mm) sharply defined nodules of interstitial disease

A. INHALATIONAL DISEASE
1. Silicosis + coal-worker's pneumoconiosis
2. Berylliosis
3. Siderosis
4. Extrinsic allergic alveolitis (chronic phase)
B. GRANULOMATOUS DISEASE
1. Eosinophilic granuloma
2. Sarcoidosis (with current / previous adenopathy)
C. INFECTIOUS DISEASE
1. Tuberculosis
2. Fungus: histoplasmosis, coccidioidomycosis, blastomycosis, aspergillosis (rare), cryptococcosis (rare)
3. Bacteria: salmonella, nocardiosis
4. Virus: varicella (more common in adults)
D. METASTASES
Thyroid carcinoma, melanoma, adenocarcinoma of breast, stomach, colon, pancreas
E. ALVEOLAR MICROLITHIASIS (rare)
F. BRONCHIOLITIS OBLITERANS
G. GAUCHER DISEASE

mnemonic: "TEMPEST"
Tuberculosis + fungal disease
Eosinophilic granuloma
Metastases (thyroid, lymphangitic carcinomatosis)
Pneumoconiosis, **P**arasites
Embolism of oily contrast
Sarcoidosis
Tuberous sclerosis

Micronodular disease
1. Granulomatous disease (miliary tuberculosis, histoplasmosis)
2. Hypersensitivity (organic dust)
3. Pneumoconiosis (inorganic dust, thesaurosis = prolonged hair spray exposure)
4. Sarcoidosis
5. Metastases (thyroid, melanoma)
6. Histiocytosis X
7. Chickenpox

Fine nodular disease in afebrile patient
1. Inhalational disease
2. Eosinophilic granuloma
3. Sarcoidosis

4. Metastases
5. Fungal infection (late stage)
6. Miliary tuberculosis (rare)

Fine nodular disease in febrile patient
1. Tuberculosis
2. Fungal infection (early stage)
3. Pneumocystis
4. Viral pneumonia

Macronodular disease
√ nodules >5 mm in diameter
mnemonic: "GAMMA WARPS"
Granuloma (EG, fungus)
Abscess
Metastases
Multiple myeloma
AVM
Wegener granulomatosis
Amyloidosis
Rheumatoid lung
Parasites (Echinococcus, Paragonimus)
Sarcoidosis

Chronic infiltrates in childhood
mnemonic: "ABC'S"
Asthma, **A**gammaglobulinemia, **A**spiration
Bronchiectasis
Cystic fibrosis
Sequestration, intralobar

Chronic interstitial disease simulating air space disease
A. Replacement of lung architecture by an interstitial process
   (a) Neoplastic
       Hodgkin disease, histiocytic lymphoma
   (b) Benign cellular infiltrate
       lymphocytic interstitial pneumonia, pseudolymphoma
   (c) Granulomatous disease
       alveolar sarcoidosis
   (d) Fibrosis
B. Exudative phase of interstitial pneumonia
   1. UIP
   2. Adult respiratory distress syndrome
   3. Radiation pneumonitis
   4. Drug reaction
   5. Reaction to noxious gases
C. Cellular filling of air space
   1. Desquamative interstitial pneumonia
   2. Pneumocystis carinii pneumonia

DENSE LUNG LESION

Opacification of hemithorax
mnemonic: "FAT CHANCE"
Fibrothorax
Adenomatoid malformation

Trauma (ie, hematoma)
Collapse, **C**ardiomegaly
Hernia
Agenesis of lung
Neoplasm (ie, mesothelioma)
Consolidation
Effusion

Atelectasis
A. TUMOR
   1. Bronchogenic carcinoma (2/3 of squamous cell carcinoma occur as endobronchial mass with persistent / recurrent atelectasis or recurrent pneumonia)
   2. Bronchial carcinoid
   3. Metastases: renal cell carcinoma, breast carcinoma, melanoma
   4. Lymphoma (usually as a late presentation)
   5. Lipoma, granular cell myoblastoma, amyloid tumor, fibroepithelial polyp
B. INFLAMMATION
   1. Tuberculosis (endobronchial granuloma, broncholith, bronchial stenosis)
   2. Right middle lobe syndrome (chronic right middle lobe atelectasis)
   3. Sarcoidosis (endobronchial granuloma — rare)
C. MUCUS PLUG
   1. Severe chest / abdominal pain (postoperative patient)
   2. Respiratory depressant drug (morphine; CNS illness)
   3. Chronic bronchitis / bronchiolitis obliterans
   4. Asthma
   5. Cystic fibrosis
   6. Bronchopneumonia (peribronchial inflammation)
D. OTHER
   1. Large left atrium (mitral stenosis + left lower lobe atelectasis)
   2. Foreign body (aspiration of food, endotracheal intubation)
   3. Amyloidosis
   4. Wegener granulomatosis
   5. Bronchial transection

√ local increase in lung density
√ crowding of pulmonary vessels
√ bronchial rearrangement
√ displacement of fissures
√ displacement of hilus
√ mediastinal shift
√ elevation of hemidiaphragm
√ cardiac rotation
√ approximation of ribs
√ compensatory overinflation of normal lung

A. OBSTRUCTIVE ATELECTASIS
   Resorptive Atelectasis
   Pathophysiology: sum of partial gas pressures in venous blood perfusing atelectatic region is less than atmospheric pressure, which is responsible for

gradual resorption of air trapped distal to site of obstruction; continuing secretion into small airways leads to consolidation (postobstructive pneumonitis / bacterial infection)

Cause: bronchiolar obstruction by
1. Tumor
2. Stricture
3. Foreign body
4. Mucous plug
5. Bronchial rupture
- airless collapse within minutes to hours

MR:
√ high signal intensity on T2WI in atelectatic area

B. NONOBSTRUCTIVE ATELECTASIS
Pathophysiology: pathway between bronchial system + alveoli is maintained because bronchi are less compliant than lung parenchyma + remain patent; secretions can be eliminated + convective airflow to distal bronchioles remains
- collapsed lung not completely airless (up to 40% residual air)

MR:
√ low signal intensity on T2WI in atelectatic area

Passive Atelectasis
= pleural space-occupying process
1. Pneumothorax
2. Hydrothorax / hemothorax
3. Diaphragmatic hernia
4. Pleural masses: metastases, mesothelioma

Adhesive Atelectasis
= decrease in surfactant production
1. Respiratory distress syndrome of the newborn (hyaline membrane disease)
2. Pulmonary embolism: edema, hemorrhage, atelectasis
3. Intravenous injection of hydrocarbon

Cicatrizing Atelectasis
= parenchymal fibrosis causing decreased lung volume
1. Tuberculosis / histoplasmosis (upper lobes)
2. Silicosis (upper lobes)
3. Scleroderma (lower lobes)
4. Radiation pneumonitis (nonanatomical distribution)
5. Idiopathic pulmonary fibrosis

Rounded Atelectasis
√ comet-tail sign (= converging lung markings)
√ pleural thickening
√ subpleural mass lateral / posterior chest wall
√ "swiss cheese" air bronchogram (AP tomogram)

Discoid Atelectasis
mnemonic: "EPIC"
Embolus
Pneumonia
Inadequate inspiration
Carcinoma, obstructing

Segmental + lobar densities
A. PNEUMONIA
1. Lobar pneumonia
2. Lobular pneumonia
3. Acute interstitial pneumonia
4. Aspiration pneumonia
5. Primary tuberculosis
B. PULMONARY EMBOLISM
(rarely multiple / larger than subsegmental)
C. NEOPLASM
1. Obstructive pneumonia
2. Bronchioloalveolar cell carcinoma
D. ATELECTASIS

Multifocal ill-defined densities
= densities 5 – 30 mm resulting in air-space filling

A. INFECTION
1. Bacterial bronchopneumonia
2. Fungal pneumonia:
histoplasmosis, blastomycosis, actinomycosis, coccidioidomycosis, aspergillosis, cryptococcosis, mucormycosis, sporotrichosis
3. Viral pneumonia
initially may have interstitial appearance
= tracheitis, bronchitis, bronchiolitis, peribronchial infiltrate, interstitial septa infiltrates, injury to alveolar cells, hyaline membranes, necrosis of alveolar walls with blood, edema, fibrin, macrophages in alveoli
(a) Influenza: cavitary lesion confirms superimposed infection
(b) Varicella / herpes zoster: 10% of adults; 2 – 5 days after rash
(c) Rubeola (measles) = before / with onset of rash; following overt measles = giant cell pneumonia
(d) Cytomegalic inclusion virus: features suggestive of bronchopneumonia
(e) Coxsackie, parainfluenza, adenovirus, respiratory syncytial virus
4. Tuberculosis (primary infection)
5. Rocky Mountain spotted fever
6. Pneumocystis carinii
B. GRANULOMATOUS DISEASE
1. Sarcoidosis (alveolar form secondary to peribronchial granulomas)
2. Eosinophilic granuloma
C. VASCULAR
1. Thromboembolic disease
2. Septic emboli
3. Vasculitis
(a) Wegener granulomatosis
(b) Wegener variants: limited Wegener, lymphomatoid granulomatosis
(c) Infectious vasculitis = invasion of pulmonary arteries: mucormycosis, invasive form of aspergillosis, Rocky Mountain spotted fever
(d) Goodpasture syndrome
(e) Scleroderma

D. NEOPLASTIC
1. Bronchioloalveolar cell carcinoma
   = only primary lung tumor to produce multifocal ill-defined densities with air bronchograms
2. Alveolar type of lymphoma
   = massive accumulation of tumor cells in interstitium with compression atelectasis + obstructive pneumonia
3. Metastases
   (a) Choriocarcinoma: hemorrhage (however rare)
   (b) Vascular tumors: malignant hemangiomas
4. Waldenström macroglobulinemia
5. Angioblastic lymphadenopathy
6. Mycosis fungoides
7. Amyloid tumor

E. IDIOPATHIC INTERSTITIAL DISEASE
1. Lymphocytic Interstitial Pneumonitis (LIP)
2. Desquamative Interstitial Pneumonitis (DIP)
3. Pseudolymphoma = localized form of LIP
4. Usual Interstitial Pneumonitis (UIP)

F. INHALATIONAL DISEASE
1. Allergic alveolitis: acute stage (eg, farmer's lung)
2. Silicosis
3. Eosinophilic pneumonia

G. DRUG REACTIONS

Chronic multifocal ill-defined opacities
1. Organizing pneumonia
2. Granulomatous disease
3. Allergic alveolitis
4. Bronchioloalveolar cell carcinoma
5. Lymphoma

Chronic diffuse confluent opacities
1. Alveolar proteinosis
2. Hemosiderosis
3. Sarcoidosis

Ill-defined densities with holes
A. INFECTION
1. Necrotizing pneumonias:
   Staphylococcus aureus, ß-hemolytic streptococcus, Klebsiella pneumoniae, E. coli, Proteus, Pseudomonas, anaerobes
2. Aspiration pneumonia:
   mixed Gram-negative organisms
3. Septic emboli
4. Fungus:
   histoplasmosis, blastomycosis, coccidioidomycosis, cryptococcosis
5. Tuberculosis
B. NEOPLASM
1. Primary lung carcinoma
2. Lymphoma (cavitates very rarely)
C. VASCULAR + COLLAGEN-VASCULAR DISEASE
1. Emboli with infarction
2. Wegener granulomatosis
3. Necrobiotic rheumatoid nodules
D. TRAUMA
1. Contusion with pneumatoceles

Perihilar "bat-wing" infiltrates
mnemonic: "**P**lease, **P**lease, **P**lease, **S**tudy **L**ight, **D**on't **G**et **A**ll **U**ptight"
Pulmonary edema
Proteinosis
Periarteritis
Sarcoidosis
Lymphoma
Drugs
Goodpasture syndrome
Alveolar cell carcinoma
Uremia

Peripheral "reverse bat-wing" infiltrates
mnemonic: "REDS"
Resolving pulmonary edema
Eosinophilic pneumonia
Desquamative interstitial pneumonia
Sarcoidosis

Recurrent fleeting infiltrates
1. Löffler disease
2. Bronchopulmonary aspergillosis / bronchocentric granulomatosis
3. Asthma
4. Subacute bacterial endocarditis with pulmonary emboli

Tubular density
A. Mucoid impaction
B. Vascular malformation
   1. Arteriovenous malformation
   2. Pulmonary varix

Mucoid impaction
1. Asthma (most frequent cause): esp. during acute attack or convalescent phase
2. Cystic fibrosis
3. Chronic bronchitis
4. Bronchial obstruction by neoplasm: bronchogenic carcinoma / adenoma
5. Bronchopulmonary aspergillosis: central perihilar bronchiectasis
6. Fluid-filled bronchiectasis: history of childhood pneumonia; peripheral distribution
7. Bronchial atresia

Bronchial obstruction
mnemonic: "MEATFACE"
Mucus plug
Endobronchial granulomatous disease
Adenoma
Tuberculosis
Foreign body
Amyloid, **A**tresia (bronchial)
Cancer (primary)
Endobronchial metastasis

Multiple pulmonary calcifications
A. Infection
   1. Histoplasmosis
   2. Tuberculosis
   3. Chickenpox pneumonia
B. Inhalational disease
   1. Silicosis
C. Miscellaneous
   1. Hypercalcemia
   2. Mitral stenosis
   3. Alveolar microlithiasis

PULMONARY EDEMA
Transcapillary flow dependent on (1) hydrostatic pressure
(2) colloid osmotic pressure (3) capillary permeability

A. INCREASED HYDROSTATIC PRESSURE
   (a) CARDIOGENIC (most common)
      = pulmonary venous hypertension
      1. Heart disease: left ventricular failure, mitral
         valve disease, left atrial myxoma
      2. Pulmonary venous disease: primary veno-
         occlusive disease, mediastinal fibrosis
      3. Pericardial disease: pericardial effusion,
         constrictive pericarditis (extremely rare)
      4. Drugs: antiarrhythmic drugs; drugs depressing
         myocardial contractility (beta-blocker)
   (b) NONCARDIOGENIC
      1. Renal failure
      2. IV fluid overload
      3. Hyperosmolar fluid (eg, contrast medium)
   (c) NEUROGENIC
      ? sympathetic venoconstriction in
      cerebrovascular accident, head injury, CNS tumor,
      postictal state
B. DECREASED COLLOID OSMOTIC PRESSURE
   1. Hypoproteinemia
   2. Transfusion of crystalloid fluid
   3. Rapid reexpansion of lung
C. INCREASED CAPILLARY PERMEABILITY
   Endothelial injury from
   (a) Physical trauma: parenchymal contusion,
       radiation therapy
   (b) Aspiration injury:
      1. Mendelson syndrome (gastric contents)
      2. Near drowning in sea water / fresh water
      3. Aspiration of hypertonic contrast media
   (c) Inhalation injury:
      1. Nitrogen dioxide = silo-filler's disease
      2. Smoke (pulmonary edema may be delayed by
         24 – 48 hours)
      3. Sulfur dioxide, hydrocarbons, carbon
         monoxide, beryllium, cadmium, silica,
         dinitrogen tetroxide, oxygen, chlorine,
         phosgene, ammonia, organophosphates
   (d) Injury via bloodstream
      1. Vessel occlusion: shock (trauma, sepsis,
         ARDS) or emboli (fat, amniotic fluid, thrombus)
      2. Circulating toxins: snake venom, paraquat

3. Drugs: heroin, morphine, methadone, aspirin,
   phenylbutazone, nitrofurantoin, chlorothiazide
4. Anaphylaxis: transfusion reaction, contrast
   medium reaction, penicillin
5. Hypoxia: high altitude, acute large airway
   obstruction
mnemonic: "ABCDEFGHI - PRN"
Aspiration
Burns
Chemicals
Drugs (heroin, nitrofurantoin, salicylates)
Exudative skin disorders
Fluid overload
Gram negative shock
Heart failure
Intracranial condition
Polyarteritis nodosa
Renal disease
Near drowning

Unilateral pulmonary edema
A. IPSILATERAL = on side of preexisting abnormality
   1. Prolonged lateral decubitus position
   2. Unilateral aspiration / pulmonary lavage
   3. Pulmonary contusion
   4. Rapid thoracentesis (rapid reexpansion)
   5. Bronchial obstruction (drowned lung)
   6. Unilateral venous obstruction
   7. Systemic artery-to-pulmonary artery shunt
      (Waterston, Blalock-Taussig, Pott procedure)
B. CONTRALATERAL = opposite to side of abnormality
   1. Congenital absence / hypoplasia of pulmonary
      artery
   2. Unilateral arterial obstruction
   3. Swyer-James syndrome
   4. Thromboembolism
   5. Unilateral emphysema
   6. Lobectomy
   7. Pleural disease

Interstitial pulmonary edema
√ nothing differentiates it from other interstitial lesions
√ does not necessarily develop before alveolar
   pulmonary edema
√ often marked dissociation between clinical signs +
   symptoms + roentgenographic evidence
√ NOT typical for bacterial pneumonia

Pulmonary edema with cardiomegaly
1. Cardiogenic
2. Uremic (with cardiomegaly from pericardial effusion /
   hypertension)

Pulmonary edema without cardiomegaly
mnemonic: "U DOPA"
Uremia
Drugs
Overhydration
Pulmonary hemorrhage
Acute myocardial infarction, **A**rrhythmia

Noncardiogenic pulmonary edema

mnemonic: "The alphabet"

ARDS, **A**lveolar proteinosis, **A**spiration, **A**naphylaxis
Bleeding diathesis, **B**lood transfusion reaction
CNS (increased pressure, trauma, surgery, CVA, cancer)
Drowning (near), **D**rugs
Embolus (fat, thrombus)
Fluid overload, **F**oreign body inhalation
Glomerulonephritis, **G**oodpasture syndrome, **G**astrografin aspiration
High altitude, **H**eroin, **H**ypoproteinemia
Inhalation (SO$_2$, smoke, CO, cadmium, silica)
-
Narcotics, **N**itrofurantoin
Oxygen toxicity
Pancreatitis
-
Rapid reexpansion of pneumothorax / removal of pleural effusion
-
Uremia

PNEUMONIA

"Classic" pneumonia pattern:
1. Lobar distribution : Streptococcus pneumoniae
2. Bulging fissure : Klebsiella
3. Pulmonary edema : Viral pneumonia, Pneumocystis pneumonia
4. Pneumatocele : Staphylococcus
5. Alveolar nodules : Varicella, bronchogenic spread of TB

Distribution:
- A. SEGMENTAL / LOBAR
  — Normal host: S. pneumoniae, Mycoplasma, virus
  — Compromised host: S. pneumoniae

- B. BRONCHOPNEUMONIA
  — Normal host: Mycoplasma, virus, Streptococcus, Staphylococcus, S. pneumoniae
  — Compromised host: Gram-negative, Streptococcus, Staphylococcus
  — Nosocomial: Gram-negative, Pseudomonas, Klebsiella, Staphylococcus
  — Immunosuppressed: Gram-negative, Staphylococcus, Nocardia, Legionella, Aspergillus, Phycomycetes

- C. EXTENSIVE BILATERAL
  — Normal host: virus (eg, influenza), Legionella
  — Compromised host: candidiasis, pneumocystis, tuberculosis

- D. BILATERAL LOWER LOBE
  — Normal host: anaerobic (aspiration)
  — Compromised host: anaerobic (aspiration)

- E. PERIPHERAL
  — Noninfectious eosinophilic pneumonia

Transmission:
- A. COMMUNITY-ACQUIRED PNEUMONIA
  Organisms: viruses, S. pneumoniae, Mycoplasma
- B. NOSOCOMIAL PNEUMONIA
  (a) Gram-negative organisms (>50%): Klebsiella pneumoniae, P. aeruginosa, E. coli, Enterobacter
  (b) Gram-positive organisms (10%): S. aureus, S. pneumoniae, H. influenzae

Lobar pneumonia

= ALVEOLAR PNEUMONIA
= pathogens reach peripheral air space, incite exudation of watery edema into alveolar space, centrifugal spread via small airways, pores of Kohn + Lambert into adjacent lobules + segments

√ nonsegmental sublobar consolidation
√ round pneumonia (= uniform involvement of contiguous alveoli)
  (a) Streptococcus pneumoniae
  (b) Klebsiella pneumoniae (more aggressive); in immunocompromised + alcoholics
  (c) any pneumonia in children
  (d) atypical measles
√ expansion of lobe with bulging of fissures
√ lung necrosis with cavitation
DDx: Aspiration, pulmonary embolus

Lobular pneumonia

= BRONCHOPNEUMONIA
= combination of interstitial + alveolar disease (injury starts in airways involves bronchovascular bundle, spills into alveoli, which may contain edema fluid, blood, leukocytes, hyaline membranes, organisms)
Organisms:
  (a) Staphylococcus aureus, Pseudomonas pneumoniae: thrombosis of lobular artery branches with necrosis + cavitation
  (b) Streptococcus, Klebsiella, Legionnaires' bacillus, Bacillus proteus, E. coli, anaerobes (Bacteroides + Clostridia), Nocardia, actinomycosis
  (c) Mycoplasma

√ small fluffy ill-defined acinar nodules, which enlarge with time
√ lobar + segmental densities with volume loss from airway obstruction secondary to bronchial narrowing + mucus plugging

Acute interstitial pneumonia

= NONBACTERIAL PNEUMONIA
initially predominantly affecting interstitial tissues
Organisms: viruses, mycoplasma, pneumocystis
• often subacute atypical pneumonia

√ diffuse interstitial process with peribronchial thickening
√ segmental / lobar densities (mucus plugging + damage of surfactant-producing type 2 alveolar cells)

Gram-negative pneumonia

In 50% cause of nosocomial necrotizing pneumonias
(including staphylococcal pneumonia)
predisposed: elderly, debilitated, diabetes, alcoholism,
COPD, malignancy, bronchitis, Gram-
positive pneumonia, treatment with
antibiotics, respirator therapy
Organisms:
1. Klebsiella   4. Proteus
2. Pseudomonas   5. Haemophilus
3. E. coli   6. Legionella
√ air-space consolidation (Klebsiella)
√ spongy appearance (Pseudomonas)
√ affecting dependent lobes (poor cough reflex without
clearing of bronchial tree)
√ bilateral
√ cavitation common
Cx: (1) exudate / empyema (2) bronchopleural fistula

Mycotic infections of lung

A.   In healthy subjects
1. Histoplasmosis
2. Coccidioidomycosis
3. Blastomycosis
B.   Opportunistic infection
1. Aspergillosis
2. Candidiasis
3. Mucormycosis (phycomycosis)
Growth: (a) mycelial form (b) yeast form (depending on
environment)
Source of contamination:
(a) soil (b) growth in moist areas (apart from
Coccidioides immitis) (c) contaminated bird / bat excreta

Cavitating pneumonia

1. Staphylococcus aureus
2. Haemophilus influenzae
3. S. pneumoniae
other Gram-negative organisms (eg, Klebsiella)

Cavitating opportunistic infections

A.   FUNGAL INFECTIONS
1. Aspergillosis
2. Nocardiosis
3. Mucormycosis (= phycomycosis)
B.   SEPTIC EMBOLI
1. Anaerobic organisms
C.   STAPHYLOCOCCAL ABSCESS
D.   TUBERCULOSIS
nummular form
Δ Repeated infections in same patient are not necessarily
due to same organism!
DDx: Metastatic disease in carcinoma / Hodgkin
lymphoma

Recurrent pneumonia in childhood

A.   Immune problem
1. Immune deficiency
2. Chronic granulomatous disease of childhood
(males)

3. Alpha 1-antitrypsin deficiency
B.   Aspiration
1. Gastroesophageal reflux
2. H-type tracheoesophageal fistula
3. Disorder of swallowing mechanism
4. Esophageal obstruction, impacted esophageal
foreign body
C.   Underlying lung disease
1. Sequestration
2. Bronchopulmonary dysplasia
3. Cystic fibrosis
4. Atopic asthma
5. Bronchiolitis obliterans
6. Sinusitis
7. Bronchiectasis
8. Ciliary dysmotility syndromes
9. Pulmonary foreign body

Hypersensitivity to organic dusts

A.   TRACHEOBRONCHIAL HYPERSENSITIVITY
large particles reaching the tracheobronchial mucosa
(pollens, certain fungi, some animal / insect epithelial
emanations)
1. Extrinsic asthma
2. Hypersensitivity aspergillosis
3. Bronchocentric granulomatosis
4. Byssinosis in cottonwool workers

B.   ALVEOLAR HYPERSENSITIVITY
= HYPERSENSITIVITY PNEUMONITIS
= EXTRINSIC ALLERGIC ALVEOLITIS
small particles of <5 μ reaching alveoli

Drug-induced pulmonary damage

A.   CHEMOTHERAPEUTIC AGENTS
1. BUSULFAN = Myleran® (for CML)
Dose-dependent toxicity after 3 – 4 years on the
drug in 1 – 10%
√ diffuse linear pattern (occasionally reticulonodular
/ nodular pattern)
√ partial / complete clearing after withdrawal of
drug
DDx: pneumocystis pneumonia, interstitial
leukemic infiltrate
2. BLEOMYCIN (for squamous cell carcinoma,
lymphoma, testicular tumor)
Toxicity at doses >300 mg (in 3 – 6%);
increased toxicity with age + radiation therapy
+ high oxygen concentrations
√ subpleural linear / nodular opacities in lower lung
zones occuring after 1 – 3 months following
beginning of therapy
3. NITROSOUREAS = BCNU, CCNU (for glioma,
lymphoma, myeloma)
Incidence of 50% after doses >1500 mg/sqm
√ linear / finely nodular opacities (following
treatment of 2 – 3 years)
√ high incidence of pneumothorax
4. METHOTREXATE, PROCARBAZINE (for AML,
psoriasis, pemphigus)

Not dose-related, usually self-limited despite continuation of therapy
- blood eosinophilia (common)
- √ linear / reticulonodular process (time delay of 12 days to 5 years, usually early)
- √ acinar filling pattern (later)
- √ transient hilar adenopathy + pleural effusion (on occasion)

  DDx: Pneumocystis pneumonia

B. NITROFURANTOIN (Macrodontin®)
(a) acute disorder with fever + eosinophilia (commonest presentation)
(b) chronic reaction with interstitial fibrosis (less common), may not be associated with peripheral eosinophilia
- positive for ANA + LE cells
- √ bilateral basilar interstitial opacities
- √ prompt resolution after withdrawal from drug

C. HEROIN, PROPOXYPHENE, METHADONE
Overdose followed by pulmonary edema in 30 – 40%
- √ bilateral widespread air space consolidation
- √ aspiration pneumonia in 50 – 75%

D. SALICYLATES
- asthma
- √ pulmonary edema (with chronic ingestion)

E. INTRAVENOUS CONTRAST AGENT
- √ pulmonary edema

F. AMIODARONE (for refractory ventricular arrhythmia)
- pulmonary insufficiency after 1 – 12 months in 14 – 18% on long-term therapy
- √ alveolar + interstitial infiltrates
- √ peripheral consolidation
- √ pleural thickening adjacent to consolidation

PULMONARY MASS

Solitary nodule / mass
Incidence:
(a) roentgenographic survey of low risk population: <5% of masses are cancerous
(b) on surgical resection: 40% malignant tumors, 40% granulomas

A. INFLAMMATION / INFECTION
1. Granuloma (most common lung mass):
   Sarcoidosis (1/3), tuberculosis, histoplasmosis, coccidioidomycosis, nocardiosis, cryptococcosis, talc, Dirofilaria immitis (dog heartworm), gumma, atypical measles infection
   CT: √ gross calcification / positive phantom study (usually >164 HU)
2. Fluid-filled cavity: abscess, hydatid cyst, bronchiectatic cyst, bronchocele
3. Mass in preformed cavity: fungus ball, mucoid impaction
4. Rounded atelectasis
5. Inflammatory pseudotumor: fibroxanthoma, histiocytoma, plasma cell granuloma, sclerosing hemangioma
6. Paraffinoma = lipoid granuloma

B. MALIGNANT TUMORS
(a) Malignant primaries of lung
   1. Bronchogenic carcinoma (66%, 2nd most common mass)
   2. Lymphoma
   3. Primary sarcoma of lung
   4. Plasmacytoma (primary / secondary)
   5. Clear cell carcinoma, carcinoid, giant cell carcinoma
(b) Metastases (4th most common cause) from kidney, colon, ovary, testes, Wilms tumor, sarcoma

C. BENIGN TUMORS
(a) lung tissue: hamartoma (6%, 3rd most common lung mass)
(b) fat tissue: lipoma (usually pleural lesion)
(c) fibrous tissue: fibroma
(d) muscle tissue: leiomyoma
(e) neural tissue: schwannoma, neurofibroma, paraganglioma
(f) lymph tissue: intrapulmonary lymph node
(g) deposits: amyloid, splenosis, endometrioma, extramedullary hematopoiesis

D. VASCULAR
1. Arteriovenous malformation
2. Hemangioma
3. Hematoma
4. Organizing infarct
5. Pulmonary vein varix
6. Rheumatoid / vasculitic nodule

E. DEVELOPMENTAL
1. Bronchogenic cyst (fluid-filled)
2. Pulmonary sequestration

F. INHALATIONAL
1. Silicosis (conglomerate mass)
2. Mucoid impaction (allergic aspergillosis)

G. MIMICKING DENSITIES
1. Fluid in interlobar fissure
2. Mediastinal mass
3. Pleural mass (mesothelioma)
4. Chest wall density: nipple, rib lesion, skin tumor (mole, neurofibroma, lipoma)
5. Artifacts: buttons, snaps

DIFFERENTIAL DIAGNOSTIC FEATURES OF LUNG MASSES ON CXR
- √ corona radiata = spiculations strongly suggestive of primary malignancy
  Δ 89% of irregular / spiculated lesions are malignant
- √ lucencies / air bronchogram
  (a) cavitation
  (b) infiltrative spread with air bronchogram: bronchioloalveolar cell carcinoma, lymphoma, resolving pneumonia
- √ calcifications
  (a) central / complete: granuloma
  (b) peripheral   : granuloma, tumor
- √ decrease in size with time: benign lesion
- √ absence of growth over 2 years: benign lesion

√ increase in size with time:
masses with "doubling times" (refers to volume not diameter) of <1 month / >16 months are unlikely to be malignant
  (a) very rapid growth:
  osteosarcoma, choriocarcinoma, testicular neoplasm, organizing infectious process, infarct (thromboembolism, Wegener granulomatosis)
  (b) very slow growth:
  hamartoma, bronchial carcinoid, inflammatory pseudotumor, granuloma, low-grade adenocarcinoma, metastases from renal cell carcinoma
√ nodule >3 cm is considered indeterminate
√ lobulation
  (a) organizing mass
  (b) tumor with multiple cell types growing at different rates (eg, hamartoma)
  Δ 79% of sharply derfined marginated lesions are benign
√ bubble-like areas of low attenuation:
bronchioloalveolar cell carcinoma (in 50%)
√ vessel leading to mass: pulmonary varix, AVM

mnemonic: "**B**ig **S**olitary **P**ulmonary **M**asses **C**ommonly **A**ppear **H**opeless **A**nd **L**onely"
Bronchogenic carcinoma
Solitary metastasis, **S**equestration
Pseudotumor
Mesothelioma
Cyst (bronchogenic, neuroenteric, echinococcal)
Adenoma
Hamartoma
Abscess, **A**ctinomycosis
Lymphoma

Multiple nodules and masses
√ homogeneous masses with sharp border
√ no air alveolo- / bronchogram
A. TUMORS
  (a) malignant
    1. Metastases:
    from breast, kidney, GI tract, uterus, ovary, testes, malignant melanoma, sarcoma, Wilms tumor
    2. Lymphoma (rare)
  (b) benign
    1. Hamartoma (rarely multiple)
    2. AV malformations
    3. Amyloidosis
B. VASCULAR LESIONS
  1. Thromboemboli with organizing infarcts
  2. Septic emboli with organized infarcts
C. COLLAGEN-VASCULAR DISEASE
  1. Wegener granulomatosis: vasculitis with organizing infarcts
  2. Wegener variants
  3. Rheumatoid nodules: tendency for periphery, occasionally cavitating

D. INFLAMMATORY GRANULOMAS
  1. Fungal: coccidioidomycosis, histoplasmosis, cryptococcosis
  2. Bacterial: nocardiosis, tuberculosis
  3. Viral: atypical measles
  4. Parasites: hydatid cysts, paragonimiasis
  5. Sarcoidosis: large accumulation of interstitial granulomas
  6. Inflammatory pseudotumors: fibrous histiocytoma, plasma cell granuloma, hyalinizing pulmonary nodules, pseudolymphoma

Small pulmonary nodules
mnemonic: "**MALTS**"
Metastases (esp. thyroid)
Alveolar cell carcinoma
Lyphoma, **L**eukemia
TBC
Sarcoid

Shaggy pulmonary nodule
mnemonic: "**S**haggy **S**ue **M**ade **L**oving **A** **R**eally **W**ild **F**antasy **T**oday"
Sarcoidosis, alveolar type
Septic emboli
Metastasis
Lymphoma, **L**ung primary, **L**ymphomatoid granulomatosis
Alveolar cell carcinoma
Rheumatoid lung
Wegener granulomatosis
Fungus
Tuberculosis

Calcified pulmonary nodules
mnemonic: "**HAM TV S**tation"
Histoplasmosis, **H**amartoma
Amyloid, **A**lveolar microlithiasis
Mitral stenosis, **M**etastasis (thyroid, osteosarcoma, mucinous carcinoma)
Tuberculosis
Varicella
Silicosis

Pleura-based lung nodule
√ ill-defined / sharply defined lesion mimicking a true pleural mass
√ associated linear densities in lung parenchyma
Causes:
  1. Granuloma (fungus, tuberculosis)
  2. Inflammatory pseudotumor
  3. Metastasis
  4. Rheumatoid nodule
  5. Pancoast tumor
  6. Lymphoma
  7. Infarct: Hampton hump
  8. Atelectatic pseudotumor

Cavitating lung nodules
A. NEOPLASM
- (a) Lung primary:
    1. Squamous cell carcinoma
    2. Adenocarcinoma
    3. Bronchioloalveolar carcinoma (rare)
    4. Hodgkin disease (rare)
- (b) Metastases (4% cavitate):
    1. Squamous cell carcinoma (2/3)
       nasopharynx (males), cervix (females),
       esophagus
    2. Adenocarcinoma
    3. Melanoma
    4. Sarcoma: Ewing sarcoma, osteo-, myxo-,
       angiosarcoma
    5. Seminoma, teratocarcinoma
    6. Wilms tumor
B. COLLAGEN-VASCULAR DISEASE
    1. Wegener granulomatosis + Wegener variant
    2. Rheumatoid nodules + Caplan syndrome
    3. SLE
    4. Periarteritis nodosa (rare)
C. GRANULOMATOUS DISEASE
    1. Histiocytosis X
    2. Sarcoidosis (rare)
D. VASCULAR DISEASE
    1. Pulmonary embolus with infarction
    2. Septic emboli (Staphylococcus aureus)
E. INFECTION
    1. Bacterial: pneumatoceles from staphylococcal /
       Gram-negative pneumonia
    2. Mycobacterial: TB
    3. Fungal: nocardiosis, cryptococcosis,
       coccidioidomycosis (in 10%), aspergillosis
    4. Parasitic: echinococcosis (multiple in 20 – 30%),
       paragonimiasis
F. TRAUMA
    1. Traumatic lung cyst (after hemorrhage)
    2. Hydrocarbon ingestion (lower lobes)
G. BRONCHOPULMONARY DISEASE
    1. Infected bulla
    2. Cystic bronchiectasis
    3. Communicating bronchogenic cyst

mnemonic: "CAVITY"
  Carcinoma (squamous cell), **C**ystic bronchiectasis
  Autoimmune disease (Wegener granulomatosis,
     rheumatoid lung)
  Vascular (bland / septic emboli)
  Infection (abscess, fungal disease, TB, echinococcus)
  Trauma
  Young = congenital (sequestration, diaphragmatic
     hernia, bronchogenic cyst)

Intrathoracic mass of low attenuation
A. Cysts
    1. Bronchogenic / neurenteric / pericardial cyst
    2. Hydatid disease
B. Fatty substrate
    1. Hamartoma

2. Lipoma
3. Tuberculous lymph node
4. Lymphadenopathy in Whipple disease
C. Necrotic masses
    1. Resolving hematoma
    2. Treated lymphoma
    3. Metastases from ovary, stomach, testes

Pulmonary mass with air bronchogram
1. Bronchioloalveolar carcinoma
2. Lymphoma
3. Pseudolymphoma
4. Kaposi sarcoma
5. Blastomycosis

Pulmonary nodules + pneumothorax
1. Osteosarcoma
2. Wilms tumor
3. Histiocytosis

Pneumoconiosis with mass
Anthracosilicosis with:
    1. Granuloma (histoplasmosis, TB, sarcoidosis)
    2. Bronchogenic carcinoma (incidence same as in
       general population)
    3. Metastasis
    4. Progressive massive fibrosis
    5. Caplan syndrome (rheumatoid nodules)

Air-crescent sign
1. Invasive pulmonary aspergillosis
2. Noninvasive mycetoma
3. Septic emboli
4. Cavitating benign + malignant neoplasms
5. Echinococcal cyst
6. TB with Rasmussen aneurysms (most are too small to
   be identified on CXR)

Benign lung tumor
A. CENTRAL LOCATION
    1. Bronchial polyp
    2. Bronchial papilloma
    3. **Granular cell myoblastoma**
       = cell of origin from neural crest
       Age: middle-aged, esp. black women
       √ endobronchial lesion in major bronchi

B. PERIPHERAL LOCATION
    1. Hamartoma
    2. Leiomyoma
       benign metastasizing leiomyoma, history of
       hysterectomy
    3. Amyloid tumor
       not associated with amyloid of other organs /
       rheumatoid arthritis / myeloma
    4. Intrapulmonary lymph node
    5. Arteriovenous malformation
    6. Endometrioma, fibroma, neural tumor,
       chemodectoma

C. CENTRAL / PERIPHERAL
1. Lipoma: (a) subpleural (b) endobronchial
D. PSEUDOTUMOR
1. Fibroxanthoma / xanthogranuloma
2. Plasma cell granuloma
3. Sclerosing hemangioma
middle-aged woman, RML / RLL (most commonly),
may be multiple
4. Pseudolymphoma
5. Round atelectasis

LUCENT LUNG LESIONS

Hyperlucent lung
Bilateral hyperlucent lung
A. FAULTY RADIOLOGIC TECHNIQUE
1. Overpenetrated film
B. DECREASED SOFT TISSUES
1. Thin body habitus
2. Bilateral mastectomy
C. CARDIAC CAUSE of decreased pulmonary blood
flow
1. Right-to-left shunt:
Tetralogy of Fallot (small proximal pulmonary
vessels), pseudotruncus, truncus type IV,
Ebstein malformation, tricuspid atresia
2. Eisenmenger physiology of left-to-right shunt:
ASD, VSD, PDA (dilated proximal pulmonary
vessels)
D. PULMONARY CAUSE of decreased pulmonary
blood flow
(a) Decrease of vascular bed:
1. Pulmonary embolism
bilaterality is rare; localized areas of
hyperlucency (Westermark sign)
(b) Increase in air space:
1. Air trapping (reversible changes):
acute asthmatic attack, acute bronchiolitis
(pediatric patient)
2. Emphysema
3. Bulla
4. Bleb
5. Interstitial emphysema

Unilateral hyperlucent lung
A. FAULTY RADIOLOGIC TECHNIQUE
1. Rotation of patient
B. CHEST WALL DEFECT
1. Mastectomy
2. Absent pectoralis muscle (Poland syndrome)
C. INCREASED PULMONARY AIR SPACE
with decreased pulmonary blood flow
(a) Large airway obstruction with air trapping
@ Bronchial compression:
hilar mass (rare), cardiomegaly
compressing LLL bronchus
@ Endobronchial obstruction with air trapping
(collateral air drift):
foreign body, broncholith, bronchogenic
carcinoma, carcinoid, bronchial mucocele

(b) Small airway obstruction
1. Bronchiolitis obliterans
2. Swyer-James / Macleod syndrome
3. Emphysema (particularly bullous
emphysema)
4. Emphysema + unilateral lung transplant
(c) Pneumothorax (in supine patient)
D. PULMONARY VASCULAR CAUSE of decreased
pulmonary blood flow
1. Pulmonary artery hypoplasia
2. Pulmonary embolism
3. Congenital lobar emphysema
4. Compensatory overaeration

Localized lucent lung defect
A. CAVITY = tissue necrosis with bronchial drainage
(a) INFECTION
Bacterial pneumonia
1. Pyogenic infection = abscess = necrotizing
pneumonia
Staphylococcus, Klebsiella, Pseudomonas,
anaerobes, β-hemolytic streptococcus,
E. coli, mixed Gram-negative organisms
2. Aspiration pneumonia = gravitational
pneumonia:
mixed Gram-negative organisms, anaerobes
Granulomatous infection
1. Tuberculosis
cavitation indicates active infectious disease
with risk for hematogenous / bronchogenic
dissemination
2. Fungal infection:
nocardiosis (in immunocompromised),
coccidioidomycosis (any lobe, desert
Southwest), histoplasmosis, blastomycosis,
mucormycosis, sporotrichosis, aspergillosis
cryptococcosis
√ very thin-walled cavities less likely to
follow apical distribution of TB /
histoplasmosis
3. Sarcoidosis (stage IV, upper lobe
predominance)
4. Angioinvasive organism (septic lung
infarction followed by cavity formation):
Aspergillus, Mucorales, Candida, Torulopsis,
P. aeruginosa
Parasitic infestation: hydatid disease
(b) NEOPLASM
Primary lung tumor: 16% of peripheral lung
cancers (in particular in squamous cell
carcinoma (30%); also in bronchioloalveolar cell
carcinoma
Metastasis (usually multiple)
1. Squamous cell carcinoma (nasopharynx,
esophagus, cervix) in 2/3
2. Adenocarcinoma (lung, breast, GI)
3. Osteosarcoma (rare)
4. Melanoma
5. Lymphoma (rare): with adenopathy; cavities
often secondary to opportunistic infection with

nocardiosis + cryptococcosis
(c) VASCULAR OCCLUSION
1. Infarct (thromboembolic, septic)
2. Pulmonary vasculitis (Wegener granulomatosis
3. Rheumatoid arthritis
(d) INHALATIONAL
1. Silicosis with coal-worker's pneumoconiosis
— complicating tuberculosis
— ischemic necrosis of center of conglomerate
mass (rare)

B. CYSTS
(a) Cystic bronchiectasis
1. Cystic fibrosis (more obvious in upper lobes)
2. Agammaglobulinemia (predisposed to recurrent
bacterial infections)
3. Recurrent bacterial pneumonias
√   multiple thin-walled lucencies with air-fluid
levels in lower lobes
4. Childhood infection: tuberculosis, pertussis
5. Allergic bronchopulmonary aspergillosis (in
asthmatic patients)
√   involvement of proximal perihilar bronchi
6. Kartagener syndrome (ciliary dismotility)
(b) Pneumatoceles
in area of previous pneumonia / posttraumatic
hematoma
(c) Congenital lesions (rare)
1. Multiple bronchogenic cysts
2. Intralobar sequestration:
multicystic structure in lower lobes
3. Congenital cystic adenomatoid malformation
(CCAM) Type I
4. Diaphragmatic hernia (congenital / traumatic)
(d) Centrilobular / bullous emphysema
(e) Honeycomb lung

Multiple lucent lung lesions

for details see causes of localized lucent lung defect
A. CAVITIES
(a) Infection
1. Bacterial pneumonia = necrotizing pneumonia
2. Granulomatous infection: TB,
coccidioidomycosis
3. Parasites (hydatid disease)
4. Angioinvasive organism (septic lung infarction
followed by cavity formation): Aspergillus,
Mucorales, Candida, Torulopsis, P. aeruginosa
(b) Neoplasm
(c) Vascular
1. Thromboembolic + septic infarcts
2. Wegener granulomatosis
3. Rheumatoid arthritis
B. CYSTS
(a) Cystic bronchiectasis
1. Cystic fibrosis (more obvious in upper lobes)
2. Agammaglobulinemia (predisposed to
recurrent bacterial infections)
3. Recurrent bacterial pneumonias
4. Tuberculosis
5. Allergic bronchopulmonary aspergillosis (in

asthmatic patients)
(b) Pneumatoceles
(c) Congenital lesions (rare)
1. Multiple bronchogenic cysts
2. Intralobar sequestration:
multicystic structure in lower lobes
3. Congenital cystic adenomatoid malformation
(CCAM) Type I
4. Diaphragmatic hernia (congenital / traumatic)
(d) Centrilobular / bullous emphysema
(e) Honeycomb lung
(f) Juvenile pulmonary polyposis

Multiple pulmonary cysts

1. Lymphangiomyomatosis
√   randomly scattered cysts in otherwise normal lung
2. Pulmonary tuberous sclerosis
√   randomly scattered cysts in otherwise normal lung
3. Histiocytosis X
√   combination of nodules ± cavitation with cysts
√   predominant distribution in upper lung zones
4. Bronchiectasis
√   related to bronchi
√   thick walls, often containing fluid secretions
5. Centrilobular emphysema
√   focal areas of decreased attenuation lacking a
discernible wall
6. Honeycombing of pulmonary fibrosis
√   small thick irregular walled cavities surrounded by
abnormal lung parenchyma
√   predominantly peripheral + basilar distribution

Cyst-like pulmonary lesions

mnemonic: "C.C., I BAN WHIPS"
Coccidioidomycosis
Cystic adenomatoid malformation
Infection
Bronchogenic cyst, **B**ronchiectasis, **B**owel
Abscess
Neoplasm
Wegener granulomatosis
Hydatid cyst, **H**istiocytosis X
Infarction
Pneumatocele
Sequestration

Mass within cavity

1. Mycetoma = aspergilloma
2. Tissue fragment within carcinoma
3. Necrotic lung within abscess
4. Disintegrating hydatid cyst
5. Intracavitary blood clot

Pulmonary cyst

A. CONGENITAL CYST
1. Cystic adenomatoid malformation
2. Congenital lobar emphysema
3. Bronchial atresia
4. Bronchogenic cyst

5. Sequestration

B. ACQUIRED CYST
1. Pneumatocele (traumatic / infectious)
2. Pseudocyst (from interstitial emphysema)
3. Hydatid disease
4. **Bleb** = cystic air collection within visceral pleura; mostly apical with narrow neck; associated with spontaneous pneumothorax
5. **Bulla** = cystic air collection within lung parenchyma due to destruction of alveoli; associated with emphysema

Multiple thin-walled cavities
mnemonic: "BITCH"
Bullae + pneumatoceles
Infection (TB, cocci, staph)
Tumor (squamous cell carcinoma)
Cysts (traumatic, bronchogenic)
Hydrocarbon ingestion

Pneumothorax
Etiology:
1. Neonatal disease: meconium aspiration, respirator therapy for hyaline membrane disease
2. Malignancy: primary lung cancer, lung metastases (esp. osteosarcoma, pancreas, adrenal, Wilms tumor)
3. Pulmonary infections: coccidioidomycosis, hydatid disease, acute bacterial pneumonia, staphylococcal septicemia
4. Cx of honeycomb lung: sarcoidosis, histiocytosis X, rheumatoid lung, idiopathic pulmonary hemosiderosis, pulmonary alveolar proteinosis
5. Marfan syndrome
6. Spasmodic asthma, diffuse emphysema
7. Pulmonary infarction
8. **Catamenial pneumothorax** = recurrent spontaneous pneumothorax during menstruation associated with endometriosis of the diaphragm; R >> L
9. Lymphangiomyomatosis + tuberous sclerosis

mnemonic: "THE CHEST SET"
Trauma
Honeycomb lung, **H**amman-Rich syndrome
Emphysema, **E**sophageal rupture
Chronic obstructive pulmonary disease
Hyaline membrane disease
Endometriosis
Spontaneous, **S**cleroderma
Tuberous sclerosis
Sarcoma (osteo-), **S**arcoidosis
Eosinophilic granuloma
Tuberculosis + fungus

Spontaneous Pneumothorax
result of rupture of subpleural bleb / bulla
Age: 3rd + 4th decade; M:F = 8:1, esp. in patients with tall thin stature
- chest pain (69%)
- dyspnea

Prognosis: recurrence in 30% on same side, in 10% on contralateral side

Traumatic Pneumothorax
(a) secondary to rib fractures / contusion / laceration
(b) iatrogenic: tracheostomy, central venous catheter, PEEP ventilator

Tension Pneumothorax
= intrapleural pressure exceeds atmospheric pressure in lung during expiration (check-valve mechanism)
√ displacement of mediastinum / anterior junction line
√ diaphragmatic inversion
√ total / subtotal lung collapse
√ collapse of SVC / IVC / right heart border (decreased systemic venous return)

RADIOGRAPHIC SIGNS OF PNEUMOTHORAX IN SUPINE POSITION
1. Anteromedial pneumothorax (earliest location)
   √ sharp delineation of mediastinal contours (SVC, azygos vein, left subclavian artery, anterior junction line, superior pulmonary vein, heart border, IVC, deep anterior cardiophrenic sulcus, pericardial fat pad)
   √ outline of medial diaphragm under cardiac silhouette
2. Subpulmonic pneumothorax (second most common location)
   √ hyperlucent upper abdominal quadrant
   √ deep lateral costophrenic sulcus
   √ visualization of anterior costophrenic sulcus
   √ visualization of inferior surface of lung
   √ sharply outlined diaphragm in spite of parenchymal disease
3. Apicolateral pneumothorax (least common location)
   √ visualization of visceral pleural line
4. Posteromedial pneumothorax (in presence of lower lobe collapse)
   √ lucent triangle with vertex at hilum
   √ V-shaped base delineating costovertebral sulcus
5. Pneumothorax outlines pulmonary ligament

MEDIASTINUM
Pneumomediastinum
A. SPONTANEOUS PNEUMOMEDIASTINUM (common)
   Age: neonates (0.05-1%), 2nd – 3rd decade
   Causes:
   (a) rupture of marginally situated alveoli from sudden rise in intraalveolar pressure (acute asthma, aspiration pneumonia, hyaline membrane disease, measles, giant cell pneumonia, coughing, vomiting, strenuous exercise, parturition, diabetic acidosis)
   (b) Tumor erosion of trachea / esophagus
   (c) Pneumoperitoneum / retropneumoperitoneum
   Cx: **Air block** = build-up of pressure impeding blood flow in low pressure veins particularly common in neonatal period

B. TRAUMATIC PNEUMOMEDIASTINUM (rare)
1. Pulmonary interstitial emphysema
   = disruption of marginal alveoli with gas traveling toward mediastinum due to positive pressure ventilation
2. Ruptured bronchus
   √ commonly associated with pneumothorax
3. Ruptured esophagus (diabetic acidosis, alcoholic, Boerhaave syndrome)
4. Iatrogenic - accidental
   neck / chest / abdominal surgery, subclavian vein catheterization, mediastinoscopy, bronchoscopy, gastroscopy, recto-sigmoido-colonoscopy, electrosurgery with intestinal gas explosion, positive pressure ventilation, intubation, barium enema

Mediastinal shift

= displacement of heart, trachea, aorta, hilar vessels
Δ expiration film, lateral decubitus film (expanded lung down), fluoroscopy help to determine side of abnormality

A. DECREASED LUNG VOLUME
1. Atelectasis
2. Postoperative (lobectomy, pneumothorax)
3. Hypoplastic lung / lobe
   √ small pulmonary artery + small hilum
   √ decreased peripheral pulmonary vasculature
   √ irregular reticular vascular pattern (bronchial origin) without converging on the hilum
4. Bronchiolitis obliterans = Swyer-James syndrome

B. INCREASED LUNG VOLUME = air trapping
@ Major bronchus
   1. Foreign body obstructing main stem bronchus (common in children) with ball valve mechanism + collateral air drift
      √ contralateral mediastinal shift increasing with expiration
@ Emphysema
   1. Bullous emphysema (localized form)
      √ large avascular areas with thin lines
   2. Congenital lobar emphysema: only in infants
   3. Interstitial emphysema
      √ pattern of diffuse coarse lines;
        Cx of positive pressure ventilation therapy
@ Cysts / masses
   1. Bronchogenic cyst: with bronchial connection + check valve mechanism
   2. Cystic adenomatoid malformation
   3. Large mass (pulmonary, mediastinal)

C. PLEURAL SPACE ABNORMALITY
1. Large unilateral pleural effusion:
   opaque hemithorax through empyema, congestive failure, metastases
2. Tension pneumothorax:
   not always complete collapse of lung

3. Large diaphragmatic hernia:
   usually detected in neonatal period
4. Large mass

D. Partial absence of pericardium / pectus excavatum
   √ shift of heart without shift of trachea, aorta, or mediastinal border

Acute mediastinal widening

1. Rupture of aorta / brachiocephalic arteries
2. Venous hemorrhage: traumatic / iatrogenic (malpositioning of central venous line)
3. Congestive heart failure (venous dilatation)
4. Rupture of esophagus
5. Rupture of thoracic duct

MEDIASTINAL MASS

(excluding hyperplastic thymus glands, granulomas, lymphoma, metastases)
1. Neurogenic tumors   (28%)   : malignant in 16%
2. Teratoid lesions   (19%)   : malignant in 15%
3. Enterogenous cysts (16%)
4. Thymomas   (13%)   : malignant in 46%
5. Pericardial cysts   (7%)

Δ 75% of all mediastinal tumors are benign (in all age groups)
Δ 1/3 diagnosed on routine chest X-ray
Δ 2/3 found in association with symptoms (pain, cough, shortness of breath)
Δ 80% of malignant tumors are symptomatic

Thoracic inlet lesions

1. Thyroid mass
   1 – 3% of all thyroidectomies have a mediastinal component; 1/3 of goiters are intrathoracic
   Location: anterior (80%) / posterior (20%) mediastinum
   √ displacement of trachea posteriorly + laterally (anterior goiter)
   √ displacement of trachea anteriorly + esophagus posteriorly + laterally (posterior goiter)
   √ inhomogeneous density (cystic spaces, high-density iodine contents)
   √ focal calcifications are common
   √ marked + prolonged contrast enhancement
   √ connection to thyroid gland
   √ vascular compression
   NUC (rarely helpful as thyroid tissue may be nonfunctioning):
      √ ± uptake on I-123 / I-131 scan (pertechnetate sufficient with modern gamma cameras, SPECT imaging may be helpful)
2. Cystic hygroma
   3 – 10% involve mediastinum; childhood
3. Lymphoma
4. Other tumors: adenoma, carcinoma, ectopic thymoma

Anterior mediastinal mass

mnemonic: "4 T's"

Thymoma
Teratoma
Thyroid tumor / goiter
Terrible lymphoma

A. SOLID THYMIC LESIONS
　1. Thymoma (benign, malignant): most common
　2. Normal thymus (neonate)
　3. Thymic hyperplasia (child)
　4. Thymolipoma
　5. Lymphoma
B. SOLID TERATOID LESIONS
　1. Teratoma
　2. Embryonal cell carcinoma
　3. Choriocarcinoma
　4. Seminoma
C. THYROID / PARATHYROID
　1. Substernal thyroid / intrathoracic goiter
　2. Thyroid adenoma / carcinoma
　3. Ectopic parathyroid adenoma:
　　ectopia in 10% (62% in anterior mediastinum,
　　30% within thyroid tissue,
　　8% in posterior superior mediastinum)
D. LYMPH NODES
　1. Lymphoma (Hodgkin, NHL): may arise in thymus,
　　more common in young adults
　2. Metastases
　3. Benign lymph node hyperplasia
　4. Angioblastic lymphadenopathy
　5. Mediastinal lymphadenitis: sarcoidosis /
　　granulomatous infection
E. CARDIOVASCULAR
　1. Tortuous brachiocephalic artery
　2. Aneurysm of ascending aorta
　3. Aneurysm of sinus of Valsalva
　4. Dilated SVC
　5. Cardiac tumor
　6. Epicardial fat pad
F. CYSTS
　1. Cystic hygroma
　2. Bronchogenic cyst
　3. Extralobar sequestration
　4. Thymic cysts / dermoid cysts
　5. Pericardial cyst:　(a) true cyst
　　　　　　　　　　　　(b) pericardial diverticulum
　6. Pancreatic pseudocyst
G. OTHERS
　1. Neural tumor (vagus, phrenic nerve)
　2. Paraganglioma
　3. Hemangioma / lymphangioma
　4. Mesenchymal tumor (fibroma, lipoma)
　5. Sternal tumors
　　(a) metastases from breast, bronchus, kidney,
　　　thyroid
　　(b) malignant primary (chondrosarcoma, myeloma,
　　　lymphoma)
　　(c) benign primary (chondroma, aneurysmal bone
　　　cyst, giant cell tumor)
　6. Primary lung / pleural tumor
　　(invading mediastinum)

7. Mediastinal lipomatosis:　(a) Cushing disease
　　　　　　　　　　　　　　(b) Corticosteroid therapy
8. Morgagni hernia / localized eventration
9. Abscess

Middle mediastinal mass
mnemonic: "HABIT[5]"
Hernia, **H**ematoma
Aneurysm
Bronchogenic cyst / duplication cyst
Inflammation (sarcoidosis, histoplasmosis,
　coccidioidomycosis, primary TB in children)
Tumors - remember the 5 L's:
　Lung, especially oat cell carcinoma
　Lymphoma
　Leukemia
　Leiomyoma
　Lymph node hyperplasia

A. LYMPH NODES
　Δ　90% of masses in the middle mediastinum are
　　malignant
　(a) NEOPLASTIC ADENOPATHY
　　1. Lymphoma (Hodgkin: NHL = 2 : 1)
　　2. Leukemia (in 25%): lymphocytic > granulocytic
　　3. Metastasis (bronchus, lung, upper GI, prostate,
　　　kidney)
　　4. Angioimmunoblastic lymphadenopathy
　(b) INFLAMMATORY ADENOPATHY
　　1. Tuberculosis / histoplasmosis (may lead to
　　　fibrosing mediastinitis)
　　2. Blastomycosis (rare) / coccidioidomycosis
　　3. Sarcoidosis (predominant involvement of
　　　paratracheal nodes)
　　4. Viral pneumonia (particularly measles + cat
　　　scratch fever)
　　5. Infectious mononucleosis / pertussis
　　　pneumonia
　　6. Amyloidosis
　　7. Plague / tularemia
　　8. Drug reaction
　　9. Giant lymph node hyperplasia
　　　= Castleman disease
　　10. Connective tissue disease (rheumatoid, SLE)
　　11. Bacterial lung abscess
　(c) INHALATIONAL DISEASE ADENOPATHY
　　1. Silicosis (eggshell calcification also in
　　　sarcoidosis + tuberculosis)
　　2. Coal-worker's pneumoconiosis
　　3. Berylliosis
B. FOREGUT CYST
　1. Bronchogenic / respiratory cyst: cartilage,
　　respiratory epithelium
　2. Enteric cyst = esophageal duplication cyst
　3. Extralobar sequestration (anomalous feeding
　　vessel)
　4. Hiatal hernia
C. PRIMARY TUMORS (infrequent)
　1. Carcinoma of trachea
　2. Bronchogenic carcinoma
　3. Esophageal tumor:

leiomyoma, carcinoma, leiomyosarcoma
4. Mesothelioma
5. Granular cell myoblastoma of trachea (rare)
D. VASCULAR LESIONS
1. Aneurysm
2. Distended veins (SVC, azygous vein)
3. Hematoma

Posterior mediastinal mass
A. NEOPLASM
1. <u>Neurogenic tumor</u> (largest group): 30% malignant
(a) Tumor of peripheral nerve origin
- more common in adulthood
- √ 80% appear as round masses with sulcus
- √ lower attenuation than muscle (in 73%)
1. Schwannoma = neurilemoma (32%): derived from sheath of Schwann without nerve cells
2. Neurofibroma (10%): contains Schwann cells + nerve cells, 3rd + 4th decade
3. Malignant schwannoma
(b) Tumor of sympathetic ganglia origin
- more common in childhood
- √ 80% are elongated with tapered borders
1. Ganglioneuroma (25%): benign tumor from mature ganglion cells
2. Neuroblastoma (15%): highly malignant undifferentiated small round cell tumor originating in sympathetic ganglia, <10 years of age
3. Ganglioneuroblastoma (14%): both features, spontaneous maturation possible
(c) Tumors of paraganglia origin (rare)
1. Chemodectoma = paraganglioma (4%)
2. Pheochromocytoma
√ rib spreading, erosion, destruction
√ enlargement of neural foramina (dumbbell lesion)
√ scalloping of posterior aspect of vertebral body
√ scoliosis
CT: √ low density soft tissue mass (lipid contents)
2. Spine tumor: Metastases (eg, bronchogenic carcinoma, multiple myeloma), ABC, chordoma, chondrosarcoma, Ewing sarcoma
3. Lymphoma
4. Invasive thymoma
5. Mesenchymal tumor (fibroma, lipoma, leiomyoma)
6. Hemangioma
7. Lymphangioma
8. Thyroid tumor

B. INFLAMMATION / INFECTION
1. Infectious spondylitis: pyogenic, tuberculous, fungal
√ destruction of endplates + disc space
√ paravertebral soft tissue mass
2. Mediastinitis
3. Lymphoid hyperplasia
4. Sarcoidosis (in 2%, typically asymptomatic patient)
5. Pancreatic pseudocyst
C. VASCULAR MASS

1. Aneurysm of descending aorta (curvilinear calcification; elderly)
2. Enlarged azygos + accessory hemiazygos vein
3. Esophageal varices
4. Congenital vascular anomalies: aberrant subclavian artery, double aortic arch, pulmonary sling, interruption of IVC with azygos / hemiazygos continuation
D. TRAUMA
1. Aortic aneurysm / pseudoaneurysm
2. Hematoma
3. Loculated hemothorax
4. Traumatic pseudomeningocele
E. FOREGUT CYST
√ cysts may demonstrate peripheral rimlike calcifications
1. Bronchogenic cyst
2. Enteric cyst
3. Neurenteric cyst
4. Extralobar sequestration
F. FATTY MASS
1. Bochdalek hernia
2. Mediastinal lipomatosis
3. Fat-containing tumors: lipoma, liposarcoma, teratoma (rare)
G. OTHER
1. Loculated pleural effusion
2. Pancreatic pseudocyst
3. Lateral meningocele (neurofibromatosis; enlarged neural foramen)
4. Extramedullary hematopoiesis: in chronic bone marrow deficiency; paraspinal area rich in RES-elements
√ splenomegaly; widening of ribs
5. "Pseudomass" of the newborn

Mediastinal cysts
= 21% of all primary mediastinal tumors, mostly developmental
1. Pericardial cyst
2. Thymic cyst
3. FOREGUT CYST
(a) Bronchogenic cyst (54 –63%)
(b) **Esophageal duplication cyst**
arise from foregut
Histo: contains no cartilage, lined by gastrointestinal tract epithelium
Location: adjacent to esophagus / within esophageal musculature at any level, lower posterior mediastinum in paraspinal position (in up to 60%)
Cx: peptic ulceration, perforation + bleeding (gastric mucosa)
(c) **Neurenteric cyst** (least common)
connected to meninges through midline defect
√ vertebral body anomalies (hemivertebrae, butterfly vertebrae, scoliosis) at the same level
√ air-fluid level (if communicating with GI-tract)
4. **Lateral meningocele**
= outpouching of leptomeninges through

intervertebral foramen
Etiology: in 75% neurofibromatosis
√ spinal abnormalities (kyphoscoliosis, scalloping of dorsal vertebrae, enlargement of intervertebral foramen, pedicle erosion, thinning of ribs)
5. **Hydatid cyst**
Location: paravertebral gutter
√ erosion of ribs + vertebrae
6. **Thoracic duct cyst**
rare, filled with chyle
Etiology: degenerative / lymphangiomatous
7. Traumatic lymphocele
8. Parathyroid cyst
uncommon as mediastinal mass

Low-attenuation mediastinal mass
A. FLUID
1. Foregut cyst
2. Lymphocele
3. Seroma
4. Hematoma
5. Abscess
6. Hydatid disease
B. LYMPH NODE
1. Tuberculous lymph nodes
2. Metastasis from thyroid / testicular tumor
3. Lymphoma: treated / untreated
C. PRIMARY NEOPLASM
1. Neurogenic tumor
2. Fat-containing neoplasm

Mediastinal fat
A. Mediastinal lipomatosis
B. Fat herniation
= omental fat herniating into chest
1. Foramen of Morgagni
= cardiophrenic angle mass, R >> L side
2. Foramen of Bochdalek
= costophrenic angle mass, almost always on left
3. Paraesophageal hernia = perigastric fat through phrenicoesophageal membrane
CT: √ fat with fine linear densities (= omental vessels)
C. Lipoma
un- / encapsulated with variable amount of fibrous septa
√ smooth + sharply defined boundaries
DDx: Liposarcoma, lipoblastoma (infancy), fat-containing teratoma, thymolipoma (inhomogeneous, higher CT numbers, poor demarcation, ± invasion of surrounding structures)
D. Multiple symmetrical lipomatosis
rare entity without involvement of anterior mediastinal / cardiophrenic / paraspinal areas
√ compression of trachea
√ periscapular lipomatous masses

Tracheal tumor
- asthma symptomatology
- hoarseness, cough
- wheeze (inspiratory with extrathoracic lesion, expiratory with intrathoracic lesion)
- hemoptysis
A. BENIGN
1. Cartilaginous tumor (hamartoma)
2. Squamous cell papilloma
3. Fibroma / lipoma
4. Hemangioma
5. Granular cell myoblastoma
6. Granuloma (inflammatory, TB, fungus)
7. Amyloid tumor
B. MALIGNANT
1. Squamous-cell carcinoma (commonest primary)
2. Adenoid cystic carcinoma = cylindroma
3. Metastasis from renal cell carcinoma, colon cancer, malignant melanoma
4. Lymphoma
5. Plasmacytoma

Enlargement of azygos vein
A. COLLATERAL CIRCULATION
1. Portal hypertension
2. SVC obstruction / compression
3. IVC obstruction / compression
4. Azygos continuation of IVC
5. Partial anomalous venous return (rare)
B. RIGHT ATRIAL HYPERTENSION
1. Right heart failure
2. Constrictive pericarditis
3. Large pericardial effusion

Hilar mass
A. LARGE PULMONARY ARTERIES
√ enlargement of main pulmonary artery
√ abrupt change in vessel caliber
√ enlarged pulmonary artery compared with bronchus (in same bronchovascular bundle)
√ cephalization
√ enlargement of right ventricle (RAO 45°, LAO 60°)
Cause:
1. Chronic obstructive disease (emphysema)
2. Chronic restrictive interstitial lung disease (idiopathic fibrosis, cystic fibrosis, rheumatoid arthritis, sarcoidosis)
3. Pulmonary embolic disease (acute massive / chronic)
4. Idiopathic pulmonary hypertension
5. Left-sided heart failure + mitral stenosis
6. Congenital heart disease with left-to-right shunt
(a) acyanotic: ASD, VSD, PDA
(b) cyanotic (admixture lesions): transposition of great vessels, truncus arteriosus

B. DUPLICATION CYST

C. UNILATERAL HILAR ADENOPATHY
(a) NEOPLASTIC
1. Bronchogenic carcinoma (most common)
2. Metastases (lack of mediastinal involvement exceptional)

3. Lymphoma
(b) INFLAMMATORY
   1. Tuberculosis (primary) in 80%
   2. Fungal infection: histoplasmosis, coccidioidomycosis, blastomycosis
   3. Viral infections: atypical measles
   4. Infectious mononucleosis
   5. Drug reaction
   6. Sarcoidosis (in 1 – 3%)
   7. Bilateral lung abscess

mnemonic: "**F**at **H**ila **S**uck"
   Fungus
   Hodgkin disease
   Squamous / oat cell carcinoma

D. BILATERAL HILAR ADENOPATHY
   (a) NEOPLASTIC
      1. Lymphoma (50% in Hodgkin disease)
      2. Metastases
      3. Leukemia
      4. Primary bronchogenic carcinoma
      5. Plasmacytoma
   (b) INFLAMMATORY
      1. Sarcoidosis (in 70 – 90%)
      2. Silicosis
      3. Histiocytosis X
      4. Idiopathic pulmonary hemosiderosis
      5. Chronic berylliosis
   (c) INFECTIOUS
      1. Rubella, ECHO virus, varicella, mononucleosis

mnemonic: "**P**lease **H**elen **L**ick **M**y **P**opsicle **St**ick"
   Primary TB
   Histoplasmosis
   Lymphoma
   Metastases
   Pneumoconiosis
   Sarcoidosis

Eggshell calcification of nodes

A. Pneumoconiosis
   1. Silicosis (5%)
   2. Coal worker's pneumoconiosis (1.3 – 6%)
      not seen in: asbestosis, berylliosis, talcosis, baritosis
B. Sarcoidosis (5%)
C. Fungal + bacterial infection (rare):
   1. Tuberculosis
   2. Histoplasmosis
   3. Coccidioidomycosis
D. Lymphoma following radiation therapy

Right cardiophrenic angle mass

1. Epicardial fat pad / lipoma (most common cause)
   √ triangular opacity in cardiophrenic angle less dense than heart
   √ increase in size under corticosteroid treatment
2. Pericardial cyst

3. Aneurysm
4. Dilated right atrium
5. Diaphragmatic hernia
6. Diaphragmatic lymph node (esp. in Hodgkin disease + breast cancer)
7. Primary lung mass
8. Anterior mediastinal mass

THYMUS
Thymic mass
1. Thymoma
2. Thymolipoma
3. Thymic cyst

Diffuse thymic enlargement
1. Thymic hyperplasia
2. Thymic infiltration
   by leukemia, Hodgkin lymphoma, non-Hodgkin lymphoma, histiocytosis
   • presence of adenopathy elsewhere
   √ no pleural implants

PLEURA
Pleural Effusion
A. TRANSUDATE (protein level of 1.5 – 2.5 g/dl)
   (a) Increased hydrostatic pressure
      1. Congestive heart failure (in 65%)
         bilateral (88%); right-sided (8%); left-sided (4%); least amount on left side due to cardiac movement, which stimulates lymphatic resorption
      2. Constrictive pericarditis (in 60%)
   (b) Decreased colloid-oncotic pressure
      — decreased protein production
         1. Cirrhosis with ascites (in 6%): right-sided (67%)
      — protein loss / hypervolemia
         1. Nephrotic syndrome (21%), overhydration, glomerulonephritis (55%), peritoneal dialysis
         2. Hypothyroidism
   (c) Chylous effusion

B. EXUDATE (protein level >3 g/dl)
   (a) Infection
      1. **Empyema** (anaerobic bacteria most frequent)
         • gross pus
         • WBC >15,000/ccm
         • positive Gram stain
         • pH <7.2
         • LDH >1000 U/l
         • glucose <40 mg/dl
      2. Parapneumonic exudate (in 40%)
      3. Tuberculosis (in 1%):
         high protein content (75 g/dl), lymphocytes > 70%, positive culture (only in 20 – 25%)
      4. Fungi: actinomyces, nocardia
      5. Parasites: amebiasis (secondary to liver abscess in 15 – 20%), echinococcus
      6. Mycoplasma, rickettsia (in 20%)

(b) Malignant disease (in 60%)
lung cancer (26 – 49%), breast cancer (8 – 24%),
lymphoma (10 – 28%, in 2/3 chylothorax), ovarian
cancer (10%), malignant mesothelioma (hyaluronic
acid)
Pathogenesis:
— pleural metastases (increase pleural
permeability)
— lymphatic obstruction (pleural vessels,
mediastinal nodes, thoracic duct disruption)
— bronchial obstruction (loss of volume +
resorptive surface)
— hypoproteinema (secondary to tumor cachexia)

(c) Vascular
Pulmonary emboli (in 15 – 30% of all embolic
events): often serosanguinous

(d) Abdominal disease
1. Pancreatitis / pancreatic pseudocyst (in 2/3):
usually left-sided pleural effusion
2. Boerhaave syndrome: left-sided esophageal
perforation
3. Subphrenic abscess
√ pleural effusion (79%)
√ elevation + restriction of diaphragmatic
motion (95%)
√ basilar platelike atelectasis / pneumonitis
(79%)
4. Abdominal tumor with ascites
5. **Meigs-Salmon syndrome**
= primary pelvic neoplasms (ovarian fibroma,
thecoma, granulosa cell tumor, Brenner
tumor, cystadenoma, adenocarcinoma,
fibromyoma of uterus) cause pleural effusion
in 2 – 3%; ascites + hydrothorax resolve
with tumor removal
6. Endometriosis
7. Bile fistula

(e) Collagen-vascular disease
1. Rheumatoid arthritis (in 3%):
unilateral; R > L (in 75%), recurrent alternating
sides; pleural effusion relatively unchanged in
size for months; predominantly in men; LOW
GLUCOSE content of 20 – 50 mg/dl (in 70 –
80%) without increase following IV infusion of
glucose
(DDx: TB, metastatic disease, parapneumonic
effusion)
2. SLE (in 15 – 74%)
most common collagenosis to give pleural
effusion, bilateral in 50%; L > R
√ enlargement of cardiovascular silhouette (in
35 – 50%)
3. Wegener granulomatosis (in 50%)
4. Sjögren syndrome
5. Mixed connective tissue disease
6. Periarteritis nodosa
7. Postmyocardial infarct syndrome

(f) Traumatic
hemorrhagic, chylous, esophageal rupture, thoracic
/ abdominal surgery, intrapleural infusion, radiation
pneumonitis
(g) Miscellaneous
1. Sarcoidosis
2. Uremic pleuritis (in 20% of uremic patients)
3. Drug-induced effusion
CXR:
√ first 300 ml not visualized on PA view (collect in
subpulmonic region first, then spill into posterior
costophrenic sinus)
√ lateral decubitus views may detect as little as 25 ml
√ hemidiaphragm + costophrenic sinuses obscured
√ extension upward around posterior > lateral > anterior
thoracic wall (mediastinal portion fixed by pulmonary
ligament + hilum)
√ meniscus-shaped semicircular upper surface with
lowest point in midaxillary line
√ associated collapse of ipsilateral lung
Massive pleural effusion:
√ enlargement of ipsilateral hemithorax
√ displacement of mediastinum to contralateral side
√ severe depression / flattening / inversion of
ispsilateral hemidiaphragm
√ visible air bronchogram
Subpulmonic / subdiaphragmatic / infrapulmonary
pleural effusion:
√ peak of dome of pseudodiaphragm laterally
positioned
√ acutely angulated costophrenic angle
√ increased distance between stomach bubble and
lung
√ blunted posterior costophrenic sulcus
√ thin triangular paramediastinal opacity (mediastinal
extension of pleural effusion)
√ flattened pseudodiaphragmatic contour anterior to
major fissure (on lateral CXR)
CT:
√ fluid outside diaphragm
√ fluid elevating crus of diaphragm
√ indistinct fluid-liver interface
√ fluid posteromedial to liver (= bare area of liver)
CAVE: "central oval" sign of ascites may be seen in
subpulmonic effusion with inverted diaphragm

Unilateral pleural effusion
1. Neoplasm
2. Infection: TB
3. Collagen vascular disease
4. Subdiaphragmatic disease
5. Pulmonary emboli
6. Trauma: fractured rib
7. Chylothorax

Left-sided pleural effusion
1. Spontaneous rupture of the esophagus
2. Dissecting aneurysm of the aorta
3. Traumatic rupture of aorta distal to left subclavian
artery

4. Transection of <u>distal</u> thoracic duct
5. Pancreatitis: left-sided (68%), right-sided (10%), bilateral (22%)
6. Pancreatic + gastric neoplasm

Right-sided pleural effusion
1. Congestive heart failure
2. Transection of <u>proximal</u> thoracic duct
3. Pancreatitis

Pleural effusion + large cardiac silhouette
1. Congestive heart failure (most common)
   √   cardiomegaly
   √   prominence of upper lobe vessels + constriction of lower lobe vessels
   √   prominent hilar vessels
   √   interstitial edema (fine reticular pattern, Kerley lines, perihilar haze, peribronchial thickening)
   √   alveolar edema (perihilar confluent ill-defined densities, air bronchogram)
   √   "phantom tumor" = fluid localized to interlobar pleural fissure (in 78% in right horizontal fissure)
2. Pulmonary embolus with right-sided heart enlargement
3. Myocarditis / pericarditis with pleuritis
   (a) viral infection
   (b) tuberculosis
   (c) rheumatic fever (poststreptococcal infection)
4. Tumor: metastatic, mesothelioma
5. Collagen-vascular disease
   (a) SLE (pleural + pericardial effusion)
   (b) rheumatoid arthritis

Pleural effusion + subsegmental atelectasis
1. Postoperative (thoracotomy, splenectomy, renal surgery) secondary to thoracic splinting + small airway mucous plugging
2. Pulmonary embolus
3. Abdominal mass
4. Ascites
5. Rib fractures

Pleural effusion + lobar densities
1. Pneumonia with empyema
2. Pulmonary embolism
3. Neoplasm
   (a) bronchogenic carcinoma (common)
   (b) lymphoma
4. Tuberculosis

Pleural effusion + hilar enlargement
1. Pulmonary embolus
2. Tumor
   (a) bronchogenic carcinoma
   (b) lymphoma
   (c) metastasis
3. Tuberculosis
4. Fungal infection (rare)
5. Sarcoidosis (very rare)

Pleural solitary mass
= density with incomplete border and tapered superior + inferior borders, difficult to distinguish from chest wall mass (rib destruction reliable sign of chest wall mass)
1. Loculated pleural effusion ("vanishing tumor")
2. Organized empyema
3. Metastasis
4. Local benign mesothelioma
5. Subpleural lipoma: may erode adjacent rib
6. Hematoma
7. Mesothelial cyst
8. Neural tumor: schwannoma, neurofibroma
9. **Fibrin bodies** = 3 – 4 cm large tumorlike concentrations of fibrin forming in serofibrinous pleural effusions; usually near lung base

Multiple pleural densities
√ diffuse pleural thickening with lobulated borders
1. Loculated pleural effusion: infectious, hemorrhagic, neoplastic
2. Metastasis (most common cause): predominantly adenocarcinoma
3. Diffuse malignant mesothelioma almost always unilateral, associated with asbestos exposure
4. Malignant thymoma (rare)
   √ contiguous spread, invasion of pleura, spreads around lung
   √ NO pleural effusion
5. **Thoracic splenosis**
   = autotransplantation of splenic tissue to pleural space following thoracoabdominal trauma; discovered 10 – 30 years later
   √ positive Tc-99m sulfur colloid scan

mnemonic: "**M**ary **T**yler **M**oore **L**ikes **L**emon"
Metastases (especially adenocarcinoma)
Thymoma (malignant)
Malignant mesothelioma
Loculated pleural effusion
Lymphoma

Pleural thickening
A. TRAUMA
   1. **Fibrothorax** (most common cause)
      = organizing effusion / hemothorax / pyothorax
      √ dense fibrous layer of approx. 2 cm thickness almost always on visceral pleura
      √ frequent calcification on inner aspect of pleural peel
B. INFECTION
   1. Chronic empyema: over bases; history of pneumonia; parenchymal scars
   2. Tuberculosis / histoplasmosis: lung apex; associated with apical cavity
   3. Aspergilloma: in preexisiting cavity concomitant with pleural thickening
C. COLLAGEN-VASCULAR DISEASE
   1. Rheumatoid arthritis: pleural effusion fails to resolve
D. INHALATIONAL DISORDER

1. Asbestos exposure: lower lateral chest wall; basilar interstitial disease (<25%); thickening of parietal pleura with sparing of visceral pleura
2. Talcosis

E. NEOPLASM
  (a) Metastases: often nodular appearance; may be obscured by effusion
  (b) Diffuse malignant mesothelioma
  (c) Pancoast tumor

F. OTHER
  1. **Pleural hyaloserositis**
     Path: hyaline sclerotic tissue = cartilagelike whitish sugar icing appearance (Zuckerguss) with occasional calcification
  2. Mimicked by extrathoracic musculature, 1st + 2nd rib companion shadow, subpleural fat, focal scarring around old rib fractures

Apical cap

1. Inflammatory process: TB, healed empyema
2. Postradiation fibrosis
3. Neoplasm
4. Vascular abnormality
5. Mediastinal hemorrhage
6. Mediastinal lipomatosis
7. Peripheral upper lobe collapse

Pleural calcification

A. INFECTION
  1. Healed empyema
  2. Tuberculosis (and Rx for TB: pneumothorax / oleothorax), histoplasmosis

B. TRAUMA
  1. Healed hemothorax = fibrothorax:
     • Hx of significant chest trauma
     √ irregular plaques of calcium usually in visceral pleura
     √ healed rib fracture
  2. Radiation therapy

C. PNEUMOCONIOSIS
  1. Asbestos-related pleural disease (most common):
     √ combination of basilar reticular interstitial disease (<1/3) + pleural thickening
     √ calcifications of parietal pleura frequently diagnostic (diaphragmatic surface of pleura, bilateral but asymmetric)
  2. Talcosis: similar to asbestos-related disease
  3. Bakelite
  4. Muscovite mica

D. HYPERCALCEMIA
  1. Pancreatitis
  2. Secondary hyperparathyroidism in chronic renal failure / scleroderma

E. MISCELLANEOUS
  1. Mineral oil aspiration
  2. Pulmonary infarction

mnemonic: "TAFT"
  Tuberculosis
  Asbestosis

Fluid (effusion, empyema, hematoma)
Talc

DIAPHRAGM
Bilateral diaphragmatic elevation

A. Shallow inspiration (most frequent)
B. Abdominal causes
   Obesity, pregnancy, ascites, large abdominal mass
C. Pulmonary causes
   (1) Bilateral atelectasis
   (2) Restrictive pulmonary disease (SLE)
D. Neuromuscular disease
   (1) Myasthenia gravis
   (2) Amyotrophic lateral sclerosis

Unilateral diaphragmatic elevation

1. Subpulmonic pleural effusion
   √ dome of pseudodiaphragm migrates toward the costophrenic angle and flattens
2. Altered pulmonary volume
   (a) Atelectasis
       √ associated pulmonary density
   (b) Postoperative lobectomy / pneumectomy
       √ rib defects, metallic sutures
   (c) Hypoplastic lung
       √ small hemithorax (more often on the right), crowding of ribs, mediastinal shift, absent / small pulmonary artery, frequently associated with dextrocardia + anomalous pulmonary venous return
3. Phrenic nerve paralysis
   (a) Primary lung tumor
   (b) Malignant mediastinal tumor
   (c) Iatrogenic
   (d) Idiopathic
   √ paradoxic motion on fluoroscopy (patient in lateral position sniffing)
4. Abdominal disease
   (a) Subphrenic abscess: history of surgery, accompanied by pleural effusion
   (b) Distended stomach / colon
   (c) Interposition of colon
   (d) Liver mass (tumor, echinococcal cyst, abscess)
5. Diaphragmatic hernia
6. Eventration of diaphragm
7. Traumatic rupture of diaphragm
   Associated with rib fractures, pulmonary contusion, hemothorax
8. Diaphragmatic tumor
   Mesothelioma, fibroma, lipoma, lymphoma, metastases

CHEST WALL

Chest wall lesions

A. EXTERNAL
   1. Cutaneous lesion: moles, neurofibroma
   2. Nipples
   3. Artifact
B. NEOPLASTIC

1. Mesenchymal tumor
   Muscle tumor, fibroma, desmoid tumor, lipoma
   (common; growing between ribs presenting as
   intrathoracic + subcutaneous mass; CT diagnostic)
2. Neural tumor
   Schwannoma, neurofibroma (may erode ribs
   inferiorly with sclerotic bone reaction),
   neuroblastoma
3. Vascular tumor
   Hemangioma, hemangiopericytoma
4. Malignant bone tumor = rib tumor
   Δ in adult: metastasis, multiple myeloma
   Δ in child: Ewing sarcoma, metastatic
      neuroblastoma, chondrosarcoma (calcified
      matrix), osteosarcoma (rare), fibrosarcoma
5. Benign bone tumor
   Benign cortical defect, fibrous dysplasia,
   hemangioma of bone

C. TRAUMATIC
   1. Hematoma
   2. Rib fracture
D. INFECTIOUS
   1. Actinomycosis (parenchymal infiltrate, pleural
      effusion, chest wall mass, rib destruction,
      cutaneous fistulas)
   2. Aspergillosis, nocardiosis, blastomycosis,
      tuberculosis (rare)

√ incomplete border sign
√ smooth tapering borders (tangential views)
√ rib destruction (metastases / small round cell tumors /
   aggressive granulomatous infections)
√ inferior rib erosion + sclerosis (neurofibroma,
   schwannoma)

Lung disease with chest wall extension

A. Infectious
   1. Actinomycosis
   2. Nocardia
   3. Blastomycosis
   4. Tuberculosis
B. Malignant tumor
   1. Bronchogenic carcinoma
   2. Lymphoma
   3. Metastases
   4. Mesothelioma
   5. Breast carcinoma
   6. Internal mammary node
C. Benign tumor
   1. Capillary hemangioma of infancy
   2. Cavernous hemangioma
   3. Extrapleural lipoma
   4. Abscess
   5. Hematoma

Malignant tumors of chest wall in children

1. Ewing Sarcoma of rib (most common)
   (a) older child: rib involvement in 7%, predominant
      involvement of pelvis + lower extremity
   (b) child <10 years: rib involvement in 30%

2. Rhabdomyosarcoma
   relatively common in children + adolescents
   √ sclerosis / destruction / scalloping of cortex (local
      extension to contiguous bone)
   √ may calcify
   Metastases to: lung, occasionally lymph nodes
   Prognosis: infiltrative growth with high risk of local
      recurrence
3. Neuroblastoma
   10% present as chest wall mass
   √ may calcify
4. **Askin tumor**
   = uncommon tumor probably arising from intercostal
      nerves in young Caucasian females
   Path: neuroectodermal small cell tumor containing
      neuron-specific enolase (may also be found in
      neuroblastoma)
   √ rib destruction
   √ pleural effusion
   Metastases to: bone, CNS, liver, adrenal
   DDx: Chest wall hamartoma in infancy

PULMONARY MALFORMATION

= SEQUESTRATION SPECTRUM
1. Congenital lobar emphysema
2. Bronchogenic cyst
3. Congenital cystic adenomatoid malformation
4. Bronchopulmonary sequestration
5. Hypogenetic lung syndrome
6. Pulmonary arteriovenous malformation

NEONATAL LUNG DISEASE
Mediastinal shift + abnormal aeration

A. SHIFT TOWARD LUCENT LUNG
   1. Diaphragmatic hernia
   2. Chylothorax
   3. Cystic adenomatoid malformation
B. SHIFT AWAY FROM LUCENT LUNG
   1. Congenital lobar emphysema
   2. Persistent localized pulmonary interstitial
      emphysema
   3. Obstruction of main stem bronchus (by
      anomalous or dilated vessel / cardiac chamber)

Reticulogranular densities in neonate

1. Respiratory distress syndrome (90%): premature
   infant, inadequate surfactant
2. Immature lung: premature infant, normal surfactant
3. Transient tachypnea of the newborn
4. Neonatal group-B streptococcal pneumonia
5. Idiopathic hypoglycemia
6. Congestive heart failure
7. Early pulmonary hemorrhage
8. Infant of diabetic mother

Hyperinflation in newborn

1. Fetal aspiration syndrome
2. Neonatal pneumonia
3. Pulmonary hemorrhage
4. Congenital heart disease

5. Transient tachypnea (mild)

Hyperinflation in child
mnemonic: "BUMP FAD"
Bronchiectasis
Upper airway obstruction
Mucoviscidosis
Pneumonia (esp. staph)
Foreign body (ball valve mechanism)
Asthma
Dehydration (diarrhea, acidosis)

Pulmonary hemorrhage
A. WITHOUT RENAL DISEASE
　1. Bleeding diathesis: leukemia
　2. Anticoagulation therapy
　3. Disseminated intravascular coagulation
　4. Blunt trauma
　5. Idiopathic pulmonary hemosiderosis
　6. Limited Wegener granulomatosis
　7. Infectious diseases
　8. Exogenous agents: D-penicillamine, lymphangiography
B. WITH RENAL DISEASE

1. Goodpasture syndrome = anti-basement membrane antibody disease
2. Collagen vascular disease + systemic vasculitides: SLE, Wegener granulomatosis, polyarteritis nodosa, Henoch-Schönlein purpura, Behçet disease
3. Rapidly progressive glomerulonephritis ± immune complexes
C. HEMORRHAGIC PNEUMONIA
　1. Bacteria: Legionnaires' disease
　2. Viruses: CMV, herpes
　3. Fungi: Aspergillosis, mucormycosis

Hemoptysis
A. Tumor
　1. Carcinoma
　2. Bronchial adenoma
B. Bronchial wall injury
　1. Foreign body erosion
　2. Bronchoscopy / biopsy
C. Vascular
　1. COPD
　2. Pulmonary embolus with infarction
　3. Venous hypertension (most common)
　4. AV fistula
D. Infection
　1. Chronic bronchitis
　2. Bronchiectasis (mouthful)
　3. Tuberculosis (Rasmussen aneurysm)
　4. Aspergillosis

FUNCTION AND ANATOMY OF LUNG

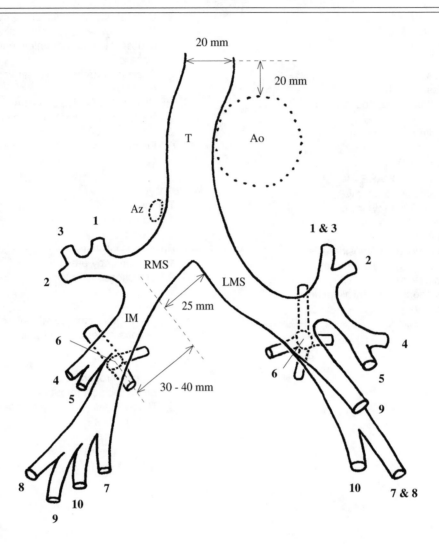

Bronchopulmonary Anatomy

Ao = aortic arch   RMS = right main stem bronchus
Az = azygos vein   LMS = left main stem bronchus
T = trachea   IM = intermediate bronchus

RUL   LUL
  1 = apical   1&3 = apicoposterior
  2 = anterior   2 = anterior
  3 = posterior   4 = superior lingula
RML   5 = inferior lingula
  4 = lateral
  5 = medial
RLL   LLL
  6 = superior   6 = superior
  7 = mediobasal   7&8 = anteromedial
  8 = anterobasal   9 = laterobasal
  9 = laterobasal   10 = posterobasal
 10 = posterobasal

Order of lower lobe bronchi in frontal projection from lateral to medial:
   mnemonic "ALPm" = **A**nterior-**L**ateral-**P**osterior-medial

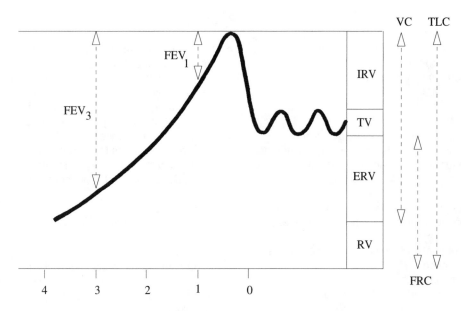

Secondary pulmonary lobule

= anatomic + functional lung unit appearing as an irregular polyhedron measuring 10 – 30 mm on each side; separated from each other by thin fibrous interlobular septa; supplied by 3 – 5 terminal bronchioles

Contents:
- — centrally: branches of terminal bronchioles + pulmonary arterioles
- — peripherally (in interlobular septa): pulmonary veins + lymph vessels

HRCT:
- √ fine peripheral lines of increased attenuation in contact with pleura (= interlobular septa)
- √ dots / Y-shaped lines with branching points 3 – 5 mm from pleura (= pulmonary arterioles)

Lung volumes & capacities

1. Tidal volume (**TV**)
   = amount of gas moving in and out with each respiratory cycle
2. Residual volume (**RV**)
   = amount of gas remaining in the lung after a maximal expiration
3. Total lung capacity (**TLC**)
   = gas contained in lung at the end of a maximal inspiration
4. Vital capacity (**VC**)
   = amount of gas that can be expired after a maximal inspiration without force
5. Functional residual capacity (**FRC**)
   = volume of gas remaining in lungs at the end of a quiet expiration

Changes in lung volumes

A. DECREASED VC:
1. Reduction in functioning lung tissue due to
   (a) space-occupying process (eg, pneumonia, infarction)
   (b) surgical removal of lung tissue
2. Process reducing overall volume of the lungs (eg, diffuse pulmonary fibrosis)
3. Inability to expand lungs due to
   (a) muscular weakness (eg, poliomyelitis)
   (b) increase in abdominal volume (eg, pregnancy)
   (c) pleural effusion
B. INCREASED FRC and RV:
   characteristic of air trapping and overinflation (eg, asthma, emphysema)
   Associated with increased TLC
C. DECREASED FRC and RV:
1. Process reducing overall volume of lungs (eg, diffuse pulmonary fibrosis)
2. Process that occupies volume within alveoli (eg, alveolar microlithiasis)
3. Process that elevates diaphragm (eg, ascites, pregnancy), usually associated with decreased TLC

Flow rates

A. Spirometric measurements:
1. Forced expiratory volume (FEV)
   = amount of air expired during a certain time period (usually 1 + 3 sec);
   Normal values: $FEV_1 = 83\%$; $FEV_3 = 97\%$
2. Maximal midexpiratory flow rate (MMFR)
   = amount of gas expired during the middle half of forced expiratory volume curve (largely effort independent)
   Indicator of small airway resistance
3. Flow-volume loop
   = gas flow is plotted against the actual volume of lung at which this flow is occurring
   Useful in identifying obstruction in large airways
B. Resistance in small airways
   Closing volume = lung volume at which dependent lung zones cease to ventilate because of airway closure in small airway disease or loss of lung elastic recoil

- decrease in FEV, MMFR, MBC:
  - (a) expiratory airway obstruction (reversible as in spasmodic asthma / irreversible as in emphysema)
  - (b) respiratory muscle weakness

Diffusing capacity

= rate of gas transfer across the alveolocapillary membrane in relation to a constant pressure difference across it; measured by the carbon monoxide diffusion method

Reduction:

1. Ventilation / perfusion inequality: less CO is taken up by poorly ventilated or poorly perfused areas (eg, emphysema)
2. Reduction of total surface area (eg, emphysema, surgical resection)
3. Reduction in permeability from thickening of alveolar membrane (eg, cellular infiltration, edema, interstitial fibrosis)
4. Anemia with lack of hemoglobin

Arterial blood gas abnormalities

- decreased pulmonary arterial O_2:
  1. alveolar hypoventilation
  2. impaired diffusion
  3. abnormal ventilation/perfusion ratios
  4. anatomic shunting
- elevated pulmonary arterial CO_2:
  1. alveolar hypoventilation
  2. impaired ventilation / perfusion ratios

V/Q inequality

A. normal:
  - (a) blood flow decreases rapidly from base to apex
  - (b) ventilation decreases less rapidly from base to apex
  - Δ V/Q is low at base and high at apex
  - Δ Pulmonary arterial O_2 is substantially higher at apex
  - Δ Pulmonary arterial CO_2 is substantiallly higher at base

B. abnormal:
  chiefly resulting from non- / underventilated lung regions (non- / underperfused   regions do not result in blood gas disturbances)

Compliance

= relationship of the change in intrapleural pressure to the volume of gas that moves into the lungs

A. Decreased compliance:
   edema, fibrosis, granulomatous infiltration
B. Increased compliance:
   emphysema (faulty elastic architecture)

√ height of diaphragm at TLC can provide some indication of lung compliance, particularly valuable in sequential roentgenograms for comparison in:
  1. Diffuse interstitial pulmonary edema
  2. Diffuse interstitial pulmonary fibrosis

Surfactant

= surface-active material essential for normal pulmonary function

Substrate:
  phospholipids (phosphatidylcholine, phosphatidylglycerol), other lipids, cholesterol, lung-specific proteins

Production:
  type II pulmonary alveoli synthesize + transport + secrete lung surfactant; earliest production around 18th week of gestation (in amniotic fluid by 22nd week of gestation)

Action:
  increases lung compliance, stabilizes alveoli, enhances alveolar fluid clearance, reverses surface tension, protects against alveolar collapse during respiration, protects epithelial cell surface, reduces opening pressure + precapillary tone

THYMUS

Origin: 3rd (and possibly 4th) branchial pouch migrating from pharynx to anterior mediastinum during embryogenesis; residual thymic tissue in neck in 1.8 – 21%

Thymic weight:
  increases from birth to age 11 – 12 years (22 ± 13 g in neonate, 34 ± 15 g at puberty); ratio of thymic weight to body weight decreases with age (involution after puberty, total fatty replacement after age 60)

√ measurement (perpendicular to axis of aortic arch): <18 mm before age 20; <13 mm after age 20
√ convex borders, triangular, vaguely bilobed with muscular density (before puberty)
√ flat / concave borders with abundant fat (after puberty)
Δ atrophies under stress (due to increase in endogenous steroids)

CHEST DISORDERS

ACTINOMYCOSIS

Organism: Actinomyces israelii, Gram-positive anaerobic pleomorphic small bacterium with proteolytic activity, superficially resembling the morphology of a hyphal fungus; closely related to mycobacteria

Histo: mycelial form in tissue; rod-shaped bacterial form in oropharynx

Occurrence: rod-shaped form in dental caries, gingival margins, tonsillar crypts, GI tract

Predisposed: individuals with very poor dental hygiene, immunosuppressed patients

- "sulfur granules" in sputum / exudate = colonies of organisms arranged in circular fashion = mycelial clumps with thin hyphae 1 – 2 mm in diameter

Organ involvement: mandibulofacial > intestinal > lung

@ Mandibulofacial actinomycosis
   √ osteomyelitis of mandible
@ Abdominal actinomycosis
   √ fold thickening (resembling Crohn disease)
   √ rupture of abdominal viscus (usually appendix)
   √ fistula formation
@ Pleuropulmonary actinomycosis
   √ consolidation extending across interlobar fissures (acute air-space pneumonia rare)
   √ cavitary lesion (abscess)
   √ empyema
   √ osteomyelitis of ribs
   √ draining chest wall sinuses (spread through fascial planes)

Rx: surgical debridement + penicillin

AIDS

= Acquired immune deficiency syndrome
= ultimately fatal disease characterized by HIV seropositivity, specific opportunistic infections, specific malignant neoplasms (Kaposi sarcoma, Burkitt lymphoma, primary lymphoma of brain)

AIDS-related complex (ARC)
   = GENERALIZED LYMPHADENOPATHY SYNDROME
   = prodromal phase of HIV seropositivity, generalized lymphadenopathy, CNS diseases other than those associated with AIDS

- weight loss, malaise, diarrhea
- fever, night sweats, lymphadenopathy
- lymphopenia with selective decrease in helper T-cells

Organism: human immunodeficiency virus (HIV)
   = human T-cell lymphotropic virus type III (HTLV III) = lymphadenopathy-associated virus (LAV)

Groups at risk:
1.   Homosexual males (74%)
2.   IV drug abusers (16%)
3.   Contaminated blood products (3%)
4.   Sexual partner of drug abuser + bisexual man
5.   Infants born to woman infected with AIDS virus
Δ   HIV antibodies present in >50% of homosexuals + 90% of IV drug abusers!

Clinical classification:
group I   acute HIV infection with seroconversion
group II   asymptomatic HIV infection
group III   persistent generalized lymphadenopathy
group IV   other HIV disease
   — subgroup A   constitutional disease
   — subgroup B   neurologic disease
   — subgroup C   secondary infectious disease
   — subgroup D   secondary cancers
   — subgroup E   other conditions

A.   LYMPHADENOPATHY
   Cause: reactive follicular hyperplasia (50%), NHL (20%), mycobacterial infection (17%), Kaposi sarcoma (10%), metastatic tumor, opportunistic infection with multiple organisms, drug reaction
   Location: mediastinum, axilla, retrocrural
B.   OPPORTUNISTIC INFECTION
   accounts for majority of pulmonary disease, recurrent in 20 – 40%
   1. Pneumocystis carinii pneumonia (up to 85%)
      >60% develop at least 1 episode during disease
      - subacute insidious onset with malaise, minimal cough
      Prognosis: in 25% fatal
   2. CMV pneumonia
      most frequent infection found at autopsy
   3. Mycobacterium (20%): M. avium-intracellulare (83%), M. tuberculosis (9%)
   4. Nocardia pneumonia (<5%)
      usually occurs in cavitating pneumonia
   5. Cryptococcal pneumonia (2 – 15%)
   6. Pyogenic bacteria (10%)
C.   TUMOR
   1. Metastatic Kaposi sarcoma (25%)
      Location: widespread skin + organ involvement, lung (20%)
      √ numerous fluffy nodules of peribronchial distribution
      √ pleural effusion
   2. Lymphoma
      primarily immunoblastic NHL, occasionally Hodgkin disease
      Location: pulmonary involvement (<9%), CNS, GI tract, liver, spleen, bone marrow
D.   Lymphocytic interstitial pneumonitis (especially in children)
E.   Septic emboli
F.   Premature development of bullae (40%) with disposition to spontaneous pneumothorax

ADULT RESPIRATORY DISTRESS SYNDROME
= SHOCK LUNG = POSTTRAUMATIC PULMONARY
   INSUFFICENCY = HEMORRHAGIC LUNG
   SYNDROME = RESPIRATOR LUNG = STIFF LUNG
   SYNDROME = PUMP LUNG = CONGESTIVE
   ATELECTASIS = OXYGEN TOXICITY
= severe unexpected life-threatening acute respiratory
  distress characterized by abrupt onset of marked
  dyspnea, increased respiratory effort, severe hypoxemia
  associated with widespread air-space consolidation

Histo:
(a) up to 12 hours: fibrin + platelet microemboli
(b) 12 – 24 hours: interstitial edema
(c) 24 – 48 hours: capillary congestion, extensive
    interstitial + alveolar proteinaceous edema +
    hemorrhage, widespread microatelectasis,
    destruction of type I alveolar epithelial cells
(d) 5 – 7 days: extensive hyaline membrane formation,
    hypertrophy + hyperplasia of type II alveolar lining
    cells
(e) 7 – 14 days: extensive fibroblastic proliferation in
    interstitium + within alveoli, rapidly progressing
    collagen deposition + fibrosis; almost invariably
    associated with infection

Predisposed:
   Hemorrhagic / septic shock, massive trauma (pulmonary
   / general body), acute pancreatitis, aspiration of liquid
   gastric contents, heroine / methadone intoxication,
   massive viral pneumonia, traumatic fat embolism, near-
   drowning, conditions leading to pulmonary edema

   mnemonic: "DICTIONARIES"
   Disseminated intravascular coagulation
   Infection
   Caught drowning
   Trauma
   Inhalants: smoke, phosgene, NO_2
   O₂ toxicity
   Narcotics + other drugs
   Aspiration
   Radiation
   Includes pancreatitis
   Emboli: amniotic fluid, fat
   Shock: septic, hemorrhagic, cardiogenic, anaphylactic

CXR:
√ NO cardiomegaly / pleural effusion
— up to 12 hours:
   √ characteristic 12-hour delay between clinical onset
      of respiratory failure and CXR abnormalities
— 12 – 24 hours:
   √ patchy ill-defined opacities throughout both lungs
— 24 – 48 hours:
   √ massive air-space consolidation of both lungs
— 5 – 7 days:
   √ consolidation becomes inhomogeneous (resolution
      of alveolar edema)
   √ local areas of consolidation (pneumonia)
— >7 days:

√ reticular / bubbly lung pattern (diffuse interstitial +
   air-space fibrosis)
Complication of continuous positive pressure ventilation:
√ diffuse interstitial emphysema, pneumothorax ,
   pneumomediastinum

ALPHA-1 ANTITRYPSIN DEFICIENCY
= rare autosomal recessive disorder
Alpha-1 antitrypsin (glycoprotein) is synthesized in liver +
released into serum
   Action: proteolytic inhibitor of trypsin, chymotrypsin,
             elastase, plasmin, thrombin, kallikrein,
             leukocytic + bacterial proteases; neutralizes
             circulating proteolytic enzymes
   Mode of injury from deficiency: PMNs + alveolar
      macrophages sequester into lung during recurrent
      bacterial infections + release elastase, which digests
      basement membrane
Age: early age of onset (20 – 30 years);   M:F = 1:1
• rapid + progressive deterioration of lung function
√ severe panacinar emphysema with basilar
   predominance
√ reduction in size + number of pulmonary vessels in
   lower lobes
√ redistribution of blood flow to unaffected upper lung
   zones
√ bullae at both lung bases
√ marked flattening of diaphragm
√ minimal diaphragmatic excursion
Cx: hepatic cirrhosis (in homozygotic individuals)

ALVEOLAR MICROLITHIASIS
= very rare disease of unknown etiology characterized by
  myriad of calcispherytes (= tiny calculi) within alveoli
Age peak: 30 – 50 years; begins in early life; has been
             identified in utero
M:F = 1:1; in 50% familial (restricted to siblings)
• usually asymptomatic (70%)
• dyspnea on exertion (reduction in residual volume)
• cyanosis, clubbing of fingers
• striking discrepancy between striking radiographic
  findings and mild clinical symptoms
• NORMAL serum calcium + phosphorus levels
√ very fine, sharply defined, sand-like micronodulations
   (<1 mm)
√ diffuse involvement of both lungs
√ intense uptake on bone scan
Prognosis:
(a) late development of pulmonary insufficiency
    secondary to interstitial fibrosis
(b) disease may become arrested
(c) microliths may continue to form / enlarge
DDx: "Mainline" pulmonary granulomatosis = IV abuse
         of talc-containing drugs such as methadone
         (rarely as numerous + scarring + loss of volume)

ALVEOLAR PROTEINOSIS
= PULMONARY ALVEOLAR PROTEINOSIS (PAP)
= accumulation of PAS positive phospholipid material in
  alveoli (= surfactant)

Etiology: ?; associated with dust exposure (eg, silicoproteinosis is histologically identical to PAP), immunodeficiency, hematologic + lymphatic malignancies, AIDS, chemotherapy

Pathophysiology:
(a) overproduction of surfactant by granular pneumocytes
(b) defective clearance of surfactant by alveolar macrophages

Histo: alveoli filled with proteinaceous material (the ONLY pure air-space disease), normal interstitium

Age peak: 30 – 50 years (age range 2 – 70 years); M:F = 3:1

- asymptomatic (10 – 20%)
- gradual onset of dyspnea + cough
- weight loss, weakness, hemoptysis
- defect in diffusing capacity

√ "bat-wing" consolidation of ground-glass pattern, predominant at bases
√ small acinar nodules + coalescence + consolidation
√ patchy peripheral / primarily unilateral infiltrates (rare)
√ reticular / reticulonodular / linear interstitial pattern with Kerley B lines (late stage)
√ slow clearing over weeks or months
√ slow progression (1/3), remaining stable (2/3)
√ NO adenopathy, NO cardiomegaly, NO pleural effusion

Cx: Infections (frequently secondary to poorly functioning macrophages + excellent culture medium): Nocardia asteroides (most common), mycobacterial, fungal, pneumocystis, CMV

Prognosis:
Highly variable course with clinical and radiologic episodes of exacerbation + remissions
(a) 50% improvement / recovery
(b) 30% death within several years under progression

Rx: bronchopulmonary lavage

DDx:
(a) during acute phase: pulmonary edema, diffuse pneumonia, ARDS
(b) in chronic stage:
  1. Idiopathic pulmonary hemosiderosis (boys, symmetric involvement of mid + lower zones, progression to nodular + linear pattern)
  2. Hemosiderosis (bleeding diathesis)
  3. Pneumoconiosis
  4. Hypersensitivity pneumonitis
  5. Goodpasture syndrome (more rapid changes, renal disease)
  6. Desquamative interstitial pneumonia ("ground glass" appearance, primarily basilar + peripheral)
  7. Pulmonary alveolar microlithiasis (widespread discrete intraalveolar calcifications primarily in lung bases, rare familial disease)
  8. Sarcoidosis (usually with lymphadenopathy)
  9. Lymphoma
  10. Bronchioloalveolar cell carcinoma (more focal, slowly enlarging with time)

AMNIOTIC FLUID EMBOLISM
= most common cause of maternal peripartum death
- dyspnea
- shock during / after labor + delivery

Pathogenesis:
Amniotic debris enters maternal circulation resulting in (1) pulmonary embolization (2) anaphylactoid reaction (3) DIC
√ usually fatal before radiographs obtained
√ may demonstrate pulmonary edema

AMYLOIDOSIS
= disease characterized by an extracellular deposit of proteinaceous twisted ß-pleated sheet fibrils of great chemical diversity

Histo: protein (immunoglobulin) / polysaccharide complex
- asthmalike symptoms
- hemoptysis

1. PRIMARY AMYLOIDOSIS
   lung involvement in up to 70%
   not associated with specific disease
2. SECONDARY AMYLOIDOSIS
   most common; lung involvement rare
   associated with: rheumatoid arthritis, multiple myeloma
@ Lung involvement
   A. Tracheobronchial type (most common)
      √ multiple nodules protruding from wall of trachea
      √ prominent bronchovascular markings
      √ destructive pneumonitis
   B. Nodular type
      Age: >60 years of age
      √ mediastinal / hilar adenopathy
      √ solitary / multiple parenchymal nodules in a peripheral / subpleural location ± central calcification / ossification; slow growth over years
      √ ± pleural effusion
   C. Diffuse parenchymal type
      √ widespread interstitial involvement

ANKYLOSING SPONDYLITIS
Incidence: 1% of patients with ankylosing spondylitis
Histo: interstitial + pleural fibrosis with foci of dense collagen deposition, NO granulomas
- bone manifestations obvious + severe
Location: apices / upper lung fields
√ uni- / bilateral, coarse, linear shadows + cavities
√ bronchiectasis may be present
√ superinfection, especially with aspergillosis (mycetoma formation) / atypical mycobacteria
DDx: other causes of pulmonary apical fibrosis (primary infection by fungi / mycobacteria; cancer)

ASBESTOS-RELATED DISEASE
Substances: length of fiber's 100 μ
(a) relatively benign:
   (1) Chrysotile (white asbestos) in Canada
   (2) Anthophyllite in Finland, North America
   (3) Tremolite

(b) relatively malignant:
  (1) Crocidolite (blue / black asbestos) in South Africa, Australia
  (2) Amosite (brown asbestos)
Δ Very fine fibers (crocidolite) associated with largest number of pleural disease!
Occupational exposure:
(a) asbestos mining + milling
(b) insulation, textile manufacturing, construction, ship building, gaskets, brake linings

Pulmonary Asbestosis

= (term asbestosis reserved for) chronic progressive diffuse interstitial fibrosis
Incidence: in 49 – 52% of industrial asbestos exposure
Histo: interstitial fibrosis begins in peribronchiolar areas, then progresses to involve adjacent alveoli
Diagnostic criteria:
1. reliable history of exposure
2. appropriate time interval between exposure + detection
3. CXR evidence
4. restrictive pattern of lung impairment
5. abnormal diffusing capacity
6. bilateral crackles at posterior lung bases, not cleared by cough
• dyspnea
• restrictive pulmonary function tests
Location: more severe in lower subpleural zones (concentration of asbestos fibers under pleura)
√ small irregular opacities (NOT rounded as in coal / silica)
√ confined to lung bases, progressing superiorly
√ septal lines (= fibrous thickening around secondary lobules)
√ "shaggy" heart border = obscuration secondary to parenchymal + pleural changes
√ ill-defined outline of diaphragm
√ honeycombing (uncommon)
√ rarely massive fibrosis, predominantly at lung bases without migration toward hilum (DDx from silicosis / CWP)
√ NO hilar adenopathy
√ Ga-67 uptake gives a quantitative index of inflammatory activity
HRCT:
  √ curvilinear subpleural lines parallel to + within 1 cm of pleura (30%) = multiple subpleural dotlike reticulonodularities connected to the most peripheral branch of pulmonary artery
  √ parenchymal fibrous bands = linear opacities contacting pleural surface
  √ subpleural pulmonary arcades = branching linear structures most prominent posteriorly
  √ reticulation = network of linear densities, usually posteriorly at lung bases
  √ honeycombing = multiple cystic spaces <1 cm in diameter with thickened wall

√ thickened interlobular septal lines
√ thickened intralobular lines

Asbestos-Related Pleural Disease

1. Focal Pleural Plaques (65%)
= hyalinized collagen in submesothelial layer of parietal pleura
Incidence: most common manifestation of exposure; 6% of general population will show plaques
Latent period: in 10% after 20 years; in 50% after 40 years
Location: bilateral; posterolateral midportion of chest wall between 7 – 10th rib; aponeurotic portion of diaphragm; mediastinum; following rib contours; visceral pleura + apices + costophrenic angles typically spared
√ usually circumscribed thickening with edges thicker than central portions of plaque; in 48% only finding; in 41% with parenchymal changes
√ no hilar adenopathy
√ usually not calcified
DDx: chest wall fat, rib fractures, rib companion shadows

2. Diffuse Pleural Thickening (17%)
= diffuse thickening of parietal pleura (visceral pleura involved in 90%, but difficult to demonstrate)
• may cause restriction of pulmonary function
May be associated with rounded atelectasis
√ bilateral process with "shaggy heart" appearance (20%)
√ smooth; difficult to assess when viewed en face
√ thickening of interlobar fissures
√ commonly obliterates costophrenic angles

3. Pleural Calcification (21 – 50%)
Overall incidence: 20%
Latent period: 40% after 40 years
√ dense lines paralleling the diaphragm (most common, PATHOGNOMONIC), chest wall, mediastinum, cardiac border
√ calcium deposits may form within center of plaques
DDx: talc exposure, hemothorax, empyema, therapeutic pneumothorax for TB (often unilateral, extensive sheet-like, on visceral pleura)

4. Benign Pleural Effusion (21%)
Earliest asbestos-related pleural abnormality, frequently followed by diffuse pleural thickening + rounded atelectasis
Prevalence: 3% (increases with increasing levels of asbestos exposure)
Latent period: 8 – 10 years after exposure
• may be associated with chest pain (1/3)
• usually small sterile, serous / hemorrhagic exudate
√ recurrent bilateral effusions ± plaque formation
DDx: TB, mesothelioma

Atelectatic Asbestos Pseudotumor
= ROUNDED ATELECTASIS = "FOLDED LUNG"
= infolding of redundant pleura accompanied by segmental / subsegmental atelectasis

Location: posteromedial / posterolateral lower lobe (most common); frequently bilateral
√ 2.5 – 8 cm subpleural mass related to a site of pleural abnormality
√ size + shape show little progression, occasionally decrease in size
CT:
  √ rounded / lentiform / wedge-shaped outline
  √ contiguous to areas of diffuse pleural thickening
  √ partial interposition of lung between pleura + mass
  √ volume loss in adjacent lung
  √ "crow's feet" = linear bands radiating from mass into lung parenchyma (54%)
  √ "comet tail" = vessels + bronchi bundled together and converging toward mass
  √ air bronchogram (18%)

Lung Cancer in Asbestos-Related Disease
Occurrence related to:
  (a) cumulated dose of asbestos fibers
  (b) smoking (synergistic carcinogenic effect)
    Δ Increased risk by factor of up to 90 in smokers versus a factor of 5 in non-smokers!
    Δ Up to 25% of asbestos workers who smoke develop lung cancer!
  (c) preexisting interstitial disease
  (d) occupational exposure to known carcinogen

Latent period: >20 years
Associated with increased incidence of gastric carcinoma
Histo: bronchogenic carcinoma (adenocarcinoma + squamous cell), bronchioloalveolar cell carcinoma
Location: at lung base / in any location if associated with smoking

ASPERGILLOSIS
Organism: Aspergillus fumigatus = ubiquitous soil fungus, commonly in sputum of normal persons, ability to invade arteries + veins facilitating hematogenous dissemination
M:F = 3:1

Predisposed:
  (a) preexisting lung disease (tuberculosis, bronchiectasis)
  (b) impairment of immune system (alcoholism, advanced age, malnutrition, concurrent malignancy, poorly controlled diabetes, cirrhosis, sepsis)
Cx: dissemination to heart, brain, kidney, GI tract, liver, thyroid, spleen

SAPROPHYTIC COLONIZATION
= commensal existence in upper respiratory tract

Noninvasive Aspergillosis
= noninvasive colonization of preexisting cavity / cyst [tuberculosis, bronchiectasis, sarcoidosis (common), bullous lung disease, carcinoma]
• sputum blood-streaked or severe hemoptysis (45 – 70%)
√ aspergilloma = solid round mass within spherical / ovoid thin-walled cavity
  Histo: mycetoma = intertwined hyphae matted together with fibrin, mucus, cellular debris
√ fungus ball moves with positioning
√ crescent-shaped air space separates fungus ball from cavity wall
√ fungus ball may calcify in scattered / rimlike fashion
√ pleural thickening, may be first sign of mycetoma in preexisting lung cyst / cavity

Semi-invasive Aspergillosis
= chronic cavitary slowly progressive disease in patients with preexisting lung injury (COPD, radiation therapy), mild immune suppression, or debilitation (alcohol, diabetes)
√ consolidation (usually upper lobe)
√ development of air crescent and fungus ball

Invasive Pulmonary Aspergillosis
= often fatal form in severely immunocompromised patients (most commonly in lymphoma / leukemia patients with prolonged granulocytopenia)
Histo: endobronchial fungal proliferation followed by transbronchial vascular invasion eventually causing thrombosis of pulmonary arterioles + ischemic necrosis; fungus ball = devitalized sequestrum of lung infiltrated by fungi
• Hx of series of bacterial infections + unremitting fever
• pleuritic chest pain (mimicking emboli)
• progression of pulmonary infiltrates despite broad spectrum antibiotics
  (a) early signs:
    √ halo sign = single / multiple nodules with halo of low attenuation
    √ patchy localized bronchopneumonia
  (b) signs of progression
    √ enlargement of nodules into diffuse bilateral consolidation
    √ development into large wedge-shaped pleural-based lesions
    √ air-crescent sign = cavitation of existing nodule (air crescent between sequestrum and lung) 1 – 3 weeks after increase in white cell count
      Δ has better prognosis than consolidation without cavitation (feature of resolution phase)

Allergic Bronchopulmonary Aspergillosis
= hypersensitivity towards aspergilli in patients with long-standing asthma
A. ACUTE ALLERGIC BRONCHOPULMONARY ASPERGILLOSIS
    Type I reaction = immediate hypersensitivity (IgE-mediated)

Histo: alveoli filled with eosinophils
B.   CHRONIC ALLERGIC BRONCHOPULMONARY
        ASPERGILLOSIS
        Type III reaction = delayed immune complex
            response = Arthus reaction (IgG-mediated)
Histo: bronchial damage secondary to
            aspergillus antigen reacting with IgG
            antibodies, immune complexes activate
            complement leading to tissue injury
(a)   Primary diagnostic criteria:
        1. asthma (84%)
        2. blood eosinophilia
        3. immediate skin reaction to aspergillus
        4. precipitating antibodies against aspergillus (70%)
        5. elevated serum IgE
        6. proximal central bronchiectasis
        7. history of transient or fixed pulmonary infiltrates
(b)   Secondary diagnostic criteria:
        1. Aspergillus mycelia in sputum
        2. expectoration of brown plugs in sputum (54%)
        3. late skin reactivity to Aspergillus antigen

√ alveolar fleeting patchy subsegmental / lobar
    infiltrates: upper lobes (50%), lower lobes (20%),
    middle lobe (7%), both lungs (65%), may persist for
    >6 months
√ "tram-like" bronchial walls (edema)
√ central bronchiectasis = 1 – 2 cm ring shadows
    around hilum + upper lobes
√ "finger-in-glove", "toothpaste shadow" = V- or Y-
    shaped central mucus plugs in 2nd order bronchi of
    2.5 – 6 cm in length remaining for months + growing
    in size
√ lobar consolidation (32%)
√ atelectasis (14%) with collateral air drift
√ hyperinflation (due to bronchospasm)
√ cavitation in 14% (secondary to postobstructive
    abscess)
√ pulmonary fibrosis + retraction
√ NORMAL peripheral bronchi
    unusual are mycetoma in cavity, empyema,
    pneumothorax
DDx: tuberculosis, lipoid pneumonia, Löffler
            syndrome, bronchogenic carcinoma

Pleural Aspergillosis
= Aspergillus empyema in patients with pulmonary
    tuberculosis, bacterial empyema, bronchopleural
    fistula
√ pleural thickening

ASPIRATION OF SOLID FOREIGN BODY
Age: in 50% <3 years
Source: in 85% vegetable origin (peanut, barley grass)
Location: almost exclusively in lower lobes; R:L = 2:1
√ obstructive overinflation (68%) + reflex vasoconstriction
√ collapse (14 – 53%)
√ infiltrate (11%)
√ radiopaque foreign body (9%)
√ air trapping (expiratory / lateral decubitus film)

NUC:
    √ ventilation defect (initial breath) + retention (wash-out)
Cx: bronchiectasis (from long retention)
DDx: impacted esophageal foreign body

ASPIRATION PNEUMONIA
Predisposing conditions:
    (1)   CNS disorders / intoxication: alcoholism, mental
            retardation, seizure disorders, recent anesthesia
    (2)   Swallowing disorders: esophageal motility
            disturbances, head + neck surgery
• low grade fever
• productive cough
• choking on swallowing
Location:
    gravity-dependent portions of lung, posterior segments
    of upper lobes + lower lobes in bedridden patients,
    frequently bilateral, right middle + lower lobe with
    sparing of left lung is common
A.   ACUTE ASPIRATION PNEUMONIA
    Cause: mixed organisms (anaerobic) from GI tract
    √ segmental consolidation in dependent portion
B.   CHRONIC ASPIRATION PNEUMONIA
    Cause: repeated aspiration of foreign material from
                GI tract over long time / mineral oil
                (eg, in laxatives)
    Associated with: Zenker diverticulum, esophageal
            stenosis, achalasia, TE fistula, neuromuscular
            disturbances in swallowing
    √ recurring segmental consolidation
    √ progression to interstitial scarring (= localized
        honeycomb appearance)
    √ bronchopneumonic infiltrates of variable location
        over months / years
    √ residual peribronchial scarring
    Upper GI:
        √ abnormal swallowing / aspiration

ASTHMA
= episodic reversible bronchoconstriction secondary to
    hypersensitivity to a variety of stimuli
A.   INTRINSIC ASTHMA
    Age: middle age
    Pathogenesis: probably autoimmune phenomenon
            caused by viral respiratory infection and often
            provoked by infection, exercise, pharmaceuticals; no
            environmental antigen
B.   EXTRINSIC ASTHMA = ATOPIC ASTHMA
    Pathogenesis: secondary to antigens producing an
            immediate hypersensitivity response (type I); reagin
            sensitizes mast cells to release histamine followed
            by increased vascular permeability, edema, small
            muscle contraction; effects primarily bronchi causing
            airway obstruction
    Nonoccupational allergens: pollens, dog + cat fur,
            tamarind seed powder, castor bean, fungal spores,
            grain weevil
    Occupational allergens:
        (a)   natural substances: wood dust, flour, grain,
                beans

(b) pharmaceuticals: antibiotics, ASA
(c) inorganic chemicals: nickel, platinum
Path: bronchial plugging with large amounts of viscid tenacious mucus (eosinophils, Charcot-Leyden crystals), edematous bronchial walls, hypertrophy of mucous glands + smooth muscle

ACUTE SIGNS:
- during asthmatic attack low values for FEV + MMFR and abnormal V/Q ratios
- normal diffusing capacity
- √ hyperexpansion of lungs = severe overinflation + air trapping
  - √ flattened diaphragmatic dome
  - √ deepened retrosternal air space
- √ peribronchial cuffing

CHRONIC CHANGES:
Normal chest x-ray in 73%, findings of abnormalities depend on
  (a) age of onset (<15 years of age in 31%; >30 years of age in none)
  (b) on severity of asthma
- √ central ring shadows = bronchiectasis
- √ scars (from recurrent infections)

Cx: (1) Pneumonia (2 x as frequent as in nonasthmatics)
  - √ peripheral pneumonic infiltrates (secondary to blocked airways)
(2) Atelectasis (5 – 15%) from mucoid impaction
(3) Pneumomediastinum (5%), pneumothorax, subcutaneous emphysema; predominantly in children
(4) Emphysema
(5) Mucous plugging with secondary aspergillosis

ATYPICAL MEASLES PNEUMONIA
= clinical syndrome in patients who have been previously inadequately immunized with killed rubeola vaccine and are subsequently exposed to the measles virus (= type III immune complex hypersensitivity); noted in children who have received live vaccine before 13 months of age
- 2- to 3-day prodrome of headache, fever, cough, malaise
- maculopapular rash beginning on wrists + ankles (sometimes absent)
- postinfectious migratory arthralgias
- history of exposure to measles
- √ extensive nonsegmental consolidation, usually bilateral
- √ hilar adenopathy (100%)
- √ pleural effusion (0 – 70%)
- √ nodular densities of 0.5–10 cm in diameter in peripheral location, may calcify and persist up to 30 months

ATYPICAL TUBERCULOSIS
Organisms:
M. kansasii: lung infection in subjects with good immune status
M. marinum: "swimming pool granuloma"

M. ulcerans: "Buruli ulcer" in tropical areas
M. scrofulaceum: cervical lymphadenitis in infants
M. avium intracellulare : esp. in AIDS
Histo: lesions indistinguishable from M. tuberculosis
- weekly positive tuberculin skin test

Location: apicoposterior segment of LUL
- √ multiple thin-walled cavities with little surrounding reaction
- √ absence of significant pleural reaction
- √ nodule formation infrequent
- √ typically NO hilar elevation
- Δ Unfavorable response to antituberculous therapy is suspicious for atypical TB!

BARITOSIS
= inhalation of nonfibrogenic barium sulfate
- asymptomatic
- normal pulmonary function (benign course)
- √ bilateral nodular / patchy opacities, denser than bone (high atomic number)
- √ similar to calcified nodules
- √ NO cor pulmonale, NO hilar adenopathy
- √ regression if patient removed from exposure

BEHÇET DISEASE
- mouth / genital ulceration
- iritis, arthritis, skin rashes, encephalitis, thrombophlebitis
- √ aneurysm of large arteries (eg, pulmonary artery)
- √ large vein obstruction; may cause SVC syndrome

BERYLLIOSIS
= ? delayed hypersensitivity reaction after exposure to acid salts from extraction of beryllium oxide
Substance: one of the lightest metals (atomic weight 9), marked heat resistance, great hardness, fatigue resistance, no corrosion
Occupational exposure: fluorescent lamp factories

A. ACUTE BERYLLIOSIS (25%)
- √ pulmonary edema following an overwhelming exposure
B. CHRONIC BERYLLIOSIS
widespread systemic disease of liver, spleen, lymph nodes, kidney, myocardium, skin, skeletal muscle; removed from lungs + excreted via kidneys
Latent period: 5 – 15 years
- √ fine nodularity (granulomas similar to sarcoidosis)
- √ irregular opacities, particularly sparing apices + bases
- √ hilar + mediastinal adenopathy (may calcify)
- √ emphysema in upper lobes + interstitial fibrosis
- √ pneumothorax in 10%
DDx: (1) Nodular pulmonary sarcoidosis (indistinguishable)
(2) Asbestosis without hilar adenopathy

BLASTOMYCOSIS
= NORTH AMERICAN BLASTOMYCOSIS
= mixed pyogenic + granulomatous fungal infection

Organism:

soil-born dimorphic fungus Blastomyces dermatitidis, mycelial phase in soil + budding yeast form in mammals

Geographic distribution:

endemic in central + southeastern United States (Ohio + Mississippi River valleys, vicinity of Great Lakes), Africa, Central + South America (acquired through activities in woods)

Predisposed: elderly, immunocompromised

Histo:

(a)   exudative phase: accumulation of numerous neutrophils with infecting organism

(b)   proliferative phase: proliferation of epitheloid + giant cells to form granulomas with central microabscesses containing neutrophils and yeast forms

- mouth ulcers
- √ alveolar consolidation in acute illness (26 – 61%)
- √ multiple irregular nodular masses / satellite lesions
- √ air bronchogram in area of consolidation / mass (87%)
- √ interstitial disease
- √ cavitation if communicating with airway (13%)
- √ hilar / mediastinal lymph node enlargement (<25%)

Prognosis: disease may reactivate for up to 3 years

DDx: other pneumonias (ie, bacterial, tuberculous, fungal), pseudolymphoma, malignant neoplasm (ie, alveolar cell carcinoma, lymphoma, Kaposi sarcoma)

BRONCHIAL ADENOMA

= misnomer secondary to locally invasive features, tendency for recurrence, and occasional metastasis to extrathoracic sites (10%) = low-grade malignancy

Incidence: 6 – 10% of all primary lung tumors

Age: mean age of 35 – 45 years (range 12 – 60 years); 90% occur <50 years of age; most common primary lung tumor under age 16; M:F = 1:1; whites:blacks = 25:1

Path: arises from duct epithelium of bronchial mucous glands (predominant distribution of Kulchitsky cells at bifurcations of lobar bronchi)

Types:

mnemonic: "CAMP"

Carcinoid	90%
Adenoid cystic carcinoma = Cylindroma	6%
Mucoepidermoid carcinoma	3%
Pleomorphic carcinoma	1%

Location: most commonly near / at bifurcation of lobar / segmental bronchi;

central : peripheral = 4 : 1

— 48% on right: RLL (20%), RML (10%), RUL (7%), main right bronchus (8%), intermediate bronchus (3%)

— 32% on left :   LLL (13%), LUL (12%), main left bronchus (6%), lingular bronchus (1%)

- hemoptysis (40 – 50%)
- atypical asthma
- persistent cough
- recurrent obstructive pneumonia
- asymptomatic (10%)

- √ complete obstruction / air trapping in partial obstruction (rare) / nonobstructive (10 – 15%)
- √ obstructive emphysema
- √ recurrent postobstructive infection: pneumonitis, bronchiectasis, abscess
- √ atelectasis / consolidation of a lung / lobe / segment (78%)
- √ collateral air drift may prevent atelectasis
- √ solitary round / oval slightly lobulated pulmonary nodule (19%) of 1 – 10 cm in size
- √ hilar enlargement / mediastinal widening
= central endo- / exobronchial mass

CT:

- √ well-marginated sharply defined mass
- √ in close proximity to an adjacent bifurcation with splaying of bronchus
- √ coarse peripheral calcifications in 1/3 (cartilaginous / bony transformation)
- √ may exhibit marked homogeneous enhancement

Biopsy: risky secondary to high vascularity of tumor

Prognosis: 95% 5-year survival rate, 75% 15-year survival rate after resection

Carcinoid

= slow-growing low-grade malignant tumor

Incidence: 12 – 15% of all carcinoid tumors in the body; 1 – 4% of all bronchial neoplasms

Age peak: 5th decade (range of 2nd – 9th decade); mild female predominance; very uncommon in blacks

Path:

originates from neurosecretory cells of bronchial mucosa (= Kulchitsky cells = argentaffine cells) just as small cell cancer; part of APUD (amine precursor uptake and decarboxylation) system = chromaffin paraganglioma, which produces serotonin, ACTH, and bradykinin

Pathologic classification:

(KCC = Kulchitsky cell carcinoma)

KCC   I = classic carcinoid; endobronchial growth; usually <2.5 cm in size; younger patient; M:F = 1:10; lymph node metastases in 3%

KCC   II = atypical carcinoid (25% of carcinoid tumors); usually >2.5 cm; older patient; M:F = 3:1; lymph node metastases in 40 – 50%

KCC   III = small cell carcinoma

Δ Rarely cause for carcinoid syndrome or Cushing syndrome!

- recurrent / persistent pneumonia, hemoptysis
- wheezing, cough, dyspnea, chest pain
- carcinoid syndrome (rare) = flushing, fever, nausea + vomiting, diarrhea, hypotension, wheezing, respiratory distress from bronchospasm, left-sided endocardial damage (cardiac valve fibrosis)

- endobronchial exophytic mass at endoscopy

Location:
  58 – 90% central in lobar / segmental bronchi, 10 – 42% peripheral; located in submucosa; endobronchial / along bronchial wall / exobronchial
  √ polypoid tumor with average size of 2.2 cm
  √ most extend through bronchial wall thus involving bronchial lumen + parenchyma (= collar button lesion)
  √ calcification / ossification (26 – 33%): central carcinoid (43%), peripheral carcinoid (10%)
  √ vascular tumor supplied by bronchial circulation
  √ cavitation (rare)
  √ segmental / lobar atelectasis
  √ obstructive pneumonitis
  √ bronchiectasis + pulmonary abscess
Malignant potential: low
Metastases:
  (a) regional lymph nodes in 25%
  (b) distantly in 5% (adrenal, liver, brain, skin, osteoblastic bone metastases)
Prognosis:
  95% 5-year survival rate for classic carcinoids; 57 – 66% 5-year survival rate for atypical carcinoids

Cylindroma

= ADENOID CYSTIC CARCINOMA (7%)
Second most common primary tumor of trachea
Path: mixed serous + mucous glands; resembles salivary gland tumor
Histo:
  Grade 1: tubular + cribriform; no solid subtype
    √ entirely intraluminal
  Grade 2: tubular + cribriform; <20% solid subtype
    √ predominantly intraluminal
  Grade 3: solid subtype >20%
    √ predominantly extraluminal
Age peak: 4 – 5th decade
- typical Hx of refractory "asthma"
- hemoptysis, cough, stridor, wheezing
- dysphagia, hoarseness
√ endotracheal mass with extratracheal extension
Malignant potential:
  more aggressive than carcinoid with propensity for local invasion + distant metastases (lung, bone, brain, liver) in 25%
Rx: tracheal resection + adjunctive radiotherapy
Prognosis: 8.3 years mean survival

Mucoepidermoid Carcinoma

Path: squamous cells + mucus-secreting columnar cells; resembles salivary gland tumor
√ may involve trachea = locally invasive tumor
√ sessile / polyploid endobronchial lesion

Pleomorphic Adenoma

= MIXED TYPE = extremely rare

BRONCHIAL ATRESIA

= local obliteration of proximal lumen of a segmental bronchus

Proposed causes:
  (a) local interruption of bronchial arterial perfusion late in fetal life
  (b) tip of primitive bronchial bud separates from bud and continues to develop
Path: bronchial tree distal to obstruction patent containing mucous plugs, alveoli distal to obstruction air-filled through collateral air drift
- minimal symptoms, apparent later in childhood (most by age 15) / adult life

Location: apicoposterior segment of LUL (>>RUL / ML)
√ decreased perfusion
√ overexpanded segment (collateral air drift with expiratory air-trapping)
√ finger-like opacity lateral to hilum (= mucous plug distal to atretic lumen) is CHARACTERISTIC
Rx: no treatment because mostly asymptomatic
DDx: Congenital lobar emphysema (no mucous plug)

BRONCHIECTASIS

= localized irreversible dilatation of bronchial tree
Etiology:
  A. Congenital
    1. Structural defect of bronchi: Williams-Campbell syndrome (= bronchial cartilage deficiency), bronchial atresia
    2. Abnormal mucociliary transport: Kartagener syndrome
    3. Abnormal secretions: mucoviscidosis = cystic fibrosis
  B. Congenital / acquired immune deficiency (usually IgG deficiency):
    chronic granulomatous disease of childhood, alpha 1-antitrypsin deficiency
  C. Postinfectious: measles, whooping cough, Swyer-James syndrome, allergic bronchopulmonary aspergillosis, chronic granulomatous infection (TB)
  D. Bronchial obstruction: neoplasm, inflammatory nodes, foreign body
  E. Aspiration / inhalation: gastric contents / inhaled fumes (late complication)

Classification:
  1. **Cylindrical / tubular / fusiform bronchiectasis**
     reversible if associated with pulmonary collapse
     √ 16 subdivisions of bronchi
     √ square abrupt ending with lumen of uniform diameter and same width as parent bronchus
     CT (thin-section CT is study of choice):
       √ "tram lines" (horizontal course)
       √ "signet ring" (vertical course with cross-section of dilated bronchus + branch of pulmonary artery)
  2. **Saccular / cystic bronchiectasis**
     Associated with severe bronchial infection
     √ <5 subdivisions of bronchi
     √ progressive ballooning dilatation toward periphery with diameter of saccules greater than parent bronchus

√ dilatation of bronchi on inspiration, collapse on expiration

CT:
√ string of cysts (horizontal course) / cluster of cysts
√ air-fluid level (frequent)

3. **Varicose bronchiectasis**
Rare, associated with Swyer-James syndrome
√ 4 – 8 subdivisions of bronchi
√ beaded contour with normal pattern distally

Age: predominantly pediatric disease
• cough + expectoration of purulent sputum
• shortness of breath
• hemoptysis (50%)
Location: posterior basal segments of lower lobes, bilateral (50%), middle lobe / lingula (10%), central bronchiectasis in bronchopulmonary aspergillosis
√ normal radiograph in 7%
√ increase in size of lung markings (retained secretions)
√ loss of definition of lung markings (peribronchial fibrosis)
√ crowding of lung markings (if associated with atelectasis)
√ cystic spaces ± air-fluid levels <2 cm in diameter (dilated bronchi)
√ honeycomb pattern (in severe cases)
√ compensatory hyperinflation of uninvolved ipsilateral lung
√ increased background density
√ frequent exacerbations + resolutions (due to superimposed infections)

Cx: frequent respiratory infections
DDx of CT appearance:
(1) emphysematous blebs (no definable wall thickness)
(2) "reversible bronchiectasis" = temporary dilatation during pneumonia

BRONCHIOLITIS OBLITERANS
Etiology:
(1) 1 – 3 weeks after exposure to toxic fumes (phosgene, ammonia, sulfur dioxide, chlorine)
(2) postinfectious: mycoplasma (children), virus (older individual)
(3) connective tissue disorder
(4) heart-lung transplantation (form of chronic rejection in 30 – 50%)
(5) idiopathic

Path: obliterative granulation tissue within lumen of small airways
Peak age: 40 – 60 years; M:F = 1:1
• flulike illness (fever, malaise, sore throat)
• no response to antibiotics
• persistent nonproductive cough

√ normal / hyperinflated lungs = limited disease with connective tissue plugs in airways
√ bronchiectasis

√ bilateral patchy alveolar / "ground glass" infiltrates in lung periphery (organizing pneumonia)
√ decreased vascularity (reflex vasoconstriction)

DDx: (1) Bacterial / fungal pneumonia (response to antibiotics, positive cultures)
(2) Chronic eosinophilic pneumonia (young female, eosinophilia in 2/3)
(3) Usual interstitial pneumonia (irregular opacities, decreased lung volume)

BRONCHIOLOALVEOLAR CARCINOMA
= ALVEOLAR CELL CARCINOMA
Incidence: 20 – 25% of all primary lung cancers (increasing incidence)
Etiology: development from type II alveolar epithelial cells
Age: middle age; M:F = 1:1
Path: (a) cuboidal cells resembling alveolar type II pneumocytes
(b) mucus-producing tall columnar cells similar to bronchial cells growing along alveolar walls + septa without disrupting lung architecture
Associated with: preexisting pulmonary scar, fibrosis, diffuse interstitial inflammation, scleroderma
• often asymptomatic
• cough (60%)
• abundant mucoid expectoration (25%) can produce hypovolemia + electrolyte depletion (bronchorrhea)

A.   LOCAL FORM (60 – 90%)
1. Single mass
√ well-circumscribed focal mass at peripheral / subpleural location
√ "rabbit ears" / pleural tags / triangular strand / "tail sign" (55%) = linear strands extending from nodule to pleura (desmoplastic reaction / scarring granulomatous disease / pleural indrawing)
√ irregular margins = sunburst appearance (73%)
√ air bronchogram / pseudocavitation (= dilatation of intact air spaces from desmoplastic reaction / bronchiectasis / focal emphysema) in 60%
√ heterogeneous attenuation (57%)
√ confined to single lobe
√ NO atelectasis
2. Multinodular form
B.   DIFFUSE FORM = Pneumonic form (10 – 40%)
√ acinar air space consolidation throughout both lungs (mucus secretion)
√ pleural effusion (8 – 10%)

Metastases: to local lymph nodes + distant sites
Prognosis: 4 – 15 years survival time with single nodule; worse with extensive form

BRONCHOGENIC CARCINOMA
Most frequent cause of cancer deaths in males (35%) and females (18%)

Prevalence (1982): 135:100,000 males;
61:100,000 females

Age at diagnosis: 55 – 60 years (range 40 – 80 years)

- asymptomatic (10 – 50%)
- cough (75%)
- hemoptysis (50%)
- dysphagia (2%)

Types:
1. **Squamous cell carcinoma = epidermoid carcinoma** (30 – 35%)
   Most closely associated with smoking
   Slowest growth rate, lowest incidence of distant metastases
   (a) central location (2/3)
      √ airway obstruction with atelectasis (37%)
      √ postobstructive pneumonia
      √ large central mass
   (b) peripheral nodule (1/3)
      √ characteristic cavitation (7%)
      √ invasion of chest wall

2. **Adenocarcinoma** (25 – 35%)
   almost invariably develops in periphery, intermediate malignant potential (slow growth, high incidence of early metastases), frequently found in scars (tuberculosis, infarction, pneumoconiosis)
   √ solitary peripheral mass (52%) / alveolar infiltrate / multiple nodules
   √ upper lobe distribution (69%)
   √ calcification in periphery of mass (1%)
   √ desmoplastic reaction

3. **Small cell undifferentiated carcinoma = oat cell cancer** (20 – 25%)
   Rapid growth + high metastatic potential (early metastases in 60 – 80% at time of diagnosis); should be regarded as systemic disease regardless of stage; virtually never resectable
   - hypoglycemia
   √ small lung lesion
   √ typically large hilar mass / mediastinal adenopathy
   Staging evaluation:
      CT of abdomen + head, bone scintigraphy, bilateral bone marrow biopsies

4. **Large cell undifferentiated carcinoma** (10 – 14%)
   Intermediate malignant potential; distant metastases
   √ large peripheral mass >6 cm (50%)
   √ pleural involvement

RISK FACTORS:
   (1) cigarette smoking (squamous cell carcinoma + small cell carcinoma)
   (2) industrial exposure: asbestos, uranium, arsenic, chlormethyl ether
   (3) concomitant disease: tuberculous scar (in 10% develop adenocarcinoma)

PRESENTATION
   √ solitary peripheral mass with corona radiata / pleural tail sign / satellite lesion
   √ cavitation (16%): usually thick-walled with irregular inner surface; in 4/5 secondary to squamous cell carcinoma
   √ central mass (38%): commonest for small cell carcinoma
   √ unilateral hilar enlargement (secondary to primary tumor / enlarged lymph nodes)
      Nodes on CT: 0 – 10 mm negative, 10 – 20 mm indeterminate, >20 mm positive
   √ anterior + middle mediastinal widening (suggests small cell carcinoma)
   √ segmental / lobar / lung atelectasis (37%) = "S sign of Golden" = secondary to airway obstruction, particularly in squamous cell carcinoma
   √ rat tail termination of bronchus
   √ local hyperaeration
   √ persistent peripheral infiltrate (30%) = postobstructive pneumonitis
   √ NO air bronchogram
   √ pleural effusion (8 – 15%)
   √ bone erosion of ribs / spine (9%)
   √ involvement of main pulmonary artery (18%); lobar + segmental arteries (53%)
   √ calcification in 7% on CT (histologically in 14%) usually eccentric / finely stippled
      (a) preexisting focus of calcium engulfed by tumor
      (b) dystrophic calcium within tumor necrosis
      (c) calcium deposit from secretory function of carcinoma (eg, mucinous adenocarcinoma)
   Angio: √ bronchogenic carcinoma supplied by bronchial circulation
      √ distortion / stenosis / occlusion of pulmonary arterial circulation

PARANEOPLASTIC MANIFESTATIONS
   1. Carcinomatous neuromyopathy (4 – 15%)
   2. Migratory thrombophlebitis
   3. Hypertrophic pulmonary osteoarthropathy (3 – 5%)
   4. Endocrine manifestations (15%) usually with small cell carcinoma: Cushing syndrome, inappropriate secretion of ADH, HPT, excessive gonadotropin secretion

LOCATION
   60 – 80% arise in segmental bronchi
   — central: small cell carcinoma, squamous cell carcinoma (sputum cytology positive in 70%); arises in central airway often at points of bronchial bifurcation, infiltrates circumferentially, extends along bronchial tree
   — peripheral: adenocarcinoma, large cell carcinoma
   — upper lobe: lower lobe = right lung : left lung = 3 : 2
   — most common site: anterior segment of RUL
   — Pancoast tumor (4%) = superior pulmonary sulcus tumor, frequently squamous cell carcinoma
   — SVC obstruction (5%): frequently small cell carcinoma

TNM STAGING
- T1: <3 cm in diameter, surrounded by lung / visceral pleura
- T2: >3 cm in diameter / invasion of visceral pleura / lobar atelectasis / obstructive pneumonitis / at least 2 cm from carina
- T3: tumor of any size; less than 2 cm from carina / invasion of parietal pleura, chest wall, diaphragm, mediastinal pleura, pericardium; pleural effusion
- T4: invasion of heart, great vessels, trachea, esophagus, vertebral body, carina / malignant effusion
- N1: peribronchial / ipsilateral hilar nodes
- N2: ipsilateral mediastinal nodes
- N3: contralateral hilar / mediastinal nodes

STAGING FOR SMALL CELL LUNG CANCER
Limited disease:
1. Primary in one hemithorax
2. Ipsilateral hilar adenopathy
3. Ipsilateral supraclavicular adenopathy
4. Ipsi- and contralateral mediastinal adenopathy
5. Atelectasis
6. Paralysis of phrenic + laryngeal nerve
7. Small effusion without malignant cells

Extensive disease (60 – 80%):
1. Contralateral hilar adenopathy
2. Contralateral supraclavicular adenopathy
3. Chest wall infiltration
4. Carcinomatous pleural effusion
5. Lymphangitic carcinomatosis
6. Superior vena cava syndrome
7. Metastasis to contralateral lung
8. Extrathoracic metastases to bone (38%), liver (22 – 28%), bone marrow (17 – 23%), CNS (8 – 15%), retroperitoneum (11%), other lymph nodes
   Prognosis: 7 – 11 months median survival; 15 – 20% 2-year disease-free survival rate

SPREAD
1. direct local extension
2. hematogenous (small cell ca.)
3. lymphatic spread (squamous cell ca.); tumor in 10% of normal sized lymph nodes
4. transbronchial spread – least common

DISTANT METASTASES
@ Bone
   (a) Marrow: in 40% at time of presentation
   (b) Gross lesions in 10 – 35%:
      Location: vertebrae (70%), pelvis (40%), femora (25%)
      √ osteolytic metastases (3/4)
      √ osteoblastic metastases (1/4): in small cell carcinoma / adenocarcinoma
      √ occult metastases in 36% of bone scans
@ Adrenals: in 37% at time of presentation
@ Brain: asymptomatic metastases on brain scan in 7% (30% at autopsy), in 2/3 multiple

@ Kidney, GI tract, liver, abdominal lymph nodes, contralateral lung

Cx:
1. Horner syndrome (enophthalmus, miosis, ptosis, anhidrosis) with Pancoast tumor
2. Diaphragmatic elevation (phrenic nerve paralysis)
3. Hoarseness (laryngeal nerve involvement, left > right)
4. SVC obstruction (5%): lung cancer is cause of all SVC obstructions in 90%
5. Pleural effusion (10%): malignant, parapneumonic, lymphoobstructive
6. Dysphagia: enlarged nodes, esophageal invasion

Prognosis:
mean survival time <6 months; <10% overall 5-year survival; survival at 40 months: squamous cell 30% > large cell 16% > adenocarcinoma 15% > oat cell 1%

BRONCHOGENIC CYST
= budding / branching abnormality of primitive foregut (ventral segment = tracheobronchial tree; dorsal segment = esophagus)
Incidence: most common intrathoracic foregut cyst (54 – 63% in surgical series)
Histo: thin-walled cyst filled with mucoid material, lined with columnar respiratory epithelium, mucous glands, cartilage, elastic tissue, smooth muscle
- contains mucus / clear or turbid fluid
√ sharply outlined round / oval mass
√ may contain air-fluid level
CT: √ cyst contents of water density (50%) / higher density (50%)

A. MEDIASTINAL BRONCHOGENIC CYST (86%)
   Associated with: spinal abnormalities
   M:F = 1:1
   - usually asymptomatic
   - stridor, dysphagia
   Location: pericarinal (52%), paratracheal (19%), esophageal wall (14%), retrocardiac (9%); usually on right
   √ may communicate with tracheal lumen
   √ may show esophageal compression

B. INTRAPULMONARY BRONCHOGENIC CYST (14%)
   M > F
   - infection (75%)
   - dyspnea, hemoptysis (most common)
   Location: lower:upper lobe = 2:1; usually medial third
   √ 36% will eventually contain air
   DDx: solitary pulmonary nodule, cavitated neoplasm, cavitated pneumonia, lung abscess

BRONCHOPULMONARY DYSPLASIA
= RESPIRATOR LUNG = complication of prolonged respirator therapy of intermittent PEEP with high oxygen concentration = oxygen toxicity + barotrauma

Stage I (2 – 3 days) : √ RDS pattern of hyaline
membrane disease

Stage II (4 – 10 days) : √ complete opacification with
air bronchogram;
√ associated with congestive
failure from PDA

Stage III (10 – 20 days) : √ "spongy" / "bubbly" coarse
linear densities, esp. in upper
lobes;
√ hyperaeration of lung
√ lower lobe emphysema

Stage IV (after 1 month) : √ same pattern;
40% mortality if not resolved
by 1 month

Cx: (1) abnormal pulmonary function
(2) increased frequency of lower respiratory tract
infections

Prognosis:
(1) complete clearing over months / years (1/3)
(2) retained linear densities in upper lobe
emphysema (29%)

DDx: (1) Diffuse neonatal pneumonia (2) Meconium
aspiration (3) Total anomalous pulmonary venous
return (4) Congenital pulmonary lymphangiectasia
(5) Cystic fibrosis (6) Idiopathic pulmonary fibrosis
(7) Pulmonary interstitial emphysema (8) Wilson-
Mikity syndrome

BRONCHOPULMONARY FISTULA
= communication between the bronchial system + pleural
space

Causes:
A. Trauma
1. Complication of resectional surgery
B. Inflammation
1. Putrid lung abscess
2. Pneumonia: Klebsiella, H. influenzae,
Staphylococcus, Streptococcus, tuberculosis
3. Bronchiectasis (very rare)
C. Tumor
1. Carcinoma

Dx: (1) Introduction of methylene blue into pleural
space, in 65% dye appears in sputum
(2) Sinography (3) Bronchography

BRONCHOPULMONARY SEQUESTRATION
= congenital bronchopulmonary foregut malformation
consisting of
(1) nonfunctioning lung segment (2) no communication
with tracheobronchial tree (3) systemic artery supply

Etiology:
development of an accessory tracheobronchial foregut
bud in which
(a) early appearance leads to incorporation forming
intralobar sequestration
(b) late appearance leads to separate pleural
investment

Incidence: 0.1 – 1.7%
Age of discovery: 1st decade (majority), occasionally
in infants / in utero
Path: homogeneous bronchopulmonary mass

• cough + sputum production
• hemoptysis, pain, infection
• respiratory distress + CHF in newborn (due to shunting
of blood)

Location: LLL:RLL = 2:1; posterior basal segment of
lower lobe; rarely upper lung / within fissure
√ usually >6 cm in size
√ round / oval, smooth, well-defined solid homogeneous
mass near diaphragm
√ occasionally fingerlike appendage posteriorly +
medially (anomalous vessel)
√ multiple / single air-fluid levels if infected
√ surrounded by recurrent pulmonary consolidation in a
lower lobe that never clears completely
√ may communicate with esophagus / stomach

A. INTRALOBAR SEQUESTRATION (75 – 86%)
= enclosed by visceral pleura of affected pulmonary
lobe
Age at presentation: adulthood (50% >20 years);
M:F = 1:1
Associated with congenital anomalies in 14%:
skeletal deformities (4%), other foregut anomalies
(4%), diaphragmatic anomaly (3%), cardiac, renal,
cerebral anomalies
• acute lower lobe pneumonia

Location: posterobasal segments, L:R = 3:2
√ usually single large artery from distal thoracic aorta
(65%) / proxima abdominal aorta (22%) coursing
through pulmonary ligament
√ venous drainage via pulmonary veins to
(a) L atrium (L-to-L shunt) in 95%
(b) R atrium in 5%
√ communication with bronchial network (rare)
CT:
√ single / multiple cysts containing air / mucus / pus
√ emphysema bordering normal lung (37%)
√ homogeneous / inhomogeneous dense mass
√ irregular enhancement (rare)
√ one / two anomalous systemic arteries arising
from aorta (DDx: AVM, interrupted pulmonary
artery, isolated anomaly, chronic infection /
inflammation of lung or pleura, surgically created
shunt)
√ premature atherosclerosis of anomalous arteries
OB-US:
√ spherical homogeneous highly echogenic mass
√ anomalous systemic artery seen by color Doppler

B. EXTRALOBAR SEQUESTRATION (14 – 25%)
= with own pleural sheath (prevents collateral air drift
= airless round mass)
Age: neonatal presentation; M:F = 8:1

Associated with congenital anomalies in 60%:
diaphragmatic defect (28%) resulting in eventration / hernia, cystic adenomatoid malformation, lobar emphysema, anomalous pulmonary venous return, cardiac / pericardial anomalies (8%), epiphrenic diverticula (2%), TE fistula (1.5%), duplication of GI tract, renal anomaly
- asymptomatic (rarely becomes infected)

Location: L:R = 4:1, often in association with left hemidiaphragm; may be below diaphragm (5%) / within mediastinum
√ masslike lesion
  √ segmental / subsegmental consolidation
  √ solid paraspinal mass
  √ ± air-fluid level
√ arterial supply variable from small aortic branches / pulmonary artery
√ venous drainage via systemic veins to R heart (IVC, azygos, hemiazygos, portal vein)
√ NO communication with bronchial tree, may connect with GI tract
OB-US:
  √ conical / triangular highly echogenic homogeneous mass
  √ hydrothorax (obstructed lymphatics + veins in torsed sequestration)

DDx:
bronchiectasis, lung abscess, empyema, bronchial atresia, lobar emphysema, cystic adenomatoid malformation, intrapulmonary bronchogenic cyst, Swyer-James syndrome, pneumonia, arteriovenous fistula, primary / metastatic neoplasm, hernia of Bochdalek

CASTLEMAN DISEASE
= GIANT LYMPH NODE HYPERPLASIA
= ANGIOMATOUS LYMPHOID HAMARTOMA
= LYMPHOID HAMARTOMA = ANGIOFOLLICULAR LYMPH NODE HYPERPLASIA

= benign masses of lymphoid tissue of unknown etiology
Age: range of 8 – 66 years, <30 years (70%); M:F = 1:1

Types:
A. Hyaline-vascular type (80 – 90%)
   Path: vascular proliferation + hyalinization with small follicle centers penetrated by capillaries, capillary proliferation in interfollicular areas
   - cough, dyspnea, hemoptysis
   - lassitude, weight loss, fever
   - asymptomatic in 97%
   - growth retardation
   - refractory microcytic anemia
B. Plasma cell type (10 – 20%)
   Path: sheets of plasma cells between normal / enlarged follicles
   - fever, anemia, elevated sedimentation rate

- IgG, IgM, IgA hypergammaglobulinemia (50%)

Location:
  @ Chest: middle / posterior mediastinum (70%), within lung (rare)
  @ Extrathoracic: neck, axilla, shoulder, mesentery, pelvis, within muscle, retroperitoneum (rare)
Size: up to 16 cm in diameter
CT: √ well-defined mass of muscle density
       √ spotty central calcification
       √ enhancing rim (vascular capsule)
       √ marked enhancement almost equal to aorta (in hyalin-vascular type)
       √ slight enhancement (in plasma cell type)
Angio: √ mass with multiple feeding vessels
       √ dense homogeneous blush (hyalin-vascular type)
       √ some hypervascularity (plasma cell type)
DDx: indistinguishable from lymphoma

CHRONIC EOSINOPHILIC PNEUMONIA
= numerous eosinophils, macrophages, histiocytes, lymphocytes, PMNs within lung interstitium + alveolar sacs
Etiology: unknown
Age: middle-age; M < F
- common history of atopia (may occur during therapeutic desensitization procedure)
- adult onset asthma (wheezing)
- high fever, malaise, dyspnea (DDx to Löffler syndrome)
- peripheral blood eosinophilia (with rare exceptions)
√ homogeneous alveolar lung infiltrates with distribution at lung periphery = "photographic negative" of pulmonary edema
√ frequently bilateral nonsegmental
√ unchanged for many days / weeks (DDx to Löffler syndrome)
√ fast regression of infiltrates under steroids
Rx: dramatic response to steroid therapy (within 3 – 10 days)

CHYLOTHORAX
= leakage of chyle from thoracic duct or its branches into pleural space secondary to obstruction / disruption of thoracic duct (in 2%)
Route of thoracic duct:
enters thorax through esophageal foramen, ascends in right prevertebral location (between azygos vein + descending aorta), swings to left at T4 – 6, terminates 3 – 5 cm above clavicle at venous angle

Etiology:
1. Neoplasm (54%): disruption by lymphoma
2. Trauma (25%): latent period of 10 days blunt / penetrating trauma (birth trauma), surgery, subclavian venous catheter
3. Esophageal / cardiovascular surgery (0.5%)
4. Inflammatory disease
5. Idiopathic (15%)
6. Lymphangiomatosis (rare): mediastinal / thoracic cystic hygroma of neck growing into mediastinum

7. Tuberous sclerosis
8. Filariasis (rare)
9. Restrictive pulmonary disease

Age: in full-term infants; may be present in utero;
    M:F = 2:1
Incidence: 1:10,000 deliveries
May be associated with: Trisomy 21, TE-fistula,
    extralobar lung sequestration, congenital pulmonary
    lymphangiectasia
- high in neutral fat + fatty acid (low in cholesterol)
- milky viscoid fluid after ingestion of milk / formula

√ usually unilateral loculated pleural effusion, most
  commonly on right side
√ polyhydramnios (? result of esophageal compression)

Cx: (1) Pulmonary hypoplasia
         (2) Hydrops (congestive heart failure secondary to
              impaired venous return)
Rx: (1) Thoracocentesis (leading to loss of calories,
              lymphocytopenia, hypogammaglobulinemia)
         (2) Thoracic duct ligation
         (3) Pleuroperitoneal shunt

COAL WORKER'S PNEUMOCONIOSIS

= CWP = ANTHRACOSIS = ANTHRACOSILICOSIS
= coal dust inhalation taken up by alveolar macrophages,
  in part cleared by mucociliary action (particle size >5 μ),
  in part deposited around bronchioles + alveoli, coal dust
  in itself is inert, but admixed silica is fibrogenic

Simple CWP

= aggregates of coal dust = coal macules (usually
  <3 mm)
NO progression in absence of further exposure
Histo: development of reticulin fibers associated with
            bronchiolar dilatation (focal emphysema) +
            bronchiolar artery stenosis (decreased capillary
            perfusion)
- poor correlation between symptoms, physiologic
  findings + roentgenogram
√ small round 1 – 5 mm opacities, frequently in upper
  lobes (radiographically only seen through
  superposition after an exposure of >10 years)
√ nodularity correlates with amount of collagen (NOT
  amount of coal dust)
Cx :   (1) Chronic obstructive bronchitis
          (2) Focal emphysema
          (3) Cor pulmonale

COCCIDIOIDOMYCOSIS

Organism: soil fungus Coccidioides immitis, spores live
    in dry dust with spread by wind; endemic in southwest
    desert of USA (San Joaquin Valley, central Southern
    Arizona, western Texas, southern New Mexico) similar
    to histoplasmosis

A.   PRIMARY COCCIDIOIDOMYCOSIS
      - 60 – 80% asymptomatic

- arthralgias, erythema nodosum / multiforme
  (5 – 20%)
√ patchy infiltrates mainly in lower lobes (46 – 80%)
√ hilar adenopathy (20%)
√ pleural effusion (10%)
B.   DISSEMINATED COCCIDIOIDOMYCOSIS
      Incidence: 1: 6,000 infections
      √ meningeal spread
      √ micronodular lung pattern
C.   CHRONIC COCCIDIOIDOMYCOSIS
      - hemoptysis in 50%
      √ one / several well-defined nodules of 5 – 30 mm in
        size (5%)
      √ "grape skin" thin-walled cavities (10 – 15%), in
        90% solitary, 70% in anterior segment of upper
        lobes (DDx: TB), 3% rupture into pleural space due
        to subpleural location (pneumothorax / empyema)
      √ mediastinal adenopathy (10 – 20%)

CONGENITAL LOBAR EMPHYSEMA

= progressive overdistension of one / multiple lobes
M:F = 3 :1
Etiology:
    (a) deficiency / dysplasia / immaturity of bronchial
         cartilage
    (b) endobronchial obstruction (mucosal fold / web,
         prolonged endotracheal intubation, inflammatory
         exudate, inspissated mucus)
    (c) bronchial compression (PDA, aberrant left
         pulmonary artery, pulmonary artery dilatation)
    (d) polyalveolar / macroalveolar hyperplasia
Associated with   CHD in 15% (PDA, VSD)

- respiratory distress (90%) + progressive cyanosis
  within first 6 months of life
Location: LUL (42 – 43%), RML (32 – 35%), RUL (20%),
             two lobes (5%)
√ hazy masslike opacity immediately following birth
  (delayed clearance of lung fluid in emphysematous lobe
  over 1 – 14 days)
√ air trapping
√ hyperlucent expanded lobe (after clearing of fluid)
√ compression collapse of adjacent lobes
√ contralateral mediastinal shift
√ widely separated vascular markings
Mortality: 10%
Rx: surgical resection

CONGENITAL LYMPHANGIECTASIA

1. PRIMARY PULMONARY LYMPHANGIECTASIA (2/3)
   = abnormal development of lungs between 14 – 20th
     week of GA characterized by anomalous dilatation of
     pulmonary lymph vessels
   Path: subpleural cysts, ectatic tortuous lymph
              channels in pleura, interlobular septa + along
              bronchoarterial bundles; NO obstruction
   Age: usually manifest at birth; 50% stillborn; M = F
   May be associated with   total anomalous pulmonary
              venous return, hypoplastic left heart, Noonan
              syndrome

- respiratory distress within few hours of birth

Site: diffuse involvement of both lungs, occasionally only in one / two lobes (with good prognosis)
- √ marked prominence of coarse interstitial markings (simulating interstitial edema)
- √ hyperinflation
- √ scattered radiolucent areas (dilated airways)
- √ patchy areas of pneumonia + atelectasis
- √ pneumothorax

Prognosis: in diffuse form invariably fatal at <2 months of age

2. GENERALIZED LYMPHANGIECTASIA

= DIFFUSE LYMPHANGIOMA
= proliferation of mainly lymphatic vascular spaces with relentless systemic progression

Age: children, young adults

Location: widespread visceral + skeletal involvement
- √ diffuse pulmonary interstitial disease
- √ chylous effusions in pleural + pericardial spaces
- √ ± lytic bone lesions
- √ lymphangiographic pooling of contrast material in dilated lymphatic channels / lymph nodes

3. LOCALIZED LYMPHANGIOMA

= rare benign usually cystic lesion

Histo: collection of dilated + proliferated lymph vessels (? hamartoma / benign neoplasm / focal sequestration of ectatic lymph tissue)

Age: first 3 years of life; M = F
- asymptomatic (33%)
- dyspnea (from tracheal compression)

Location: neck (80%), mediastinum, axilla, extremity
- √ discrete featureless mass
- √ may have chylous / pleural effusion
- √ may have lytic lesion in contiguous skeleton

Prognosis: propensity for local recurrence

DDx: hemangioma

4. SECONDARY LYMPHANGIECTASIA

Secondary to elevated pulmonary venous pressure in CHD (TAPVR)

CRYPTOCOCCOSIS

= TORULOSIS = EUROPEAN BLASTOMYCOSIS

Organism: Cryptococcus neoformans, spherical single-budding yeast cell with thick capsule, stains with India ink, often in soil contaminated with pigeon excreta, opportunistic invader

Histo: granulomatous lesion with caseous necrotic center

Predisposed: diabetics, immunocompromised
- low grade meningitis (affinity to CNS); M:F = 4:1

- √ well-circumscribed mass (40%) of 2 – 10 cm in diameter, usually peripheral location
- √ lobar / segmental consolidation (35%)
- √ cavitation (15%)
- √ hilar / mediastinal adenopathy (12%)
- √ calcifications (extremely rare)

CYSTIC ADENOMATOID MALFORMATION

= CAM = hamartoma of lung characterized by an intralobar mass of disorganized pulmonary tissue communicating with bronchial tree + having normal vascular supply + drainage

Cause: arrest of normal bronchoalveolar differentiation between 4 – 10th week of gestation with overgrowth of distal bronchiolar structures

Path:

proliferation of bronchial structures at the expense of alveolar saccular development, modified by intercommunicating cysts of various size (adenomatoid overgrowth of terminal bronchioles, proliferation of smooth muscle in cyst wall, absence of cartilage)

TYPE I (50%):
   Histo: single / multiple large cyst(s) >20 mm lined by ciliated pseudostratified columnar epithelium, mucus-producing cells in 1/3
   Prognosis: excellent following resection
TYPE II (40%):
   Histo: multiple cysts <12 mm lined by ciliated cuboidal / columnar epithelium
   Prognosis: poor secondary to associated abnormalities
TYPE III (10%):
   Histo: solitary firm mass of bronchuslike structures lined by ciliated cuboidal epithelium with microscopic cysts
   Prognosis: poor secondary to pulmonary hypoplasia / hydrops

In 25% associated with abnormalities of kidneys, GI tract, chromosomes

Age of detection: children, neonates, fetus; M:F = 1:1

- respiratory distress + severe cyanosis in first week of life (2/3) due to compression of normal lung + airways
- asymptomatic, incidental finding later in life (1/3)

Location: equal frequency in all lobes (middle lobe rarely affected); more than one lobe involved in 20%

CXR:
- √ proper position of abdominal viscera
- √ almost always unilateral mass with well-defined margins (80%)
- √ compression of adjacent lung
- √ contralateral shift of mediastinum (87%)
- √ multiple air-filled cysts / occasionally fluid-filled cysts
- √ hypoplastic ipsilateral lung

CT:
- √ solitary / multiple fluid or air-fluid filled cysts with thin walls
- √ surrounding focal emphysematous changes

OB-US:
- √ single large cyst / multiple large cysts of 2 – 10 cm in diameter (Type I)
- √ multiple small cysts of <12 mm in diameter (Type II)
- √ large homogeneously echogenic mass (Type III)
- √ contralateral mediastinal shift (89%)

√ polyhydramnios (66 – 68%, ? from esophageal compression) / normal fluid (28%) / oligohydramnios (6%)
√ fetal ascites (62 – 71%)
√ fetal hydrops in 8 – 62% (decreased venous return from compression)
Cx: Pulmonary hypoplasia
Prognosis: 50% premature, 25% stillborn,
Δ Polyhydramnios, ascites, hydrops indicate a poor outcome!
DDx: (1) Congenital lobar emphysema
(2) Diaphragmatic hernia
(3) Bronchogenic cyst (small solitary cyst near midline)
(4) Bronchopulmonary sequestration (less frequently associated with polyhydramnios / hydrops)
(5) Pericardial teratoma

CYSTIC FIBROSIS

= MUCOVISCIDOSIS
= autosomal recessive disease with (a) dysfunction of exocrine glands forming a thick tenacious material obstructing conducting system (b) reduced mucociliary transport
Incidence: 1:2000; almost exclusively in Caucasians (1:20 heterozygous); unusual in Blacks, Orientals, Polynesians
• elevated concentrations of sodium + chloride in sweat

@ Lung
• chronic cough, recurrent pulmonary infections
• progressive respiratory insufficiency
• infertility in males
√ "fingerlike" mucus plugging (mucoid impaction in dilated bronchi)
√ subsegmental / segmental / lobar atelectasis with right upper lobe predominance (10%)
√ progressive cylindrical / cystic bronchiectasis (in 100% at >6 months of age) ± air-fluid levels due to prolonged mucus plugging
√ parahilar linear densities + peribronchial cuffing
√ focal / generalized hyperinflation secondary to collateral air drift
√ hilar adenopathy
√ large pulmonary arteries (pulmonary arterial hypertension)
√ recurrent local pneumonitis (staphylococcus, pseudomonas)
CT:
√ bronchiectasis
√ peribrochial thickening
√ bronchiectatic sacculations (= bronchus directly leading into sacculation)
√ bulla (= peripheral air space with long pleural attachment + without communication to bronchus)
√ emphysema
√ mucus plugs = tubular structures ± branching pattern
√ subsegmental / segmental collapse / consolidations

NUC:
√ matched patchy areas of decreased ventilation + perfusion
Cx: (1) Pneumothorax (rupture of bulla / bleb), common + recurrent
(2) Hemoptysis
(3) Cor pulmonale
(4) Hypertrophic pulmonary osteoarthropathy (rare)
Cause of death: massive mucus plugging (95%)

@ GI tract
• steatorrhea + malabsorption (pancreatic insufficiency in 80 – 90%)
• rectal prolapse (23%)
• failure to thrive
√ meconium ileus (10 – 15%), earliest finding
√ meconium ileus equivalent
√ fatty liver
√ focal biliary cirrhosis with signs of portal hypertension (clinically rare, autoptic in up to 50%)
√ gallstones
√ echogenic pancreas (pancreatic cirrhosis due to recurrent acute pancreatitis)

@ Skull
√ sinusitis with opacification of well-developed maxillary, ethmoid, sphenoid sinuses
√ hypoplastic frontal sinuses

DIAPHRAGMATIC HERNIA
Congenital Diaphragmatic Hernia
= absence of closure of the pleuroperitoneal fold by 9th week of gestational age
Incidence: 1: 2,200 – 2,500 livebirths (0.04%); M:F = 2:1; most common intrathoracic fetal anomaly
Δ delayed onset following group B streptococcal infection
Etiology:
(1) delayed fusion of diaphragm (spontaneous self-correction may occur)
(2) insult that inhibits / delays normal migration of the gut + closure of the diaphragm between 8 – 12th week of embryogenesis
Associated anomalies (in 20% of liveborn, in 90% of stillborn fetuses):
1. CNS (28%): neural tube defects
2. Gastrointestinal (20%): particularly malrotation, oral cleft, omphalocele
3. Cardiovascular (13 – 23%)
4. Genitourinary (15%)
5. Chromosomal abnormalities
6. IUGR (with concurrent major abnormality in 90%)
Location: L:R = 9:1

(1) Bochdalek Hernia (85 – 90%)
= posterolateral defect caused by maldevelopment / defective fusion of the cephalic fold of the pleuroperitoneal membranes

Incidence: 1:2,200 – 12,500 livebirths
Location: left (80%), right (15%), bilateral (5%)
Herniated organ
  (a) on left: omentl fat (6%), bowel, spleen,
     left lobe of liver, stomach (rare), kidney,
     pancreas
  (b) on right: part of liver
mnemonic: "4 B's"
   Bochdalek
   Back (posterior location)
   Babies (age at presentation)
   Big (usually large)
(2) Morgagni Hernia (1 – 2%)
  = anteromedial parasternal defect (space of Larrey)
  caused by maldevelopment of septum
  transversum; R > L
  Herniated organ: liver
  Often associated with pericardial deficiency
  (a) abdominal viscera / fat may herniate into
     pericardial sac
  (b) heart may herniate into upper abdomen
mnemonic: "4 M's"
   Morgagni
   Middle (anterior + central location)
   Mature (present in older children)
   Minuscule (usually small)
(3) Septum Transversum Defect = defect in central
  tendon
(4) Hiatal Hernia = congenitally large esophageal
  orifice
(5) Eventration (5%) = upwa displacement of
  abdominal contents secondary to a congenitally thin
  hypoplastic diaphragm
  Location: anteromedial on right, total involvement
     on left side; R:L = 5:1
  √ small diaphragmatic excursions
  √ often lobulated diaphragmatic contour

• respiratory distress in neonatal period (life-threatening
  deficiency of small airways + alveoli)
• scaphoid abdomen
Herniated organs:
  small bowel (90%), stomach (60%), large bowel
  (56%), spleen (54%), pancreas (24%), kidney
  (12%), adrenal gland, liver, gallbladder
√ bowel loops in chest
√ contralateral shift of mediastinum + heart
√ complete / partial absence of diaphragm
√ absence of stomach, small bowel in abdomen
√ passage of nasogastric tube under fluoroscopic
  control entering intrathoracic stomach
√ incomplete rotation + anomalous mesenteric
  attachment of bowel
OB-US (diagnosis possible by 18 weeks GA):
  √ solid / multicystic / complex chest mass
  √ peristalsis of bowel within fetal chest (inconsistent)
  √ displacement of fetal heart
  √ paradoxical motion of diaphragm with fetal
   breathing (defect in diaphragm sonographically not
   visible)

√ scaphoid fetal abdomen with reduced abdominal
  circumference
√ fetal stomach at level of fetal heart
√ nonvisualization of fetal stomach (GI obstruction /
  CNS abnormality)
√ polyhydramnios (common, ? secondary to bowel
  obstruction) / oligohydramnios / normal fluid volume
√ swallowed fetal intestinal contrast appears in chest
  (CT amniography confirms diagnosis)

Cx: (1) Bilateral pulmonary hypoplasia
   (2) Postsurgical pulmonary hypertension
Prognosis:
  (1) Stillbirth (35%)   (2) Neonatal death (35%)

Mortality:
  in 10% death before surgery; 40 – 50% operative
  mortality;
  60% mortality with intrathoracic stomach,
  6% mortality with intraabdominal stomach,
  89% mortality with polyhydramnios,
  45% mortality with normal amount of fluid
DDx: Congenital adenomatoid malformation,
   mediastinal cyst (bronchogenic, neuroenteric,
   thymic)

Traumatic Diaphragmatic Hernia

5% of all diaphragmatic hernias, but 90% of all
strangulated diaphragmatic hernias
Etiology:
  (a) blunt trauma (5 – 50%) due to marked increase in
     intraabdominal pressure: motor vehicle accident,
     fall from height, bout of hyperemesis
  (b) penetrating trauma (50%): knife, bullet, repair of
     hiatus hernia

Contents in order of frequency:
  stomach, colon, small bowel, omentum, spleen,
  kidney, pancreas
• may be asymptomatic for months / years following
  trauma, onset of symptoms may be so long delayed
  that traumatic event is forgotten
• virtually all become ultimately symptomatic, most in <
  3 years
• **Bergqvist triad**:
  (1) rib fractures (2) fracture of spine / pelvis
  (3) diaphragmatic hernia

Location: left side in 90 – 98%; central + posterior
     portion of diaphragm; 2 – 10% on right side
Size: most tears are >10 cm in length
√ diaphragm cannot be traced / abnormal contour of
  hemidiaphragm
√ cephalad margin of bowel may simulate an elevated
  diaphragm (look for haustra)
√ lower lobe mass / consolidation (herniated solid organ
  / omentum / airless bowel loop)
√ inhomogeneous mass with air-fluid level in left
  hemithorax
√ displacement of mediastinum + lung

√ mushroomlike mass of herniated liver in right hemithorax

√ "hourglass" constriction of afferent + efferent bowel loops at orifice

√ hydrothorax / hematothorax indicates strangulation

√ nasogastric tube first dips below diaphragm (rent spares esophageal hiatus)

√ location of diaphragm may be documented by
1. gas-filled bowel constricted at site of diaphragmatic laceration
2. barium study

Associated injuries:
√ fractures of lower ribs
√ perforation of hollow viscus
√ rupture of spleen

Cx: life-threatening strangulation occurs in majority (90% of strangulatedhernias are traumatic in origin)

DDx: eventration, diaphragmatic paralysis

EMPHYSEMA

= permanent enlargement of air spaces distal to terminal bronchiole with destruction of air space walls

• expiratory airflow obstruction (due to decreased elastic recoil from parenchymal destruction)

• decreased carbon monoxide diffusing capacity

A. CENTRILOBULAR EMPHYSEMA (more common)
= abnormal enlargement of air spaces in central part of secondary pulmonary lobule + destruction of respiratory bronchioles in center of lobe / eccentric

Predisposed: smokers
• blue bloater

Site: tendency for upper lobes
√ increased pulmonary vascular markings

B. PANACINAR / PANLOBULAR EMPHYSEMA
= destruction of lung distal to terminal bronchiole,
May be associated with alpha-1 antitrypsin deficiency

Age: older patients
• pink puffer

Site: panacinar emphysema more severe at bases
√ decreased pulmonary vascular markings

CXR (40 – 60% correct):
√ flattened diaphragm (most reliable sign)
√ centralization of pulmonary vasculature (pulmonary arterial hypertension)
√ right-side heart enlargement
√ bullae

HRCT:
√ well-defined areas of abnormally decreased attenuation without definable wall

EMPYEMA

Stage
I   "exudaive" stage = sterile exudate
• elevated number of PMNs
• pH >7.20; glucose >40 mg/dl (2.2 mmol/l)

II   "fibropurulent" stage
— early stage II empyema
• increase in WBCs, but no gross pus
• pH between 7.0 and 7.2
• glucose level >40 mg/dl
— late stage II empyema
• gross pus
• pH <7.0
• glucose level <40 mg/dl
Cx: multiloculation

III   "organization" stage with fibroblast infiltration forming "pleural peel"
Cx: limited expansion of lung
Rx: decortication

CT:
√ thickening of parietal pleura in 60% on NECT, in 86% on CECT
√ increased thickness + density of paraspinal subcostal tissue (inflammatory infiltrate of subpleural fat)
√ curvilinear enhancement of chest wall boundary in 96% (inflammatory hyperemia of pleura)

DDx: Malignant effusion after sclerotherapy, malignant invasion of chest wall, mesothelioma, pleural tuberculosis, reactive mesothelial hyperplasia, pleural effusion of rheumatoid disease

EOSINOPHILIC GRANULOMA

= variant of histiocytosis X localized to lung + bones
Pathogenesis:
smoking-related lung damage with accumulation + activation of Langerhans cells (90% smokers)
Path:
granulomatous infiltration centered on walls of bronchioles (= bronchiolitis) often extending into surrounding alveolar interstitium with subsequent bronchiolar destruction; thick-walled cysts presumably caused by check-valve bronchial obstruction
Histo:
Langerhans cell containing unique cytoplasmatic inclusion body known as Birbeck granule (identifiable only with electron microscopy), foamy histiocytes, eosinophils with deposition of reticulin + collagen
Age: most frequently in 3rd – 4th decade (range 3 months to 69 years); M:F = 3:2; Caucasians >> Blacks

@ Lung involvement
Δ CXR abnormalities more severe than clinical symptoms + pulmonary function tests!
• asymptomatic (up to 25%)
• nonproductive cough (75%)
• combination of obstructive + restrictive pulmonary function: presenting with pneumothorax in 15%
• fatigue, weight loss, fever (15 – 30%)
• dyspnea (40%)
• chest pain (25%) from pneumothorax / eosinophilic granuloma in rib
• diabetes insipidus (10 – 25%)

Location: usually bilaterally symmetric, upper lobe
predominance, sparing of costophrenic
angles
√ ill-defined / stellate nodules 3 – 10 mm (granuloma
stage)
√ diffuse fine reticular / reticulonodular pattern (cellular
infiltrate)
√ "honeycomb lung" = multiple 1 – 5 cm cysts +
subpleural blebs (fibrotic stage)
√ increased lung volumes in 1/3 (most other fibrotic
lung diseases have decreased lung volumes!)
√ pleural effusion (8%), hilar adenopathy (unusual)
√ cavitation of large nodules (rare)
√ thymic enlargement
HRCT (combination virtually diagnostic):
√ thin-walled cysts <5 mm in size equally distributed
in central + peripheral lung zones
√ centrilobular peribronchiolar nodules
DDx for nodules:
sarcoidosis, hypersensitivity pneumonitis,
berylliosis, TB, atypical TB, metastases, silicosis,
coal-worker pneumoconiosis
DDx for cysts:
emphysema, bronchioectasis, idiopathic
pulmonary fibrosis, lymphangiomyomatosis
Cx:
1. Recurrent pneumothoraces in 25% (from rupture
of subpleural cysts) CHARACTERISTIC
2. Pulmonary hypertension
3. Superimposed Aspergillus fumigatus infection

@ Bone involvement:
√ lytic bone lesions (skull, ribs, pelvis)
√ vertebra plana

@ Other organs: lymph nodes, skin, endocrine glands

Prognosis:
poor with multisystem disease + organ dysfnction
(especially with skin lesions); complete / partial
regression (13 – 55%), progression (7 – 21%);
2 – 25% mortality

Rx: cessation of smoking, chemotherapy (vincristine
sulfate, prednisone, methotrexate,
6-mercaptopurine)

EXTRAMEDULLARY HEMATOPOIESIS
= compensatory response to deficient bone marrow blood
cell production
Etiology: (NO hematologic disease in 25%)
1. Thalassemia
2. Hereditary spherocytosis
3. Myelosclerosis
4. Carcinomatous / lymphomatous replacement of bone
marrow
5. Iron deficiency anemia
6. Pernicious anemia
7. Acquired hemolytic anemia
• chronic anemia

Sites:
@ spleen, liver, lymph nodes
@ adrenal glands
@ cartilage, broad ligaments
@ thrombi, adipose tissue
@ mediastinum
√ frequently bilateral paraspinal lobulated masses in mid-
to lower thorax
√ splenomegay / absent spleen
√ lack f calcification / bone erosion

EXTRAMEDULLARY PLASMACYTOMA
Uncommon form; relatively benign course (dissemination
may be found months / ears later or not at all);
questionable if precursor to multiple myeloma
Age : 35 – 40 years; M:F = 2:
Location: air passages (50%) predominantly in upper
nose and oral cavity; conjunctiva (37%); lymph
nodes (3%)
• usually not associated with increased immunoglobulin
titer or amyloid deposition
√ mass of one to several cm in size with well-defined
lobulated border

Classification:
1. Medullary plasmacytoma
2. Multiple myeloma:
(a) scattered involvement of bone
(b) myelomatosis of bone
3. Extramedullary plasmacytoma

DDx:
(1) MULTIPLE MYELOMA
= malignant course with soft tissue involvement in
50 – 73%:
(a) microscopic infiltration
(b) enlargement of organs
(c) formation of tumor mass (1/3)
• usually associated with protein abnormalities
• may have amyloid deposition
Age incidence: 50 – 85 years
Δ tends to occur late in the course of the disease
and indicates a poor prognosis (0 – 6% 5-year
survival)

EXTRINSIC ALLERGIC ALVEOLITIS
= HYPERSENSITIVITY PNEUMONITIS
= exposure to organic dust of <5 μ particle size
• asymptomatic (10 – 40%)
• recurrent episodes of fever, chills, dry cough, dyspnea
following exposure after 6-hour interval
• resolution of episodic symptoms after cessation of
exposure, abate spontaneously over 1 – 2 days
• insidious onset of gradually progressive dyspnea
• reduction in vital capacity, diffusing capacity, arterial
PO_2
• intracutaneous injection of antigen results in delayed
hypersensitivity reaction
• presence of serum precipitins against antigen
• positive aerosol provocation inhalation test

Specific antigens for immune complex disease (Type III = Arthus reaction):

1. **Farmer's lung** from moldy hay (Thermoactinomyces vulgaris or Micropolyspora faeni)
2. Hypersensitivity pneumonitis from forced-air equipment = **Pandora's pneumoniti**s with heating / humidifying / air conditioning systems (thermophilic actinomycetes)
3. **Bird-fancier's lung**, pigeon breeder's lung from protein in bird serum / droppings / feathers
4. **Mushroom worker's lung** from mushroom compost (Thermoactinomyceslgaris or Micropolyspora faen
5. **Bagassosis** from moldy sugar cane in sugar mill (contamination with Thermoactinomyces sacchari / vulgaris and Micropolyspora faeni)
6. **Malt worker's lung** from malt dust (Aspergillus clarvatus)
7. **Maple bark disease** from moldy maple bark in saw mill (Cryptostroma corticale)
8. **Suberosis** from moldy cork dust (Penicillium frequentans)
9. **Sequoiosis** from redwood dust (Graphium species)

Location: predominantly midlung zones, occasionally lower lung zones, rarely upper lung zones

A. ACUTE EXTRINSIC ALLERGIC ALVEOLITIS
= heavy exposure to inciting antigen
√ No CXR abnormalities in 30 – 95%
√ diffuse acinar consolidative pattern (edema + exudate filling alveoli) resolving within a few days
√ lymph node enlargement (unusual, more common with recurrence)
CT:
   √ small + medium rounded opacities (large active granulomas)
   √ diffuse dense air-space consolidation (confluent collections of intraalveolar histiocytes, interstitial + intraalveolar edema)

B. SUBACUTE EXTRINSIC ALLERGIC ALVEOLITIS
√ changes may be completely reversible if present less than 1 year
√ interstitial nodular / reticulonodular pattern
CT:
   √ small rounded poorly marginated opacities (cellular bronchiolitis + granulomas)
   √ patchy soft air-space opacification (obstructive pneumonitis, filling of alveoli by large mononuclear cell infiltrates)

C. CHRONIC EXTRINSIC ALLERGIC ALVEOLITIS
= occurs months – years after initial exposure
Path: proliferation of epithelial cells + elaboration of reticulum fibers
√ irregular linear opacities (fibrosis)
√ loss of lung volume (cicatrization atelectasis)
√ pleural effusion (rare)
√ lymph node enlargement may occur

FAT EMBOLISM
= obstruction of pulmonary vessels by fat globules followed by chemical pneumonitis from unsaturated plasma fatty acids producing hemorrhage / edema
Incidence: in necropsy series in 67 – 97% of patients with major skeletal trauma, however, symptomatic fat embolism syndrome in <10% (M > F)
Onset: 24 – 72 hours after trauma

• dyspnea (progressive pulmonary insufficiency)
• fever
• systemic hypoxemia
• mentation changes
• petechiae (50%) from coagulopathy (release of tissue thromboplastin)

√ initial chest film usually negative
√ platelike atelectasis
√ diffuse alveolar infiltrates
√ consolidation
NUC:
   √ mottled peripheral perfusion defects (1 – 4 days after injury), later enlarging secondary to pneumonic infiltrates

FIBROSING MEDIASTINITIS
Etiology:
  (a) Granulomatous: histoplasmosis (most frequent), tuberculosis, actinomycosis
  (b) Sclerosing: autoimmune disease, methysergide-induced
May be associated with retroperitoneal fibrosis, orbital pseudotumor, Riedel struma
• cough, dyspnea, hemoptysis
• dysphagia
• superior vena cava syndrome
• cor pulmonale

√ increase in size of upper half of mediastinum, right > left
√ lobulated mediastinal / hilar fibrous masses, often calcified
√ lymphadenopathy (frequent)
NUC:
   √ decreased / absent perfusion with normal ventilation

Cx: (1) Compression of SVC (64%) + pulmonary veins (4%)
   (2) Chronic obstructive pneumonia (narrowing of trachea / central bronchi) in 5%
   (3) Esophageal stenosis (3%)
   (4) Pulmonary infarcts + fibrosis (narrowing of pulmonary artery)
   (5) Prominent intercostal arteries (narrowing of pulmonary artery)

DDx: (1) Swyer-James syndrome
   (2) Congenital absence of pulmonary artery
   (3) Embolus to main pulmonary artery
   (4) Bronchogenic carcinoma

FRACTURE OF TRACHEA / BRONCHUS

Location: (a) main stem bronchus 1 – 2 cm distal to
                  carina80%); R > L
           (b) just above carina (20%)
√ fracture of first 3 ribs (53 – 91%), rare in children
√ pneumothorax (70%)
√ mediastinal ± subcutaneous emphysema
√ absence of pleural effusion
√ collapsed lung falling to dependent position (loss of
  anchoring support in bronchial transsection)
√ atelectasis (may be late development)
√ inadequate reexpansion of lung despite chest tube (due
  to large air leak)

Prognosis: 30% mortality (in 15% within 1 hour)

GOODPASTURE SYNDROME

= autoimmune disease characterized by
  (1) glomerulonephritis (2) circulating antibodies against
  glomerular + alveolar basement membrane
  (3) pulmonary hemorrhage
Pathogenesis:
  cytotoxic antibody-mediated disease = Type II
  hypersensitivity; alveolar basement membrane becomes
  antigenic (perhaps viral etiology); IgG / IgM antibody
  with complement activation causes cell destruction +
  pulmonary hemorrhage, leads to hemosiderin deposition
  and pulmonary fibrosis
Age peak: 26 years (range 17 – 78 years); M:F = 7:1
• iron-deficiency anemia
• hepatosplenomegaly
• systemic hypertension

@ Lung
• preceding upper respiratory infection (in 2/3) + renal
  disease
• mild hemoptysis (72%) with hemosiderin-laden
  macrophages in sputum, commonly precedes the
  clinical manifestations of renal disease by several
  months
• cough, dyspnea, basilar rales
√ patchy alveolar filling pattern with predominance in
  perihilar area + lung bases
√ air bronchogram
√ consolidation at lung bases + central lung fields
√ gradually interstitial pattern (due to septal thickening)
  = organization of hemorrhage
√ hilar lymph nodes may be enlarged during acute
  episodes

@ Kidney
• glomerulonephritis with IgG deposits in characteristic
  linear pattern in glomeruli
• hematuria

Prognosis: death within 3 years (average 6 months)
               because of renal failure
Rx: cytotoxic chemotherapy, plasmapheresis, bilateral
        nephrectomy
DDx: idiopathic pulmonary hemosiderosis

GRANULOMA OF LUNG

constitutes the majority of solitary pulmonary nodules
√ central nidus of calcification in a laminated / diffuse
  pattern
√ absence of growth for at least 2 years
CT (most effective in nodules ≤3 cm of diameter with
    smooth discrete margins):
  √ 50 – 60% of pulmonary nodules demonstrate
    unsuspected calcification by CT

DDx: Carcinoma (in 10% eccentric calcification in
        preexisting scar / nearby granuloma / true intrinsic
        stippled calcification in larger lesion)

HAMARTOMA OF CHEST WALL

= MESENCHYMOMA (incorrect as it implies neoplasm)
= focal overgrowth of normal skeletal elements with a
  benign self-limited course; extremely rare
Age: 1st year of life
√ moderate / large extrapleural well-circumscribed mass
  affecting one / more ribs
√ ribs near center of mass partially / completely destroyed
√ ribs at periphery deformed / eroded
√ significant amount of calcification / ossification (DDx:
  aneurysmal bone cyst)
√ mass compresses underlying lung
Rx: resection curative

HAMARTOMA OF LUNG

= composed of tissues normally found in this location in
  abnormal quantity, mixture, and arrangement
Incidence: 0.25% in population (autopsy); 6 – 8% of all
               solitary pulmonary lesions; most common
               benign lung tumor
Etiology:
  1. Congenital malformation of a displaced bronchial
     anlage
  2. Hyperplasia of normal structures
  3. Cartilaginous neoplasm
  4. Response to inflammation
Path: columnar, cuboidal, ciliated epithelium, fat, bone,
          cartilage (predominates), muscle, vessels, fibrous
          tissue, calcifications, plasma cells originating in
          fibrous connective tissue beneath mucous
          membrane of bronchial wall
Age peak: 5th + 6th decade; M:F = 3:1
• mostly asymptomatic
• hemoptysis (rare)
• cough, vague chest pain, fever (with postobstructive
  pneumonitis)

Location: 2/3 peripheral; endobronchial in 10%;
           multiplicity (rare)
√ round smooth lobulated mass <4 cm (averages 2.5 cm)
√ calcification in 15% (almost pathognomonic if of
  "popcorn" type)
√ fat in 50% (detection by CT)
√ cavitation (extremely rare)
√ growth patterns: slow / rapid / stable with later growth
√ usually 5 mm increase in diameter per year

CT (thin-section):
√ fat density alone in 34% (-80 to -120 HU); calcium +
fat (19%)
DDx: Lipoid pneumonia (ill-defined mass / lung infiltrate)

HISTOPLASMOSIS OF LUNG
Organism: Histoplasma capsulatum, dimorphic fungus,
widespread in soil of central North America
(Ohio, Mississippi, St. Lawrence river valley)
Dx: (1) Culture from infected tissues
(2) Identification of yeast forms stained with PAS /
Gomori methenamine silver
(3) Complement fixation / serum immunodiffusion

A. PRIMARY HISTOPLASMOSIS
• mostly subclinical + self-limited
• fever, cough, malaise
√ nonsegmental bronchopneumonic pattern with
tendency to clear in one area + appear in another
√ multiple nodules changing into hundreds of
punctate calcifications (3 – 4 mm)
√ histoplasmoma (= one / several noncalcifying
nodules <3 cm)
√ "target lesion" = central calcification is
PATHOGNOMONIC
√ hilar / mediastinal lymph node enlargement (DDx:
acute viral / bacterial pneumonia)
√ "popcorn" calcification of mediastinal lymph nodes
CT:
√ paratracheal / subcarinal mass with regions of
low attenuation (necrosis) + enhancing septa
Cx:
(1) Mediastinal granuloma (uncommon)
Histo: involved nodes with varying degrees
of central caseation ± calcification
√ lobulated mass of lymph nodes several cm in
thickness surrounded by a thin capsule
(2) Mediastinal fibrosis (very uncommon) with
obstruction of SVC, azygos vein, pulmonary
arteries + veins, bronchi, esophagus
(3) Pericarditis (rare)
Rx: ketoconazole

B. CHRONIC HISTOPLASMOSIS
(reinfection / endogenous dispersion)
• in individuals with chronic obstructive pulmonary
disease
√ upper lobe cavitation with considerable fibrosis
(similar to TB)
√ sclerosing mediastinitis with obstruction of SVC,
pulmonary arteries + veins, esophageal narrowing,
constrictive pericarditis

C. DISSEMINATED HISTOPLASMOSIS
Predisposed: infants + elderly; massive inoculum
• rapidly fatal / chronic illness
√ may show pulmonary consolidation
√ hilar + mediastinal adenopathy +
hepatosplenomegaly
√ splenic calcifications (40%)

Dx: (1) Complement fixation test (titers of ≥ 1:32 or 4
fold increase on repeat testing suggest active /
recent infection)
(2) Agar gel diffusion test (H precipitin band)
Cx: Fibrosing mediastinitis (most common cause)

HYDATID DISEASE
= ECHINOCOCCOSIS
• asymptomatic
• eosinophilia (<25%)
• cough, expectoration, fever
• positive Casoni skin test in 60%
• hypersensitivity reaction (if cyst rupture occurs)

√ solitary (75%) / multiple (25%) sharply circumscribed
spherical / ovoid masses
√ size of 1 – 10 cm in diameter (16 – 20 weeks doubling
time)
√ cyst communicating with bronchial tree
√ "meniscus sign", "double arch sign", "moon sign",
"crescent sign" (5%) = rupture of pericyst with air
dissection between peri- and exocyst
√ "water lily sign", "sign of the camalote" = collapsed
cyst membrane floating on the fluid
√ air-fluid level = rupture of all cyst walls
√ hydropneumothorax
√ calcification of cyst wall (<6%)
√ rib + vertebral erosion (rare)
√ mediastinal cyst: posterior (65%), anterior (26%),
middle (9%) mediastinum

HYPOGENETIC LUNG SYNDROME
= PULMONARY VENOLOBAR SYNDROME
= SCIMITAR SYNDROME
= unique form of lung hypoplasia / aplasia affecting one /
more lobes accompanied by partial anomalous
pulmonary venous return; M:F = 1:1.4
Associated with:
(1) Vascular anomalies: hypoplastic artery, anomalous
venous return, systemic arterial supply
(2) Anomalies of hemidiaphragm on affected side:
√ retrosternal band (= "accessory hemidiaphragm")
on lateral CXR due to mediastinal rotation
√ phrenic cyst
√ diaphragmatic hernia
(3) Hemivertebrae + scoliosis
(4) CHD: ASD, VSD, tetralogy of Fallot, PDA,
coarctation of aorta, persistent left SVC,
pulmonary stenosis
• asymptomatic (40%)
• may have dyspnea / recurrent infections

Location: right-sided predominance
√ hypoplasia / aplasia of one / more lobes of the lung with
errors of lobation (bilateral left bronchial branching
pattern / horseshoe lung)
√ "scimitar vein" (90%) = partial anomalous pulmonary
venous return (commonly infradiaphragmatic into IVC /
portal vein / hepatic vein / R atrium), on CXR seen only
in 1/3

√ systemic arterial supply to abnormal segment my be present from thoracicorta (bronchial, intercostal, transpleural) or abdominal aorta (celiac artery, transdiaphragmatic)
√ reticular densities (enlarged bronchial / transpleural arterial collaterals)
√ small hilus (absent / small pulmonary artery)
√ small right hemithorax + mediastinal shift
√ haziness of right heart border
√ cardiac dextroposition (in right lung hypoplasia)
√ anomalies of bony thorax / thoracic soft tissues
　√ absent inferior vena cava
　√ rib hypoplasia / malsegmentation
　√ rib notching
CT:
　√ small hemithorax + mediastinal shift
　√ abnormalities of bronchial branching
　√ anomalously located pulmonary fissure
　√ discontinuity of hemidiaphragm
　√ pulmonary arterial hypoplasia
　√ hyparterial right bronchus (instead of eparterial)
　√ one / more vessels increasing in diameter toward diaphragm
　√ rind of subpleural fatty tissue in affected hemithorax
　√ lack of normal venous confluence of right lung
DDx:　Meandering pulmonary vein, dextrocardia, hypoplastic lung, Swyer-James syndrome

HORSESHOE LUNG
= uncommon variant of hypogenetic lung syndrome in which RLL crosses midline between esophagus and heart + fuses with opposite lung
√ oblique fissure in left lower hemithorax (if both lungs separated by pleural layers)
√ pulmonary vessels + bronchi crossing midline

IDIOPATHIC PULMONARY HEMOSIDEROSIS
= IPH = probable autoimmune process with clinical + radiological remissions + exacerbations characterized by eosinophilia + mastocytosis, immunoallergic reaction, pulmonary hemorrhage, iron deficiency anemia
Age:　(a)　Chronic form: most commonly <10 years of age
　　　(b)　Acute form (rare): in adults; M:F = 2:1
• iron deficiency anemia
• clubbing of fingers
• hepatosplenomegaly (25%)
• bilirubinemia
• recurrent episodes of severe hemoptysis

√ bilateral patchy alveolar-filling pattern (= blood in alveoli); initially for 2 – 3 days with return to normal in 10 - 12 days unless episode repeated
√ reticular pattern (= deposition of hemosiderin in interstitial space) later
√ moderate fibrosis after repeated episodes
√ hilar lymph nodes may be enlarged during acute episodes
Prognosis:　death within 2 – 20 years (average survival 3 years)

DDx:　SECONDARY PULMONARY HEMOSIDEROSIS caused by mitral valve disease
　　　√ septal lines (NOT in idiopathic form)
　　　√ lung ossifications (NOT in idiopathic form)

INTERSTITIAL PNEUMONIA
= ORGANIZING INTERSTITIAL PNEUMONIA
= CHRONIC DIFFUSE SCLEROSING ALVEOLITIS
= HAMMAN-RICH SYNDROME

Usual Interstitial Pneumonia
= UIP = IDIOPATHIC PULMONARY FIBROSIS (IPF)
= MURAL TYPE OF FIBROSING ALVEOLITIS
= commonest form of diffuse interstitial pneumonia
Etiology:　50% idiopathic; 25% familial; drug exposure (bleomycin, cyclophosphamide (Cytoxan®), busulfan, nitrofurantoin); serologic abnormalities associated with collagen vascular disease
Age peak:　5 – 6th decade; M:F = 1:1
Path:
　proteinaceous exudate in interstitium + hyaline membrane formation in alveoli; necrosis of alveolar lining cells followed by cellular infiltration of mono- and lymphocytes + regeneration of alveolar lining; proliferation of fibroblasts + deposition of collagen fibers + smooth muscle proliferation; progressive disorganization of pulmonary architecture
• progressive dyspnea
• "Velcro" rales = crepitations
• clubbing of fingers (83%)
• lymphocytosis on lavage

√ occasionally ground glass pattern in early stage of alveolitis (alveolar wall injury, interstitial edema, proteinaceous exudate, hyaline membranes, infiltrate of monocytes + lymphocytes)
√ diffuse linear / small iregular reticulations (60%); predominance at bases
√ reticulonodular pattern = superimposition of linear opacities
√ heart border "shaggy"
√ honeycombing (numerous cystic spaces)
√ elevated diaphragm (progressive loss of lung volume)
√ pleural effusion (4%), pleural thickening (6%)
√ pneumothorax in 7% (in late stages)
HRCT:
　Location:　predominantly subpleural regions + lung bases
　√ reticular pattern (irregular fibrosis + honeycomb cysts)
　√ small peripheral convoluted cysts (traction bronchiectasis)
　√ patchy areas of air-space consolidation (diffuse inflammatory mononuclear cell infiltrates of active disease)
Cx:　bronchogenic carcinoma (more frequent occurrence)
Prognosis:　average survival of 4 – 6 years; 87% mortality rate

Desquamative Interstitial Pneumonia

= DIP = DESQUAMATIVE TYPE OF FIBROSING ALVEOLITIS

= second commonest form of interstitial pneumonia with more benign course than UIP, may be self-limited disease or lead to UIP

Age: approximately 8 years younger than in UIP

Path: alveoli lined by large cuboidal cells + filled with heavy accumulation of mononuclear cells; preservation of normal lung architecture; minimal fibrosis

- asymptomatic
- weight loss
- dyspnea + noproductive cough
- clubbing of fingers
√ normal chest X-ray (15 – 20%)
√ "ground-glass" alveolar pattern sparing costophrenic angles (20%)
√ linear irregular opacities (60%), predominantly at bases
√ progressive loss of lung volume (not as severe as in UIP)

Prognosis: better response to corticosteroid Rx than UIP; 16% mortality rate

KARTAGENER SYNDROME

= IMMOTILE / DYSMOTILE CILIA SYNDROME

Incidence: 1:40,00; high familial incidence

Etiology: abnormal mucociliary function secondary to generalized deficiency of dynein arms of cilia affecting respiratory epithelium, auditory epithelium, sperm

Triad: (1) Situs inversus (50%)
     (2) Sinusitis
     (3) Bronchiectasis

- deafness
- infertility (abnormal sperm tails)

Associated anomalies:

Transposition of great vessels, tri- / bilocular heart, pyloric stenosis, postcricoid web, epispadia

KLEBSIELLA PNEUMONIA

Most common cause of Gram-negative pneumonias; community acquired

Incidence: responsible for 5% of adult pneumonias

Organism: Friedländer bacillus = encapsulated, nonmotile, Gram-negative rod

Predisposed: elderly, debilitated, alcoholic, chronic lung disease, malignancy

- bacteremia in 25%

√ propensity for posterior portion of upper lobe / superior portion of lower lobe
√ dense lobar consolidation
√ bulging of fissure (large amounts of inflammatory exudate) CHARACTERISTIC but unusual
√ empyema (one of the most common causes)
√ patchy bronchopneumonia may be present
√ uni- / multilocular cavities (50%) appearing within 4 days

√ pulmonary gangrene = infarcted tissue (rare)

Cx: meningitis, pericarditis

Prognosis: mortality rate 25 – 50%

DDx: Acute pneumococcal pneumonia (bulging of fissures, abscess + cavity formation, pleural effusion / empyema frequent)

LEGIONELLA PNEUMONIA

Organism: Legionella pneumophila, Gram-negative, weakly acid-fast, silver-impregnation stain

Predisposed: middle-aged / elderly, immunosuppressed, alcoholism, chronic obstructive lung disease, diabetes, cancer, cardiovascular disease, chronic renal failure

Clue: involvement of other organs with
- diarrhea, myalgia, toxic encephalopathy
- liver + renal disease

Location: unilateral / bilateral (less frequent); lobar / segmental

√ patchy bronchopneumonia
√ pleural effusion (rare)
√ cavitation (rare)

LIPOID PNEUMONIA

Etiology: aspiration of vegetable / animal / mineral oil (most common)

Predisposed: elderly, debilitated, neuromuscular disease, swallowing abnormalities

Path: pool of oil surrounded by giant cell foreign body reaction (mineral oil) / initially hemorrhagic bronchopneumonia (animal fat)

- mostly asymptomatic
- fever, constitutional symptoms

Location: predilection for RML + lower lobes

√ homogeneous segmental consolidation (most common)
√ acinar alveolar consolidation
√ reticulonodular pattern (rare)
√ paraffinoma = circumscribed peripheral mass (granulomatous reaction + fibrosis)
√ slow progression / no change

LÖFFLER SYNDROME

= disorder of unknown etiology characterized by local areas of transient parenchymal consolidation associated with blood eosinophilia

Path: interstitial + alveolar edema containing a large number of lymphocytes

- no / mild symptoms
- eosinophilia
- history of atopia

√ single / multiple areas of homogeneous ill-defined consolidation
√ uni- or bilateral, nonsegmental distribution, predominantly in lung periphery
√ transient + shifting in nature (changes within one to several days)

Prognosis: may undergo spontaneous remission

LYMPNGIOMYOMATOSIS

= rare disorder of women in child-bearing age characterized by (1) gradually progressive diffuse interstitial lung disease (2) recurrent chylous pleural effusions (3) recurrent pneumothoraces

Age: 17 – 50 years, exclusively in young women

Histo: proliferation of atypical smooth muscle in pulmonary lymphatic vessels, blood vessels and airways

Pathogenesis:

proliferated smooth muscle obstructs (a) bronchioles (trapping of air, overinflation, formation of cysts, pneumothorax), (b) venules (pulmonary edema, hemorrhage, hemoiderosis), (c) lymphatics (thickening of lymphatics, chylothorax)

May be associated with: Tuberous sclerosis (lung involvement in 1%)

- increasing shortness of breath
- disease aggravated by birth control pills
- hemoptysis (30 – 40%), chyloptysis
- radiologic-physiologic discrepancy = severe airflow obstruction despite relatively normal findings on CXR

Classic signs:
  √ coarse reticular interstitial pattern
  √ recurrent large chylothorax (50 – 75%)
  √ recurrent pneumothorax (40%)
√ increasing lung volume (only interstitial disease to develop increasing lung volumes)
√ Kerley-B lines
√ pulmonary cysts + honeycombing
√ occasionally chylous ascites
CT:
  √ numerous randomly scattered thin-walled cysts of various sizes surrounded by normal lung parenchyma
  √ bronchovascular bundles at periphery of cyst walls

Prognosis: death within 10 years
DDx:
(1) Histiocytosis (cyst walls more variable in thickness, nodularity common)
(2) Emphysema (lobular architecture preserved with bronchovascular bundle in central position, areas of lung destruction without arcuate contour)

LYMPHANGITIC CARCINOMATOSIS

= INTERSTITIAL CARCINOMA
= tumor cell accumulation within connective tissue (bronchovascular bundles, interlobular septa, subpleural space, pulmonary lymphatics) from tumor embolization of blood vessels followed by lymphatic obstruction, interstitial edema, and collagen deposition (fibrosis from desmoplastic reaction when tumor cells extend into adjacent pulmonary parenchyma)

Incidence: 7% of all pulmonary metastases

Tumor origin: bronchogenic carcinoma, carcinoma of breast (56%), stomach (46%), thyroid, pancreas, larynx, cervix

mnemonic: "**C**ertain **C**ancers **S**pread **B**y **P**lugging **T**he **L**ymphatics"
  Cervix
  Colon
  Stomach
  Breast
  Pancreas
  Thyroid
  Larynx

Path: (1) interstitial edema (2) interstitial fibrotic changes (3) lymphatic dilatation (4) tumor cells within connective tissue planes
- dyspnea (often preceding radiographic abnormalities)
- rarely dry cough + hemoptysis

Location: bilateral; unilateral if secondary to lung primary
CXR (accuracy 23%):
  √ normal chest radiograph
  √ reticular densities
  √ coarsened bronchovascular markings
  √ Kerley A + B lines
  √ small lung volume
  √ hilar adenopathy (20 – 50%)
HRCT:
  √ circumferentially thickened linear irregular / nodular "beaded" densities forming a reticular network
  √ well-defined polygonal structures (= thickened interlobular septa of secondary pulmonary lobule)
  √ central dot within secondary pulmonary lobule = thickened bronchovascular bundle
  √ pleural fluid + thickening
  √ ± nodules, hilar / mediastinal lymphadenopathy
Prognosis: death within 1 yea
DDx:
(1) Fibrosing alveolitis (peripheral predominance)
(2) Extrinsic allergic alveolitis (no polygonal structures, pleural changes rare)
(3) Sarcoidosis (nodules of irregular outline more frequent in upper lobes, polygonal structures uncommon)

LYMPHOID INTERSTITIAL PNEUMONIA

= LYMPHOCYTIC INTERSTITIAL PNEUMONITIS
= LIP = lymphocytic infiltration of pulmonary interstitium of unknown etiology with frequently chronic + progressive course

Histo: diffuse interstitial infiltrate of lymphocytes, histiocytes, plasma cells; difficult to distinguish from lymphoma
- dyspnea + cough
- cyanosis + clubbing (50%)
- enlargement of salivary glands (20%)
- NO lymphocytosis or history of atopia
- monoclonal gammopathy (usually IgM)
√ fine reticular changes in both lungs
√ resembling air space disease (in severe form)
√ nodular pattern

Localized form = PSEUDOLYMPHOMA

LYMPHOMA
7th leading cause of death from cancer in United States
Pathogenesis: ? viral cause
HD: contiguous spread requires scanning of abnormal area only
NHL: noncontiguous spread requires scanning of chest, abdomen, pelvis

@ Thorax
  Δ Hodgkin disease more common in thorax than NHL (especially nodular sclerosing type) in 85% versus 40 – 50%
  1. Lymph adenopathy
     anterior mediastinal, pretracheal, hilar, subcarinal, axillary, periesophageal, paracardiac, superior diaphragmat internal mammary lymph nodes
  2. Lung parenchyma involvement (HD in 12%, NHL in 4%)
  3. Pleural + subpleural lymphoma (up to 30%)

@ Abdomen
  1. Periaortic adenopathy ....HD in 25%
                                                      NHL in 49%
  2. Mesenteric adenopathy ....HD in 4%
                                                      NHL in 51%
  3. Liver involvement ....HD in 8%
                                                      NHL in 14%
     √ hepatomegaly with involvement ....HD in <30%
                                                      NHL in 57%
     HD: commonly diffuse infiltrating process
     NHL: diffuse infiltrating / discrete tumor nodules
  4. Splenic involvement ....HD in 37%
                                                      NHL in 41%
     HD: most common site of abdominal involvement
     NHL: 3rd mos common site of abdominal involvement; may be initial manifestation in large cell NHL
     Δ Staging laparotomy necessary as 2/3 of tumor nodules <1 cm in size

5. Gastrointestinal involvement
   in 10% of patients with abdominal lymphoma (uncommon in HD, common in histiocytic NHL); NHL accounts for 80% of all gastric lymphomas
6. Renal involvement
   late manifestation, most commonly in NHL
7. Adrenal involvement
   more common in NHL
8. Extranodal involvement
   more frequent with histologically diffuse forms of NHL

Hodgkin Disease
40% of all lymphomas; disease of T cells
Age: bimodal distribution at 25 – 30 years + >70 years
• asymptomatic unilateral cervical adenopathy
Histo: Reed-Sternberg cell characteristic
  1. lymphocyte predominance: uncommon, localized, excellent prognosis, majority <35 years
  2. nodular sclerosis: most common, localized, good prognosis; greatest adenopathy in anterior mediastinum
  3. mixed cellularity: more commonly abdominal than mediastinal, less favorable prognosis
  4. lymphocyte depletion: uncommon, disseminated, older patients, rapidly fatal

Ann Arbor Staging Classification:
Stage I   = limited to one / two contiguous anatomic regions on same side of diaphragm
  I_E = single extralymphatic organ / site
Stage II   = >2 anatomic regions / two noncontiguous regions on same side of diaphragm
  II_E = with extralymphatic organ / site
Stage III = on both sides of diaphragm, not extending beyond lymph nodes, spleen (Stage III_S), Waldeyer's ring
  III_E = with extralymphatic organ / site

Histologic Classification of Non-Hodgkin Lymphoma	
International Working Formulation	Rappaport Classification
Low grade	
A. Small lymphocytic	Well-differentiated lymphocytic
B. Follicular, predominantly small cleaved cell	Nodular, poorly differentiated lymphocytic
C. Follicular, mixed small and large cell	Nodular, mixed
Intermediate grade	
D. Follicular, predominantly large cell	Nodular, histiocytic
E. Diffuse, small cleaved cell	Diffuse, poorly differentiated lymphocytic
F. Diffuse, mixed small and large cell	Diffuse, mixed
G. Diffuse, large cell, cleaved or noncleaved	...
High grade	
H. Diffuse large cell, immunoblastic	...
I. Small, noncleaved cell	...
J. Lymphoblastic	Undifferentiated

Stage IV   = organ involvement (bone marrow, bone, lung, pleura, liver, kidney, GI tract, skin) ± lymph node involvement
Substage A = absence of systeic symptoms
Substage B = fever, night sweats, pruritus, ≥10% weight loss

@ CHEST INVOLVEMENT
at presentation: 67% with intrathoracic disease
Sites of lyphoid aggregates:
1. Lymph nodes in mediastinum
2. Lymph nodes at bifurcation of 1st + 2nd order bronchi
3. Encapsulated lymphoid collections on thoracic surface deep to parietal pleura
4. Unencapsulated nodules at points of divisions of more distally situated bronchi, bronchioles, and pulmonary vessels
5. Unencapsulated lymphoid aggregates within peribronchial connective tissue
6. Small accumulations of lymphocytes in interlobular septa + lymphatic channels

(a) INTRAPULMONARY MANIFESTATIONS
     in 15 – 40% during disease duration; most commonly in nodular sclerosing type; invariably subsequent to hilar adenopathy

     1. Bronchovascular form (most common type of involvement):
        √ coarse reticulonodular pattern contiguous with mediastinum = direct extension from mediastinal nodes along lymphatics
        √ nodular parenchymal lesions
        √ miliary nodules
        √ endobronchial involvement
        √ lobar atelectasis secondary to endobronchial obstruction (rare)
        √ cavitation secondary to necrosis (rare)
     2. Subpleural form
        √ circumscribed subpleural masses
        √ pleural effusion (20 – 50%) from lymphatic obstruction
     3. Massive pneumonic form (68%)
        √ diffuse nonsegmental infiltrate (pneumonic type)
        √ massive lobar infiltrates (30%)
        √ homogeneous confluent infiltrates with shaggy borders
        √ air bronchogram
     4. Nodular form
        √ multiple nodules <1 cm in diameter (DDx: metastatic disease)

(b) EXTRAPULMONARY MANIFESTATIONS

     1. Mediastinal + Hilar Lymphadenopathy
        Most common manifestation, present in 90 – 99%

Location:
     anterior mediastinal + retrosternal nodes commonly involved (DDx: sarcoidosis); 20% with mediastinal nodes have hilar lymph adenopathy also; enlargement of a single lymph node group in 5%, bilateral in 50%
     √ CXR: on initial film adenopathy identified in 50%
     √ necrotic lymph nodes (commonly nodular sclerosing type)
     √ lymph nodes may calcify following radiation / chemotherapy
     2. Pleural Effusion (30%)
     3. Pleural Masses + Plaques (direct invasion from mediastinum)
Cx:
     1. Superimposed infection
        √ consolidation with bulging borders: necrotizing bacterial pneumonia
        √ multiple nodular foci: aspergillosis + nocardiosis
        √ bilateral diffuse consolidation: Pneumocystis carinii
        √ rapidly developing cavitation within consolidation: anaerobes / fungus
        Dx: by culture, sputum cytology, lung biopsy
     2. Drug toxicity

@ BONE INVOLVEMENT (15%)
     √ frequently osteoblastic (28%), eg, ivory vertebrae
     √ osteolysis of sternum / ribs (direct invasion)

Cx: increased risk for other malignancies from aggressive therapy (acute leukemia, NHL, radiation-induced sarcoma)

Non-Hodgkin Lymphoma
= NHL = disease of B cells
Incidence: 3% of all newly diagnosed cancers; 3rd most common cancer in childhood (behind leukemia + CNS neoplasms); 4 times more common than Hodgkin disease

Predisposed: (40 – 100 times greater risk) congenital immunodeficiency syndromes, organ transplant patients undergoing immunosuppression, patients with HIV infection, collagen vascular diseases
Age: all ages; median age of 55 years; M:F = 1.4:1

Modified Rappaport Classification:
A. Nodular
    (a) Poorly differentiated lymphocytic (PDL)
    (b) Mixed lymphocytic / histiocytic (mixed cell)
    (c) Large cell (histiocytic)
B. Diffuse
    (a) well-differentiated lymphocytic (WDL)
    (b) intermediate-differentiated lymphocytic (IDL)
    (c) poorly differentiated lymphocytic (PDL)

(d) mixed lymphocytic / histiocytic large cell (histiocytic) (DLCL); undifferentiated Burkitt lymphoma; undifferentiated Non-Burkitt lymphoma (pleiomorphic); lymphoblastic (LBL); unclassified

Working Formulation Classification:
A. Low grade
   (a) small lymphocytic (3.6%)
       median age 61 years, 59% 5-year survival
   (b) follicular, small cleaved cell (22.5%)
       median age 54 years, 70% 5-year survival
   (c) follicul, mixed (7.7%)
       median age 56 years, 50% 5-year survival
B. Intermediate grade
   (a) follicular, large cell (3.8%)
       median age 55 years, 45% 5-year survival
   (b) diffuse, small cleaved cell (6.9%)
       median age 58 years, 33% 5-year survival
   (c) diffuse, mixed (6.7%)
       median age 58 years, 38% 5-year survival
   (d) diffuse, large cell (19.7%)
       median age 57 years, 35% 5-year survival
C. High grade
   (a) large cell, immunoblastic (7.9%)
       median age 51 years, 32% 5-year survival
   (b) lymphoblastic (4.2%)
       median age 17 years, 26% 5-year survival
   (c) small noncleaved cell (5%)
       median age 30 years, 23% 5-year survival
D. Miscellaneous (12%)
   composite, mycosis fungoides, histiocytic, extramedullary plasmacytoma
Staging: same Ann Arbor system as for Hodgkin disease

Extranodal involvement:
@ GI tract:
   stomach (3%), small bowel (5%), large bowel (2%), pancreas (0.7%), peritoneal nodules + ascites (1.4%)
@ Chest:
   lung (6%), pleural fluid (3.3%), pericardial fluid (0.7%), heart (0.2%)
@ GU tract (10%):
   kidneys (6%), testes (1.2%), ovaries (1.8%), uterus (1.2%)
@ Bone (3.8%)
@ CNS (2.4%)
@ Breast (1.2%)
@ Skin (6.4%)
@ Head and neck (1.7%)
@ Liver (14%)
@ Spleen (41%)

Nodal involvement:
@ Paraaortic lymph nodes (49%)
@ Mesenteric lymph nodes (51%)
@ Splenic hilar lymph nodes (53%)
Δ Lymphography 89% sensitive + 86% specific

Intrathoracic disease (40 – 50%):
√ hilar + mediastinal adenopathy (DDx: sarcoidosis; anterior nodes favor lymphoma)
√ isolated lymph nodes may enhance (DDx: Castleman disease)
√ lung nodules + air bronchograms
√ pleural effusion
Prognosis: unfavorable

MECONIUM ASPIRATION SYNDROME
= most common cause of neonatal respiratory distress in full term / postmature infants (hyaline membrane disease most common cause in premature infants)
Etiology: fetal circulatory accidents / placental insufficiency / postmaturity result in perinatal hypoxia + fetal distress with meconium defecated in utero
Pathogenesis: meconium produces bronchial obstruction + chemical pneumonitis
Incidence: 10% of all deliveries have meconium-stained amniotic fluid, 1% of all deliveries have respiratory distress
• cyanosis (rare)
√ large infant
√ bilateral diffuse grossly patchy opacities (atelectasis + consolidation)
√ hyperinflation with areas of emphysema (air trapping)
√ spontaneous pneumothorax + pneumomediastinum (25%) requiring no therapy
√ small pleural effusions (20%)
√ NO air bronchograms
√ rapid clearing usually within 48 hours
Cx: morbidity from anoxic brain damage is high

MEDIASTINAL LIPOMATOSIS
= excess unencapsulated fat deposition
Etiology:
(a) Exogenous steroids (average daily dose of >30 mg prednisone): (1) chronic renal disease, renal transplant (5%) (2) collagen vascular disease, vasculitis (3) hemolytic anemia (4) asthma (5) dermatitis (6) Crohn disease (7) myasthenia gravis
(b) Endogenous steroid elevation:
    (1) adrenal tumor (2) pituitary tumor / hyperplasia = Cushing disease (3) ectopic ACTH-production (carcinoma of the lung)
(c) Obesity
• moon facies
• buffalo hump
• supraclavicular + episternal fat
Location: upper mediastinum (common), cardiophrenic angles + paraspinal areas (less common)
√ upper mediastinal widening
√ paraspinal widening
√ increase in epicardial fat pads
√ symmetric slightly lobulated extrapleural deposits extending from apex to 9th rib laterally
OTHER FEATURES:
√ osteoporosis
√ fractures

√ aseptic necrosis
√ increased rectosacral distance

MESOTHELIOMA

Benign Mesothelioma

= LOCALIZED FIBROUS MESOTHELIOMA
= FIBROUS TUMOR OF THE PLEURA
No direct connection to asbestos; arises from visceral
> parietal pleura
Age: 3rd – 8th decade; mean age of 40 – 50 years
Histo: tumor originates from submesothelial
  mesenchal cells, lined by layer of mesothelial cells
  (a) relatively acellular fibrous tissue
  (b) rounded spindle-shaped densely packed cells
  (c) resembling hemangiopericytoma of lung

• asymptomatic in 50%
• cough, fever, dyspnea, chest pain (larger mass)
• digital clubbing + hypertrophic pulmonary
  osteoarthropathy in 20%
• episodic hypoglycemia (rare)

√ sharply circumscribed lobular mass of 2 – 30 cm in
  diameter located near lung periphery / adjacent to
  pleural surface / within fissure
√ obtse angle with chest wall
√ sessile (common) / pedunculated (rare, benign
  feature)
√ tumor may change in shape + location (if
  pedunculated)
√ areas of hemorrhage / necrosis may be present
  (favors malignancy)
√ ipsilateral pleural effusion (rare) containing
  hyaluronic acid
DDx: metastatic deposit
Rx: excision is curative

Malignant Mesothelioma

Δ Occupational exposure of asbestos found in 80% of
  all cases!
Δ 5 – 10% of occupationally exposed subjects will
  develop mesothelioma risk factor of 300 compared
  with general population)
Δ No relation to duration / degree of exposure or
  smoking history
Carcinogenic potential: crocidolite > amosite >
  chrysotile > antophyllite
Latent period: 20 – 40 years
Peak age: 6 – 7th decade
Histo: (a) epithelial (b) mesenchymal (c) mixed;
  intracellular asbestos fibers in 25%
Associated with   peritoneal mesothelioma
• dyspnea, chest pain

√ extensive irregular lobulated bulky pleural-based
  masses / pleural thickening
√ exudative / hemorrhagic pleural effusion without
  mediastinal shift (fixation by pleural rind of neoplastic
  tissue) in 80 – 100% containing hyaluronic acid
√ associated with pleural plaques in 50%

√ circumferential encasement = involvement of all
  pleural surfaces (mediastinum, pericardium, fissures)
  as late manifestation
√ may show rib destruction
√ ascites (peritoneum involved in 35%)
Metastases to:
  ipsilateral lung (60%), hilar + mediastinal nodes,
  contralateral lung + pleura (rare), extension
  through chest wall + diaphragm
Prognosis: survival <2 years

METASTASES TO LUNG

Pulmonary metastases occur in 30% of all malignancies;
mostly hematogenous
Age: >50 years (in 87%)

FREQUENCY:

Origin of pulmonary mets		Probability of pulmonary mets	
1. Breast	22%	Kidney	in 75%
2. Kidney	11%	Osteosarcoma	in 75%
3. Head and neck	10%	Choriocarcinoma	in 75%
4. Colorectal	9%	Thyroid	in 65%
5. Uterus	6%	Melanoma	in 60%
6. Pancreas	5%	Breast	in 55%
7. Ovary	5%	Prostate	in 40%
8. Prostate	4%	Head and neck	in 30%
9. Stomach	4%	Esophagus	in 20%

Incidence of pulmonary metastases:
  mnemonic: "CHEST"

Choriocarcinoma	60%
Hypernephroma / Wilms tumor	30 / 20%
Ewing sarcoma	18%
Sarcoma (rhabdomyo- / osteosarcoma)	21 / 15%
Testicular tumor	12%

√ multiple nodules (in 75%) of varying sizes (most
  typical), 82% subpleural
√ fine micronodular pattern: highly vascular tumor (renal
  cell, breast, thyroid, prostate carcinoma, bone sarcoma,
  choriocarcinoma)
√ pneumothorax (2%): especially in children with bone
  tumors
CT:
  √ noncalcified multiple (>10) round lesions >2.5 cm
    likely to be metastatic
  √ connection to pulmonary arterial branches (75%)

SOLITARY METASTATIC NODULE
  Δ A solitary lung nodule represents a primary lung
    tumor in 62% in patients with known Hx of neoplasm
  Δ 5% of all solitary nodules are metastatic;
    most likely origin: colon carcinoma (30 – 40%),
    osteosarcoma, renal cell carcinoma, testicular tumor,
    breast carcinoma

CALCIFYING METASTASES (<1%)
  mnemonic: "BOTTOM"
    Breast
    Osteo- / chondrosarcoma

Thyroid (papillary)
Testicular
Ovarian
Mucinous adenocarcinoma
+ lung metastases following radiation / chemotherapy

CAVITATING METASTASES (4%):
mnemonic: "**S**quamous **C**ell **M**etastases **T**end to
Cavitate"
Squamous cell carcinoma, **S**arcoma
Colon
Melanoma
Transitional cell carcinoma
Cervix, under **C**hemotherapy

HEMORRHAGIC METASTASES
√ ill-defined nodules
1. Choriocarcinoma
2. Renal cell carcinoma
3. Melanoma
4. Thyroid carcinoma

ENDOBRONCHIAL METASTASES
√ segmental / subsegmental atelectasis
1. Bronchogenic carcinoma
2. Lymphoma
3. Renal cell carcinoma
4. Breast cancer
5. Colon carcinoma

MUCORMYCOSIS
= PHYCOMYCOSIS = caused by a variety of
phycomycetes (soil fungi) leading to severe vascular
obstruction
Organisms: Mucor (most common), Absidia, Rhizopus,
Predisposed: diabetics, immunocompromised patients
(lymphoma, leukemia)
Opportunistic infection in:
1. Lymphoproliferative malignancies and leukemia
2. Acidotic diabetes mellitus
3. Immunosuppression through steroids, antibiotics,
immunosuppressive drugs (rare)
A. RHINOCEREBRAL FORM
= involvement of paranasal sinuses (frontal sinus
usually spared) with extension into:
(a) orbit = orbital cellulitis
(b) base of skull = meningoencephaliti + cerebritis
B. PULMONARY FORM
Histo: invasion of blood vessels
√ segmental homogeneous consolidation
√ cavitation
√ nodules (from arterial thrombi + infarction)
DDx: aspergillosis

MYCOPLASMA PNEUMONIA
= PRIMARY ATYPICAL PNEUMONIA (PAP)
commonest cause of nonbacterial pneumonia with a
mild course (only 2% require hospitalization), usually
lasts 2 – 3 weeks; only 10% of infected subjects
develop pneumonia

Incidence: 10 – 33% of all pneumonias; autumn peak
Organism: Eaton agent = pleuropneumonia-like
organism (PPLO)
Age: most common in ages 5 – 20 years (esp. in closed
populations)
• mild symptoms of cough + low fever, malaise, otitis
• mild leukocytosis (20%)
• most common respiratory cause of cold agglutinin
production (60%)

√ radiologic findings often diverge from clinical condition
√ pulmonary infiltrates show a significant lag time
√ fine interstitial infiltration from hilum into lower lobe
(earliest change)
√ alveolar infiltrates: unilateral (L > R) air-space
consolidation in segmental lower lobe in 50%, bilateral
in 10 – 40%
√ small pleural effusions in 20%
√ hilar adenopathy (rare)

Cx: (1) Meningoencephalitis
(2) Erythema nodosum, erythema multiforme,
Stevens-Johnson syndrome
Prognosis: 20% with recurrent symptoms of pharyngitis
+ bronchitis ± infiltrations

NEAR DROWNING
1. SEA WATER DROWNING
• hemoconcentration, hypovolemia
2. FRESH WATER DROWNNG
• hemodilution, hypervolemia
• hemolysis
3. SECONDARY DROWNING
(a) pneumonia with toxic debris
(b) progressive pulmonary edema
4. DRY DROWNING (20 – 40%)
= laryngeal spasm prevents water from entering
√ no roentgenographic abnormality
Similarities of all 4 types:
• hypoxemia
• metabolic acidosis
√ pulmonary edema
√ hyaline membrane formation = considerable loss of
protein from blood

NEONATAL PNEUMONIA
Pathogenesis:
(a) in utero infection (ascending from premature
rupture of membranes or prolonged labor /
transplacental route)
(b) aspiration of infected vaginal secretions during
delivery
(c) infection after birth
Organism:
(1) Group B streptococcus (GBS): in low birth-weight
premature infants; 50% mortality
√ radiographic picture may be identical to RDS (in
52%)
√ appearance suggesting retained lung fluid / focal
infiltrates (35%)

√ normal CXR (13%)
√ cardiomegaly
√ pleural effusions (in 2/3, but RARE in RDS)
√ delayed onset diaphragmatic hernia (evidenced by clinical deterioration)
  (2) Pneumococci: RDS-like
  (3) Listeria: RDS-like
  (4) Candida: progressive consodation + cavitatin
  (5) Chlamydia: bronchopneumonic pattern
• afebrile
• ower ventilatory pressure requirements
√ bilateral focal / diffuse reas of opacities (may initially appear similar to fetal aspiration syndrome)
√ hyperaration
√ may cause lobar atelectasis
√ may cause pneumothorax / pneumomediastinum
√ pleural effusion (exceedingly rare)

NOCARDIOSIS
Organism: Gram-positive acid-fast bacterium resembling fungus
Predisposed: immunocompromised
√ multiple poorly / well-defid nodules ± cavitation
√ lobar consolidation
√ empyema without sinus tracts
√ SVC obstruction (rare)

PERICARDIAL CYST
secondary to defect in embryogenesis of coelomic cavities; M = F
Histo: lined by single layer of mesothelial cells
Location: 75% at cardiophrenic gle (R:L = 3:1), 25% higher; may extend into major fissure
√ mass of 3 – 8 cm (range 1 – 28 cm) in diameter
√ change in size + shape with respiration / body position

POLYARTERITIS NODOSA
= PERIARTERITIS NODOSA = systemic vasculitis of small + medium-sized arteries + arterioles characterized by necrotizing granulomas of all wall layers
Usually in male adults
• associated with hepatitis B antigenemia
• systemic hypertension

@ Renal involvement (80%): aneurysms
@ Chest involvement (70%)
√ cardiac enlargement / pericardial effusion (14%)
√ pleural effusion (14%)
√ pulmonary venous engorgement (21%)
√ massive pulmonary edema (4%)
√ linear densities / plate-like atelectasis (10%)
√ wedge-shaped / round peripheral infiltrates of nonsegmental distribution (14%) (simulating thromboembolic disease with infarction)
√ cavitation may occur
√ interstitial lower lung field pneumonitis

PNEUMATOCELE
= cystic air collection within lung parenchyma due to obstructive overinflation

Δ does not indicate destruction of lung parenchyma
Δ occurs during healing phase
Δ appears to enlarge while patient improves
Δ frequently multiple

Developmental theories:
  (1) result of severe distension of small bronchioles secondary to check-valve endobronchial / peribronchial obstruction
  (2) communication between ruptured peribronchial abscess + bronchus with check-valve obstruction
  (3) subpleural collection of air formed by dissection of air from ruptured alveoli / bronchioles

A. PNEUMATOCELE ASSOCIATED WITH INFECTION
    Organism: Pneumococci, E. coli, Klebsiella, Staphylococcus (in childhood)
    √ appears within 1st week, disappears within 6 weeks
    √ thin-walled + completely air-filled cavity
    √ ± air-fluid level + wall thickening (during infection)
    √ pneumothorax
    √ spontaneous resolution (in most)

B. TRAUMATIC PNEUMATOCELE = PNEUMATOCYST
    (a) appearance within hours after blunt chest trauma with lung hematoma
    (b) hydrocarbon (furniture polish, kerosene) inhalation
    √ single / multiple pneumatoceles
    √ spontaneous resolution over several weeks to months

PNEUMOCOCCAL PNEUMONIA
Most common Gram-positive pneumonia
90% community-acquired, 10% nosocomial
Incidence: 15% of all adulthood pneumonias, uncommon in child; peaks in winter + early spring; increased during influenza epidemics
Organism: Streptococcus pneumoniae (formerly Diplococcus pneumoniae), Gram-positive, in pairs / chains, encapsulated, capsular polysaccharide responsible for virulence + serotyping
Susceptible: elderly, debilitated, alcoholics, CHF, COPD, multiple myeloma, hypogammaglobulinemia, functional / surgical asplenia
• rusty blood-streaked sputum
• left-shift leukocytosis
• impaired pulmonary function

Location: usually involves one lobe only; bias for lower lobes + posterior segments of upper lobes (bacteria flow under gravitational influence to most dependent portions as in aspiration)
√ extensive air-space consolidation abutting against visceral pleura (lobar / beyond confines of one lobe through pores of Kohn) CHARACTERISTIC
√ slight expansion of involved lobes
√ prominent air bronchograms (20%)

√ patchy bronchopneumonic pattern (in some)
√ pleural effusion (parapneumonic transsudate) uncommon with antibiotic thepy
√ cavitation (rare, with Type III)
Variations (modified by bronchopulmonary disease, eg, chronic bronchitis, emphysema):
 √ bronchopneumonia-like pattern
 √ effusion may be only presentation (esp. in COPD)
 √ empyema (with persistent fever)
Δ in childrn:
 √ round pneumonia = sharply defined rond lesion
Prognosis: prompt response to antibiotics (if without complications); 5% mortality rate
Dx: blood culture (positive in 30%)
Cx: meningitis, endocarditis, septic arthritis, empyema (now rarely seen)

PNEUMOCYSTOSIS

Most common cause of interstitial pneumonia in immuno-compromised patiens, which quickly leads to air space disease
Organism: protozoan Pneumocystis carinii; often associated with simultaneous infection by CMV, Mycobacterium avium-intracellulare, Herpes simplex
Predisposed:
 (1) debilitated premature infants, children with hypogammaglobulinemia (12%)
 (2) immunocompromised patients: congenital immunodeficiency syndrome, AIDS (60 – 80%), lymphoproliferative disorders, organ transplant recipients (renal transplant patients in 10%), patients on long-term corticosteroid therapy (nephrotic syndrome, collagen vascular disease), patients on cytotoxic drugs [under therapy for leukemia (40%), lymphoma (16%)]
 • severe dyspnea + cyanosis
 • WBC slightly elevated (PMNs)
 • lymphopenia (50%) heralds poor prognosis

√ bilateral + diffuse changes of perihilar + basilar distribution with sparing of apices (CHARACTERISTIC central location)
√ linear / reticular pattern (early changes)
√ "ground glass" = eventual progression to diffuse alveolar homogeneous consolidation (DDx: pulmonary edema)
√ air bronchogram
√ patchy localized consolidation (occasional presentation)
√ pleural effusion (uncommon)
√ NO hilar lymphadenopathy
CT:
 √ patchwork pattern (56%)
 = bilateral asymmetric patchy mosaic appearance with sparing of segments / subsegments of pulmonary lobe
 √ ground glass pattern (26%)
 = bilateral diffuse symmetric air space disease (fluid + inflammatory cells in alveolar space)
 √ interstitial pattern (18%)
 = bilateral symmetric / asymmetric, linear / reticular markings (thickening of lobular septa)

√ bullae + thin-walled cysts (38%)
√ pneumothorax (13%)
√ lymph adenopathy (18%)
√ pleural effusion (18%)
√ pulmonary nodules usually due to malignancy (leukemia, lymphoma, Kaposi sarcoma, metastasis) / septic emboli
√ pulmonary cavities usually due to superimposed fungal / mycobacterial infection
NUC:
 √ bilateral and diffuse Ga-67 uptake without mediastinal involvement prior to roentgenographic changes
 DDx: TB / MAI infection (with mediastinal involvement)

Dx: (1) sputum collection (2) bronchoscopy with lavage (3) transbronchial / transthoracic / open lung Bx
Prognosis: rapid fulminant disease; death within 2 weeks

PNEUMONECTOMY CHEST

Early signs (within 24 hours):
 √ partial filling of thorax
 √ ipsilateral mediastinal shift + diaphragmatic elevation
Late signs (after 2 months):
 √ complete obliteration of space
N.B.: Depression of diaphragm / shift of mediastinum to contralateral side indicates a bronchopleural fistula / empyema / hemorrhage!

POSTOBSTRUCTIVE PNEUMONIA

= chronic inflammatory disease distal to bronchial obstruction
Causes:
 1. Bronchogenic carcinoma (most commonly)
 2. Bronchial adenoma
 3. Granular cell myoblastoma (almost always tracheal lesion)
 4. Bronchostenosis
Histo: "golden pneumonia" = cholesterol pneumonia = endogenous lipid pneumonia = mixture of edema, atelectasis, round cell infiltration, bronchiectasis, liberation of lipid material from alveolar pneumocytes secondary to inflammatory reaction
√ frequently associated with some degree of atelectasis
√ persists unchanged for weeks
√ recurrent pneumonia in same region after antibiotic treatment

PROGRESSIVE MASSIVE FIBROSIS

= (PMF) = COMPLICATED PNEUMOCONIOSIS
= CONGLOMERATE ANTHRACOSILICOSIS
May develop / progress after cessation of dust exposure
Path: avascular amorphous central mass of insoluble proteins stabilized by cross-links + ill-defined bundles of coarse hyalinized collagen at periphery
Location: almost exclusively restricted to posterior segment of upper lobe / superior segment of lower lobe

√ large >1 cm opacities initially in middle + upper lung zones at periphery of lung

√ discoid contour (44%) = mass flat from front to back (thin opacity on lateral view, large opacity on PA view), medial border often ill-defined, lateral borders sharp + parallel trib cage

√ migration toward hila starting at lung periphery; bilateral symmetry

√ apparent decrease in nodularity (incorporation of nodules from surroundings)

√ cavitation (occasionally) due to ischemic necrosis / superimposed TB infection

√ bullous scr emphysema

√ pulmonry hypertension

PSEUDOLYMPHMA

= reactive benign lesion resembling lymphoma histologically without lymph node involvement
= localized form of lymphocytic interstitial pneumonitis (LIP); no progression to lymphoma

associated with: Sjögren syndrome

• mostly asymptomatic

√ well-demarcated dense infiltrate

√ infiltrate typically in central location extending to visceral pleura

√ prominent air bronchogram

√ NO lymadenopathy

Prognosis: occasionally progression to non-Hodgkin lymphoma

Rx: most patients respond well to steroids initially

PSEUDOMONAS PNEUMONIA

= mt dreaded nosocomial infectiobecause of resistance to antibiotics in patients with debilitating diseases on multiple antibiotics + corticosteroids; rare in community

Organism: Pseudomonas aeruginosa, Gram-negative

• bradycardia

• temperature with morning peaks

√ widespread patchy bronchopneumonia (secondary to bacteremia; unlike other Gram-negative pneumonias)

√ predilection for lower lobes

√ extensive bilateral consolidation

√ "sponge-like pattern" with multiple nodules >2 cm (= extensive necrosis with formation of multiple abscesses)

√ small pleural effusions

PULMONARY APLASIA

= rudimentary bronchus in blind pouch with absence of parenchyma + vessels

Agenesis = complete absence of tissue

Aplasia = bronchus without lung tissue

Hypoplasia = bronchus with rudimentary lung tissue

Incidence: 1:10,000; R:L = 1:1

Associated malformations:

1. Hypoplasia of contralateral lung
2. Diaphragmatic hernia
3. Surrounding calcified pleura

• asymptomatic

√ dense small hemithorax with marked mediastinal shift + herniation of contralateral lung

CT:

√ absence of ipsilateral pulmonary artery + bronchus ending blindly

√ absence of ipsilateral pulmonary tissue

PULMONARY ARTERIAL MALFORMATION

= PAVM = PULMONARY ARTERIOVENOUS ANEURYSM = PULMONARY ARTERIOVENOUS FISTULA = PULMONARY ANGIOMA = PULMONARY TELANGIECTASIA

= abnormal vascular communication between pulmonary artery and vein (95%) or systemic artery and pulmonary vein (5%)

Etiology:

(a) congenital defect of capillary structure

(b) acquired in cirrhosis (hepatogenic pulmonary angiodysplasia), cancer, trauma, surgery, actinomycosis, schistosomiasis

Path: hemangioma of cavernous type

Pathophysiology:

low-resistance extracardiac R-to-L shunt; quantification with Tc-99m labeled albumin microspheres by measuring fraction of dose reaching kidneys

Age: 3 – 4th decade; manifest in adult life, 10% in childhood

Occurrence:

(a) isolated abnormality (40%)

(b) associated with Rendu-Osler-Weber syndrome (in 30 – 88%) = hereditary hemorrhagic telangiectasia; only 15% of patients with Rendu-Osler-Weber disease have pulmonary AVMs

• family history

• epistaxis

• telangiectasia of skin / mucous membranes

• GI bleeding

Types:

1. Simple type (79%)

= single feeding artery empties into a bulbous nonseptated aneurysmal segment with a single draining vein

2. Complex type (21%)

= more than one feeding artery empties into septated aneurysmal segment with more than one draining vein

• asymptomatic in 56% (until 3 – 4th decade) if AVM single and <2 cm

• orthodeoxia (= increased hypoxemia with PaO_2 <85 mm Hg in erect position due to gravitational shift of pulmonary blood flow to base of lung)

• cyanosis with normal-sized heart (R-to-L shunt) in 25 – 50%, clubbing

• bruit over lesion (increased during inspiration)

• dyspnea on exertion (60 – 71%)

• epistaxis (79%)

• palpitation, chest pain

• No CHF

Location: lower lobes (65 – 70%) > middle lobe > upper lobes; medial third of lung; often subpleural; bilateral (8 – 20%)
√ sharply defined, lobulated oval / round mass (90%) of 1 to several cm in size ("coin lesion")
√ cordlike bands from mass to hilum (feeding artery + draining veins)
√ in 2/3 single lesion, in 1/3 multiple lesions
√ enlargement with advancing age
√ change in size with Valsalva / Mueller maneuver / erect vs. recumbent position (decrease with Valsalva maneuver)
√ phleboliths (occasionally)
√ increased pulsations of hilar vessels
CT (98% detection rate):
√ homogeneous circumscribed noncalcified nodule / serpiginous mass up to several cm in diameter
√ vascular connection of mass with enlarged feeding artery + draining vein
√ sequential enhancement of feeding artery + aneurysmal part + efferent vein on dynamic CT
MR: (if contraindication to contrast / slow flow due to partial thrombosis / follow-up)
√ signal void on standard spin echo / high sgnal intensity on GRASS images
Angio (diagnostic standard)

Cx: (1) Cerebrovascular accident: stroke (18%), transient ischemic attack (37%) secondary to paradoxical bland emboli
(2) Brain abscess (5 – 9%) secondary to loss of pulmonary filter function for septic emboli
(3) Hemoptysis (13%) secondary to rupture of PAVM into bronchus, most common presenting symptom
(4) Hemothorax (9%) secondary to rupture of subpleural PAVM
(5) Polycythemia

Prognosis: 26% morbidity, 11% mortality
DDx: solitary / multiple pulmonary nodules
Rx: embolization with coils / detachable balloons

PULMONARY CONTUSION
= most common manifestation of blunt chest trauma, esp. deceleration trauma
Path: exudation of edema + blood into air space + interstitium
Time of onset: apparent within 6 hours after trauma
• clinically inapparent
• hemoptysis (50%)

Location: directly deep to site of impact / contrecoup
√ irregular patchy / diffuse homogeneous extensive consolidation
√ opacity may enlarge for 48 – 72 hours
√ rapid resolution beginning 24 – 48 hours, complete within 2 – 10 days
√ overlying rib fractures (frequent)
DDx: fat embolism (1 – 2 days after injury)

PULMONARY HYPOPLASIA
= completely formed but small bronchus affecting one lobe / entire lung with rudimentary parenchyma + small vessels
Causes:
(a) Extrathoracic compression
1. Oligohydramnios
2. Fetal ascites
3. Membranous diaphragm
(b) Thoracic cage compression
1. Thoracic dystrophies
2. Muscular disease
(c) Intrathoracic compression
1. Diaphragmatic defect
2. Excess pleural fluid
3. Large intrathoracic cyst / tumor
(d) Primary hypoplasia
= idiopathic
• respiratory distress at birth
√ poorly expanded lungs
√ contralateral mediastinal shift (in unilateral process)

PULMONARY INTERSTITIAL EMPHYSEMA
= PIE = complication of respirator therapy with PEEP
Pathogenesis:
gas escapes from overdistended alveolus, dissects into perivascular sheath surrounding arteries, veins, and lymphatics, tracks into mediastinum forming clusters of blebs; **air block** = compression + obstruction of pulmonary veins + mediastinal structures by interstitial pulmonary emphysema / pneumomediastinum / pneumothorax (obstruction esp. during expiration)
• sudden deterioration in patient's condition during respiratory therapy
√ elongated lucencies following distribution of bronchovascular tree
√ circular densities
√ bilateral, symmetrical distribution
√ lobar overdistension (occasionally)

Cx: pneumomediastinum, pneumothorax, subcutaneous emphysema, pneumopericardium, intracardiac air, pneumoperitoneum, pneumatosis intestinalis

PULMONARY MAINLINE GRANULOMATOSIS
= pulmonary embolism in drug addicts from IV injection of oral medication
Drugs: amphetamines, methylphenidate hydrochloride ("West coast"), tripelennamine ('blue velvet'), methadone hydrochloride, dilaudid, meperidine, pentazocine, propylhexedrine, hydromorphone hydrochloride
Δ added talc (= magnesium silicate) particles incite a granulomatous foreign body reaction + subsequent fibrosis in perivascular distribution
• angiothrombotic pulmonary hypertension + cor pulmonale
√ widespread micronodularity of "pinpoint" size (1 mm) with perihilar / basilar predominance

√ loss of lung volume
√ coalescent opacities similar to progressive massive fibrosis (DDx: in silicosis away from hila)

PULMONARY THROMBOEMBOLIC DISEASE= PULMONARY EMBOLISM (PE)

Incidence: 600,000 cases/year; in 9 – 56% of deep venous thrombosis; diagnosed in 1% of all hospitalized patients; in 12 – 64% at autopsy
Age peak: >70 years
Cause: deep vein thrombosis (DVT)

Pathophysigy:
Class 1 = <20% of pulmonary arteries occluded
  • asymptomatic
  • normal arterial blood gas levels
  • normal pulmonary + systemic hemodynamics
Class 2 = 20 – 30% of pulmonary arteries occlude
  • anxiety, hyperventilation
  • arterial PO_2 <80 torr
  • PCO_2 <35 torr
Class 3 = 30 – 50% of pulmonary arteries occluded
  • dyspnea, collapse
  • arterial PO_2 <65 torr
  • arterial PCO_2 <30 torr
  • elevated central venous pressure
Class 4 = >50% of pulmonary arteries occluded
  • shock, dyspnea
  • arterial PO_2 <50 torr
  • arterial PCO_2 <30 torr
  • elevated central venous pressure
  • mean PA pressure >20 mm Hg
  • systolic blood pressure <100 mm Hg

• Classic triad (<33%):
  (1) hemoptysis (25 – 34%) (2) pleural friction rub (3) thrombophlebitis
  Δ only 10 – 33% of patients with fatal PE are symptomatic for DVT
  Δ DVT diagnosed ante mortem in <30%
  Δ clinically suspected diagnosis accurate in 26 – 45%
  Δ 30% of patients with angiographically detected PE have negative bilateral venograms ("big bang" theory = clot embolizes in toto to lung leaving no residual in leg veins)
• may be asymptomatic
• false-positive clinical diagnosis in 62%
• dyspnea (81 – 86%)
• pleuritic chest pain (58 – 72%)
• apprehension (59%)
• cough (54 – 70%)
• tachycardia, tachypnea
• accentuated 2nd heart sound
• ECG changes (83%), mostly nonspecific
• bronchospasm (histamine-mediated), bronchial plugging, rales (loss of surfactant)

Sites of PE: lower lobes (>50%), upper lobes (10%); bilateral (42%); multiple (65%)

RESOLUTION OF PE
(through thrombolysis + fragmentation):
in 8% by 24 hours, in 56% by 14 days, in 77% by 7 months; complete in 65%, partial in 23%, no resolution in 12%
Δ Resolution less favorable with increasing age + cardiac disease
Δ Resolution improved with urokinase > heparin within first week (after 1 year 80% for both)

A. EMBOLISM WITHOUT INFARCTION (90%)
  Histo: hemorrhage + edema
  √ normal chest film common (>29%), abnormal CXR in 40 – 93%
  √ platelike atelectasis
  √ focal oligemia (vasoconstriction) distal to embolus (Westermark sign in 2%)
  √ "knuckle sign" = abrupt tapering of an occluded vessel distally
  √ local widening of artery by impaction of embolus
  √ segmental / lobar consolidation
  √ pleural effusion

B. EMBOLISM WITH INFARCTION (10 – 15%)
  = any opacity developing as a result of thromboembolic disease; more likely to develop in presence of cardiopulmonary disease with obstruction of pulmonary venous outflow (diagnosed in retrospect)
  Histo: (1) reversible hemorrhagic congestion
       (2) hemorrhagic infarction with necrosis

  √ segmentally distributed wedge-shaped consolidation (54%)
  √ ± cavitation
  √ Hampton hump = pleural-based shallow consolidation in form of a truncated cone with base against pleural surface
  √ pleural effusion (54%)
  √ thoracentesis: bloody (65%), predominantly PMNs (61%), exudate (65%)
  √ NO air-bronchogram (hemorrhage into alveoli)
  √ "melting sign" = within few days to weeks regression from periphery toward center
  √ Fleischner lines = long-line shadows (fibrotic scar) from invagination of pleura at the base of the collapse resulting in pseudofissure
  √ platelike atelectasis (27%)
  √ cardiomegaly / CHF (17%)
  √ elevated hemidiaphragm (17%)
  √ subsequent nodular / linear scar

CT:
  √ pleural-based triangular appearance of lesion
  √ vascular connection to a branch of pulmonary artery
  √ peripheral rim-like contrast enhancement
NUC (V/Q scan = guide for angiographic evaluation)
  √ V/Q scans interpreted in reference to Biello or PIOPED criteria (see page 662)

Angio (indicated within 24 hours of indeterminate NUC scan):
- √ intraluminal defect (94%)
- √ abrupt termination of pulmonary arterial branch
- √ pruning + attenuation of branches
- √ wedge-shaped parenchymal hypovascularity
- √ absence of draining vein in affected segment
- √ tortuous arterial collaterals

Cx of pulmonary angiography (4%): arrhythmia, endocardial injury, cardiac perforation, cardiac arrest, contrast reaction

Mortality: 3:1,000 surgical procedures; 7% of all autopsies; 26% if untreated; 8% if treated; fatal if >60% o pulmonary bed obstructed
Fatality rate: 0.2%
Rx:
1. Heparin IV: 10,000 – 15,000 units as initial dose; 8,000 – 10,000 units/hour during diagnostic evaluation; continued for 10 – 14 days
2. Streptokinase: better results with massive PE
3. Urokinase: slightly etter than streptokinase
4. Coumadin: maintained for at least 3 months

Acute thromoembolic pulmonary arterial hypertension
Hypertension disappears as emboli lyse
- sudden onset of chest pain
- acute dyspnea
- hemoptysis occasionally
Prognosis: healthy patients may survive obstruction of 50 – 60% of vascular bed

Chronic thromboembolic pulmonary arterial hypertension
- history of previous embolic episodes
- may be clinically silent

PULMONARY VARIX
= abnormal tortuosity + dilatation of pulmonary vein just before entrance into left atrium
Etiology: congenital / associated with pulmonary venous hypertension
Location: medial third of either lung below hila
- √ well-defined lobulated round / oval mass
- √ change in size during Valsalva / Mueller maneuver

RADIATION PNEUMONITIS
= damage to lungs following radiation therapy dependent on:
(a) irradiated lung volume
(b) radiation dose: unusual if <2000 R given in 2 – 3 weeks; common if >6000 R given in 5 – 6 weeks
(c) fractionation of dose
(d) concurrent / later chemotherapy
Pathologic phases:
(1) Exudative phase = edema fluid + hyaline membranes
(2) Organizing phase

(3) Fibrotic phase = interstitial fibrosis
Time of onset: usually 4 – 6 months after treatment
Location: confined to radiation port

1. ACUTE RADIATION PNEUMONITIS
(within 1 – 8 weeks after radiation therapy)
Path: depletion of surfactant (1 week to 1 month later), plasma exudation, desquamation of alveolar + bronchial cells
- asymptomatic (majority)
- nonproductive cough, shortness of breath, weakness, fever (insidious onset)
- acute respiratory failure (rare)
- √ changes usually within portal entry fields
- √ patchy / confluent consolidation, may persist up to 1 month (exudative reaction)
- √ atelectasis + air bronchogram
- √ spontaneous pneumothorax (rare)
CT:
- √ homogeneous slight increase in attenuation (2 – 4 months after therapy)
- √ patchy consolidation (1 – 12 months after therapy)
- √ nonuniform discrete consolidation (most common; 3 months to 10 years after therapy)
Prognosis: recovery / progression to death / fibrosis
Rx: steroids

2. CHRONIC RADIATION DAMAGE
(9 – 12 months after radiation therapy)
Histo: permanent damage of endothelial + type I alveolar cells
May be associated with:
(1) thymic cyst
(2) calcified lymph nodes (in Hodgkin disease)
(3) pericarditis + effusion (within 3 years)
- √ severe loss of volume
- √ dense fibrous strands from hilum to periphery
- √ thickening of pleura
- √ pericardial effusion
CT:
- √ solid consolidation (radiation fibrosis) + bronchiectasis (stabilized by 1 year after therapy)

RESPIRATORY DISTRESS SYNDROME OF NEWBORN
= RDS = HYALINE MEMBRANE DISEASE
= acute pulmonary disorder characterized by generalized atelectasis, intrapulmonary shunting, ventilation-perfusion abnormalities, reduced lung compliance
Cause:
immature surfactant production (usually begins at 18 – 20 weeks of gestational age) causing acinar atelectasis + dilatation of terminal airways
Predisposed:
perinatal asphyxia, cesarean section, infants of diabetic mothers, premature infants (<1000 g in 66%; 1000 g in 50%; 1500 g in 16%; 2000 g in 5%; 2500 g in 1%)
Onset: <2 – 5 hours after birth, increasing in severity from 24 to 48 hours, gradual improvement after 48 – 72 hours; M:F = 1.8:1

- abnormal retraction of chest wall
- cyanosis (carbon dioxide retention)
- expiratory grunting
- increased respiratory rate

√ hypoaeration with loss of lung volume (counteracted by respirator therapy)
√ reticulogranular pattern (coincides with onset of clinical signs)
√ prominent air bronchograms (distension of compliant airways)
√ bilateral + symmetrical distribution
Prognosis: spontaneous clearing within 7 – 10 days (mild course in untreated survivors); death in 18%

ACUTE COMPLICATIONS
(a) Barotrauma with air-block phenomena
1. Parenchymal pseudocyst
2. Pulmonary interstitial emphysema
3. Pneumomediastinum, -thorax, -pericardium, -peritoneum -retroperitoneum
4. Subcutaneous emphysema
5. as embolism
(b) Diffuse opacity
1. Worsening RDS
2. Superimposed pneumonia
3. Massive aspiration
4. Pulmonary hemorrhage
5. Congestive heart failure (PDA, fluid overload)
(c) Persistent patency of ductus arteriosus
oxygen stimulus is missing to close duct; gradual decrease in pulmonary resistance (by end of 1st week) leads to L-to-R shunt through PDA
(d) Hemorrhage
1. Pulmonary hemorrhage
2. Intracranial hemorrhage
(e) Necrotizing enterocolitis
(f) Acute renal failure

CHRONIC COMPLICATIONS
1. Lobar emphysema
2. Localized interstitial emphysema
3. Delayed onset of diaphragmatic hernia
4. Recurrent inspiratory tract infections
5. Hyperinflation
6 Bronchopulmonary dysplasia (10 – 20%)
7. Retrolental fibroplasia
8. Subglottic stenosis (intubation)

Rx: exogenous surfactant intratracheally

RHEUMATOID LUNG
Type III hypersensitivity = delayed hypersensitivity
= immune complex disease
= formation of antigen-antibody complexes with complement fixation
Incidence: 2 – 54% of patients with rheumatoid arthritis; M >> F
(incidence of rheumatoid arthritis: M < F)

- rheumatoid arthritis
- subcutaneous nodules
- rheumatoid factor = IgM-antibody (positive in most) (DDx: in 5% of normals, in 25% of asbestos workers with fibrosing alveolitis)
- antinuclear antibodies (positive in many)
- LE cells (positive in some)
Stage 1: multifocal ill-defined alveolar infiltrates
Stage 2: fine interstitial reticulations (histio- and lymphocytes)
Stage 3: honeycombing

A. Pleural abnormalities (most frequent manifestation)
- Hx of pleurisy (21%)
√ pleural effusion (3%): unilateral (92%), with little change over months; M:F = 9:1; most often without other pulmonary changes, may antedate rheumatoid arthritis
- high in protein content (>4 g/dl)
- low in sugar content (<30 mg/dl) without rise during glucose infusion (75%)
- high in lymphocytes
- positive for rheumatoid factor, LDH, RA cells
√ pleural thickening, usually bilateral

B. Diffuse interstitial fibrosis (30%)
- restrictive ventilatory defect
Location: lower lung fields
√ punctate / nodular densities (mononuclear cell infiltrates in early stage)
√ reticulonodular densities
√ medium to coarse reticulations (mature fibrous tissue in later stage)
√ honeycomb lung (uncommon in late stage)

C. Necrobiotic nodules (rare)
= well-circumscribed nodular mass in lung, pleura, pericardium identical to subcutaneous nodules associated with advanced rheumatoid arthritis
Path: central zone of fibrinoid necrosis surrounded by palisading fibroblasts
Associated with interstitial lung disease
√ well-circumscribed usually multiple nodules of 3 – 70 mm in size
√ commonly located in lung periphery
√ cavitation with thick symmetric walls + smooth inner lining (common)

D. Caplan syndrome
= RHEUMATOID PNEUMOCONIOSIS
= pneumoconiosis + rheumatoid arthritis in coal workers with rheumatoid disease;
= hypersensitivity reaction to irritating dust particles in lungs of rheumatoid patients
Incidence: 2 – 6% of all men affected by pneumoconioses
Path: disintegrating macrophages deposit a pigmented ring of dust surrounding the central necrotic core + zone of fibroblasts palisading the zone of necrosis

Δ NOT necessarily evidence of long-standing pneumoconiosis
- concomitant with joint manifestation (most frequent) / may precede arthritis by several years
- concomitant with systemic rheumatoid nodules
√ rapidly developing well-defined nodules of 5 – 50 mm in size with a tendency to appear in crops predominantly in upper lobes + in periphery of lung
√ nodules may remain unchaned / increase in number / calcify
√ background of pneumoconiosis
√ pleural effusion (may occur)

E. Pulmonary arteritis
= fibroelastoid intimal proliferation of pulmonary arteries
- pulmonary arterial hypertension
- cor pulmonale

F. Obliterative bronchitis — may be transient

G. Cardiac enlargement (pericarditis + carditis / congestive heart failure)

ROUND PNEUMONIA
= NUMMULAR PNEUMONIA = fairly spherical pneumonia caused by pyogenic organisms
Organism: Haemophilus influnzae, Streptococcus, Pneumococcus
Age: children >> adults
- cough, chest pain, fever
Location: always posterior, usually in lower lobes
√ spherical infiltrate with slightly fluffy borders + air bronchogram
√ triangular infiltrate abutting a pleural surface (usually seen on lateral view)
√ rapid change in size and shape

SARCOIDOSIS
= BOECK SARCOID = immunologically mediated widespread formation of noncaseating granulomas of unknown etiology
Prevalence: 1:10,000
Age peak: 20 – 40 years; M:F = 1:3; Blacks:Caucasians = 14:1
- angiotensin-converting enzyme (ACE) elevated in 70%
- hypercalcemia in 2 – 15% from enhanced sensitivity to vitamin D
- Kveim test positive (70%), rarely used today
- functional impairment: VC + FRC reduced, diffusing capacity decreased, reduction in compliance (even with NO radiographic abnormality)

A. ACUTE FORM = **Löfgren Syndrome**
bilateral hilar adenopathy + fever (17%), erythema nodosum (13%), arthralgia of large joints

B. CHRONIC FORM
- asymptomatic (50%)
- fever, malaise, weight loss

- dry cough + shortness of breath (25%)
- hemoptysis in 4% (from endobronchial lesion / vascular erosion / cavitation)

Prognosis:
75% complete resolution of hilar adenopathy
33% complete resolution of parenchymal disease
30% improve significantly
20% irreversible pulmonary fibrosis (may persist unchanged for >15 years)
10% mortality (cor pulmonale / CNS / lung fibrosis / liver cirrhosis)
25% relapse (in 50% detected by CXR)

@ Bone (6 – 15%)   : √ phalangeal sclerosis of hands
                       √ lytic cystic lesions with lacelike trabecular pattern
@ Liver   (25 – 70%): √ hepatomegaly
                       √ scattered nodular lesions
@ Spleen   (25 – 70%): √ splenomegaly
                       √ scattered nodular lesions
@ Stomach   : √ polypoid / nodular mass ± ulcer
                       √ loss of antral compliance
@ Skin   (10 – 60%): erythema nodosum, lupus pernio (slightly raised purplish nodules)
@ Muscle   (25%)   : myopathy
@ Eyes   (10 – 25%): uveitis
@ Myocardium (6 – 20%): paroxysmal arrhythmia, heart block, cardiomyopathy
@ CNS   (9%)   : hypothalamus, basal granulomatous meningitis, facial nerve palsy
@ Salivary gland (4%): bilateral parotid enlargement
@ Involved peripheral lymph nodes (30%)

@ THORACIC DISEASE (90%)
Associated with tuberculosis in up to 13%
— adenopathy alone (43%)
— adenopathy + parenchymal disease (41%)
— parenchymal disease alone (16%)
√ intrathoracic lymphadenopathy (80%)
Location:
  (a) "1-2-3 sign" = Garland triad = right paratracheal, right + left hilar groups most frequent combination (in 75 – 90%)
  (b) unilateral hilar enlargement (3 – 8%)
  (c) mediastinal nodes are regularly enlarged on CT
Prognosis:
  adenopathy commonly decreases as parenchymal disease gets worse; subsequent parenchymal disease in 32%; adenopathy does not develop subsequent to parenchymal disease
√ eggshell calcification of lymph nodes (5%) in long-standing sarcoidosis >10 years
√ parenchymal disease (60%); without adenopathy in 16 – 20%
Δ Parenchymal granulomas are invariably present on open lung biopsy!
Site: predominantly mid-zone involvement

√ reticulonodular pattern (46%)
√ acinar pattern (20%) = ill-defined 6 – 7 mm
  opacities / coalescence
√ "alveolar / acinar sarcoidosis" = multiple large
  nodules >10 mm (2 – 10%) ± air bronchogram
  (coalescence of numerous interstitial granulomas)
√ progressive fibrosis with upper lobe retraction +
  bullae (20%)
√ endstage lung (11%)

ATYPICAL MANIFESTATIONS (25%):
  √ pleural effusion (2%) = exudate with predominance
    of lymphocytes
  √ focal pleural thickening
  √ solitary / multiple pulmonary nodules
  √ cavitation of nodules (0.6%)
  √ mycetoma formation (common complication of
    advanced sarcoidosis)
  √ isolated hilar / mediastinal nodal enlargement
  √ bronhostenosis (2% with lobar / segmental
    atelectasis
  √ pulmonary arterial hypertension (periarterial
    granulomatosis without extensive pulmonary
    fibrosis)

Cx: √ pneumothorax secondary to chronic lung
          fibrosis (rare)
        √ cardiomegaly from cor pulmonale (rare)

ASSESSMENT OF ACTIVITY
(1) ACE titer (= angiotensin I converting enzyme)
(2) Bronchopulmonary lavage: 20 – 50% lymphocytes
     with number of T-suppressor lymphocytes 4 – 20
     times above normal
(3) Gallium scan
     √ uptake in lymph nodes + lung parenchyma +
       salivary glands (correlates with alveolitis +
       disease activity); monitor of therapeutic response
       (indicator of macrophage activity)

SCLERODERMA
= PROGRESSIVE SYSTEMIC SCLEROSIS = PSS
= collagen disease characterized by atrophy + sclerosis of
  many organ systems
Age: 4 – 6th decade; M:F = 1:3

• thickened inelastic waxy skin most prominent about face
  + extremities
• slightly productive cough + progressive dyspnea
• rheumatoid factor (35%)
• LE cells (5%)
• antinuclear antibodies (30 – 80%)

@ Pulmonary involvement (evident in 10 – 25%):
  Histo: thickening of basement membrane of alveoli
             + small arteries and veins
  • pulmonary function abnormalities in the absence of
    frank roentgenographic changes (typical
    dissociation of clinical, functional, and radiologic
    evidence)

Location: most prominent at lung bases (where
              blood flow greatest)
√ fine / coarse reticulations / diffuse interstitial
  infiltrates
√ alveolar changes (secondary to aspiration from
  disturbed esophageal motility)
√ formation of subpleural fibrocystic spaces
  (honeycombing)
√ progressive volume loss
√ air esophagogram (DDx: achalasia, mediastinitis)
√ pleural reaction / effusion distinctly uncommon
Cx: increased incidence of lung cancer
@ Gastrointestinal tract
  √ esophageal dilatation + aperistalsis (>50%)
  √ hiatus hernia + GE reflux + esophagitis + distal
    esophageal stricture
  √ irregular dilatation + disturbed motility of small +
    large bowel
  √ pseudosacculations in colon
@ Musculoskeletal
  • arthralgia (50 – 80%)
  • Raynaud phenomenon
  √ resorption of distal phalanges of hand (63%)
  √ arthritis of interphalangeal joints of hands (25%)
  √ calcinosis of finger tips + over pressure areas
    (elbows)
  √ erosion of superior aspect of ribs
@ Heart: sclerosis of cardiac muscle ± cor pulmonale
@ Renal involvement (25%)

PROGRESSIVE SYSTEMIC SCLEROSIS (PSS) divided
into:
A. DIFFUSE SCLERODERMA
    interstitial pulmonary fibrosis common
B. CREST: vasculitis with pulmonary arterial
    hypertension; more common
    Calcinosis of skin
    Raynaud phenomenon
    Esophageal dysmotility
    Sclerodactyly
    Telangiectasia

Prognosis: 50 – 67% 5-year survival rate

SEPTIC PULMONARY EMBOLI
= lodgement of an infected thrombus in a pulmonary
  artery
Organism: S. aureus, Streptococcus
Predisposed: IV drug abusers, alcoholism,
                immunodeficiency, CHD, dermal
                infection (cellulitis, carbuncles)
Source:
(a) infected venous catheter / pacemaker wires,
     arteriovenous shunts for hemodialysis, drug abuse
     producing septic thrombophlebitis (eg, heroin
     addicts), pelvic thrombophlebitis, peritonsillar
     abscess, osteomyelitis
(b) tricuspid valve endocarditis (most common cause in
     IV drug abusers)
Age: majority <40 years

- sepsis, cough, dyspnea, chest pain
- shaking chills, high fever, severe sinus tachycardia

Location: predilection for lung bases
√ multiple nondescript pulmonary infiltrates (initially)
√ migratory infiltrates (old ones heal, new ones appear)
√ cavitation (frequent), usually thin-walled
√ pleural effusion (rare)
CT (more sensitive than CXR):
   √ multiple peripheral parenchymal nodules ± cavitation / air bronchogram (83%)
   √ wedge-shaped subpleural lesion with apex of lesion directed toward pulmonary hilum (50%)
   √ feeding vessel sign = pulmonary artery leading to nodule (67%)
   √ cavitation (50%), esp. in staphylococcal emboli
   √ air bronchogram within pulmonary nodule (28%)
Cx: empyema (39%)

SIDEROSIS
= inert iron oxide / metallic iron deposits
Path: iron phagocytosed by macroges in alveoli / respiratory bronchioles, elimination from lung by lymphatic circulation
Occupational exposure:
   arc welding, cutting / burning of steel, foundry workers, grinders, fettlers, polishers (jewelry industry)

√ reticulonodular pattern (may disappear after exposure discontinued)
√ small round opacities (indistinguishable from silica / coal)
√ NO secondary fibrosis + NO hilar adenopathy (unless mixed dust inhalation as in sidero-silicosis)

SILICOSIS
= inhalation of silicon dioxide; most prevalent silicosis of progressive nature after termination of exposure; similar to CWP (because of silica component in CWP)

Substance: Crystalline silica (quartz); one of the most widespread elements on earth
Occupational exposure: tunneling, mining, quarrying, sandblasting, ceramic industry

Path: small particles engulfed by macrophages; liberation of silica results in cell death; 2 – 3 mm nodules with layers of laminated connective tissue around smaller vessels

A. ACUTE SILICOPROTEINOSIS
   = acute silicosis of sandblasters; exposure may be <1 year
   Associated with   increased risk to develop autoimmune disease
   √ diffuse air space disease

B. CHRONIC SIMPLE SILICOSIS
   At least 10 – 20 years of dust exposure before appearance of roentgenographic abnormality

√ small 1 – 10 mm rounded opacities, beginning in upper + middle lung zones
√ may calcify centrally in 5 – 10% (rather typical for silicosis)
√ hilar lymphadenopathy, may calcify in 5% ("eggshell pattern")
√ ± reticulonodular pattern
HRCT:
   √ nodules of 3 – 10 mm in size
   √ thickened intra- and interlobular lines
   √ subpleural curvilinear lines (peribronchiolar fibrosis)
   √ ground-glass pattern = mild thickening of alveolar wall + interlobular septa (fibrosis / edema)
   √ parenchymal fibrous bands
   √ pleura-based nodular irregularities
   √ traction bronchiectasis
   √ honeycombing

C. COMPLICATED SILICOSIS
   √ conglomerate masses of nonsegmental distribution in middle + upper lung zones
   √ progressive massive fibrosis = sausage-shaped masses with ill-defined margins (in advanced stages)
   √ compensatory emphysema in unaffected portion
   √ slow change over years
   √ may cavitate

D. SILICOTUBERCULOSIS
   Doubtful synergistic relationship between silicosis + tuberculosis
   √ little change over years with intermittently positive sputa

E. CAPLAN SYNDROME
   More common in coal worker's pneumoconiosis

Cx: predisposes to tuberculosis

SJÖGREN SYNDROME
= MYOEPITHELIAL SIALADENITIS
= poorly understood chronic systemic inflammatory disorder of unknown etiology characterized by dryness of mucous membranes

A. PRIMARY SJÖGREN SYNDROME
   without underlying systemic autoimmune disease
   (a) recurrent parotitis in children
   (b) SICCA SYNDROME = Mikulicz disease
      = xerophthalmia + xerostomia

B. SECONDARY SJÖGREN SYNDROME
   Associated with:
   (a) connective tissue diseases
      1. Rheumatoid arthritis (55%)
      2. Systemic lupus erythematosus (2%)
      3. Progressive systemic sclerosis (0.5%)
      4. Psoriatic arthritis, primary biliary cirrhosis (0.5%)

  (b) lymphoproliferative disorders
    1. Lymphocytic interstitial pneumonitis (LIP)
    2. Pseudolymphoma
    3. Lymphoma (44 x increased risk)
    4. Waldenström macroglobulinemia

Mean age: 57 years; M:F = 1:9
Path: benign lymphoepithelioma = lymphoid
   infiltrates in lacrimal glands, mucous glands of
   conjunctivae, nasal cavity, pharynx, larynx,
   trachea, bronchi

- Xerophthalmia = dryness of eyes
  = keratoconjunctivitis sicca = desiccation of cornea +
  conjunctiva
- Xerostomia dryness of mouth + lips from diminished
  saliva
- Xerorhinia = dryness of nose
- Swelling of parotid gland: usually unilateral, recurrent

CXR:
 √ reticulonodular pattern (3 – 33%)
 √ patchy consolidation + atelectasis
 √ pneumonitis (secondaryto dryness of respitory
  tract)
 √ ± pleural effusion
Sialogram:
 √ nonobstructive punctate / globular / cavitary
  sialectasia (ducts + acini destroyed by lymphocytic
  infiltrates / infection)
US of parotid gland:
 √ multiple scattered cysts bilaterally
MR:
 √ inhomogeneous pittd honeycomblike iternal
 pattern (= areas of low intensity between nodular
 parenchyma of high signal intensity) on T2WI / Gd-
 enhanced T1WI

STAPHYLOCOCCAL PNEUMONIA
Most common cause of bronchopneumonia
 (a) common nosocomial infection (patients on antibiotic
   drugs most susceptible)
 (b) accounts for 5% of community-acquired
   pneumonias (esp. in infants + elderly)
Δ secondary invader to influenza (commonest cause of
 death during influenza epidemics)

Organism: Staphylococcus aureus, Gram-positive,
     appears in clusters, coagulase-producing

√ rapid spread through lungs
√ empyema (esp. in children)
√ pneumothorax, pyopneumothorax
√ abscess formation
√ bronchopleural fistula

A. in CHILDREN:
 √ rapidly developing lobar / multilobar consolidation
 √ pleural effusion (90%)
 √ pneumatocele (40 – 60%)

B. in ADULTS:
 √ patchy often confluent bronchopneumonia of
  segmental distribution, bilateral in >60%
 √ segmental collapse (air bronchograms absent)
 √ late development of thick-walled lung abscess
  (25 – 75%)
 √ pleural effusion / empyema (50%) (DDx from other
  pneumonias)

Cx: meningitis, metastatic abscess to brain / kidneys,
   acute endocarditis

STREPTOCOCCAL PNEUMONIA
Incidence: 1 – 5% of bacterial pneumonias (rarely
     seen); most common in winter months
Organism: Group A ß-hemolytic streptococcus
     = Streptococcus pyogenes, Gram-positive
     cocci appearing in chains
Predisposed: newborns, following infection with measles
Associated with: delayed onset of diaphragmatic hernia
       (in newborns)
- rarely follows tonsillitis + pharyngitis
√ patchy bronchopneumonia
√ lower lobe predominance (similar to staphylococcus)
√ empyema
Cx: (1) Residual pleural thickening (15%)
  (2) Bronchiectasis
  (3) Lung abscess
  (4) Glomerulonephritis

SWYER-JAMES SYNDROME
= MACLEOD SYNDROME
= UNILATERAL LOBAR EMPHYSEMA
= IDIOPATHIC UNILATERAL HYPERLUCENT LUNG
Etiology: probably childhood adenoviral infection with
    acute obliterative bronchiolitis, bronchiectasis,
    distal air space destruction (develops in
    7 – 30 months)
- asymptomatic
- dyspnea on exertion
- history of repeated lower respiratory tract infections
  during childhood

Location: one / both lungs (usually entire lung,
     occasionally lobar / subsegmental)
√ increased radiolucency of affected lung
√ small hemithorax with decreased / normal volume
 (collateral air drift)
√ air trapping (expiration radiograph!)
 DDx: no air trapping with proximal interruption of
    pulmonary artery (no hilum), hypogenetic lung
    syndrome, pulmonary embolus
√ mild cylindrical bronchiectasis with paucity of bronchial
 subdivisions (cut-off at 4 – 5th generation = "pruned
 tree" bronchogram)
√ small ipsilateral hilum (diminuted hilar vessels +
 attenuated arteries)
√ diminutive pulmonary vasculature
Angio:
 √ "pruned tree appearance"

NUC:
- √ decreased perfusion
- √ decreased ventilation + delayed washout

SYSTEMIC LUPUS ERYTHEMATOSUS

= most prevalent of the potentially grave collagen diseases characterized by involvement of vascular system, skin, serous + synovial membranes (type III immune complex phenomenon)

Incidence: 1:2,000; Blacs:Caucasians = 3:1
*Age:*women in child-bear age; M:F = 1:10

- chronic fse-positive Wasserman test for syphilis (24%)
- LE cells (= antigen-antibody complexes engulfed by PMNs) in 78%
- Sjögren syndrome (frequent)
- antinuclear DNA antibodies (87%)
- hypergammaglobulinemia (77%)
- positive rheumatoid factor (21%)
- anemia (78%)
- leukopenia (66%)
- thrombocytopenia (19%)

@ Skin changes (81%)
- "butterfly rash" (= facial erythema), discoid lupus erythematosus, alopecia, photosensitivity
- Raynaud phenomenon (15%)

@ Thoracic involvement (30 – 70%)
- dyspnea, pleuritic chest pain (35%)
- (a) Pulmonary changes
  - √ Lupus pneumonitis (acute form) = poorly defined patchy areas of increased density peripherally at lung bases (alveolar pattern) secondary to infection / uremia in 10%
  - √ interstitial reticulations in lower lung fields (chronic form) in 3%
  - √ fleeting patelike atelectasis in both bases (? infarction due to vasculitis)
  - √ cavitating nodules (vasculitis)
  - √ elevated sluggish diaphragms (progressive volume loss)
  - √ hilar + mediastinal lymphadenopathy (extremely rare)
- (b) Pleural changes (most common manifestation)
  - √ recurrent bilateral pleural effusions (70%) from pleuritis
  - √ pleural thickening
- (c) Cardiovascular changes
  - √ pericardial effusion (from pericarditis)
  - √ cardiomegaly (primary lupus cardiomyopathy)

@ Joints
- arthralgia (95%)
- √ arthritis without deformity

@ Abdomen
- renal failure (fibrinoid thickening of basement membrane)
- √ splenomegaly

Prognosis: 60 – 90% 10-year survival; death from renal failure / CNS involvement / myocardial infarction

DRUG-INDUCED LUPUS ERYTHEMATOSUS = DIL

(temporary phenomenon):
Agents: procainamide, hydralazine, isoniazid, phenytoin account for 90%
- √ pulmonary + pleural disease more common than in SLE

TALCOSIS

= prolonged inhalation of magnesium silicate dust containing amphibole fibers (tremolite and anthophyllite) and silica

Talcosis resembles:
- (1) Asbestosis (indistinguishable)
  - √ massive and bizarre pleural plaques
  - √ may encase lung with calcification
- (2) Silicosis
  - √ small rounded + large opacities
  - √ fibrogenic process (NO regression after removal of patient from exposure)

TERATOID TUMOR OF MEDIASTINUM

= GERM CELL NEOPLASM = arising from primordial germ cells

Age: 20 – 40 years, may be present at birth; M:F = 1:1.5
Incidence: 10 – 15% of all mediastinal tumors; 16 – 28% of all mediastinal cysts
Δ Occurs in same frequency as the usually larger thymoma
Δ 1/3 of primary neoplasms in this area are in children

- sebaceous material, hair, teeth
Physiologic activity:
- thyroid hormone
- alpha fetoprotein
- hCG (may be associated with gynecomastia)
- amylase
- insulin

Location: 5% of all teratomas occur in mediastinum; mediastinum is 3rd most common site for teratoid lesions (after gonadal + sacrococcygeal location); posterior mediastinal location in only 1%
√ often inseparable from thymus gland

A. BENIGN TERATOID TUMOR (80 – 86%)
1. Epidermoid = ectodermal derivatives (52%)
2. Dermoid = ecto- + mesodermal derivatives (27%)
3. Teratoma = ecto- + meso- + endodermal derivatives (21%)
- √ well-demarcated smooth mass bulging into right / left hemithorax
- √ contains densities of fat, water, soft tissue, calcium, bone, teeth
- √ may be homogeneous (indistinguishable from lymphoma / thymoma)

√ calcifications (25 – 40%); 4 x more common in benign lesions
√ often inseparable from thymic gland

B. MALIGNANT TERATID TUMOR (14 – 20%)
1. Choriocarcinoma
2. Seminoma (most common)
3. Embryonal carcinoma
4 Yolk sac / endodermal sinus tumr
5. Mixed germ cell tumor
6. Teratocarcinoma
M > F
√ lobulation suggests malignancy
√ invasion of mediastinal structures (SVC obstruction is ominous)
Δ Absence of primary testicular tumor / retroperitoneal mass proves primary!

Cx:
(1) Hemorrhage
(2) Pneumothorax (from bronchial obstruction with air trapping + alveolar rupture)
(3) Respiratory distress (rapid increase in size from fluid production) with compression of trachea / SVC
(4) Fistula formation to aorta, SVC, esophagus
(5) Rupture into bronchus (trichoptysis in 5 – 14%), pericardium, pleural cavity

THYMIC CYST
Incidence: 1 – 2% of mediastinal tumors
Etiology:
(1) Congenital cyst (persistent tubular remnants of 3rd pharyngeal pouch, develops during 5th – 8th week of gestation)
(2) Inflammatory cyst
(3) Neoplastic cyst (cytic teratoma, cystic degeneration within a thymoma), S/P radiation therapy for Hodgkin disease
Associated with
(1) Hodgkin disease (? thymic involvement / treatment-induced cystic degeneration)
(2) myasthenia gravis (rare)
• commonly asymptomatic
• symptomatic when hemorrhage occurs

Location: anterior mediastinum / lateral neck
√ multiloculated
√ may show partial wall calcification (rare)
√ low-density fluid (0 – 10 HU), may be higher depending on cyst contents
US: √ typically anechoic

DDx: Benign thymoma, teratoma, dermoid cyst, Hodgkin disease, non-Hodgkin lymphoma, pleural fibroma

THYMIC HYPERPLASIA
Most common anterior mediastinal mass in pediatric age group through puberty
Age: particular in young individual

Histo: numerous active lymphoid germinal centers
Etiology: hyperthyroidism (most common), treatment of primary hypothyroidism, idiopathic thyromegaly, Graves disease, myasthenia gravis (65%), rebound growth in children recovering from stress (eg, from burns), acromegaly, Addison disease

√ normal thymus visible in 50% of neonates 0 – 2 years of age
√ notch sign = indentation at junction of thymus + heart
√ sail sign = triangular density extending from superior mediastinum
√ wave sign = rippled border due to indentation from ribs
√ shape changes with respiration + position

THYMOLIPOMA
Incidence: 2 – 9% of thymic tumors; M > F
Histo: well-encapsulated benign adult adipose tissue interspersed with areas of normal / hyperplastic / atrophic thymus tissue

√ grows downward from cardiac base bilaterally, envelops heart
√ may be very large with enlargement of cardiac silhouette (68% >500 g, may weigh up to 3000 g)
√ NO compression / invasion of adjacent structures

THYMOMA
Most common primary neoplasm of anterior superior mediastinum

Age: majority >40 years; 70% occur in 5th – 6th decade; less frequent in young adults, rare in children; M:F = 1:1

Associated with: parathymic syndromes (40%) such as
• **Myasthenia gravis**:
  = neuromuscular disorder characterized by weakness + fatigability of skeletal muscles (from antibodies against acetylcholine receptors)
  Δ 15 – 25% of patients with myasthenia gravis have a thymoma (in 65% due to thymic hyperplasia)
  Δ 7 – 54% of patients with thymoma have myasthenia gravis; removal of thymic tumor often results in symptomatic improvement; myasthenia gravis may develop after surgical excision of a thymoma
• Pure red cell aplasia = aregenerative anemia
  = almost total absence of marrow erythroblasts + blood reticulocytes resulting in severe normochromic normocytic anemia
  Δ 50% of patients with red cell aplasia have thymoma
  Δ 5% of patients with thymoma have red cell aplasia
• Acquired hypogammaglobulinemia
  Δ 5% of patients with hypogammaglobulinemia have thymoma
  Δ 10% of patients with thymoma have hypogammaglobulinemia
• Paraneoplastic syndromes occur with thymic carcinoid (10%): eg, Cushing syndrome (ACTH production)

Histo:
round / ovoid slow-growing primary epithelial neoplasm with smooth / lobulated surface divided into lobules by fibrous septa; areas of hemorrhage + necrosis may form cysts; completely encapsulated (thick fibrous capsule ± calcifications) / locally invasive (microscopic foci outside capsule)
(a) biphasic thymoma (most common)
= epithelial + lymphoid elements in equal amounts
(b) predominantly lymphocytic thymoma
= >2/3 of cells are lymphocytic
(c) predominantly epithelial thymoma
= >2/3 of cells are epithelial

- asymptomatic (50% discovered incidentally)
- signs of mediastinal compression (25 – 30%):
cough, dyspnea, chest pain, respiratory infection, hoarseness, dysphagia
- signs of tumor invasion (rare): SVC syndrome

Location: any anterior mediastinal location between thoracic inlet and cardiophrenic angle; rare in neck, other mediastinal compartments, lung parenchyma, tracheobronchial tree

Size: 5 – 10 cm (up to 34 cm)

(A) NONINVASIVE THYMOMA
Age peak: 5 – 6th decade, almost all are >25 years of age
√ oval / round lobulated sharply demarcated asymmetric homogeneous mass of soft tissue density, usually on one side of the midline
√ abnormally wide mediastinum
√ displacement of heart + great vessels posteriorly
√ amorphous, flocculent central / curvilinear peripheral calcification (5 – 20%)
CT:
√ homogeneous soft-tissue mass with smooth / lobulated border partially / completely outlined by fat
√ homogeneous enhancement
√ areas of decreased attenuation (fibrosis, cysts, hemorrhage, necrosis)
MRI:
√ isointense to skeletal muscle on T1WI
√ increased signal intensity (approaching that of fat) on T2WI
√ fluid characteristics of cysts with high water content

(B) INVASIVE THYMOMA (in 30% of thymomas)
Stage I : intact capsule
Stage II : pericapsular growth into mediastinal fat
Stage III: invasion of surrounding organs such as lung, pericardium, SVC, aorta
Stage IVa: dissemination in thoracic cavity (metastases to pleura + lung in 6%)
Stage IVb: distant metastases (liver, bone, lymph nodes, kidneys, brain)

√ spread by contiguity along pleural reflections, extension along aorta reaching posterior mediastinum / crus of diaphragm / retroperitoneum
√ irregular interface with lung
√ unilateral diffuse nodular circumferential pleural thickening / pleural masses
Rx: radical excision ± adjuvant radiation therapy
Prognosis: 5-year survival of 93% for stage I, 86% for stage II, 70% for stage III, 50% for stage IV

TRACHEOBRONCHOMEGALY
= MOUNIER-KUHN SYNDROME = primary atrophy / dysplasia of supporting structures of trachea + major bronchi with abrupt transition to normal bronchi at 4 – 5th division
Incidence: 0.5 – 1.5%
Age: discovered in 3rd – 5th decade
- cough with copious sputum
- shortness of breath on exertion
- long history of recurrent pneumonias
May be associated with: Ehlers-Danlos syndrome
√ marked dilatation of trachea (>29 mm), right (>20 mm) + left (>15 mm) main stem bronchi
√ sacculated outline / diverticulosis of trachea on lateral CXR (= protrusion of mucous membrane between rings of trachea)
√ may have emphysema, bullae in perihilar region

TRANSIENT TACHYPNEA OF THE NEWBORN
= NEONATAL WET LUNG DISEASE = TRANSIENT RESPIRATORY DISTRESS OF THE NEWBORN
= RETAINED FETAL LUNG FLUID
Incidence: 6%; most common cause of respiratory distress in newborn
Causes: cesarean section, precipitous delivery, breech delivery, prematurity, maternal diabetes
Pathophysiology: delayed resorption of fetal lung fluid (normal clearance occurs through capillaries (40%), lymphatics (30%), thoracic compression during vaginal delivery (30%)
Onset: within 6 hours of life; peak at day 1 of age
- increasing respiratory rates during first 2 – 6 hours of life
- intercostal + sternal retraction
- normal blood gases during hyperoxygenation
√ linear opacities + perivascular haze + thickened fissures + interlobular septal thickening (interstitial edema)
√ mild hyperaeration
√ mild cardiomegaly
√ small amount of pleural fluid
Prognosis: resolving within 1 – 4 days (retrospective diagnosis)
DDx: (1) normal during first several hours of life (2) diffuse pneumonitis / sepsis (3) mild meconium aspiration syndrome (4) "drowned newborn syndrome" = clear amniotic fluid aspiration (5) alveolar phase of RDS (6) pulmonary venous congestion (7) pulmonary hemorrhage (8) hyperviscosity syndrome = thick blood (9) immature lung syndrome

TRAUMATIC LUNG CYST

Age: children + young adults are particularly prone
√ thin-walled air-filled cavity (50%) ± air-fluid level
  preceded by homogeneous well-circumscribed mass
  (hematoma)
√ oval / spherical lesion of 2 – 14 cm in diameter
√ single / multiple lesions; uni- or multilocular
√ usually subpleural under point of maximal injury
√ persistent up to 4 month + progressive decrease in size
  (apparent within 6 weeks)

TUBERCULOSIS

Prevalence: 10 million people worldwide, active TB
  develops in 5 – 10% of those exposed
Organism: Mycobacterium = acid-fast aerobic rods
  staining red with carbol-fuchsin;
  M. tuberculosis (95%), atypical types
  increasing: M. avium-intracellulare, M.
  kansasii, M. fortuitum
Susceptible: infants, pubertal adolescents, elderly,
  alcoholics, blacks, diabetics, silicosis,
  measles, AIDS, sarcoidosis (in up to 13%)

Pathologic phases:
  (a)   exudative reaction (initial reaction, present for 1
        month)
  (b)   caseous necrosis (after 2 – 10 weeks with onset of
        hypersensitivity)
  (c)   hyalinization = invasion of fibroblasts (granuloma
        formation in 1 – 3 week)
  (d)   calcification / ossification
  (e)   chronic destructive form in 10% (<1 year of age,
        adolescents, young adults)

Spread: regional lymph nodes, hematogenous
  dissemination, pleura, pericardium, upper
  lumbar vertebrae
Mortality: 1:100,000

Positive PPD test: 3 weeks after infection
Negative PPD test:
  1.   Overwhelming tuberculous infection (miliary TB)
  2.   Sarcoidosis
  3.   Corticosteroid therapy
  4.   Pregnancy
  5.   Infection with atypical Mycobacterium

ENDOBRONCHIAL TUBERCULOSIS
Path: ulceration of bronchial mucosa followed by
  fibrosis leads to
  (a)   bronchial stenosis (lobar consolidation)
  (b)   bronchiectasis
  (c)   acinar nodules reflecting airway spread

TUBERCULOMA
= manifestation of primary / postprimary TB
√ round / oval smooth sharply defined mass
√ 0.5 – 4 cm in diameter remaining stable for a long
  time
√ lobulated mass (25%)

√ satellite lesions (80%)
√ may calcify

CAVITARY TUBERCULOSIS
= hallmark of reactivation tuberculosis
= semisolid caseous material is expelled into bronchial
  tree after lysis
√ moderately thick-walled cavity with smooth inner
  surface
Cx:
  (1)   dissemination to other bronchial segments
        √ multiple small acinar shadows remote from
          massive consolidation
  (2)   colonization with Aspergillus
        √ aspergilloma

Primary Pulmonary Tuberculosis
Mode of infection: inhalation of infected airborne
  droplets
Age: usually in childhood, becoming commoner in
  adults
• asymptomatic (91%)
• symptomatic (5 – 10%)
Location: lower lobes, middle lobe, anterior segment of
  upper lobes
√ one / more areas of homogeneous ill-defined air
  space consolidation of 1 – 7 cm in diameter (requires
  several weeks for complete clearing with
  antituberculous therapy)
√ cavitation (rare in children, up to 29% in adults)
√ massive hilar (60%) / paratracheal (40%) / subcarinal
  lymphadenopathy (particularly common in children),
  in 80% on right side
√ atelectasis (30%), esp. in right lung (anterior segment
  of upper lobe / medial segment of middle lobe)
  secondary to
  (a)   endobronchial tuberculosis
  (b)   bronchial / tracheal compression by enlarged
        lymph nodes (68%)
√ pleural effusion (10% in childhood, 40% in
  adulthood) most commonly 3 – 7 months after initial
  exposure (from subpleural foci rupturing into pleural
  space)
√ pneumonic reaction (mid or lower lung zones) with
  segmental / lobar consolidation
√ calcified lung lesion (17%) / parenchymal scar <5 mm
  = **Ghon lesion**
√ calcified lymph node (36%) in hilus / mediastinum
√ **Ranke complex** = Ghon lesion + calcified lymph
  node (22%)
√ **Simon focus** = healed site of primary infection in lung
  apex
CT:
  √ tuberculous adenopathy may demonstrate necrotic
    center with low attenuation after enhancement
Outcome of primary infection:
  1. Immunity prevents multiplication of organism
     (containment of initial infection by delayed
     hypersensitivity response + granuloma formation in
     1 – 3 weeks)

2. Progressive primary TB (inadequate immune mechanism with local progression)
3. Miliary tuberculosis (uncontrolled massive hematogenous dissemination overwhelming host defense system)
4. Postprimary TB = reactivation TB (reactivation of dormant organisms after asymptomatic years)

Prognosis: 3.6% mortality rate
Cx: (1) Bronchopleural fistula + empyema
    (2) Fibrosing mediastinitis

Postprimary Pulmonary Tuberculosis

= REACTIVATION TB = infection under the influence of acquired hypersensitivity and immunity secondary to longevity of bacillus + impairment of cellular immunity

Etiology: (a) reactivation of focus acquired in childhood
    (b) initial infection in individual vaccinated with BCG
    (c) continuation of initial infection = progressive primary tuberculosis (rare)

Path: foci of caseous necrosis with surrounding edema, hemorrhage, mononuclear cell infiltration; formation of tubercles = accumulation of epithelioid cells + Langhans giant cells; bronchial perforation leads to intrabronchial dissemination

Age: predominantly in adulthood
Site: 85% in apical + posterior segments of upper lobe, 10% in superior segment of lower lobe, 5% in mixed locations (anterior + contiguous segments of upper lobe)
R > L
(DDx: histoplasmosis tends to affect anterior segment)

A. LOCAL EXUDATIVE TB
√ chronic patchy / confluent ill-defined areas of acinar consolidation
√ thin-walled cavitation with smooth inner surface (present in more advanced disease), cavity under tension (air influx + obstructed efflux), air-fluid level is strong evidence for superimposed bacterial / fungal infection
√ accentuated drainage markings toward ipsilateral hilum

B. LOCAL FIBROPRODUCTIVE TB
√ sharply circumscribed irregular + angular mass-like fibrotic lesion (in up to 7%)
√ thick-walled irregular cavitation (HALLMARK) secondary to expulsion of caseous necrosis into airways, esp. in apical / posterior segments of upper lobes
√ reticular pulmonary scars
√ cicatrization atelectasis = volume loss in affected lobe
√ bronchiectasis in apical / posterior segments of upper lobes
√ pleural thickening

√ apical cap = pleural rind = thickening of layer of extrapleural fat (3 – 25 mm) + pleural thickening (1 – 3 mm)
√ tuberculous lymphadenitis
√ calcified hilar / mediastinal nodes
√ Rasmussen aneurysm

Miliary Pulmonary Tuberculosis

= massive hematogenous dissemination of organisms any time after primary infection
Cause:
    (1) severe immunodepression during postprimary state of infection
    (2) impaired defenses during primary infection = PROGRESSIVE PRIMARY TB
Incidence: 2 – 3.5% of TB infections
√ chronic focus often not identifiable
√ radiographically recognizable after 6 weeks post hematogenous dissemination
√ generalized granulomatous interstitial small foci of pinpoint to 2 – 3 mm size
√ rapid complete clearing with appropriate therapy
CT (earlier detection than CXR):
    √ diffusely scattered discrete 1 – 2 mm nodules

Cx: dissemination via bloodstream affecting lymph nodes, liver, spleen, skeleton, kidneys, adrenals, prostate, seminal vesicles, epididymis, fallopian tubes, endometrium, meninges

UNILATERAL PULMONARY AGENESIS

= one-sided lack of primitive mesenchyme
Associated with
anomalies in 60% (higher if right lung involved): PDA, anomalies of great vessels, Tetralogy of Fallot (left-sided pulmonary agenesis), bronchogenic cyst, congenital diaphragmatic hernia, bone anomalies
• may be asymptomatic
• respiratory infections

√ complete opacity of hemithorax
√ ipsilateral absence of pulmonary artery + vein
√ absent ipsilateral main stem bronchus
√ symmetrical chest cage with approximation of ribs
√ overdistension of contralateral lung
√ ipsilateral shift of mediastinum + diaphragm

VARICELLA-ZOSTER PNEUMONIA

Incidence: 14% overall; 50% in hospitalized adults
Age: >19 years (90%); 3rd – 5th decade (75%); contrasts with low incidence of varicella in this age group
• vesicular rash
√ patchy diffuse air space consolidation
√ tendency for coalescence near hila + lung bases
√ widespread nodules (30%) representing scarring
√ tiny 2 – 3 mm calcifications widespread throughout both lungs (2%)
Cx: unilateral diaphragmatic paralysis
Prognosis: 11% mortality rate

VIRAL PNEUMONIA

Organisms: Rhinovirus (43%), respiratory syncytial
virus (12%), Mycoplasma (10%),
Para-influenza virus, adenovirus, Influenza-
virus

Path: necrosis of ciliated epithelial cells, goblet cells,
bronchial mucous glands with frequent
involvement of peribronchial tissues + interlobular
septae

Age: most common cause of pneumonia in children
under 5 years of age

Distribution: usually bilateral

√ hyperaeration + air trapping
√ "dirty chest" = peribronchial cuffing + opacification
√ perihilar linear densities (bronchial wall thickening)
√ interstitial pattern
√ air space pattern (from hemorrhagic edema) in 50%
√ pleural effusion (20%)
√ hilar adenopathy (3%)
√ striking absence of pneumatoceles, lung abscess,
pneumothorax
√ radiographic resolution lags 2 – 3 weeks behind clinical

Cx: bronchiectasis; unilateral hyperlucent lung

Δ Atypical measles pneumonia does NOT show the typical
radiographic findings of viral pneumonias!

WEGENER GRANULOMATOSIS

= probably autoimmune disease characterized by
systemic necrotizing granulomatous process with
destructive angiitis

Path: peribronchial necrotizing granulomas + vasculitis
not intimately related to arteries

Age peak: 5th decade (range of all ages); M:F = 2:1

@ Respiratory tract (100% involvement)
(a) Upper respiratory tract (similar to midline
granuloma)
• rhinorrhea, sinusitis
• bleeding mucosal ulcers of nose
√ thickening of mucous membranes of paranasal
sinuses
√ may progress to destruction of cartilage + bone
(b) Pulmonary disease
• intractable cough, occasionally with hemoptysis
√ patchy alveolar infiltrates (with acute air space
pneumonia)

√ widely distributed multiple irregular masses /
nodules of varying sizes (up to 9 cm), especially
in lower lung fields
√ thick-walled cavities with irregular shaggy inner
lining (25 – 50%)
√ pleural effusion in 25%
√ lymphadenopathy exceedingly rare

@ Other organ involvement:
(a) Urinary tract (83%): focal glomerulonephritis
(b) Joints (56%): migratory polyarthropathy
(c) Skin + muscle (44%): inflammatory skin lesions
(d) Eyes + middle ear (29%): proptosis, otitis media
(e) Heart + pericardium (28%): myocardial infarction
(vasculitis)
(f) CNS (22%): central / peripheral neuritis

Cx: (1) Hypertension (2) Uremia
Dx: lung / renal biopsy
Prognosis: death within 2 years from renal failure (83%)
/ respiratory failure
Rx: corticosteroids, cytotoxic drugs, renal
transplantation

LIMITED WEGENER GRANULOMATOSIS

= Wegener granulomatosis WITHOUT renal
involvement

MIDLINE GRANULOMA

= mutilating granulomatous + neoplastic lesions limited
to nose + paranasal sinuses with very poor prognosis;
considered a variant of Wegener granulomatosis
WITHOUT the typical granulomatous + cellular
components

WILSON-MIKITY SYNDROME

= PULMONARY DYSMATURITY = similarity to
bronchopulmonary dysplasia in patients breathing room
air; rarely encountered anymore

Predisposed: premature infants <1500 g who are
initially well

• gradual onset of respiratory distress between 10 – 14
days
√ hyperinflation
√ reticular pattern radiating from both hila
√ small bubbly lucencies throughout both lungs (identical
to bronchopulmonary dysplasia)

Prognosis: resolution over 12 months

DIFFERENTIAL DIAGNOSIS OF BREAST DISORDERS

ASYMMETRIC BREAST DENSITY
A. OBVIOUS PATHOLOGIC LESION
   1. Stellate lesion
   2. Circular / ovoid lesion
   3. Calcifications
   4. Combination
B. PARENCHYMA
   1. Nodular densities + fat
      (a) normal TDLU – *Terminal ductal lobular unit*
      (b) adenosis
   2. Linear densities + fat
   3. Fibrosis + fat
   4. Accessory breast
C. FIBROSIS
   1. Postinflammatory fibrosis
   2. Posttraumatic fibrosis
   3. Desmoplastic reaction

OVAL-SHAPED BREAST LESION
Mammographic evaluation of breast masses
True mass or pseudomass?
A. SIZE
   — well-defined nodules <1.0 cm are of low risk for cancer
   — "most likely benign" nodules approaching 1 cm should be considered for ultrasound / aspiration / biopsy
B. SHAPE
   — increase in probability of malignancy: round < oval < lobulated < irregular < architectural distortion
C. MARGIN (most important factor)
   — well-circumscribed mass with sharp abrupt transition from surrounding tissue is almost always benign
   — "halo" sign of apparent lucency = optical illusion of Mach effect is almost always benign but not pathognomonic for benignity
   — microlobulated margin worrisome for cancer
   — obscured margin may represent infiltrative cancer
   — irregular ill-defined margin has a high probability of malignancy
   — spiculated margin due to (a) fibrous projections extending from main cancer mass (b) previous surgery (c) sclerosing duct hyperplasia (radial scar)
D. LOCATION
   — intramammary lymph node typically in upper outer quadrant (in 5% of all mammograms)
   — large hamartoma + abscess common in retro- / periareolar location
   — sebaceous cyst in subcutaneous tissue
E. X-RAY ATTENUATION = DENSITY
   — fat-containing lesions are never malignant
   — high-density mass suspicious for carcinoma (higher density than equal volume of fibroglandular tissue due to fibrosis)

F. NUMBER
   — multiplicity of identical lesions decreases risk
G. INTERVAL CHANGE
   — enlarging mass needs biopsy
H. PATIENT RISK FACTORS
   — increasing age increases risk for malignancy
   — positive family history
   — history of previous abnormal breast biopsy
   — history of extramammary malignancy

Well-circumscribed breast mass
Δ Well-defined nonpalpable lesions have a 4% risk of malignancy!
A. BENIGN
   1. Cyst (45%)
   2. Fibroadenoma
   3. Sclerosing adenoma
   4. Papilloma
   5. Galactocele
   6. Sebaceous cyst
B. MALIGNANT
   1. Medullary / mucinous / intracystic / papillary carcinoma
   2. Invasive ductal cancer not otherwise specified (rare)
   3. Pathologic intramammary lymph node
   4. Metastases to breast: melanoma, lymphoma / leukemia, lung cancer, hypernephroma

WELL-CIRCUMSCRIBED DE NOVO MASS IN WOMAN >40 YEARS OF AGE
   1. Cyst
   2. Papilloma
   3. Carcinoma
   4. Sarcoma (rare)
   5. Fibroadenoma (exceedingly rare)
   6. Metastasis (extremely rare)

Bilateral pathologic axillary lymph nodes
   1. Rheumatoid arthritis
   2. Sarcoidosis
   3. Lymphoproliferative disorders

Fat-containing breast lesion
Fat contained within a lesion proves benignity!
   1. Lipoma
   2. Galactocele
      = fluid with high lipid content (last phase)
      • during / shortly after lactation
   3. Traumatic lipid cyst = fat necrosis = oil cyst
      • site of prior surgery / trauma
   4. Focal collection of normal breast fat

MIXED FAT- AND WATER-DENSITY LESION
1. Intramammary lymph node
2. Hamartoma = lipofibroadenoma = fibroadenolipoma
3. Galactocele
4. Small superficial hematoma

Breast lesion with halo sign
A. HIGH DENSITY LESION
   = vessels + parenchymal elements not seen in superimposed lesion
   1. Cyst
   2. Sebaceous cyst
   3. Wart
B. LOW DENSITY LESION
   = vessels + parenchyma seen superimposed on lesion
   1. Fibroadenoma
   2. Galactocele
   3. Cystosarcoma phylloides

STELLATE BREAST LESION
Risk of malignancy:
— 75% for nonpalpable spiculated masses
— 32% for nonpalpable irregular masses
A. PSEUDOSTELLATE STRUCTURE
   caused by summation; unveiled by coned-down compression views ± microfocus magnification technique
B. "BLACK STAR"
   √ groups of fine fibrous strands bunched together
   √ circular / oval lucencies within center
   √ change in appearance on different views
   1. Radial scar = sclerosing duct hyperplasia
   2. Posttraumatic fat necrosis
C. "WHITE STAR"
   √ individual straight dense spicules
   √ central solid tumor mass
   √ little change in different views
   1. Invasive ductal carcinoma = scirrhous carcinoma
      = desmoplastic reaction + secondary retraction of surrounding structures
      • clinical dimensions larger than mammographic size
      √ distinct central tumor mass with irregular margins
      √ length of spicules increase with tumor size
      √ localized skin thickening / retraction when spiculae extend to skin
      √ commonly associated with malignant-type calcifications
   2. Postoperative scar
      • correlation with history + site of biopsy
      √ scar diminishes in size + density over time
   3. Postoperative hematoma
      • clinical information
      √ short-term mammographic follow-up confirms complete resolution
   4. Breast abscess
      • clinical information
      √ high density lesion with flame-like contour
   5. Hyalinized fibroadenoma with fibrosis

√ changing pattern with different projections
√ may be accompanied by typical coarse calcifications of fibroadenomas

Tumor-mimicking lesions
1. "Phantom breast tumor" = simulated mass
   (a) asymmetric density
      √ scalloped concave breast contour
      √ interspersed fatty elements
   (b) summation shadow = chance overlap of glandular breast structures
      √ failure to visualize "tumor" on more than one view
2. Silicone injections
3. Skin lesions
   (a) Dermal nevus
      √ sharp halo / fissured appearance
   (b) Skin calcifications
      √ lucent center (clue)
      √ superficial location (tangential views)
   (c) Sebacious / epithelial inclusion cyst
   (d) Neurofibromatosis
   (e) Biopsy scar
4. Lymphedema
5. Lymph nodes
   Location: axilla, subcutaneous tissue of axillary tail, lateral portion of pectoralis muscle, intramammary
   √ ovoid / bean-shaped mass with fatty notch representing hilum
   √ central zone of radiolucency (fatty replacement of center) surrounded by "crescent" rim of cortex
   √ usually <1.5 cm (up to 4 cm) in size
6. Hemangioma

BREAST CALCIFICATIONS
Indicative of focally active process; often requiring biopsy

Δ 75 – 80% of biopsied clusters of calcifications represent a benign process
Δ 10 – 30% of microcalcifications in asymptomatic patients are associated with cancers

Composition: hydroxyapatite / tricalcium phosphate / calcium oxalate

BREAST BIOPSIES FOR MICROCALCIFICATIONS
(without any other mammographic findings)
A. BENIGN LESIONS (80%)
   1. Mastopathy without proliferation 44%
   2. Mastopathy with proliferation 28%
   3. Fibroadenoma 4%
   4. Solitary papilloma 2%
   5. Miscellaneous 2%
B. MALIGNANT LESIONS (20%)
   1. Lobular carcinoma in situ 10%
      in 8% no spatial relationship to LCIS
   2. Infiltrating carcinoma 6%
   3. Ductal carcinoma in situ 4%

A. LOCATION
  (a) intramammary
      1. **Ductal microcalcifications**
         √ 0.1 – 0.3 mm in size, irregular, sometimes
           mixed linear + punctate
         Occurrence:
           secretory disease, epithelial hyperplasia,
           atypical ductal hyperplasia, intraductal
           carcinoma
      2. **Lobular microcalcifications**
         √ smooth round, similar in size + density
         Occurrence:
           cystic hyperplasia, adenosis, sclerosing
           adenosis, atypical lobular hyperplasia,
           lobular carcinoma in situ, cancerization of
           lobules (= retrograde migration of ductal
           carcinoma to involve lobules), ductal
           carcinoma obstructing egress of lobular
           contents
         N.B.: lobular and ductal microcalcifications occur
           frequently in fibrocystic disease + breast
           cancer!
  (b) extramammary: arterial wall, duct wall,
      fibroadenoma, oil cyst, skin, etc.
B. SIZE
   √ malignant calcifications usually <0.5 mm; rarely
     >1.0 mm
C. NUMBER
   √ <4 – 5 calcifications per 1 cm² have a low
     probability for malignancy
D. MORPHOLOGY
  (a) benign
      1. smooth round calcifications: formed in dilated
         acini of lobules
      2. solid / lucent-centered spheres: usually due to
         fat necrosis
      3. crescent-shaped calcifications that are concave
         on horizontal beam lateral projection =
         sedimented milk of calcium at bottom of cyst
      4. lucent-centered calcifications: around
         accumulated debris within ducts / in skin
      5. solid rod-shaped calcifications / lucent-centered
         tubular calcifications: formed within / around
         normal / ectatic ducts
      6. eggshell calcifications in rim of breast cysts
      7. calcifications with parallel track appearance =
         vascular calcifications
  (b) malignant
      √ calcifications varying in size + shape distributed
        in linear / branching pattern: calcified cellular
        secretion / necrotic cancer cells within ducts
E. DISTRIBUTION
   1. clustered heterogeneous calcifications: adenosis,
      peripheral duct papilloma, hyperplasia, cancer
   2. segmental calcifications within single duct network:
      suspect for multifocal cancer within lobe
   3. regional / diffusely scattered calcifications with
      random distribution throughout large volumes of
      breast: almost always benign
F. DENSITY

Malignant calcifications

1. **Granular calcifications** = resembling fine grains of
   salt
   √ amorphous, dotlike / elongated, fragmented
   √ grouped very closely together
   √ irregular in form, size and density

2. **Casting calcifications** = fragmented cast of
   calcifications within ducts
   √ variable in size + length
   √ great variation in density within individual
     particles + among adjacent particles
   √ jagged irregular contour
   √ ± Y-shaped branching pattern
   √ clustered (>5 per focus within an area of 1 cm²)

Benign calcifications

1. Lobular calcifications = arise within a spherical
   cavity of cystic hyperplasia, sclerosing adenosis,
   atypical lobular hyperplasia
   √ sharply outlined, homogeneous, solid, spherical
     "pearl"-like
   √ little variation in size
   √ numerous + scattered
   √ associated with considerable fibrosis
   (a) adenosis
       √ diffuse calcifications involving both breasts
         symmetrically
   (b) periductal fibrosis
       √ diffuse / grouped calcifications + irregular
         borders, simulating malignant process
2. Sedimented milk of calcium
   Frequency: 4%
   √ multiple, bilateral, scattered / occasionally
     clustered calcifications within microcysts
     √ smudge-like particles at bottom of cyst on
       vertical beam
     √ crescent-shaped on horizontal projection
       = "teacup-like"
3. Plasma cell mastitis = periductal mastitis
   √ sharply marginated calcifications of uniform
     density = intraductal form
   √ sharply marginated hollow calcifications =
     periductal form
4. Eggshell calcifications
   (a) with radiolucent lesion
       — liponecrosis micro- / macrocystica calcificans
         (= fatty acids precipitate as calcium soaps at
         capsular surface) as calcified fat necrosis /
         calcified hematoma
   (b) with radiopaque lesion
       — degenerated fibroadenoma
       — macrocyst
   √ high uniform density in periphery
   √ usually subcutaneous
   √ no associated fibrosis
5. Papilloma
   √ solitary raspberry configuration in size of duct
   √ central / retroareolar

6. Degenerated fibroadenoma
   √ bizarre, coarse, sharply outlined "popcorn-like" very dense calcification within dense mass (= central myxoid degeneration)
   √ eggshell type calcification (= subcapsular myxoid degeneration)
7. Arterial calcifications
   √ parallel lines of calcifications
8. Dermal calcifications
   Site: sebaceous glands
   √ hollow radiolucent center
   √ polygonal shape
   √ peripheral location (may project deep within breast even on 2 views at 90° angles)
   √ linear orientation when caught in tangent
   √ same size as skin pores
   Proof: superficial marking technique

NIPPLE

Nipple retraction
1. Positional
2. Relative to inflammation / edema of periareolar tissue
3. Congenital
4. Acquired (carcinoma, ductal ectasia)

Nipple discharge
Δ The most significant discharge comes from one breast + one orifice!
Δ The most common cause of bloody / serosanguinous discharge is intraductal papilloma!
Type of discharge:
   (a) lactating breast: galactorrhea
   (b) nonlactating breast:
      — normal: white, yellowish, greenish-gray
      — abnormal: clear serous (cancer 7%, papilloma 35%, fibrocystic change 36%, ductectasia 11%), bloody (cancer 13%, papilloma 61%, fibrocystic change 12%, ductectasia 2%)
• exfoliative cytology not helpful (true positive in 11%)
Site of origin:
   A. Lobules + terminal duct lobular unit:
      1. Galactorrhea
      2. Fibrocystic changes
   B. Larger lactiferous ducts (collecting duct, segmental duct, subsegmental duct)
      1. Solitary papilloma
      2. Papillary carcinoma
      3. Ductectasia
Galactography:
   injection of 0.1 – 0.3 cm³ of water-soluble contrast material through blunt 27-gauge pediatric sialography needle (0.4 – 0.6 mm outer diameter, tip bent 90°)
DDx of intraductal defects:
   gas bubble, clot, inspissated secretions, solitary intraductal papilloma, epithelial hyperplastic lesion, duct carcinoma

Secretory disease
1. Retained lactiferous secretions
   result of incomplete / prolonged involution of lactiferous ducts
   √ branching pattern of fat density in dense breast (high lipid content)
2. Prolonged inspissation of secretion + intraductal debris
   √ duct dilatation
   √ calcifications with linear orientation towards subareolar area a few mm long: rod-shaped / sausage-shaped / spherical with hollow center
3. Galactocele
4. Plasma cell mastitis

Skin thickening of breast
Normal skin thickness: 0.8 – 3 mm; may exceed 3 mm in inframammary region
A. Localized skin thickening
   1. Trauma (prior biopsy)
   2. Carcinoma
   3. Abscess
   4. Nonsuppurative mastitis
   5. Dermatologic conditions
B. Generalized skin thickening
   Δ Skin is thickened initially and to the greatest extent in the lower dependent portion of breast!
   √ overall increased density with coarse reticular pattern (= dilated lymph vessels + interstitial fluid triggering fibrosis)
   (a) Axillary lymphatic obstruction
      1. Primary breast cancer
         — advanced breast cancer
         — invasive comedocarcinoma in large area
         Δ Primary breast cancer not necessarily seen due to small size / hidden location (axillary tail, behind nipple)!
      2. Primary malignant lymphatic disease (eg, lymphoma)
   (b) Intradermal + intramammary obstruction of lymph channels
      1. Lymphatic spread of breast cancer from contralateral side
      2. Inflammatory breast carcinoma = diffusely invasive ductal carcinoma
   (c) Mediastinal lymphatic blockage
      1. Sarcoidosis
      2. Hodgkin disease
      3. Advanced bronchial / esophageal carcinoma
      4. Actinomycosis
   (d) Advanced gynecological malignancies from thoraco-epigastric collaterals
      1. Ovarian cancer
      2. Uterine cancer
   (e) Inflammation
      1. Acute mastitis
      2. Retromamillary abscess
      3. Fat necrosis
      4. Radiation therapy
      5. Reduction mammoplasty

(f) Right heart failure
may be unilateral (R>L) / migrating with change in patient position (to avoid decubitus ulcer)
(g) Nephrotic syndrome, anasarca
1. Dialysis
2. Renal transplant
(h) Subcutaneous extravasation of pleural fluid following thoracentesis

Diffuse increase in breast density
√ generalized increased density
√ skin thickening
√ reticular pattern in subcutis
A. Cancer
  1. "Inflammatory" breast cancer (angiolymphatic spread)
     • rapid development of diffuse swelling, induration, skin redness + peau d'orange edema over 1/3 of breast surface
     Dx: skin biopsy
  2. Diffuse primary noninflammatory breast cancer
  3. Diffuse metastatic breast cancer
  4. Lymphoma / leukemia
     due to obstructive lymphedema of breast
B. Infectious mastitis
   usually in lactating breast
C. Radiation
   (a) diffuse exudative edema within weeks after beginning of radiation therapy
   (b) indurational fibrosis months after radiation therapy
D. Edema
  1. Lymphatic obstruction: extensive axillary / intrathoracic lymphadenopathy, mediastinal / anterior chest wall tumor, axillary surgery
  2. Generalized body edema: congestive heart failure (breast edema may be unilateral if patient in lateral decubitus position), hypoalbuminemia (renal disease, liver cirrhosis)

E. Hemorrhage
  1. Posttraumatic
  2. Anticoagulation therapy
  3. Bleeding diathesis
F. Accidental infusion of fluid into subcutaneous tissue

MAMMOGRAPHY REPORTS (Marc J. Homer)
Provide answers for:
  1. Is mammogram normal?
  2. If it is abnormal, must biopsy be done?
  3. If it is abnormal but biopsy not indicated, what must be done?

NORMAL REPORT
  "No dominant mass or suspicious calcification."
DENSE NORMAL REPORT
  "The breasts are very dense limiting the sensitivity of the examination. A mass could be easily hidden."
MUST BIOPSY REPORT
  "There is a *(description)* in the *(location)* quadrant. These are characteristics highly suggestive of cancer. Biopsy is mandatory to rule out breast cancer."
MULTIPLICITY REPORT
  "There are *masses / multiple asymmetric densities / multiple microcalcifications.* No one area appears more suspicious to merit biopsy at this time. I recommend a repeat examination within *(3)* months to assess the stability of these areas."
NEUTRAL REPORT
  "There is a *(description)* in the *(location)* quadrant. This has a high probability of being benign. It can be localized prior to biopsy to establish histology. If biopsy is deferred, I recommend a follow-up examination within 6 months to assess its stability."
DISCLAIMER for lawyers
  "The false-negative rate of mammography is approximately 10%. Management of a palpable abnormality must be based upon clinical grounds."

	Malignant	v/s	benign
1° signs → density	high		relatively low
	non-homogeneous		homogeneous
Outline	Irregular opacity, long thin spicules.		Smooth
2° signs →	Comet-tail appearance.		
architecture	disruption		distortion
Vascularity	usually ↑		Ⓝ / occasional hyper
Perifocal haziness	+		rare
Size	Rad size < clinical		Same / larger than clinical

BREAST ANATOMY AND MAMMOGRAPHIC TECHNIQUE

Lobes

6 – 15 lobes disposed radially around nipple, each lobe has a main duct with an opening in the central portion of nipple

Main duct: branches dicotomously eventually forming terminal ductal lobular units

Histo: epithelial cells, myoepithelial cells surrounded by extralobular connective tissue with elastic fibers

Terminal ductal lobular unit (TDLU)

(1) Extralobular terminal duct
   Histo: lined by columnar cells + prominent coat of elastic fibers
(2) Lobule
   (a) intralobular terminal duct
      Histo: lined by cuboidal cells
   (b) ductules / acini
   (c) intralobular connective tissue
Size: 1 – 8 mm (most 1 – 2 mm) in diameter
Change:
   (a) reproductive age: cyclic proliferation (up to time of ovulation) + cyclic involution (during menstruation)
   (b) post menopause: regression with fatty replacement
Significance:
   TDLU is site of fibroadenoma, epithelial cyst, apocrine metaplasia, adenosis (= proliferation of ductules + lobules), epitheliosis (= proliferation of mammary epithelial cells within preexisting ducts + lobules), ductal + lobular carcinoma in situ, infiltrating ductal + lobular carcinoma

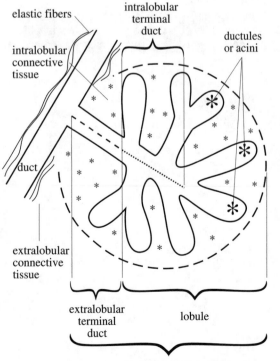

terminal ductal lobular unit

Components of normal breast parenchyma

1. Nodular densities surrounded by fat
   (a) 1 – 2 mm = normal lobules
   (b) 3 – 9 mm = adenosis
2. Linear densities
   = ducts and their branches + surrounding elastic tissue
3. Structureless ground-glass density
   = stroma / fibrosis with concave contours

Parenchymal Breast Pattern (László Tabár)

Pattern I
   named QDY = quasi dysplasia (for Wolfe classification)
   √   concave contour from Cooper's ligaments
   √   evenly scattered 1 – 2 mm nodular densities
       (= normal terminal ductal lobular units)
   √   oval-shaped / circular lucent areas (= fatty replacement)
Pattern II
   similar to N1 (Wolfe)
   √   total fatty replacement
   √   NO nodular densities
Pattern III
   similar to P1 (Wolfe)
   √   normal parenchyma occupying <25% of breast volume in retroareolar location
Pattern IV = adenosis pattern
   similar to P2 (Wolfe)
   Cause: hypertrophy + hyperplasia of acini within lobules
   Histo: small ovoid proliferating cells with rare mitoses
   √   scattered 3 – 7 mm nodular densities (= enlarged terminal ductal lobular units) = adenosis
   √   thick linear densities (= periductal elastic tissue proliferation with fibrosis) = fibroadenosis
   √   no change with increasing age (genetically determined)
Pattern V
   similar to DY (Wolfe)
   √   uniformly dense parenchyma with smooth contour (= extensive fibrosis)

Parenchymal Breast Pattern (Wolfe)

   Classification of little practical value because
   (a) >72% of breast cancers are found in the low-risk group of N1 + P1
   (b) risk in N1 + P1 delayed by about 15 years
   N1   = no proliferation
        breast composed primarily of fat, prominent trabeculation is present that appears curvilinear and often branches, no ducts visible
   P1   = little proliferation
        minor ducts occupy 1/4 or less of the breast volume, ducts have a definite cross-sectional diameter and often a nodular component

P2 = severe proliferation
severe ducting occupying more than 1/4 of the breast volume, strong tendency to form a central triangular density, ducts are coalescent

DY = dysplasia
severe mammary dysplasia, nearly completely homogeneous breasts without discernible linearity or nodularity, interspersed are irregular collections of fat

Age (years)	Breast cancer prevalence per 1,000	
	N1 and P1	P2 and DY
40 – 49	0.9	5.3
50 – 59	2.8	8.8
60 – 69	7.4	15.4
≥70	12.2	25.5

Mammographic Film Reading Technique
1. Compare with earlier films
2. Scan "forbidden" areas
   (a) "Milky Way" = 2 – 3 cm wide area parallel with the edge of the pectoral muscle on MLO projection
   (b) "No man's land" = fatty replaced area between posterior border of parenchyma + chest wall on CC projection
   (c) Medial half of breast on CC view
3. Look for increased retroareolar density
4. Look for parenchymal contour retraction
5. Look for architectural distortion
6. Look for straight lines superimposed on normal scalloped contour
7. Compare left with right side
8. Don't stop looking after one lesion is found

Mammographic Technique
Beam quality
Molybdenum target material with characteristic emission peaks of 17.9 + 19.5 keV (lower average energy than tungsten)

Focal spot
0.1 – 0.4 mm (0.1 mm for magnification views)
Tube output
80 – 100 mA
Exposure
(a) without grid: 25 kV (optimum between contrast + penetration), exposure time of 1.0 seconds
(b) with grid: 26 – 27 kV; exposure time of 2.3 seconds
(c) microfocus magnification: 26 – 27 kV; 1.5 – 2.0 times magnification with 16 – 30 cm air gap
(d) specimen radiography: 22 – 24 kV
Filter
(a) beryllium window (absorbs less radiation than glass tube)
(b) molybdenum filter (0.03 mm): allows more of lower energy radiation to reach breast

Reduction of scatter radiation
(1) adequate compression (also improves contrast + decreases radiation dose)
(2) beam collimation to <8 – 10 cm
(3) air gap with microfocus magnification (greater spatial resolution, 2 – 3-fold increase in radiation exposure)
(4) Moving grid
grid if compressed breast >5 cm / very dense breast (facilitates perception, 2 – 3-fold increase in radiation exposure)
Screen-film combination
(1) Intensifying screen phosphor single screen systems
(2) Film-screen contact
(3) Mammography film with minimal base fog, suffcient maximum density + contrast
Film processing
(1) Processing time of 3 minutes (42 – 45 seconds in developing fluid) superior to 90-second processor for double-emulsion film (which creates underdevelopment + compensatory higher radiation exposure)

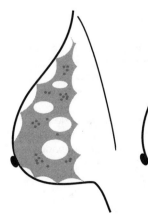 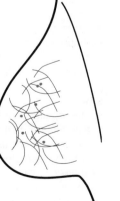 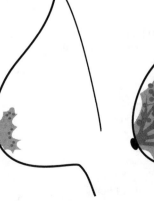 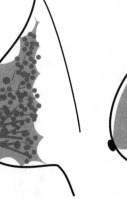 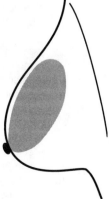

Parenchymal Breast Pattern

Pattern I **Pattern II** **Pattern III** **Pattern IV** **Pattern V**

(2) Developing temperature of 35° C (95° F)
(3) Developing fluid replenishment rate:
     450 – 500 ml replenisher per square meter of film

Quality control
(1) Processor (daily)
     with sensito- / densitometric measurements
     (a) base fog <0.16 – 0.17
     (b) maximum density >3.50
     (c) contrast >1.9 – 2.0
(2) X-ray unit (semiannually)
     (a) beam quality
     (b) phototimer

Average glandular dose: <0.6 mGy per breast for
nonmagnification film-screen mammogram (ACR
accreditation requirement)
Screen/film technique (molybdenum target; 0.03 mm
molybdenum filter, 28 kVp):
     mean absorbed dose: 0.05 rad for CC view
                            0.06 rad for LAT view

Effective dose equivalent H_e:
screen-film mammography ....0.11 mSv
xeroradiographic mammography ....0.78 mSv
chest ....0.05 mSv
skull ....0.15 mSv
abdomen...1.40 mSv
lumbar spine ....2.20 mSv

ADVANTAGES OF MAGNIFICATION MAMMOGRAPHY
1. Sharpness effect = increased resolution
2. Noise effect = noise reduced by a factor equal to
    the degree of magnification
3. Air-gap effect = increased contrast by reduction in
    scattered radiation
4. Visual effect = improved perception and analysis of
    small detail

Factors Affecting Mammographic Image Quality

A. RADIOGRAPHIC SHARPNESS
    = subjective impression of distinctness / perceptibility
       of structure boundary / edge
    1. **Radiographic contrast**
        = magnitude of optical density difference between
           structure of interest + surroundings
           influenced by
        (a) subject contrast
             = ratio of x-ray intensity transmitted through one
                part of the breast to that transmitted through a
                more absorbing adjacent part
                affected by
                — absorption differences in the breast
                  (thickness, density, atomic number)
                — radiation quality (target material, kilovoltage,
                  filtration)
                — scattered radiation (beam limitation, grid,
                  compression)
        (b) receptor contrast
             = component of radiographic contrast that
                determines how the X-ray intensity pattern will
                be related to the optical density pattern in the
                mammogram

    affected by
    — film type
    — processing (chemicals, temperature, time,
      agitation)
    — photographic density
    — fog (storage, safelight, light leaks)

    2. **Radiographic blurring**
        = lateral spreading of a structural boundary
           (= distance over which the optical density
           between the structure and its surrounding
           changes)
        (a) motion
             reduced by compression + short exposure time
        (b) geometric blurring
             affected by
             — focal spot: size, shape, intensity distribution
             — focus-object distance (= cone length)
             — object-image distance
        (c) receptor blurring
             = light diffusion (= spreading of the light emitted
                by the screen) affected by
             — phosphor thickness + particle size
             — light-absorbing dyes + pigments
             — screen-film contact

B. RADIOGRAPHIC NOISE
    = unwanted fluctuation in optical density

    1. **Radiographic mottle**
        = optical density variations consist of
        (a) receptor graininess
             = optical density variation from random
                distribution of finite number of silver halide
                grains
        (b) quantum mottle (principal contributor to mottle)
             = variation in optical density from random
                spatial distribution of X-ray quanta absorbed
                in image receptor
                affected by
                — film speed + contrast
                — screen absorption + conversion efficiency
                — light diffusion
                — radiation quality
        (c) structure mottle
             = optical density fluctuation from nonuniformity
                in the structure of the image receptor (eg,
                phosphor layer of intensifying screen)

    2. **Artifacts**
        = unwanted optical density variations in the form of
           blemishes on the mammogram
        (a) improper film handling (static, crimp marks,
             fingerprints, scratches)
        (b) improper exposure (fog)
        (c) improper processing (streaks, spots,
             scratches)
        (d) dirt + stains

BREAST DISORDERS

BREAST CANCER
Origin: terminal ductal lobular unit

A. NONINVASIVE BREAST CANCER
= malignant transformation of epithelial cells lining mammary ducts + lobules confined within boundaries of basement membrane

1. **Ductal carcinoma in situ** (DCIS)
= intraductal carcinoma
Incidence: 10 – 20% in screening population
- may persist for years without palpatory abnormality

   (a) Low nuclear grade DCIS ("noncomedo type")
   Precursor stages:
   (1) normal typical cells
   (2) ductal epithelial hyperplasia (= epitheliosis)
   (3) atypical ductal hyperplasia with slight / moderate / severe atypia
   (4) low nuclear grade DCIS
   Characteristics:
   } nuclear grade: monomorphic small round nuclei, few / no mitoses
   } growth pattern: predominantly micropapillary / cribriform; atypically solid cell proliferation
   } necrosis: not present in classic micropapillary / cribriform growth pattern
   } calcifications: laminated / psammoma-like in classic micropapillary / cribriform DCIS
   √ fine granular "cotton ball" calcifications in micropapillary / cribriform growth pattern
   √ coarse granular "crushed stone" / "broken needle tip" / "arrowhead" calcifications in solid growth pattern
   √ palpable dominant mass without calcifications (intracystic papillary carcinoma, multifocal papillary carcinoma in situ)
   √ nonpalpable asymmetric density with architectural distortion
   √ occasionally serous / bloody nipple discharge + ductal filling defects on galactography
   Risk of recurrence: 2%

   (b) High nuclear grade DCIS ("comedo type")
   One stage development; no precursor lesions known
   Characteristics:
   } nuclear grade: large / intermediate nuclei, numerous mitoses
   } growth pattern: predominantly solid cell proliferation; atypically micropapillary / cribriform
   } necrosis: extensive

   } calcifications: dystrophic / amorphous within necrosis in center of dilated ductal system outlining most of the lobe in classic solid growth pattern
   √ ductal system enlarged to 300 – 350 μ
   √ large solid high-density casting calcifications (fragmented, coalesced, irregular) in solid growth pattern
   √ "snake skin"-like / "birch tree flower"-like dotted casting calcifications within necrosis of micropapillary / cribriform growth pattern
   √ palpable dominant mass without calcifications (very unusual)
   √ nipple discharge (rare)
   Risk of recurrence: 25% within 26 months in immediate vicinity of biopsy site

   Δ 50% of DCIS are >5 cm in size
   Δ Histologic size of DCIS is independent of histologic subgroup
   Δ Mammography underestimates the size of DCIS, especially in "non-comedo" type
   Δ Almost all "comedo" type DCIS contain significant microcalcifications
   Δ DCIS often involves the nipple + subareolar ducts

2. **Lobular carcinoma in situ** (LCIS)
= arises in epithelium of blunt ducts of mammary lobules
Incidence: 0.8 – 3.6% in screening population; high during reproductive age; decreasing with age
Histo: monomorphous cell population filling + expanding lobule
- not palpable
√ mammographically occult
Dx: incidental microscopic finding depending on accident of biopsy (performed for unrelated reasons + findings)
Prognosis:
20 – 30% develop invasive carcinoma with high frequency of multicentricity + equal frequency for both breasts; LCIS serves as a marker of increased risk
Rx: recommendations range from observation to unilateral / bilateral mastectomy

3. **Intracystic papillary carcinoma in situ** (0.5 – 2%)
= rare form of ductal cancer
Age: average of 51 years
- well-circumscribed + freely movable
- aspiration may yield bloody fluid (cytology negative in 80%)
√ intracystic mass on pneumocystography
√ solid intracystic mass on US
√ round benign appearing mass on mammography
Prognosis: favorable

B. INVASIVE BREAST CANCER
1. **Infiltrating ductal carcinoma** (65%)
   Histo: grade I = well-differentiated
             grade II = moderately differentiated
             grade III = poorly differentiated
   • larger by palpation than on mammogram
   √ dense mass of variable size surrounded by spiculations
   √ malignant calcifications common
2. **Invasive lobular carcinoma** (10 – 13%)
   2nd most common type of breast cancer; 30 – 50% of patients will develop a second primary in same / opposite breast within 20 years
   Δ Most frequently missed breast cancer (difficult to detect mammographically)!
   Histo: 20% grade I, 64% grade II, 16% grade III
   • may be palpable
   √ asymmetric density without definable margins (most frequent) = (1/3)
     Histo: single file of cells around non-neoplastic ducts resulting in subtle changes in architecture ("Indian files")
   √ dense tissue with radiating spicules (1/3)
   √ round / ovoid mass (1/3)
3. **Tubular carcinoma** (6 – 8%)
   (a) low grade: bilateral in 1:3
   (b) high grade: bilateral in 1:300
   Associated with lobular carcinoma in situ in 40%
   Mean age: 40 – 49 years
   • positive family history in 40%
4. **Medullary carcinoma** (2%)
   Δ Fastest growing breast cancer!

Path: well-circumscribed mass with nodular architecture + lobulated contour; central necrosis is common in larger tumors; reminiscent of medullary cavity of bone
Histo: intense lymphoplasmocytic reaction (reflecting host resistance); propensity for syncytial growth; no glands
Incidence: 11% of breast cancers in women <35 years of age; 40 – 50% of medullary cancers in women <50 years of age
Mean age: 46 – 54 years
• softer than average breast cancer
√ well-defined round / oval noncalcified uniformly dense mass (hemorrhage) with lobulated margin
√ may have partial / complete halo sign
US:
  √ hypoechoic mass with some degree of through transmission
  √ distinct / indistinct margins
  √ large central cystic component
DDx: fibroadenoma
Prognosis: 70% 10-year survival rate
5. **Mucinous / colloid carcinoma** (2%)
   Path: contains gelatinous / colloid fluid
   Age: more frequent in older women
   • slow growth rate
   √ may enlarge fast (through mucin production)
   Prognosis: favorable
6. **Papillary carcinoma** (2 – 4%)
   Histo: multilayered papillary projections extending from vascularized stalks
   • palpable mass (67%)

Distribution of Breast Cancers in Screening Population

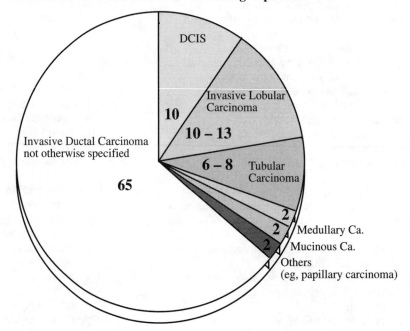

- nipple discharge (25 – 35%)
- √ multinodular pattern of increased density (55%)
- √ solitary well-circumscribed nodule
- √ associated microcalcifications in 60%
- √ usually confined to single quadrant
  Prognosis: 90% 5-year survival after mastectomy

C. Paget carcinoma of the nipple (5%)
- eczemalike crusting + erosion of nipple and areola
- nipple discharge + itching
  Associated with intraductal subareolar / remote carcinoma
  Histo: Paget cell

Epidemiology of Breast Cancer
Incidence:
2 – 5 breast cancers/1,000 women; in USA >142,000 new cases per year; 1 of 10 women will develop breast cancer during her life; 25% of all female malignancies
Age: 1.5 – 2% in women <30 years of age;
15% in women <40 years of age;
85% in women >30 years of age

Mortality: 43,000 deaths per year

RISK FACTORS (increasing risk):
A. DEMOGRAPHIC FACTORS
- increasing age (66% of cancers in women >50 years): age 40 in 80/100,000, age 50 in 180/100,000, age 60 in 240/100,000
- whites > blacks after age 40
- Jewish women + nuns
- upper > lower social class
- unmarried > married women
B. REPRODUCTIVE VARIABLES
- nulliparous > parous
- first full-term pregnancy after age 35: 2 x risk
- low parity > high parity
- early age at menarche (<12 years) + late age at menopause
- bilateral oophorectomy under age 40 decreases risk
C. MULTIPLE PRIMARY CANCERS
- 4 – 5 x increase in risk for cancer in contralateral breast
- increased risk after ovarian + endometrial cancer
D. FAMILY HISTORY
- breast cancer in first-degree relative
  — 2-fold increase if mother / sister had cancer
  — 3-fold increase if mother + sister had cancer
- 25% of patients with carcinoma have a positive family history
- carcinoma tends to affect successive generations approx. 10 years earlier
E. BENIGN BREAST DISEASE
- 2 – 4 x increased risk with atypical hyperplasia / epithelial hyperplasia)

F. MAMMOGRAPHIC FEATURES
- prominent duct pattern + extremely dense breasts
  N1 (0.14%), P1 (0.52%), P2 (1.95%), DY (5.22%)
G. RADIATION EXPOSURE
excess risk of 3.5 – 6 cases per 1,000,000 women per year per rad after a minimum latent period of 10 years (atomic bomb, fluoroscopy during treatment of tuberculosis, irradiation for postpartum mastitis)
H. GEOGRAPHY
- Western + industrialized nations (highest incidence)
- Asia, Latin America, Africa (decreased risk)

Breast cancer evaluation
A. PRIMARY = LOCALIZING SIGNS OF BREAST CANCER
1. <u>Dominant mass</u> seen on two views with
   (a) *spiculation* = stellate / star burst appearance (= fine linear strands of tumor extension + desmoplastic response) "scirrhus" caused by:
   (1) infiltrating ductal carcinoma (75% of all invasive cancers)
   (2) invasive lobular carcinoma (occasionally)
   √ mass feels larger than its mammographic / sonographic size
   DDx: prior biopsy / trauma / infection
   (b) *smooth border*
   (1) intracystic carcinoma (rare): subareolar area; bloody aspiration
   (2) medullary carcinoma: soft tumor
   (3) mucinous / colloid carcinoma: soft tumor
   (4) papillary carcinoma
   √ "telltale" signs: lobulation, small comet tail, flattening of one side of the lesion, slight irregularity
   √ halo sign (= Mach band) may be present
   DDx: cyst (sonographic evaluation)
   (c) *lobulation*
   Appearance similar to fibroadenoma (only characteristic calcifications may exclude malignancy)
   Δ the likelihood of malignancy increases with number of lobulations
   - clinical size of mass > radiographic size (Le Borgne's law)
2. <u>Asymmetric density</u> = <u>star-shaped lesion</u>
   √ distinct central tumor mass with volumetric rather than planar appearance (additional coned compression views!)
   √ denser relative to other areas (= vessels + trabeculae cannot be seen within high-density lesion)
   √ fat does not traverse density
   √ corona of spicules
   √ in any quadrant (but fatty replacement occurs last in upper outer quadrant)

DDx: postsurgical fibrosis, traumatic fat
necrosis, sclerosing duct hyperplasia

3. Microcalcifications
Associated with malignant mass
mammographically in 40%, pathologically with
special stains in 60%, on specimen radiography
in 86%
Δ 20% of clustered microcalcifications
represent a malignant process!
(a) *shape:* fragmented, irregular contour,
polymorphic, casting rod-shaped without
polarity, Y-shaped branching pattern,
granular "salt and pepper" pattern, reticular
pattern
(b) *density:* various densities
(c) *size:* 100 – 300 μ (usually); rarely up to 2 mm
(d) *distribution:*   tight cluster over an area of 1
cm² or less is most suggestive; coursing
along ductal system seen in ductal carcinoma
with comedo elements

4. Architectural distortion
due to desmoplastic reaction
√   ragged irregular border
DDx: postsurgical fibrosis

5. Interval change
(a) neodensity = de novo developing density (in
6% malignant)
(b) enlarging mass (malignant in 10 – 15%)

6. Enlarged single duct
(low probability for cancer in asymptomatic
woman with normal breast palpation)
√   solitary dilated duct >3 cm long
DDx: inspissated debris / blood, papilloma

7. Diffuse increase in density (late finding)
Cause: (1) plugging of dermal lymphatics with
tumor cells (2) less flattening of sclerotic
+ fibrous elements of neoplasm in
comparison with more compressible
fibroglandular breast tissue

B. SECONDARY = NONLOCALIZING SIGNS OF
BREAST CANCER
1. Asymmetric thickening
2. Asymmetric ducts, especially if discontinuous
with subareolar area
3. Skin changes
(a) retraction = dimpling of skin
from desmoplastic reaction causing
shortening of Cooper ligaments / direct
extension of tumor to skin
DDx: trauma, biopsy, abscess, burns
(b) skin thickening secondary to blocked
lymphatic drainage / tumor in lymphatics
• peau d'orange
DDx: normal in inframammary region
4. Nipple / areolar abnormalities
(a) retraction / flattening of nipple
DDx: normal variant
(b) Paget disease = eczematoid appearance of
nipple + areola in ductal carcinoma
Associated with ductal calcifications toward
the nipple
DDx: nipple eczema
(c) nipple discharge
• spontaneous persistent discharge
• need not be bloody
DDx : lactational discharge
5. Abnormal veins
venous diameter ratio of >1.4:1 in 75% of
cancers; late sign + thus not very important
6. Axillary nodes (sign of advanced / occult cancer)
√   >1.5 cm without fatty center
DDx: reactive hyperplasia

LOCATION OF BREAST MASSES
benign + malignant masses are of similar distribution
@   upper outer quadrant (54%)
@   upper inner quadrant (14%)
@   lower outer quadrant (10%)

PREDICTIVE VALUES OF RADIOGRAPHIC SIGNS FOR MALIGNANCY

1. Classic mammographic findings of malignancy + palpable abnormality 100%
   only 3% of cancers present this way
2. Classic mammographic findings of malignancy + NO palpable finding 74%
   only 6% of cancers present this way
3. Indeterminate mammographic features + palpable mass 11%
4. Indeterminate mass + no palpable finding 5%
5. Mammographically benign mass 2%
6. Asymmetric density (mass questionable) + clinical finding 4%
7. Asymmetric density (mass questionable) + NO clinical finding 0%
8. Microcalcifications + clinical abnormality 25%
9. Microcalcifications + NO clinical abnormality 21%
   (>3 punctate irregular microcalcifications in area <1 cm²)
10. Vein dilatation 0%
11. Skin thickening 0%
12. Duct dilatation 0%

@ lower inner quadrant (7%)
@ retroareolar (15%)
Δ Mediolateral oblique view is important part of screening because it includes largest portion of breast tissue + considers most common location of cancers!

METASTATIC BREAST CANCER
@ Axillary lymph adenopathy
Incidence: 40 – 74%
risk for positive nodes: 30% if primary >1 cm, 15% if primary <1 cm
@ Bone
@ Liver
Incidence: 48 – 60%
US: √ hypoechoic (83%) / hyperechoic (17%) masses

Screening of asymptomatic patients
Guidelines of American Cancer Society, American College of Radiology, American Medical Association, National Cancer Institute:
1. Breast self-examination to begin at age 20
2. Breast examination by physician every 3 years between 20 – 40 years, in yearly intervals after age 40
3. Baseline mammogram between age 35 – 40; follow-up screening based upon parenchymal pattern + family history
4. Initial screening at 30 years if patient has first-degree relative with breast cancer in premenopausal years; follow-up screening based upon parenchymal pattern
5. Mammography at 1-year intervals for women between 40 – 49 years
6. Mammography at yearly intervals after age 50
7. All women who have had prior breast cancer require annual follow-up

RATE OF DETECTED ABNORMALITIES
30 abnormalities in 1,000 screening mammograms:
20 – 23 benign lesions
7 – 10 cancers

VALUE OF SCREENING MAMMOGRAPHY
Indication:
decrease in cancer mortality through earlier detection + intervention when tumor size small + lymph nodes negative; tumor grade of no prognostic significance in tumors <10 mm in size
1. Health Insurance Plan (HIP) 1963 – 1969
Randomized controlled study of 62,000 women aged 40 – 64
• 25 – 30% reduction in mortality in women >50 years (followed for 18 years)
2. Breast Cancer Detection Demonstration Project (BCDDP) 1973 – 1980
4,443 cancers found in 283,000 asymptomatic volunteers
• 41.6% of cancers found by mammography alone (77% with negative nodes)
• 8.7% of cancers found by physical examination alone
• 59% of non-infiltrating cancers found by mammography alone
• 25% of cancers were intraductal (vs. 5% in previous series)
• 21% of cancers found in women aged 40 – 49 years (mammography alone detected 35.4%)
3. Two-county Swedish trial 1977 – 1990
randomized controlled study of 134,000 women
• 31% reduction in mortality in women >50 years

OCCULT VERSUS PALPABLE CANCERS
27% are occult cancers (NO age difference)
Positive axillary nodes: occult cancers (19%); palpable cancers (44%)
10-year survival: occult cancers (65%); palpable cancers (25%)

Role of mammography
OVERALL DETECTION RATE:
58 – 69%; 8% if <1 cm in size

MAMMOGRAPHIC ACCURACY:
88% correctly diagnosed by radiologist
27% detected only by mammography
8% misinterpretations
4% not detected

MAMMOGRAPHICALLY MISSED CANCERS
Incidence: approx. 10 – 30%
1. Technical error (5%):
(a) poor image quality
(b) failure to image region of interest
2. Observer error (30%): oversight, rushed interpretation, heavy caseload, extraneous distraction, eye fatigue
3. Unrecognized signs (33%): masked by dense breast parenchyma
4. Acute cancers (33%): cancers surfacing in screening interval

RADIATION-INDUCED BREAST CARCINOMA
Δ Lifetime risk with cumulative carcinogenic effect related to age!
(a) women age <35: 7.5 additional cancers per 1 million irradiated women per year per rad
(b) women age >35: 3.5 additional cancers per 1 million irradiated women per year per rad

Role of breast ultrasound
Indications:
(1) Differentiation of cystic from solid lesion (principal role)
(2) Equivocal mammogram with palpable mass / mammographic asymmetry
(3) Dense breast, particularly in adolescent patient
(4) Evaluation of breast implant

(5) Postmastectomy tissue
(6) Ultrasound-guided cyst aspiration
(7) In pregnancy
(8) "Radiophobic" patient
(9) Bedridden patient
Δ Ultrasound is no screening tool!

Accuracy: 98% accuracy for cysts; 99% accuracy for solid masses; small carcinomas have the least characteristic features

BREAST CYST
Incidence: most common single cause of breast lumps between 35 and 55 years of age; characteristically in perimenopausal age
Cause: fluid cannot be absorbed due to obstruction of extralobular terminal duct by fibrosis / intraductal epithelial proliferation
Histo: cyst wall lined by single layer of
   (a)   flattened epithelial cells; cyst fluid with Na^+/ K^+ ratio ≥3
   (b)   epithelial cells with apocrine metaplasia (secretory function); cyst fluid with Na^+/K^+ ratio <3
Δ Patients with apocrine cysts are at greater risk to develop breast cancer!
• size changes over time
• inspection of cyst fluid:
   (a)   normal: turbid greenish / grayish / black fluid
   (b)   abnormal: straw-colored clear fluid / dark blood

√ solitary / multiple
√ well-defined oval / round mammographic mass + surrounding halo (DDx: well-defined solid mass)
√ needle aspiration of fluid (proof) + postaspiration mammogram as new baseline
US:
   √ anechoic lesion + well-defined posterior wall + acoustic enhancement (98 – 100% accuracy)
   √ occasionally loculated
Pneumocystography (for palpable / symptomatic cysts):
   √ air remains mammographically detectable for up to 3 weeks
   √ diagnosis of intracystic tumor in 2% (1% benign, 1% malignant)
   √ therapeutic effect of air insufflation: no cyst recurrence in 94% (40 – 45% cyst recurrence without air insufflation)
Cx: intracystic carcinoma in 0.3% of all breast cancers

CARCINOMA OF MALE BREAST
Incidence: 0.2%
Δ 3.7% of males with breast carcinoma have Klinefelter syndrome (20-fold risk over normals)!
Peak age: 60 – 69 years
Associated with: high incidence of breast cancer in family members

√ resembles scirrhous carcinoma of female breast
√ usually located eccentrically

√ calcifications fewer + more scattered + more round + larger
√ enlarged axillary nodes

CHRONIC ABSCESS OF BREAST
= COLD ABSCESS usually seen in lactating women
• fever, pain, increased WBC (clinical diagnosis)
• rapid response to antibiotics
Location: most commonly in central / subareolar area
√ ill-defined mass of increased density with flame-like contour
√ secondary changes common: architectural distortion, nipple + areolar retraction, lymphedema, skin thickening, pathologic axillary nodes
√ liquefied center can be aspirated
US:
   √ anechoic / nearly anechoic area with posterior enhancement

CYSTOSARCOMA PHYLLOIDES
= GIANT FIBROADENOMA = ADENOSARCOMA
= usually benign giant form of intracanalicular fibroadenoma
Incidence: 1: 6,300 examinations; 0.3% of all breast tumors; 3% of all fibroadenomas
Mean age: 45 years
Histo:
similar to fibroadenoma with anaplasia, fibroepithelial tumor with leaflike (phyllodes) growth pattern
= branching projections of tissue into cystic cavities; cystic degeneration + hemorrhage; cavernous structures contain mucus; cellular connective tissue stroma with wide variations in size, shape, differentiation

• rapidly enlarging breast mass
• sense of fullness
• huge, firm, mobile, discrete, lobulated, smooth mass
• discoloration of skin, wide veins, shining skin
√ large noncalcified mass with smooth polylobulated margins mimicking fibroadenoma
√ rapid growth to large size (>6 – 8 cm), may fill entire breast

Prognosis: limited invasion frequently seen; 15 – 20% recurrence rate if not completely excised
Cx: in 5 – 10% malignant degeneration into malignant fibrous histiocytoma / fibrosarcoma / liposarcoma / chondrosarcoma / osteosarcoma with local invasion + hematogenous metastases to lung, pleura, bone (axillary metastases quite rare)

FAT NECROSIS OF BREAST
= TRAUMATIC LIPID CYST = OIL CYST = aseptic saponification of fat by tissue lipase after local destruction of fat cells with release of lipids + hemorrhage + fibrotic proliferation
Etiology: direct external trauma, breast biopsy, reduction mammoplasty, irradiation, nodular panniculitis (Weber-Christian disease), ductal ectasia of chronic mastitis

Incidence: 0.5% of breast biopsies
Histo: cavity with oily material surrounded by "foam cells" (= lipid-laden macrophages)
- history of trauma in 40% (eg, prior surgery, radiation >6 months ago, reduction mammoplasty, lumpectomy)
- firm, slightly fixed mass
- skin retraction (50%)
- yellowish fatty fluid on aspiration
Location: anywhere; more common in areolar region; near biopsy site / surgical scar
√ ill-defined irregular spiculated dense mass (indistinguishable from carcinoma if associated with distortion, skin thickening, retraction)
√ well-circumscribed mass with translucent areas at center (= homogeneous fat density of oil cyst) surrounded by thin pseudocapsule (in old lesions)
√ may calcify (= **liponecrosis macrocystica calcificans**)
√ occasionally curvilinear / eggshell calcification in wall
√ fine spicules of low density vary with projection
√ localized skin thickening / retraction possible
US:
√ hypo- / anechoic mass with ill- / well-defined margins ± acoustic shadowing

Weber-Christian Disease
= nonsuppurative panniculitis with recurrent bouts of inflammation = areas of fat necrosis, involving subcutaneous fat + fat within internal organs
- accompanied by fever + nodules over trunk and limbs

FIBROADENOMA
= estrogen-induced benign tumor; forms during adolescence; pregnancy + lactation are growth stimulants; regression after menopause (mucoid degeneration, hyalinization, involution of epithelial components, calcification)
Incidence: 3rd most common type of breast lesion after fibrocystic disease + carcinoma, most common benign solid tumor in women of child-bearing age
Age: mean age of 39 years (range 13 – 80 years); usually after puberty + before age 30; most common breast tumor under age 25 years; regresses after menopause; may occur in postmenopausal women receiving estrogen replacement therapy
Histo: mixture of proliferated fibrous stroma + secondarily increased epithelial ductal structures
  (a) intracanalicular fibroadenoma
  (b) pericanalicular fibroadenoma
  (c) combination
- firm, smooth, sometimes lobulated, freely moveable mass
- in 35% not palpable
- NO skin fixation
- rarely tender / painful
- clinical size = radiographic size

Size: 1 – 5 cm (in 60%); multiple in 10 – 20%; bilateral in 4%

√ circular / oval-shaped lesion of low density
√ nodular / lobulated contour when larger (areas with different growth rates)
√ smooth, discrete margins (indistinguishable from cysts when small)
√ often with "halo" sign
√ smoothly contoured calcifications of high + fairly equal density in 3% due to necrosis from regressive changes in older patients:
  (a) peripheral subcapsular myxoid degeneration
  (b) central myxoid degeneration = "popcorn" type of calcification (PATHOGNOMONIC)
Δ Calcifications enlarge as soft tissue component regresses!
US:
√ round (3%) / oval mass (96%) with length-to-depth ratio of >1.4 (in carcinomas usually <1.4)
√ hypoechoic (80 – 96%) / hyperechoic / mixed pattern / anechoic / isoechoic compared with adjacent fibroglandular tissue
√ homogeneous (48 – 89%) / inhomogeneous texture
√ regular (57%) / lobulated / irregular (6 – 58%) contour
√ intratumoral bright echoes (10%) = macrocalcifications
√ posterior acoustic enhancement (17 – 25%) / acoustic shadow without calcifications (6%)
√ echogenic halo (capsule) with lateral shadowing

GIANT FIBROADENOMA
= fibroadenoma >6 cm; usually occurring in adolescents / young adults

JUVENILE FIBROADENOMA
= rapidly growing tumor in young girls during puberty
√ may grow to huge size, enlarging the breast

DDx: medullary / mucinous / papillary carcinoma / carcinoma within fibroadenoma

FIBROCYSTIC CHANGES
= Mazoplasia = mastitis fibrosa cystica = chronic cystic mastitis = cystic disease = generalized breast hyperplasia = desquamated epithelial hyperplasia
= fibroadenomatosis = mammary dysplasia
= Schimmelbusch disease = fibrous mastitis
= mammary proliferative disease
Δ Not a disease since found in 72% of screening population >55 years of age
Δ The College of American Pathologists suggests to use the term "fibrocystic changes / condition" in mammography reports!

Incidence: most common diffuse breast disorder; in 51% of 3,000 autopsies
Age: 35 – 55 years
Etiology: exaggeration of normal cyclical proliferation + involution of the breast with production + incomplete absorption of fluid by apocrine cells
- asymptomatic in macrocystic disease
- fullness, tenderness, pain in microcystic disease

- palpable nodules + thickening
- symptoms occur with ovulation; regression with pregnancy + menopause

Histo:
(1) overgrowth of fibrous connective tissue = stromal fibrosis, fibroadenoma
(2) cystic dilatation of ducts + cyst formation (in 100% microscopic, in 20% macroscopic)
(3) hyperplasia of ducts + lobules + acini = adenosis; ductal papillomatosis

√ individual round / ovoid cysts with discrete smooth margins
√ lobulated multilocular cyst
√ enlarged nodular pattern (= fluid-distended lobules + extensive extralobular fibrous connective tissue overgrowth)
√ "teacup"-like curvilinear thin calcifications with horizontal beam + low-density round calcifications in craniocaudal projection = milk of calcium (4%)
√ "oyster pearl"-like / psammoma-like calcifications
√ "involutional type" calcifications = very fine punctate calcifications evenly distributed within one / more lobes against a fatty background (from mild degree of hyperplasia in subsequently atrophied glandular tissue)

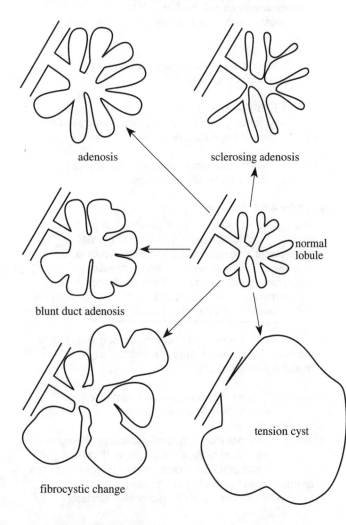

adenosis

sclerosing adenosis

blunt duct adenosis

normal lobule

fibrocystic change

tension cyst

US:
√ ductal pattern, ductectasia, cysts, ill-defined focal lesions

ADENOSIS
= hyperplasia + hypertrophy of glandular elements
√ increase in size of lobules to 3 – 7 mm
√ "snowflake pattern" of widespread ill-defined nodular densities

SCLEROSING ADENOSIS
= adenosis + reactive fibrosis = proliferating acinar structure maintaining a lobular configuration
√ adenosis + diffusely scattered calcifications (calcifications in cystically dilated acinar structure)
√ dense breast

FIBROSIS
√ round / oval clustered microcalcifications with smooth contours + associated fine granular calcifications filling lobules

ATYPICAL LOBULAR HYPERPLASIA
= proliferative cells not distending lobules (as in lobular carcinoma in situ)
√ round dense microcalcifications in a loose cluster, some variability in size

INTRADUCTAL PAPILLOMATOSIS
= hyperplastic polypoid lesions within a duct
Age: perimenopausal
- spontaneous bloody / serous / serosanguinous nipple discharge (most common cause of nipple discharge)
√ small retroareolar opacity (= dilated duct) extending 2 – 3 cm into breast
√ intraluminal filling defect on galactography

Risk for Invasive Breast Carcinoma
A. No increased risk:
   1. Fibroadenoma
   2. Nonproliferative lesions: adenosis, florid adenosis, apocrine metaplasia without atypia, macro- / microcysts, duct ectasia, fibrosis, mild hyperplasia (more than 2 but not more than 4 epithelial cells deep), mastitis, periductal mastitis, squamous metaplasia
B. Slightly increased risk (1.5 – 2 times):
   1. Moderate + florid solid / papillary hyperplasia
   2. Papilloma with fibrovascular core
   3. Sclerosing adenosis
C. Moderately increased risk (5 times):
   Ductal / lobular atypical hyperplasia (borderline lesion with some features of carcinoma in situ)
D. High risk (8 – 11 times):
   1. Atypical hyperplasia + family history of breast cancer
   2. Ductal / lobular carcinoma in situ

GALACTOCELE
= retention of fatty material in areas of cystic duct dilatation appearing during / shortly after lactation
Cause: ? abrupt suppression of lactation
Age: occurs during / shortly after lactation
- thick inspissated milky fluid (colostrum)

Location: retroareolar area
√ large radiopaque lesion of water density (1st phase)
√ smaller lesion of mixed density + fat-water level with horizontal beam (2nd phase)
√ small radiolucent lesion resembling lipoma
√ ± fluid-calcium level

GRANULAR CELL MYOBLASTOMA OF BREAST
= tumor originating from ? Schwann cell, smooth muscle, or undifferentiated mesenchymal cell
Age : 20 – 59 years; more common in blacks
Locations: tongue, skin, bronchial wall, subcutaneous breast tissue (6%)
• asymmetric lump with slow growth, hardness, skin fixation, ulceration
√ well-circumscribed mass with stellate extensions (tumor insinuating itself into surrounding breast tissue)
√ may exhibit acoustic shadow

GYNECOMASTIA
Causes:
(1) Hormonal
  (a) puberty: high estradiol levels
  (b) older men: decline in serum testosterone levels
  (c) hypogonadism (Klinefelter syndrome, testicular neoplasm)
  (d) tumors: adrenal carcinoma, pituitary adenoma, testicular tumor, hyperthyroidism
(2) Systemic disorders
  advanced alcoholic cirrhosis, hemodialysis in chronic renal failure, chronic pulmonary disease (emphysema, TB), malnutrition
(3) Drug-induced
  estrogen treatment for prostate cancer, digitalis, cimetidine, thiazide, spironolactone, reserpine, isoniazid, ergotamine, marijuana
(4) Neoplasm: hepatoma (with estrogen production)
(5) Idiopathic
mnemonic: "CODES"
  Cirrhosis
  Obesity
  Digitalis
  Estrogen
  Spironolactone
Incidence: 85% of all male breast masses
Age: adolescent boys (40%), men >50 years (32%)
Histo: increased number of ducts, proliferation of duct epithelium, periductal edema, fibroplastic stroma, adipose tissue
• palpable firm mass >2 cm in subareolar region
Location: bilateral (63%), left-sided (27%), right-sided (10%)
Types: (a) focal type
  (b) diffuse type
DDx: Pseudogynecomastia (= fatty proliferation)

HAMARTOMA OF BREAST
= FIBROADENOLIPOMA = LIPOFIBROADENOMA = ADENOLIPOMA
Incidence: 2 – 16:10,000 mammograms

Mean age: 45 (27 – 88) years
Histo: normal / dysplastic mammary tissue composed of dense fibrous tissue + variable amount of fat, delineated from surrounding tissue without a true capsule
• soft, often nonpalpable (60%)
Location: retroareolar (30%),
  upper outer quadrant (35%)
√ round / ovoid well-circumscribed mass usually > 3 cm
√ mixed density with mottled center (secondary to fat) = "slice of sausage" pattern
√ thin smooth pseudocapsule (= thin layer of surrounding fibrous tissue)
√ peripheral radiolucent zone
√ may contain calcifications
DDx: liposarcoma

Cowden Disease = multiple hamartoma syndrome
1. Cutaneous + oral verrucous papules (lips, gingiva, tongue)
2. Endodermal, ectodermal, mesodermal dysplasia with tumors of skin, breast, GI tract, thyroid gland
3. Malignant tumors of breast + thyroid

HEMATOMA OF BREAST
Causes:
(1) surgery / biopsy (most common)
(2) blunt trauma
(3) coagulopathy (leukemia, thrombocytopenia)
(4) anticoagulant therapy
√ well-defined ovoid mass (= hemorrhagic cyst)
√ ill-defined mass with diffuse increased density (edema + hemorrhage)
√ adjacent skin thickening / prominence of reticular structures
√ regression within several weeks leaving (a) no trace (b) architectural distortion (c) incomplete resolution
√ calcifications (occasionally)
US:
  √ hypoechoic mass with internal echoes

JUVENILE PAPILLOMATOSIS
Path: many aggregated cysts with interspersed dense stroma
Histo: cysts lined by flat duct epithelium / epithelium with apocrine metaplasia, sclerosing adenosis, duct stasis; marked papillary hyperplasia of duct epithelium with often extreme atypia
Mean age: 23 years (range of 12 – 48 years)
• localized palpable tumor
• family history of breast cancer in 28% (affected first-degree relative in 8%; in one / more relatives in 28%)
Prognosis: development of synchronous (4%) / metachronous (4%) breast cancer after 8 – 9 years
DDx: fibroadenoma

LIPOMA OF BREAST
= usually solitary asymptomatic slow-growing lesion
Mean age: 45 years + postmenopause

- soft, freely moveable, well delineated
√ usually >2 cm
√ radiolucent lesion easily seen in dense breast; almost invisible in fatty breast
√ discrete thin radiopaque line (= capsule), seen in most of its circumference
√ displacement of adjacent breast parenchyma
√ calcification with fat necrosis (extremely rare)

DDx: fat lobule surrounded by trabeculae / suspensory ligaments

LYMPHOMA OF BREAST
A. Primary lymphoma: 0.3% incidence
B. Metastatic lymphoma

- axillary nodes involved in 35%
Location: right-sided predominance; 13% bilateral
√ round / oval mass
√ infiltrate with poorly defined borders

PSEUDOLYMPHOMA
= lymphoreticular lesion as an overwhelming response to trauma

MASTITIS
A. PUERPERAL MASTITIS
  = usually interstitial infection during lactational period
    (a) through infected nipple cracks
    (b) hematogenous
    (c) ascending via ducts = galactophoritis
  Organism: staphylococcus, streptococcus
  - tender swollen red breast (DDx: inflammatory carcinoma)
  - enlarged painful axillary lymph nodes
  - ± febrile, elevated ESR, leukocytosis
  √ diffuse increased density
  √ diffuse skin thickening
  √ swelling of breast
  √ enlarged axillary lymph nodes
  √ rapid resolution under antibiotic therapy
B. NONPUERPERAL MASTITIS
  1. Infected cyst
  2. Purulent mastitis with abscess formation
  3. Plasma cell mastitis
  4. Nonspecific mastitis
C. GRANULOMATOUS MASTITIS
  1. Foreign body granuloma
  2. Specific disease (TB, sarcoidosis, leprosy, syphilis, actinomycosis, typhus)
  3. Parasitic disease (hydatid disease, cysticercosis, filariasis, schistosomiasis)

METASTASES TO BREAST
Incidence: 1%
Mean age: 43 years
Primaries: (1) Malignant melanoma
          (2) Ovarian carcinoma
          (3) Leukemia / lymphoma
√ solitary mass (85%), esp. in upper outer quadrant

√ skin adherence (25%)
√ axillary node involvement (40%)

PAPILLOMA OF BREAST
= usually benign proliferation of ductal epithelial tissue
Age: 30 – 77 years (juvenile papillomatosis = 20 – 26 years)
Histo: hyperplastic proliferation of ductal epithelium; lesion may be pedunculated / broad-based; connective tissue stalk covered by epithelial cells proliferating in the form of apocrine metaplasia / solid hyperplasia may cause duct obstruction + distension to form an intracystic papilloma

A. CENTRAL SOLITARY PAPILLOMA (more common)
  Location: subareolar within major duct
  NOT premalignant
  - spontaneous bloody / serous / clear nipple discharge (52 – 100%)
    Δ Most common cause of serous / sanguinous nipple discharge!
  - "trigger point" = nipple discharge produced upon compression of area with papilloma
  - intermittent mass disappearing with discharge
  √ negative mammogram / intraductal nodules in subareolar area
  √ asymmetrically dilated single duct
  √ subareolar amorphous coarse calcifications
  √ dilated duct with obstructing / distorting intraluminal filling defect on ductography (= galactography)
  Cx: 0 – 14% frequency of carcinoma development

B. PERIPHERAL MULTIPLE PAPILLOMAS
  Location: within terminal ductal lobular unit; bilateral in up to 14%
  In 10 – 38% associated with
    atypical ductal hyperplasia, lobular carcinoma in situ, papillary + cribriform intraductal cancers, radial scar
  - nipple discharge (20%)
  √ round / oval / slightly lobulated well-circumscribed nodules
  √ segmental distribution with dilated ducts extending from beneath the nipple (20%)
  √ may be associated with coarse microcalcifications
  Cx: 5% frequency of carcinoma development; increased risk dependent on degree of cellular atypia
  Prognosis: in 24% recurrence after surgical treatment

DDx: invasive papillary carcinoma

PLASMA CELL MASTITIS
= CHRONIC MASTITIS
= rare aseptic inflammation of subareolar area
Etiology:
  ? sequelae of secretory disease secondary to stasis of intraductal secretion + extravasation of inspissated material that is rich in fatty acids + incites an aseptic chemical mastitis = nontraumatic fat necrosis

Age: elderly women
Histo: ductal ectasia, heavily calcified ductal secretions; infiltration of plasma cells + giant cells + eosinophils
• often asymptomatic
Location: subareolar, often bilateral + symmetric; may be unilateral + focal
√ dense triangular mass with apex toward nipple
√ distended ducts connecting to nipple
√ periphery blending with normal tissue
√ multiple often bilateral dense round / oval calcifications with lucent center + polarity (= orientation towards nipple)
  (a) periductal
      √ oval / elongated calcified ring around dilated ducts with very dense periphery (surrounding deposits of fibrosis + fat necrosis)
  (b) intraductal
      √ fairly uniform linear, often "needle-shaped" calcifications of wide caliber, occasionally branching (within ducts / confined to duct walls)
√ nipple retraction / skin thickening may occur

RADIAL SCAR

= SCLEROSING DUCT HYPERPLASIA = INDURATIVE MASTOPATHY = FOCAL FIBROUS DISEASE = BENIGN SCLEROSING DUCTAL PROLIFERATION
= benign proliferative breast lesion (malignant potential is controversial); "scar" = sclerotic center with surrounding contracted ducts + lobules
Incidence: 1 – 2/1,000 screening mammograms; 16% in mastectomy specimens

Histo:
  central core of elastosis (= acellular connective tissue and abundant deposits of elastin); one / more ducts obliterated by connective tissue; entrapped tubules in sclerotic center surrounded by a corona of contracted ducts + lobules (sclerosing adenosis) and papillomatosis
May be associated with tubular carcinoma, comedo carcinoma, invasive lobular carcinoma + contralateral breast cancer
Δ Avoid frozen section
• rarely palpable
√ irregular noncalcified mass often with architectural distortion
√ variable appearance in different projections
√ oval / circular translucent areas at center
√ very thin long spicules, clumped together centrally
√ radiolucent linear structures paralleling spicules
√ no skin thickening / retraction
Rx: surgical excision required for definite diagnosis
DDx : carcinoma

SARCOMA OF BREAST

Incidence: 1% of malignant mammary lesions
Age: 45 – 55 years
Histo: fibrosarcoma, rhabdomyosarcoma, osteogenic sarcoma, mixed malignant tumor of the breast, malignant fibrosarcoma and carcinoma, liposarcoma
• rapid growth
√ smooth / lobulated large dense mass
√ well-defined outline
√ palpated size similar to mammographic size

DIFFERENTIAL DIAGNOSIS OF CARDIOVASCULAR DISORDERS

CONGENITAL HEART DISEASE
Classification of CHD

	acyanotic	cyanotic
Increased PBF + increased CT ratio	*L-R shunts* 　VSD 　ASD 　PDA 　ECD 　PAPVR	*T-lesions* 　Transposition 　Truncus arteriosus 　TAPVR 　"Tingles" (single ventricle / atrium) 　Tricuspid atresia (without RVOT obstruction)
Normal PBF + normal CT ratio	*LV outflow obstruction* 　AS 　Coarctation 　Interrupted aortic arch 　Hypoplastic left heart 　PS *LV inflow obstruction* 　Obstructed TAPVR 　Cor triatriatum 　Pulmonary vein atresia 　Congenital MV stenosis *Muscle disease* 　Cardiomyopathy 　Myocarditis 　Anomalous LCA	
Decreased PBF + normal CT ratio Cardiomegaly		*VSD present* 　Tetralogy of Fallot 　Tricuspid atresia (with PS + nonrestrictive ASD) 　Pulmonary atresia + VSD *Intact ventricular septum* 　Pulmonary atresia without VSD 　Ebstein anomaly

Incidence of CHD in liveborn infants
Overall incidence: 8 – 9:1000 livebirths
- most common CHD: mitral valve prolapse (5 – 20%), bicuspid aortic valve (2%) [usually not recognized before late infancy / childhood]
- ASD + VSD + PDA account for 45% of all CHD
- 12 lesions account for 89% of all CHD

Ventricular septal defect	30.3%
Patent ductus arteriosus	8.6%
Pulmonary stenosis	7.4%
Septum secundum defect	6.7%

Coarctation of aorta	5.7%
Aortic stenosis	5.2%
Tetralogy of Fallot	5.1%
Transposition	4.7%
Endocardial cushion defect	3.2%
Hypoplastic right ventricle	2.2%
Hypoplastic left heart	1.3%
TAPVR	1.1%
Truncus arteriosus	1.0%
Single ventricle	0.3%
Double outlet right ventricle	0.2%

High risk pregnancy:
  (1) Previous sibling with CHD   :   2 – 5%
  (2) Previous 2 siblings with CHD: 10 – 15%
  (3) One parent with CHD: 2 – 10%

Most common causes for CHF + PVH in neonate:
  1. Left ventricular failure due to outflow obstruction
  2. Obstruction of pulmonary venous return

CHD with relatively long life

Congenital lesions compatible with a relative long life are:
  1. Mild tetralogy: mild pulmonic stenosis + small VSD
  2. Valvular pulmonic stenosis: with relatively normal
      pulmonary circulation
  3. Transposition of great vessels: some degree of
      pulmonic stenosis + large VSD
  4. Truncus arteriosus: delicate balance between
      systemic + pulmonary circulation
  5. Truncus arteriosus type IV: large systemic collaterals
  6. Tricuspid atresia + transposition + pulmonic stenosis
  7. Eisenmenger complex
  8. Ebstein anomaly
  9. Corrected transposition without intracardiac shunt

Juxtaposition of atrial appendages

  1. Tricuspid atresia with transposition
  2. Complete transposition
  3. Corrected transposition of great arteries
  4. DORV

Continuous heart murmur

  1. PDA
  2. AP window
  3. Ruptured sinus of Valsalva aneurysm
  4. Hemitruncus
  5. Coronary arteriovenous fistula

Congestive heart failure + cardiomegaly

mnemonic: "Ma McCae & Co."
  Myocardial infarction
  anemia
  Malformation
  cardiomyopathy
  Coronary artery disease
  aortic insufficiency
  effusion
  Coarctation

Neonatal cardiac failure

  A. OBSTRUCTIVE LESIONS
      1. Coarctation of the aorta
      2. Aortic valve stenosis
      3. Asymmetrical septal hypertrophy / hypertrophic
          obstructive cardiomyopathy
  B. VOLUME OVERLOAD
      1. Congenital mitral valve incompetence
      2. Corrected transposition with left (= tricuspid) AV
          valve incompetence
      3. Congenital tricuspid insufficiency
      4. Ostium primum ASD
  C. MYOCARDIAL DYSFUNCTION / ISCHEMIA
      1. Nonobstructive cardiomyopathy
      2. Anomalous origin of LCA from pulmonary trunk
      3. Primary endocardial fibroelastosis
      4. Glycogen storage disease (Pompe disease)
      5. Myocarditis
  D. NONCARDIAC LESIONS
      1. AV fistulas: hemangioendothelioma of liver, AV
          fistula of brain, vein of Galen aneurysm, large
          pulmonary AV fistula
      2. Transient tachypnea of the newborn
      3. Intraventricular / subarachnoid hemorrhage
      4. Neonatal hypoglycemia (low birth weight, infants
          of diabetic mothers)
      5. Thyrotoxicosis (transplacental passage of LATS
          hormone)

Presenting age in CHD

AGE	SEVERE PVH	PVH + SHUNT VASCULARITY
0 – 2 days	Hypoplastic left heart Aortic atresia TAPVR below diaphragm Myocardiopathy in IDM	Hypoplastic left heart TAPVR above diaphragm Complete transposition
3 – 7 days		PDA in preterm infant
7 – 14 days	CoA + VSD / PDA Aortic valve stenosis Peripheral AVM Endocardial fibroelastosis Anomalous left coronary artery	Coarctation of aorta (CoA) AVM

Syndromes with CHD

5 p – (Cri-du-chat) syndrome
Incidence of CHD: 20%

DiGeorge syndrome (thymic agenesis)
1. Conotruncal malformation
2. Interrupted aortic arch

Down syndrome = MONGOLISM = TRISOMY 21
1. Endocardial cushion defect (25%)
2. Membranous VSD
3. Ostium primum ASD
4. AV communis
5. Cleft mitral valve
6. PDA
7. 11 rib pairs (25%)
8. Hypersegmented manubrium (90%)

Ellis-van Creveld syndrome
Incidence of CHD: 50%
- polydactyly
√ single atrium

Holt-Oram syndrome
= UPPER LIMB-CARDIAC SYNDROME
Incidence of CHD: 50%
1. ASD
2. VSD
3. Valvular pulmonary stenosis
4. Radial dysplasia

Hurler syndrome
Cardiomyopathy

Ivemark syndrome
Incidence of CHD: 100%
- asplenia
√ complex cardiac anomalies

Klippel-Feil syndrome
Incidence of CHD: 5%
1. Atrial septal defect
2. Coarctation

Marfan syndrome = ARACHNODACTYLY
1. Aortic sinus dilatation
2. Aortic aneurysm
3. Aortic insufficiency
4. Pulmonary aneurysm

Noonan syndrome
1. Pulmonary stenosis
2. ASD
3. Hypertrophic cardiomyopathy

Osteogenesis imperfecta
1. Aortic valve insufficiency
2. Mitral valve insufficiency
3. Pulmonic valve insufficiency

Postrubella syndrome
- low birth weight
- deafness
- cataracts
- mental retardation
1. Peripheral pulmonic stenosis
2. Valvular pulmonic stenosis
3. Supravalvular aortic stenosis
4. PDA

Trisomy 13 – 15
VSD, Tetralogy of Fallot, DORV

Trisomy 16 – 18
VSD, PDA, DORV

Turner syndrome (XO) = OVARIAN DYSGENESIS
Incidence of CHD: 35%
1. Coarctation of the aorta (in 15%)
2. Bicuspid aortic valve
3. Dissecting aneurysm of aorta

Williams syndrome = IDIOPATHIC HYPERCALCEMIA
- peculiar elfin-like facies
- mental + physical retardation
- hypercalcemia (not in all patients)
1. Supravalvular aortic stenosis (33%)
2. ASD, VSD
3. Valvular + peripheral pulmonary artery stenosis
4. Aortic hypoplasia, stenoses of more peripheral arteries

SHUNT EVALUATION

Evaluation of L-to-R shunts
A. AGE
  — Infants:
    (1) Isolated VSD
    (2) VSD with CoA / PDA / AV canal
    (3) PDA
    (4) Ostium primum
  — Children / adults:
    (1) ASD
    (2) Partial AV canal with competent mitral valve
    (3) VSD / PDA with high pulmonary resistance
    (4) PDA without murmur
B. SEX
  99% chance for ASD / PDA in female patient
C. CHEST WALL ANALYSIS
  √ 11 pair of ribs + hypersegmented manubrium:
    Down syndrome
  √ pectus excavatum + straight back:
    prolapsing mitral valve
D. CARDIAC SILHOUETTE
  √ absent pulmonary trunk:
    corrected transposition with VSD; pink tetralogy
  √ left-sided ascending aorta:
    corrected transposition with VSD
  √ tortuous descending aorta:
    aortic valve incompetence + ASD

√ huge heart:
persistent complete AV canal (PCAVC); VSD + PDA; VSD + mitral valve incompetence
√ enlarged left atrium:
intact atrial septum; mitral regurgitation (endocardial cushion defect, prolapsing mitral valve + ASD)

DIFFERENTIAL DIAGNOSIS OF L-R SHUNTS

	RA	RV	PA	LA	LV	Prox. Ao
ASD	inc	inc	inc	nl	nl	nl
VSD	nl	inc	inc	inc	inc	nl
PDA	nl	nl	inc	inc	inc	often inc

Shunt with normal left atrium
A. Precardiac shunt
   1. Anomalous pulmonary venous connection
B. Intracardiac shunt
   1. ASD (8%)
   2. VSD (25%)
C. Postcardiac
   1. PDA (12%)

Aortic size in shunts
A. Extracardiac shunts
   √ aorta enlarged + hyperpulsatile
   1. PDA
B. Pre- and intracardiac shunts
   √ aorta small but not hypoplastic
   1. Anomalous pulmonary venous return
   2. ASD
   3. VSD
   4. Common AV canal

Abnormal heart chamber dimensions
A. LEFT VENTRICULAR VOLUME OVERLOAD
   1. VSD
   2. PDA
   3. Mitral incompetence
   4. Aortic incompetence
B. LEFT VENTRICULAR HYPERTROPHY
   1. Coarctation
   2. Aortic stenosis
C. RIGHT VENTRICULAR VOLUME OVERLOAD
   1. ASD
   2. Partial APVR / total APVR
   3. Tricuspid insufficiency
   4. Pulmonary insufficiency
   5. Congenital / acquired absence of pericardium
   [6. Ebstein anomaly] – not truly RV
D. RIGHT VENTRICULAR HYPERTROPHY
   1. Pulmonary valve stenosis
   2. Pulmonary hypertension
   3. Tetralogy of Fallot
   4. VSD
E. Fixed subvalvular aortic stenosis
F. Hypoplastic left / right ventricle, common ventricle
G. Congestive cardiomyopathy

Cardiomegaly in newborn
A. NONCARDIOGENIC
   1. Metabolic:
      (a) ion imbalance in serum levels of sodium, potassium, and calcium
      (b) hypoglycemia
   2. Decreased ventilation
      (a) asphyxia
      (b) transient tachypnea
      (c) perinatal brain damage
   3. Erythrocyte function
      (a) anemia
      (b) erythrocythemia
   4. Endocrine
      (a) glycogen storage disease
      (b) thyroid disease: hypo- / hyperthyroidism
   5. Infant of diabetic mother
   6. Arteriovenous fistula
      (a) vein of Galen aneurysm
      (b) hepatic angioma
      (c) chorioangioma
B. CARDIOGENIC
   1. Arrhythmia
   2. Myo- / pericarditis
   3. Cardiac tumor
   4. Myocardial infarction
   5. Congenital heart disease

CYANOTIC HEART DISEASE
Chemical cyanosis = $PaO_2 \leq 94\%$
Clinical cyanosis = $PaO_2 \leq 85\%$
Δ Decrease in hemoglobin delays detectability!
Most common cause of cyanosis
— in newborn is transposition of great vessels
— in child is tetralogy of Fallot!

A. OVERCIRCULATION VASCULARITY
   mnemonic: "5 T's + CAD"
   1. **T**ransposition, complete
   2. **T**ricuspid atresia with transposition
   3. **T**runcus arteriosus
   4. **T**APVR above diaphragm
   5. **T**ingle ventricle
   6. **C**ommon atrium
   7. **A**ortic atresia
   8. **D**ORV

B. DECREASED VASCULARITY (with R-to-L shunt)
   (a) at ATRIAL LEVEL
      1. Isolated pulmonary stenosis / atresia
      2. Tricuspid atresia without transposition with pulmonary stenosis
      3. Ebstein / Uhl malformation
      4. Congenital tricuspid regurgitation
      5. Pericardial effusion
   (b) at VENTRICULAR LEVEL
      1. Tetralogy of Fallot
      2. Single ventricle
      3. Tricuspid atresia without transposition without pulmonary stenosis

4. DORV
5. Asplenia syndrome
6. Corrected transposition + VSD

C. PULMONARY VENOUS HYPERTENSION
1. Atresia of common pulmonary vein
2. TAPVR below diaphragm
3. Aortic atresia
N.B.: tricuspid atresia = the great mimicker

Increased pulmonary blood flow with cyanosis
= ADMIXTURE LESIONS = bidirectional shunt with 2 components:
(a) mixing of saturated blood (L-R shunt) and unsaturated blood (R-L shunt)
(b) NO obstruction to pulmonary blood flow

Evaluation process:
√ PA segment absent = transposition
√ PA segment present:
(a) L atrium normal (= extracardiac shunt) = TAPVR
(b) L atrium enlarged (= intracardiac shunt) = truncus arteriosus

N.B.: Overcirculation + cyanosis = complete transposition until proven otherwise!

ADMIXTURE LESIONS = T-LESIONS
mnemonic: "5 **T**'s + **CAD**"
Transposition of great vessels = complete TGV ± VSD (most common cause for cyanosis in neonate)
Tricuspid atresia with or without transposition + VSD (2nd most common cause for cyanosis in neonate)
Truncus arteriosus
Total anomalous pulmonary venous return (TAPVR) above diaphragm
(a) supracardiac
(b) cardiac (coronary sinus / right atrium)
"**T**ingle" = single ventricle
Common atrium
Aortic atresia
Double-outlet right ventricle (DORV type I) / Taussig-Bing anomaly (DORV type II)

Clues:
√ skeletal anomalies: Ellis-van Creveld syndrome (truncus / common atrium)
√ polysplenia: common atrium
√ R aortic arch: persistent truncus arteriosus
√ ductus infundibulum: aortic atresia
√ pulmonary trunk seen: supracardiac TAPVR; DORV; tricuspid atresia; common atrium
√ ascending aorta with leftward convexity: single ventricle
√ dilated azygous vein: common atrium + polysplenia + interrupted IVC; TAPVR to azygous vein
√ left-sided SVC: vertical vein of TAPVR
√ "waterfall" right hilum: single ventricle + transposition

√ large left atrium (rules out TAPVR)
√ prominent L heart border: single ventricle with inverted rudimentary R ventricle; levoposition of R atrial appendage (tricuspid atresia + transposition)
√ age of onset ≤2 days: aortic atresia

Decreased pulmonary blood flow with cyanosis
= two components of (a) impedance of blood flow through right heart due to obstruction / atresia at pulmonary valve / infundibulum (b) R-to-L shunt; pulmonary circulation maintained through systemic arteries / PDA

A. SHUNT AT VENTRICULAR LEVEL
1. Tetralogy of Fallot
2. Tetralogy physiology (associated with pulmonary obstruction):
— Complete / corrected transposition
— Single ventricle
— DORV
— Tricuspid atresia (PS in 75%)
— Asplenia syndrome
√ prominent aorta with L / R aortic arch; inapparent pulmonary trunk
√ NORMAL R atrium (without tricuspid regurgitation)
√ NORMAL-sized heart (secondary to escape mechanism into aorta)
Clues:
1. Skeletal anomaly (eg, scoliosis): tetralogy (90%)
2. Hepatic symmetry: asplenia
3. Right aortic arch: tetralogy, complete transposition, tricuspid atresia
4. Aberrant right subclavian artery: tetralogy
5. Leftward convexity of ascending aorta: single ventricle with inverted right rudimentary ventricle, corrected transposition, asplenia, JAA (tricuspid valve atresia)

B. SHUNT AT ATRIAL LEVEL
1. **P**ulmonary stenosis / atresia with intact ventricular septum
2. **E**bstein malformation + Uhl anomaly
3. **T**ricuspid atresia (ASD in 100%)
√ moderate to severe cardiomegaly
√ R atrial dilatation
√ R ventricular enlargement (secondary to massive tricuspid incompetence)
√ inapparent aorta
√ left aortic arch

ACYANOTIC HEART DISEASE
Increased pulmonary blood flow without cyanosis
= indicates L-R shunt with increased pulmonary blood flow (shunt volume >40%)
A. WITH LEFT ATRIAL ENLARGEMENT
Indicates shunt distal to mitral valve = increased volume without escape defect
1. VSD (25%): small aorta in intracardiac shunt
2. PDA (12%): aorta + pulmonary artery of equal size in extracardiac shunt
3. Ruptured sinus of Valsalva aneurysm (rare)

4. Coronary arteriovenous fistula (very rare)
5. Aortopulmonary window (extremely rare)
B. <u>WITH NORMAL LEFT ATRIUM</u>
Indicates shunt proximal to mitral valve = volume increased with escape mechanism through defect
1. ASD (8%)
2. Partial anomalous pulmonary venous return (PAPVR) + sinus venosus ASD
3. Endocardial cushion defect (ECD) (4%)

Normal pulmonary blood flow without cyanosis
A. OBSTRUCTIVE LESION
  (a) <u>Right ventricular outflow obstruction</u>
    1. at level of pulmonary valve:
       subvalvular / valvular / supravalvular pulmonic stenosis
    2. at level of peripheral pulmonary arteries:
       peripheral pulmonary stenosis
  (b) <u>Left ventricular inflow obstruction</u>
    1. at level of peripheral pulmonary veins:
       pulmonary vein stenosis / atresia
    2. at level of left atrium: cor triatriatum
    3. at level of mitral valve:
       supravalvular mitral stenosis, congenital mitral stenosis / atresia, "parachute" mitral valve
  (c) <u>Left ventricular outflow obstruction</u>
    1. at level of aortic valve:
       anatomic subaortic stenosis, functional subaortic stenosis (IHSS), valvular aortic stenosis, hypoplastic left heart, supravalvular aortic stenosis
    2. at level of aorta:
       interruption of aortic arch, coarctation of aorta
B. CARDIOMYOPATHY
  1. Endocardial fibroelastosis
  2. Hypertrophic cardiomyopathy
  3. Glycogen storage disease
C. HYPERDYNAMIC STATE
  1. Noncardiac AVM (cerebral AVM, vein of Galen aneurysm, large pulmonary AVM, hemangioendothelioma of liver)
  2. Thyrotoxicosis
  3. Anemia
  4. Pregnancy
D. MYOCARDIAL ISCHEMIA
  1. Anomalous left coronary artery
  2. Coronary artery disease (CAD)

PULMONARY VASCULARITY
Increased pulmonary vasculature
A. <u>Overcirculation</u> = shunt vascularity = arterial + venous overcirculation
  (a) Congenital heart disease (most common)
    (1) L-R shunts
    (2) Admixture lesions / cyanotic lesions
  (b) High-flow syndromes
    (1) Thyrotoxicosis (2) Anemia (3) Pregnancy
    (4) Peripheral arteriovenous fistula
  √ diameter of right descending pulmonary artery larger than trachea just above aortic knob

√ increased size of veins + arteries with size larger than accompanying bronchus (= "kissing cousin" sign), best seen just above hila on AP view
√ enlarged hilar vessels (lateral view)
√ visualization of vessels below 10th posterior rib
B. <u>Pulmonary venous hypertension</u>
  √ redistribution of flow (not seen in younger children)
  √ indistinctness of vessels with Kerley lines (= interstitial edema)
  √ alveolar edema
  √ fine reticulated pattern
C. <u>Precapillary hypertension</u>
  √ enlarged main + right and left pulmonary arteries
  √ abrupt tapering of pulmonary arteries
D. <u>Prominent systemic / aortopulmonary collaterals</u>
  1. Tetralogy of Fallot with pulmonary atresia (= pseudotruncus)
  2. VSD + pulmonary atresia (single ventricle, complete transposition, corrected transposition)
  3. Pulmonary-systemic collaterals
  √ coarse vascular pattern with irregular branching arteries (from aorta / subclavian arteries)
  √ small central vessels despite apparent increase in vascularity

Decreased pulmonary vascularity
= obstruction to pulmonary flow
√ vessels reduced in size and number
√ hyperlucent lungs
√ small hilar vessels + pulmonary artery segment

Normal pulmonary vascularity + normal-sized heart
mnemonic: "MAN"
  Myocardial ischemia
  Afterload (= pressure overload problems)
  Normal

Pulmonary arterial hypertension
= PAH = pulmonary arterial pressure in systole >30 mm Hg, in diastole >15 mm Hg, mean pressure >20 mm Hg
Pathogenesis:
A. PRIMARY PAH (rare) = plexogenic pulmonary arteriopathy = unknown cause / mechanism
B. SECONDARY PAH (more common)
  (a) primary pleuropulmonic disease
    1. <u>Parenchymal pulmonary disease</u> = **cor pulmonale**: COPD, emphysema, chronic bronchitis, asthma, bronchiectasis, malignant infiltrate, granulomatous disease, cystic fibrosis, end-stage fibrotic lung, S/P lung resection, idiopathic hemosiderosis, alveolar proteinosis, alveolar microlithiasis
    2. <u>Alveolar hypoventilation</u> = hypoxic pulmonary arterial hyperperfusion: chronic high altitude, sleep apnea, hypoventilation due to neuromuscular disease / obesity

3. Pleural disease + chest deformity
fibrothorax, thoracoplasty, kyphoscoliosis
(b) primary vascular disease
1. Congenital heart disease
— increased flow: large L-R shunt
(Eisenmenger syndrome)
— decreased flow: tetralogy of Fallot
2. Capillary obliteration: chronic pulmonary
thromboembolism, persistent fetal circulation,
arteritides (eg, Takayasu)
3. Venous obliteration: pulmonary
venoocclusive disease
(c) pulmonary venous hypertension

Histo:
Grade I = hypertrophy of media of muscular
pulmonary arteries + arterioles
Grade II = hypertrophy of muscle cells + proliferation
of intima cells in small muscular arteries +
arterioles
Grade III = muscular hypertrophy + intimal thickening
+ subendothelial fibrosis
Grade IV = occlusion of vessels with progressive
dilatation of small arteries nearby;
muscular hypertrophy less apparent
Grade V = tortuous channels within proliferation of
endothelial cells (= plexiform +
angiomatoid lesions) + intraalveolar
macrophages
Grade VI = thrombosis + necrotizing arteritis

√ dilatation of pulmonary trunk, main pulmonary arteries,
intermediate arteries
√ "pruning" of pulmonary arteries = rapid tapering of
pulmonary arteries with narrowed peripheral pulmonary
vessels
√ NO increase of pulsations in middle third of lung
√ calcification of central pulmonary vessels
(PATHOGNOMONIC)
√ normal-sized heart / right heart enlargement

Pulmonary venous hypertension
= INCREASED VENOUS PULMONARY PRESSURE
= VENOUS CONGESTION
= pulmonary capillary wedge pressure (PCWP) >15 mm
Hg
Causes:
A. LEFT VENTRICULAR INFLOW TRACT
OBSTRUCTION
√ normal-sized heart with right ventricular
hypertrophy
√ prominent pulmonary trunk
@ proximal to mitral valve:
√ normal-sized left atrium
1. TAPVR below the diaphragm
2. Primary pulmonary veno-occlusive disease
3. Stenosis of individual pulmonary veins
4. Atresia of common pulmonary vein
5. Cor triatriatum
6. Left atrial tumor / clot

7. Supravalvular ring of left atrium
8. Fibrosing mediastinitis
9. Constrictive pericarditis
@ at mitral valve level
√ enlarged left atrium
1. Rheumatic mitral valve stenosis ±
regurgitation (99%)
√ enlarged left atrial appendage
2. Congenital mitral valve stenosis
3. Parachute mitral valve (= single bulky
papillary muscle)

B. LEFT VENTRICULAR FAILURE
(a) ABNORMAL PRELOAD with secondary mitral
valve incompetence (= volume overload)
1. Aortic valve regurgitation
2. Eisenmenger syndrome (= R-to-L shunt in
VSD)
3. High-output failure:
Noncardiac AVM (cerebral AVM, vein of
Galen aneurysm, large pulmonary AVM,
hemangioendothelioma of liver, iatrogenic),
thyrotoxicosis, anemia, pregnancy
(b) ABNORMAL AFTERLOAD
(= pressure overload) = LV outflow tract
obstruction
1. Hypoplastic left heart syndrome
2. Aortic stenosis (supravalvular, valvular,
anatomic subaortic)
3. Interrupted aortic arch
4. Coarctation of the aorta
(c) DISORDERS OF CONTRACTION AND
RELAXATION
1. Endocardial fibroelastosis
2. Glycogen storage disease (Pompe disease)
3. Cardiac aneurysm
4. Cardiomyopathy
(a) congestive (alcohol)
(b) hypertrophic obstructive cardiomyopathy
(HOCM), particularly in IDM
— asymmetric septal hypertrophy (ASH)
— idiopathic hypertrophic subaortic
stenosis (IHSS)
(d) MYOCARDIAL ISCHEMIA
1. Anomalous left coronary artery
2. Coronary artery disease (CAD)

√ moderate redistribution (PCWP 13 – 15 mm Hg)
√ redistribution (PCWP 15 – 18 mm Hg)
√ indistinct vessel margins due to interstitial edema
(PCWP 18 – 25 mm Hg)
√ alveolar pulmonary edema (PCWP >30 mm Hg)

Pulmonary artery-bronchus ratios
= ratio of diameters of end-on segmental pulmonary
artery + accompanying end-on bronchus
A. ERECT CHEST FILM
1. Normal: upper lung zone 0.85 ± 0.15
lower lung zone 1.34 ± 0.25
= effect of gravity

2. Pulmonary plethora:

    upper lung zone 1.62 ± 0.31

    lower lung zone 1.56 ± 0.28

    = balanced engorgement

3. Decompensated CHF:

    upper lung zone 1.50 ± 0.25

    lower lung zone 0.87 ± 0.20

    = redistribution from left-sided CHF

B. SUPINE CHEST FILM

1. Normal: upper lung zone 1.01 ± 0.13

           lower lung zone 1.05 ± 0.13

    = gravitational effect lost

2. Decompensated CHF:

    upper lung zone 1.49 ± 0.31

    lower lung zone 0.96 ± 0.31

    = inverted pattern / plethora pattern

AORTA
Enlarged aorta

A. INCREASED VOLUME LOAD
1. Aortic insufficiency
2. PDA

B. POSTSTENOTIC DILATATION
1. Valvular aortic stenosis

C. INCREASED INTRALUMINAL PRESSURE
1. Coarctation
2. Systemic hypertension

D. MURAL WEAKNESS / INFECTION
1. Cystic media necrosis: Marfan / Ehlers-Danlos syndrome
2. Congenital aneurysm
3. Syphilitic aortitis
4. Mycotic aneurysm
5. Atherosclerotic aneurysm (compromised vasa vasorum)

E. LACERATION OF AORTIC WALL
1. Traumatic aneurysm
2. Dissecting hematoma

Double Aortic Arch

Common cause of vascular ring

Incidence: 55% of all vascular rings

• usually asymptomatic
• stridor, dyspnea, recurrent pneumonia
• dysphagia (less common than respiratory symptoms, more common after starting baby on solids)

Location: in 75% left descending aorta, in 25% right descending aorta; smaller arch anterior in 80%; right arch larger + higher than left in 80%

√ two separate arches arise from single ascending aorta

√ each arch joins to form a single descending aorta

√ impressions may be present on both sides of trachea: usually R > L

√ broad posterior impression on esophagus

√ small anterior impression on trachea

CT:

√ "four-artery sign" = each arch gives rise to 2 dorsal subclavian + 2 ventral carotid arteries evenly spaced around trachea on section cephalad to aortic arch

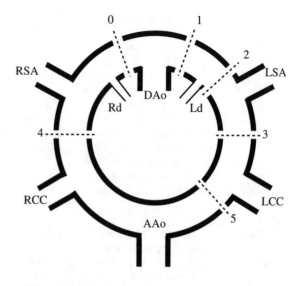

Hypothetical double aortic arch of Edwards

RSA = right subclavian a.   AAo = ascending aorta

LSA = left subclavian a.   DAo = descending aorta

RCC = right common carotid a.   Rd = right ductus

LCC = left common carotid a.   Ld = left ductus

0 = normal left aortic arch

1 = right aortic arch with mirror-image branching; ductus from pulmonary a. to left brachiocephalic / subclavian a. = no vascular ring

2 = right aortic arch with mirror-image branching; ductus from pulmonary a. to descending aorta = complete vascular ring

3 = right aortic arch with aberrant left subclavian a.; ductus from pulmonary a. to descending aorta (most common complete vascular ring)

4 = left aortic arch with aberrant right subclavian a.

5 = right aortic arch with aberrant left brachiocephalic artery; ductus from pulmonary a. to descending aorta (very uncommon)

2 + 3 = right aortic arch with isolated left subclavian a. (very uncommon)

DDx: right arch with aberrant left subclavian artery (indistinguishable by esophagram when dominant arch on right side)

Right aortic arch

Incidence: 1 – 2%

INCIDENCE OF RIGHT AORTIC ARCH IN CONGENITAL HEART DISEASE

1. Truncus arteriosus	35%
2. Tetralogy of Fallot	25%
3. TGV	10%
4. Tricuspid atresia	5%
5. Large VSD	2%

Rare anomalies:

1. Corrected transposition	50%
2. Pseudotruncus	50%
3. Asplenia	30%
4. Pink tetralogy	15%

mnemonic: "TRU TETRA TRIC"
  TRUncus arteriosus
  TEtralogy of Fallot
  TRAnsposition
  TRICuspid atresia

Right aortic arch
with aberrant left subclavian artery

= interruption of embryonic left arch between left CCA and left subclavian artery; most common type of right aortic arch anomaly: 35 – 72%

Incidence: 1:2,500

Associated with congenital heart disease in 12%:
  1. Tetralogy of Fallot   (2/3 = 8%)
  2. ASD ± VSD   (1/4 = 3%)
  3. Coarctation   (1/12 = 1%)
• usually asymptomatic (loose ring around trachea + esophagus)

• may be symptomatic in infancy / early childhood provoked by bronchitis + tracheal edema
• may be symptomatic in adulthood provoked by torsion of aorta
√ left common carotid artery is first branch of ascending aorta
√ left subclavian artery arises from descending aorta
√ retroesophageal aortic diverticulum (= diverticulum of Kommerell = remnant of embryonic left arch)
  √ small rounded density lateral to trachea
  √ impression on left side of esophagus simulating a double aortic arch
√ vascular ring (= left ductus extends from aortic diverticulum to left pulmonary artery)
  √ right aortic arch impression on tracheal air shadow
  √ broad posterior impression on esophagus (left subclavian artery)
  √ small anterior impression on trachea

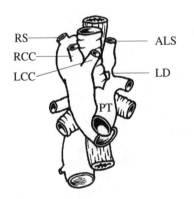

Right aortic arch with aberrant left subclavian
  RS/LS =   right / left subclavian a.
  LD   =   left ductus arteriosus

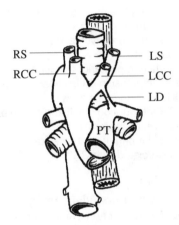

Right aortic arch with mirror image branching
  RCC / LCC = right / left common carotid a.
  ALS   = aberrant left subclavian a.

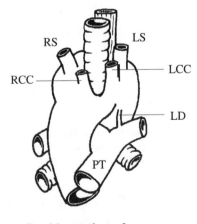

Double aortic arch
  RS / LS =   right / left subclavian a.
  LD   =   left ductus arteriosus
  PT   =   pulmonary trunk

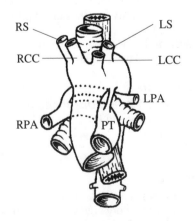

Aberrant left pulmonary artery
  RCC / LCC =   right / left common carotid a.
  RPA / LPA =   right / left pulmonary a.

√ aorta descends on right side

Right aortic arch with mirror image branching

2nd most common aortic arch anomaly: 24 – 60%
= interruption of embryonic left arch between left
   subclavian artery and descending aorta; dorsal to left
   ductus arteriosus

(a) Type 1 = interruption of left aortic arch distal to
    ductus arteriosus (common)
    Associated with cyanotic congenital heart disease
    in 98%:
    1. Tetralogy of Fallot   (87%)
    2. Multiple defects   (7.5%)
    3. Truncus arteriosus   (2 – 6%)
    4. Transposition   (1 – 10%)
    5. Tricuspid atresia   (5%)
    6. ASD ± VSD   (0.5%)
    Δ 25% of patients with tetralogy have right
       aortic arch!
    Δ 37% of patients with truncus arteriosus have
       right aortic arch!
    √ NO vascular ring, NO retroesophageal
      component
    √ NO structure posterior to trachea
    √ R arch impression on tracheal air shadow
    √ NORMAL barium swallow
(b) Type 2 = interruption of left aortic arch proximal to
    ductus arteriosus (rare)
    true vascular ring (if duct persists)
    rarely associated with CHD

Right aortic arch with isolated left subclavian artery

3rd most common right aortic arch anomaly: 2%
= interruption of embryonic left arch between
   (a) left CCA and left subclavian artery and
   (b) left ductus and descending aorta
   resulting in a connection of left subclavian artery with
   left pulmonary artery
Associated with: Tetralogy of Fallot
√ left common carotid artery arises as the first branch
√ left subclavian artery attaches to left pulmonary artery
  through PDA
√ NO vascular ring, NO retroesophageal component
• congenital subclavian steal syndrome

Right aortic arch with aberrant left brachiocephalic artery

Similar in appearance to R aortic arch + aberrant L
subclavian artery

Left aortic arch

Left aortic arch with aberrant right subclavian artery

= right subclavian artery arises as 4th branch from
   proximal descending aorta
Incidence: 0.4 – 2.3%; most common congenital arch
              anomaly; in 37% of Down syndrome
              children with CHD

Associated with: (1) Absent recurrent pharyngeal nerve
                    (2) CHD in 10 – 15%

Course: (a) behind esophagus (80%)
         (b) between esophagus + trachea (15%)
         (c) anterior to trachea (5%)

√ radiolucent band crossing the esophagus obliquely
  upward toward the right shoulder
√ dilated origin of aberrant subclavian artery (in up to
  60%) = diverticulum of Kommerell = remnant of
  embryonic right arch
√ unilateral L-sided rib notching (if aberrant R
  subclavian artery arises distal to coarctation)

Anomalous innominate artery compression syndrome

= origin of R innominate artery to the left of trachea
  coursing to the right
√ anterior tracheal compression

Symptomatic vascular rings

(a) Usually symptomatic lesions:
    1. Double aortic arch with R descending aorta +
       L ductus arteriosus
    2. R aortic arch with R descending aorta + aberrant L
       subclavian artery + persistent L ductus /
       ligamentum teres
    3. L arch with L descending aorta + R ductus /
       ligamentum
    4. Aberrant L pulmonary artery = "pulmonary sling"
(b) Occasionally symptomatic lesions:
    1. Anomalous innominate
    2. Anomalous L common carotid artery / common
       trunk
    3. R aortic arch with L descending aorta + L ductus /
       ligamentum
(c) Usually asymptomatic lesions:
    1. L aortic arch + aberrant R subclavian artery
    2. L aortic arch with R descending aorta
    3. R aortic arch with R descending aorta + mirror
       image branching
    4. R aortic arch with R descending aorta + aberrant L
       subclavian artery
    5. R aortic arch with R descending aorta + isolation
       of L subclavian artery
    6. R aortic arch with L descending aorta + L ductus /
       ligamentum

Abnormal left ventricular outflow tract

LVOT = area between IVS + aML from aortic valve cusps
to mitral valve leaflets

1. Membranous subaortic stenosis
   = crescent-shaped fibrous membrane extending
      across LVOT + inserting at aML
   √ diffuse narrowing of LVOT
   √ abnormal linear echoes in LVOT space
      (occasionally)
2. Prolapsing aortic valve vegetation

Pattern of vascular compression of esophagus and trachea

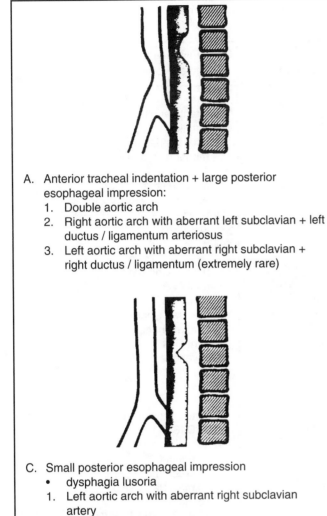

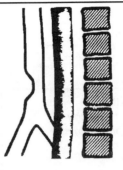

A. Anterior tracheal indentation + large posterior esophageal impression:
    1. Double aortic arch
    2. Right aortic arch with aberrant left subclavian + left ductus / ligamentum arteriosus
    3. Left aortic arch with aberrant right subclavian + right ductus / ligamentum (extremely rare)

B. Anterior tracheal indentation
    1. Compression by innominate artery with origin more distal along arch
    2. Compression by left common carotid with origin more proximal on arch
    3. Common origin of innominate and left common carotid artery

C. Small posterior esophageal impression
    •   dysphagia lusoria
    1. Left aortic arch with aberrant right subclavian artery
    2. Right aortic arch with aberrant left subclavian artery (very rare)

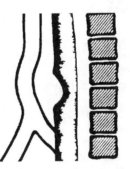

D. Posterior tracheal indentation + anterior esophageal impression
    1. Aberrant left pulmonary artery

3. <u>Narrowed LVOT</u> (<20 mm)
    (a) Long-segment subaortic stenosis
        √ aortic valve closure in early systole with coarse fluttering
        √ high frequency flutter of mitral valve in diastole (aortic regurgitation)
        √ symmetric LV hypertrophy
    (b) ASH / IHSS
        √ asymmetrically thickened septum bulging into LV + LVOT
        √ systolic anterior motion of aML (SAM)
    (c) Mitral stenosis
    (d) Endocardial cushion defect

PULMONARY ARTERY
Invisible main pulmonary artery
A. Underdeveloped = RVOT obstruction
    1. Tetralogy of Fallot

    2. Hypoplastic right heart syndrome (tricuspid / pulmonary atresia)
B. Misplaced pulmonary artery
    1. Complete transposition of great vessels
    2. Persistent truncus arteriosus

Unequal pulmonary blood flow
1. Tetralogy of Fallot
    √ diminished flow on left side (hypoplastic / stenotic pulmonary artery in 40%)
2. Persistent truncus arteriosus (esp. Type IV)
    √ diminished / increased blood flow to either lung
3. Pulmonary valvular stenosis
    √ increased flow to left lung secondary to jet phenomenon

Dilatation of pulmonary trunk
1. Idiopathic dilatation of pulmonary artery

HETEROTAXIA

= CARDIOSPLENIC SYNDROMES = sporadic disorders with abnormal relationship between abdominal organs + tendency toward symmetric development of organs within trunk + associated cardiac anomalies

	Asplenia bilateral R sidedness	Polysplenia bilateral L sidedness
CLINICAL		
Presenting age	newborn / infant	infant / adult
Sex predominance	male	female
Cyanosis	severe	usually absent
Heart disease	severe	moderate / none
Howell-Jolly bodies	present	absent
Spleen scan	no spleen	multiple small spleens
Characteristic ECG	none	abnormal P wave vector
Prognosis	poor	good
Mortality	high	low
PLAIN FILM		
Lung vascularity	decreased	normal / increased
Aortic arch	right / left	right / left
Cardiac apex	right / left / midline	right / left
Bronchi	bilateral eparterial	bilateral hyparterial
Minor fissure	possibly bilateral	normal / none
Stomach	midline / right / left	right / left
Liver	symmetrical / R / L	in various positions
Malrotation of bowel	yes	yes
CARDIOGRAPHY		
Coronary sinus	usually absent	sometimes absent
Atrial septum	common atrium (100%)	ASD (84%)
AV valve	atresia / common valve	normal / abnormal MV
Single ventricle	44%	infrequent
IVS	VSD	VSD common
Great vessels	d- / l-transposition (72%)	normal relationship
Pulmonary stenosis	the rule	frequent
Pulmonary veins	TAPVR	PAPVR (42%) TAPVR (6%)
Single coronary artery	19%	
SVC	bilateral (53%)	bilateral (33%)
IVC-aorta relationship	same side of spine	normal
IVC	normal	interrupted (84%) / normal
Azygos vein	inapparent	continuation R / L

2. Pulmonic valve stenosis
   √ poststenotic dilatation of trunk + left pulmonary artery
3. Pulmonary regurgitation
   (a) severe pulmonic valve insufficiency
   (b) absence of pulmonic valve (may be associated with tetralogy)

SITUS

= term describing the position of atria, tracheobronchial tree, pulmonary arteries, thoracic + abdominal viscera
A. SITUS SOLITUS = normal situs
   = position of morphologic LA is the same as that of the aortic arch + stomach bubble + hyparterial

bronchus + bilobed lung; the position of the morphologic RA is the same as that of the eparterial bronchus + trilobed lung
1. Abdominal situs solitus
   √ liver + IVC are right-sided
   √ stomach, spleen, abdominal aorta are left-sided
2. Cardiac situs solitus
   √ morphologic right atrium is right-sided
   √ morphologic left atrium is left-sided
Associated with:
   (a) levocardia : <1% chance for CHD
   (b) dextrocardia : 95% chance for CHD
B. SITUS INVERSUS
   = mirror-image position of normal

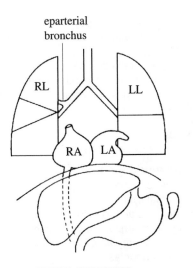

eparterial
bronchus

SITUS SOLITUS
anterior view

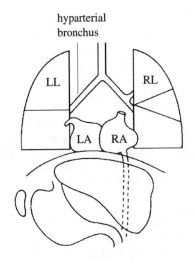

hyparterial
bronchus

SITUS INVERSUS
anterior view

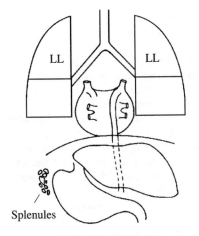

Splenules

LEFT ISOMERISM
posterior view

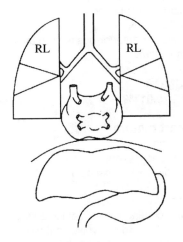

RIGHT ISOMERISM
posterior view

1. <u>Abdominal situs inversus</u>
   √ mirror-image position of abdominal organs
2. <u>Cardiac situs inversus</u>
   √ morphologic right atrium is left-sided
   √ morphologic left atrium is right-sided
   Associated with:
   (a) dextrocardia = situs inversus totalis (usual variant): 3 – 5% chance for CHD, eg, Kartagener syndrome
   (b) levocardia (extremely rare): 95% chance for CHD
C. SITUS INDETERMINATUS / INDETERMINUS / AMBIGUUS
   = ambiguous relationship

1. <u>Abdominal situs ambiguus</u>
   √ liver may be midline + symmetric
   √ bowel malrotations are typical

2. <u>Cardiac situs ambiguus</u>
   √ atrial morphology indeterminate / bilateral right atria (right atrial isomerism) / bilateral left atria (left atrial isomerism)

Associated with:
   (a) bilateral right isomerism / sidedness
       = Asplenia syndrome
   (b) bilateral left isomerism / sidedness
       = Polysplenia syndrome

Cardiac position

= determined by base-apex axis; no assumption is made regarding cardiac chamber / vessel arrangement

A. POSITION OF CARDIAC APEX
1. Levocardia = apex directed leftward
2. Dextrocardia = apex directed rightward
3. Mesocardia = vertical / midline heart (usually with situs solitus)
√ atrial septum characteristically bowed into left atrium in cardiac situs solitus with dextrocardia + cardiac situs inversus with levocardia (DDx: juxtapositioned atrial appendages)

B. CARDIAC DISPLACEMENT
by extracardiac factors (eg, lung hypoplasia, pulmonary mass)
1. Dextroposition
suggests hypoplasia of ipsilateral pulmonary artery (PAPVR implies scimitar syndrome)
2. Levoposition
3. Mesoposition

C. CARDIAC INVERSION
= alteration of normal relationship of chambers
1. D-bulboventricular loop
2. L-bulboventricular loop

D. TRANSPOSITION
= alteration of anterior-posterior relationship of great vessels

CARDIAC TUMOR

Prevalence: 0.017%

Malignant heart tumors

1. Angiosarcoma
2. Multiple cardiac myxomas
3. Metastatic disease: most commonly breast, lung, melanoma
4. Lymphoma
   Incidence: cardiac involvement in 29% on autopsy; pericardial involvement more frequent
   • intractable congestive heart failure
   • chest pain
   √ SVC obstruction

Benign heart tumor

1. Myxoma (most common cardiac tumor)
2. Rhabdomyoma:
   associated with tuberous sclerosis
3. Hydatid cyst (uncommon):
   √ localized bulge of left cardiac contour
   √ curvilinear / spotty calcifications (resembling myocardial aneurysm)
   Cx: may rupture into cardiac chamber / pericardium

Congenital cardiac tumor

Incidence: 1:10,000
1. Rhabdomyoma (58%)
   Associated with: tuberous sclerosis (in 50 – 86%)
   • supraventricular tachycardia (accessory conductive pathways within tumor)

√ often multiple
√ tendency to involve septum
2. Teratoma (20%): intrapericardiac, extracardiac
3. Fibroma (12%):
   √ may be pedunculated, may calcify
4. Myxoma, hemangioma, mesothelioma:
   √ mass-occupying lesion impinging upon cardiac cavities

PERICARDIUM

Cardiophrenic angle mass

A. Lesion of pericardium
1. Pericardial cyst
2. Intrapericardiac bronchogenic cyst
3. Benign intrapericardiac neoplasm: teratoma, leiomyoma, hemangioma, lipoma
4. Malignant neoplasm: mesothelioma, metastasis (lung, breast, lymphoma, melanoma)

B. Cardiac lesion: aneurysm
C. Others: masses arising from lung, pleura, diaphragm, abdomen

Pericardial effusion

= pericardial fluid >50 ml
Etiology:

A. SEROUS FLUID = transudate
Congestive heart failure, hypoalbuminemia, irradiation

B. BLOOD = hemopericardium
(a) iatrogenic: cardiac surgery / catheterization, anticoagulants, chemotherapy
(b) trauma: penetrating / nonpenetrating
(c) acute myocardial infarction / rupture
(d) rupture of ascending aorta / pulmonary trunk
(e) coagulopathy
(f) neoplasm: mesothelioma, sarcoma, teratoma, fibroma, angioma, metastasis (lung, breast, lymphoma, leukemia, melanoma)

C. LYMPH
neoplasm, congenital, cardiothoracic surgery, obstruction of hilum / SVC

D. FIBRIN = exudate
(a) infection: viral, pyogenic, TB
(b) uremia: 18% in acute uremia; 51% in chronic uremia; dialysis patient
(c) collagen disease: rheumatoid arthritis, SLE, acute rheumatic fever
(d) hypersensitivity

CXR:
√ normal with fluid <250 ml / in acute pericarditis
√ "water bottle configuration" = symmetrically enlarged cardiac silhouette
√ loss of retrosternal clear space
√ "fat pad sign" = separation of retrosternal from epicardial fat line >2 mm (15%)
√ rapidly appearing cardiomegaly + normal pulmonary vascularity

√ "differential density sign" = increase in lucency at heart margin secondary to slight difference in contrast between pericardial fluid + heart muscle

√ diminished cardiac pulsations

ECHO: √ separation of epi- and pericardial echoes extending into diastole (rarely behind LA)

Volume estimates by M-mode:
 (a) separation only posteriorly = <300 ml
 (b) separation throughout cardiac cycle = 300 – 500 ml
 (c) plus anterior separation = >1000 ml

VENA CAVA
Vena cava anomalies

1. <u>Retrocaval ureter</u> = <u>circumcaval ureter</u>
2. <u>Duplicated IVC</u>
   Incidence: 0.2 – 3%
   Etiology: persistence of right + left supracardinal veins
   √ small / equal-sized left IVC formed by left iliac vein
   √ crossover to right IVC via left renal vein / or more inferiorly
   √ crossover usually anterior / rarely posterior to aorta
3. <u>Transposition of IVC</u> = <u>solitary left IVC</u>
   Incidence: 0.2 – 0.5%
   Etiology: persistence of left + regression of right supracardinal vein
   √ left IVC usually crosses over via left renal vein / or more inferiorly
   √ crossover usually anterior / rarely posterior to aorta
4. <u>Retroaortic left renal vein</u>
   Incidence: 1.8 – 2.4%
   Etiology: persistence of posterior intersupracardinal anastomosis + regression of anterior intersubcardinal anastomosis
   √ crossover usually below / occasionally at level of right renal vein
5. <u>Circumaortic left renal vein</u>
   Incidence: 1.5 – 8.7%
   Etiology: persistence of anterior intersubcardinal + posterior intersupracardinal anastomosis
   √ venous collar encircling aorta
6. <u>Interrupted IVC with azygos / hemiazygos continuation</u>
   Incidence: 0.6%
   Etiology: failure to form subcardinohepatic anastomosis
   May be associated with: congenital heart disease, indeterminate situs, polysplenia, asplenia (rare)
   √ enlarged azygos arch + paravertebral and retrocrural portions of azygos + hemiazygos veins
   √ NO definable intrahepatic IVC
   √ drainage of hepatic veins directly into right atrium via posthepatic segment of IVC
   √ drainage of iliac + renal veins via azygos / hemiazygos vein
7. <u>Left SVC</u>
   Incidence: 0.3%
   Etiology: persistence of left anterior cardinal vein
   √ left SVC drains into coronary sinus

√ simultaneously present right SVC (82 – 90%) draining into right atrium

√ anastomosis between right + left anterior cardinal veins (in 35%)

IVC obstruction
INTRINSIC OBSTRUCTION
A. NEOPLASTIC (most frequent)
  1. Renal cell carcinoma (in 10%), Wilms tumor
  2. Adrenal carcinoma, pheochromocytoma
  3. Pancreatic carcinoma, hepatic adenocarcinoma
  4. Metastatic disease to retroperitoneal lymph nodes (carcinoma of ovary, cervix, prostate)
B. NON-NEOPLASTIC
  1. Idiopathic
  2. Proximally extending thrombus from femoroiliac veins
  3. Systemic disorders: coagulopathy, Budd-Chiari syndrome, dehydration, infection (pelvic inflammatory disease), sepsis, CHF
  4. Postoperative / traumatic phlebitis, ligation, plication, clip, cava filter, severe exertion

INTRINSIC CAVAL DISEASE
A. NEOPLASTIC
  1. Leiomyoma, leiomyosarcoma, endothelioma
B. NONNEOPLASTIC
  1. Congenital membrane

EXTRINSIC COMPRESSION
A. NEOPLASTIC
  1. Retroperitoneal lymphadenopathy (adults) due to metastatic disease, lymphoma, granulomatous disease (TB)
  2. Renal + adrenal tumors (children)
  3. Hepatic masses
  4. Pancreatic tumor
  5. Tumor-induced desmoplastic reaction (eg, metastatic carcinoid)
B. NONNEOPLASTIC
  1. Hepatomegaly
  2. Tortuous aorta / aortic aneurysm
  3. Retroperitoneal hematoma
  4. Massive ascites
  5. Retroperitoneal fibrosis

FUNCTIONAL OBSTRUCTION
1. Pregnant uterus
2. Valsalva maneuver
3. Straining / crying (in children)
4. Supine position with large abdominal mass

COLLATERAL PATHWAYS
1. Deep pathway: ascending lumbar veins to azygos vein (right) + hemiazygos vein (left) + intravertebral, paraspinal, extravertebral plexus (Batson plexus)
2. Intermediate pathway: via periureteric plexus + left gonadal vein to renal vein
3. Superficial pathway: external iliac vein to inferior epigastric vein + superior epigastric vein + internal mammary vein into subclavian vein

4. Portal pathway: retrograde flow through internal iliac vein + hemorrhoidal plexus into inferior mesenteric vein + splenic vein into portal vein

SURGERY
Surgical procedures
AORTICOPULMONARY WINDOW SHUNT
  = side-to-side anastomosis between ascending aorta and left pulmonary artery (reversible procedure)
  Δ Tetralogy of Fallot
BLALOCK-HANLON PROCEDURE
  = surgical creation of ASD
  Δ Complete transposition
BLALOCK-TAUSSIG SHUNT
  = end-to-side anastomosis of subclavian artery to pulmonary artery, performed ipsilateral to innominate artery / opposite to aortic arch
  Modified Blalock-Taussig shunt uses synthetic graft material such as polytetrafluoroethylene (Gore-Tex®) in an end-to-side anastomosis between subclavian artery + ipsilateral branch of pulmonary artery
  Δ Tetralogy of Fallot, Tricuspid atresia with pulmonic stenosis
FONTAN PROCEDURE
  = (1) external conduit from right atrium to pulmonary trunk (= venous return enters pulmonary artery directly) (2) closure of ASD: floor constructed from flap of atrial wall and roof from piece of prosthetic material
  Δ Tricuspid atresia
GLENN SHUNT
  = end-to-side shunt between distal end of right pulmonary artery and SVC; reserved for patients with cardiac defects in which total correction is not anticipated
  Δ Tricuspid atresia

POTT SHUNT
  = side-to-side anastomosis between descending aorta + left pulmonary artery
  Δ Tetralogy of Fallot
MUSTARD PROCEDURE
  (1) removal of atrial septum (b) pericardial baffle placed into common atrium such that systemic venous blood is rerouted into left ventricle and pulmonary venous return into right ventricle and aorta
  Δ Complete transposition
RASHKIND PROCEDURE = balloon atrial septostomy
  Δ Complete transposition
RASTELLI PROCEDURE
  external conduit (Dacron) with porcine valve connecting RV to pulmonary trunk
  Δ Transposition
WATERSTON-COOLEY SHUNT
  = side-to-side anastomosis between ascending aorta and right pulmonary artery; (a) extrapericardial (WATERSTON) (b) intrapericardial (COOLEY)
  Δ Tetralogy of Fallot

Postoperative thoracic deformity
on RIGHT SIDE:
  1. Systemic-PA shunt: Blalock-Taussig shunt, Waterston-Cooley shunt, Glenn shunt, Central conduit shunt
  2. Atrial septectomy: Blalock-Hanlon procedure through RA
  3. VSD repair:
  4. Mitral valve commissurotomy

on LEFT SIDE:
  1. PDA
  2. Coarctation
  3. PA banding

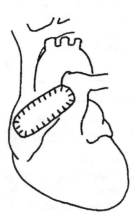

Fontan Procedure

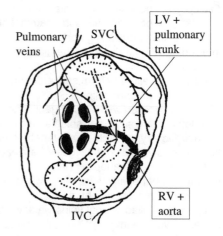

Mustard Procedure
(lateral view into opened right atrium)

4. Mitral valve commissurotomy
5. Systemic-PA shunt: Blalock-Taussig shunt, Pott shunt

Heart valve prosthesis
1. Starr-Edwards
   √ caged ball
   Δ predictable performance from large long-term experience
2. Bjørk-Shiley / Lillehei-Kaster / St. Jude
   √ tilting disc
   Δ excellent hemodynamics, very low profile, durable
3. Hancock / Carpentier-Edwards (= porcine xenograft) Ionescu-Shiley (= bovine xenograft)
   Δ low incidence of thromboembolism, no hemolysis, central flow, inaudible

CARDIAC CALCIFICATIONS
best detected fluoroscopically at low beam energies ≤75 kVp
@ Coronary arteries

@ Cardiac valves
1. Aortic valve
   • usually indicates significant aortic stenosis
   Cause: bicuspid valve, syphilis, healed bacterial endocarditis, ankylosing spondylitis
   √ above + anterior to a line connecting carina + anterior costophrenic angle (lateral view)
   √ usually extensive + dense calcifications
   √ may extend onto septal leaflet of mitral valve / ventricular septum
2. Mitral valve leaflet
   Cause: rheumatic heart disease, mitral valve prolapse
   √ inferior to a line connecting carina + anterior costophrenic angle (on lateral view)
   √ delicate calcification similar to coronary arteries (DDx: calcium in RCA / LCX)
   √ superior-to-inferior motion
3. Mitral valve annulus
   Cause: physiologic in elderly
   May be associated with mitral valve prolapse + regurgitation
   √ dense calcification frequently forming a "C" / "J"
4. Pulmonic valve
   Cause: tetralogy of Fallot, pulmonary stenosis, atrial septal defect

@ Left atrium
   Cause: rheumatic mitral valve disease, myxoma

@ Endocardium
   Cause: cardiac aneurysm, thrombus, endocardial fibroelastosis

@ Myocardium
   Cause: infarction, aneurysm, rheumatic fever, myocarditis
   √ curvilinear / amorphous

@ Pericardium
   Cause: idiopathic pericarditis, rheumatoid arthritis (5%), tuberculosis, viral, chronic renal failure, radiotherapy of mediastinum
   Cx: constrictive pericarditis

@ Pulmonary artery
   Cause: pulmonary arterial hypertension, syphilis

Coronary artery calcification
= due to (1) arteriosclerosis of intima (2) Mönckeberg medial sclerosis (exceedingly rare)
Histo: calcified subintimal plaques

CXR: (detection rate up to 42%) indicating more severe coronary artery disease
Fluoroscopy: (promoted as inexpensive screening test)
— calcifications in 34% in asymptomatic male individuals
— in 54% of symptomatic patients with ischemic heart disease
— in 35% of patients with calcifications exercise test will be positive (without calcifications only in 4% positive)
— calcifications indicate >50% stenosis with 72 – 76% sensitivity, 78% specificity); frequency of coronary artery calcifications with normal angiogram increases with age; predictive values in population <50 years as good as exercise stress test
Location:
"coronary artery calcification triangle" = triangular area along mid left heart border, spine, and shoulder of LV containing left main coronary artery, proximal portions of LAD + LCX calcifications at autopsy:
   LAD (93%), LCX (77%), left main CA (70%), RCA (69%)
√ parallel calcified lines (lateral view)

Prognosis: 58% 5-year survival rate with and 87% without calcifications

Vasculitis
A. Immune complex deposition
   (a) systemic necrotizing vasculitis
       1. Polyarteritis nodosa
       2. Allergic angiitis + granulomatosis
   (b) hypersensitivity vasculitis
       1. Serum-sickness vasculitis
       2. Henoch-Schönlein purpura
       3. Collagen vascular disease with vasculitis
       4. Hypocomplemenic vasculitis
       5. Malignancy with vasculitis
       6. Mixed cryoglobulinemia
B. Cell-mediated round cell granuloma formation
   1. Giant cell arteritis
       (a) Temporal arteritis
       (b) Takayasu arteritis
   2. Wegener granulomatosis
   3. Lymphomatoid granulomatosis

C. Miscellaneous
   1. Kawasaki disease = mucocutaneous lymph node syndrome
   2. Thromboangiitis obliterans = Buerger disease
   3. Behçet disease
   4. Cogan syndrome
   5. Sweet syndrome
   6. Erythema nodosum
   7. Bowel bypass dermatitis

Pulsus alternans

= alternating arterial pulse height with regular cardiac rhythm
   1. Intrinsic myocardial abnormality
      severe left ventricular dysfunction (CHF, aortic valvular disease, hypothermia, hypocalcemia, hyperbaric stress, ischemia)
   2. Alternating end-diastolic volumes
      abnormalities in venous filling + return (obstructed venous return, IVC balloon)

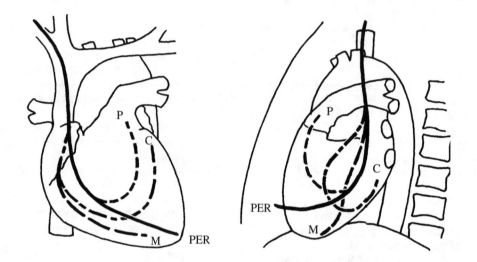

Central Venous Line Positions
C = coronary sinus, M = middle cardiac vein, P = main pulmonary artery, PER = perforation

CARDIOVASCULAR ANATOMY AND ECHOCARDIOGRAPHY

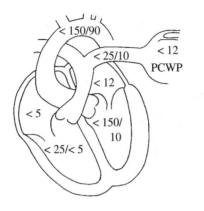

Normal Blood Pressures

PCWP = pulmonary capillary wedge pressure

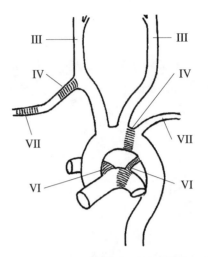

Development of Major Blood Vessels

numbers refer to embryologic aortic arches
most portions of aortic arches I, II, V regress

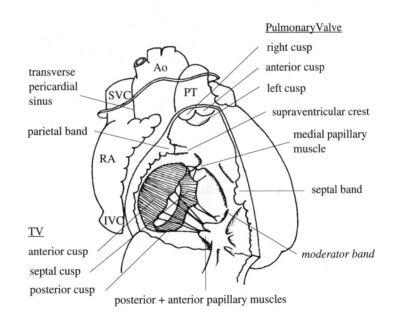

Right Ventricle Viewed From Front

Demarcation between posteroinferior inflow portion and anterosuperior outflow portion
by prominent muscular bands forming an almost circular orifice
— parietal band
— crista supraventricularis
— septomarginal trabeculae (= septal band + moderator band)
Anterior papillary muscle originates from moderator band!

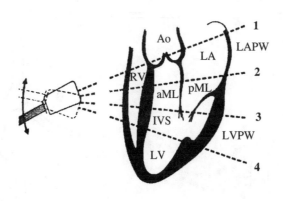

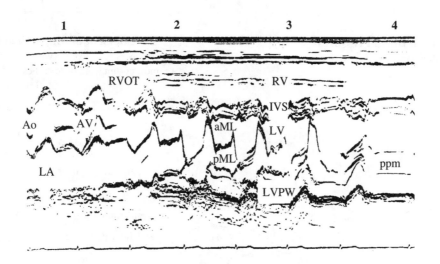

Sweep of Transducer from Aorta toward Apex

Area 1:   recognized by parallel motion of both aortic walls (a) toward the transducer during systole (b) away from the transducer during diastole. Left atrial posterior wall (LAPW) does not move because of mediastinal attachment by pulmonary veins.
<u>Aortic valve</u> cusps (right coronary + noncoronary / left cusps) are positioned in middle of aorta during diastole, open abruptly during systole at onset of ventricular ejection in a "box-like" fashion.
<u>Aortic + LA dimension</u> are similar in most cases.

Area 2:   <u>Aortic-septal continuity</u> = anterior aortic wall becomes interventricular septum
<u>Aortic-mitral continuity</u> = posterior aortic wall becomes anterior mitral valve leaflet
<u>Mitral valve</u> with typical "M" configuration during diastole; motion of aML toward transducer during systole secondary to movement of whole mitral valve apparatus

Area 3:   posterior mitral valve leaflet (pML) = reciprocal "W-shaped" configuration; left ventricular posterior wall (LVPW) shows anterior motion during systole.

Area 4:   Chordae tendineae in continuity with mitral valve leaflets merge with a thick posterior band of echoes representing the posteromedial papillary muscle (ppm).

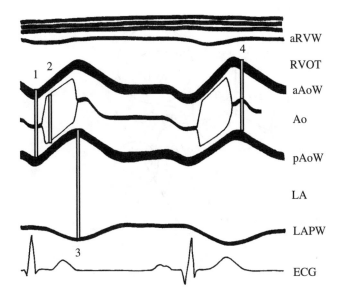

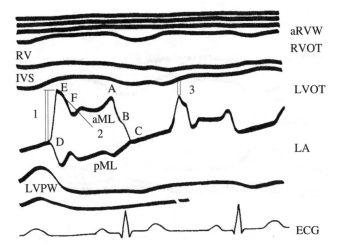

Echocardiogram of Aortic Root

1	=	aortic root diameter at end-diastole at R-wave of ECG = 20 – 37 mm
2	=	aortic cusp separation = 15 – 26 mm
3	=	left atrial dimension at moment of mitral valve opening = 15 – 40 mm
4	=	eccentricity index of aortic valve cusps = ratio of anterior to posterior dimension <1.3 (rarely used)
aRVW	=	anterior right ventricular wall
RVOT	=	right ventricular outflow tract
aAoW	=	anterior aortic wall
Ao	=	aorta
pAoW	=	posterior aortic wall
LA	=	left atrium
LAPW	=	left atrial posterior wall
ECG	=	electrocardiogram

Echocardiogram of Mitral Valve

1	=	opening amplitude of anterior leaflet of mitral valve (DE amplitude) ≥16 mm
2	=	early diastolic posterior motion of anterior leaflet (EF slope) ≥75 mm/sec
3	=	E point septal separation ≤10 mm
RV	=	right ventricle
IVS	=	interventricular septum
LVPW	=	left ventricular posterior wall
aML	=	anterior mitral valve leaflet
pML	=	posterior mitral valve leaflet
aRVW	=	anterior right ventricular wall
RVOT	=	right ventricular outflow tract
LVOT	=	left ventricular outflow tract
LA	=	left atrium
ECG	=	electrocardiogram
A	=	point of atrial contraction
C	=	closure point
DE	=	opening secondary to passive ventricular filling
CD	=	systole with steady anterior drift of coapted leaflets (passive movement secondary to movement of entire heart toward chest wall)

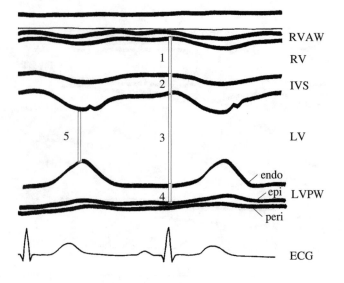

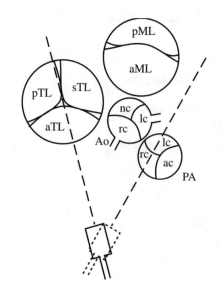

Echocardiogram of Right and Left Ventricle

1	=	RV end-diastolic dimension (RVEDD) at R-wave of ECG ≤ 30 mm
2	=	end-diastolic IVS thickness at R wave of ECG = 6 – 12 mm
3	=	LV end-diastolic dimension (LVEDD) at R-wave of ECG = 39 – 56 mm
4	=	end-diastolic LVPW thickness at R-wave of ECG = 6 – 12 mm
5	=	LV end-systolic dimension (LVESD)
RVAW	=	right ventricular anterior wall
RV	=	right ventricle
IVS	=	interventricular septum
LV	=	left ventricle
LVPW	=	left ventricular posterior wall
endo	=	endocardium
epi	=	epicardium
peri	=	pericardium

Fractional shortening (FS) = [(end-diastolic size - systolic size) / end-diastolic size] x 100

Δ	for LV	= 25 – 42%
Δ	for IVS	= 28 – 62%
Δ	for LVPW	= 36 – 70%

Diagram Showing the Relationship of the Four Cardiac Valves in Cross-section

aTL, pTL, sTL	=	anterior, posterior, septal tricuspid valve leaflets
aML, pML	=	anterior, posterior mitral valve leaflets
rc, lc, nc (Ao)	=	right, left, non-coronary cusps of aorta
rc, lc, ac (PA)	=	right, left, anterior cusps of pulmonary artery

Normal Echocardiographic Values in Adults

	range (mm)
Aortic root dimension (end-diastolic)	20 – 37
Aortic cusp separation	15 – 26
Left atrial dimension	15 – 40
Mitral valve excursion	≥16
E point septal separation	≤10
RV dimension (end-diastolic)	<30
IVS thickness (end-diastolic)	6 – 12
LVPW thickness (end-diastolic)	6 – 12
IVS:LVPW thickness	<1.3
Left ventricular dimension (end-diastolic)	39 – 56
Fractional shortening	0.25 – 0.42

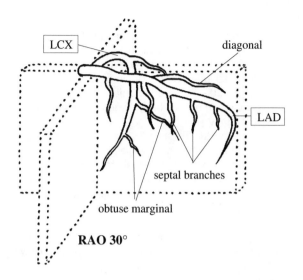

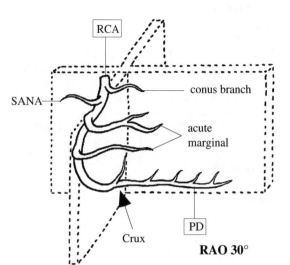

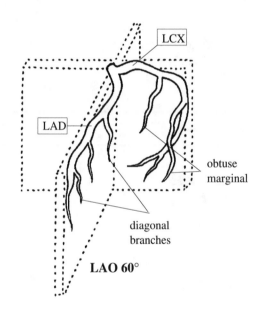

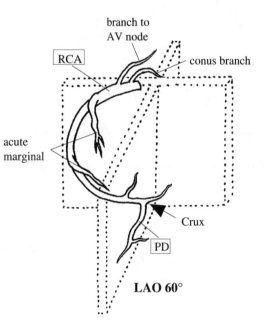

Anatomy of Left Coronary Artery

Marginals emanate from vessels in the AV groove (RCA, LXR)
    — on left side called obtuse marginal arteries
    — on right side called acute marginal arteries

Diagonals emanate from vessel in the interventricular groove
    (LAD)
    Note: **D**iagonals from LA**D**

Coronary Dominance
    the dominant vessel is the one that supplies the
    inferolateral wall of LV

AV-node branch from RCA (in 90%) = conus branch (1st
    branch in 50%)

SA-node branch from RCA (in > 50%)

Anatomy of Right Coronary Artery

Arteries in atrioventricular plane:
    RCA = right coronary artery
    LCX = left circumflex artery

Arteries in interventricular plane:
    LAD = left anterior descending artery
    PD   = posterior descending artery
    SANA = sinoatrial node artery

CORONARY ARTERIES
Coronary arteriography
CONTRAST AGENTS:
1. Monomeric ionic contrast material:
   (a) negative inotropic = depression of myocardial contractility due to hyperosmolality of sodium + decrease in total calcium
   (b) peripheral vasodilatation
2. Meglumine diatrizoate (contains small quantities of sodium citrate + EDTA)
3. Nonionic contrast material = slight increase in LV contractility

Mortality: 0.05%
Risk factors associated with death:
1. multiple ventricular premature contractions
2. congestive heart failure
3. systemic hypertension
4. severe triple-vessel coronary artery disease (highest risk)
5. LV ejection fraction <30%
6. Left main coronary artery stenosis

PROJECTIONS:
(a) LAO + 20 – 30° caudocranial angulation
   proximal 1/3 of LAD + origin of first diagonal branch

(b) LAO + 20 – 30° craniocaudal angulation = "spider view"
   Left main coronary artery, proximal LCX, first marginal / diagonal branches
(c) RAO + 20 – 30° craniocaudal angulation
   Proximal 1/3 of LCX + origin of its branches
(d) RAO + 20 – 30° caudocranial angulation
   Separation of LAD from diagonal branches
False-negative interpretation:
(1) eccentric lesion in 75%
(2) foreshortening of vessel
(3) overlap of other vessels remedied by angulated projections: improved diagnosis (50%), upgrade to more significant stenosis (30%), lesion unmasked (20%)

Coronary artery dominance
= vessel that supplies the inferior portion of left ventricle
RCA in 80%
LCA in 10%
RCA + LCA (codominance with balanced supply) in 10%

Coronary artery collaterals
A. INTRACORONARY COLLATERALS
   = filling of a distal portion of an occluded vessel from the proximal portion

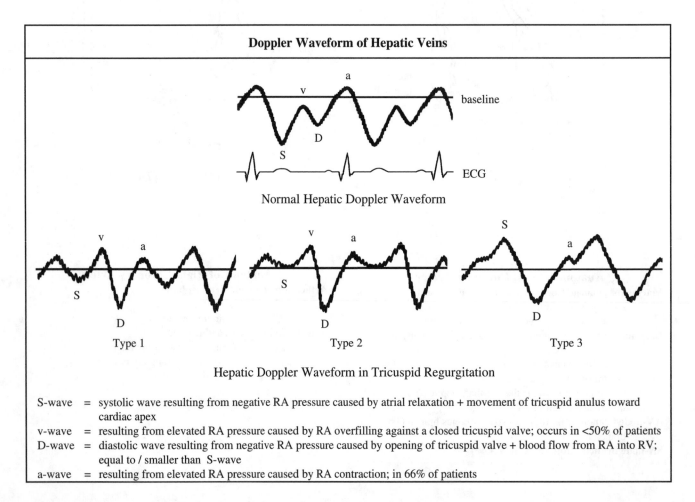

Doppler Waveform of Hepatic Veins

Normal Hepatic Doppler Waveform

Type 1   Type 2   Type 3

Hepatic Doppler Waveform in Tricuspid Regurgitation

S-wave = systolic wave resulting from negative RA pressure caused by atrial relaxation + movement of tricuspid anulus toward cardiac apex
v-wave = resulting from elevated RA pressure caused by RA overfilling against a closed tricuspid valve; occurs in <50% of patients
D-wave = diastolic wave resulting from negative RA pressure caused by opening of tricuspid valve + blood flow from RA into RV; equal to / smaller than S-wave
a-wave = resulting from elevated RA pressure caused by RA contraction; in 66% of patients

√ tortuous course outside the normal path

B. INTERCORONARY COLLATERALS
= between different coronary arteries / between branches of the same artery

Location: on epicardial surface, in atrial / ventricular septum, in myocardium

1. proximal RCA to distal RCA
   (a) by way of acute marginal branches
   (b) from sinoatrial node artery (SANA) to atrioventricular node artery (AVNA) = Kugel collateral
2. RCA to LAD
   (a) between PDA and LAD through ventricular septum / around apex
   (b) conus artery (1st branch of RCA) to proximal part of LAD
   (c) acute marginals of RCA to right ventricular branches of LAD
3. distal RCA to distal LCX
   (a) posterolateral segment artery of RCA to distal LCX (in AV groove)
   (b) AVNA of RCA to LCX (through atrial wall)
   (c) posterolateral branch of RCA to obtuse marginal branches of LCX (over left posterolateral ventricular wall)
4. proximal LAD to distal LAD
   (a) proximal diagonal to distal diagonal artery of LAD
   (b) proximal diagonal to LAD directly
5. LAD to obtuse marginal of LCX

VENOUS SYSTEM OF LOWER EXTREMITY

Deep Veins of Leg

3 paired stem veins of the calf accompany the arteries as venae commitantes + anastomose freely with each other:

1. **Anterior tibial veins**
   draining blood from dorsum of foot, running within extensor compartment of lower leg close to interosseous membrane
2. **Posterior tibial veins**
   formed by confluence of superficial + deep plantar veins behind ankle joint
3. **Peroneal veins**
   directly behind + medial to fibula
4. Calf veins
   (a) **Soleal muscle veins**
       baggy valveless veins in soleus muscle (= sinusoidal veins); draining into posterior tibial + peroneal veins or lower part of popliteal vein
   (b) **Gastrocnemius veins**
       thin straight veins with valves; draining into lower + upper parts of popliteal vein
5. **Popliteal vein**
   formed by stem veins of lower leg
6. **Superficial femoral vein**
   continuation of popliteal vein; receives deep femoral vein about 9 cm below inguinal ligament

7. **Deep femoral vein**
   draining together with superficial femoral vein into common femoral vein; may connect to popliteal vein (38%)
8. **Common femoral vein**
   formed by confluence of deep + superficial femoral vein; becomes external iliac vein as it passes beneath inguinal ligament

Superficial Veins of Leg

1. **Greater saphenous vein**
   formed by union of veins from medial side of sole of foot with medial dorsal veins; ascends in front of medial malleolus; passes behind medial condyles of tibia + femur
   (a) Posterior arch vein
       connected to deep venous system by communicating veins
   (b) **Anterior superficial tibial vein**
   (c) **Posteromedial superficial thigh vein**
       often connects with upper part of lesser saphenous vein
   (d) **Anterolateral superficial thigh vein**
   (e) Tributaries in fossa ovalis
       — superficial inferior epigastric vein
       — superficial external pudendal vein
       — superficial circumflex iliac vein

2. **Lesser saphenous vein**
   originates at outer border of foot behind lateral malleolus as continuation of dorsal venous arch; enters popliteal vein between heads of gastrocnemius in popliteal fossa within 8 cm of knee joint (60%) or joins with greater saphenous vein via posteromedial / anterolateral superficial thigh veins (20%)

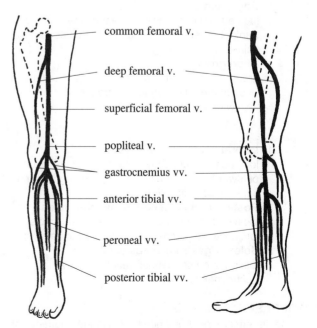

Deep Venous System of Lower Extremity

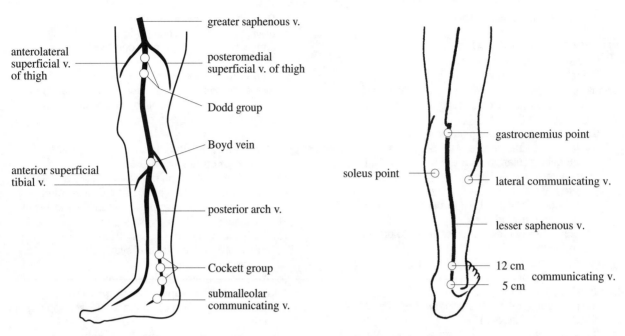

Superficial Venous System of Lower Extremity

Communicating = perforating veins
>100 veins in each leg
(a) medial
1. Submalleolar communicating vein
2. **Cockett group**
group of 3 veins located 7, 12, 18 cm above the tip of medial malleolus connecting posterior arch vein with posterior tibial vein
3. **Boyd vein**
located 10 cm below knee joint connecting main trunk of greater saphenous vein to posterior tibial veins
4. **Dodd group**
group of 1 or 2 veins passing through Hunter canal (= subsartorial canal) to join greater saphenous vein with superficial femoral vein

(b) lateral
1. **Lateral communicating vein**
located from just above lateral malleolus to junction of lower-to-mid thirds of calf connecting lesser saphenous vein with peroneal veins
2. **Posterior mid-calf communicating veins**
located posteriorly 5 + 12 cm above os calcis joining lesser saphenous vein to peroneal veins
3. **Soleal + gastrocnemius points**
joining short saphenous vein to soleal / gastrocnemius veins

DOPPLER PRINCIPLE
Doppler effect = phenomenon by which the frequency of a backscattered wave reflected from a moving target is shifted in frequency from that of the source

Doppler equation:
$$\Delta f = (2\, f_t\, v \cos \theta)/c$$

$$v = \Delta f\, c\, /\, (2\, f_t \cos \theta)$$

Δf = Doppler frequency shift (Hz)
f_t = ultrasound transmitter frequency (Hz)
v = velocity of blood cells (m/sec)
θ = angle between transmitted sound beam and direction of blood flow
c = velocity of sound in soft tissue (1540 m/sec)

$+\Delta f$ = blood flow toward transducer
$-\Delta f$ = blood flow away from transducer

Doppler signal constitutes a variety of spectrum frequencies due to
— different velocities of RBCs across vessel lumen
— variations in blood cell interspace
— divergence of sound beam resulting in variations in incident angle θ
— nonuniformity

Power of received signal dependent on
— amount of backscattering of insonant energy
— amount absorbed by tissues
— transmitter frequency (backscatter + sound absorption increase with higher frequency)
— number of reflectors (low numbers of RBCs as in anemia decrease backscatter)
— motion of vessel wall (high-amplitude low-frequency signal)

Display:
Spectral line (= amplitude versus frequency) is displayed every 2.5 msec providing 400 spectral lines per second
1. frequency (Y-axis)
2. time (X-axis)
3. amplitude = gray-scale intensity

A. LAMINAR FLOW
= narrow range of Doppler shift frequencies, esp. during systole, due to blunt velocity profile
√ window below spectral trace in systole (small sample volume located in center of vessel)

B. DISTURBED FLOW
= breakdown of laminar flow with a wide range of Doppler shifts secondary to velocity vectors whose direction varies
  (a) vortex formation = rotating flow elements form secondary to increase in velocity during upstroke of systole
  (b) turbulence = shed vortices travel downstream
    Cause: stenosis / tortuosity of vessel
√ increase in velocity
√ spectral broadening = reduction of size of window
√ simultaneous forward + reversed flow
√ fluctuations of flow velocity with time

DECREASE IN LUMEN DIAMETER VS. CROSS-SECTIONAL AREA

decrease in lumen diameter	decrease in cross-sectional area
20%	36%
40%	64%
60%	84%
80%	96%

PULSATILITY
= assessment of vascular resistance (increased resistance reduces diastolic flow)
Δ Can be assessed in vessels too small / tortuous to be imaged (Doppler angle unnecessary)!
Index should be calculated for each of several cardiac cycles (5 heartbeats adequate) and an average value taken

  S = A = maximal systolic shift
  D = B = end-diastolic frequency shift

1. Full pulsatility index of Gosling (PI_F) = $1/A_0^2 \sum A_i^2$
2. Simplified pulsatility index (PI)
  = (S - D)/mean
3. Resistance index (RI) = Pourcelot index
  = (S - D)/S or 1 - (D/S)
4. Stuart index = A/B ratio = S/D ratio
5. B/A ratio = B(100%)/A

Pelvic Arterial Anatomy (right side)

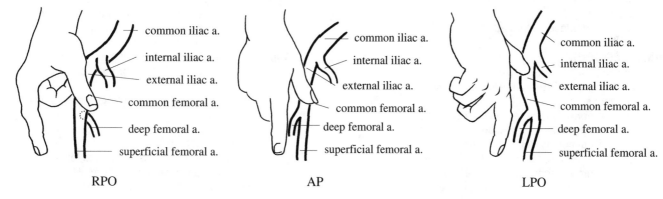

RPO   AP   LPO

- common iliac a.
- internal iliac a.
- external iliac a.
- common femoral a.
- deep femoral a.
- superficial femoral a.

CARDIOVASCULAR DISORDERS

ABERRANT LEFT PULMONARY ARTERY
= PULMONARY SLING = failure of development / obliteration of left 6th aortic arch followed by development of a collateral branch of right pulmonary artery to supply the left lung

Site: left PA passes above right main stem bronchus + between trachea and esophagus on its way to left lung

Age at presentation: neonate / infant / child

Associated with:
  (1)   "napkin-ring trachea" = absent pars membranacea (50%)
  (2)   PDA (most common), ASD, persistent left SVC
- stridor (most common), wheezing, apneic spells, cyanosis
- respiratory infection
- feeding problems
√ deviation of trachea to left
√ "inverted T" appearance of main stem bronchi
  = horizontal course secondary to lower origin of right main stem bronchus
√ anterior bowing of right main stem bronchus
√ "carrot-shaped trachea" = narrowing of tracheal diameter in caudad direction resulting in functional tracheal stenosis
√ obstructive emphysema / atelectasis of RUL + LUL
√ low left hilum
√ separation of trachea + esophagus at hilum by soft tissue mass
√ anterior indentation on esophagogram

AMYLOIDOSIS
= extracellular deposits of insoluble fibrillar protein
- asymptomatic / CHF (restrictive cardiomyopathy), arrhythmia

CXR: √ normal / generalized cardiomegaly
       √ pulmonary congestion
       √ pulmonary deposits of amyloid

NUC: √ striking uptake of Tc-99m pyrophosphate greater than bone (50 – 90%)

ECHO: √ granular sparkling appearance of myocardium
       √ LV wall thickening
       √ decreased LV systolic + diastolic function

ANOMALOUS LEFT CORONARY ARTERY
= left coronary artery arises from pulmonary trunk (left sinus of Valsalva)

Hemodynamics: with postnatal fall in pulmonary arterial pressure perfusion of LCA drops (ischemic left coronary bed), collateral circulation from RCA with flow reversal in LCA
  — adequate collateral circulation   = life-saving
  — inadequate collateral circulation   = myocardial infarction
  — large collateral circulation = L–R shunt with volume overload of heart

- episodes of sweating, ashen color (angina symptomatology)
- ECG: anterolateral infarction
- continuous murmur (if collaterals large)
√ dilatation of LV
√ enlargement of LA
√ normal pulmonary vascularity / redistribution

Rx:
  (1)   Ligation of LCA at its origin from pulmonary trunk
  (2)   Ligation of LCA + graft of left subclavian artery to LCA
  (3)   Creation of an AP window + baffle from AP window to ostium of LCA

DDx: Endocardial fibroelastosis, viral cardiomyopathy (NO shock-like symptoms)

ANOMALOUS PULMONARY VENOUS RETURN
Total Anomalous Pulmonary Venous Return
= TAPVR = anomalous connection between pulmonary veins and systemic veins secondary to embryologic failure of the common pulmonary vein to join the posterior wall of the left atrium

Associated with: ASD (necessary for survival)

A. SUPRADIAPHRAGMATIC TAPVR
  Type I   =   SUPRACARDIAC TAPVR (52%)
         =   drainage into left innominate vein / right + left persistent SVC / azygos vein; <10% obstructed
  Type II   =   CARDIAC TAPVR (30%)
         =   drainage into RA / coronary sinus

Hemodynamics:
  — functional L-to-R shunt from pulmonary veins to right atrium
  — increased pulmonary blood flow (= overcirculation)
  — ASD restores oxygenated blood to left side
  — normal systemic venous pressure with increased flow through widened SVC
  — after birth CHF secondary to (a) mixture of systemic + pulmonary venous blood in RA (b) volume overload of RV
- neck veins undistended (shunt level distally)
- R ventricular heave (= increased contact of enlarged RV with sternum)
- systolic ejection murmur (large shunt volume)
√ "figure of 8" / "snowman" configuration of cardiac silhouette (= dilated SVC + left vertical vein)
√ pretracheal density on lateral film (= left vertical vein)
√ enlargement of RA + RV (= volume overload)
√ normal LA (= ASD acts as escape valve)
√ increased pulmonary blood flow (= overcirculation)
√ absent connection of pulmonary veins to LA

B. <u>INFRACARDIAC TAPVR</u> (12%) = Type III
   = drainage into IVC / portal vein / hepatic vein with constriction of descending pulmonary vein by diaphragm en route through esophageal hiatus leading to pulmonary venous hypertension + RV pressure overload; >90% obstructed
   • intense cyanosis + respiratory distress (R-to-L shunt through ASD)
   Prognosis: death within a few days of life
   Associated with: asplenia syndrome (80%), polysplenia
   √ unique appearance of pulmonary edema with normal-sized heart (DDx: hyaline membrane disease)
   √ low anterior indentation on barium-filled esophagus

C. <u>MIXED TYPE</u> (6%) = Type IV
   = with various connections to R side of heart (6%)

Overall Prognosis: 75% mortality rate within 1 year of birth if untreated

Partial Anomalous Pulmonary Venous Return
   = PAPVR
   May be associated with hypogenetic lung syndrome (= partial / total hypoplasia of right lung + pulmonary artery)
   (a) RUL pulmonary vein enters SVC / RA
      frequently associated with: sinus venosus type ASD (90%)
      √ RUL vein courses in a horizontal direction
   (b) LUL pulmonary vein enters innominate vein
      frequently associated with: ostium secundum type ASD
      √ vertical density along left upper border of mediastinum
   CECT:
      √ nodular / tubular opacity (= anomalous vein), which opacifies in phase with pulmonary vein

AORTIC ANEURYSM
   Causes:
   1. Atherosclerosis (73 – 80%): descending aorta
   2. Traumatic (15 – 20%): following transection
   3. Congenital (2%): aortic sinus, post coarctation, ductus diverticulum
   4. Syphilis: ascending aorta + arch
   5. Mycotic = bacterial dissection
   6. Cystic media necrosis (Marfan / Ehlers-Danlos syndrome, annuloaortic ectasia)
   7. Inflammation of media + adventitia:
      Takayasu arteritis, giant cell arteritis, relapsing polychondritis, rheumatic fever, rheumatoid arthritis, ankylosing spondylitis, Reiter syndrome, psoriasis, ulcerative colitis, systemic lupus erythematosus, scleroderma, Behçet disease, radiation
   8. Increased pressure: systemic hypertension, aortic valve stenosis
   9. Abnormal volume load: severe aortic regurgitation

TRUE ANEURYSM
   = permanent dilatation of all layers of weakened but intact wall

FALSE ANEURYSM
   = focal perforation with all layers of wall disrupted; escaped blood contained by adventitia / perivascular connective tissue + organized blood

FUSIFORM ANEURYSM = circumferential involvement
SACCULAR ANEURYSM = involvement of portion of wall

Abdominal Aortic Aneurysm
   = focal widening >3 cm
   Age: >60 years; M:F = 5:1
   Associated with:
   (a) visceral + renal artery aneurysm (2%)
   (b) isolated iliac + femoral artery aneurysm (16%):
      common iliac (89%), internal iliac (10%), external iliac (1%)
   (c) stenosis / occlusion of celiac trunk / SMA (22%)
   (d) stenosis of renal artery (22 – 30%)
   (e) occlusion of inferior mesenteric artery (80%)
   (f) occlusion of lumbar arteries (78%)
   Growth rate of aneurysm of 3 – 6 cm in diameter: 0.39 cm / year
   • asymptomatic (30%)
   • abdominal mass (26%)
   • abdominal pain (37%)
   Site: infrarenal (91%) with extension into iliac arteries (66%)
   Plain film: √ mural calcification (86%)
   CT: √ perianeurysmal fibrosis (10%), may cause ureteral obstruction
   US: √ >98% accuracy in size measurement
   Angio:
      √ focally widened aortic lumen >3 cm
      √ normal-sized lumen secondary to mural thrombus (11%)
      √ mural clot (80%)
      √ slow antegrade flow of contrast medium
      Contained rupture = extraluminal hematoma / cavity
      √ absent parenchymal stain = avascular halo
      √ displacement + stretching of aortic branches
   Cx:
   (1) Rupture (25%)
      (a) into retroperitoneum: commonly on left
      (b) into GI tract: massive GI hemorrhage
      (c) into IVC: rapid cardiac decompensation
         Incidence: aneurysm <4 cm in 10%, 4 – 5 cm in 23%, 5 – 7 cm in 25%, 7 – 10 cm in 46%, >10 cm in 60%
   (2) Peripheral embolization
   (3) Infection
   (4) Spontaneous occlusion of aorta
   Prognosis: 17% 5-year survival without surgery, 50 – 60% 5-year survival with surgery
   Postoperative Cx: (1) Left colonic ischemia (1.6%) with 10% mortality
                        (2) Renal failure (14%)

Atherosclerotic Aneurysm

Incidence: leading cause of thoracic aortic aneurysm
Histo: diseased intima with secondary degeneration + fibrous replacement of media; ultimately wall of aneurysm composed of acellular + avascular connective tissue
Pathophysiology:
   increasing lateral hydrostatic pressure as the velocity of blood flow diminishes leading to compromise of mural vascular nutrition with further degeneration + progressive dilatation
Age: elderly; M>F
Location:
   (1)   descending thoracic aorta distal to left subclavian artery
   (2)   infrarenal aorta (associated with thoracic aneurysm in 29%)
   (3)   thoracoabdominal
√ fusiform (80%), saccular (20%)
Cx: rupture (cause of death in 50%): usually unrestrained + fatal in thoracic location

Degenerative Aneurysm

= medial degeneration
Most common cause of aneurysm in ascending aorta
Cause:
   (1)   genetically transmitted metabolic disorder: Marfan syndrome, Ehlers-Danlos syndrome
   (2)   acquired: result of repetitive aortic injury + repair associated with aging

Mycotic Aneurysm

Incidence: 2.6% of all abdominal aneurysms
A. PRIMARY MYCOTIC ANEURYSM (rare)
   unassociated with any demonstrable intravascular inflammatory process
B. SECONDARY MYCOTIC ANEURYSM
   = aneurysm due to nonsyphilitic infection
   Predisposing factors:
      (1) IV drug abuse (2) bacterial endocarditis (12%) (3) immunocompromise (malignancy, alcoholism, steroids, chemotherapy, autoimmune disease, diabetes) (4) atherosclerosis (5) aortic trauma caused by accidents / aortic valve surgery / coronary artery bypass surgery / arterial catheterization
   Mechanism:
      (a)   septicemia with abscess formation via vasa vasorum
      (b)   septicemia with abscess formation via vessel lumen
      (c)   direct extension of contiguous infection
      (d)   preexisting intima laceration (trauma, atherosclerosis, coarctation)

Organism:
   S. aureus (53%), Salmonella (33-50%), nonhemolytic Streptococcus, Pneumococcus, Gonococcus, Mycobacterium (contiguous spread from spine / lymph nodes)

Histo: loss of intima + destruction of internal elastic lamella; varying degrees of destruction of muscularis of media + adventitia
• frequently insidious
Site: ascending aorta > abdominal visceral artery > intracranial artery > lower / upper extremity artery
√ true aneurysm (majority)
√ saccular structure arising eccentrically from aortic wall with rapid enlargement
√ interrupted ring of aortic wall calcification
√ periaortic gas collection
√ adjacent vertebral osteomyelitis
√ adjacent reactive lymph node enlargement
Cx:
   (1)   life-threatening rupture + hemorrhage (75%)
   (2)   uncontrolled sepsis if untreated
Prognosis: 67% overall mortality

Syphilitic Aneurysm

Spectrum:
   1.   Uncomplicated syphilitic aortitis
   2.   Syphilitic aortic aneurysm (mostly saccular)
   3.   Syphilitic aortic vasculitis (aortic regurgitation)
Incidence: 12% of patients with untreated syphilis
Onset: 10 – 30 years after initial spirochete infection
Histo: chronic inflammation of aortic adventitia + media beginning at vasa vasorum + leading to obstruction of vasa vasorum followed by nutritional impairment of media + loss of elastic fibers + smooth muscle fibers
• positive venereal disease research laboratory (VDRL) test
• positive microhemagglutination assay - Treponema pallidum (MHA-TP) test
Location: ascending aorta (36%), aortic arch (34%), proximal descending aorta (25%), distal descending aorta (5%), aortic sinuses (<1%)
√ asymmetric enlargement of aortic sinuses (DDx to medial degeneration with symmetric enlargement)
√ saccular (75%) / fusiform (25%) aneurysm
√ pencil-thin dystrophic aortic wall calcification (up to 40%) most severe in ascending aorta, frequently obscured by thick coarse irregular calcifications of secondary atherosclerosis
Prognosis: death in 2%, rupture in up to 40%; death within months of onset of symptoms if untreated

Thoracic Aortic Aneurysm

Most common vascular cause of mediastinal mass!
Average diameter of thoracic aorta (<4 – 5 cm wide):
   —   aortic root: 3.6 cm
   —   ascending aorta 1 cm proximal to arch: 3.5 cm
   —   proximal descending aorta   2.6 cm
   —   middle descending aorta: 2.5 cm
   —   distal descending aorta: 2.4 cm
Associated with: hypertension, coronary artery disease, abdominal aneurysm
Mean age: 65 years; M:F = 3:1

- substernal / back / shoulder pain (26%)
- SVC syndrome (venous compression)
- dysphagia (esophageal compression)
- stridor, dyspnea (tracheobronchial compression)
- hoarseness (recurrent laryngeal nerve compression)
√ wide tortuous aorta
√ curvilinear peripheral calcifications (75%)
√ circumferential / crescentic mural thrombus
√ Angio: may show normal caliber secondary to mural thrombus
Cx:
  (1) Rupture into mediastinum, pericardium, either pleural sac, extrapleural space
       √ high-attenuation fluid
  (2) Aortobronchopulmonary fistula
       √ consolidation of lung adjacent to aneurysm
  Δ Most aneurysms rupture when >10 cm in size
Prognosis: 1-year survival 57%, 3-year survival 26%, 5-year survival 19% (60% die from ruptured aneurysm, 40% die from other causes)
Surgical mortality: 10%

Traumatic Pseudoaneurysm
= CHRONIC AORTIC PSEUDOANEURYSM
2nd most common form of thoracic aortic aneurysm; most common type occurring in young patients
Incidence: 2.5% of patients who survive initial trauma of acute aortic transection
√ usually calcified
√ may contain thrombus
Cx: (1) progressive enlargement
      (2) rupture (even years after insult)

AORTIC DISSECTION
= spontaneous longitudinal separation of media of aortic wall produced by hemorrhage
Path: hemorrhage of vasa vasorum leading to
      (a) transverse tear in weakened intima (95 – 97%) when hematoma breaks into aortic lumen
      (b) no intimal tear (3 – 5%)
Incidence: 3:1,000 (more common than all ruptures of thoracic + abdominal aorta combined)
Peak age: 60 years (range 13 – 87 years); M:F = 3:1
Predisposed: (cystic medial necrosis / disease of aortic wall)
Δ Starts in fusiform aneurysms in 28%
Δ Does not occur in aneurysms <5 cm in diameter
1. Hypertension (60 – 90%)
2. Marfan syndrome (16%)
3. Ehlers-Danlos syndrome
4. Turner syndrome
5. Valvular aortic stenosis
6. Relapsing polychondritis
7. Coarctation
8. Bicuspid aortic valve
9. S/P prosthetic valve
10. Trauma (rare)
11. Pregnancy
NOT syphilis

- sharp tearing intractable anterior / posterior chest pain (75 – 95%)
- murmur, bruit (65%) from aortic regurgitation
- asymmetric peripheral pulses (59%)

- absent femoral pulses (25%), reappearing after reentry
- hemodynamic shock (25%)
- neurologic deficits (25%): hemiplegia, paraparesis
- persistent oliguria
- congestive heart failure
- recurrent arrhythmias / right bundle branch block
- signs of pericardial tamponade: clouded sensorium, extreme restlessness, dyspnea, distended neck veins

Types:
DeBakey Type I   (29 – 34%) = dissection involving entire aorta
DeBakey Type II (12 – 21%) = dissection involving ascending aorta only
DeBakey Type III (50%)   = dissection involving descending aorta only
  Subtype IIIA   = up to diaphragm
  Subtype IIIB   = below diaphragm
Stanford Type A (70%)   = ascending aorta ± aortic arch involved
Stanford Type B (20 – 30%) = confined to descending aorta

Location of dissection (following heliceal flow pattern):
— on lateral wall of ascending aorta just distal to aortic valve (65%)
— on superior + posterior wall of transverse aortic arch (10%)
— on posterior + left wall of upper descending aorta (20%)
— more distal aorta (5%) usually terminating in left iliac artery (80%) / right iliac artery (10%) (involvement of left renal artery in 50%)

CXR (best assessment from comparison with serial films):
√ mediastinal widening (40 – 80%) due to hemorrhage / large false channel
√ cardiac enlargement (LV hypertrophy / hemopericardium)
√ irregular wavy contour / indistinct outline of aorta
√ "calcification sign" = inward displacement of atherosclerotic plaque by 4 – 10 mm from outer aortic contour (7%), can only be applied to contour of descending aorta secondary to projection, may be misleading in presence of periaortic soft tissue mass / hematoma
√ left pleural effusion (27%)
√ atelectasis of lower lobe
√ displacement of trachea / endotracheal tube
ECHO (transesophageal approach preferred):
√ pericardial fluid
√ aortic insufficiency
√ aortic flap
Angio (1st choice because of contrast limitation):
Superior to any other technique in demonstrating
    — entry + reentry points (in 50%)
    — branch vessel involvement + coronary arteries
    — aortic insufficiency
√ abnormal catheter position outside anticipated aortic course

√ linear radiolucency within opacified aorta (= intimal / medial flap)

√ "double barrel aorta" (87%) = opacification of second channel

√ compression of true lumen by false channel (72 – 85%)

√ aortic valvular regurgitation (30%)

√ increase in aortic wall thickness >6 – 10 mm

√ obstruction of aortic branches: left renal artery (25 – 30%)

√ slower blood flow in false lumen

CT: within 4 hours (if patient responds rapidly to medical Rx); detection as accurate as angio

√ crescentic high-attenuation clot within aortic wall

√ internally displaced intimal calcification (DDx: calcification of thrombus on luminal surface or within)

√ intimal flap + two aortic lumens

Cx: (1) Retrograde dissection
        (a) aortic valve malfunction
        (b) occlusion of coronary artery (8%)
        (c) rupture into pericardial sac / pleural space: 70% mortality
        (d) rupture into RV, LA, vena cava, pulmonary artery producing large L-to-R shunt
    (2) occlusion / transient obstruction of major aortic branches (30%)
    (3) rupture of aorta
    (4) development of saccular aneurysm requiring surgery (15%)

Prognosis:
  immediate death (3%);
  death within: 1 day (20 – 30%), 1 week (50 – 62%),
                3 weeks (60%), 3 months (80%), 1 year
                (80 – 95%)
  5 – 10% mortality rate following timely surgery

Rx:
  (1) Immediate surgical reinforcement of aortic wall (Type I, II = A) preventing proximal extension
  (2) Reducing peak systolic pressure to 120 – 70 mm Hg (Type III = B rarely progresses proximally): death from rupture of aortic aneurysm in 46% of hypertensive + 17% of normotensive patients

DDx: Penetrating ulcer of thoracic aorta (= atherosclerotic lesion of middle descending aorta with ulceration extending through intima into aortic media)

AORTIC GRAFT INFECTION

Classification:
  (1) PERIGRAFT INFECTION (2 – 6%)
     • fever, chills, leukocytosis
     • groin swelling / drainage
  (2) AORTOENTERIC FISTULA (0.6 – 2%)
     • acute / chronic GI bleeding (may be occult)
     • sepsis

Normal postoperative course:
  Δ complete resolution of hematoma by 2 – 3 months
  Δ disappearance of ectopic gas by 3 – 4 weeks

CT (94% sensitive, 85% specific, 91% accurate):
  √ perigraft soft tissue

√ ectopic gas (fistulous communication with bowel / gas-producing organism)

√ focal bowel wall thickening (indicates fistula)

√ >5 mm soft tissue between graft + surrounding wrap (beyond 7th postoperative week)

√ focal discontinuity of calcified aneurysmal wrap

False positives:
  perigraft hematoma in early postoperative period, pseudoaneurysm (in 15 – 20%)

Prognosis: 17 – 75% mortality; 30 – 50% morbidity

AORTIC REGURGITATION

Cause:
  A. Intrinsic aortic valve disease
    1. Congenital bicuspid valve
    2. Rheumatic endocarditis
    3. Bacterial endocarditis (perforation / prolapse of cusp)
    4. Myxomatous valve associated with cystic medial necrosis
    5. Prosthetic valve: mechanical break, thrombosis, paravalvular leak
  B. Primary disease of ascending aorta
    (a) Dilatation of aortic annulus
      1. Syphilitic aortitis
      2. Ankylosing spondylitis (5 – 10%)
      3. Reiter disease
      4. Rheumatoid arthritis
      5. Cystic medial necrosis: Marfan syndrome
    (b) Laceration
      1. Decelerating trauma
      2. Hypertension

Pathogenesis:
  progressive enlargement of diastolic + systolic LV dimensions result in increase in myocardial fiber length + increase in stroke volume; decompensation occurs if critical limit of fiber length is reached

• "water-hammer pulse" = twin-peaked pulse

• systolic ejection murmur + high-pitched diastolic murmur

• Austin Flint murmur = soft mid-diastolic or presystolic bruit

√ LV enlargement (cardiothoracic ratio >0.55) + initially normal pulmonary vascularity (DDx: congestive cardiomyopathy, pericardial effusion)

√ normal aorta (in intrinsic valve disease)

√ dilatation ± calcification of ascending aorta (in aortic wall disease)

√ tortuous descending aorta

√ increased pulsations along entire aorta

ECHO:
  √ increased dimension of aortic root
  √ high frequency diastolic flutter of aML, IVS (uncommon)
  √ LV dilatation + large amplitude of LV wall motion (volume overload, increased ejection fraction)
  √ premature closure of mitral valve (high diastolic LV pressure)

Doppler:
  √ slope of peak diastolic to end-diastolic velocity decrease >3 m/sec^2 in severe aortic regurgitation

√ area of color Doppler regurgitant flow
√ ratio of width of regurgitant beam to width of aortic root is good predictor of severity (color Doppler)

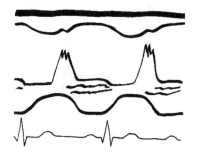

Mitral Valve in Severe Aortic Regurgitation

The valve is almost completely closed before onset of ventricular systole. Atrial contraction has little effect in reopening the valve. Complete closure occurs with ventricular systole. A high velocity flutter of aML is present in diastole.

AORTIC STENOSIS

Aortic valve area decreased to <0.8 cm² = 0.4 cm²/m² BSA (normal 2.5 – 3.5 cm²)

A. Acquired aortic stenosis
 1. Rheumatic valvulitis (almost invariably associated with mitral valve disease)
 2. Senile calcific valve degeneration
B. Congenital aortic stenosis (most common)
 = most frequent CHD associated with IUGR
 1. Subvalvular AS (30%)
 2. Valvular AS (70%): degeneration of bicuspid valve most common cause
 3. Supravalvular AS

Pathogenesis:
increased gradient across valve produces LV hypertrophy and diminished LV compliance; increased muscle mass may outstrip coronary blood supply (subendocardial myocardial ischemia with angina); LV decompensation leads to LV dilatation + pulmonary venous congestion

• asymptomatic for many years
• angina, syncope, heart failure
• systolic murmur
• carotid pulsus parvus et tardus
• diminished aortic component of 2nd heart sound
• sudden death in severe stenosis (20%) after exercise (diminished flow in coronary arteries causes ventricular dysrhythmias + fibrillation)
√ poststenotic dilatation of ascending aorta (in 90% of acquired, in 70% of congenital AS)
√ normal-sized / enlarged LV (small LV chamber with thick walls)
@ in adults >30 years
 √ calcification of aortic valve (best seen on RAO); indicates gradient >50 mm Hg
 √ discrete enlargement of ascending aorta (NO correlation with severity of stenosis)
 √ calcification of mitral annulus

√ "left ventricular configuration" = concavity along mid-left lateral heart border + increased convexity along lower left lateral heart border
@ in children / young adults
 √ prominent ascending aorta
 √ left ventricular heart configuration
@ in infancy:
 √ left ventricular stress syndrome
ECHO:
 √ multiple dense cusp echoes throughout cardiac cycle; if thickened cusp echoes only in diastole then consider DDx of calcification of aortic annulus in elderly, calcified coronary artery ostium
 √ decreased separation of leaflets in systole with reduced opening orifice (13 – 14 mm = mild AS; 8 – 12 mm = moderate AS; <8 mm = severe AS)
 √ dilated aortic root
 √ increased thickness of LV wall (concentric LV hypertrophy)
 √ hyperdynamic contraction of LV (in compensated state)
 √ thickened + calcified aortic valve with restrictive motion ± doming in systole
 √ increased aortic valve gradient (Doppler)
 √ decreased aortic valve area by continuity equation
Prognosis: depends on symptomatology (angina, syncope, CHF)

Subvalvular Aortic Stenosis
= SUBAORTIC STENOSIS
(a) Anatomic / fixed subaortic stenosis
 Associated with cardiac defects in 50% (usually VSD)
 Type I : thin 1 – 2 mm membranous diaphragmatic stenosis, usually located within 2 cm or less of valve annulus
 Type II : thick collar-like stenosis
 Type III : irregular fibromuscular stenosis
 Type IV : "tunnel subaortic stenosis" = fixed tunnel-like narrowing of LVOT = excessive thickening of only upper ventricular septum with normal mitral valve motion
(b) Functional / dynamic subaortic stenosis
 1. Asymmetric septal hypertrophy (ASH)
 2. Idiopathic hypertrophic subaortic stenosis (IHSS)
 3. Hypertrophic obstructive cardiomyopathy (HOCM)
 may occur in infants of diabetic mothers
 √ asymmetrically thicker ventricular septum than free wall of LV (95%)
 √ normal / small left + right ventricular cavities (95%)
 √ systolic anterior motion of mitral valve
 √ lucent subaortic filling defect in systole
ECHO:
 √ coarse systolic flutter of valve cusps
 √ opening of leaflets followed by rapid inward move in mid-systole, leaflets may remain in partially closed position through latter portion of systole (to appose borders of the flow jet)

Cx: mitral regurgitation (secondary to abnormal position of anterolateral papillary muscle preventing complete closure of MV in systole)

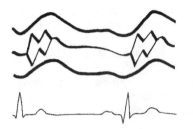

Aortic Valve in Hypertrophic Subaortic Stenosis
during midsystole the aortic valve closes secondary to subvalvular obstruction

Valvular Aortic Stenosis
= fusion of commissures between cusps
Congenital types:
(a) bicuspid / unicuspid (in 95%): in 1 – 2% of population; M > F; commonly associated with coarctation of the aorta
(b) tricuspid (5%)
(c) dysplastic thickened aortic cusps
√ valvular calcifications (in 60% of patients >24 years of age)

@ IN INFANT with critical aortic stenosis:
• intractable CHF in first days / weeks of life with severe dyspnea
• may simulate neonatal sepsis
Associated with L-R shunts (ASD, VSD)
√ marked cardiomegaly (thickened wall of LV)
√ pulmonary venous hypertension
√ decreased ejection fraction
√ doming of thickened valve cusps
√ dilated ascending aorta
Rx: emergency surgical dilatation
@ IN CHILD:
• asymptomatic until late in life
√ normal pulmonary vascularity
√ LV configuration with normal size of heart
√ large posterior noncoronary cusp, smaller fused right + left cusps
√ doming of thickened valve cusps
√ eccentric jet of contrast
√ poststenotic dilatation of ascending aorta

ECHO:
√ increase in echoes from thickened deformed leaflets (maximal during diastole)
√ decrease in leaflet separation

Supravalvular Aortic Stenosis
Types:
(a) localized hourglass narrowing just above aortic sinuses

(b) discrete fibrous membrane above sinuses of Valsalva
(c) diffuse tubular hypoplasia of ascending aorta + branching arteries
Associated with: peripheral PS, valvular + discrete subvalvular AS, Marfan syndrome, Williams syndrome

√ dilatation + tortuosity of coronary arteries (may undergo early atherosclerotic degeneration secondary to high pressure)
ECHO:
√ narrowing of supravalvular aortic area (normal root diameter: 20 – 37 mm)
√ normal movement of cusps

AORTIC TRANSECTION
= TRAUMATIC AORTIC RUPTURE = aortic laceration / rupture from sudden horizontal deceleration injury
Site: (a) Aortic isthmus (88 – 95%)
            brachiocephalic arteries + ligamentum arteriosum fix aorta in this region
       (b) Aortic arch with avulsion of brachiocephalic trunk (4.5%)
       (c) Ascending aorta immediately above aortic valve (1%)
            Cx: cardiac tamponade; NO mediastinal hematoma
       (d) Descending aorta (1.8%)
Extent of injury:
(a) transverse intimal tear
(b) tear of intima + media with subadventitial accumulation of blood (40%) = false aneurysm

• interscapular severe chest pain, dyspnea
• hypertension in upper extremities = acute traumatic coarctation
• alteration in peripheral pulses
• systolic murmur in 2nd left parasternal interspace

CXR:
√ normal admission CXR in 28% (radiographic signs may not develop until 6 – 36 hours)
√ mediastinal width >8 cm at level of aortic knob (75%)
√ mediastinal width to chest width >0.25
√ poorly defined irregular aortic contour (75%)
√ deviation of nasogastric tube to right of spinous process at T4 (67%)
√ tracheal compression + displacement towards right (61%)
√ depression of left main stem bronchus anteroinferiorly + towards right (53%)
√ right / left "apical cap" sign = extrapleural hematoma (37%)
√ opacification of aortopulmonary window
√ partial obliteration of descending aorta
√ rapidly accumulating commonly left-sided hemothorax without evident rib fracture (break in mediastinal pleura)
√ fractures of 1st + 2nd rib (17%)

√ widening of right / left paraspinal line
√ widening of right paratracheal stripe >5 mm
Angio (definite means for diagnosis):
√ traumatic false aneurysm
√ intimal tear (5 – 10%)
√ posttraumatic dissection (11%)
√ posttraumatic coarctation
DDx: ductus diverticulum (in 10% of normals)
Prognosis:
15 – 20% initial survival rate (due to formation of periaortic hematoma + false aneurysm contained by adventitia ± surrounding connective tissue)
(a) with surgical repair: 15% survive
(b) no intervention: 80% dead within 1 hour; 85% dead within 24 hours, 98% dead within 10 weeks; chronic false aneurysm may develop in 5% at isthmus / descending aorta

Chronic Traumatic Aortic Pseudoaneurysm
= aneurysm existing for >3 months (amount of wall fibroplasia following rupture usually not sufficient to prevent subsequent rupture until at least 3 months after initial traumatic episode)
Incidence: 5% of patients surviving aortic transection >24 – 48 hours
• symptom-free period of months to years (in 11% >10 years)
• delayed clinical symptoms: chest pain, back pain, dyspnea, cough, hoarseness, dysphagia
Prognosis: enlargement + eventual rupture

AORTOPULMONIC WINDOW
= defect in septation process characterized by large round / oval communication between left wall of ascending aorta + right wall of pulmonary trunk
• clinically resembles PDA
CXR:
√ shunt vascularity
√ cardiomegaly (LA + LV enlarged)
√ diminutive aortic knob
√ prominent pulmonary trunk
Angio (left ventriculogram / aortogram in AP / LAO projection):
√ defect several mm above aortic valve
√ pulmonary valve identified (DDx to truncus arteriosus)

ARTERIOSCLEROSIS OBLITERANS
= ASO = hardening of the arteries
Prevalence:
2.4 million people in U.S.; in 1978 12% of autopsies had ASO as leading cause of death (excluding MI)
Etiology: unknown
Contributing factors:
aging, diabetes (16 – 44%), hypertension, atherosclerosis
Effect of hyperlipidemia:
(a) High-density lipoproteins (HDL) have a protective effect: carry 25% of blood cholesterol
(b) Low-density lipoproteins (LDL): carry 60% of blood cholesterol

Histo:
deposition of lipids, blood products, carbohydrates, begins as disruption of intimal surface; fatty streaks (as early as childhood); fibrous plaques (as early as 3rd decade); thrombosis, ulceration, calcification, aneurysm
Age: 50 – 70 years; M>F (after menopause)
Clinical classification:
(1) ischemic symptoms with exercise = intermittent claudication: calf, thigh, hip, buttock
(2) ischemic symptoms at rest (indicative of multisegment disease)
• cramping / burning / aching pain
• cold extremity
• paresthesia
• trophic changes: hair loss, thickened nails
• ulcer, gangrene
• decreased / absent pulses
Location:
medium + large arteries; frequently at bifurcations; most frequent:
— superficial femoral artery in adductor canal (diabetics + nondiabetics)
— aortoiliac segment (nondiabetics)
— tibioperoneal trunk (diabetics)

Prognosis:
accelerated by diabetes (34% will require amputation), hypertension, lipoprotein abnormalities, heart disease (decreased cardiac output resulting in increased blood viscosity from polycythemia), chronic addiction to tobacco (11.4% will require amputation), intermittent claudication (5 – 7% require amputation if nondiabetic = 1 – 2% per year), ischemic ulcer / rest pain (19.6% require amputation)

ASPLENIA SYNDROME
= BILATERAL RIGHT-SIDEDNESS
= IVEMARK SYNDROME
Incidence: 1:1,750 to 1:40,000 livebirths; M > F
Associated with:
(a) CHD (in 50%):
TAPVR (almost 100%), endocardial cushion defect (85%), single ventricle (51%), TGA (58%), pulmonary stenosis / atresia (70%), dextrocardia (42%), mesocardia, VSD, ASD, absent coronary sinus, common atrium, bilateral right atrial appendages, bilateral SVC, common hepatic vein
(b) GI anomalies:
Partial / total situs inversus, annular pancreas, agenesis of gallbladder, ectopic liver, esophageal varices, duplication + hypoplasia of stomach, Hirschsprung disease, hindgut duplication, imperforate anus
(c) GU anomalies (15%):
Horseshoe kidney, double collecting system, hydroureter, cystic kidney, fused / horseshoe adrenal, absent left adrenal, bilobed urinary bladder, bicornuate uterus
(d) Cleft lip / palate, scoliosis, single umbilical artery, lumbar myelomeningocele

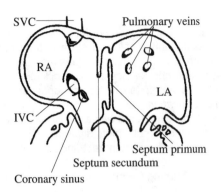

Normal Newborn Heart

atrial septum consists of two components

(a) right side: septum secundum (muscular, firm) with posterior opening = foramen ovale

(b) left side: septum primum (fibrous, thin) with anterior opening = ostium secundum

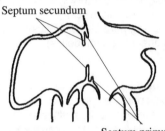

Ostium Secundum Defect

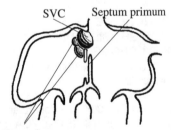

Sinus Venosus Defect

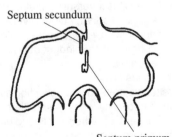

Ostium Primum Defect

- cyanosis in neonatal period / infancy (if severe cyanotic CHD)
- Howell-Jolly bodies = RBC inclusions in patients with absent spleen

√ absent spleen
@ Lung
 √ bilateral trilobed lungs = bilateral minor fissures (SPECIFIC)
 √ bilateral eparterial bronchi (tomogram)
 √ diminished pulmonary vascularity / pulmonary venous hypertension (TAPVR below diaphragm)
 √ bilateral SVC
 √ right atrial isomerism
@ Abdomen
 √ centrally located liver = hepatic symmetry
 √ stomach on right / left side / in central position
 √ abdominal aorta + IVC located on same side of spine (aorta usually posterior) (ALMOST PATHOGNOMONIC)
Prognosis: 80% mortality by end of 1st year of life

ATRIAL SEPTAL DEFECT

Most common congenital cardiac defect in subjects >20 years of age

Incidence: 8 – 14% of all CHD; M:F = 1:4

Age: presentation frequently > age 40 secondary to benign course

(a) mildly symptomatic (60%): dyspnea, fatigue, palpitations

(b) severely symptomatic (30%): cyanosis, heart failure

Embryology:

1. Septum primum = membrane growing from atrial walls toward endocardial cushion

2. Ostium primum = temporary orifice between septum primum + endocardial cushion, which becomes obliterated by 5th week

3. Ostium secundum = multiple small coalescing perforations in septum primum

4. Septum secundum = membrane developing on right side of septum primum + covering part of ostium secundum

5. Foramen ovale = orifice limited by septum secundum + septum primum

6. Foramen ovale flap = lower edge of septum primum (foramen ovale patent in 6%, probe-patent in 25%; not considered an ASD)

1. OSTIUM SECUNDUM ASD (60 – 70%)
     = exaggerated resorptive process of septum primum leads to absence / fenestration of the foramen ovale flap
    Location: in the body of the atrial chamber at fossa ovalis
    Size: large defect of 1 – 3 cm in diameter
    May be associated with:
      Prolapsing mitral valve, pulmonary valve stenosis, tricuspid atresia, TAPVR, hypoplastic left heart, interrupted aortic arch

2. OSTIUM PRIMUM ASD (30%)
= defect of atrioventricular endocardial cushion
Location: inferior to fossa ovalis at outlet portion of
atrial septum
Almost always associated with: Endocardial cushion
defects, cleft mitral valve, anterior fascicular block

3. SINUS VENOSUS ASD (5%)
= defect of the superior inlet portion of the atrial septum
Location: superior to fossa ovalis near entrance of
superior vena cava (SVC straddles ASD)
Associated with:
Partial anomalous pulmonary venous return in 90%
(RUL pulmonary veins connect to SVC / right atrium),
Holt-Oram syndrome, Ellis-van Creveld syndrome

LUTEMBACHER SYNDROME = ASD + mitral stenosis

Hemodynamics:
no hemodynamic perturbance in the fetus; after birth
physiologic increase in LA pressure creates a L-R shunt
(shunt volume may be 3 – 4 times that of systemic blood
flow) with volume overload of RV leading to RV
dilatation, right heart failure, pulmonary hypertension;
diastolic pressure differences in atria determine direction
of shunt; pulmonary pressure remains normal for
decades before Eisenmenger syndrome sets in;
pulmonary hypertension in young adulthood (6%)
• repeated respiratory infections
• feeding difficulties
• arrhythmias
• thromboembolism
• asymptomatic; occasionally discovered by routine CXR
• right ventricular heave
• fixed splitting of second heart sound with accentuation
of pulmonary component
• ECG: right axis deviation + some degree of right bundle
branch block
• exertional dyspnea after development of pulmonary
arterial hypertension (= Eisenmenger syndrome)
• cyanosis may occur (shunt reversal to R-L shunt),
typically during 3rd – 4th decade
• right heart failure in patients >40 years
CXR:
√ normal (if shunt <2 x systemic blood flow)
√ "hilar dance" = increased pulsations of central
pulmonary arteries (DDx: other L-to-R shunts)
√ overcirculation (if pulmonary-to-systemic blood flow ≥
2 : 1)
√ loss of visualization of SVC (= clockwise rotation of
heart due to RV hypertrophy)
√ small appearing aorta with normal aortic knob
√ normal size of LA after shunt reversal (due to
immediate decompression into RA) in
EISENMENGER SYNDROME
√ enlargement of pulmonary trunk + arteries
√ RV enlargement
ECHO:
√ paradoxical interventricular septal motion (due to
volume overload of RV)

√ direct visualization of ASD (= lack of echoes of atrial
septum) in subcostal view
√ diastolic blood flow from interatrial septum crossing
RA + tricuspid valve observed by color Doppler
Angio:
√ RA fills with contrast shortly after LA is opacified (on
levophase of pulmonary angio in AP or LAO
projection)
√ injection into RUL pulmonary vein to visualize exact
size + location of ASD (LAO 45° + C-C 45°)

Prognosis:
(1) Mortality: 0.6% in 1st decade; 0.7% in 2nd decade;
2.7% in 3rd decade; 4.5% in 4th decade; 5.4% in
5th decade; 7.5% in 6th decade; median age of
death is 37 years
(2) Spontaneous closure: 22% in infants <1 year;
33% between ages 1 and 2 years; 3% in children
>4 years
Cx: (1) Tricuspid insufficiency (secondary to dilatation
of AV ring)
(2) Mitral valve prolapse
(3) Atrial fibrillation (in 20% 1st presenting
symptom in patients > age 40)
Rx: (if vascular changes still reversible = resistance of
pulmonary-to-systemic system ≤0.7); 1% surgical
mortality
1. Surgical patch closure
2. Rashkind foam + stainless steel prosthesis

BENEFICIAL ASD
= secundum type ASD serves an essential
compensatory function in:
1. Tricuspid atresia
RA blood reaches pulmonary vessels via ASD +
PDA; improvement through Rashkind procedure
2. TAPVR
significant shunt volume only available through ASD
(VSD / PDA much less reliable)
3. Hypoplastic left heart
systemic circulation maintained via RV with
oxygenated blood from LA through ASD into RA

AZYGOS CONTINUATION OF IVC
= development failure of hepatic / infrahepatic segment of
IVC
Incidence: 2% of CHD
Associated with: Polysplenia syndrome (more common),
asplenia syndrome (rare)
√ enlargement of arch of azygos
√ enlarged paraspinal + retrocrural azygos + hemiazygos
vein
√ absence of hepatic ± infrahepatic IVC

BACTERIAL ENDOCARDITIS
Predisposed:
1. Rheumatic valve disease
2. Mitral valve prolapse with mitral regurgitation
3. Aortic stenosis, mitral stenosis, aortic regurgitation,
mitral regurgitation

4. Most CHD (VSD, TOF) except ostium secundum ASD
5. Previous endocarditis
6. Drug addicts:
   endocarditis of tricuspid valve causes multiple septic pulmonary emboli
7. Bicuspid aortic valve:
   responsible for 50% of aortic valvular bacterial endocarditis
8. Prosthetic valve:
   4% incidence of bacterial endocarditis
   √ exaggerated valve motion (= disintegration of suture line + regurgitation)

Valve Vegetations
ECHO:
   √ usually discrete focal echodensities with sharp edges; may show fuzzy / shaggy nonuniform thickening of cusps (vegetations) in systole + diastole
   √ may appear as shaggy echoes that prolapse when the valve is closed

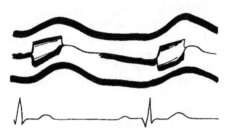

Aortic Valve Endocarditis

BUERGER DISEASE
= THROMBANGIITIS OBLITERANS
= idiopathic recurrent segmental obliterative vasculitis of small + medium-sized peripheral arteries + veins (panangiitis)
Incidence: <1% of all chronic vascular diseases; more common in Israel, Orient, India
Etiology: unknown
Histo:
   (a) acute stage: multiple microabscesses within fresh / organizing thrombus; all layers of vessel wall inflamed but intact; internal elastic lamina may be damaged; multinucleated giant cells within microabscesses (PATHOGNOMONIC)
   (b) subacute stage: thrombus organization with little residual inflammation
   (c) chronic stage: lumen filled with organized recanalized thrombus, fibrosis of adventitia binds together artery, vein and nerve
Associated with   cigarette smoking (95%)
• instep claudication ± distal ulceration (symptoms abate on cessation of smoking + return on its resumption)
• Raynaud phenomenon (33%)
Location: legs (80%), arms (10 – 20%)

Site: starts in palmar + plantar vessels with proximal progression
√ superficial + deep migratory thrombophlebitis (20 – 33%)
√ arterial occlusions, tapered narrowing of arteries
√ abundant corkscrew-shaped collaterals
√ direct collateral following the path of the original artery (Martorell sign) in 80%
√ skip lesions = multiple segments involved with portions of arterial wall remaining unaffected
√ absence of generalized arteriosclerosis / arterial calcifications (90%)

CARDIAC TAMPONADE
= significant compression of heart by fluid contained within pericardial sac causing compromise of diastolic filling of ventricles

• pulsus paradoxus = exaggeration of normal pattern = drop in systolic arterial pressure >10 mm Hg during inspiration (secondary to increase in right heart filling during inspiration at the expense of left heart filling)
• elevated jugular venous pressure
• distant heart sounds / friction rub
• ECG: reduced voltage, ST elevation, PR depression, nonspecific T wave abnormalities

√ normal lung fields + normal pulmonary vascularity
√ rapid enlargement of heart size
ECHO: √ diastolic collapse of RV
        √ cyclical collapse of either atrium

CARDIOMYOPATHY
Congestive Cardiomyopathy
= DILATED CARDIOMYOPATHY
Etiology:
   (a) Myocarditis: viruses, bacteria
   (b) Endocardial fibroelastosis = thickened endocardium + reduced contractility
   (c) Infants of diabetic mothers
   (d) Inborn error of metabolism: glycogenosis, mucolipidosis, mucopolysaccharidosis
   (e) Coronary artery disease: myocardial infarction, anomalous origin of left coronary artery, coronary calcinosis
   (f) Muscular dystrophies
• tendency for CHF

√ cardiomegaly + poor contractility of ventricular wall
√ global heart enlargement
√ LA enlargement without enlargement of LA appendage
ECHO:
   √ enlarged LV with global hypokinesis
   √ IVS and LVPW of equal thickness with decreased amplitude of motion
   √ low profile / "miniaturized" mitral valve
   √ mildly enlarged LA (elevated end-diastolic LV pressure)
   √ enlarged hypokinetic right ventricle

Hypertrophic Cardiomyopathy

= OBSTRUCTIVE CARDIOMYOPATHY
1. SYMMETRIC / CONCENTRIC HYPERTROPHY (uncommon)
   (a) midventricular (b) diffuse (c) apical
2. IDIOPATHIC HYPERTROPHIC SUBAORTIC STENOSIS (IHSS) = ASYMMETRIC SEPTAL HYPERTROPHY (ASH) is part of IHSS
   Etiology: autosomal dominant transmission
   √ prominent left midheart border (septal hypertrophy)
   ECHO:
   √ IVS >14 mm thick; IVS:LVPW thickness >1.3:1
   √ systolic anterior movement of mitral valve (SAM) causing narrowed LVOT in systole
   √ midsystolic closure of aortic valve
   √ increased LVOT gradient with late systolic peaking on Doppler

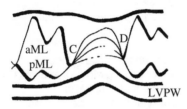

Systolic Anterior Motion (SAM) of MV in IHSS

mitral valve leaflets move abruptly toward septum at a rate greater than the endocardium of the posterior wall; responsible for obstruction to blood ejected from LV

Restrictive Cardiomyopathy

Etiology: (a) infiltrative disease: amyloid, glycogen, hemochromatosis
   (b) constrictive pericarditis

CHRONIC VENOUS STASIS DISEASE

= CHRONIC VENOUS INSUFFICIENCY
= insufficiency / incompetence of venous valves in deep venous system of lower extremity
Cause:
   (a) postphlebitic valvular incompetence: destruction of valve apparatus results in short thickened valves secondary to scar formation
   (b) primary valvular incompetence: shallow elongated redundant valve cusps prevent effective closure
Associated with incompetent venous valves in the calf (secondary to pressure dilatation from stasis in deep venous system) leading to superficial vein varicosities
• edema, induration (= fluid exudation from increased capillary pressure)
• ulceration (from minor trauma + decreased diffusion of oxygen secondary to fibrin deposits around capillaries)
• skin hyperpigmentation (= breakdown products of exudated RBCs)
• aching pain

√ venous reflux on descending venography with Valsalva
   (a) 82% in deep venous system alone
   (b) 2% in saphenous vein alone
   (c) 16% in both
   bilateral in 75%
   Grade
   1 = minimal incompetence = to level of upper thigh
   2 = mild incompetence = to level of lower thigh
   3 = moderate incompetence = to level of knee
   4 = severe incompetence = to level of calf veins

COARCTATION OF AORTA

M:F = 4:1; rare in Blacks
A. <u>LOCALIZED COARCTATION</u> [former classification = ADULT / POSTDUCTAL / JUXTADUCTAL TYPE] (most common type)
   = short discrete narrowing close to ligamentum arteriosum
   Δ Coexistent cardiac anomalies uncommon!
   Location: most frequent in juxtaductal portion of arch
   • incidental finding late in life
   • ductus usually closed
   √ shelf-like lesion at any point along the aortic arch
   √ narrow isthmus above the lesion
   √ poststenotic aortic dilatation distally

B. <u>TUBULAR HYPOPLASIA</u> [former classification = INFANTILE / PREDUCTAL / DIFFUSE TYPE]
   = hypoplasia of long segment of aortic arch after origin of innominate artery
   Δ Coexistent cardiac anomalies common!
   • CHF in neonatal period (in 50%)

Hemodynamics:
   fetus : no significant change because only 10% of cardiac output flows through aortic isthmus
   neonate : determined by how rapidly the ductus closes; without concurrent VSD overload of LV leads to CHF in 2nd / 3rd week of life
Collateral circulation via subclavian artery and its branches:
   — intercostals   — internal mammary
   — anterior spinal artery   — scapular artery
   — lateral thoracic   — transverse cervical artery
Associated with (in 50%):
1. Bicuspid aortic valve (in 25 – 50%), which may result in calcific aortic valve stenosis (after 25 years of age) + bacterial endocarditis

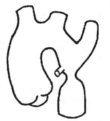 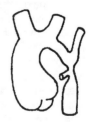

Localized Coarctation   **Tubular Hypoplasia**

2. Intracardiac malformations:
   PDA (33%), VSD (15%), aortic stenosis, aortic insufficiency, ASD, TGV, ostium primum defect, truncus arteriosus, double outlet right ventricle
3. Noncardiac malformations (13%):
   Turner syndrome (13 – 15%)
4. Cerebral berry aneurysms
5. Mycotic aneurysm distal to CoA

Prognosis: 11% mortality prior to 6 months of age

SYMPTOMATIC CoA

Second most common cause of CHF in neonate (after hypoplastic left heart)
Time: (a) toward the end of 1st week of life in "critical stenosis"
      (b) more commonly presents in older child
- lower extremity cyanosis (in tubular hypoplasia)
- left ventricular failure (usually toward end of 1st week of life)
√ generalized cardiomegaly
√ increased pulmonary vascularity (L-to-R shunt through PDA / VSD)
√ pulmonary venous hypertension

ASYMPTOMATIC CoA

- headaches (from hypertension)
- claudication (from hypoperfusion)
√ "figure 3 sign" = indentation of lateral margin of aortic arch with poststenotic dilatation at site of coarctation
√ "reverse 3 sign" on barium esophagogram
√ elevated left ventricular apex (secondary to hypertrophy)
√ linear wavy opacity behind sternum (= dilated internal mammary arteries)
√ dilatation of brachiocephalic vessels + aorta proximal to stenosis
√ rib notching in ribs 3 – 8 (in 75%, unusual before age 6)
    (a) bilateral
    (b) rib notching on left side: anomalous right subclavian artery
    (c) rib notching on right side: CoA proximal to left subclavian artery

Rx: ages 3 – 5 years are ideal time for operation (late enough to avoid restenosis + early enough before irreversible hypertension occurs); surgical correction past 1 year of age decreases operative mortality drastically; 3 – 11% perioperative mortality

Procedures:
1. Resection + end-to-end anastomosis
2. Patch angioplasty
3. Subclavian flap (Waldhausen procedure) using left subclavian artery as a flap

Postsurgical Cx:
1. Residual coarctation (in 32%)
2. Subsequent obstruction (rare)
3. Mesenteric arteritis: 2 – 3 days after surgery secondary to paradoxical hypertension from increased plasma renin
   - abdominal pain, loss of bowel control
4. Chronic persistent hypertension

CONGENITAL ABSENCE OF PULMONARY VALVE

Massive regurgitation between pulmonary artery and RV
Associated with (in 90%):
    VSD, tetralogy of Fallot (50%)
- cyanosis (not in immediate newborn period)
- repeated episodes of respiratory distress
- continuous murmur
- ECG: right ventricular hypertrophy
√ prominent main, right, and left pulmonary artery
√ RV dilatation (increased stroke volume)
√ partial obstruction of right / left main stem bronchus (compression by vessel)
√ right-sided aorta (33%)

CONGESTIVE HEART FAILURE

= elevation of microvascular pressure of lung; most common cause of interstitial + air-space edema of lungs
Cause:
    (a) back pressure from LV: long-standing systemic hypertension, aortic valve disease, coronary artery disease, cardiomyopathy, myocardial infarction
    (b) obstruction proximal to LV: mitral valve disease, LA myxoma, cor triatriatum
Histo:
    (a) Interstitial phase: fluid in loose connective tissue around conducting airways and vessels + engorgement of lymphatics
    (b) Alveolar phase: increase in alveolar wall thickness
    (c) Alveolar air-space phase: alveoli filled with fluid + loss of alveolar volume; pulmonary fibrosis upon organization of intra-alveolar fibrin (if chronic)
√ large heart
√ vascular congestion

1. **Interstitial pulmonary edema** (invariably precedes alveolar edema)
   - NO abnormal physical finding
   - hypoxemia (ventilation-perfusion inequality)
   √ loss of sharp definition of vascular markings
   √ thickening of interlobular septa (pulmonary venous wedge pressure 17 – 20 mm Hg)
   √ poorly defined increased bronchial wall thickness
   √ thickening of interlobar fissures (due to fluid in subpleural connective tissue layer)
2. **Air-space edema** (when volume of capillary filtration exceeds that of lymphatic drainage)
   - severe dyspnea / orthopnea
   - tachypnea + cyanosis
   - dry cough / copious frothy sputum
   - hypoxemia (vascular shunting)
   √ poorly defined patchy acinar opacities
   √ coalescence of acinar consolidation, particularly in medial third of lung
   √ butterfly / bat-wing distribution of consolidation (= consolidated hilum + uninvolved lung cortex)

CONSTRICTIVE PERICARDITIS

= fibrous thickening of pericardium interfering with filling of ventricular chambers through restriction of heart motion
Age: 30 – 50 years; M:F = 3:1

Etiology:
1. Idiopathic (most common)
2. Viral (Coxsackie B)
3. Tuberculosis (formerly most common)
4. Chronic renal failure
5. Rheumatoid arthritis
6. Neoplastic involvement
7. Radiotherapy to mediastinum

- dyspnea
- abdominal enlargement (ascites + hepatomegaly)
- peripheral edema
- pericardial knock sound = loud early-diastolic sound
- neck vein distension
- Kussmaul sign = failure of venous pressure to fall with inspiration
- prominent X and Y descent on venous pressure curve

√ linear / plaque-like pericardial calcifications (50%): predominantly over RV, posterior surface of LV, in atrioventricular groove
√ dilatation of SVC, azygos vein
√ small atria
√ normal / small-sized heart (enlargement only due to preexisting disease)
√ normal pulmonary vascularity / pulmonary venous hypertension
√ straightening of right + left heart borders
√ increase in ejection fraction (small EDV)
CT:
√ epicardium = visceral pericardium >2 mm thick
√ dilatation of SVC + IVC
√ reflux of contrast into coronary sinus
√ flattening of right ventricle + curvature of interventricular septum toward left
√ pleural effusion + ascites
ECHO (nonspecific features):
√ thickening of pericardium
√ rapid early filling motion followed by flat posterior wall motion during diastasis period (= period between early rapid filling and atrial contraction)

Cx: protein-losing enteropathy (increased pressure in IVC + portal vein)
DDx: Cardiac tamponade, restrictive cardiomyopathy (eg, amyloid)

CORONARY ARTERY FISTULA
= single / multiple fistulous connections between a coronary artery (R > L) and other heart structures
Abnormal communication with (>90% right heart):
RV > RA > pulmonary trunk > coronary sinus > SVC
Hemodynamics: L-R shunt; pulmonary:systemic blood flow = <1.5:1 (usually)

√ may have normal CXR (in small shunts)
√ cardiomegaly + shunt vascularity (in large shunts)
Angio:
√ dilated tortuous coronary artery with anomalous connection

COR TRIATRIATUM
= rare congenital anomaly in which a fibromuscular septum with a single stenotic / fenestrated / large opening separates the embryologic common pulmonary vein from the left atrium:
(1) proximal / accessory chamber lies posteriorly receiving pulmonary veins
(2) distal / true atrial chamber lies anteriorly connected to left atrial appendage + emptying into LV through mitral valve
Etiology: failure of common pulmonary vein to incorporate normally into left atrium
Associated with: ASD, PDA, anomalous pulmonary venous drainage, left SVC, VSD, tetralogy of Fallot, atrioventricular canal
- dyspnea, heart failure, failure to thrive
- clinically similar to mitral valve stenosis
√ pulmonary venous distention + interstitial edema + dilatation of pulmonary trunk and pulmonary arteries (in severe obstruction)
√ enlarged RA + RV
√ mild enlargement of LA
Angio:
√ dividing membrane on levophase of pulmonary arteriogram
Prognosis (if untreated):
usually fatal within first 2 years of life; 50% 2-year survival; 20% 20-year survival
Rx: surgical excision of obstructing membrane

DEEP VEIN THROMBOSIS
= DVT
Incidence:
140,000 – 250,000 new cases per year in United States with an estimated sole / major cause of 50,000 – 200,000 deaths per year (15% of in-hospital deaths); 6 – 7 million stasis skin changes; in 0.5% cause of skin ulcers
Etiology:
1. Hypercoagulability
2. Decreased blood flow / stasis
3. Intimal changes
4. Decreased fibrinolytic potential of veins
5. Platelet aggregation
Risk factors:
1. Surgery, esp. on legs / pelvis: orthopedic (45 – 50%) especially total hip replacement >50%), gynecologic (7 – 35%), neurosurgery (18 – 20%), urologic (15 – 35%), general surgery (20 – 25%)
2. Severe trauma
3. Prolonged immobilization: hemiplegic extremity, paraplegia + quadriplegia, casting / orthopedic appliances
4. Obesity (risk factor 1.5)
5. Diabetes
6. Pregnancy (risk factor 5.5)
7. Medication: birth control pills, estrogen replacement, tamoxifen (risk factor 3.2)
8. Smoking
9. Malignancy (risk factor 2.5)

10. Decreased cardiac function: congestive heart failure, myocardial infarction (20 – 50%; risk factor 3.5)
11. Varicose veins / history of previous DVT / PE
12. Polycythemia
13. Patients with blood group A > blood group O
14. Age >40 years (risk factor 2.2)
15. Previous DVT (risk factor 2.5)

Location:
1. Dorsal veins of calf (± ascending thrombosis)
2. Iliofemoral veins (± descending thrombosis)
3. Peripheral + iliofemoral veins simultaneously
4. rare: internal iliac v., ovarian v., ascending lumbar vv.

L:R = 7:3 due to compression of left common iliac v. by left common iliac a. (arterial pulsations lead to chronic endothelial injury with formation of intraluminal spur, which is present in 22% of autopsies + in 90% of patients with DVT)

- Local symptoms due to obstruction / phlebitis usually only when (a) thrombus occlusive (b) clot extends into popliteal / more proximal vein (14 – 78% sensitivity, 4 – 21% specificity)
  - warmth
  - swelling (measurement of circumference)
  - blanching of skin (phlegmasia dolens alba) / blue leg with complete obstruction (phlegmasia cerulea dolens)
  - deep crampy pain in affected extremity, worse in erect position, improved while walking
  - tenderness along course of affected vein
  - Homans sign = calf pain with dorsal flexion of foot
  - Payr sign = pain upon compression of sole of foot
  - Δ 2/3 of deep vein thromboses are clinically silent
  - Δ Clinically suspected DVT only in 50% confirmed
  - Δ DVT symptomatology due to other causes in 15 – 35% of patients
  - Δ Negative bilateral venograms in 30% of patients with angiographically detected pulmonary emboli (big bang theory = clot embolizes in toto to the lung leaving no residual)

Venography (89% sensitivity, 97% specificity):
false negative in 11%, false positive in 5%;
study aborted / nondiagnostic in 5%
  Risk: postvenography phlebitis, contrast reaction, contrast material-induced skin slough, nephropathy

B-mode US (88 – 100% sensitivity, 92 – 100% specificity, >90% accuracy for DVT in thigh and popliteal veins):
  √ lack of complete luminal collapse with venous compression (DDx: deformity + scarring from prior DVT; technical difficulties in adductor canal + distal deep femoral vein)
  √ visualization of clot within vein (DDx: slow flowing blood; machine noise)
  √ <75% increase in diameter of common femoral vein during Valsalva
  √ venous diameter at least twice that of adjacent artery suggests thrombus <10 days old

Doppler US:
  √ absence of spontaneity (= any waveform recording), not reliable in peripheral veins
  √ continuous venous signal = absence of phasicity (= no cyclic variation in flow velocity with respiration, ie, decrease in expiration + increase in inspiration) is suspicious for proximal obstruction
  √ attenuation / absence of augmentation (= no increase in flow velocity with distal compression) indicates venous occlusion / compression in intervening venous segments
  √ pulsatile venous flow is a sign of congestive heart failure / pericardial effusion / cardiac tamponade / pulmonary embolism with pulmonary hypertension

Venous Occlusion Plethysmography :
(a) 87 – 100% sensitivity, 92 – 100% specificity for above-knee DVT
(b) 17 – 33% sensitivity for below-knee DVT
= temporary obstruction of venous outflow by pneumatic cuff around mid-thigh inflated above venous pressure leads to progressive increase in blood volume in lower leg; upon release of cuff limb quick return to resting volume with prompt venous runoff; limb blood volume changes are measured by *impedance plethysmography* in which a weak alternating current is passed through the leg; the electrical resistance varies inversely with blood volume; the current strength is held constant and voltage changes directly reflect blood volume changes
  √ initial rise in venous volume (= venous capacitance) diminished
  √ delay in venous outflow = "fall" measured at 3 seconds
False positives (6%): severe cardiopulmonary disease, pelvic mass

Cx:
(1) Pulmonary embolism (50%): in 90% from lower extremity / pelvis; in 60% with proximal "free-floating" / "widow-maker" thrombus; occurs usually between 2nd to 4th day of thrombosis
  Source of pulmonary emboli:
    multiple sites (1/3), cryptogenic in 50%;
    (a) lower extremity   (46%)
    (b) inferior vena cava   (19%)
    (c) pelvic veins   (16%)
    (d) mural heart thrombus   (4.5%)
    (e) upper extremity   (2%)
  Likelihood of pulmonary embolism: 77% for iliac veins, 35 – 67% for femoropopliteal vein, 0 – 46% for calf veins
(2) Postphlebitic syndrome (PPS) in 20% of cases with DVT (= recanalization to a smaller lumen, focal wall changes) due to valvular incompetence
(3) Phlegmasia cerulea / alba dolens (= severely impaired venous drainage resulting in gangrene)

Prognosis:
Tibial / peroneal venous thrombi resolve spontaneously in 40%, stabilize in 40%, propagate into popliteal vein in 20%

Rx:
(1) Systemic anticoagulation for ≥3 months decreases risk of recurrent DVT in initial 3 months from 50% to 3% + fatal pulmonary embolism from 30% to 8%; necessity for anticoagulation in DVT of calf veins is controversial
(2) Caval filter (10 – 15%) in patients with contra-indication / complication from anticoagulation or progression of DVT / PE despite adequate anticoagulation

DOUBLE-OUTLET RIGHT VENTRICLE
= DORV = TAUSSIG-BING HEART = most of the aorta + pulmonary artery arise from the RV secondary to maldevelopment of conotruncus
Type 1 = aorta posterior to pulmonary artery + spiraling course (most frequent)
Type 2 = Taussig-Bing heart = aorta posterior to pulmonary artery + parallel course
Type 3 = aorta anterior to pulmonary artery + parallel course
Hemodynamics:
  fetus   : no CHF in utero (in absence of obstructing other anomalies)
  neonate : ventricular work overload leads to CHF
Associated with: VSD (100%), pulmonary stenosis (50%), PDA
√ aorta overriding the interventricular septum with predominant connection to RV
√ aorta posterior / parallel / anterior to pulmonary artery
√ LV enlargement (volume overload)

EBSTEIN ANOMALY
= downward displacement of septal + posterior leaflets of dysplastic tricuspid valve with ventricular division into
(a) a large superior atrialized portion and
(b) a small inferior functional chamber
Etiology: chronic maternal lithium intake (10%)
Hemodynamics:
tricuspid valve insufficiency leads to tricuspid regurgitation ("Ping-Pong" volume); may be followed by CHF in utero / in neonate (50%); survival into adulthood if valve functions normally
Associated with: PDA, ASD (R-L shunt)
• cyanosis in neonatal period (R-L shunt), may improve / disappear postnatally with decrease in pulmonary arterial pressure
• systolic murmur (tricuspid insufficiency)
• Wolff-Parkinson-White syndrome (10%) = paroxysmal supraventricular tachycardia / right bundle branch block (responsible for sudden death)
√ "boxlike / funnellike" cardiomegaly (enlargement of RA + RV)
√ extreme RA enlargement (secondary to insufficient tricuspid valve)
√ IVC + azygos dilatation (secondary to tricuspid regurgitation)
√ hypoplastic aorta + pulmonary trunk (the ONLY cyanotic CHD to have this feature)
√ normal LA

√ calcification of tricuspid valve may occur
ECHO:
√ large "sail-like" tricuspid valve structure within dilated right heart
√ tricuspid regurgitation identified by Doppler ultrasound

Prognosis: 50% infant mortality; 13% operative mortality
Rx: 1. Digitalis + diuretics
2. Tricuspid valve prosthesis

EISENMENGER COMPLEX
= EISENMENGER DEFECT
= (1) high VSD ± overriding aorta with hypoplastic crista supraventricularis
(2) RV hypertrophy
and as consequence of increased pulmonary blood flow:
(3) dilatation of pulmonary artery + branches
(4) intimal thickening + sclerosis of small pulmonary arteries + arterioles
• cyanosis appears in 2nd + 3rd decade with shunt reversal

EISENMENGER SYNDROME
= EISENMENGER REACTION
= development of high pulmonary vascular resistance after many years of increased pulmonary blood flow secondary to L-R shunt (ASD, PDA, VSD), which leads to a bidirectional (= balanced) shunt and ultimately to R-L shunt
Etiology:
pulmonary microscopic vessels undergo reactive muscular hypertrophy, endothelial thickening, in situ thrombosis, tortuosity + obliteration; once initiated, pulmonary hypertension accelerates the vascular reaction, thus increasing pulmonary hypertension in a vicious cycle with RV failure + death

√ pronounced dilatation of central pulmonary arteries (pulmonary trunk, main pulmonary artery, intermediate branches)
√ pruning of peripheral pulmonary arteries
√ enlargement of RV
√ LA + LV return to normal size (with decrease of L-R shunt)
√ pulmonary veins NOT distended (NO increase in pulmonary blood flow)
√ NO redistribution of pulmonary veins (normal venous pressure)
Dx: measurement of pulmonary artery pressure + flow via catheter

ENDOCARDIAL CUSHION DEFECT
= ECD = ATRIOVENTRICULAR SEPTAL DEFECT
= PERSISTENT OSTIUM ATRIOVENTRICULARE COMMUNE = PERSISTENT COMMON ATRIOVENTRICULAR CANAL
= persistence of primitive atrioventricular canal + anomalies of AV valves

Associated with:
(1) Down syndrome:
in 25% of trisomy 21 an ECD is present;
in 45% of ECD trisomy 21 is present
(2) Asplenia, polysplenia

A. INCOMPLETE / PARTIAL ECD
= (1) Ostium primum ASD
(2) Cleft in anterior mitral valve leaflet / trileaflet
(3) Accessory short chordae tendineae arising from anterior MV leaflet insert directly into crest of deficient ventricular septum
√ left atrioventricular valve usually has 3 leaflets with a wide cleft between anterior + septal leaflet
√ "gooseneck" deformity secondary to downward attachment of anterior MV leaflet close to interventricular septum by accessory chordae tendineae
√ communication between LA–RA or LV–RA, occasionally LV–RV
√ right atrioventricular valve usually normal

B. TRANSITIONAL / INTERMEDIATE ATRIOVENTRICULAR CANAL
(uncommon)
= (1) Ostium primum ASD
(2) High membranous VSD
(3) Wide clefts in septal leaflets of both AV valves
(4) Bridging tissue between anterior + posterior common leaflet of both AV valves

C. COMPLETE ECD = AV COMMUNIS = COMMON AV CANAL
= (1) Ostium primum ASD above
(2) Posterior VSD below
(3) One AV valve common to RV + LV with 5 – 6 leaflets
(a) anterior common "bridging" leaflet
(b) two lateral leaflets
(c) posterior common "bridging" leaflet
Type 1 = chordae tendineae of anterior bridging leaflet attached to both sides of ventricular septum
Type 2 = chordae tendineae of anterior leaflet attached medially to anomalous papillary muscle within RV, but unattached to septum
Type 3 = free floating anterior leaflet with chordae attachments to septum; only type becoming symptomatic in infancy !
√ common atrioventricular orifice
√ oval septal defect consisting of a low ASD + high VSD
√ atrial septum secundum usually spared ("common atrium" if absent)
√ frequently associated with mesocardia / dextrocardia

Hemodynamics:
fetus : atrioventricular valves frequently incompetent leading to regurgitation + CHF

neonate : L-R shunt after decrease of pulmonary vascular resistance resulting in pulmonary hypertension
• incomplete right bundle branch block (distortion of conduction tissue)
• left-anterior hemiblock
CXR:
√ increased pulmonary vascularity (= shunt vascularity)
√ redistribution of pulmonary blood flow (mitral regurgitation)
√ enlarged pulmonary artery
√ diminutive aorta (secondary to L-R shunt)
√ cardiac enlargement out of proportion to pulmonary vascularity (L-R shunt + mitral insufficiency)
√ enlarged RV + LV
√ enlarged RA (LV blood shunted to RA)
√ normal-sized LA (secondary to ASD)
ECHO:
√ visualization of ASD + VSD + valve + site of insertion of chordae tendineae
√ paradoxical anterior septal motion (secondary to ASD)
√ atrioventricular insufficiency + shunts identified by Doppler ultrasound
Angio:
AP projection:
√ gooseneck deformity of LVOT (in diastole)
√ cleft in anterior leaflet of mitral valve (in systole)
√ mitral regurgitation
Hepatoclavicular projection in 45° LAO + C-C 45° (= 4 chamber view):
√ best view to demonstrate LV-RA shunt
√ best view to demonstrate VSD (inflow tract + posterior portion of interventricular septum in profile)
LAT projection:
√ irregular appearance of superior segment of anterior mitral valve leaflet over LVOT
Prognosis:
54% survival rate at 6 months, 35% at 12 months, 15% at 24 months, 4% at 5 years; 91% long-term survival with primary intracardiac repair, 4 – 17% operative mortality

ENDOCARDIAL FIBROELASTOSIS
= diffuse endocardial thickening of LV + LA from deposition of collagen + elastic tissue
Etiology:
(1) ? viral infection
(2) Secondary endocardial fibroelastosis
= subendocardial ischemia in critical LVOT obstruction: aortic stenosis, coarctation, hypoplastic left heart syndrome
• sudden onset of CHF during first 6 months of life
√ mitral insufficiency:
(a) involvement of valve leaflets
(b) shortening + thickening of chordae tendineae
(c) distortion + fixation of papillary muscles
√ enlarged LV = dilatation of hypertrophied LV from mitral regurgitation

√ restricted LV motion
√ enlarged LA
√ pulmonary venous congestion + pulmonary edema
√ LLL atelectasis (= compression of left lower lobe
  bronchus by enlarged LA)
Prognosis: mortality almost 100% by 2 years of age

FLAIL MITRAL VALVE
Cause:
  (1) ruptured chordae tendineae in rheumatic heart
       disease, ischemic heart disease, bacterial
       endocarditis
  (2) rupture of head of papillary muscle in acute
       myocardial infarction, chest trauma
Location: chordae to leaflet from posteromedial papillary
            muscle (single vessel blood supply)
√ deep holosystolic posterior movement
√ random anarchic motion pattern of flail parts in diastole
√ excessively large amplitude of opening of aML

GLYCOGEN STORAGE DISEASE
= POMPE DISEASE = abnormal metabolism with
  enlargement of myocardial cells due to glycogen
  deposition; similar to endocardial fibroelastosis
√ massive cardiomegaly with CHF
Prognosis: sudden death in 1st year of life (conduction
               abnormalities); survival rarely beyond infancy

HYPOPLASTIC LEFT HEART SYNDROME
= SHONE SYNDROME = AORTIC ATRESIA
= underdevelopment of left side of heart characterized by
  (a) aortic valve atresia (b) hypoplastic ascending aorta
  (c) hypoplastic / atretic mitral valve (d) endocardial
  fibroelastosis giving rise to small LA + small LV + small
  ascending aorta
Incidence: most common cause of CHF in neonate;
               responsible for 25% of all cardiac deaths in
               1st week of life
Hemodynamics:
  pulmonary venous return is diverted from LA to RA
  through herniated foramen ovale / ASD (L–R shunt); RV
  supplies (a) pulmonary artery (b) ductus arteriosus
  (c) descending aorta (antegrade flow) (d) aortic arch +
  ascending aorta + coronary circulation (retrograde flow)
  leading to RV work overload + CHF

• characteristically presents within first few hours of life
• ashen gray color (inadequate atrial L–R shunt with
  systemic underperfusion)
• myocardial ischemia (decreased perfusion of aorta +
  coronary arteries)
• cardiogenic shock, metabolic acidosis
• CHF (RV volume + pressure overload)
OB-US:
  √ small left ventricular cavity (apex of LV and RV should
    be at same level)
  √ hypoplastic ascending aorta + aortic arch
  √ aortic coarctation (in 80%)
ECHO:
  √ normal / enlarged LA

√ small LV
√ enlarged RA
√ herniation + prolapse of foramen ovale flap into RA
√ small / absent aortic root
√ absent / grossly distorted mitral valve echoes
Angio:
  √ retrograde flow in ascending aorta + aortic arch +
    coronary arteries via PDA
  √ string-like ascending aorta <6 mm in diameter
  √ massive enlargement of RV + RVOT

Prognosis: almost 100% fatal by 6 weeks
Rx: (1) Norwood procedure = palliative attempt
        (2) Cardiac transplant

HYPOPLASTIC RIGHT VENTRICLE
= PULMONARY ATRESIA WITH INTACT VENTRICULAR
  SEPTUM
= underdeveloped right ventricle due to pulmonary atresia
  in the presence of an intact interventricular septum
Type I   =   small RV secondary to competent tricuspid
             valve (more common)
Type II =   normal / large RV secondary to incompetent
             tricuspid valve
Hemodynamics:
  fetus   : L–R atrial shunt through foramen ovale;
              retrograde flow through ductus arteriosus
              into pulmonary vascular bed
  neonate :   closure of ductus results in cyanosis,
              acidosis, death
√ small right ventricular cavity (apex of RV + LV should be
  at same level)
√ atresia of pulmonary valve
√ hypoplastic proximal pulmonary artery
√ secundum atrial septal defect (frequently associated)
Rx: prostaglandin E1 infusion + valvotomy + systemic-
        pulmonary artery shunt

IDIOPATHIC DILATATION OF PULMONARY ARTERY
= CONGENITAL ANEURYSM OF PULMONARY
  ARTERY
Age: adolescence;   M < F
• systolic ejection murmur (in most cases)
√ dilated main pulmonary artery
√ normal peripheral pulmonary vascularity
√ normal pulmonary arterial pulsations
√ NO lateralization of pulmonary flow

Dx per exclusion:
  1. Absence of shunts, CHD, acquired disease
  2. Normal RV pressure
  3. No significant pressure gradient across pulmonic
     valve
DDx: (1) Marfan syndrome
        (2) Takayasu arteritis

INTERRUPTION OF AORTIC ARCH
= rare congenital anomaly as a common cause of death in
  the neonatal period

Trilogy: 1. Interrupted aortic arch
            2. VSD
            3. PDA (pulmonary blood supplies lower part of
                body)
Associated with (in 1/3):
    1. Transposition
    2. Truncus arteriosus
    3. Complete anomalous pulmonary venous return
•   presents with CHF
Location:
    Type A: distal to left subclavian artery (42%)
    Type B: between left CCA and subclavian artery (53%)
    Type C: between innominate and left CCA (4%)
√ dilatation of right atrium + ventricle
√ dilatation of pulmonary artery
√ ascending aorta much smaller than pulmonary artery
√ arch formed by pulmonary artery + ductus arteriosus
    gives the appearance of a low aortic arch
√ aortic knob absent
√ trachea in midline
√ NO esophageal impression
√ retrosternal clear space increased (small size of
    ascending aorta)
√ increased pulmonary vascularity (L-to-R shunt)
Prognosis: 76% dead at end of 1st month

INTERRUPTION OF PULMONARY ARTERY

= pulmonary trunk continues only as one large artery to
one lung while systemic aortic collaterals supply the
other side
Associated with CHD (particularly if interruption on left
side):
    1. Tetralogy of Fallot
    2. Scimitar syndrome = Congenital pulmonary
        venolobar syndrome
    3. PDA, VSD
    4. Pulmonary hypertension
Collateral supply:
    1. Arteries arising from arch + ascending aorta
    2. Bronchial vessels
    3. Intercostal vessels
    4. Branches from subclavian artery
Location: usually opposite from aortic arch;
             R + L pulmonary artery equally involved
CXR:
√ hypoplastic ipsilateral lung
√ mediastinal shift toward involved lung
√ hemidiaphragm may be elevated
√ small hyperlucent ipsilateral chest with narrowed
    intercostal spaces
√ "comma-shaped" small distorted hilar shadow
√ asymmetry of pulmonary vascularity
√ normal respiratory motion (normal aeration of
    hypoplastic lung)
NUC: √ absent perfusion with normal aeration
Angio: √ absent pulmonary artery
Rx: Surgical anastomosis between proximal + distal
        pulmonary artery (to prevent progressive pulmonary
        hypertension with dyspnea, cyanosis, hemoptysis,
        death)

DDx: (1) Hemitruncus
        (2) Swyer-James syndrome (ipsilateral air
             trapping, reduced ventilation + perfusion)

INTRAVENOUS DRUG ABUSE

Complications secondary to:
    (a) direct toxic effects of drugs or drug combinations
         (eg, heroin + cocaine / Talwin)
    (b) direct toxic effects of adulterants [eg, heroin is
         mixed ("cut") with quinine, baking soda, sawdust]
    (c) septic preparation
    (d) injection technique
    (e) choice of injection site (eg, "groin hit" into femoral
         vein; "pocket shot" into jugular, subclavian,
         brachiocephalic vein)

A. Cardiovascular complications
    1. Arterial pseudoaneurysm
        may be followed by rupture with exsanguination /
        loss of limb
    2. Arteriovenous fistula
    3. Arterial occlusion
        (a) at injection site due to intimal damage,
             thrombosis, spasm
        (b) distal to injection site due to embolization,
             spasm
    4. Venous thrombosis
    5. Intravenous migration of needle to heart / lungs
    6. Embolization of infectious agent / foreign body / air
        through inadvertent arterial injection ("hit the pink")
    7. Endocarditis (most commonly S. aureus)
B. Soft tissue complications
    1. Hematoma / abscess
    2. Foreign bodies
    3. Lymphadenopathy
    4. Cellulitis
C. Skeletal complications
    1. Osteomyelitis
        (a) direct contamination: eg, pubic bone ("groin
             hit") / clavicle ("pocket shot")
        (b) hematogenous: spine most commonly affected
    2. Septic arthritis: sacroiliac, sternoclavicular,
        symphysis pubis, hip, knee, wrist
D. Pleuropulmonary complications
    1. Pneumothorax ("pocket shot")
    2. Hemo- / pyothorax
    3. Septic pulmonary emboli
E. Gastrointestinal complications
    1. Severe colonic ileus
    2. Colonic pseudoobstruction
    3. Necrotizing enterocolitis
    4. Liver abscess
F. Genitourinary complications
    1. Focal / segmental glomerulosclerosis (heroin
        abuser)
    2. Amyloidosis
G. CNS complications
    1. Spinal epidural abscess in 5 – 18% (from vertebral
        osteomyelitis)
    2. Cord compression (from collapsed vertebral body)

3. Cerebral infarction (from subacute bacterial endocarditis, toxic effect of drug, spasm, intimal damage from "pocket shot")
4. Intracranial hemorrhage (from trauma, hypertension, injection of anticholinergic drugs, vasculitis, rupture of mycotic aneurysm)
5. Meningitis, cerebral abscess

ISCHEMIC HEART DISEASE

CXR: √ often normal
√ coronary artery calcification
√ pulmonary venous hypertension following acute infarction (40%)
√ LV aneurysm

ECHO:
√ region of dilatation with disturbance of wall movement
(1) Akinesis = no wall motion
(2) Hypokinesis = reduced wall motion
(3) Dyskinesis = paradoxical systolic expansion
(4) Asynchrony = disturbed temporal sequence of contraction

MARFAN SYNDROME

= autosomal dominant connective tissue disease with variable penetrance, 15% new mutations
Cardiovascular abnormalities (60 – 98%):
affecting mitral valve, ascending aorta, pulmonary artery, splenic + mesenteric arteries (occasionally)

@ Sinus of Valsalva + ascending aorta
√ "tulip bulb aorta" = dilatation of aortic sinuses of Valsalva slightly extending into ascending aorta
√ fusiform aneurysm of ascending aorta, rarely beyond innominate artery
√ aortic wall calcification rare
Cx: (1) Aortic regurgitation:
in 81% if root diameter >5 cm,
in 100% if root diameter >6 cm
(2) Annuloaortic ectasia = combination of aneurysm of aortic root + aortic valve regurgitation
(3) Aortic dissection
@ Mitral valve
Myxomatous degeneration of valve leads to redundancy + laxness
• mid-to-late systolic murmur + one / more clicks
√ prolapse of mitral valve + regurgitation
Cx: rupture of chordae tendineae (rare)
@ Coarctation (mostly not severe)
@ Cor pulmonale (secondary to chest deformity)

Prognosis: cardiovascular abnormalities are cause of death in 93%; aortic disease is cause of death in 55%

MITRAL REGURGITATION

Causes:
1. Rheumatic heart disease
(a) isolated: frequently seen in children
(b) uncommon in adults (mostly combined with stenosis)
2. Bacterial endocarditis
3. Myocardial infarction with involvement of papillary muscle
4. Congenital (short / abnormally inserted chordae tendineae)
5. Marfan syndrome
6. Corrected transposition with Ebstein-like anomaly
7. Idiopathic hypertrophic subaortic stenosis (IHSS)
8. Persistent ostium primum ASD with cleft mitral valve
9. Mitral valve prolapse syndrome
10. Functional / secondary
(from dilatation of mitral ring in any condition with dilatation of LV)

Pathogenesis:
backward flow of blood from LV into LA during LV systole; increased volume of blood under elevated pressure causes dilatation of LA; marked increase in LV diastolic volume with little increase in LV diastolic pressure
√ mild pulmonary venous hypertension (less than with mitral stenosis)
√ LA + LV enlargement (cardiothoracic ratio >0.55)
√ enlarged LA appendage (with history of previous rheumatic heart disease)
√ mitral annular calcification (frequent)

ECHO:
√ LA + LV enlargement
√ bulging of interatrial septum to the right
√ Doppler is diagnostic + allows assessment of severity

MITRAL STENOSIS

Acquired causes:
principal cause: rheumatic heart disease
rare cause: mass obstructing LV inflow (tumor, myxoma, thrombus)

M:F = 1:8

Pathogenesis:
rise in left atrial + pulmonary vascular pressure throughout systole and into diastole; development of medial hypertrophy + intimal sclerosis in pulmonary arterioles leads to pulmonary arterial hypertension, RV hypertrophy, tricuspid regurgitation, RV dilatation, right heart failure
• history of rheumatic fever (in 50%)
• atrial fibrillation
• systemic embolization from thrombosis of atrial appendage

Stages (according to degree of pulmonary venous hypertension):
Stage 1 : loss of hilar angle, redistribution
Stage 2 : interstitial edema
Stage 3 : alveolar edema
Stage 4 : hemosiderin deposits + ossification
√ calcification of valve leaflets (calcification of mitral annulus is a feature of age)
√ prominent pulmonary artery segment (precapillary hypertension)

√ small aorta (if forward cardiac output decreased)
√ enlarged LA ± wall calcification
   √ "double density" seen through right upper cardiac border (AP view)
   √ bulge of superior posterior cardiac border below carina (lateral view)
   √ esophagus displaced toward right + posteriorly
√ dilated left atrial appendage (not present with retracting clot)
√ hypertrophy of RV
√ dilatation of RV (tricuspid insufficiency / pulmonary hypertension)
   √ increase in cardiothoracic ratio
   √ diminution of retrosternal clear space
   √ IVC pushed backwards (lateral view)
√ redistribution of pulmonary blood flow to upper lobes (postcapillary pressure 16 – 19 mm Hg)
√ interstitial pulmonary edema (postcapillary pressure 20 – 25 mm Hg)
√ alveolar edema (postcapillary pressure 25 – 30 mm Hg)

ECHO:
   √ thickening of leaflets (fibrosis, calcification)
   √ commissural fusion
      √ restricted diastolic excursion of aML
      √ flattening of EF slope (early diastolic closing velocity) <50 mm/sec in 90%
      √ anterior tracking of pML in 80% (secondary to pull by aML)
      √ doming in diastole possible
   √ restricted mobility
      √ DE opening amplitude reduced to <16 mm (DDx: low cardiac output state)
      √ absent A-wave common (atrial fibrillation)
      √ slowed LV filling pattern
   √ dilatation of LA (>5 cm increases risk of atrial fibrillation + left atrial thrombus)
   √ increase in valve gradient + pressure half-time on Doppler
   DDx: Cor triatriatum, myxoma of LA (identical findings)

LUTEMBACHER SYNDROME = rheumatic mitral valve stenosis + ASD

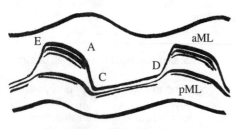

Classic Mitral Valve Stenosis

MITRAL VALVE PROLAPSE
= "Floppy Mitral Valve" = elongation of cusps + chordae leading to redundant valve tissue, which prolapses into LA during systole

Incidence: 2 – 6% of general population;
               5 – 20% of young women;
               ? autosomal dominant inheritance
Age: commonly 14 – 30 years
Associated with:
  (1) Skeletal abnormalities: scoliosis, straightening of thoracic spine, narrow anteroposterior chest dimension, pectus excavatum deformity of sternum
    (a) Barlowe syndrome = straight back syndrome
    (b) Marfan syndrome
  (2) Tricuspid valve prolapse
  (3) Long-standing ASD
• arrhythmias, palpitation, chest pain, light-headedness, syncope
• responsible for midsystolic click + late systolic murmur (when associated with mitral regurgitation)
√ LA not enlarged (unless associated with significant mitral regurgitation)
ECHO:
   √ interruption of CD line with bulge toward left atrium
      √ abrupt mid-systolic posterior buckling of both leaflets (classic pattern)
      √ "hammocklike" pansystolic posterior bowing of both leaflets
   √ multiple scallops on leaflets
   √ valve leaflets may appear thickened (myxomatous degeneration + valve redundancy)
   √ amount of mitral valve leaflets passing posterior to plane of mitral annulus >2 mm

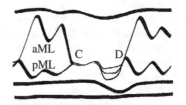

Mid-systolic Mitral Valve Prolapse

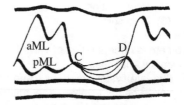

Holo-systolic Mitral Valve Prolapse

MYOCARDIAL INFARCTION
• atrioventricular block (common with inferior wall infarction as AV nodal branch originates from RCA); complete heart block has worse prognosis because it indicates a large area of infarction
CXR:
   √ normal-sized heart (84 – 95%) in acute phase if previously normal

√ cardiomegaly: high incidence of congestive heart failure in anterior wall infarction, multiple myocardial infarctions, double- and triple-vessel CAD, LV aneurysm

CECT:
√ perfusion defect within 60 – 90 seconds after bolus injection
√ delayed enhancement of infarcted tissue peaking at 10 – 15 minutes (due to accumulation of iodine in ischemic cells), size of enhanced area correlates well with size of infarct

Cx: (myocardium is prone to rupture during 3rd – 14th day post infarction)
(1) LEFT VENTRICULAR FAILURE (60 – 70%)
 • "cardiac shock" = systolic pressure <90 mm Hg
 Δ Signs of pulmonary venous hypertension are a good predictor of mortality (>30% if present, <10% if absent)
 √ progressive enlargement of heart
 √ haziness + indistinctness of pulmonary arteries
 √ increase in size of right descending pulmonary artery >17 mm
 √ pleural effusion
 √ septal lines
 √ perihilar ± peripheral parenchymal clouding
 √ alveolar pulmonary edema
 Mortality: 30 – 50% with mild LV failure; 44% with pulmonary edema; 80 – 100% with cardiogenic shock; 8% in absence of LV failure
(2) ANEURYSM (12 – 15% of survivors)
(3) MYOCARDIAL RUPTURE (3.3%)
 • occurs usually on 3rd – 5th day post MI
 √ enlargement of heart (slow leakage of blood into pericardium)
 Prognosis: cause of death in 13% of all infarctions; almost 100% mortality
(4) RUPTURE OF PAPILLARY MUSCLE (1%)
 from infarction of posteromedial papillary muscle in inferior MI (common) / anterolateral papillary muscle in anterolateral MI (uncommon)
 • sudden onset of massive mitral insufficiency
 • unresponsive to medical management
 √ abrupt onset of severe persistent pulmonary edema
 √ minimal LV enlargement / normal-sized heart
 √ NO dilatation of LA (immediate decompression into pulmonary veins)
 Prognosis: 70% mortality within 24 hours; 80 – 90% within 2 weeks
(5) RUPTURE OF INTERVENTRICULAR SEPTUM (0.5 – 2%)
 • occurs usually within 4 – 21 days with rapid onset of L–R shunt
 • Swan-Ganz catheterization: increase in oxygen content of RV, capillary wedge pressure may be within normal limits
 √ right-sided cardiac enlargement
 √ engorgement of pulmonary vasculature

√ NO pulmonary edema (DDx to ruptured papillary muscle)
Prognosis: 24% mortality within 24 hours; 87% within 2 months; >90% in 1 year
(6) DRESSLER SYNDROME (<4%)
 = POSTMYOCARDIAL INFARCTION SYNDROME
 Etiology: autoimmune reaction
 Onset: 2 – 3 weeks (range 1 week – several months) following infarction
 • relapses occur as late as 2 years after initial episode
 • fever
 √ pericarditis + pericardial effusion
 √ pleuritis + pleural effusion
 √ pneumonitis

Right Ventricular Infarction
Right ventricle involved in 33% of left inferior myocardial infarction
√ decreased RV ejection fraction
√ accumulation of Tc-99m pyrophosphate
Prognosis: in 50% RV ejection fraction returns to normal within 10 days
Cx: (1) cardiogenic shock (unusual)
 (2) elevation of RA pressure
 (3) decrease of pulmonary artery pressure

MYXOMA
Most common benign primary intracardiac tumor in adults, 40% of all cardiac tumors
Age: 30 – 60 years
May be associated with skin lesions, myxoid breast fibroma, pituitary adenoma, testicular tumor, Cushing disease
• short history + rapid progression
• fever, myalgia, arthralgia, weight loss
• leukocytosis, anemia, elevated ESR
• tachyarrhythmia, murmur (change with position)
• syncope
• dyspnea, chest pain
Location: LA:RA = 4:1; ventricles (exceptional); attached to atrial septum by small stalk; may protrude into ventricle causing partial obstruction of atrioventricular valve
√ generalized cardiac enlargement
√ atrial obstruction
√ persistent defect in atrium / diastolic defect in ventricle
A. LEFT ATRIAL MYXOMA
 with obstruction of mitral valve:
 √ enlargement of LA
 √ pulmonary venous hypertension
 √ ossific lung nodules
 √ NO enlargement of atrial appendage
 Cx: systemic emboli (27%) in 50% to CNS (stroke / "mycotic" aneurysm)
B. RIGHT ATRIAL MYXOMA
 with obstruction of tricuspid valve:
 √ enlargement of RA
 √ prominent SVC, IVC, azygos vein

√ decreased pulmonary vascularity
  Cx: pulmonary emboli
ECHO: (2D-ECHO is study of choice)
  Δ M-mode findings of only historical interest!
    √ dense echoes appearing posterior to aML soon
      after onset of diastole
    √ pML obscured
    √ tumor echoes can be traced into LA
    √ dilated LA
    √ reduced E-F slope
  DDx: (1) Thrombus (most commonly in LA + LV)
         (2) Other cardiac tumors: sarcoma, malignant
              mesenchymoma, metastasis

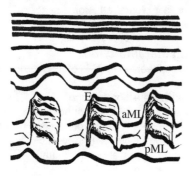

Atrial Myxoma Prolapsing into Mitral Valve Orifice
Note the interval between the opening of aML and pML and the
moment that the tumor reaches its maximal anterior excursion at
point E when a slight additional opening of the aML results; aML
stays open during entire diastole as a result of obstruction to left
atrial emptying.

PATENT DUCTUS ARTERIOSUS
  = PDA = persistence of left 6th aortic arch
  Incidence: 9% of all CHD; M:F = 1:2
  Associated with:
    prematurity, birth asphyxia, high altitude births, rubella
    syndrome, coarctation, VSD, trisomy 18 + 21
  Normal physiology in mature infant:
    increase in arterial oxygen pressure leads to constriction
    + closure of duct
    Δ functional closure due to muscular contraction within
      10 – 15 hours
    Δ anatomic closure due to subintimal fibrosis +
      thrombosis: in 35% by 2 weeks; in 90% by 2 months;
      in 99% by 1 year

• mostly asymptomatic
• congestive heart failure (rare) usually by 3 months of
  age if L–R shunt is large
• continuous murmur
• bounding peripheral pulses (intraaortic pressure run-off
  through PDA)
CXR (mimics VSD):
  √ LA enlargement
  √ enlarged pulmonary artery segment

√ increase of pulmonary vasculature (less flow directed
  to LUL)
√ enlarged RV + LV
√ enlarged ascending aorta + aortic arch (thymus may
  obscure this)
√ prominent ductus infundibulum (diverticulum)
  = prominence between aortic knob + pulmonary artery
  segment
√ obscured aortopulmonary window
√ "railroad track" = calcified ductus arteriosus

ECHO:
  √ LA:Ao ratio = >1.2:1 (signalizes significant L–R shunt)
Angio:
  √ catheter course from RA to RV, main pulmonary
    artery, PDA, descending aorta
  √ communication from aorta (distal to left subclavian
    artery) to left pulmonary artery on AP / LAT / LAO
    aortogram

PDA IN PREMATURE INFANT
  Premature infant not subject to medial muscular
  hypertrophy of small pulmonary artery branches (which
  occurs in normal infants subsequent to progressive
  hypoxia in 3rd trimester)
• CHF
  Cause:
    (a) pulmonary artery pressure remains low without
         opposing any L–R shunts (PDA / VSD)
    (b) ductus arteriosus remains open secondary to
         hypoxia in RDS
√ recurrence of alveolar air-space filling after resolution
  of RDS
√ granular pattern of hyaline membrane disease
  becomes more opaque
√ enlargement of heart (masked by positive pressure
  ventilation)
Rx:
  (a) Medical therapy:
    (1) supportive oxygen, diuretics, digitalis
    (2) avoid fluid overload (not to increase shunt
         volume)
    (3) antiprostaglandins = indomethacin opposes
         prostaglandins, which are potent duct
         dilators
  (b) Surgical ligation

BENEFICIAL PDA = compensatory effect of PDA in:
  1. Tetralogy of Fallot
     cyanosis usually occurs during closure of duct
     shortly after birth
  2. Eisenmenger pulmonary hypertension
     PDA acts as escape valve shunting blood to
     descending aorta
  3. Interrupted aortic arch
     supply of lower extremity via PDA

NONBENEFICIAL PDA
  in L–R shunts (VSD, aortopulmonic window) a PDA
  increases shunt volume

PENETRATING AORTIC ULCER

= characterized by ulceration of atheromatous plaque that disrupts the internal elastic lamina + results in hemorrhage into media / rupture through wall of aorta

Location:　middle of descending thoracic aorta

Angio:
√ ulcerated atherosclerotic plaque
√ aortic wall thickening

CECT:
√ focally ulcerated plaque
√ intramural hematoma cannot be differentiated from intraluminal thrombus / atherosclerotic plaque

MR:
√ deeply ulcerated aortic plaque
√ subacute hematoma in aortic wall indicated by high signal intensity on T1WI + T2WI (methemoglobin) either localized or mimicking type 3 dissection
√ aortic rupture with contained hematoma

DDx:
(1) Aortic dissection (intimal flap, patent false lumen)
(2) Atheroma / thrombus (low signal intensity on T1WI + T2WI)

PERICARDIAL CYST

M:F = 3:2
• asymptomatic
Location:　(a)　costophrenic angle, R:L = 3:2
　　　　　　(b)　mediastinum (rare)
√ round / ovoid cyst usually 3 – 8 cm in diameter
√ attenuation values of 20 – 40 HU, occasionally higher

PERICARDIAL DEFECT

= failure of pericardial development secondary to premature atrophy of the left duct of Cuvier (cardinal vein), which fails to nourish the left pleuropericardial membrane

Incidence:　1:13,000;　M:F = 3:1

Age at detection:　newborn – 81 years (mean 21 years)

Location:
(a) foraminal defect on left side　　(35%)
(b) complete absence on left side　　(35%)
(c) diaphragmatic pericardial aplasia (17%)
(d) total bilateral absence　　　　(9%)
(e) foraminal defect on right side　(4%)

Associated with (in 30%):
(1) Bronchogenic cyst (30%)
(2) VSD, PDA, mitral stenosis
(3) Diaphragmatic hernia, sequestration
• mostly asymptomatic
• ECG: right axis deviation, right bundle branch block
• palpitations, tachycardia, dyspnea, dizziness, syncope
• positional discomfort while lying on left side
• nonspecific intermittent chest pain (lack of pericardial cushioning, torsion of great vessels, tension on pleuropericardial adhesions, pressure on coronary arteries by rim of pericardial defect)
√ size:　— small foraminal defect = no abnormality
　　　　— large defect　　= herniation of cardiac structures / lung
　　　　— complete absence　= levoposition of heart

√ absence of left pericardial fat pad
√ levoposition of heart with lack of visualization of right heart border
√ prominence / focal bulge in the area of RVOT, main pulmonary artery, left atrial appendage
√ sharp margination + elongation of left heart border
√ insinuation of lung between heart + left hemidiaphragm
√ insinuation of lung between aortic knob + pulmonary artery
√ increased distance between heart + sternum secondary to absence of sternopericardial ligament (cross-table lateral projection)
√ pneumopericardium following pneumothorax
√ NO tracheal deviation

Rx:　Foraminal defect requires surgery because of (a) herniation + strangulation of left atrial appendage (b) herniation of LA / LV
　　　(1)　closure of defect with pleural flap
　　　(2)　resection of pericardium

PERSISTENT FETAL CIRCULATION

= PERSISTENT PULMONARY HYPERTENSION OF THE NEWBORN

= delay in transition from intra- to extrauterine pulmonary circulation

Cause:　primary disorder related to birth asphyxia, concurrent parenchymal lung disease (meconium aspiration, pneumonia, pulmonary hemorrhage, hyaline membrane disease, pulmonary hypoplasia), concurrent cardiovascular disease, hypoxic myocardial injury, hyperviscosity syndromes)

• labile PO_2
√ structurally normal heart

POLYARTERITIS NODOSA

= PERIARTERITIS NODOSA = necrotizing vasculitis of small + medium-sized muscular arteries

Incidence:　rare (2 new cases/million/year)

Etiology:　? deposition of immune complexes

Histo:
polymorphonuclear cell infiltrate in all layers of arterial wall + perivascular tissue (acute phase), mononuclear cell infiltrate, fibrinoid necrosis, intimal proliferation, thrombosis, perivascular inflammation (chronic stage)

Associated with:　hepatitis B antigen
• fever, myalgia, arthralgias, malaise, weight loss
• abdominal pain, peripheral neuropathy
• painless hematuria
• tender subcutaneous nodules (15%)
• elevated ESR, thrombocytosis, anemia

Location:　all organs may be involved, kidney (85%), heart (65%), liver (50%), pancreas, bowel, CNS (cerebrovascular accident, seizure)

Angiography (61% sensitivity, 80% true-positive rate):
√ 1 – 5 mm saccular aneurysms of small + medium-sized arteries in 60 – 75% as a result of necrosis of the internal elastic lamina (HALLMARK)
√ luminal irregularities + stenoses of arteries
√ arterial occlusions + small tissue infarctions

Cx: Hypertension, renal failure, hemorrhage secondary to aneurysm rupture, organ infarction due to vessel thrombosis, gangrene of fingers / toes
Rx: Steroids (50% 5-year survival rate)

POLYSPLENIA SYNDROME

= BILATERAL LEFT-SIDEDNESS
Age: presentation in infancy / adulthood; M < F

Associated with:
  (a) Low incidence of CHD:
      APVR (70%), dextrocardia (37%), ASD (37%), ECCD (43%), pulmonic valvular stenosis (23%), TGA (13 – 17%), DORV (13 – 20%)
  (b) GI abnormalities:
      esophageal atresia, TE fistula, gastric duplication, preduodenal portal vein, duodenal webs + atresia, short bowel, mobile cecum, malrotation, semiannular pancreas, biliary atresia, absent gallbladder
  (c) GU anomalies (15%): renal agenesis, renal cysts, ovarian cysts
  (d) Vertebral anomalies, common celiac trunk–SMA
• heart murmur, CHF, occasional cyanosis
• leftward / superiorly directed P wave vector
• extrahepatic biliary obstruction

@ Lung
  √ bilateral morphologic left lungs (68%), normal (18%), bilateral R-sided lungs (7%)
  √ bilateral hyparterial bronchi
  √ normal / increased pulmonary vascularity
  √ bilateral SVC (50%)
  √ azygos / hemiazygos continuation with interruption of hepatic segment of IVC (70%)
  √ large azygos vein (MOST SPECIFIC sign) may mimic aortic arch
@ Abdomen
  √ presence of ≥2 spleens (usually two major + indefinite number of splenules) located on both sides of the mesogastrium (esp. greater curvature of stomach)
  √ hepatic symmetry
  √ stomach on right / left side
  √ malrotation of bowel (80%)
OB-US:
  √ interrupted IVC
  √ aorta anterior to spine in midline
  √ azygos vein on left / right side of spine

Prognosis: 50 – 60% mortality within 1st year of life; 75% mortality by 5 years; 90% mortality by midadolescence

POPLITEAL ARTERY ENTRAPMENT SYNDROME

= anomalous development of medial head of gastrocnemius muscle, which attaches to medial femoral condyle after development of primitive popliteal artery in 20 mm embryo; bilateral in 30%
Incidence: 35 cases in American surgical literature

Cause: abnormal course of medial head of gastrocnemius muscle slinging around lateral aspect of popliteal a.
Pathophysiology:
  flow unimpeded when muscle relaxed; increased arterial angulation with muscle contraction (early); progressive intimal hyperplasia ("atheroma" = misnomer) in area of compression with ultimately occlusion (late)
Age: usually <35 years
• intermittent claudication (early) esp. during periods of prolonged standing
• acute ischemia of leg with permanent occlusion of popliteal a. (late)
  √ posterior tibial pulse obliterated during active plantar flexion against resistance
  √ PVR has 40% false-positive results
  √ ankle-arm index reduced during active muscle contraction
  √ Doppler waveforms of posterior tibial a. diminished during muscle contractions
Dx:
  √ arteriography with typical medial deviation of popliteal a. before + after gastrocnemius contraction
  √ popliteal a. thrombosis / occlusion
Cx: Popliteal a. aneurysm
DDx: Cystic adventitial disease of popliteal a., arterial embolism, premature arteriosclerosis, popliteal aneurysm with thrombosis, popliteal a. trauma, popliteal a. thrombosis, spinal cord stenosis (= neurogenic claudication)

PRIMARY PULMONARY HYPERTENSION

= PLEXOGENIC PULMONARY ARTERIOPATHY
Diagnosis per exclusion:
  clinically unexplained progressive pulmonary arterial hypertension without evidence for thromboembolic disease + pulmonary venoocclusive disease
Histo: plexiform + angiomatoid lesions = tortuous channels within proliferation of endothelial cells
Age: 3rd decade; M < F
• dyspnea on exertion, syncope
• easy fatigability
• hyperventilation
• chest pain
• hemoptysis

PSEUDOCOARCTATION

= AORTIC KINKING = elongation of thoracic aorta with redundancy + kinking just distal to origin of left subclavian artery at lig. arteriosum
= variant of coarctation without a pressure gradient
Age: 12 – 64 years
Associated with:
  Bicuspid aortic valve, PDA, VSD, aortic / subaortic stenosis, single ventricle, ASD, anomalies of aortic arch branches
• asymptomatic
• ejection murmur
• NO pressure gradient across the buckled segment

√ mediastinal widening (elongation of ascending aorta + aortic arch)

√ anteromedial deviation of aorta

√ "chimney-shaped" high aortic arch (in children)

√ rounded / oval mass in left upper mediastinum above aortic arch (in adults)

√ anterior displacement of esophagus

√ NO rib notching / dilatation of brachiocephalic arteries / LV enlargement / poststenotic dilatation

Angio:

√ high position of aortic arch

√ "figure 3 sign" = notch in descending aorta at attachment of short ligamentum arteriosum

DDx: True coarctation, aneurysm, mediastinal mass

PULMONARY ATRESIA

= CONGENITAL ABSENCE OF PULMONARY ARTERY

= atretic pulmonary valve with underdeveloped pulmonary artery distally

√ small hemithorax of normal radiodensity

√ mediastinal shift to affected side

√ elevation of ipsilateral diaphragm

√ rib notching from prominence of intercostal arteries

PULMONARY ATRESIA WITH INTACT
INTERVENTRICULAR SEPTUM

Associated with ASD (R-L shunt)

Type I : no remaining RV, no tricuspid regurgitation
√ moderately enlarged RA (depending on size of ASD)

Type II : normal RV with tricuspid regurgitation
√ massive enlargement of RA

√ cardiomegaly (LV, RA)

√ concave / small pulmonary artery segment

√ diminished pulmonary vascularity

PULMONARY VENOOCCLUSIVE DISEASE

= fibrous narrowing of intrapulmonary veins in the presence of a normal left heart characterized by pulmonary arterial hypertension, pulmonary edema, normal wedge pressures

Age: children, adolescents; M:F = 1:1

Histo: fibrous narrowing + thrombosis in up to 95% of pulmonary veins

√ pulmonary edema

√ pleural effusions

√ delayed filling of normal main pulmonary veins + left heart

Prognosis: poor (no effective therapy)

PULMONIC STENOSIS

Pulmonary artery stenosis without VSD = 8% of all CHD

• mostly asymptomatic

• cyanosis / heart failure

• loud systolic ejection murmur

√ systolic doming of pulmonary valve (= incomplete opening)

√ normal / diminished / increased pulmonary vascularity (depending on presence + nature of associated malformations)

√ enlarged pulmonary trunk + left pulmonary artery (poststenotic dilatation)

√ prominent left pulmonary artery + normal right pulmonary artery

√ hypertrophy of RV with reduced size of RV chamber

√ elevation of cardiac apex

√ increased convexity of anterior cardiac border on LAO

√ diminution of retrosternal clear space

√ cor pulmonale

√ mild enlargement of LA (reason unknown)

√ calcification of pulmonary valves in older adults (rare)

Prognosis: death at mean age of 21 years if untreated

Subvalvular Pulmonic Stenosis

A. INFUNDIBULAR PULMONIC STENOSIS
typically in tetralogy of Fallot

B. SUBINFUNDIBULAR PULMONIC STENOSIS
= hypertrophied anomalous muscle bundles crossing portions of RV

Associated with: VSD (73 – 85%)

(a) low type:
courses diagonally from low anterior septal side to crista posteriorly

(b) high type:
horizontal defect across RV below infundibulum

Valvular Pulmonic Stenosis

1. CLASSIC / TYPICAL PULMONIC VALVE STENOSIS (95%)
= commissural fusion of pulmonary cusps

Age of presentation: childhood

• pulmonic click

• ECG: hypertrophy of RV

√ thickened dome-shaped valve

√ dilated main + left pulmonary artery

√ jet of contrast

Rx: balloon valvuloplasty

2. DYSPLASTIC PULMONIC VALVE STENOSIS (5%)
= thickened redundant distorted cusps, immobile secondary to myxomatous tissue

• NO click

√ NO poststenotic dilatation

Rx: surgical resection of redundant valve tissue

CXR: √ normal pulmonary vascularity
√ normal-sized heart

Angio: √ increase in trabecular pattern of RV
√ hypertrophied crista supraventricularis (lateral projection)

TRILOGY OF FALLOT (infantile presentation)

(1) severe pulmonic valvular stenosis

(2) hypertrophy of RV

(3) ASD with R-L shunt (increased pressure in RA forces foramen ovale open)

Supravalvular Pulmonic Stenosis
60% of all pulmonary valve stenoses
Site of narrowing: pulmonary trunk, pulmonary
  bifurcation, one / both main pulmonary arteries, lobar
  pulmonary artery, segmental pulmonary artery
Shape of narrowing:
  (a) localized with poststenotic dilatation
  (b) long tubular hypoplasia
May be associated with:
  (1) Valvular pulmonic stenosis, supravalvular aortic
     stenosis, VSD, PDA, systemic arterial stenoses
  (2) Familial peripheral pulmonic stenoses +
     supravalvular aortic stenosis
  (3) Williams-Beuren syndrome: PS, supravalvular
     AS, peculiar facies
  (4) Ehlers-Danlos syndrome
  (5) Postrubella syndrome: peripheral pulmonic
     stenoses, valvular pulmonic stenosis, PDA, low
     birth weight, deafness, cataract, mental
     retardation
  (6) Tetralogy of Fallot / critical valvular pulmonic
     stenosis

RAYNAUD SYNDROME
= episodic digital ischemia in response to cold / emotional
  stimuli
Pathogenesis:
  (1) increase in vasoconstrictor tone
  (2) low blood pressure
  (3) slight increase in blood viscosity
  (4) immunologic factors (4 – 81%)
  (5) cold provocation
• exaggerated response of digit to cold / emotional stress:
  • numbness + loss of tactile perception
  • demarcated pallor / cyanosis
• hyperemic throbbing during rewarming
• sclerodactyly
• small painful ulcers at tip of digit

A. **Raynaud disease** = PRIMARY VASOSPASM
  = SPASTIC FORM
  = exaggerated cold-induced constriction of smooth
    muscle cells in otherwise normal artery
  Cause: ? acquired adrenoreceptor hypersensitivity
  May be associated with early stages of autoimmune
                           disorders
  Age: most common in young women
  • usually affects all fingers of both hands equally
  √ normal segmental arm + digit pressures at room
    temperature
  √ peaked digit volume pulse = rapid rise in systole,
    anacrotic notch just before the peak, dicrotic notch
    high on the downslope
  PPG:
    √ flat line tracing at low temperatures (10° – 22°C)
      with sudden reappearance of normal waveform at
      24 – 26°C = "threshold phenomenon"
B. **Raynaud phenomenon**
  = SECONDARY VASOSPASM WITH OBSTRUCTION
  = OBSTRUCTIVE FORM

= digital artery occlusion due to stenotic process in
  normally constricting artery / associated with an
  abnormally high blood viscosity
Cause:
  1. Atherosclerosis (most frequent)
    (a) embolization from an upstream lesion
    (b) occlusion of major arteries supplying arm
  2. Arterial trauma
  3. <u>End stage</u> of many autoimmune disorders: eg,
    scleroderma, rheumatoid arthritis, systemic lupus
    erythematosus
  4. Takayasu disease
  5. Buerger disease
  6. Drug intoxication (ergot, methysergide)
  7. Dysproteinemia
  8. Primary pulmonary hypertension
  9. Myxedema
• normal vasoconstrictive response to cold
√ reduced segmental arm + digit pressures at room
  temperature
PPG (76% sensitivity, 92% specificity):
  √ flat line / barely detectable tracing at low
    temperature with gradual increase of amplitude
    upon rewarming
Hand magnification angiography:
  1. Baseline angiogram with ambient temperature
  2. Stress angiogram immediately following immersion
    of hand in ice water for 20 seconds

SINGLE VENTRICLE
= UNIVENTRICULAR HEART
= DOUBLE INLET SINGLE VENTRICLE
= failure of development of interventricular septum ±
  absence of one atrioventricular valve (mitral / tricuspid
  atresia) ± aortic / pulmonic stenosis
• conduction defect (aberrant anatomy of conduction
  system)
√ two atrioventricular valves connected to a main
  ventricular chamber
√ the single ventricle may be a LV (85%) / RV /
  undetermined
√ a second rudimentary ventricular chamber may be
  present, which is located anteriorly (in left univentricle) /
  posteriorly (in right univentricle)
√ rudimentary chamber ± connection to one great artery
√ may be associated with tricuspid / mitral atresia

SINUS OF VALSALVA ANEURYSM
= deficiency between aortic media + annulus fibrosis of
  aortic valve resulting in distension + eventual aneurysm
  formation
Age: puberty to 30 years of age
Site: right sinus / noncoronary sinus (>90%)
    Δ Right sinus usually ruptures into RV, occasionally
     into RA
    Δ Noncoronary sinus ruptures into RA
• sudden retrosternal pain, dyspnea, continuous murmur
√ shunt vascularity
√ cardiomegaly
√ prominent ascending aorta

SPLENIC ARTERY ANEURYSM

= most frequent of visceral artery aneurysms

Etiology: medial degeneration with superimposed atherosclerosis, congenital, mycotic, pancreatitis, trauma, portal hypertension

Predisposed: women with ≥2 pregnancies (88%)

May be associated with fibromuscular disease (in 20%)

M:F = 1:2

- usually asymptomatic
- pain, GI bleeding

Location: intra- / extrasplenic

√ calcified wall of aneurysm (2/3)

Cx: Rupture of aneurysm (6 – 9%, higher during pregnancy) with up to 76% mortality

DDx: renal artery aneurysm, tortuous splenic artery

SUBCLAVIAN STEAL SYNDROME

= stenosis / obstruction of subclavian artery near its origin with flow reversal in ipsilateral vertebral artery at the expense of the cerebral circulation

Incidence: 2.5% of all extracranial arterial occlusions

Etiology:
(a) congenital: interruption of aortic arch, preductal infantile coarctation, hypoplasia of left aortic arch, hypoplasia / atresia / stenosis of an anomalous left subclavian artery with right aortic arch, coarctation with aberrant subclavian artery arising distal to the coarctation
(b) acquired: atherosclerosis (94%), dissecting aneurysm, chest trauma, embolism, tumor thrombosis, inflammatory arteritis (Takayasu, syphilitic), ligation of subclavian artery in Blalock-Taussig shunt, complication of coarctation repair, radiation fibrosis

Age: average 59 – 61 years; M:F = 3:1; Whites:Blacks = 8:2

Associated with additional lesions of extracranial arteries in 81%

- lower systolic blood pressure by >20 – 40 mm Hg on affected side
- delayed weak / absent pulse in ipsilateral extremity
- Signs of vertebrobasilar insufficiency (40%):
  - syncopal episodes initiated by exercising the ischemic arm
  - headaches, nausea, vertigo, ataxia
  - mono-, hemi-, para-, quadriparesis, paralysis
  - diplopia, dysphagia, dysarthria, paresthesias around mouth
  - uni- / bilateral homonymous hemianopia
- Signs of brachial insufficiency (3 – 10%):
  - intermittent / constant pain in affected arm precipitated by increased activity of that arm
  - paresthesia, weakness, coolness, numbness, burning in fingers + hand
  - fingertip necrosis

Location: L:R = 3:1

Color Doppler:

√ reversal of vertebral artery flow, augmented by reactive hyperemia (blood pressure cuff inflated above systolic pressure for 5 minutes) / arm exercise

Angio:

√ subclavian stenosis / occlusion (aortic arch injection)

√ reversal of vertebral artery flow (selective injection of contralateral subclavian / vertebral artery)

CAVE: "false steal" = transient retrograde flow in contralateral vertebral artery caused by high pressure injection

PARTIAL STEAL SYNDROME

= retrograde flow in systole + antegrade flow in diastole

OCCULT STEAL SYNDROME

= reverse flow seen only after provocative maneuvers, ie, ipsilateral arm exercise of 5 minutes / 5 minutes inflation of sphygmomanometer > systolic blood pressure levels

Rx: Bypass surgery, PTA (good long-term results)

SUPERIOR VENA CAVA SYNDROME

= obstruction of SVC with development of collateral pathways

Etiology:
(a) Malignant lesion (80 – 90%)
   1. Bronchogenic carcinoma (>50%)
   2. Lymphoma
(b) Benign lesion
   1. Granulomatous mediastinitis (usually histoplasmosis, sarcoidosis, TB)
   2. Substernal goiter
   3. Ascending aortic aneurysm
   4. Pacer wires / central venous catheters (23%)
   5. Constrictive pericarditis

Collateral routes:
1. Esophageal venous plexus = "downhill varices" (predominantly upper 2/3)
2. Azygos + hemiazygos veins
3. Accessory hemiazygos + superior intercostal veins = "aortic nipple" (visualization in normal population in 5%)
4. Lateral thoracic veins + umbilical vein
5. Vertebral veins

- head and neck edema (70%)
- cutaneous enlarged venous collaterals
- headache, dizziness, syncope
- with benign etiology: slower onset + progression, both sexes, 25 – 40 years of age
- with malignancy: rapid progression within weeks, mostly males, 40 – 60 years of age
- proptosis, tearing
- dyspnea, cyanosis, chest pain
- hematemesis (11%)

√ superior mediastinal widening (64%)

√ encasement / compression / occlusion of SVC

√ dilated cervical + superficial thoracic veins (80%)

√ SVC thrombus

NUC:
√ increased tracer uptake in quadrate lobe + posterior aspect of medial segment of left lobe (umbilical pathway toward liver when injected in upper extremity)

SYPHILITIC AORTITIS

Incidence: in 10 – 15% of untreated patients (accounts for death in 1/3)

Path: periaortitis (via lymphatics), mesoaortitis (via vasa vasorum)

Site: ascending aorta (36%), aortic arch (24%), descending aorta (5%), sinus of Valsalva (1%), pulmonary artery

√ thick aortic wall (fibrous + inflammatory tissue)
√ saccular (75%) / fusiform (25%) dilatation of ascending aorta
√ small saccular aneurysms often protrude from fusiform aneurysm
√ fine pencil-like calcifications of intima (15%) in ascending aorta, late in disease

Cx: (1) Stenosis of coronary ostia (intimal thickening)
         (2) Aortic regurgitation (syphilitic valvulitis), rare

TAKAYASU ARTERITIS

= PULSELESS DISEASE = AORTITIS SYNDROME = AORTOARTERITIS = IDIOPATHIC MEDIAL AORTOPATHY = AORTIC ARCH SYNDROME

= chronic inflammatory panarteritis of unknown pathogenesis affecting segments of aorta + main aortic branches + pulmonary arteries

Etiology: probably cell-mediated inflammation

Incidence: 2.6 new cases/million/year;
                2.2% (at autopsy)

Age: 15 – 41 years; M:F = 1:8; especially in Orientals

Histo:
(a) Acute stage: granulomatous infiltrative process focused on elastic fibers of arterial wall consisting of multinucleate giant cells, lymphocytes, histiocytes, plasma cells
(b) Fibrotic stage (weeks to years): progressive fibrosis of vessel wall resulting in constriction from intimal proliferation / thrombotic occlusion / aneurysm formation

Δ Morphologically indistinguishable from temporal arteritis!

• prepulseless phase of a few months to a year = nonspecific systemic signs + symptoms of fever, weight loss, myalgia, arthralgia
• pulseless phase = signs + symptoms of ischemia of limb (claudication, pulse deficit, bruits) + renovascular hypertension
• erythrocyte sedimentation rate (ESR) >20 mm/hour in 80%

Location:
Type I: aortic arch + brachiocephalic arteries
Type II: thoracic aorta distal to arch, abdominal aorta + its major branches
Type III: combination of type I + II

Type IV: any portion of aorta with its branches + pulmonary artery

Commonly involved: left subclavian artery, left common carotid artery, brachiocephalic trunk, renal artery, celiac trunk, superior mesenteric artery, pulmonary artery (>50%)

Infrequently involved: axillary, brachial, vertebral, iliac arteries (usually bilaterally)

CXR:
√ widened supracardiac shadow >3.0 cm
√ contour irregularities of lateral margin of descending aorta
√ aortic calcification (15%) commonly in aortic arch + descending aorta
√ focal decrease of pulmonary vascularity

Angiography:
√ long + diffuse / short + segmental irregular stenosis / occlusion of major branches of aorta near their origins
√ stenotic lesions of thoracic aorta > abdominal aorta
√ frequent skip areas
√ abundant collateralization
√ fusiform aortic aneurysms + ectasia (10 – 15%)

US:
√ diffuse homogeneous circumferential thickening of vessel wall in proximal common carotid artery
√ increase in flow velocity + turbulence
√ distal CCA, ICA, ECA spared with dampened waveforms

DDx: Atherosclerosis, temporal arteritis (CCA not involved), fibromuscular dysplasia (in ICA not CCA), idiopathic carotid dissection (ICA)

Rx: Steroids, angioplasty after decline of active inflammation

TEMPORAL ARTERITIS

= CRANIAL / GRANULOMATOUS ARTERITIS
= POLYMYALGIA RHEUMATICA = GIANT CELL ARTERITIS (poor choice because Takayasu disease is also a giant cell arteritis)

= systemic granulomatous vasculitis limited to persons >50 years of age

Incidence: 1.7 new cases/million/year

Histo:
(a) acute stage: granulomatous infiltrative process focused on elastic fibers of arterial wall consisting of multinucleate giant cells, lymphocytes, histiocytes, plasma cells
(b) fibrotic stage (weeks to years): progressive fibrosis of vessel wall resulting in constriction from intimal proliferation / thrombotic occlusion / aneurysm formation

Δ Morphologically indistinguishable from Takayasu arteritis!

Age peak: 65 – 75 years; M:F = 1:3
• prodromal phase of flu-like illness of 1 – 3 weeks:
  • malaise, low-grade fever, weight loss, myalgia
  • unilateral headache (50 – 90%)

- chronic stage:
  - jaw claudication (while chewing + talking)
  - palpable tender temporal artery
  - neuro-ophthalmic manifestations: visual impairment / diplopia / blindness
  - polymyalgia rheumatica (50%) = intense myalgia of shoulder + hip girdles
- erythrocyte sedimentation rate (ESR) of 40 – 140 mm/hour (HALLMARK)

Location:
any artery of the body; mainly medium-sized branches of aortic arch (10%), external carotid artery branches (particularly temporal artery);
extracranial arteries below neck (9%): subclavian > axillary > brachial > profunda femoris > forearm > calf; commonly bilateral + symmetrical
√ long smooth stenotic arterial segments with skip areas
√ smooth tapered occlusions with abundance of collateral supply
√ absence of atherosclerotic changes
√ aortic root dilatation + aortic valve insufficiency

Dx: Biopsy of palpable temporal artery
Prognosis: disease may be self-limiting (1 – 2 years); 10% mortality within 2 – 3 years

TETRALOGY OF FALLOT
= underdevelopment of pulmonary infundibulum secondary to unequal partitioning of the conotruncus
Incidence: 8% of all CHD; most common CHD with cyanosis after 1 year of life
TETRAD:
1. Obstruction of right ventricular outflow tract: usually at pulmonary infundibulum, occasionally at pulmonic valve
2. VSD
3. Right ventricular hypertrophy
4. Aorta overriding the interventricular septum
Hemodynamics:
fetus: pulmonary blood flow supplied by retrograde flow through ductus arteriosus with absence of RV hypertrophy / IUGR
neonate: R–L shunt bypassing pulmonary circulation with decrease in systemic oxygen saturation (cyanosis); pressure overload + hypertrophy of RV secondary to pulmonic-infundibular stenosis
Associated with:
1. Bicuspid pulmonic valve (40%)
2. Stenosis of left pulmonary artery (40%)
3. Right aortic arch (25%)
4. TE fistula
5. Down syndrome
6. Forked ribs, scoliosis
7. Anomalies of coronary arteries in 10% (single RCA / LAD from RCA)
- cyanosis by 3 – 4 months of age (concealed at birth by PDA)
- dyspnea on exertion, clubbing of fingers and toes

- "squatting position" when fatigued (increases pulmonary blood flow)
- "episodic spells" = loss of consciousness
- polycythemia, lowered PO_2 values, systolic murmur in pulmonic area

√ pronounced concavity in region of pulmonary artery trunk (small / absent PA)
√ coeur en sabot (boot-shaped heart) = enlargement of right ventricle
√ right-sided aortic arch in 25%
√ marked reduction in caliber + number of pulmonary vessels
√ asymmetric pulmonary vascularity
√ reticular pattern with horizontal course usually in periphery (= prominent collateral circulation of pleuropulmonary connections)
OB-US:
√ dilated aorta overriding the interventricular septum
√ usually perimembranous VSD
√ mildly stenotic RV outflow tract
√ NO RV hypertrophy in midtrimester
ECHO:
√ discontinuity between anterior aortic wall + interventricular septum (= overriding of the aorta)
√ small left atrium
√ RV hypertrophy with small right ventricular outflow tract
√ widening of the aorta
√ thickening of right ventricular wall + interventricular septum

Prognosis: spontaneous survival without surgical correction in 50% up to age 7; in 10% up to age 21
Rx: Surgery in early childhood
(a) Palliative
1. Blalock-Taussig shunt = end-to-side anastomosis of subclavian to pulmonary artery opposite aortic arch (64% survival rate at 15 years, 55% at 20 years)
2. Pott operation on left = anastomosis of left PA with descending aorta
3. Waterston-Cooley procedure = anastomosis between ascending aorta + right pulmonary artery
4. Central shunt = Rastelli procedure = tubular synthetic graft between ascending aorta + pulmonary artery
(b) Corrective open cardiac surgery = VSD-closure + reconstruction of RV outflow tract by excision of obstructing tissue (82% survival rate at 15 years)
Operative mortality: 3 – 10%

PINK TETRALOGY = infundibular hypertrophy in VSD (3%)
PENTALOGY OF FALLOT = tetralogy + ASD
TRILOGY OF FALLOT = pulmonary stenosis + RV hypertrophy + patent foramen ovale

THORACIC OUTLET SYNDROME
= compression of nerves, veins and arteries between chest and arm

Causes:
A. CONGENITAL
1. Cervical rib
    = elevation of floor of scalene triangle with decrease of costoclavicular space
    Incidence: 0.5 – 1% of population
    Δ 5 – 10% of complete cervical ribs cause symptoms
    Δ 10 – 20% of symptomatic patients have a responsible cervical rib
    Cx: aneurysmal dilatation of subclavian a.
2. Scalenus minimus muscle (rare) extending from transverse process of 7th cervical vertebra to 1st rib with insertion between brachial plexus + subclavian artery
3. Anterior scalene muscle = scalenus anticus syndrome (most common) = wide / abnormal insertion / hypertrophy of muscle
4. Anomalous 1st rib = unusually straight course with narrowing of costoclavicular space
B. ACQUIRED
1. Muscular body habitus
    = arterial compression in pectoralis minor tunnel
2. Slender body habitus
    with long neck, sagging shoulders
3. Fracture of clavicle / 1st rib (34%)
    with nonanatomic alignment / exuberant callus
4. Supraclavicular tumor / lymphadenopathy

- pain in forearm + hand which increases upon elevation of arm
- paresthesias of hand + fingers (numbness, "pins and needles") in 95%
- decreased skin temperature, discoloration of hand
- intermittent claudication of fingers (from ischemia)
- hyperabduction maneuver with obliteration of radial pulse (34%)
- Raynaud phenomenon (40%): episodic constriction of small vessels
- supraclavicular bruit (15 – 30%)

Bidirectional Doppler:
1. Adson maneuver (for scalenus anticus muscle) = hold deep inspiration while neck is fully extended + head turned toward ipsilateral and opposite side
2. Costoclavicular maneuver (compression between clavicle + 1st rib) = exaggerated military position with shoulders drawn back and downward
3. Hyperabduction maneuver (compression by humeral head / pectoralis minor muscle) = extremity monitored through range of 180° abduction
    √ complete cessation of flow in one position

Photoplethysmography:
1. Photo pulse transducer secured to palmar surface of one fingertip of each hand

2. Arterial pulsations recorded with arm in
    (a) neutral position
    (b) extended 90° to side
    (c) 180° over the head
    (d) in "military" position with arms at 90° + shoulders pressed back
    √ complete disappearance of pulse in one position
Angio:
√ abnormal course of distal subclavian artery
√ focal stenosis / occlusion
√ poststenotic dilatation of distal subclavian artery
√ aneurysm
√ stress test: band-like / concentric constriction
√ mural thrombus ± distal embolization
√ venous thrombosis / obstruction
DDx: Cervical disc disease, radiculopathy, spinal cord tumor, trauma to brachial plexus, arthritis, carpal tunnel syndrome, Pancoast tumor, peripheral arterial occlusive disease, aneurysm, thromboembolism, Raynaud disease, vasculitis, causalgia

TRANSPOSITION OF GREAT ARTERIES
Complete Transposition of Great Arteries
= TGA = D-TRANSPOSITION = failure of the aorticopulmonary septum to follow a spiral course characterized by (1) aorta originating from RV (2) pulmonary artery originating from LV (3) normal position of atria + ventricles
Incidence: 10% of all CHD
VARIATIONS:
1. Complete TGA + intact interventricular septum
2. Complete TGA + VSD: CHF due to VSD
3. Complete TGA + VSD + PS: PS prevents CHF
   = longest survival
Hemodynamics:
fetus: no hemodynamic compromise with normal birth weight
neonate: mixing of the 2 independent circulations necessary for survival

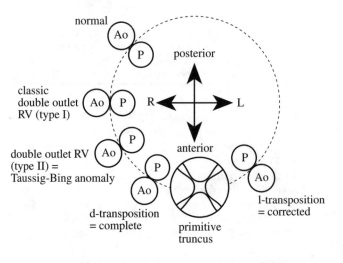

Admixture of blood from both circulations via:
  (1) PDA + patent foramen ovale (when PDA closes worst prognosis)
  (2) VSD (in 50%)
- cyanosis (most common cause for cyanosis in neonate) 2nd most common cause of cyanosis after tetralogy of Fallot
- symptomatic 1 – 2 weeks following birth

CXR:
  √ "egg-on-its-side" appearance of heart = narrow superior mediastinum secondary to hypoplastic thymus + hyperaeration + abnormal relationship of great vessels
  √ cardiac enlargement beginning 2 weeks after birth
  √ right heart enlargement
  √ enlargement of LA (with VSD)
  √ absent pulmonary trunk (99%) = PA located posteriorly in midline
  √ increased pulmonary blood flow (if not associated with PS)
  √ midline aorta (30%) / ascending aorta with convexity to the right
  √ right aortic arch in 3% (difficult assessment due to midline position + small size)
OB-US:
  √ great arteries arise from ventricles in a parallel fashion
  √ aorta anterior + to right of pulmonary artery (in 60%; rarely side by side)

Prognosis: overall 70% survival rate at 1 week, 50% at 1 month, 11% at 1 year by natural history
Rx:
  (1) Prostaglandin E1 administration to maintain ductal patency
  (2) Rashkind procedure = balloon septostomy to create ASD
  (3) Blalock-Hanlon procedure = surgical creation of ASD
  (4) Mustard operation (corrective) = removal of atrial septum + creation of intraatrial baffle directing the pulmonary venous return to RV + systemic venous return to LV; 79% 1-year survival rate; 64 – 89% 5-year survival

Corrected Transposition of Great Arteries
= CONGENITALLY CORRECTED TRANSPOSITION
= L-TRANSPOSITION
= anomalous looping of the primordial ventricles associated with lack of spiral rotation of conotruncal septum characterized by
  (1) Transposition of great arteries
  (2) Inversion of ventricles (LV on right side, RV on left side):
      (a) RA connected to morphologic LV
      (b) LA connected to morphologic RV
  (3) AV valves + coronary arteries follow their corresponding ventricles

Hemodynamics: functionally corrected abnormality
Associated with:
  (1) usually perimembranous VSD (in >50%)
  (2) pulmonic stenosis (in 50%)
  (3) anomaly of left (= tricuspid) atrioventricular valves (Ebstein-like)
  (4) dextrocardia (high incidence)
- atrioventricular block (malalignment of atrial + ventricular septa)

CXR:
  √ abnormal convexity / straightening in upper portion of left heart border (ascending aorta arising from inverted RV)
  √ inapparent aortic knob + descending aorta (overlying spine)
  √ inapparent pulmonary trunk (rightward posterior position) = PREMIER SIGN
  √ humped contour of lower left heart border with elevation above diaphragm (anatomic RV)
  √ apical notch (= septal notch)
  √ increased pulmonary blood flow (if shunt present)
  √ pulmonary venous hypertension (if left-sided AV valve incompetent)
  √ LA enlargement
Angio:
  √ original LV on right side: smooth-walled, cylinder- / cone-shaped with high recess emptying into aorta (= venous ventricle)
  √ original RV on left side: bulbous, triangular shape, trabeculated chamber with infundibular outflow tract into pulmonary trunk (= arterial ventricle)
OB-US:
  √ great arteries arise from ventricles in a parallel fashion
  √ aortic valve separated from tricuspid valve by a complete infundibulum
  √ fibrous continuity between pulmonic valve + mitral valve
Prognosis: (unfavorable secondary to additional cardiac defects) 40% 1-year survival rate, 30% 10-year survival rate

TRICUSPID ATRESIA
2nd most common cause of pronounced neonatal cyanosis (after transposition) characterized by absent tricuspid valve, ASD, and small VSD (in most patients)
Incidence: 1.5% of all CHD
1. TRICUSPID ATRESIA WITHOUT TRANSPOSITION (80%)
   (a) without PS (b) with PS (c) with pulmonary atresia
2. TRICUSPID ATRESIA WITH TRANSPOSITION
   (a) without PS (b) with PS (most favorable combination) (c) with pulmonary atresia
Δ Usually small VSD + PS (75%) restrict pulmonary blood flow
- progressive cyanosis from birth on, increasing with crying = OUTSTANDING FEATURE (inverse relationship between degree of cyanosis + volume of pulmonary blood flow)

- pansystolic murmur (VSD)
- ECG: left-axis deviation

CXR (typical cardiac contour):
- √ left rounded contour = enlargement + hypertrophy of LV
- √ right rounded contour = enlarged RA
- √ flat / concave pulmonary segment
- √ normal / decreased pulmonary vascularity
- √ typical flattening of right heart border with transposition (in 15%)

Prognosis: may survive well into early adulthood
Rx:
1. Blalock-Taussig procedure (if pulmonary blood flow decreased in infancy)
2. Glenn procedure = shunt between IVC + right PA (if total correction not anticipated)
3. Fontan procedure = external conduit from RA to pulmonary trunk + closure of ASD (if pulmonary vascular disease has not developed)

TRUNCUS ARTERIOSUS
= PERSISTENT TRUNCUS ARTERIOSUS
= SINGLE OUTLET OF THE HEART
= abnormal septation of the conotruncus characterized by
(1) one great artery arising from the heart giving rise to the coronary, pulmonary, and systemic arteries, straddling
(2) large VSD

Incidence: 2% of all CHD
Types:

Type I   (50%)   = main PA + aorta arise from common truncal valve

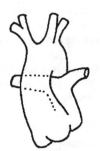

Type I

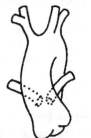

Type II

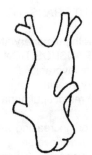

Type III

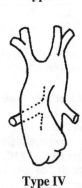

Type IV

Type II   (25%)   = both pulmonary arteries arise from back of trunk

Type III (10%)   = both pulmonary arteries arise from side of trunk

Type IV   = "Pseudotruncus" = absence of pulmonary arteries; pulmonary supply from systemic collaterals arising from descending aorta

Subtype A   = infundibular VSD present
Subtype B   = VSD absent

Associated with:
(1) Right aortic arch (in 35%)
    cyanosis + shunt vascularity + right aortic arch = TRUNCUS
(2) Forked ribs

Hemodynamics:
fetus: CHF only with incompetent valve secondary to massive regurgitation from truncus to ventricles
neonate: L–R shunt after decrease in pulmonary resistance (massive diversion of flow to pulmonary district) leads to CHF (ventricular overload) / pulmonary hypertension with time

- moderate cyanosis, apparent with crying
- severe CHF within first days / months of life (in large R–L shunt)
- systolic murmur

CXR:
- √ cardiomegaly (increased LV volume)
- √ enlarged LA (50%) secondary to increased pulmonary blood flow
- √ large "aortic shadow" = truncus arteriosus
- √ "waterfall / hilar comma sign" = elevated right hilum (30%); elevated left hilum (10%)
- √ concave pulmonary segment (50%) (Type I has left convex pulmonary segment)
- √ markedly increased pulmonary blood flow, may be asymmetric

ECHO:
- √ single arterial vessel overriding the interventricular septum (DDx: tetralogy of Fallot)
- √ frequently dysplastic + incompetent single semilunar valve with 3 – 6 leaflets (most commonly 3 leaflets)

Prognosis: 40% 6-months survival rate, 20% 1-year survival rate
Rx: Rastelli procedure (30% no longer operable at 4 years of age) = (a) artificial valve placed high in RVOT and attached via a Dacron graft to main pulmonary artery (b) closure of VSD

Hemitruncus
= rare anomaly characterized by
(a) one pulmonary artery (commonly right PA) arising from trunk
(b) one pulmonary artery arising from RV / supplied by systemic collaterals

Associated with: PDA (80%), VSD, tetralogy (usually isolated to left PA)
- acyanotic

Pseudotruncus Arteriosus
= TRUNCUS TYPE IV = severe form of tetralogy of Fallot with atresia of the pulmonary trunk; entire pulmonary circulation through bronchial collateral arteries (NOT a form of truncus arteriosus in its true sense); characterized by (1) pulmonary atresia (2) VSD with R–L shunt (3) RV hypertrophy
Associated with: right aortic arch in 50%
- cyanosis
- √ concavity in area of pulmonary segment
- √ comma-like abnormal appearance of pulmonary artery
- √ absent normal right and left pulmonary artery (lateral chest film)
- √ esophageal indentation posteriorly (due to large systemic collaterals)
- √ prominent hilar + intrapulmonary vessels (= systemic collaterals)
- √ "coeur en sabot" = RV enlargement
- √ prominent ascending aorta with hyperpulsations

VENTRICULAR ANEURYSM
A. CONGENITAL LEFT VENTRICULAR ANEURYSM rare, young black adult
  - (a) Submitral type: √ bulge at left middle / upper cardiac border
  - (b) Subaortic type: √ small + not visualized
    - √ heart greatly enlarged (from aortic insufficiency)
B. ACQUIRED LEFT VENTRICULAR ANEURYSM
  = complication of myocardial infarction, Chagas disease
  - may be asymptomatic + well tolerated for years
  - occasionally associated with persistent heart failure, arrhythmia, peripheral embolization

True Aneurysm
= circumscribed noncontractile outpouching of ventricular cavity with broad mouth + localized dyskinesis
Cause: sequela of transmural myocardial infarction
Location:
  - (a) left anterior + anteroapical: readily detected (anterior + LAO views)
  - (b) inferior + inferoposterior: less readily detected (steep LAO + LPO views)
Detection rate: 50% by fluoroscopy; 96% by radionuclide ventriculography; frequently not visible on CXR
- √ localized bulge of heart contour = "squared-off" appearance of mid-left lateral margin of heart border
- √ localized paradoxical expansion during systole (CHARACTERISTIC)
- √ rim of calcium in fibrotic wall (chronic), rare
- √ akinetic / severely hypokinetic segment
- √ left ventriculography in LAO, RAO is diagnostic

- √ wide communication with heart chamber (no neck)
Cx: wall thrombus with embolization
Prognosis: rarely ruptures

Pseudoaneurysm
= FALSE ANEURYSM = left ventricular rupture contained by fused layers of visceral + parietal pericardium / extracardiac tissue
  - (a) cardiac rupture with localized hematoma contained by adherent pericardium; typically in the presence of pericarditis
  - (b) subacute rupture with gradual / episodic bleeding
Etiology: trauma, myocardial infarction
Location: typically at posterolateral / diaphragmatic wall of LV
- √ left retrocardiac double density
- √ diameter of mouth smaller than the largest diameter of the globular aneurysm
- √ delayed filling
Cx: high risk of delayed rupture (infrequent in true aneurysms)

VENTRICULAR SEPTAL DEFECT
Most common CHD (25 – 30%): (a) isolated in 20% (b) with other cardiac anomalies in 5%;
Δ Acyanotic L-R shunt + right aortic arch (in 2 – 5%) = VSD
1. MEMBRANOUS = PERIMEMBRANOUS VSD (75 – 80%)
   Location: posterior + inferior to crista supraventricularis near commissure between right and posterior (= noncoronary) aortic valve cusps
   May be associated with small aneurysms of membranous septum commonly leading to decrease in size of membranous VSD (their presence does not necessarily predict eventual complete closure)

2. SUPRACRISTAL = CONAL VSD (5 – 8%)
   Δ Crista supraventricularis = inverted U-shaped muscular ridge posterior + inferior to pulmonary valve
   (a) RV view = VSD just beneath pulmonary valve with valve forming part of superior margin of defect
   (b) LV view = VSD just below commissure between R + L aortic valve cusps

   Cx: right aortic valve cusp may herniate into VSD (= aortic insufficiency)

3. MUSCULAR VSD (5 – 10%)
   May consist of multiple VSDs; bordered entirely by myocardium
   Location: (a) inlet portion (b) trabecular portion (c) infundibular / outlet portion

4. ATRIOVENTRICULAR CANAL TYPE = ENDOCARDIAL CUSHION TYPE = POSTERIOR VSD (5 – 10%)
   Location: adjacent to septal + anterior leaflet of mitral valve; rare as isolated defect

Hemodynamics:
small bidirectional shunt during fetal life (similar pressures in RV + LV); after birth a decrease in pulmonary arterial pressure + increase in systemic arterial pressure occurs with development of L-R shunt
(a) small VSD: little / no hemodynamic significance
(b) large VSD: pulmonary vascular disease + hypertension will increase RV pressure; eventually leads to shunt reversal (R-L shunt)
(c) very large VSD: gross right ventricular overload creates CHF soon after birth

NATURAL HISTORY OF VSD causing reduction in pulmonary blood flow:
1. Spontaneous closure
   in 40% within first 2 years of life; 60% by 5 years (65% with muscular VSD, 25% with membranous VSD); with large VSD in 10%; with small VSD in 50%
2. Eisenmenger syndrome
   = progressive increase in pulmonary vascular resistance through intima + medial hyperplasia; occurs in 10% of large VSDs by 2 years of age
3. RVOT obstruction
   infundibular hypertrophy in 3% = pink tetrad
4. Prolapse of right aortic valve cusp
   = aortic valve insufficiency

CLASSIFICATION:
Group I: "maladie de Roger" = small shunt with defect <1 cm; normal pulmonary artery pressure, normal pulmonary vascular resistance; spontaneous closure
   • asymptomatic
   • heart murmur
   √ normal plain film
Group II: moderate shunt with defect of 1 – 1.5 cm; intermediate pulmonary artery pressure; normal pulmonary vascular resistance; spontaneous closure in large percentage
   • respiratory infections, mild dyspnea
   √ slight prominence of pulmonary vessels (45% shunt)
   √ slight enlargement of LA
Group III: nonrestrictive large shunt with size equal to aortic valve orifice; pulmonary artery pressure approaching systemic levels; slightly increased pulmonary vascular resistance; pulmonary blood flow 2 – 4 x systemic flow
   • bouts of respiratory infections
   • feeding problems, failure to thrive

√ prominent pulmonary segment + vessels (= shunt vascularity)
√ enlargement of LA + LV
√ normal / small aorta
Group IV: Eisenmenger syndrome with shunt reversal into R–L shunt; irreversible increase in pulmonary vascular resistance (when pulmonary vascular resistance >0.75 of systemic vascular resistance)
   • cyanotic, but less symptomatic; CHF rare
   √ decrease of pulmonary vessel caliber
   √ decrease in size of LA + LV

CXR (with increase in size of VSD):
√ enlargement of LA
√ enlargement of pulmonary artery segment
√ enlargement of LV
√ RV hypertrophy
√ increase in pulmonary blood flow (>45% of pulmonary blood flow from systemic circulation)
√ Eisenmenger reaction
ECHO:
√ lack of echoes in region of interventricular septum with sharp edges (DDx: artifactual dropout with sound beam parallel to septum); muscular VSD difficult to see
√ LA enlargement
√ prolapse of aortic valve cusp (in supracristal VSD)
√ deformity of aortic cusp (in membranous VSD)
Angio:
Projections:
   (a) LAO 60° C-C 20° for membranous + anterior muscular VSD
   (b) LAO 45° C-C 45° (hepatoclavicular) for posterior endocardial cushion + posterior muscular VSD
   (c) RAO for supracristal VSD + assessment of RVOT
√ RVOT / pulmonary valve fill without filling of RV chamber (in supracristal VSD)
Rx:
   (a) Large VSD + left heart failure at 3 months of age: aim is to delay closure until child is 18 months of age; pulmonary-to-systemic blood flow >2:1 requires surgery before pulmonary hypertension becomes manifest
      1. Digitalis + diuretics
      2. Pulmonary artery banding
      3. Patching of VSD: surgical approach through RA / through RV for supracristal VSD
   (b) Small VSDs without increase in pulmonary arterial pressure are followed

DIFFERENTIAL DIAGNOSIS OF HEPATIC, BILIARY, PANCREATIC, AND SPLENIC DISORDERS

LIVER
Diffuse hepatic enlargement
NORMAL LIVER SIZE:
  (craniocaudad measurement in midclavicular line)
        <13 cm = normal
  13.0 – 15.5 cm = indeterminate (in 25% of patients)
     >15.5 cm = hepatomegaly (87% accuracy)

A. METABOLIC
1. Fatty infiltration
2. Amyloid
3. Wilson disease
4. Gaucher disease
5. Von Gierke disease
6. Niemann-Pick disease
7. Weber-Christian disease
8. Galactosemia
B. MALIGNANCY
1. Lymphoma
2. Diffuse metastases
3. Diffuse HCC
4. Angiosarcoma
C. INFLAMMATION / INFECTION
1. Hepatitis
2. Mononucleosis
3. Miliary TB, histoplasmosis, sarcoid
4. Malaria
5. Syphilis
6. Leptospirosis
7. Chronic granulomatous disease of childhood
D. VASCULAR
1. Passive congestion
E. OTHERS
1. Early cirrhosis
2. Polycystic liver disease

Increased liver attenuation
Abnormal deposits of substances with high atomic
  numbers
1. IRON
(a) Primary hemochromatosis (b) Transfusional
hemosiderosis (c) Bantu siderosis = excessive dietary
iron from food preparation in iron containers (Kaffir
beer)
2. COPPER
Wilson disease = hepatolenticular degeneration
= increased copper deposits in liver + basal ganglia
3. IODINE
Amiodarone (= antiarrhythmic drug with 37% iodine by
weight)
√ 95 – 145 HU (range of normal for liver 30 – 70 HU)
4. GOLD
Colloidal form of gold for therapy of rheumatoid arthritis
5. THOROTRAST
Alpha-emitter with atomic number of 90

6. THALLIUM
Accidental / suicidal ingestion of rodenticides (lethal
dose is 0.2 – 1.0 gram)
7. ACUTE MASSIVE PROTEIN DEPOSITS
8. GLYCOGEN STORAGE DISEASE

Generalized increased liver echogenicity
1. Fatty infiltration
2. Cirrhosis
3. Chronic hepatitis
4. Vacuolar degeneration

Focal liver lesion
A. SOLITARY
  (a) benign
    1. Simple cyst / echinococcal cyst
    2. Cavernous hemangioma
    3. Abscess
    4. Hematoma / traumatic cyst
    5. Adenoma
    6. Focal nodular hyperplasia
    7. Fatty change
  (b) malignant
    1. Hepatoma
    2. Metastasis
    3. Peripheral cholangiocarcinoma
B. MULTIPLE
  (a) benign
    1. Simple cysts
    2. Cavernous hemangioma
    3. Polycystic disease
    4. Multiple abscesses
    5. Caroli disease
    6. Adenoma
    7. Regenerating hepatic nodules
  (b) malignant
    1. Metastases (most common malignant liver
       tumor)
    2. Multifocal hepatoma
    3. Lymphoma

Primary benign liver tumor
A. EPITHELIAL TUMORS
  (a) hepatocellular
    1. Nodular transformation
    2. Focal nodular hyperplasia
    3. Hepatocellular adenoma
  (b) cholangiocellular
    1. Bile duct adenoma
    2. Biliary cystadenoma
B. MESENCHYMAL TUMORS
  (a) tumor of adipose tissue
    1. Lipoma
    2. Myelolipoma
    3. Angiomyolipoma

(b) <u>tumor of muscle tissue</u>
  1. Leiomyoma
(c) <u>tumor of blood vessels</u>
  1. Infantile hemangioendothelioma
  2. Hemangioma
(d) <u>mesothelial tumor</u>
  1. Benign mesothelioma
C. MIXED TISSUE TUMOR
  1. Mesenchymal hamartoma
  2. Benign teratoma
D. MISCELLANEOUS
  1. Adrenal rest tumor
  2. Pancreatic rest

Primary malignant liver tumor
A. EPITHELIAL TUMOR
  (a) <u>hepatocellular</u>
    1. Hepatoblastoma (7%)
    2. Hepatocellular carcinoma (75%)
  (b) <u>cholangiocellular</u> (6%)
    1. Cholangiocarcinoma
    2. Cystadenocarcinoma
B. MESENCHYMAL TUMOR
  (a) <u>tumor of blood vessels</u>
    1. Angiosarcoma
    2. Hemangioendothelioma
  (b) <u>other tumor</u>
    1. Embryonal sarcoma
    2. Fibrosarcoma
C. TUMOR OF MUSCLE TISSUE
  1. Leiomyosarcoma
  2. Rhabdomyosarcoma
D. MISCELLANEOUS
  1. Carcinosarcoma
  2. Teratoma
  3. Yolk sac tumor
  4. Carcinoid
  5. Squamous carcinoma
  6. Primary lymphoma

Solitary echogenic liver mass
mnemonic: "Hyperechoic **F**ocal **M**asses **A**ffecting the
             Liver"
Hepatoma, **H**emangioma, **H**emochromatosis
Fatty infiltration, **F**ocal nodular hyperplasia, **F**ibrosis
Metastasis
Adenoma
Lipoma

Hepatic lesion with central scar
1. Focal nodular hyperplasia
2. Hepatic adenoma
3. Giant cavernous hemangioma
4. Fibrolamellar hepatocellular carcinoma

Low-density mass in porta hepatis
1. Choledochal cyst
2. Hepatic cyst
3. Pancreatic pseudocyst
4. Enteric duplication

5. Hepatic artery aneurysm
6. Biloma

Low-density hepatic mass with enhancement
1. Hepatoma
2. Hypervascular metastases (lesions that may be obscured after contrast injection: pheochromocytoma, carcinoid, melanoma)
3. Cavernous hemangioma
4. Focal nodular hyperplasia with central fibrous scar
5. Hepatic adenoma

Portal venous gas
Δ Should be considered a life-threatening event and sign of bowel infarction + gangrene until proved otherwise!
Composition of colonic gas:
  methane, carbon dioxide, oxygen, nitrogen, hydrogen
Etiology:
  (1) Bowel infarction
  (2) Ulcerative colitis
  (3) Necrotizing enterocolitis
  (4) Small bowel obstruction
  (5) Intraabdominal abscess
  (6) Gastric ulcer
  (7) Pneumonia
  (8) Iatrogenic injection of air during endoscopy
Pathogenesis:
  1. gas-forming organisms traverse intestinal wall into portal venous system
  2. gas infiltrates directly through damaged intestinal wall into intestinal venules (bowel obstruction, ulcer)
√ branching linear gas densities in periphery of liver
√ gas in mesenteric vessels
√ pneumatosis of intestinal wall
US:
  √ intensely hyperechoic foci within lumen of portal vein + liver parenchyma
Doppler:
  √ tall sharp bidirectional spikes (overloading of Doppler receiver from strong reflection of gas bubble in bloodstream) superimposed on normal portal vein spectrum
Prognosis: often fatal within 1 week of diagnosis
DDx: biliary gas (closer to liver hilum)

Hepatic calcification
A. INFECTION
  1. Tuberculosis (48%), histoplasmosis, gumma, brucellosis
  2. Echinococcal cyst (in 33%)
  3. Chronic granulomatous disease of childhood
  4. Old pyogenic / amebic abscess
B. VASCULAR
  1. Hepatic artery aneurysm
  2. Portal vein thrombosis
  3. Hematoma
C. BILIARY
  1. Intrahepatic calculi
D. BENIGN TUMORS
  1. Congenital cyst

2. Cavernous hemangioma
3. Capsule of regenerating nodules
4. Infantile hemangioendothelioma
E. PRIMARY MALIGNANT TUMOR
1. Hepatoblastoma (10 – 20%)
2. Cholangiocellular carcinoma
F. METASTATIC TUMOR
1. Mucinous carcinoma of colon, breast, stomach
2. Ovarian carcinoma (psammomatous bodies)
3. Melanoma, pleural mesothelioma, osteosarcoma, carcinoid, leiomyosarcoma

PANCREAS
Pancreatic calcification
1. CHRONIC PANCREATITIS
   Numerous irregular stippled calcifications of varying size; predominantly intraductal
   (a) Alcoholic pancreatitis (in 20 – 50%):
       √ calcifications limited to head / tail in 25%
   (b) Biliary pancreatitis (in 2%)
   (c) Hereditary pancreatitis (in 35 – 60%):
       √ round calcifications throughout gland
   (d) Idiopathic pancreatitis
   (e) Pancreatic pseudocyst
2. NEOPLASM
   (a) Microcystic adenoma (in 33%):
       √ "sunburst" appearance of calcifications
   (b) Macrocystic cystadenoma:
       √ rounded cystic areas
   (c) Adenocarcinoma (in 2%): with "sunburst" pattern
   (d) Cavernous lymphangioma / hemangioma:
       √ multiple   phleboliths
   (e) Metastases from colon cancer
3. INTRAPARENCHYMAL HEMORRHAGE
   (a) Old hematoma / abscess / infarction
   (b) Rupture of intrapancreatic aneurysm
4. HYPERPARATHYROIDISM (in 20%):
   50% of patients develop chronic pancreatitis, concomitant nephrocalcinosis indistinguishable from alcoholic pancreatitis
5. CYSTIC FIBROSIS
   Fine granular calcifications imply advanced pancreatic fibrosis
6. HEMOCHROMATOSIS
7. KWASHIORKOR = tropical pancreatitis:
   indistinguishable from alcoholic pancreatitis

Fatty replacement + atrophy of pancreas
1. Main pancreatic duct obstruction
2. Cystic fibrosis
3. Schwachman syndrome
4. Hemochromatosis
5. Viral infection
6. Malnutrition

Pancreatic masses
A. NEOPLASTIC
1. Adenocarcinoma
2. Islet cell tumor
3. Cystadenoma / -carcinoma

4. Solid and papillary neoplasm
5. Lymphoma
B. INFLAMMATORY
1. Acute pancreatitis
2. Pseudocyst
3. Pancreatic abscess

Pancreatic cyst
1. Pseudocyst (90%): secondary to obstructive tumor / trauma / acute pancreatitis (in 2 – 4%), chronic pancreatitis (in 10 – 15%) [develop within 10 – 20 days, consolidated after 6 – 8 weeks]
2. Cystic neoplasm (5 – 15%):
   <5% of all pancreatic tumors
   (a) Microcystic adenoma
   (b) Mucinous cystic neoplasm
   (c) Solid and papillary epithelial neoplasm
3. Congenital cyst (rare)
   (a) solitary
   (b) multiple (when associated with cystic disease of the liver / other organs):
       Adult polycystic kidney disease (hepatic cysts in 90% at autopsy); von Hippel-Lindau disease (pancreatic cysts in 72% at autopsy; in only 25% on CT)
4. Acquired cyst: retention cyst (= exudate within bursa omentalis), parasitic cyst

Pancreatic neoplasm
A. EPITHELIAL ORIGIN
1. Ductal adenoma, intraductal papilloma
   <1% of epithelial cell neoplasms
2. Serous cystadenoma
3. Mucinous cystadenoma
4. **Ductectatic mucinous tumor**
   √ mass usually in uncinate portion of pancreatic head = cystic dilatation of pancreatic duct + branches
   √ grape-like clusters of cysts containing thick mucinous secretions
   √ surrounded by thin rim of normal pancreatic parenchyma
5. Solid and papillary neoplasm

B. ACINAR CELL ORIGIN
1. Solid and papillary neoplasm of pancreas
2. **Acinar cell carcinoma**
   in elderly patients
   • increased serum lipase ± amylase
   • disseminated subcutaneous + intraosseous fat necrosis
   √ lobulated mass of 2 – 15 cm in diameter
   √ moderately vascular tumor + neovascularity + arterial and venous encasement
   Prognosis: median survival of 7 months

C. NONEPITHELIAL ORIGIN
1. Lymphoma
   (a) Primary lymphoma:
       <1% of pancreatic neoplasms

(b) Secondary lymphoma
- √ large homogeneous solid mass, infrequently with central cystic area
- √ peripancreatic nodal masses
- √ peripancreatic vessels displaced + stretched

2. Metastases
melanoma, lung cancer, breast cancer, ovarian cancer, hepatocellular carcinoma, renal cell carcinoma, sarcoma

Hypervascular pancreatic tumors
A. PRIMARY
Islet cell tumor, microcystic adenoma, solid and papillary epithelial neoplasm
B. METASTASES from
angiosarcoma, leiomyosarcoma, melanoma, carcinoid, renal cell carcinoma, adrenal carcinoma, thyroid carcinoma

Hyperamylasemia
A. PANCREATIC
1. Acute / chronic pancreatitis
2. Pancreatic trauma
3. Pancreatic carcinoma
B. GASTROINTESTINAL
1. Perforated peptic ulcer
2. Intestinal obstruction
3. Peritonitis
4. Acute appendicitis
5. Afferent loop syndrome
6. Mesenteric infarction
C. TRAUMA
1. Burns
2. Cerebral trauma
3. Postoperative
D. OBSTETRICAL
1. Pregnancy
2. Ectopic
E. RENAL
1. Transplantation
2. Renal insufficiency
F. METABOLIC
1. Diabetic ketoacidosis
2. Drugs
G. PNEUMONIA
H. SALIVARY GLAND LESION
1. Facial trauma

BILE DUCTS

Obstructive jaundice in adult
Etiology:
A. BENIGN DISEASE (76%)
1. Traumatic / operative stricture (44%)
2. Calculi (21%)
3. Pancreatitis (8%)
4. Sclerosing cholangitis (1%)
5. Recurrent pyogenic cholangitis

6. Parasitic disease (ascariasis)
7. Liver cysts
8. Aortic aneurysm
B. MALIGNANCY (24%)
1. Pancreatic carcinoma (18%)
2. Ampullary / duodenal carcinoma (8%)
3. Cholangiocarcinoma (3%)
4. Metastatic disease (2%)
from stomach, pancreas, lung, breast, colon, lymphoma

INCIDENCE OF INFECTED BILE IN BILE DUCT OBSTRUCTION
(a) incomplete / partial obstruction in 64%
(b) complete obstruction in 10%
Δ Infection twice as high with biliary calculi than with malignant obstruction!
Organisms: E. coli (21%), Klebsiella (21%), Enterococci (18%), Proteus (15%)

TEST SENSITIVITY OF COMMON BILE DUCT OBSTRUCTION
1. Intravenous cholangiography
depends on level of bilirubin: <1 mg/dl in 92%; <2 mg/dl in 82%; <3 mg/dl in 40%; >4 mg/dl in <10%
False-negative rate: 45%
Cx: adverse reactions in 4 – 10%
2. US
88 – 90% sensitivity with dilatation of CBD
Δ in 27 – 95% correct level of obstruction determined by US
Δ in 23 – 81% correct cause of obstruction determined by US
False-negative: not dilated in acute obstruction (in 70%), sclerosing cholangitis, intermittent obstruction from choledocholithiasis
√ "double channels" = dilated intrahepatic bile ducts
√ "Swiss cheese sign" = abundance of fluid-filled structures in liver sections
3. CT
100% visualization in tumorous obstruction, 60% in non-tumorous obstruction
4. NUC
√ delayed / nonvisualization of biliary system (93% specificity)
√ vicarious excretion of tracer through kidneys
DDx: Hepatocellular dysfunction (delayed clearance of cardiac blood pool)

Neonatal obstructive jaundice
= severe persistent jaundice in a child beyond 3 – 4 weeks of age
Causes:
A. INFECTION
(a) bacterial: E. coli, syphilis, Listeria monocytogenes
(b) viral: TORCH, hepatitis B, Coxsackie, echovirus, adenovirus

B. METABOLIC
   (a) inherited: alpha 1-antitrypsin deficiency, cystic fibrosis, galactosemia, hereditary tyrosinemia
   (b) acquired: inspissated bile syndrome (= cholestasis due to erythroblastosis); cholestasis due to total parenteral nutrition
C. BILIARY TRACT ABNORMALITIES
   (a) extrahepatic: biliary obstruction / hypoplasia / atresia, choledochal cyst, spontaneous perforation of bile duct, "bile plug" syndrome
   (b) intrahepatic: ductular hypoplasia / atresia
D. IDIOPATHIC NEONATAL HEPATITIS

mnemonic: "CAN"
   Choledochal cyst
   Atresia
   Neonatal hepatitis

NUC – imaging regimen:
   (1) Premedication with phenobarbital (5 mg/kg/day) over 5 days to induce hepatic microsomal enzymes which enhance uptake and excretion of certain compounds and increase bile flow
   (2) IDA scintigraphy (50 µCi/kg; minimum of 1 mCi)
   (3) Imaging at 5 minute intervals for 1 hour + at 2, 4, 6, 8, 24 hours

Large nonobstructed CBD
   1. Passage of stone (return to normal after days to weeks)
   2. Common duct surgery (return to normal in 30 – 50 days)
   3. Post-cholecystectomy dilatation (in up to 16%)
   4. Intestinal hypomotility
   5. Normal variant (aging)
   Fatty-meal sonography (to differentiate from obstruction)
   Method: peroral Lipomul (1.5 ml/kg) followed by 100 ml of water [cholecystokinin causes contraction of gallbladder, relaxation of sphincter of Oddi, increase in bile secretion], CBD measured before and 45 / 60 minutes after stimulation
   √ little change / decrease in size = normal response
   √ increase in size >2 mm = partial obstruction

Filling defect in bile ducts
A. ARTIFACT
   1. Pseudocalculus = contracted sphincter of Boyden + Oddi with smooth arcuate contour
   2. Air bubble: confirmed by positional changes
   3. Blood clot: spheroid configuration, spontaneous resolution with time
B. BILIARY CALCULI
C. MIRIZZI SYNDROME
D. NEOPLASM
   1. Cholangiocarcinoma: irregular stricture, intraluminal polypoid mass

   2. Others: ampullary carcinoma, hepatoma, villous tumor, hamartoma, carcinoid, adenoma, papilloma, fibroma, lipoma, neuroma, cystadenoma, granular cell myoblastoma, sarcoma botryoides
E. PARASITES
   1. Ascaris lumbricoides: long linear filling defect / discrete mass if coiled
   2. Liver fluke (Clonorchis sinensis, Fasciola hepatica): intrahepatic epithelial hyperplasia, periductal fibrosis, cholangitis, liver abscess, hepatic duct stones, common duct obstruction
   3. Hydatid cyst: after erosion into biliary tree

Gas in biliary tree
   mnemonic: "SITS"
   Stone
   Inflammation (emphysematous cholecystitis)
   Tumor with fistula
   Surgery

Bile duct narrowing
A. BENIGN STRICTURE (44%)
   (a) Inflammation
       1. Sclerosing cholangitis
       2. Recurrent pyogenic cholangitis
       3. Acute / chronic pancreatitis
       4. Pancreatic pseudocyst
       5. Perforated duodenal ulcer
       6. Erosion by biliary calculus
       7. Gallstones + cholecystitis
       8. Abscess
       9. Radiation therapy
       10. Papillary stenosis
   (b) Congenital
       1. Choledochal cyst
   (c) Trauma
       1. Postoperative stricture (99%)
       2. Blunt / penetrating trauma
       3. Hepatic artery embolization
       4. Infusion of chemotherapeutic agents
B. MALIGNANT STRICTURE
   1. Pancreatic carcinoma
   2. Ampullary carcinoma
   3. Cholangiocarcinoma
   4. Compression by enlarged lymph node

Congenital cystic dilatation of bile ducts
   1. Choledochal cyst (87%)
   2. Choledochocele (6%)
   3. Choledochal diverticulum (3%)
   4. Caroli disease
   5. Multiple hepatic cysts

   TYPE A = anomalous pancreaticobiliary duct system causing cystic dilatation of CBD, involving papilla of Vater = CHOLEDOCHAL CYST (most common type)
   TYPE B = true diverticulum of CBD
   TYPE C = true diverticulum of hepatic duct

TYPE D = CHOLEDOCHOCELE = intraduodenal portion of CBD analogous to ureterocele

Classification of Biliary Tree Anomalies:
I. Common bile duct
   A. Choledochal cyst
   B. Segmental dilatation
   C. Diffuse dilatation
II. Diverticulum of extrahepatic ducts
III. Choledochocele
IV. Multiple cysts
   A. in intra- and extrahepatic ducts
   B. in extrahepatic ducts
V. Intrahepatic cysts

GALLBLADDER

Nonvisualization of gallbladder on OCG
Peak opacification of gallbladder: 14 – 19 hours
(13 – 35% of dose excreted in urine)

A. EXTRABILIARY CAUSES
   1. Failure to ingest contrast
   2. Fasting
   3. Failure to reach absorptive surface of bowel
      (a) vomiting, nasogastric suction
      (b) esophageal / gastric obstruction
      (c) hiatal, umbilical, inguinal hernias
      (d) Zenker, epiphrenic, gastric, duodenal, jejunal diverticula
      (e) gastric ulcer, gastrocolic fistula
      (f) malabsorption, diarrhea
      (g) postoperative ileus, severe trauma
      (h) inflammation: acute pancreatitis, acute peritonitis
   4. Deficiency of bile salts
      Crohn disease, surgical resection of terminal ileum, liver disease, cholestyramine therapy, abnormal communication between biliary system and gastrointestinal tract
B. INTRINSIC GALLBLADDER DISEASE
   1. Cholecystectomy
   2. Anomalous position
   3. Obstruction of cystic duct
   4. Chronic cholecystitis

ORAL CHOLECYSTOGRAM (OCG)
Dose: 6 x 0.5 g tablets 2 hours after evening meal
A. PATIENT SELECTION
   • bilirubin <5 mg% (not necessary if due to hemolysis)
   Δ Contraindicated in serious liver disease!
   Δ Relative contraindications in peritonitis, postoperative ileus, acute pancreatitis!
B. TOXICITY
   1. Nausea + vomiting (also noted in 29% on placebo)
   2. Immediate anaphylactic response
   3. Delayed hypotensive reaction (increased risk in cirrhosis)

4. Renal failure
5. Precipitation of hyperthyroidism

High density bile
1. Hemorrhagic cholecystitis
2. Hemobilia
3. Prior contrast administration
   (a) vicarious excretion of urographic agent
   (b) cholecystopaque
4. Milk of calcium bile

Displaced gallbladder
A. NORMAL IMPRESSION
   by duodenum / colon (positional change)
B. HEPATIC MASS
   hepatoma, hemangioma, regenerating nodule, metastases, intrahepatic cyst, polycystic liver, hydatid disease, hepar lobatum (tertiary syphylis), granuloma, abscess
C. EXTRAHEPATIC MASS
   1. Retroperitoneal tumor (renal, adrenal)
   2. Polycystic kidney
   3. Lymphoma
   4. Lymph node metastasis to porta hepatis
   5. Pancreatic pseudocyst

Alteration in gallbladder size
A. ENLARGED GALLBLADDER
   = CHOLECYSTOMEGALY
   (a) OBSTRUCTION
      1. Cystic duct obstruction (40%)
         (a) Hydrops: chronic cystic duct obstruction + distension with clear sterile mucus (white bile)
         (b) Empyema: acute / chronic obstruction with superinfection of bile
      2. Cholelithiasis causing obstruction (37%)
      3. Cholecystitis with cholelithiasis (11%)
      4. Courvoisier phenomenon (10%) = secondary to neoplastic process in pancreas / duodenal papilla / ampulla of Vater / common bile duct
      5. Pancreatitis
   (b) UNOBSTRUCTED (mostly neuropathic)
      1. S/P vagotomy
      2. Diabetes mellitus
      3. Alcoholism
      4. Appendicitis (in children)
      5. Narcotic analgesia
      6. WDHA syndrome
      7. Hyperalimentation
      8. Acromegaly
      9. Kawasaki syndrome
      10. Anticholinergics
      11. Bedridden patient with prolonged illness
      12. AIDS (in 18%)
   (c) NORMAL (2%)
B. SMALL GALLBLADDER
   1. Chronic cholecystitis
   2. Cystic fibrosis: in 30 – 50% of patients
   3. Congenital hypoplasia / multiseptate gallbladder

Focal gallbladder wall thickening

A. METABOLIC
   1. Metachromatic sulfatides
   2. Hyperplastic cholecystoses
B. BENIGN TUMOR
   1. Adenoma: glandular elements (0.2%)
   2. Papilloma: fingerlike projections (0.2%)
   3. Fibroadenoma
   4. Cystadenoma: ? premalignant
   5. Neurinoma, hemangioma
   6. Carcinoid tumor
C. MALIGNANT TUMOR
   1. Carcinoma of gallbladder: adenocarcinoma / squamous cell carcinoma
   2. Leiomyosarcoma
   3. Metastases: from malignant melanoma (15%), lung, kidney, esophagus
D. INFLAMMATION / INFECTION
   1. Inflammatory polyp: in chronic cholecystitis
   2. Parasitic granuloma: Ascaris lumbricoides, Paragonimus westermani, Clonorchis, filariasis, Schistosoma, Fasciola
   3. Intramural epithelial cyst / mucinous retention cyst
   4. Xanthogranulomatous cholecystitis
E. WALL-ADHERENT GALLSTONE = embedded calculus
F. HETEROTOPIC MUCOSA
   1. Ectopic pancreatic tissue
   2. Ectopic gastric glands
   3. Ectopic intestinal glands
   4. Ectopic hepatic tissue
   5. Ectopic prostatic tissue

FIXED FILLING DEFECTS IN GALLBLADDER
   mnemonic: "PANTS"
   Polyp
   Adenomyomatosis
   Neurinoma
   Tumor, primary / secondary
   Stone, wall-adherent

Diffuse gallbladder wall thickening

= anterior wall of gallbladder >3 mm
A. INTRINSIC
   1. Acute cholecystitis
   2. Chronic cholecystitis (10 – 25%)
   3. Hyperplastic cholecystosis
   4. Gallbladder perforation
   5. Sepsis
   6. Gallbladder carcinoma
   7. AIDS (average of 9 mm in up to 55%)
B. EXTRINSIC
   1. Hepatitis (in 80%)
   2. Hypoalbuminemia
   3. Renal failure
   4. Right heart failure
   5. Ascites
   6. Multiple myeloma
   7. Portal node lymphatic obstruction
   8. Cirrhosis
   9. Acute myelogenous leukemia
   10. Brucellosis
   11. Graft-versus-host disease
   12. Systemic venous hypertension
C. PHYSIOLOGIC
   = contracted gallbladder after eating

Comet-tail artifact in liver and gallbladder

A. LIVER
   1. Foreign metallic body (eg, surgical clip)
   2. Intrahepatic clacification
   3. Pneumobilia
   4. Multiple bile duct hamartoma = von Meyenburg complex
B. GALLBLADDER
   1. Rokitansky-Aschoff sinus
   2. Intramural stone
   3. Cholesterolosis of gallbladder

SPLEEN

Splenomegaly

Normal size (in children):
   Formula for length = 5.7 + 0.31 x age (in years)
Normal weight: 150 g

A. CONGESTIVE SPLENOMEGALY
   Heart failure, portal hypertension, cirrhosis, cystic fibrosis, portal / splenic vein thrombosis
B. NEOPLASM
   Leukemia, lymphoma, metastases, primary neoplasm
C. STORAGE DISEASE
   Gaucher disease, Niemann-Pick disease, amyloidosis, diabetes mellitus, histiocytosis, hemochromatosis, gargoylism
D. INFECTION
   Hepatitis, malaria, infectious mononucleosis, leishmaniosis, brucellosis, TB, typhoid, syphilis, echinococcosis
E. HEMOLYTIC ANEMIA
   Hemoglobinopathy, hereditary spherocytosis, primary neutropenia, thrombotic thrombocytopenic purpura
F. EXTRAMEDULLARY HEMATOPOIESIS
   Osteopetrosis, myelofibrosis
G. COLLAGEN VASCULAR DISEASE
   Systemic lupus erythematosus, rheumatoid arthritis, Felty syndrome
H. TRAUMA
   Intrasplenic laceration / fracture, subcapsular hematoma
I. OTHERS
   Sarcoidosis, hemodialysis

Small spleen

1. Hereditary hypoplasia
2. Irradiation
3. Infarction
4. Polysplenia syndrome
5. Atrophy

Splenic calcification
A. DISSEMINATED
   1. Phlebolith
   2. Granuloma: histoplasmosis, TB, brucellosis
B. CAPSULAR & PARENCHYMAL
   1. Pyogenic / tuberculous abscess
   2. Infarction (multiple)
   3. Hematoma
C. VASCULAR
   1. Splenic artery calcification
   2. Splenic artery aneurysm
   3. Splenic infarct
D. CALCIFIED CYST WALL
   1. Congenital cyst
   2. Posttraumatic cyst
   3. Echinococcal cyst
   4. Cystic dermoid
   5. Epidermoid
E. GENERALIZED INCREASED DENSITY
   1. Sickle cell anemia (in 5% of sicklers)
   2. Hemochromatosis
   3. Thorotrast
   4. Lymphangiography

mnemonic: "HITCH"
   Histoplasmosis (most common)
   Infarct (sickle cell disease)
   Tuberculosis
   Cyst (Echinococcus)
   Hematoma

Hyperechoic splenic spots
   1. Granulomas: miliary tuberculosis, histoplasmosis
   2. Phleboliths
   3. Lymphoma / leukemia
   4. Myelofibrosis
   5. Sinus hyperplasia of portal hypertension

Cystic splenic lesion
A. CONGENITAL
   1. Epidermoid cyst = epithelial cyst = primary cyst
   Average age at detection: 18 years
B. VASCULAR
   1. Splenic laceration / fracture
   2. Hematoma
   3. Posttraumatic cyst
   4. Cystic degeneration of infarct (embolic / local thrombosis)

C. INFECTION / INFLAMMATION
   1. Pyogenic abscess
      Incidence: 0.1 – 0.7%
      Predisposed: infarction (10%), trauma, neoplasm, sickle cell disease
   2. Microabscesses
      Organism: fungus (especially Candida)
      Predisposed: immunocompromised
   3. Parasitic cyst
   4. Pancreatic pseudocyst
D. CYSTIC NEOPLASM
   1. Cavernous hemangioma
      Most common benign splenic tumor; autopsy
      Incidence: 0.03 – 14%
      Age: 20 – 50 years
   2. Lymphangiomatosis
   3. Necrotic metastasis (malignant melanoma; ovarian, pancreatic, endometrial, colonic, mammary carcinoma; chondrosarcoma; lymphoma)

Solid splenic lesion
A. MALIGNANT TUMOR
   1. Metastasis (7%)
      melanoma (34%), breast carcinoma (12%), bronchogenic carcinoma (9%), colon carcinoma (4%), renal cell carcinoma (3%), ovary, prostate, stomach, pancreas, endometrium cancer
   2. Lymphoma (Hodgkin disease, non-Hodgkin lymphoma)
      Spleen involved in 70%
      √ splenomegaly (from diffuse infiltration)
      √ miliary nodules
      √ large 2 – 10 cm nodules (10 – 25%)
      √ nodes in splenic hilum (50%) in NHL; uncommon in Hodgkin disease
   3. Angiosarcoma
      May be associated with liver angiosarcoma
      Age: 50 – 60 years; poor survival rate
B. BENIGN TUMOR
   1. Hamartoma = SPLENOMA
   2. Hemangioma
   3. Hematopoietic
   4. Sarcoidosis
   5. Gaucher disease (islands of RES cells laden with glucosylceramide)
C. SPLENIC INFARCTION

ANATOMY OF LIVER, BILE DUCTS, AND PANCREAS

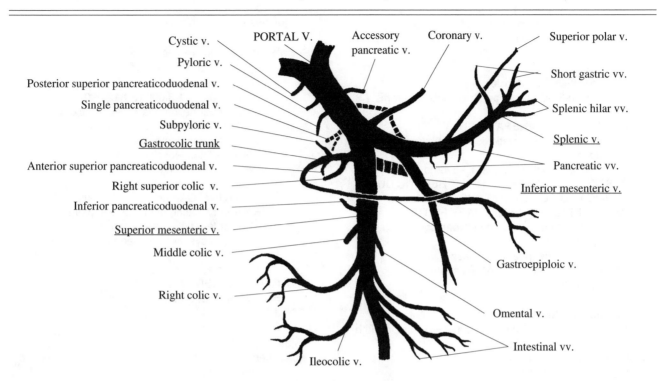

Extrahepatic Portal Vein Tributaries

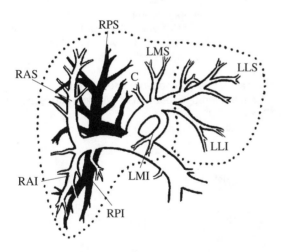

Intrahepatic Portal Vein Branches

RAI	=	right anterior inferior
RAS	=	right anterior superior
RPS	=	right posterior superior
RPI	=	right posterior inferior
C	=	caudate lobe
LMI	=	left median inferior
LMS	=	left median superior
LLS	=	left lateral superior
LLI	=	left lateral inferior

Functional segmental liver anatomy

based on distribution of 3 major hepatic veins (Couinaud):
- (a) middle hepatic vein divides liver into right + left lobe
- (b) right hepatic vein divides right lobe into medial + lateral sections
- (c) left hepatic vein divides left lobe into medial + lateral sections

Each of the four sections is divided by an imaginary transverse line drawn through the portal vein into anterior + posterior segments; the segments are numbered counterclockwise from IVC:

LEFT LOBE

segment I	= caudate lobe segment
segment II	= left posterior segment
segment III	= left anterior segment
segment IV	= left medial segment

RIGHT LOBE

segment V	= right medial-anterior segment
segment VI	= right lateral-anterior segment
segment VII	= right lateral-posterior segment
segment VIII	= right medial-posterior segment

Normal size of bile ducts

- @ CBD at point of maximum diameter:
  ≤ 5 mm = normal; 6 – 7 mm = equivocal;
  ≥ 8 mm = dilated
- @ CHD at porta hepatis + CBD in head of pancreas:
  5 mm
- @ right intrahepatic duct just proximal to CHD:
  2 – 3 mm

@   Cystic duct diameter: 1.8 mm
average length of 1 – 2 cm
distal cystic duct posterior to CBD (in 95%),
anterior to CBD (in 5%)

Bile duct variants
Incidence: 2.4% of autopsies;
in 5 – 13% of operative cholangiograms

1. ABERRANT INTRAHEPATIC DUCT
may join CHD, CBD, cystic duct, right hepatic duct,
gallbladder
Cx: postoperative bile leak if severed
2. CYSTIC DUCT ENTERING RIGHT HEPATIC DUCT
3. DUPLICATION OF CYSTIC DUCT / CBD
4. CONGENITAL TRACHEOBILIARY FISTULA
= fistulous communication between carina and left
hepatic duct
• infants with respiratory distress
• productive cough with bilious sputum
√ pneumobilia

Gallbladder measurements
Size: 7 – 10 cm in length; 2 – 3.5 cm in width
Capacity: 30 – 50 ml
Wall thickness: 2 – 3 mm

Congenital gallbladder anomalies

Agenesis of gallbladder
Incidence: 0.04 - 0.07 % (autopsy)
Associated with
common: rectovaginal fistula, imperforate anus,
hypoplasia of scapula + radius, intracardiac shunt
rare: absence of corpus callosum, microcephaly,
atresia of external auditory canal, tricuspid atresia,
TE fistula, dextroposition of pancreas + esophagus,
absent spleen, high position of cecum, polycystic
kidney

Hypoplastic gallbladder
(a) congenital
(b) associated with cystic fibrosis

Septations of gallbladder
A. LONGITUDINAL SEPTA
1. Duplication of gallbladder
Incidence: 1:3,000 to 1:12,000
= two separate lumens + two cystic ducts
2. Bifid gallbladder = double gallbladder
= two separate lumens with one cystic duct
3. Triple gallbladder (extremely rare)
B. TRANSVERSE SEPTA
1. Isolated transverse septum
2. PHRYGIAN CAP (2 – 6 % of population)
= kinking / folding of fundus ± septum
3. Multiseptated gallbladder (rare)
= multiple cyst-like compartments connected by
small pores
Cx: stasis + stone formation
C. GALLBLADDER DIVERTICULUM
= persistence of cystohepatic duct

Gallbladder ectopia
Most frequent locations:
(1) beneath the left lobe of the liver > (2) intrahepatic
> (3) retrohepatic
Rare locations:
(4) within falciform ligament (5) within interlobar
fissure (6) suprahepatic (lodged between superior
surface of right hepatic lobe + anterior chest wall)
(7) within anterior abdominal wall (8) transverse
mesocolon (9) retrorenal (10) near posterior spine +
IVC (11) intrathoracic GB (inversion of liver)
Associated with   eventration of diaphragm
"Floating GB"
= gallbladder with loose peritoneal reflections, may
herniate through foramen of Winslow into lesser sac
"Torqued GB"
= results in hydrops

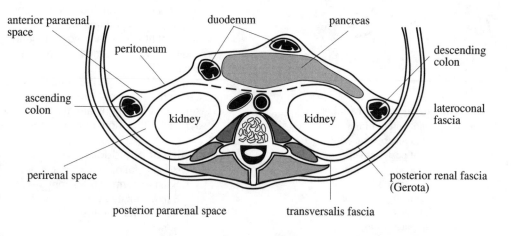

Extraperitoneal Spaces

DISORDERS OF LIVER, BILIARY TRACT, PANCREAS, AND SPLEEN

ACCESSORY SPLEEN
= failure of coalescence of several small mesodermal buds in the dorsal mesogastrium, which comprise the spleen
Incidence: 10 – 30% of population; multiple in 10%
Δ Undergoes hypertrophy after splenectomy and is responsible for recurrence of hematologic disorders (idiopathic thrombocytopenic purpura, hereditary spherocytosis, acquired autoimmune hemolytic anemia, hypersplenism)
Location: splenic hilum (most common), gastrosplenic ligament, other suspensory ligaments of spleen, rare in pancreas / pelvis
NUC (Tc-99m sulfur colloid scan / spleen-specific Tc-99m denatured RBCs):
  √ usually <1 cm in diameter
  √ <10% identified when normal spleen present

ANNULAR PANCREAS
= uncommon congenital anomaly wherein a ring of normal pancreatic tissue encircles the duodenum secondary to abnormal migration of ventral pancreas (head + uncinate); most common congenital anomaly of pancreas
Age at discovery: childhood (50%); adulthood (50%)
Associated with other congenital anomalies (in 75%): esophageal atresia, TE fistula, duodenal atresia / stenosis, duodenal diaphragm, imperforate anus, malrotation, Down syndrome
Location: 2nd portion of duodenum (85%); 1st / 3rd portion of duodenum (15%)
• mostly asymptomatic with incidental discovery
• neonate : persistent vomiting
• adult : nausea, vomiting (60%), abdominal pain (70%), hematemesis (10%), jaundice (50%)
√ polyhydramnios (in utero)
√ "double bubble" = dilated duodenal bulb + stomach
√ enlargement of pancreatic head
UGI:
  √ eccentric narrowing with lateral notching + medial retraction of 2nd part of duodenum
  √ concentric narrowing of mid-descending duodenum
  √ reverse peristalsis, pyloric incompetency
ERCP (most specific):
  √ pancreatic duct originates on anterior left + passes posteriorly around duodenum
Cx: increased incidence of periampullary peptic ulcers + pancreatitis
Rx: gastrojejunostomy / duodenojejunostomy

ASCARIASIS
Organism: Ascaris lumbricoides, 25 – 35 cm long as adult worm; life span of 1 year
Country: 644 million humans harbor the roundworm; 70 – 90% in America; in United States endemic in: Appalachian range, southern + Gulf coast states

Incidence: 12% in blacks, 1% in whites
Cycle:
  ingestion of contaminated soil / vegetable; larvae penetrate intestinal wall; migrate into mesenteric lymphatics + veins; reach lung via right heart + pulmonary artery; mature in pulmonary capillary bed to 2 – 3 mm length; burrow into alveoli; ascend in respiratory tract; are swallowed and remain in GI tract
√ barium study
√ cholangiography (49%)
√ plain film
Cx: (1) Intestinal obstruction
  (2) Intermittent biliary obstruction
  (3) Liver abscess (rare)
  (4) Granulomatous stricture of extrahepatic bile ducts (rare)

BANTI SYNDROME
= NONCIRRHOTIC IDIOPATHIC PORTAL HYPERTENSION = NONCIRRHOTIC PORTAL FIBROSIS = HEPATOPORTAL SCLEROSIS
= syndrome characterized by (1) splenomegaly (2) hypersplenism (3) portal hypertension

Etiology: increased portal vascular resistance possibly due to portal fibrosis + obliterative venopathy of intrahepatic portal branches
Histo: slight portal fibrosis, dilatation of sinusoids, intimal thickening with eccentric sclerosis of peripheral portal vein walls
Age: middle-aged women; rare in America + Europe but common in India + Japan
• elevated portal vein pressure (without cirrhosis, parasites, venous occlusion)
• normal liver function tests
• cytopenia (due to hypersplenism)
• normal / slightly elevated hepatic venous wedge pressure
√ esophageal varices
√ patent hepatic veins
√ patent extrahepatic portal vein + multiple collaterals
Prognosis: 90% 5-year survival; 55% 30-year survival

BILIARY CYSTADENOMA
= BILE DUCT CYSTADENOMA
= rare benign tumor resembling mucinous cystic neoplasms of the pancreas; <5% of all intrahepatic cysts of bile duct origin
Age: >30 years (82%); M:F = 1:4
Histo: single layer of biliary-type epithelium with papillary projections, subepithelial stroma resembles that of the ovary
Location: intrahepatic bile ducts (85%); extrahepatic bile ducts (15%); right lobe (50%); both lobes (30%); left lobe (20%)
√ mass of 1.5 – 30 cm in size
√ papillary excrescences + mural nodules

US: √ ovoid complex mass with irregular margins +
single / multiple septations
√ may contain fluid-fluid levels
CT: √ multiloculated mass of near water density with
septations
Angio: √ avascular mass with small clusters of peripheral
abnormal vessels
√ stretching + displacement of vessels
√ thin subtle blush of neovascularity in septa + wall
Aspirated fluid: mucinous, serous, containing
hemosiderin / cholesterol / necrosis

Cx: malignant transformation into cystadenocarcinoma
DDx: echinococcal cyst, necrotic hepatic metastasis,
cystic hamartoma, hepatic abscess

BILIARY-ENTERIC FISTULA
Incidence: 5% at cholecystectomy; 0.5% at autopsy
Etiology:
cholelithiasis (90%), acute / chronic cholecystitis, biliary
tract carcinoma, regional invasive neoplasm,
diverticulitis, inflammatory bowel disease, peptic ulcer
disease, echinococcal cyst, trauma, congenital
communication
Communication with:
duodenum (70%), colon (26%), stomach (4%),
jejunum, ileum, hepatic artery, portal vein (caused death
of Ignatius Loyola), bronchial tree, pericardium, renal
pelvis, ureter, urinary bladder, vagina, ovary

A. CHOLECYSTODUODENAL FISTULA (51 – 70%)
1. Perforated gallstone (90%):
associated with gallstone ileus in 20%
2. Perforated duodenal ulcer (10%)
3. Surgical anastomosis
4. Gallbladder carcinoma
B. CHOLECYSTOCOLIC FISTULA (13 – 21%)
C. CHOLEDOCHODUODENAL FISTULA (13 – 19%)
due to perforated duodenal ulcer disease
D. MULTIPLE FISTULAE (7%)

√ branching tubular radiolucencies, more prominent
centrally
√ barium filling of biliary tree
√ multiple hyperechoic foci with dirty shadowing

DDx: patulous sphincter of Oddi, ascending cholangitis,
surgery (choledochoduodenostomy,
cholecystojejunostomy, sphincterotomy)

BUDD-CHIARI SYNDROME
= global / segmental obstruction of hepatic venous outflow
Causes:
A. IDIOPATHIC (66%)
B. THROMBOSIS
(a) Hypercoagulable state: polycythemia rubra
vera (1/3), oral contraceptives, pregnancy +
postpartum state, paroxysmal nocturnal
hemoglobulinuria (successive thrombosis of
small veins), sickle cell disease

(b) Injury to vessel wall: phlebitis, trauma, hepatic
radiation injury, chemotherapeutic + immunosuppressive drugs in patients with bone marrow
transplants, veno-occlusive disease from
pyrrolizidine alkaloids (Senecio) found in
medicinal bush teas in Jamaica
C. NONTHROMBOTIC OBSTRUCTION
(a) Tumor growth into IVC / hepatic veins (renal
cell carcinoma, hepatoma, adrenal carcinoma,
metastasis, primary leiomyosarcoma of IVC)
(b) Membranous obstruction of suprahepatic IVC
= IVC diaphragm (believed to be a congenital
web or an acquired lesion from long-standing
IVC thrombosis); common cause in Oriental +
Indian population
(c) Right atrial tumor
(d) Constrictive pericarditis
(e) Right heart failure

M < F
Location:
Type I : occlusion of IVC ± hepatic veins
Type II : occlusion of major hepatic veins ± IVC
Type III : occlusion of small centrilobar veins
√ nonvisualization of hepatic veins (75%)
√ enlargement + hypodensity of hepatic veins (18%)
√ enlargement of caudate lobe (88%)
√ hypodensity in atrophic areas / periphery (82%) with
inversion of portal blood flow
√ patchy enhancement (85%) with normal portal blood
flow
CT:
√ enhancement of enlarged caudate lobe
√ hypodense nonenhancing regions (from infarction)
MRI:
√ reduction in caliber / complete absence of hepatic
veins
US:
√ hepatic veins not visualized / reduced in size / filled
with thrombus
Doppler:
√ absent / reversed / flat flow / loss of phasicity in
hepatic veins
√ reversed flow in IVC + flat flow in hepatic veins
NUC (Tc-99m sulfur colloid):
√ central region of normal activity (hot caudate lobe)
surrounded by greatly diminished activity (venous
drainage of hypertrophied caudate lobe into IVC)
√ colloid shift to spleen + bone marrow
√ wedge-shaped focal peripheral defects
Angio:
√ absence of main hepatic veins
√ spider weblike appearance of collaterals + small
hepatic veins
√ stretching + draping of intrahepatic arteries with
hepatomegaly
√ inhomogeneous prolonged intense hepatogram with
fine mottling
√ large lakes of sinusoidal contrast accumulation
√ bidirectional / hepatofugal portal vein flow

ACUTE STAGE (1/3)
- rapid onset of abdominal pain (liver congestion)
- insidious onset of intractable ascites
√ hepatomegaly without derangement of liver function
√ ascites (97%)
CT:
  √ diffuse hypodensity on NECT
  √ early enhancement of caudate lobe + central portion around IVC with decreased enhancement peripherally
  √ hypodense lumina of hepatic veins on CECT
  √ decreased attenuation of enhancing areas with patchy inhomogeneous enhancement in liver periphery on delayed scans

CHRONIC STAGE (2/3)
- insidious onset of jaundice, intractable ascites
- portal hypertension, variceal bleeding
√ enlargement of caudate lobe + atrophy of affected lobes of liver (due to extensive fibrosis)

CANDIDIASIS OF LIVER
= almost exclusively seen in immunocompromised patients (leukemia, chronic granulomatous disease of childhood, renal transplant, chemotherapy for myeloproliferative disorders)
√ hepatomegaly
US: √ "target" / "bull's eye" sign = multiple small hypoechoic masses with echogenic centers
NUC: √ uniform uptake / focal photopenic areas
       √ diminished Ga-67 uptake
DDx: Metastases, lymphoma, leukemia, septic emboli

CAROLI DISEASE
= COMMUNICATING CAVERNOUS ECTASIA OF INTRAHEPATIC DUCTS
= rare probably autosomal recessive disorder characterized by congenital segmental saccular cystic dilatation of major intrahepatic bile ducts
Etiology: (a) ? perinatal hepatic artery occlusion
           (b) ? hypoplasia / aplasia of fibromuscular wall components
Age: childhood + 2nd – 3rd decade, occasionally in infancy; M:F = 1:1

Associated with: medullary sponge kidney (in 80%), infantile polycystic kidney disease, renal tubular ectasia, choledochal cyst (rare), congenital hepatic fibrosis
- recurrent cramplike abdominal pain
- NO cirrhosis / portal hypertension

√ multiple cystic structures converging toward porta hepatis as either localized / diffusely scattered cysts communicating with bile ducts (DDx: polycystic liver disease)
√ segmental saccular / beaded appearance of intrahepatic bile ducts extending to periphery of liver
√ portal radicles completely surrounded by dilated bile ducts = central dot sign on CT
√ bridge formation across dilated lumina

√ intraluminal bulbar protrusions
√ frequent ectasia of extrahepatic ducts + CBD
√ sludge / calculi in dilated ducts
Cx: (1) Bile stasis with recurrent cholangitis (2) Biliary calculi (3) Liver abscess (4) Septicemia (5) Increased risk for cholangiocarcinoma

CHOLANGIOCARCINOMA
Intrahepatic Cholangiocarcinoma
= CHOLANGIOCELLULAR CARCINOMA
Incidence: 1/3 of all malignancies originating in the liver; 8 – 13% of all cholangiocarcinomas; 2nd most common primary hepatic tumor after hepatoma

Types:
  (1) Massive / nodular type
  (2) Diffuse (sclerosing cholangitis) type
       Δ cannot be depicted by cross-sectional imaging
- abdominal pain (47%)
- palpable mass (18%)
- weight loss (18%)
- painless jaundice (12%)
Spread: (1) local extension along duct (2) local infiltration of liver substance (3) metastatic spread to regional lymph nodes (in 15%)

√ mass of 5 – 20 cm in diameter
√ satellite nodules in 65%
√ punctate / chunky calcifications in 18%
√ calculi in biliary tree
NUC:
  √ cold lesion on sulfur colloid / IDA scans
  √ segmental biliary obstruction
  √ may show uptake on gallium scan
US:
  √ dilated biliary tree
  √ predominantly homo- / heterogeneous mass
  √ hyper- (75%) / iso- / hypoechoic (14%) mass
CT:
  √ single predominantly homogeneous round / oval hypodense mass with irregular borders
  √ no / peripheral / central enhancement
Angiography:
  √ avascular / hypo- / hypervascular mass
  √ stretched / encased arteries
  √ neovascularity in 50%
  √ lack of venous invasion
Prognosis: <20% resectable; 30% 5-year survival

Extrahepatic Cholangiocarcinoma
= BILE DUCT CARCINOMA
Age peak: 6 – 7th decade, M:F = 3:2
Incidence: <0.5% of autopsies; 90% of all cholangiocarcinomas; more frequent in Far East
Histo: well-differentiated sclerosing adenocarcinoma (2/3), anaplastic carcinoma (11%), cystadenocarcinoma, adenoacanthoma, malignant adenoma, squamous cell = epidermoid carcinoma, leiomyosarcoma

Predisposed:
(1) Inflammatory bowel disease (10 x increased risk); incidence of 0.4 – 1.4% in ulcerative colitis; latent period of 15 years; tumors usually multicentric + predominantly in extrahepatic sites; GB involved in 15% (simultaneous presence of gallstones is rare)
(2) Sclerosing cholangitis (10%)
(3) Caroli disease (due to chronic biliary stasis)
(4) Clonorchis sinensis infestation (Far East); most common cause worldwide
(5) Thorotrast exposure
(6) History of other malignancy (10%)
(7) Previous surgery for choledochal cyst / congenital biliary atresia
(8) Alpha-1-antitrypsin deficiency
(9) Autosomal dominant polycystic disease
(10) Cholecystolithiasis (20 – 50%), probably coincidental
(11) Papillomatosis of bile ducts
• gradual onset of fluctuating painless jaundice
• cholangitis (10%)
• weight loss, fatigability
• intermittent epigastric pain
• elevated bilirubin + alkaline phosphatase
• enlarged tender liver
Growth pattern:
(1) Obstructive type (70 – 85%)
 √ U- / V-shaped obstruction with nipple, rattail, smooth / irregular termination
(2) Stenotic type (10 – 25%)
 √ strictured rigid lumen with irregular margins + prestenotic dilatation
(3) Polyploid / papillary type (5 – 6%)
 √ intraluminal filling defect with irregular margins
Spread:
(a) lymphatic spread: cystic + CBD nodes (>32%), celiac nodes (>16%), peripancreatic nodes, superior mesenteric nodes
(b) infiltration of liver (23%)
(c) peritoneal seeding (9%)
(d) hematogenous (extremely rare): liver, peritoneum, lung
Location:

left / right hepatic duct	in 8 – 13%
confluence of hepatic ducts (Klatskin tumor)	in 10 – 26%
common hepatic duct	in 14 – 37%
proximal CBD	in 15 – 30%
distal CBD	in 30 – 50%
cystic duct	in 6%

UGI:
√ infiltration / indentation of stomach / duodenum
Cholangiography (PTC or ERC best modality to depict bile duct neoplasm):
√ exophytic intraductal tumor mass (46%), 2 – 5 mm in diameter
√ frequently long / rarely short concentric focal stricture in infiltrating sclerosing cholangitic type with wall irregularities
√ prestenotic diffuse / focal biliary dilatation (100%)
√ progression of ductal strictures (100%)
US / CT:
√ dilatation of intrahepatic ducts without extrahepatic duct dilatation
√ failure to demonstrate the confluence of L + R hepatic ducts
√ mass within / surrounding the ducts at point of obstruction (21% visible on US, 40% visible on CT)
√ infiltrating tumor visible as highly attenuating lesion in 22% on CT, in 13% on US
√ exophytic tumor visible in 100% on CT as low-attenuation mass, in 29% on US
√ polypoid intraluminal tumor visible as isoechoic mass within surrounding bile in 100% on US, in 25% on CT
Angiography:
√ hypervascular tumor with neovascularity (50%)
√ arterioarterial collaterals along the course of bile ducts associated with arterial obstruction
√ poor / absent tumor stain
√ displacement / encasement / occlusion of hepatic artery + portal vein

Cx: (1) Obstruction leading to biliary cirrhosis
      (2) Hepatomegaly
      (3) Intrahepatic abscess (subdiaphragmatic, perihepatic, septicemia)
      (4) Biliary peritonitis
      (5) Portal vein invasion
Prognosis: median survival of 5 months; 1.6% 5-year survival; 39% 5-year survival for carcinoma of papilla of Vater
DDx: Benign stricture, chronic pancreatitis, sclerosing cholangitis, edematous papilla, idiopathic inflammation of CBD

CHOLANGITIS
Acute Cholangitis
Causes:
A. Benign disease:
(1) Stricture from prior surgery (36%) (2) Calculi (30%) (3) Sclerosing cholangitis (4) Obstructed drainage catheter (5) Parasitic infestation
B. Malignant disease: ampullary carcinoma
Types:
1. ACUTE NONSUPPURATIVE ASCENDING CHOLANGITIS
 • bile remains clear
 • patient nontoxic
2. ACUTE SUPPURATIVE ASCENDING COLANGITIS (14%)
 Associated with   obstructing biliary stone or malignancy
 • septicemia, CNS depression, lethargy, mental confusion, shock (50%)
 √ purulent material fills biliary ducts

Organisms: E. coli > Klebsiella > Pseudomonas > Enterococci

- recurrent episodes of sepsis + RUQ pain
- Charcot triad (70%) : fever + chills + jaundice
- bile cultures in 90% positive for infection
Cx: miliary hepatic abscess formation
Prognosis: 100% mortality if not decompressed;
40 – 60% mortality with treatment; 13 –
16% overall mortality rate

Recurrent Pyogenic Cholangitis
= PRIMARY CHOLANGITIS = RECURRENT
PYOGENIC HEPATITIS = ORIENTAL
CHOLANGIOHEPATITIS = ORIENTAL CHOLANGITIS
= HONG KONG DISEASE = INTRAHEPATIC PIGMENT
STONE DISEASE
Etiology: ? Clonorchis infestation; endemic to
Indochina, South China, Taiwan, Japan,
Korea
Incidence: 3rd most common cause of an acute
abdomen in Hong Kong after appendicitis
and perforated ulcer
Age: 20 – 50 years; M:F = 1:1
- recurrent attacks of fever, chills, abdominal pain,
jaundice

Location: particularly in lateral segment of L lobe +
posterior segment of R lobe
√ marked dilatation of proximal intrahepatic ducts
(3 – 4 mm) in 100%
√ decreased arborization of intrahepatic radicles
√ intrahepatic bile ducts filled with pigment stones +
sludge (64%)
√ dilatation of CBD (68%) + choledocholithiasis (30%)
√ bile duct strictures (22%)
√ pneumobilia (3 – 52%)
√ segmental hepatic atrophy (36%)
Cx: liver abscess (18%), splenomegaly (14%),
biloma (4%), pancreatitis (4%)
DDx: complication of Caroli disease

Sclerosing Cholangitis
= insidious progressive disease affecting the intra- and
extrahepatic bile ducts
Histo: chronic obliterative fibrotic inflammation
(pericholangitis)
Age: <45 years (2/3); range 21 – 67 years;
M:F = 2:1
- chronic / intermittent obstructive jaundice (most
frequent)
- history of previous biliary surgery (53%) + chronic /
recurrent pancreatitis (14%)
- fatigability, abdominal pain, pruritus
- fever (1/3)
Location:
1. CBD almost always involved
2. intra- and extrahepatic ducts (68 – 89%)
3. cystic duct involved in 18%
4. intrahepatic ducts only (1 – 25%)
5. extrahepatic ducts only (3%)
US:
√ brightly echogenic portal triads

CT:
√ dilatation, stenosis, pruning, beading of intrahepatic
bile ducts (80%)
√ dilatation, stenosis, wall nodularity, duct wall
thickening, mural contrast enhancement of
extrahepatic bile ducts (100%)
√ hepatic metastases + lymph nodes in porta hepatis
Cholangiography:
√ multifocal strictures with predilection for bifurcations
+ skip lesions (uninvolved duct segments of normal
caliber)
√ "pruned tree" appearance (= opacification of central
ducts + diffuse obstruction of peripheral smaller
radicles)
√ "cobblestone" appearance (= coarse nodular mural
irregularities) in 50%
√ small saccular outpouchings (diverticula /
pseudodiverticula) = PATHOGNOMONIC
√ uncommonly "beaded appearance" (= alternating
segments of dilatation + focal circumferential
stenoses)
√ new strictures + lengthening of strictures between 6
months and 6 years (<20%)
√ marked ductal dilatation (24%)
√ polypoid mass (7%)
√ gallbladder irregularities uncommon
NUC (Tc 99m-IDA scan):
√ multiple persistent focal areas of retention in
distribution of intrahepatic biliary tree
√ marked prolongation of hepatic clearance
√ gallbladder visualized only in 70%

Cx: (1) Biliary cirrhosis
(2) Portal hypertension
(3) Cholangiocarcinoma (12%)

DDx:
(1) Sclerosing cholangiocarcinoma (progressive
cholangiographic changes within 0.5 – 1.5 years
of initial diagnosis, marked ductal dilatation
upstream from a dominant stricture, intraductal
mass >1 cm in diameter)
(2) Acute ascending cholangitis (history)
(3) Primary biliary cirrhosis (disease limited to
intrahepatic ducts, strictures less pronounced,
pruning + crowding of bile ducts, normal AMA
titer)

Primary Sclerosing Cholangitis
Etiology: idiopathic, ? hypersensitivity reaction
(speculative)
CRITERIA:
(1) progressive jaundice of obstructive type
(2) diffuse generalized involvement of extrahepatic
ducts
(3) exclusion of prior biliary tract surgery, gallstones,
bile duct carcinoma
(4) exclusion of primary biliary cirrhosis, Crohn
disease, ulcerative colitis, retroperitoneal fibrosis,
Riedel struma

Path: fibrosis + nonspecific inflammation with poorly defined aggregates of lymphocytes + plasma cells; sclerosing form resembles bile duct carcinoma

Secondary Sclerosing Cholangitis
Associated with:
(1) Inflammatory bowel disease (ulcerative colitis in 66 – 75%, occasionally Crohn disease)
  Δ 1 – 4% of patients with inflammatory bowel disease develop sclerosing cholangitis!
(2) Cirrhosis, chronic active hepatitis, pericholangitis, fatty degeneration
(3) Pancreatitis
(4) Retroperitoneal / mediastinal fibrosis
(5) Peyronie disease
(6) Riedel thyroiditis, hypothyroidism
(7) Retroorbital pseudotumor
NO association with gallstones

CHOLECYSTITIS
Acute Cholecystitis
Etiology: (a) in 80 – 95% cystic duct obstruction by impacted calculus; 85% disimpact spontaneously
    (b) in 10% acalculous cholecystitis
Pathogenesis: chemical irritation from concentrated bile, bacterial infection, reflux of pancreatic secretions
Age peak: 5 – 6th decade; M:F = 1:3
• Murphy sign = inspiratory arrest upon palpation of GB area (falsely positive in 6% of patients with cholelithiasis)
Oral cholecystography:
  √ nonvisualization / poor visualization of gallbladder
US (85 – 95% sensitivity, 64 – 100% specificity):
  √ GB wall thickening >3 mm (mean 9 mm)
  √ hazy delineation of GB wall
  √ "halo sign" = GB wall lucency (in 8%) = 3-layered configuration with sonolucent middle layer (edema)
  √ striated wall thickening (62%) = several alternating irregular discontinuous lucent + echogenic bands within GB wall (positive predictive value of 100%)
  √ GB hydrops = distension with AP diameter >5 cm
  √ sonographic Murphy sign in 85 – 88% = focal tenderness over gallbladder (63% sensitivity, 93% specificity)
  √ presence of pseudomembranes
  √ coarse nonshadowing nondependent echodensities (= sloughed necrotic mucosa / sludge / pus / clotted blood within gallbladder)
  √ crescent-shaped anechoic pericholecystic fluid (= inflammatory intraperitoneal exudate / abscess)
  √ cholelithiasis
NUC (95 – 97% sensitivity, 74 – 94% specificity , 95 – 98% accuracy):
  √ visualization of biliary tract + bowel
  √ nonvisualization of GB during 1st hour (in 83%)
  √ nonvisualization of GB by 4 hours (99% specificity)
  √ nonvisualization of GB + CBD (in 13%)

√ rim sign (34%) = increased activity in GB fossa conforming to inferior hepatic edge (= sign of hyperemia); predictive value of 57% for gangrenous GB + 94% for acute cholecystitis
√ increased perfusion to GB fossa during "arterial phase" (in up to 80%)

False-positive scans (10 – 12%) = nonvisualization of GB in absence of acute cholecystitis:
  congenital absence of GB, carcinoma of GB, chronic cholecystitis, acute pancreatitis, alcoholic liver disease, hepatocellular disease, severe intercurrent illness, total parenteral nutrition, hyperalimentation, prolonged fasting, recent feeding <4 – 6 hours prior to study
  Reduction to 2% false-positive scans through:
    (1) delayed images up to 4 hours
    (2) cholecystokinin (sincalide) injection 15 minutes prior to study
    (3) morphine IV (0.04 mg/kg) at 40 minutes + reimaging after 20 minutes (contraction of sphincter of Oddi + rise in intrabiliary pressure)
False-negative scans (4.8%): dilated cystic duct
Cx:
(1) Gangrene of gallbladder
  √ shaggy, irregular, asymmetric wall (mucosal ulcers, intraluminal hemorrhage, necrosis)
  √ hyperechoic foci within GB wall (microabscesses in Rokitansky-Aschoff sinuses)
  √ intraluminal membranes (gangrene)
(2) Perforation of gallbladder (in 2 – 20%)
    (a) acute free perforation with peritonitis causing pericholecystic abscess in 33%
    (b) subacute localized perforation causing pericholecystic abscess in 48%
    (c) chronic perforation resulting in internal biliary fistula causing pericholecystic abscess in 18%
    Location: most commonly perforation of fundus
  √ gallstone lying free in peritoneal cavity
  √ sonolucent / complex collection surrounding GB
(3) Empyema of gallbladder
  √ multiple medium / coarse highly reflective intraluminal echoes without shadowing / layering / gravity dependence (purulent exudate / debris)

Chronic Cholecystitis
Most common form of gallbladder inflammation
√ gallstones
√ smooth / irregular GB wall thickening (mean of 5 mm)
√ mean volume of 42 ml
NUC:
  √ normal GB visualization in majority of patients
  √ delayed GB visualization (1 – 4 hours)
  √ visualization of bowel prior to GB (sensitivity 45%, specificity 90%)

√ noncontractility / decreased response after CCK injection (decreased GB ejection fraction)

Acalculous Cholecystitis
Frequency: 5 – 15% of all acute cholecystitis cases
Etiology: probably caused by decreased blood flow through cystic artery
   (1) depressed motility / starvation in trauma, burns, surgery, total parenteral nutrition, anesthesia, mechanical ventilation, narcotics, shock, congestive heart failure, arteriosclerosis, polyarteritis nodosa, SLE, diabetes mellitus
   (2) obstruction of cystic duct by extrinsic inflammation, lymphadenopathy, metastases
   (3) infection from Salmonella, cholera, Kawasaki syndrome
Cx: gallbladder perforation
Prognosis: 6.5% mortality rate

Emphysematous Cholecystitis
= ischemia of gallbladder wall + infection with gas-producing organisms
Etiology: calculous (70 – 80%) / acalculous cystic duct obstruction with inflammatory edema resulting in cystic artery occlusion
Organism: Clostridium perfringens, Clostridium welchii, E. coli, Staphylococcus, Streptococcus
Age: >50 years; M:F = 5:1
Predisposed: diabetics (20 – 50%), debilitating diseases
• WBC count may be normal (1/3)
• point tenderness rare (diabetic neuropathy)

Plain film:
   √ gas appears 24 – 48 hours after onset of symptoms
   √ air-fluid level in GB lumen, air in GB wall within 24 – 48 hours after acute episode
   √ pneumobilia (rare)
US:
   √ high-level echoes outlining GB wall
Cx: gangrene (75%); gallbladder perforation (20%)
Mortality: 15%
DDx: 1. Enteric fistula
   2. Incompetent sphincter of Oddi
   3. Air-containing periduodenal abscess
   4. Periappendiceal abscess in malpositioned appendix
   5. Lipomatosis of gallbladder

CHOLEDOCHAL CYST
= CYSTIC DILATATION OF EXTRAHEPATIC BILE DUCT
= segmental aneurysmal dilatation of common bile duct; most common congenital lesion of bile ducts
Etiology: anomalous junction of pancreatic duct and CBD proximal to duodenal papilla, higher pressure in pancreatic duct and absent ductal sphincter allows free reflux of enzymes into CBD resulting in weakening of CBD wall

Classification:
   malunion of pancreaticobiliary duct
   Kimura Type I = pancreatic duct enters the proximal / mid CBD
   Kimura Type II = CBD drains into pancreatic duct

Incidence: 0.2 – 0.5:1,000,000; high incidence in Japanese
Age: <10 years (50%) + young adulthood, 80% diagnosed in childhood, occasionally detected up to 7th decade; M:F = 1:3
Histo: fibrous cyst wall without epithelial lining
Associated with:
   (1) dilatation, stenosis or atresia of other portions of the biliary tree (2%)
   (2) gallbladder anomaly (aplasia, double GB)
   (3) failure of union of left + right hepatic ducts
   (4) pancreatic duct + accessory hepatic bile ducts may drain into cyst
   (5) congenital hepatic fibrosis
   (6) polycystic liver disease
   (7) gallbladder carcinoma, bile duct carcinoma (increasing with age, up to 40% in adulthood)

• Classic triad (20 – 30% of adult patients):
   (1) intermittent jaundice (33 – 50%)
   (2) recurrent RUQ colicky pain (>75 – 90%), back pain
   (3) intermittent palpable RUQ abdominal mass (<25%)
• recurrent fever, chills, weight loss, pruritus

Location: (a) extra- and intrahepatic ducts (73%)
   (b) dilatation of L + R main intrahepatic ducts (45%)
      — unilateral (42%) involving only left lobe
      — bilateral (58%)
   (c) extrahepatic ducts only (27%) (= below entry of cystic duct)
√ Size: diameter of 2 cm up to 15 cm (largest contained 13 liters)
√ abrupt change in caliber at site of cyst
√ rounded smooth extrinsic compression of CBD
√ NO / mild peripheral intrahepatic bile duct dilatation
√ may contain stones / sludge
US:
   √ large cystic structure beneath porta hepatis separate from gallbladder, communication with hepatic ducts need to be demonstrated
   √ abrupt change of caliber at junction of dilated segment to normal ducts
   √ intrahepatic bile duct dilatation (16%) secondary to stenosis
OB-US:
   √ right-sided cyst in fetal abdomen + adjacent dilated hepatic ducts
   DDx: duodenal atresia; cyst of ovary, mesentery, omentum, pancreas, liver
NUC with HIDA:
   (excludes effectively DDx of hepatic cyst, pancreatic pseudocyst, enteric duplication, spontaneous loculated biloma)

√ photopenic area within liver that fills within 60 minutes
  + stasis of tracer within cyst
√ prominent hepatic ductal acitivity (dilatation of ducts)
UGI:
√ soft tissue mass in RUQ
√ anterior displacement of 2nd portion of duodenum +
  distal portion of stomach / inferior displacement of
  duodenum / widening of C-loop
Cx: 1. Rupture with bile peritonitis (1.8%)
     2. Cholangitis (20%)
     3. Malignant transformation into cholangio-
        carcinoma in extrahepatic bile duct + gall-
        bladder (<1% in 1st decade, 7 – 14% > age 20)
     4. Bleeding
     5. Biliary cirrhosis + portal hypertension
     6. Choledocholithiasis (8 – 50%)
     7. Recurrent pancreatitis (33%)
Rx: extensive resection to avoid possibility of malignant
     transformation
DDx: mesenteric, omental, renal, adrenal, hepatic,
     pancreatic cyst

CHOLEDOCHOCELE
= DUODENAL DUPLICATION CYST
  = ENTEROGENOUS CYST OF AMPULLA OF VATER /
  DUODENUM = INTRADUODENAL CHOLEDOCHAL
  CYST = DIVERTICULUM OF COMMON BILE DUCT
= cystic dilatation of the distal / intramural duodenal
  portion of the CBD with herniation of CBD into
  duodenum (similar to ureterocele)
Etiology:
  (1) congenital:
      (a) originates from tiny bud / diverticulum of distal
          CBD (found in 5.7% of normal population)
      (b) stenosis of ductal orifice / weakness of ductal
          wall
  (2) acquired:
      stone passage followed by stenosis + inflammation
Age: 33 years
Types: (a) CBD terminates in cyst, cyst drains into
            duodenum (common)
        (b) cyst drains into adjacent intramural portion of
            CBD (less common)
• biliary colic, episodic jaundice, nausea, vomiting

√ stones / sludge are frequently present
UGI:
√ smooth well-defined intraluminal duodenal filling
  defect in region of papilla
√ change in shape with compression / peristalsis
Cholangiography (diagnostic):
√ smooth clublike / saclike dilatation of intramural
  segment of CBD
Cx: choledocholithiasis, pancreatitis
DDx: choledochal cyst (involves more than only terminal
     portion of CBD)

CHOLELITHIASIS
Predisposing factors: "female, forty, fair, fat, fertile,
                          flatulent"

(a) Hemolytic disease
    Sickle cell disease (7 – 37%), hereditary
    spherocytosis (43 – 85%), pernicious anemia
    (16 – 20%), prosthetic cardiac valves + mitral
    stenosis (hemolysis), cirrhosis (hemolysis
    secondary to hypersplenism)
(b) Metabolic disorder
    Diabetes mellitus, obesity, pancreatic disease,
    cystic fibrosis, hypercholesterolemia,
    hemosiderosis (20%), hyperparathyroidism,
    hypothyroidism, prolonged use of estrogens /
    progesterone, pregnancy
(c) Hepatobiliary disease
    Hepatitis, Caroli disease, parasitic infection, benign
    / malignant strictures, foreign bodies (sutures,
    ascariasis)
(d) Inflammatory bowel disease
    (10 x increased risk of stone formation); Crohn
    disease (28 – 34%)
(e) Genetic predisposition
    Navaho, Pima, Chippewa Indians
(f) Others
    Muscular dystrophy

Composition:
  A. CHOLESTEROL STONE
     = main component of most calculi (70%)
     √ lucent (93%), calcified (7%)
     √ slightly hypodense compared with bile
       (a) pure cholesterol stones (10%): yellowish, soft
           √ buoyancy in contrast-enhanced bile
           √ density of <100 HU
       (b) mixture of cholesterol + calcium carbonate /
           bilirubinate (70%)
           √ laminated appearance
           √ radiopaque on plain film (15 – 20%)
  B. PIGMENT STONE (30%)
     • black = from deconjugation of bilirubin by beta-
       glucoronidase from E. coli organisms
     • brown = calcium bilirubinate
     contains <25% cholesterol
     √ multiple tiny faceted / spiculated stones (50%
       calcified on plain film)
     CT: √ usually denser than bile

Radioopacity:
  √ lucent stones (85%):
    cholesterol (85%), pigment (15%)
  √ calcified stones (15% on plain film, 60% on CT):
    cholesterol (33%), pigment (67%)
CT density:
  Δ Inverse relationship between CT attenuation
    numbers + cholesterol content
  21 – 24% undetectable by CT (<30 HU)
  ≤140 HU = pure cholesterol stone (= ≥80%
              cholesterol content)

FLOATING STONES (20 – 25%)
  (a) relatively pure cholesterol stones
  (b) gas-containing stones

(c) rise in specific gravity of bile (1.03) from oral cholecystopaques (1.06) causing stones (1.05) to float

GAS-CONTAINING STONES
Mechanism: dehydration of older stones leads to internal shrinkage + dendritic cracks + subsequent nitrogen gas-filling from negative internal pressure
√ "crow-foot" = "Mercedes-Benz" sign = radiating streaklike lucencies within stone, also responsible for buoyancy

SLUDGE
= calcium-bilirubinate granules + cholesterol crystals associated with biliary stasis secondary to prolonged fasting, hyperalimentation, hemolysis, cystic duct obstruction, acute + chronic cholecystitis
√ nonshadowing echogenic homogeneous mass shifting position slowly
√ "sludge ball" = tumefactive sludge (DDx: gallbladder cancer)
DDx: hemobilia, blood clot, parasitic infestation

Cholecystolithiasis
Incidence: 10% of population; M:F = 1:3; in 3rd decade M:F = 2%:4%; in 7th decade M:F = 10%:25%
Peak age: 5th – 6th decade
• asymptomatic (60 – 65%)
• biliary colic (at a rate of 2% per year)

√ high-level intraluminal echoes + acoustic shadowing (100% diagnostic)
√ reverberation artifact
√ nonvisualization of GB + collection of echogenic echoes with acoustic shadowing (15 – 25%)
√ "double-arc shadow" = 2 echogenic curvilinear parallel lines separated by sonolucent rim (ie, GB wall + GB lumen + stone with acoustic shadowing)
√ focal nonshadowing opacities <5 mm in diameter (in 70% gallstones)
√ infrequently adherent to wall
Cx: cholangitis, pancreatitis, fistula; cancer of GB + biliary ducts (2 – 3 x more frequent)

Cholangiolithiasis
A. CHOLEDOCHOLITHIASIS
  Δ Most common cause of bile duct obstruction!
  Etiology: (a) passed stones originating in GB
  (b) primary development in intra- / extrahepatic ducts
  Incidence:
  in 12 – 15% of cholecystectomy patients; in 3 – 4% of postcholecystectomy patients; in 75% of patients with chronic bile duct obstruction
  • recurrent episodes of jaundice, chills, fever (25 – 50%)
  • elevated transaminase (75%)
  • spontaneous passage with stones <6 mm size

Cholangiography (most specific technique):
  √ stone visualization in 92%
Peroperative cholangiography:
  prolongs operation by 30 minutes;
  4% false-negatives; 4 – 10% false-positives
US:
  √ stone visualization in 13 – 75% (more readily with CBD dilatation + good visibility of pancreatic head)
  √ dilated ducts in 64 – 77% / normal-sized duct in 36%
  √ dilatation of CBD with administration of fatty meal / cholecystokinin
  √ no stone in gallbladder (11%)
CT:
  √ stone visualization in 50 – 90%
  √ target sign = intraluminal mass with crescentic ring (= stone of soft-tissue density) in 85%
NUC:
  √ delayed bowel activity beyond 2 hours
  √ persistent hepatic + common bile duct activity to 24 hours
  √ prominent ductal activity beyond 90 minutes with visualization of secondary ducts

B. STONE IN CYSTIC DUCT REMNANT:
  retained in 0.4% after surgery for choledocholithiasis

CHRONIC GRANULOMATOUS DISEASE OF CHILDHOOD
= recessive sex-linked immunodeficiency disorder resulting in purulent infections + granuloma formation primarily involving lymph nodes, skin, lungs
Etiology: polymorphonuclear leukocyte dysfunction characterized by inability to generate hydrogen peroxide causing prolonged intracellular survival of phagocytized catalase-positive bacteria
Organisms: most commonly Staphylococcus, Serratia marcescens, Gram-negative enterococci
Path: chronic infection with granuloma formation / caseation / suppuration
Age: onset in childhood; M > F (more severe in boys)

• recurrent chronic infections: suppurative lymphadenitis, pyoderma
• chronic diarrhea
• perianal fistula + abscess
@ Chest
  √ chronic pneumonia
  √ hilar lymphadenopathy
  √ pleural effusions
@ Liver
  √ hepatosplenomegaly
  √ hepatic abscess
  √ liver calcifications
@ GI tract
  √ esophageal dysmotility, esophagitis, stricture
  √ gastric antral narrowing ± gastric outlet obstruction
@ Bone
  √ osteomyelitis

CIRRHOSIS

= chronic liver disease characterized by diffuse parenchymal destruction, fibrosis, and nodular regeneration with abnormal reconstruction of preexisting lobular architecture

Etiology:
  A. TOXIC: (1) Alcoholic liver disease (2) Drug-induced (prolonged methotrexate, oxyphenisatin, alpha-methyldopa, nitrofurantoin, isoniazid) (3) Iron overload (hemochromatosis, hemosiderosis)
  B. INFLAMMATION: Viral hepatitis
  C. BILIARY OBSTRUCTION: (1) Cystic fibrosis (2) Inflammatory bowel disease (3) Primary biliary cirrhosis (4) Obstructive infantile cholangiopathy
  D. VASCULAR: (1) Prolonged CHF (2) Hepatic venoocclusive disease
  E. NUTRITIONAL: (1) Intestinal bypass (2) Severe steatosis (3) Abetalipoproteinemia
  F. HEREDITARY: (1) Wilson disease (2) Alpha-1-antitrypsin deficiency (3) Juvenile polycystic kidney disease (4) Galactosemia (5) Type IV glycogen storage disease (6) Hereditary fructose intolerance (7) Tyrosinemia (8) Hereditary tetany (9) Osler-Weber-Rendu syndrome (10) Familial cirrhosis

Morphology: nodular regeneration
  (a) micronodular (1 – 5 mm): usually due to alcoholism
  (b) macronodular (up to several cm): usually due to hepatitis B
  (c) mixed: usually following bile duct obstruction

√ enlarged (early stage) / normal / shrunken liver
√ caudate lobe hypertrophy + shrinkage of right lobe; ratio of caudate to right lobe >0.65 on transverse images [sensitivity 43 – 84%, least sensitive in alcoholic cirrhosis, most sensitive in cirrhosis caused by hepatitis B; specificity 100%; 26% sensitivity; 84% accuracy] (DDx: Budd-Chiari syndrome)
√ thickening of fissures + porta hepatis
√ surface nodularity + indentations (regenerating nodules)
√ signs of portal hypertension
√ splenomegaly
√ ascites (failure of albumin synthesis, portal hypertension)
√ associated with fatty infiltration (in early cirrhosis)
US:
(sensitivity 65 – 80%; DDx: chronic hepatitis, fatty infiltration)
Hepatic signs:
√ hepatomegaly (63%)
√ hypertrophy of caudate lobe (26%)
√ surface irregularity (88 sensitivity, 95% specificity)
√ increased echogenicity in 66% (as a sign of superimposed fatty infiltration)
√ increased sound attenuation (9%)
√ heterogeneous coarse (usually) / fine echotexture (7%)
√ decreased / normal definition of walls of portal venules (sign of associated fatty infiltration NOT of fibrosis)

√ occasional depiction of isoechoic regenerating nodules
√ dilatation of hepatic arteries (increased arterial flow) with demonstration of intrahepatic arterial branches (DDx: dilated biliary radicles)
Extrahepatic signs:
√ splenomegaly
√ ascites
√ signs of portal hypertension
CT:
√ parenchymal inhomogeneity
√ decreased attenuation (steatosis) in early cirrhosis
√ occasionally depiction of isodense regenerating nodules
MR:
√ no alteration of liver parenchyma
√ regenerating nodules may have increased signal intensity
Angio:
√ stretched hepatic artery branches (early finding)
√ enlarged tortuous hepatic arteries = "corkscrewing" (increase in hepatic arterial flow)
√ shunting between hepatic artery and portal vein
√ mottled parenchymal phase
√ delayed emptying into venous phase
√ pruning of hepatic vein branches (normally depiction of 5th order branches) = postsinusoidal compression by developing nodules
NUC:
√ high blood pool activity secondary to slow clearance
√ colloid shift to bone marrow + spleen
√ shrunken liver with little or no activity + splenomegaly
√ mottled hepatic uptake (pseudotumors) on colloid scan with normal activity on IDA scans
√ displacement of liver + spleen from abdominal wall by ascites
Cx: (1) Ascites
     (2) Portal hypertension
     (3) Hepatocellular carcinoma (in 44% associated with macronodular cirrhosis, in 6% associated with micronodular cirrhosis)

Primary Biliary Cirrhosis

= CHRONIC NONSUPPURATIVE DESTRUCTIVE CHOLANGITIS
Histo: idiopathic progressive destructive cholangitis of interlobar and septal bile ducts, portal fibrosis, nodular regeneration, shrinkage of hepatic parenchyma
Age: 35 – 55 years; M:F = 1:9
• fatigue, pruritus
• xanthelasma / xanthoma (25%)
• hyperpigmentation (50%)
• insidious onset of pruritus (60%)
• IgM increased (95%)
• positive antimitochondrial antibodies (AMA) in 85 – 100%
√ normal extrahepatic ducts
√ cholelithiasis in 35 – 39%
√ hepatomegaly (50%)

√ tortuous intrahepatic ducts with narrowing + caliber variation / decreased arborization = "tree-in-winter" appearance

NUC:
- √ marked prolongation of hepatic Tc-99m IDA clearance
- √ uniform hepatic isotope retention
- √ normal visualization of GB and major bile ducts in 100%

DDx: (1) Sclerosing cholangitis (young men)
(2) CBD obstruction

Prognosis: mean survival 6 (range 3 – 11) years after onset of cholestatic symptoms

CLONORCHIASIS

Rarely of clinical significance

Country: Japan, Korea, Central + South China, Taiwan, Indochina

Organism: Chinese liver fluke = Clonorchis sinensis

Cycle: parasite cysts digested by gastric juice, larvae migrate up the bile ducts, remain in small intrahepatic ducts until maturity (10 – 30 mm in length), travel to larger ducts to deposit eggs

Infection: snail + fresh-water fish serve as intermediate hosts; infection occurs by eating raw fish; hog, dog, cat, humans are definite hosts

Path: (a) desquamation of epithelial bile duct lining with adenomatous proliferation of ducts + thickening of duct walls (inflammation, necrosis, fibrosis)
(b) bacterial superinfection with formation of liver abscess

- remittent incomplete obstruction + bacterial superinfection

√ multiple crescent- / stylette-shaped filling defects within bile ducts

Cx: (1) Bile duct obstruction (conglomerate of worms / adenomatous proliferation)
(2) Calculus formation (stasis / dead worms / epithelial debris)
(3) Jaundice in 8% (stone / stricture / tumor)
(4) Generalized dilatation of bile ducts (2%)

CONGENITAL BILIARY ATRESIA

Etiology: ? variation of same infectious process as in neonatal hepatitis with additional component of sclerosing cholangitis or vascular injury

Histo: proliferation of bile ducts in all portal triads

In 15% associated with: polysplenia, trisomy 18

NUC [phenobarbital-augmented cholescintigraphy] (90 – 97% sensitivity, 63 – 94% specificity, 90% accuracy):
Preparation of patient with 5 ng/kg/d phenobarbital twice a day for 3 – 7 days to stimulate biliary secretion (via induction of hepatic enzymes + increase in conjugation + excretion of bilirubin)
- √ good hepatic activity within 5 min
- √ delayed clearance from cardiac blood pool
- √ NO biliary excretion

√ NO visualization of bowel on delayed images at 6 and 24 hours

√ increased renal excretion

DDx: severe hepatocellular dysfunction

US:
- √ normal (visualization of gallbladder in 20%)

Rx: Kasai procedure (= portoenterostomy)
(a) child <60 days of age: 90% success rate
(b) child between 60 and 90 days of age: 50% success rate
(c) child >90 days of age: 17% success rate

CONGENITAL HEPATIC FIBROSIS

= congenital cirrhosis with rapid + fatal progression

Histo: fibrous tissue within hepatic parenchyma with excess numbers of distorted terminal interlobular bile ducts + cysts which rarely communicate with bile ducts

Age: usually present in childhood resulting in early death

Associated with: autosomal recessive type of polycystic kidney disease, medullary sponge kidney (80%)
- hepatosplenomegaly, portal hypertension
- predisposed to cholangitis + calculi

√ "lollipop-tree" = ectasia of peripheral biliary radicles
√ hepatosplenomegaly
√ periportal fibrosis + portosystemic collaterals

Cx: portal hypertension, hepatocellular carcinoma, cholangiocellular carcinoma

CYSTIC FIBROSIS

= autosomal recessive multisystem disorder with widespread abnormalities of mucus secreting exocrine glands

Incidence: 1:1,500 live births in Caucasians

Histo: increased pancreatic lobulation, fibrosis, replacement by fat, pancreatic atrophy, progressive dilatation of acini + ductules
- acute pancreatitis
- diabetes mellitus
- abnormal loss of electrolytes in sweat
- growth failure
- cirrhosis + portal hypertension
- rectal prolapse
- exocrine pancreatic insufficiency with malabsorption (90%) once 98% of entire pancreas is damaged
- obstructive lung disease
- chronic pulmonary infection (Pseudomonas colonization)

√ meconium peritonitis (50%)
Δ Intraperitoneal meconium may calcify within 24 hours!

@ Liver
Histo: focal biliary cirrhosis from inspissated bile (33%); mucus-containing cysts in gallbladder wall

√ portal hypertension + hepatosplenomegaly + hypersplenism
√ fatty infiltration of liver (if malabsorption untreated)
√ "microgallbladder" + cholecystolithiasis (rare)

@ Pancreas
obstruction of small pancreatic ducts as a result of precipitation of relatively insoluble proteins
√ increased pancreatic echogenicity
√ occasionally macroscopic pancreatic cysts (= dilated acini + ducts)
√ lipomatous pseudohypertrophy = complete fatty replacement of pancreas (-90 to -120 HU)
√ pancreatic calcifications

@ Small bowel
√ meconium ileus (10 – 15%) = obstruction usually at level of distal ileum
√ meconium ileus equivalent = episodes of low-grade obstruction later in life
√ thickened folds, dilatation, mucosal redundancy of duodenum
√ dilatation of Brunner glands

@ Colon
√ "microcolon" = colon of normal length but diminished caliber
√ "jejunization of colon" = coarse redundant + hyperplastic colonic mucosa (distended crypt goblet cells)
√ rectal prolapse between 6 months and 3 years in untreated patients

ECHINOCOCCAL DISEASE
Echinococcus granulosus
= HYDATID DISEASE (more common)
= E. cysticus; humans are accidental host
(a) <u>pastoral form</u>:   dog is definite host; intermediate hosts are cattle, sheep, horses, hogs; endemic in sheep-raising countries: Australia, New Zealand, North + East Africa, USSR, Mediterranean, Near + Middle East countries, Japan, Argentina, Chile, Uruguay
(b) <u>sylvatic form</u>:   wolf is definite host; intermediate hosts are deer, moose; endemic in northern Canada, Alaska

Cycle: ingestion of contaminated material; eggs hatch in duodenum; penetration of intestinal wall + mesenteric venules; larvae carried through body + deposited in capillary filters at various sites
Organs: liver (73%); lung (14%); peritoneum (12%); kidney (6%); spleen (4%); spinal cord; brain, bladder; thyroid; prostate; heart; eye; bone

Histo:
(1)   ENDOCYST (parasitic component of capsule)
    (a)   inner GERMINATIVE LAYER (resembling wet tissue paper) giving rise to brood capsules that may remain attached to cyst wall harboring up to 400,000 scolices / may detach + form sediment in cyst fluid = "hydatid sand" / may break up into numerous self-contained daughter cysts
    (b)   CYST MEMBRANE = laminated chitin-like substance

(2)   PERICYST / ECTOCYST = highly vascularized adventitial layer (resembling egg white), organized host granulation tissue replaces tissue necrosis (due to compression of expanding cyst), marginal vascular rim of 0.5 – 4 mm

• pain
• recurrent jaundice + biliary colic (transient obstruction by membrane fragments + daughter cysts expelled into biliary tree)
• blood eosinophilia (20 – 50%)
• urticaria + anaphylaxis (following rupture)
• Tests: 1. Casoni (60% sensitivity; may be falsely positive)
          2. Complement fixation double diffusion (65% sensitivity)
          3. Immunoelectrophoresis (most specific)
          4. Indirect hemagglutination (85% sensitivity)

Time to diagnosis: 11 – 81 (mean 51) years

Location: right lobe > left lobe of liver; multiple cysts in 20%
Size: up to 50 cm (average size of 5 cm), up to 16 liters of fluid
Plain film:
√ may have crescentic / ring-shaped / polycyclic calcifications (10 – 33%)
√ pneumohydrocyst (infection / communication with bronchial tree)
US:
√ complex heterogeneous mass (most common)
√ well-defined anechoic cyst (common)
√ "racemose" appearance = multiseptated cyst = daughter cysts internally and tangent to mother cyst (characteristic, but rare)
√ mass with eggshell calcification
√ floating undulating membrane / vesicles (characteristic, but rare)
CT:
√ well-demarcated low-density round mass ± internal septations
√ enhancement of cyst wall + septations
Angio:
√ avascular area with splaying of arteries
√ halo of increased density around cyst (inflammation / compressed liver)
Cholangiography:
√ cyst may communicate with bile ducts: right hepatic duct (55%), left hepatic duct (29%), CHD (9%), gallbladder (6%), CBD (1%)
Percutaneous aspiration:
• fluid analysis positive for hydatid disease in 70% (fragments of laminated membrane in 54%; scolices in 15%; hooklets in 15%)
Δ Risk of anaphylactic shock (0.5%); asthma (3%)

Cx: (1)   Compression of vital structures
        (2)   Infection
        (3)   Rupture

Echinococcus multilocularis
= E. alveolaris = less common but more aggressive
form of echinococcal disease; definite hosts are
rodents (moles, lemmings, wild mice) + domestic cat

Path: larvae proliferate by exogenous extension +
penetration of surrounding tissue (= diffuse +
infiltrative process resembling malignancy);
chronic granulomatous reaction with central
necrosis, cavitation, calcification

Location: widespread hematogenous dissemination is
not uncommon

√ geographic infiltrating lesion with ill-defined margins

√ faint / dense punctate calcifications (dystrophic
calcifications scattered throughout necrotic +
granulomatous tissue)

US:
  √ echogenic ill-defined single / multiple masses
  √ propensity of spread to liver hilum

CT:
  √ heterogeneous hypodense poorly marginated
  masses
  √ pseudocystic necrotic regions of near water density
  surrounded by hyperdense solid component

Angio:
  √ intrahepatic arterial tapering + obstruction

EPIDERMOID CYST OF SPLEEN
Histo: (1) mesothelial lining (2) squamous epithelial
lining = epidermoid cyst

Age: 2nd – 3rd decade

May be associated with polycystic kidney disease

(a) unilocular + solitary (80%)
(b) multiple + multilocular (20%)

√ average size of 10 cm

√ curvilinear calcification in wall (9 – 25%)

√ may contain cholesterol crystals, fat, blood

Cx: trauma, rupture, infection

FATTY LIVER
= FATTY INFILTRATION OF THE LIVER = HEPATIC
STEATOSIS

Causes:
(a) <u>Metabolic derangement</u>: diabetes mellitus (50%),
obesity, hyperlipidemia, acute fatty liver of
pregnancy, protein malnutrition, parenteral
hyperalimentation, malabsorption (jejunoileal
bypass), glycogen storage disease, glycogen
synthetase deficiency, cystic fibrosis, Reye
syndrome, corticosteroids, severe hepatitis, trauma,
congestive heart failure

(b) <u>Hepatotoxins</u>: alcohol (>50%), carbon chlorides,
phosphorus, chemotherapy

Histo: hepatocytes with large cytoplasmatic fat vacuoles
containing triglycerides; >5% fat of total liver
weight

• NO abnormal liver function tests

√ rapid change with time (few days to >10 months)
depending on clinical improvement (abstinence from
alcohol, improved nutrition) + degree of severity

Diffuse Fatty Infiltration
√ hepatomegaly (75 – 80%) / normal sized liver

Plain film:
  √ radiolucent liver sign = enlarged radiolucent liver

US (sensitivity >90%, accuracy 85 – 97%):
  √ increased sound attenuation (scattering of sound
  beam) = poor definition of posterior aspect of liver
  √ fine (more typical) / coarsened hyperechogenicity
  (compared with kidney)
  √ impaired visualization of borders of hepatic vessels
  √ attenuation of sound beam (feature of fat, NOT
  fibrosis)

CT:
  √ areas of lower attenuation than normal portal vein /
  IVC density
  √ reversal of liver-spleen density relationship
  (spleen is normally 6 – 12 HU below liver density)
  √ hyperdense intrahepatic vascular structures

NUC:
  Tc-99m sulfur colloid scan:
    √ diffuse heterogeneous uptake (68%)
    √ reversal of liver-spleen uptake (41%)
    √ increased bone marrow uptake (41%)
  Xe-133 ventilation scan:
    √ increased activity during wash-out phase (38%)

MR:
  √ slightly increased signal on T1WI + T2WI; relative
  insensitive (10% fat by weight will alter SE signal
  intensities by only 5 – 15%)
  √ fat turns black with Dixon technique

FAT-SPARED AREA in diffuse fatty infiltration
  √ hypoechoic ovoid / spherical / sheet-like mass
  Location: (a) quadrate lobe (anterior to portal vein
  bifurcation)
  (b) next to gallbladder bed
  (c) subcapsular skip areas
  √ NO mass effect (undisplaced course of vessels)
  DDx: tumor mass

Focal Fatty Infiltration
Etiology: ? vascular origin, focal tissue hypoxia

Distribution:
  (a) lobar / segmental uniform lesions
  (b) lobar / segmental nodular lesions
  (c) perihilar lesions
  (d) diffuse nodular lesions
  (e) diffuse patchy lesions
  predominantly in centrilobar + periportal regions,
  subcapsular distribution may be due to variants of
  blood supply (direct connections between peripheral
  portal radicles + perforating capsular / accessory
  cystic veins)

Location: right lobe, caudate lobe, perihilar region

√ fan-shaped lobar / segmental distribution with
angulated / interdigitating geographic margins

√ lesions extend to periphery of liver

√ NO mass effect (undisplaced course of vessels, no
bulging of liver contour)

US:
  √ hyperechoic area with poorly defined / sharp
    margins
  √ multiple / rarely single echogenic nodules
    simulating metastases (rare)
CT:
  √ patchy areas of decreased attenuation ranging from
    -40 to +10 HU (DDx: liver tumor)
  √ NO contrast enhancement
MR (not sensitive for fat):
  √ high signal on T1WI + low / isointense signal on
    T2WI
NUC with colloid:
  √ no significant changes on sulfur colloid images
    (SPECT imaging may detect focal fatty infiltration)
DDx: primary / secondary hepatic tumor

FOCAL NODULAR HYPERPLASIA

= rare benign congenital hamartomatous malformation or
  reparative process in areas of focal injury; probably
  develops as a result of preexisting vascular anomaly
Incidence:
  only 357 cases reported; 2nd most common benign
  tumor of liver; 4% of all primary hepatic tumors in
  pediatric population; twice as common as hepatocellular
  adenoma
Histo:
  composed of abnormally arranged hepatocytes,
  numerous bile ducts, vascularized fibrous septae,
  Kupffer cells; portal triads + central veins absent; bile
  duct proliferation within fibrous septae / between
  hepatocytes; difficult differentiation from regenerative
  nodules of cirrhosis + hepatocellular adenoma;
  frequently central fibrous scar in area of interconnection
  of fibrous bands (HALLMARK)
Age peak: 3rd – 5th decade (range: 7 months – 75
            years); M:F = 1:2 – 4
Associated with hepatic hemangioma (in 23%) if oral
                  contraceptives are used
Δ No definite association with oral contraceptives (11%)!
• initially often asymptomatic
• vague abdominal pain (10%) due to mass effect
• normal liver function
• hepatomegaly / abdominal mass
  √ size <5 cm (in 85%); right lobe:left lobe = 2:1
  √ well-circumscribed, non-encapsulated nodular cirrhotic-
    like mass in an otherwise normal liver
  √ NO calcifications
  √ pedunculated mass (in 5 – 20%)
  √ multiple masses (in 20%)
NECT:
  √ homogeneous mass of slightly decreased attenuation
CECT:
  √ transient hyperdensity on bolus injection followed
    rapidly by isodensity
  √ central stellate scar = central fibrous core with
    radiating fibrous septa (15%) (DDx: fibrolamellar
    HCC)
US:
  √ iso- / hypo- / hyperechoic (33%) homogeneous mass

  √ central scar in 18%
  √ may show high-velocity Doppler signals from
    arteriovenous shunts
NUC:
  Sulfur colloid scan:
    √ normal uptake (58 – 70%), cold spot (30 – 35%) /
      hot spot (7 – 10%); only FNH contains sufficient
      Kupffer cells to cause normal / increased uptake
      (rare DDx: hemangioma, hepatoblastoma, liver
      herniation, hepatocellular carcinoma)
  Tc-HIDA:
    √ normal / increased uptake (40 – 70%), cold spot
      (60%)
Angio:
  √ discretely marginated hypervascular mass (90%) with
    intense capillary blush / hypovascular (10%)
  √ enlargement of main feeding artery with central blood
    supply (= "spoked-wheel" pattern in 33%)
  √ homogeneous parenchymal stain
  √ decreased vascularity in central stellate fibrous scar
MR:
  √ usually nearly homogeneously isointense with liver on
    T1WI + T2WI
  √ central scar hypointense on T1WI + hyperintense on
    T2WI (bile stasis ± slow flowing blood)
Rx: resection for pedunculated mass; biopsy for
      extensive tumor
Cx: rupture with hemoperitoneum (increased incidence
      in patients on oral contraceptives — 14%)
DDx: hepatic adenoma (frequently tumor hemorrhage, no
       symptoms)

GALLBLADDER CARCINOMA

Most common biliary cancer (9 x more common than
  extrahepatic bile duct cancer);
5th most common gastrointestinal malignancy (after
  colorectal, pancreatic, gastric, esophageal carcinoma);
3% of all intestinal neoplasms
Incidence: 0.4 – 4.6% of biliary tract operations; 6,500
             deaths/year in United States
Peak age: 6 – 7th decade; M:F = 1:3 – 1:4
Histo: (a) well differentiated adenocarcinoma of
             scirrhous type (80 – 90%)
         (b) anaplastic carcinoma, squamous cell
             carcinoma, adenoacanthoma (10 – 20%)
         (c) carcinoid, sarcoma, basal cell carcinoma,
             lymphoma (extremely rare)
Predisposed: patients with porcelain gallbladder (22%);
               gallbladder polyp >2 cm is likely malignant

Associated with:
  (1) Gallstones in 65 – 98%
      Δ Gallbladder carcinoma occurs in only 1% of all
        patients with gallstones!
  (2) Porcelain gallbladder (in 22 – 60%): prevalence of
      gallbladder carcinoma in 11 – 22% of autopsies
  (3) Inflammatory bowel disease (predominantly
      ulcerative colitis, less common in Crohn disease)
  (4) Familial polyposis coli
  (5) Chronic cholecystitis

- history of past GB disease (50%)
- malaise, vomiting, weight loss
- RUQ pain (76%)
- obstructive jaundice (40 – 50%)
- abnormal liver function tests (20 – 75%)

Growth types:
- (a) replacement of gallbladder by mass (40 – 70%)
- (b) focal / diffuse asymmetric irregular thickening of GB wall (15 – 30%)
- (c) polypoid / fungating intraluminal mass with wide base (15 – 25%)

Location: usually in body / fundus; rarely in cystic duct
√ bulky tumor involving gallbladder fossa + adjacent liver + hepatoduodenal ligament
√ dilatation of biliary tree
√ liver metastases
√ enlarged regional lymph nodes (peripancreatic / in porta hepatis)
√ fine granular / punctate flecks of calcification (mucinous adenocarcinoma)

OCG:
√ non-visualization of gallbladder (2/3)

Metastases: in 75 – 77% at time of diagnosis
- (a) local invasion of liver (50 – 75%), duodenum (12%), colon (9%), stomach, bile duct, pancreas, right kidney, abdominal wall
- (b) lymphatic spread (50 – 63%): cystic duct node, CBD nodes, lesser omental nodes, superior + posterior pancreaticoduodenal nodes, periaortic nodes
- (c) intraperitoneal seeding (common)
- (d) hematogenous spread (less common): liver, lung, bones
- (e) neural spread (frequent): associated with more aggressive tumors
- (f) intraductal spread (least common): particularly in papillary adenocarcinoma

Cx: perforation of gallbladder + abscess formation
√ gallstones located within abscess
Prognosis: 75% unresectable at presentation; average survival is 6 months; 5% 1-year survival rate; 6% 5-year survival rate
DDx: (1) Xanthogranulomatous cholecystitis (lobulated mass filling gallbladder + stones)
(2) Acute / chronic cholecystitis (generalized gallbladder wall thickening <10 mm)
(3) Liver tumor invading gallbladder fossa
(4) Tumors from adjacent organs (pancreas, duodenum)
(5) Metastases (melanoma, leukemia, lymphoma)
(6) Polyps: cholesterol polyp, hyperplastic polyp, granulation polyp
(7) Adenomyomatosis

GALLSTONE ILEUS
1 – 3% of all intestinal obstructions (20% of obstruction in patients >65 years; 24% of obstructions in patients >70 years)

Incidence: develops in <1% of patients with cholelithiasis; in 1 of 6 perforations; risk increases with age; stones are commonly >2.5 cm in diameter
Age: average 65 – 75 years; M:F = 1:7
- acute colicky abdominal pain (20 – 30%)
- nausea, vomiting, fever, distension, obstipation

√ **Rigler triad** on plain film:
1. Partial / complete intestinal obstruction (usually small bowel), "string of rosary beads" = multiple small amounts of air trapped between dilated + stretched valvulae conniventes
2. Air in biliary tree
3. Ectopic calcified gallstone
√ change in position of previously identified gallstone
UGI / BE:
√ well-contained localized barium collection lateral to first portion of duodenum (barium-filled collapsed GB + possibly biliary ducts)
Fistulous communication:
cholecystoduodenal (60%), choledochoduodenal, cholecystocolic, choledochocolic, cholecystogastric
√ identification of site of obstruction: terminal ileum (60 – 70%), proximal ileum (25%), distal ileum (10%), pylorus, sigmoid, duodenum (Bouveret syndrome)

Cx: recurrent gallstone ileus in 5 – 10% (additional silent calculi more proximally)
Prognosis: high mortality

GLYCOGEN STORAGE DISEASE
= autosomal recessive diseases with varying severity and clinical syndromes
A. VON GIERKE (TYPE I)
Etiology: defect in glucose-6-phosphatase with excess deposition of glycogen in liver, kidney, intestines
Dx: failure of rise in blood glucose after glucagon administration
Age at presentation: infancy
√ hepatomegaly
US:
√ increased echogenicity (glycogen / fat)
CT:
√ increased (glycogen) / normal / decreased (fat) parenchymal attenuation
Prognosis: death in infancy, may survive into adulthood with early therapy
Cx: (1) Hepatic adenoma
(2) Hepatocellular carcinoma
B. CORI DISEASE (TYPE III)
C. ANDERSON DISEASE (TYPE IV)
D. HERS DISEASE (TYPE VI)

HEMOCHROMATOSIS
= excess iron deposition in various parenchymal organs (liver, pancreas, spleen, kidneys, heart) leading to cirrhosis with portal hypertension [HEMOSIDEROSIS = increased iron deposition without organ damage]

A. PRIMARY / IDIOPATHIC HEMOCHROMATOSIS
Cause:
   autosomal recessive disorder with mucosal defect in intestinal wall / increased absorption of intestinal iron
Incidence:
   1:220 whites of northern European ancestry; homozygote frequency up to 0.25%
Path:
   excess iron stored as crystalline iron oxide (ferric oxyhydroxide) within ferritin + hemosiderin; iron overload affects parenchymal cells (liver, pancreas, heart) NOT Kupffer cells / RE of bone marrow + spleen
- hyperpigmentation (90%)
- hepatomegaly (90%)
- arthralgias (50%)
- diabetes mellitus (30%)
- CHF + arrhythmias (15%)
- loss of libido, impotence, amenorrhea, testicular atrophy, loss of body hair
CT (60% sensitivity for iron):
   √ diffuse / rarely focal increase in liver density (up to 75 – 130 HU)
   √ depiction of hepatic veins on NECT
   √ dual energy CT (at 80 + 120 kVp) can quantitate amount of iron deposition
MR:
   √ significant signal loss in liver on T2WI with signal intensity equal to background noise
   √ pancreatic signal intensity equal to / less than muscle
Dx: liver biopsy
Cx: (1) Periportal fibrosis resulting in cirrhosis
       (2) Hepatocellular carcinoma (14 – 30%)
Rx: phlebotomies in precirrhotic stage

B. SECONDARY HEMOCHROMATOSIS
Cause:
   result of multiple blood transfusions (usually >40 units = 10 g of iron), increased absorption of normal dietary iron (eg, related to alcoholic liver disease), rhabdomyolysis, dietary iron overload (eg, Bantu siderosis)
Path:
   iron deposition initially in RES (phagocytosis of intact RBC) with sparing of parenchymal cells of pancreas; after saturation of RES storage capacity parenchymal cells of other organs accumulate iron
Age: 4 – 5th decade; M:F = 10:1
- little clinical significance
MR:
   √ signal loss in liver on T2WI with signal intensity greater than background noise (iron in Kupffer cells)
   √ splenic signal intensity less than muscle

HEPATIC ABSCESS
Etiology:
   (1) Obstructive biliary tract disease with cholangitis

(2) Portal pyemia (suppurative appendicitis, diverticular disease, colitis)
(3) Infarction from embolism
(4) Indwelling arterial catheters
(5) Direct spread from contiguous organ (cholecystitis, peptic ulcer, subphrenic sepsis)
(6) Trauma (rupture / laceration with direct contamination)
(7) Cryptogenic in 45% (invasion of cysts / dead tissue by pyogenic intestinal flora)
Types: pyogenic (88%), amebic (10%), fungal (2%)
Location: multiple in 50%
√ hepatomegaly
√ elevation of right hemidiaphragm
√ pleural effusion
√ right lower lobe atelectasis / infiltration
√ gas within abscess (esp. Klebsiella)
Cx: (1) Septicemia (2) Rupture into right subphrenic space (3) Rupture into abdominal cavity (4) Rupture into pericardium (5) Empyema (6) Common hepatic duct obstruction
Mortality: 100% if unrecognized / untreated

Pyogenic Liver Abscess
Organisms: E. coli, aerobic streptococci, S. aureus, anaerobic bacteria (45%)
Incidence: 0.016%
Etiology: (1) Ascending cholangitis (2) Portal phlebitis (3) Trauma (penetrating wounds, biopsy) (4) Direct spread from contiguous infection
Age: 6 – 7th decade; M > F
- pyrexia (79%)
- abdominal pain (68%)
- nocturnal sweating (43%)
- vomiting / malaise (39%)
- jaundice (0 – 20%)
- positive blood culture (50%)
Location: solitary abscess in right lobe (40 – 75%), in left lobe (2 – 10%); multiple abscesses in 50 – 67%
US:
   √ hypoechoic round lesion with well-defined mildly echogenic rim
   √ distal acoustic enhancement
   √ coarse clumpy debris / low-level echoes / fluid-debris level
   √ intensely echogenic reflections with reverberations (from gas) in 20 – 30%
CT:
   √ inhomogeneous hypodense single / multiloculated cavity
   √ "double target sign" = wall-enhancement + surrounding hypodense zone (30%)
NUC:
   √ photon-deficient area on sulfur colloid + IDA scan
   √ Ga-67 citrate uptake in 80%
   √ In-111 tagged WBC uptake is highly specific (since WBCs normally go to liver, may need sulfur colloid test for correlation)
Mortality: 20 – 80%

Amebic Abscess

Organism: Entamoeba histolytica
Etiology: spread of viable amebae from colon to liver via portal system
Incidence: in 1 – 25% of intestinal amebiasis
Age: 3rd – 5th decade; M:F = 4:1
- amebic dysentery
- amebic hepatitis (15%)

Location: liver abscess (right lobe) in 2 – 25%; systemic dissemination by invasion of lymphatics / portal system (rare) liver:lung:brain = 100:10:1
Size: 2 – 12 cm; multiple liver abscesses in 25%
√ nodularity of abscess wall (60%)
√ internal septations (30%)
√ not gas-containing (unless hepatobronchial / hepatoenteric fistula present)
NUC:
√ sensitivity of sulfur colloid scan is 98%
√ photon-deficient area surrounded by rim of uptake on Ga-67 scan
Aspiration:
typically opaque reddish / dirty brown / pink material ("anchovy paste / chocolate sauce"), usually sterile, parasite confined to margin of abscess

Cx: (1) Diaphragmatic disruption (rare) is strongly suggestive of amebic abscess
(2) Fistulization into colon, right adrenal gland, bile ducts, pericardium
Rx: conservative treatment with chloroquine / metronidazole (Flagyl®)

HEPATIC ADENOMA

= HEPATOCELLULAR ADENOMA = LIVER CELL ADENOMA
= rare benign neoplasm, most frequent hepatic tumor in young women after use of contraceptive steroids; not seen in males unless on anabolic steroids
Path:
no true capsule; pseudocapsule due to compression of liver tissue; high incidence of hemorrhage and necrosis; no scar
Histo:
solitary spherical benign growth of hepatocytes; sheets of hepatocytes without portal veins, central veins; scattered thin-walled vascular channels + bile canaliculi; decrease in number of abnormally functioning Kupffer cells; hepatocytes contain increased amounts of glycogen ± fat
Associated with oral contraceptives (2.5 x risk after 5-year use, 7.5 x risk after 9-year use, 25 x risk >9-year use), steroids, pregnancy, diabetes mellitus, type Ia glycogen storage disease (von Gierke) in 60%

Δ Pregnancy may increase tumor growth rate + lead to tumor rupture!
Δ Tumor remission may occur with dietary therapy leading to normal insulin, glucagon and serum glucose levels

- asymptomatic (20%)
- RUQ pain as sign of mass effect (40%) / intratumoral or intraperitoneal hemorrhage (40%)
- hepatomegaly

Location: right lobe of liver in subcapsular location (75%)
√ round well-circumscribed mass; between 6 – 30 cm in size (average size of 8 – 10 cm)
√ intraparenchymal / pedunculated (in 10%)
CT:
√ round mass of decreased density; areas of necrosis (30 – 40%)
√ hyperdense areas of fresh intratumoral hemorrhage (22 – 50%)
√ variable patterns of enhancement, does not enhance to the same degree as normal liver
US:
√ usually small well-demarcated solid echogenic / complex hyper- and hypoechoic heterogeneous mass with anechoic areas (if large)
MR:
√ inhomogeneous on all pulse sequences (indistinguishable from HCC)
√ may have hyperintense areas on T1WI (due to presence of fat)
√ isointense (sheets of hepatocytes) and hyperintense areas (necrosis, hemorrhage) on T2WI
NUC:
√ focal photopenic lesion on sulfur colloid scan (because lesion composed of hepatocytes + nonfunctioning Kupffer cells) surrounded by rim of increased uptake (due to compression of adjacent normal liver containing Kupffer cells); may show uptake equal to / slightly less than liver (23%)
√ usually increased activity on HIDA scan
√ NO gallium uptake
Angio:
√ usually hypervascular mass
√ homogeneous but not intense stain in capillary phase
√ enlarged hepatic artery with feeders at tumor periphery (50%)
√ hypo- / avascular regions (secondary to hemorrhage / necrosis)
√ neovascularity
CAVE: percutaneous biopsy carries high risk of bleeding!
Cx:
(1) Spontaneous hemorrhage with subcapsular hematoma / hemoperitoneum (41%)
(2) Malignant transformation (? contiguous development of hepatocellular carcinoma)
(3) Recurrence after resection
Rx: surgical resection
DDx: hepatocellular carcinoma

HEPATIC ANGIOSARCOMA

= HEMANGIOENDOTHELIAL SARCOMA = KUPFFER CELL SARCOMA = HEMANGIOSARCOMA
= extremely rare tumor (0.2 per million) with rapid metastatic spread

Etiology: (1) Thorotrast (latent period of 15 – 24 years)
(2) Arsenic
(3) Polyvinyl chloride (latent period of 4 – 28 years)

Age: 6 – 7th decade

Metastases to:
lung, spleen, porta hepatis nodes, portal vein, thyroid, peritoneal cavity, bone marrow (rapid metastatic spread)

√ areas of increased density in RES (liver, spleen, lymph nodes)

√ portal vein invasion

NUC:
√ cold defect on sulfur colloid sc

US:
√ solid / mixed mss with anechoic areas (hemorrage / necrosis)

CT:
√ hypodense masses with high density regions (hemorrhage / necrosis)
√ striking peripheral enhancement

Angio:
√ hypervascular stain around tumor periphery, NO arterial encasement

Prognosis: death within 1 year

HEPATIC CYST

= second most common benign hepatic lesion (22%)

A. ACQUIRED HEPATIC CYST
secondary to trauma, inflammation, parasitic infestation, neoplasia

B. CONGENITAL HEPATIC CYST
= defective development of aberrant intrahepatic bile ducts

Incidence: liver cysts detected at autopsy in 50%; in 22% detected during life

Age of detection: 5th – 8th decade

Histo: cysts surrounded by fibrous capsule + lined by columnar epithelium, related to bile ducts within portal triads

Associated with:
(1) Tuberous sclerosis
(2) Polycystic kidney disease (25 – 33% have liver cysts)
(3) Polycystic liver disease: autosomal dominant; M:F = 1:2 (50% have polycystic kidney disease)

• hepatomegaly (40%); pain (33%); jaundice (9%)

Size of cyst:
range from microscopic to huge (average 1.2 cm; in 25% largest cyst <1 cm; in 40% largest cyst >4 cm; maximal size of 20 cm); multiple cysts spread throughout liver (in 60%) / solitary cyst

√ "cold spot" on IDA, Ga-68, Tc-99m sulfur colloid scans

√ echo-free cyst, may show fluid-fluid interface

HEPATIC HEMANGIOMA
Cavernous Hemangioma of Liver

most common benign liver tumor (78%); second most common liver tumor after metastases

Incidence: 4%; autopsy incidence 0.4 – 7.3%; increased with multiparity

Age: rarely seen in young children; M:F = 1:5

Histo:
large vascular channels filled with slowly circulating blood; lined by single layer of mature flattened endothelial cells separated by thin fibrous septa; no bile ducts; thrombosis of vascular channels common resulting in fibrosis + calcifications

Associated with:
(1) Hemangiomas in other organs
(2) Focal nodular hyperplasia
(3) Rendu-Osler-Weber disease

• asymptomatic if tumor small (50 – 70%)
• may present with hemorrhage if large (5%)
• hepatomegaly
• may enlarge during pregnancy
• abdominal discomfort + pain (from thrombosis in large hemangioma)
• **Kasabach-Merritt syndrome** (= hemangioma + thrombocytopenia) rare

Location: frequently peripheral / subcapsular in posterior right lobe of liver; 20% are pedunculated; multiple in 10%

Size: <4 cm (90%); giant cavernous hemangioma of over 4 cm (10%)

√ may have central area of fibrosis = areas of nonenhancement / nonfilling / cystic space (occurrence increases with age)

√ calcifications (phleboliths / septal calcifications) are extremely uncommon

US:
√ hyperechoic (60 – 70%) / hypoechoic (20%) / mixed pattern (20%) mass with discrete margins
√ homogeneous (58 – 73%) / heterogeneous (fibrosis, thrombosis, hemorrhagic necrosis)
√ hypoechoic center possible
√ may show acoustic enhancement (37 – 77%)
√ unchanged in size / appearance (82%) on 1 – 6 year follow-up
√ no Doppler signals / signals with peak velocity of <50 cm/sec

CT (combination of precontrast images, good bolus, dynamic scanning):
√ well-circumscribed spherical / ovoid low-density mass
√ may have areas of higher / lower density within mass
√ typical pattern of low-density on NECT + peripheral enhancement + complete fill-in on delayed images 3 – 30 minutes post IV bolus (55 – 89%)
√ peripheral (72%) / central (in 8%) / diffuse dense (in 8%) enhancement
√ complete (75%) / partial (24%) / no (2%) fill-in to isodensity in delayed phase

Angio (historical gold standard):
√ dense opacification of well-circumscribed, dilated, irregular, punctate vascular lakes / puddles in late arterial + capillary phase starting at periphery in ring- / C-shaped configuration

√ normal-sized feeders; AV shunting (very rare)
√ contrast persistence late into venous phase
NUC (95% accuracy with SPECT):
Indication: lesions >2 cm (detectable in 70 – 90%)
√ delayed filling on Tc-99m labeled RBC scans (dose of 15 – 20 mCi) with increased activity on delayed images at 1 – 2 hours
√ cold defect on sulfur colloid scans
MR (90 – 95% accuracy):
√ spheroid / ovoid (87%) mass with smooth well-defined margins (87%); no capsule
√ homogeneous internal architecture if <4 cm, hypointense internal inhomogeneities if >4 cm
√ hypo- / isointense on T1WI; hyperintense "light bulb" appearance on T2WI (due to slow flowing blood) (DDx: hepatic cyst, hypervascular tumor, necrotic tumor, cystic neoplasm)
√ peripheral enhancement with subsequent fill-in toward center after gadolinium-DTPA
Bx: may be biopsied safely provided normal liver is present between tumor + liver capsule
√ nonpulsatile blood (73%)
√ endothelial cells without malignancy (27%)
Cx (rare): (1) Spontaneous rupture (4.5%)
(2) Abscess formation
(3) Kasabach-Merritt syndrome (platelet sequestration)

Infantile Hemangioendothelioma of Liver
= INFANTILE HEPATIC HEMANGIOMA = CAPILLARY / CAVERNOUS HEMANGIOMA
= most common benign hepatic tumor in infants
Histo: thick-walled endothelium-lined vascular spaces similar to cavernous hemangioma but with multiple layers and scattered bile ducts; involutional changes (infarction, hemorrhage, necrosis, scarring)
Classification:
(a) Hemangioendothelioma type 1: orderly proliferation of small blood vessels
(b) Hemangioendothelioma type 2: more aggressive histologic pattern
(c) Cavernous hemangioma: dilated vascular spaces lined by flat endothelial cells
Δ Relationship to adult cavernous hemangioma unknown!
Age at presentation: <6 months (in 85%)
M:F = 2:1
• abdominal mass secondary to hepatomegaly
• cutaneous hemangiomas (45%)
• may present with high-output CHF secondary to AV shunts (15%)
Size: several mm up to 15 cm
√ diffuse involvement of entire liver, rarely focal; single / multiple
Plain film:
√ fine speckled / fibrillary calcifications (DDx: hepatoblastoma, hamartoma, metastatic neuroblastoma)

US:
√ predominantly hypoechoic / complex / hyperechoic lesion
√ multiple sonolucent areas (= enlarging vascular channels secondary to initial rapid growth) (DDx: mesenchymal hamartoma)
CT:
√ focal areas of low attenuation with early peripheral enhancement + variable delayed central enhancement (similar to cavernous hemangioma)
MRI:
√ inhomogeneous on T1WI + T2WI (hemorrhage, necrosis, scarring)
√ varying degrees of hyperintensity on T2WI (resembling hemangioma)
NUC:
√ early appearance of tracer in liver
√ marked delay in tracer clearance
√ multiple defects on static images
Angio:
√ enlargement of celiac + hepatic arteries
√ rapid decrease in aortic caliber below celiac trunk
√ enlarged, tortuous feeding arteries and stretched intrahepatic vessels
√ hypervascular tumor with inhomogeneous stain; clusters of small abnormal vessels
√ pooling of contrast material in sinusoidal lakes with rapid clearing through early venous drainage (AV shunting)

Prognosis: tendency to involute within 6 – 8 months; reduction in size with steroids / radiotherapy
Cx: (1) Congestive heart failure
(2) Disseminated intravascular coagulopathy
(3) Thrombocytopenia (platelet trapping)

HEPATITIS
A. ACUTE HEPATITIS
US:
√ decreased parenchymal echogenicity
√ increased brightness of portal venule walls ("starry sky" pattern) = centrilobular pattern (DDx: leukemic infiltrate, diffuse lymphomatous involvement, toxic shock syndrome)

B. CHRONIC HEPATITIS
US:
√ increased liver echogenicity
√ coarsening of parenchymal texture
√ silhouetting of portal vein walls = loss of definition of portal venules
√ NO sound attenuation

HEPATOBLASTOMA
Incidence: 3rd most common abdominal tumor in children; most frequent malignant hepatic tumor in children (51%)
Incidence increased with: hemihypertrophy, Beckwith syndrome

Histo: small cells resebling embryonal / fetal liver +
mesenchymal cells (osteoid, cartilagenous,
fibrous tissue)
Age: <3 years; <18 months (in 50%); range from
newborn to 15 years; M:F = 2:1
- upper abdominal mass, weight loss, nausea, vomiting
- precocious puberty (production of endocrine
substanes)
- persistently + markedly elevated alpha-fetoprotein
(66%)
Location: right lobe of the liver
√ coarse calcifications / osseous matrix (12 – 30%)
US:
√ large heterogeneous echogenic mass, sometimes
with calcifications, occasionally cystic areas (necrosis
/ extramedullary hematopoiesis)
CT:
√ hypointense tumor with peripheral rim enhancement
MR:
√ inhomogeneously hypointense on T1WI with
hyperintense foci (hemorrhage)
√ inhomogeneously hyperintense with hypointense
bands (fibrous septae) on T2WI
NUC:
√ photopenic defect
Angio:
√ hypervascular mass with dense stain
√ marked neovascularity; NO AV-shunting
√ vascular lakes may be present
√ avascular areas (secondary to tumor necrosis)
√ may show caval involvement (= unresectable)

Prognosis: 60% resectable; 75% mortality; better
prognosis than hepatoma
DDx: hemangioendothelioma (fine granular
calcifications), metastatic neuroblastoma,
mesenchymal hamartoma, hepatocellular
carcinoma (>5 years of age, no calcifications)

HEPATOCELLULAR CARCINOMA

= HEPATOMA = most frequent primary visceral
malignancy in the world; 80 – 90% of all primary liver
malignancies; 2nd most frequent malignant hepatic
tumor in children (39%) after hepatoblastoma

Incidence: (a) in industrialized world: 0.2 – 0.8%
(b) in sub-Saharan Africa, Southeast Asia,
Japan, Greece, Italy: 5.5 – 20%
Peak age:
(a) industrialized world: 6th – 7th decade; M:F = 2.5:1
fibrolamellar subtype (in 3 – 10%) below age 40
years
(b) high incidence areas: 30 – 40 years; M:F = 5:1
(c) in children: >5 years of age; M:F = 4:3

Etiology:
1. Cirrhosis (60 – 90%)
Latent period: 8 months – 14 years from onset
of cirrhosis

Incidence of HCC:
— 44% in macronodular (= postnecrotic)
cirrhosis due to hepatitis B virus, alcoholism,
hemochromatosis
— 6% in micronodular cirrhosis due to
alcoholism
Δ 5% of alcoholic cirrhotics develop HCC!
(a) alcohol (c) cardiac
(b) hemochromatosis (d) biliary atresia
2. Chronic hepatitis B / C; 12% develop HCC
3. Carcinogens
(a) aflatoxin
(b) siderosis
(c) oral contraceptives / anabolic androgens
(d) Thorotrast
4. Inborn errors of metabolism
(a) alpha-1-antitrypsin deficiency
(b) galactosemia
(c) type I glycogen storage disease (von Gierke)
(d) Wilson disease
(e) tyrosinosis

mnemonic: "WHAT causes HCC"
Wilson disease
Hemochromatosis
Alpha-1-antitrypsin deficiency
Tyrosinosis
Hepatitis
Cirrhosis (alcoholic, biliary, cardiac)
Carcinogens (aflatoxin, sex hormones, Thorotrast)

Histo: HCC cells resemble hepatocytes in appearance +
structural pattern (trabecular, pseudoglandular,
compact, scirrhous);
(a) expansive encapsulated HCC: collapsed
portal vein branches at capsule
(b) infiltrative nonencapsulated HCC: portal
venules communicate with tumoral sinusoids
= often invasion of portal ± hepatic veins
GROWTH PATTERN:
(a) solitary massive (27 – 59%):
bulk in one (most often right) lobe involved with
satellite nodules
(b) multicentric small nodular (15 – 26%):
small foci of up to 5 cm in both hepatic lobes
(c) diffuse microscopic (15 – 51%):
tiny indistinct nodules closely resembling cirrhosis

- elevated alpha-fetoprotein (90%), negative in
cholangiocarcinoma
- elevated liver function tests
- persistent RUQ pain, hepatomegaly, ascites
- fever, weight loss, malaise
- Paraneoplastic syndromes:
(a) sexual precocity / gynecomastia
(b) hypercholesterolemia
(c) erythrocytosis (tumor produces erythropoietin)
(d) hypoglycemia
(e) hypercalcemia
(f) carcinoid syndrome

Metastases to: lung (most common = 8%), adrenal, lymph nodes, bone

√ portal vein invasion (25 – 40%)
√ invasion of hepatic vein (16%) / IVC (= Budd-Chiari syndrome)
√ occasionally invasion of bile ducts
√ NO calcifications in usual HCC; however, common in fibrolamellar (30 – 40%) and sclerosing HCC
√ hepatomegaly and ascites

NUC:
√ Sulfur colloid scan: single cold spot (70%), multiple defects (15 – 20%), heterogeneous distribution (10%)
√ Tc-HIDA scan: cold spot / atypical uptake in 4% (delayed images)
√ Gallium-scan: avid accumulation in 70 – 90%
CT (accuracy >80%):
√ hypodense mass / rarely isodense / hyperdense in fatty liver
√ circular zone of radiolucency surrounding the mass
CECT:
√ uni- / multifocal mass of decreased attenuation with inhomogeneous areas of contrast accumulation
√ enhancement during arterial phase (80%)
√ thin contrast-enhancing capsule (50%)
√ isodensity on delayed scans (10%)
CT with intraarterial Ethiodol injection:
√ hyperdense mass detectable as small as 0.5 cm
US (86 – 99% sensitivity, 90 – 93% specificity, 65 – 94% accuracy):
√ hyperechoic HCC (13%) due to fatty metamorphosis or marked dilatation of sinusoids
√ hypoechoic HCC (26%) due to solid tumor
√ HCC of mixed echogenicity (61%) due to nonliquefactive tumor necrosis
√ Doppler peak velocity signals >250 cm/sec
MR:
√ hypointense (50%) / iso- to hyperintense (with fatty metamorphosis) on T1WI
√ ring sign = well-defined hypointense capsule on T1WI (24 – 44%), double layer of inner hypointensity (fibrous tissue) + outer hyperintensity (compressed blood vessels + bile ducts) on T2WI in expansive-type of HCC
√ hyperintense on T2WI
√ Gd-DTPA enhancement peripherally (21%) / centrally (7%) / mixed (10%) / no enhancement (21%)

Angio:
√ "thread and streaks" = linear parallel vascular channels coursing along portal venous radicles seen with portal venous involvement
√ in differentiated HCC: enlarged arterial feeders, coarse neovascularity, vascular lakes, dense tumor stain, arterioportal shunts
√ in anaplastic HCC: vascular encasement, fine neovascularity, displacement of vessels + corkscrew-like vessels of cirrhosis

Fibrolamellar Hepatocellular Carcinoma
NO underlying cirrhosis or known risk factors
• alpha-fetoprotein negative
Age: 5 – 35 (mean 23) years; M:F = 1:1
Path: well-circumscribed strikingly desmoplastic tumor with calcifications + fibrous central scar
Histo: hepatocytes with granular eosinophilic cytoplasm separated by broad bands of fibrous stroma
√ partially / completely encapsulated solitary mass 4 – 17 cm in diameter
√ prominent depressed central fibrous scar
√ central stellate / trabecular calcifications (30 – 40%)
MRI:
√ heterogeneously hpointense on T1WI; hyperintense on T2WI
√ central scar hypointense on T1WI + T2WI (DDx: hyperintense scar on T2WI in FNH)

Prognosis:
>90% overall mortality; 17% resectability rate (48% for fibrolamellar subtype); 6 months average survival time (32 months for fibrolamellar subtype); 30% 5-year survival time (63% for fibrolamellar subtype)
Cx: spontaneous rupture (in 8%)
Rx: (1) Resection (2) I-131 antiferritin IgG (remission rate >40% up to 3 years)

HYPERPLASTIC CHOLECYSTOSIS
= variety of degenerative + proliferative changes of gallbladder wall characterized by hyperconcentration, hyperexcitability, and hyperexcretion
Incidence: 30 – 50% of all cholecystectomy specimens; M:F = 1:6

Cholesterolosis
= abnormal deposits of cholesterol esters in macrophages within lamina propria (foam cells) + in mucosal epithelium

1. STRAWBERRY GALLBLADDER
= LIPID CHOLECYSTITIS = CHOLESTEROSIS
= planar form = seedlike patchy / diffuse thickening of the villous surface pattern (disseminated micronodules)
Associated with cholesterol stones in 50 – 70%
• not related to serum cholesterol level
√ radiologically not demonstrable

2. CHOLESTEROL POLYP (90%)
= polypoid form
= abnormal deposit of cholesterol ester producing a villouslike structure covered with a single layer of epithelium and attached via a delicate stalk
Δ Most common fixed filling defect of GB
Location: commonly in middle 1/3 of gallbladder
√ multiple small filling defects <10 mm in diameter
DDx: papilloma, adenopapilloma, inflammatory granuloma

Adenomyomatosis of Gallbladder
= increase in number + height of mucosal folds
Histo: hyperplasia of epithelial + muscular elements
with mucosal outpouching of epithelial-lined cytic
spaces into (46%) or all the way through (30%) a
thickened muscular layer as tubules / crypts /
saccules (= intramural diverticula = Rokitansky-
Aschoff sinus); develop with increasing age

Incidence: 5% of all cholecystectomies
Age: >35 years;   M:F = 1:3
Associated with: (1) Gallstones in 25 – 75%
             (2) Cholesterolosis in 33%

(a) generalized form = ADENOMYOMATOSIS
    √ "pearl necklace gallbladder" = tiny extraluminal
    extensions of contrast on OCG (enhanced after
    contraction)
(b) segmental form
    compartmentalization most often in neck / distal 1/3
(c) localized form in fundus = ADENOMYOMA
    √ smooth sessile fundal mass in GB fundus
    = solitary adenomyoma + extraluminal
    diverticulalike formation
(d) annular form
    √ "hourglass" configuration of GB with transverse
    congenital septum

HYPOSPLENISM
= no uptake of Tc-99m sulfur colloid

A. ANATOMIC ABSENCE OF SPLEEN
   1. Congenital asplenia = Ivemark syndrome
   2. Splenectomy
B. FUNCTIONAL ASPLENIA
   = spleen anatomically present without uptake of Tc-
   99m sulfur colloid
   1. Circulatory disturbances:
   occlusion of splenic artery / vein,
   hemoglobinopathies (sickle cell disease,
   hemoglobin-SC disease, thalassemia),
   polycythemia vera, idiopathic thrombocytopenic
   purpura
   2. Altered RES activity:
   Thorotrast irradiation, combined splenic irradiation
   + chemotherapy, replacement of RES by tumor /
   infiltrate, splenic anoxia (cyanotic congenital heart
   disease), sprue
   3. Autoimmune disease
      Cx: children at risk for pneumococcal
            pneumonia (liver partially takes over
            immune response later in life)
C. FUNCTIONAL ASPLENIA + SPLENIC ATROPHY
   Ulcerative colitis, Crohn disease, celiac disease,
   tropical sprue, dermatitis herpetiformis, thyrotoxicosis,
   idiopathic thrombocytopenic purpura, Thorotrast
D. FUNCTIONAL ASPLENIA + NORMAL / LARGE
   SPLEEN
   Sarcoidosis, amyloidosis, sickle cell anemia (if not
   infarcted)

• RBC (acanthocytes, siderocytes)
• lymphocytosis, monocytosis
• Howell-Jolly bodies (intraerythrocytic inclusions)
• thrombocytosis
√ spleen not visualized on Tc-99m sulfur colloid
√ Tc-99m heat-damaged RBCs / In-111 labeled platelets
  may demonstrate splenic tissue if Tc-99m sulfur colloid
  does not
Cx: increased risk of infection (pneumococcus,
      meningococcus, influenza)

KAWASAKI SYNDROME
= MUCOCUTANEOUS LYMPH NODE SYNDROME
= acute febrile multisystem vasculitis of unknown cause
  with a predilection for the coronary arteries
Incidence: average of 1.1:100,000 population per year
Histo: panvasculitis
Age: <5 years of age (in 85%); peak age of 1 – 2 years;
      M:F = 1.5:1
• fever >5 days
• mucosal reddening (injected fissured lips, injected
  pharynx, strawberry tongue) in 99%
• cervical lymphadenopathy (82%)
• maculopapular rash on extensor surfaces (99%)
• bilateral nonpurulent conjunctivitis (96%)
• erythema of palms + soles with desquamation (88%)
Associated with:
  polyarthritis (30 – 50%), aseptic meningitis (25%),
  hepatitis (5 – 10%), pneumonitis (5 – 10%)

@ Cardiovascular system (1/3)
   1. Coronary artery abnormality (15 – 25%)
      √ coronary artery aneurysm:
      LCA (2/3), RCA (1/3); proximal segment in 70%;
      48% regress, 37% diminish in size
      √ coronary artery stenosis (39%):
      due to thrombus formation in aneurysm + intimal
      thickening
      √ coronary artery occlusion (8%) in aneurysms
      >9 mm
   2. Myocarditis (25%)
   3. Pericarditis
   4. Valvulitis
   5. Atrioventricular conduction disturbance
√ intestinal pseudoobstruction
√ transient gallbladder hydrops
Prognosis: 0.4 – 3% mortality (from myocardial
         infarction / myocarditis with congestive heart
         failure / rupture of coronary artery aneurysm)
Rx: aspirin (100 mg/kg per day) + gamma globulin

LIPOMA OF LIVER
Extremely rare
• asymptomatic
May be associated with   tuberous sclerosis
US:
   √ echogenic mass
   √ striking acoustic refraction (sound velocity in soft
   tissue 1,540 m/sec, in fat 1,450 m/sec)
Prognosis: no malignant potential

LIVER TRANSPLANT
BILIARY COMPLICATIONS (13 – 19%)
1. Biliary obstruction
   (a) stricture at anastoosis
   (b) tension mucocele of allograft cystic duct remnant
      √ extrinsic mass compressing CHD
      √ fluid collection adjacent to CHD
2. Bile leak

LYMPHOMA OF LIVER
A. Primary lymphoma (rare)
   √ solid solitary mass
B. Secondarylmphoma (common)
   Autoptic incidence of liver involvement:
      60% in Hodgkin disease
      50% in non-Hodgkin lymphoma
Pattern:
   (a) infiltrative diffuse (most common): no alteration in hepatic architecture
   (b) focal nodular: detectable by cross-sectional imaging
   (c) combination of diffuse + nodular (3%)
DETECTION RATE (for CT, MRI): <10%

MACROCYSTIC ADENOMA OF PANCREAS
= MUCINOUS CYSTIC NEOPLASM
= thick-walled uni- / multilocular benign tumor composed of large cystic spaces
Mean age: 50 years; in 50% between 40 – 60 years; M:F = 1:9
Histo: cysts lined by columnar, mucin-producing cells often in papillary arrangement, lack of cellular glycogen
   (a) cystadenoma
   (b) cystadenocarcinoma
Location: often in pancreatic tail (85%) / body, infrequently in head
√ well-demarcated thick-walled mass of 5 – 33 (mean 12) cm in diameter
√ uni- / multilocular large cysts >2 cm with septations
√ solid papillary excrescences protrude into the interior of tumor (sign of malignancy)
√ amorphous peripheral mural calcifications (15%)
√ hypovascular mass with sparse neovascularity
√ vascular encasement and splenic vein occlusion may be present
Metastases:
   √ round thick-walled cystic lesions in liver
Prognosis: invariable transformation into cystadenocarcinoma
DDx: pancreatic pseudocyst

MESENCHYMAL HAMARTOMA OF LIVER
= rare developmental cystic liver tumor
Histo: disordered arrangement of primitive mesenchyme, bile ducts, hepatic parenchyma; stromal / cystic predominance with cysts of a few mm up to 14 cm in size; no capsule
Age peak: 15 – 22 months (range from newborn to 19 years); M:F = 2:1

Location: right lobe:left lobe = 6:1; 20% pedunculated
√ 16 cm average tumor size (range of 5 – 29 cm)
√ grossly discernible cysts in 80%
US:
   √ multiple rounded cystic areas on an echogenic background
   √ may appear solid in younger infant (when cysts are still small)
CT:
   √ multiple lucencies of variable size + attenuation
NUC:
   √ one / more areas of diminished uptake on sulfur colloid scan
Angio:
   √ hypovascular mass
   √ may show patchy areas of neovascularity
   √ enlarged irregular tortuous feeding vessels

METASTASES TO LIVER
Incidence:
   liver is most common metastatic site after regional lymph nodes; incidence of metastatic carcinoma 20 x greater than primary carcinoma; metastases represent 22% of all liver tumors in patients with known malignancy; most common malignant lesion of the liver
Organ of origin: colon (42%), stomach (23%), pancreas (21%), breast (14%), lung (13%)
• hepatomegaly (70%)
• abnormal liver enzymes (50 – 75%)
Location : both lobes (77%), right lobe (20%), left lobe (3%)
Number : multiple (98%), solitary (2%)
√ involvement of liver + seen typical in lymphoma + melanoma
US: most sensitive imaging modality
NUC: 80 – 95% sensitivity in lesions >1.5 cm; lesions <1.5 cm are frequently missed; sensitivity increases with metastatic deposit size, peripheral location, and use of SPECT
NECT: important for hypervascular tumors (eg, renal cell carcinoma, carcinoid, islet cell tumors), which may be obscured by CECT
CECT:
   Technique:
      optimal is bolus technique with dynamic incremental scanning; sensitivity is decreased relative to NCCT if scans obtained during equilibrium phase of contrast administration
   √ no (35%), peripheral (37%), mixed (20%), central (8%) enhancement
   √ complete isodense fill-in on delayed scans (5%)
Δ CT-sensitivity 88 – 90%; specificity 99%; lesions of approx. 1 cm can usually be detected!
CT-Angiography:
   Indication: patients with potentially resectable isolated liver metastases / preoperative to partial hepatectomy for detection of additional metastases (additional lesions detected in 40 – 55%)

(1) CT arteriography = angiography catheter in hepatic artery, detects lesions by virtue of increased enhancement

(2) CT arterial portography = angiography catheter in SMA, detects hypodense lesions on a background of increased enhancement of normal surroundings in portal venous phase

CT-delayed iodine scanning:
= CT performed 4 – 6 hours following administration of 60 mg iodine results in detection of additional lesions in 27%

CALCIFIED LIVER METASTASES
Incidence: 2 – 3%
1. Mucinous carcinoma of GI tract (colon, rectum, stomach)
2. Endocrine pancreatic carcinoma
3. Leiomyosarcoma, osteosarcoma
4. Malignant melanoma
5. Papillary serous ovarian cystadenocarcinoma
6. Lymphoma
7. Pleural mesothelioma
8. Neuroblastoma
9. Breast cancer
10. Medullary carcinoma of the thyroid
11. Renal cell carcinoma
12. Lung carcinoma
13. Testicular carcinoma

HYPERVASCULAR LIVER METASTASES
1. Renal cell carcinoma
2. Carcinoid tumor
3. Colonic carcinoma
4. Choriocarcinoma
5. Breast carcinoma
6. Melanoma
7. Pancreatic islet cell tumor
8. Ovarian cystadenocarcinoma
9. Sarcomas
10. Pheochromocytoma

ECHOGENIC LIVER METASTASES
Incidence: 25%
1. Colonic carcinoma (mucinous adenocarcinoma) 54%
2. Hepatoma 25%
3. Treated breast carcinoma 21%

LIVER METASTASES OF MIXED ECHOGENICITY
Incidence: 37.5%
1.	Breast cancer	31%
2.	Rectal cancer	20%
3.	Lung cancer	17%
4.	Stomach cancer	14%
5.	Anaplastic cancer	11%
6.	Cervical cancer	5%
7.	Carcinoid	1%

CYSTIC LIVER METASTASES
1. Mucinous ovarian carcinoma
2. Colonic carcinoma
3. Sarcoma
4. Melanoma
5. Lung carcinoma
6. Carcinoid tumor

ECHOPENIC LIVER METASTASES
Incidence: 37.5%
1.	Lymphoma	44%
2.	Pancreas	36%
3.	Cervical cancer	20%
4.	Lung (adenocarcinoma)	
5.	Nasopharyngeal cancer	

MICROCYSTIC ADENOMA OF PANCREAS
= SEROUS CYSTADENOMA = GLYCOGEN-RICH CYSTADENOMA
= benign lobulated neoplasm composed of innumerable small cysts (1 – 20 mm) containing proteinaceous fluid separated by thin connective tissue septa

Incidence: approximately 50% of all cystic pancreatic neoplasms
Histo: cyst walls lined by cuboidal / flat glycogen-rich epithelial cells derived from centroacinar cells of pancreas (DDx: lymphangioma), thin fibrous pseudocapsule
Age: 34 – 88 years; mean age 65 years; 82% over 60 years of age;   M:F = 1:4
Associated with: von Hippel-Lindau syndrome
• pain, weight loss, jaundice
• palpable mass

Location: any part of pancreas affected, slight predominance for head
√ well-demarcated lobulated mass 4 – 25 (mean 13) cm in diameter
√ innumerable small <2 cm cysts; uncommonly larger cyst up to 8 cm in diameter
√ prominent central stellate scar
√ amorphous central calcifications (in 33% on plain film) in dystrophic area of stellate central scar ("sunburst")
√ pancreatic duct + CBD may be displaced, encased or obstructed
US:
√ solid predominantly echogenic mass with mixed hypoechoic + echogenic areas
CT:
√ attenuation values close to water
√ contrast enhancement
Angio:
√ hypervascular mass with dilated feeding arteries, dense tumor blush, prominent draining veins, neovascularity, occasional AV shunting, NO vascular encasement

Prognosis: no malignant potential
Rx: surgical excision / follow-up examinations

MILK OF CALCIUM BILE

= LIMY BILE = CALCIUM SOAP = precipitation of particulate material with high concentration of calcium carbonate, calcium phosphate, calcium bilirubinate

Associated with: chronic cholecystitis + gallstone obstruction of cystic duct

√ diffuse opacification of GB lumen with dependent layering

√ usually functionless GB on oral cholecystogram

US:
√ intermediate features between sludge + gallstones

MIRIZZI SYNDROME

= extrinsic right-sided compression of common hepatic duct by large gallstone impacted in cystic duct / gallbladder neck / cystic duct remnant; accompanied by chronic inflammatory reaction

Frequently associated with formation of fistula between gallbladder and common hepatic duct

• jaundice

√ normal CBD below level of impacted stone

√ TRIAD:
(1) gallstone impacted in GB neck
(2) dilatation of bile ducts above level of cystic duct
(3) smooth curved segmental stenosis of CHD

Cholangiography:
√ partial obstruction of CHD due to external compression on lateral side of duct / eroding stone

DDx: lymphadenopathy, neoplasm of GB / CHD

MULTIPLE BILE DUCT HAMARTOMA

= VON MEYENBURG COMPLEX

Incidence: 0.15 – 2.8% of autopsies

Etiology: failure of involution of embryonic bile ducts

Histo:
cluster of proliferated bile ducts lined by single layer of cuboidal cells embedded in fibrocollagenous tissue with single ramified lumen, communication with biliary system usually obliterated

Associated with polycystic liver disease

Size: 0.1 – 10 mm

CT:
√ multiple irregular hypodense lesions of up to 10 mm

US:
√ multiple small cysts / echogenic areas (if size not resolved) up to 10 mm ± comet-tail artifact

Angio:
√ multiple areas of abnormal vascularity in form of small grape-like clusters persisting into venous phase

DDx: metastatic liver disease

MULTIPLE ENDOCRINE NEOPLASIA

= MEN = MULTIPLE ENDOCRINE ADENOMAS (MEA)
= familial autosomal dominant adenomatous hyperplasia

Theory:
cells of involved principal organs originate from neural crest and produce polypeptide hormones in cytoplasmic granules, which allow **a**mine **p**recursors **u**ptake and **d**ecarboxylation = APUD cells

reminder:
Type I = Wermer syndrome   PPP
Type II = Sipple syndrome (Type IIA)   PMP
Type III = Mucosal neuroma syndrome (Type IIB) MPM

MEA	Type I	Type II	Type III
Pituitary adenoma	+		
Parathyroid adenoma	+	+	
Medullary thyroid carcinoma		+	+
Pancreatic island cell tumor	+		
Pheochromocytoma		+	+
Ganglioneuromatosis			+

MEN I Syndrome

= WERMER SYNDROME

Organ involvement:
1. Parathyroid (90%): mostly hyperplasia
2. Pancreatic islet cell tumor (80%):
   (a) gastrinoma = Zollinger-Ellison syndrome (most common type)
   (b) insulinoma
   (c) VIPoma = WDHH-syndrome (watery diarrhea, hypokalemia, hypochlorhydria)
3. Pituitary gland (40%): mostly adenoma
4. Combination of parathyroid + pancreas + pituitary involvement (40%)
5. Adrenal cortical tumors (40%)
6. Thyroid tumor (20%)

May be associated with carcinoid, lipoma, thymoma, buccal mucosal tumor, colonic polyposis, Ménétrièr disease

MEN II Syndrome

= SIPPLE DISEASE = MEN Type IIA

Organ involvement:
1. Medullary carcinoma of thyroid
2. Pheochromocytoma: often bilateral
3. Hyperparathyroidism

May be associated with carcinoid tumors, Cushing disease

MEN III Syndrome

= MUCOSAL NEUROMA SYNDROME = MEN Type IIB

Organ involvement:
1. Medullary carcinoma of thyroid
2. Pheochromocytoma
3. Oral + intestinal ganglioneuromatosis
   Δ Usually precedes the appearance of thyroid carcinoma + pheochromocytoma!

• Marfanoid appearance
• prognathism
• thickened lips (due to submucosal nodules)
• constipation alternating with diarrhea
@ GI tract
√ thickened / plaquelike colonic wall
√ dilated colon with abnormal haustral markings
√ alternating areas of colonic spasm + dilatation

NEONATAL HEPATITIS

Etiology: CMV, hepatitis A/B, rubella, toxoplasmosis, spirochetes, idiopathic

Path: multinucleated giant cells, bile ducts relatively free of bile

NUC:

Technique: often performed after pre-treatment with phenobarbital (5 mg/kg x 5 days) to maximize hepatic function

√ normal / decreased hepatic tracer accumulation

√ prolonged clearance of tracer from blood pool

√ bowel activity faint / delayed usually by 24 hours (best seen on lateral view; covering liver activity with lead shielding is helpful)

√ gallbladder may not be visualized

Prognosis: spontaneous remission

DDx: biliary atresia

PANCREAS DIVISUM

= failure of fusion of the ventral and dorsal anlage at 8th week of fetal life

(a) <u>dorsal anlage:</u> develops into tail, body, and cranial portion of pancreatic head; drains to the minor papilla through accessory duct of Santorini

(b) <u>ventral anlage:</u> arises between duodenum and liver bud; forms the caudal portion of the pancreatic head, uncinate process and CBD; the ventral duct of WIRSUNG drains with the CBD through ampulla of Vater and becomes the major drainage pathway for the entire pancreas after fusion with the duct of SANTORINI

Incidence: 4 – 14% in autopsy series; 1.3 – 6.7% in ERCP series; 3 – 7% in normal population; 12 – 26% in patients with idiopathic recurrent pancreatitis

Hypothesis: relative / actual stenosis of minor papilla predisposes to nonalcoholic pancreatitis in dorsal segment

Pancreatography: ONLY reliable means for diagnosis

√ contrast injection into major papilla demonstrates only short ventral pancreatic duct

CT:

√ oblique fat cleft between ventral + dorsal pancreas (25%)

√ failure to see union of dorsal + ventral pancreatic ducts (rare)

PANCREATIC DUCTAL ADENOCARCINOMA

= DUCT CELL ADENOCARCINOMA

Incidence: 80% of nonendocrine pancreatic neoplasms, 4th – 5th leading cause of cancer death in the United States

Etiology: alcohol abuse (4%), diabetes (2 x more frequent than in general population, particularly in females), hereditary pancreatitis (in 40%); cigarette smoking (risk factor 2 x)

Path: scirrhous infiltrative adenocarcinoma

Mean age at onset: 55 years; peak age in 7th decade; M:F = 2:1

Origin: – in 99% exocrine ductal epithelium
– in 1% acinar portion of pancreatic glands
– in 0.1% malignant ampullary tumor with better prognosis

STAGE I : confined to pancreas
II : + regional lymph node metastases
III : + distant spread

Extension:

(a) local extension beyond margins of organ (68%): posteriorly (96%), anteriorly (30%), into porta hepatis (15%), into splenic hilum (13%)

(b) invasion of adjacent organs (42%): duodenum > stomach > left adrenal gland > spleen > root of small bowel mesentery

Metastases:

liver (30 – 36%), regional lymph nodes >2 cm (15 – 28%), ascites from peritoneal carcinomatosis (7 – 10%), lung (pulmonary nodules / lymphangitic), pleura, bone

- weight loss, anorexia, fatigue
- pain in hypochondrium radiating to back
- obstructive jaundice (75%): most frequent cause of malignant biliary obstruction
- new onset diabetes (25 – 50%), steatorrhea
- thrombophlebitis

Location: pancreatic head (56 – 62%); body (26%); tail (12%)

Size: 2 – 10 cm (in 60% between 4 – 6 cm)

UGI:

√ "antral padding" = extrinsic indentation of the posteroinferior margin of antrum

√ "Frostberg 3" sign = inverted 3 contour to the medial portion of the duodenal sweep

√ spiculated duodenal wall + traction + fixation (neoplastic infiltration of duodenal mucosa / desmoplastic response)

√ irregular / smooth nodular mass with ampullary carcinoma

BE:

√ localized haustral padding / flattening / narrowing with serrated contour at inferior aspect of transverse colon / splenic flexure

√ diffuse tethering throughout peritoneal cavity (intraperitoneal seeding)

CT (99% detection rate for dynamic CT scan; 100% in predicting unresectability):

√ pancreatic mass (95%) / diffuse enlargement (4%) / normal scan (1%)

√ mass with central zone of diminished attenuation (75 – 83%)

√ pancreatic + bile duct obstruction without detectable mass (4%)

√ duct dilatation (58%): 3/4 biductal, 1/10 isolated to one duct; dilated pancreatic duct (67%); dilated bile ducts (38%)

√ atrophy of pancreatic body + tail (20%)

√ calcifications (2%)

√ postobstructive pseudocyst (11%)

√ obliteration of retropancreatic fat (50%)

√ thickening of celiac axis / SMA (invasion of perivascular lymphatics) in 60%
√ dilated collateral veins (12%)
√ thickening of Gerota fascia (5%)
√ local tumor extension posteriorly, into splenic hilum, into porta hepatis (68%)
√ contiguous organ invasion (duodenum, stomach, mesenteric root) in 42%

US:
√ hypoechoic pancreatic mass
√ focal / diffuse (10%) enlargement of pancreas
√ contour deformity of gland; rounding of uncinate process
√ dilatation of pancreatic ± biliary duct

Angiography (70% accuracy):
√ hypovascular tumor / neovascularity (50%)
√ arterial encasement: SMA (33%), splenic artery (14%), celiac trunk (11%), hepatic artery (11%), gastroduodenal artery (3%), left renal artery (0.6%)
√ venous obstruction: splenic vein (34%), SMV (10%)
√ venous encasement: SMV (23%), splenic vein (15%), portal vein (4%)

Cholangiography:
√ "rat tail / nipplelike" occlusion of CBD
√ nodular mass / meniscus-like occlusion in ampullary tumors

Pancreatography (abnormal in 97%):
√ irregular, nodular, rattailed, eccentric obstruction
√ localized encasement with prestenotic dilatation
√ acinar defect

Prognosis:
10% 1-year survival, 2% 3-year survival, <1% 5-year survival; 14 months medial survival after curative resection, 8 months after palliative resection, 5 months without treatment; tumors resectable in only 8 – 15% at presentation, 5% 5-year survival rate after surgery
DDx: focal pancreatitis, islet cell carcinoma, metastasis, lymphoma, normal variant

PANCREATIC ISLET CELL TUMORS
Origin: embryonic neuroectoderm, derivatives of APUD (amino precursor uptake and decarboxylation) cell line arising from islet of Langerhans (APUDOMA)
Prevalence: 1:100,000; isolated or part of MEN I syndrome
Average time from onset of symptoms to diagnosis is 2.7 years

Classification: (a)   functional (85%)
(b)   nonfunctional (below threshold of detectability) / hypofunctional
Metastases: in 60 – 90% to liver ± regional lymph nodes
√ calcifications highly suggestive of malignancy

Gastrinoma
2nd most common islet cell tumor; in alpha-cells / delta-cells
Age: 8% in patients <20 years; M > F

Path: (a)   islet cell hyperplasia (10%)
(b)   benign adenoma (30%): solitary / multiple (especially in MEN I)
(c)   malignant (60%) with metastases to liver, spleen, lymph nodes, bone
Associated with: MEN Type I (in 20 – 40%)
• Zollinger-Ellison syndrome: severe recurrent peptic ulcer disease, malabsorption, hypokalemia, gastric hypersecretion, hyperacidity / occasionally hypoacidity, diarrhea
• GI bleeding

Location: 50% solitary in head / tail; ectopic (7 – 33%) in duodenal wall / peripancreatic nodes / stomach / omentum
√ average tumor size 3.4 cm (up to 15 cm)
√ occasionally calcifications
√ successful angiographic localization in 70% (hypervascular lesion)
√ transhepatic portal venous sampling for gastrin (42%)
√ venous sampling after arterial stimulation with secretin (58%)
√ arteriography combined with intraarterial injection of secretin (77% sensitivity)
√ homogeneous hypoechoic mass (sonographic detection rate 50%)
CT:
√ transiently hyperdense on dynamic CT (majority)
√ thickening of gastric rugal folds

Glucagonoma
Uncommon tumor; derived from alpha cells; M < F
Associated with   MEN
• necrolytic erythema migrans (erythematous macules / papules on lower extremity, groin, buttocks, face)
• diarrhea, diabetes, glossitis, weight loss, anemia
Location: predominantly in pancreatic body / tail
√ tumor size 2.5 – 25 cm (mean 6.4 cm) with solid + necrotic components
√ hypervascular in 90%; successful angiographic localization in 15%
Prognosis: in 80% malignant transformation (liver metastases at time of diagnosis in 50%)

Insulinoma
Most common functioning islet cell tumor
Age: 4th – 6th decade; M:F = 2:3
Associated with: MEN Type I
Path: (a)   single benign adenoma (80 – 90%)
(b)   multiple adenomas / microadenomatosis (5 – 10%)
(c)   islet cell hyperplasia (5 – 10%)
(d)   malignant adenoma (5 – 10%)
• Whipple triad: starvation attack + hypoglycemia (fasting glucose <50 mg/dl) + relief by IV dextrose
• obesity
Location: no predilection for any part of pancreas, 2 – 5% in ectopic location; 10% multiple (especially in MEN I)
√ average tumor size 1 – 2 cm; <1.5 cm in 70%

√ solid homogeneous hypoechoic mass (intraoperative US very sensitive)

√ hypervascular tumor (66%): accurate angiographic localization in 50 – 90%

√ transhepatic portal venous sampling (correct localization in 95%)

√ venous sampling after arterial stimulation with calcium gluconate

Prognosis: malignant transformation in 5 – 10%

VIPoma

= solitary tumor liberating **V**asoactive **I**ntestinal **P**eptides relaxing vascular smooth muscle; sporadic occurrence

Histo: adenoma / hyperplasia

M:F = 1:2

- **WDHA syndrome** = **w**atery **d**iarrhea + **h**ypokalemia + **a**chlorhydria (more recently + more accurately described as) **WDHH syndrome** = **w**atery **d**iarrhea + **h**ypokalemia + **h**ypochlorhydria = "pancreatic cholera" = **Verner-Morrison syndrome**

Location:

(1) pancreas: from delta cells predominantly in pancreatic body / tail

(2) extrapancreatic: retroperitoneal ganglioblastoma, pheochromocytoma, lung, neuroblastoma (in children)

√ average size 5 – 10 cm with solid + necrotic tissue

√ mostly hypervascular tumor

√ dilatation of gallbladder

Prognosis: in 60% malignant transformation

DDx: small cell carcinoma of lung / neuroblastoma may also cause WDHH syndrome

Somatostatinoma

Somatostatin function:

suppresses release of growth hormone, TSH, insulin, glucagon, gastric acid, pepsin, secretin

Derived from delta cells

- diabetes, cholelithiasis, steatorrhea

Location: predominantly in pancreatic head

√ tumor size 0.6 – 20 cm (average >4 cm)

√ hypervascular

Prognosis: 50 – 90% malignant transformation

Nonfunctioning Islet Cell Tumors

Incidence:

3rd most common islet cell tumor after insulinoma + gastrinoma; 15 – 25% of all islet cell tumors

Derived from either alpha or beta cells

Age: 24 – 74 (mean 57) years

- mostly asymptomatic (hormonally quiescent)
- palpable mass, gastric outlet obstruction, jaundice, GI bleeding

Location: predominantly in pancreatic head

√ tumor size 6 – 20 cm (>5 cm in 72%) with solid + necrotic components

√ coarse nodular calcifications (20 – 25%)

√ CT contrast enhancement in 83%

√ hypoechoic mass

√ late dense capillary stain

√ large irregular pathological vessels with early venous filling

Prognosis: in 80 – 100% malignant transformation with metastases to liver + regional nodes; 60% 3-year survival; 44% 5-year survival

Rx: may respond to systemic chemotherapy

DDx: pancreatic ductal adenocarcinoma (hypovascular, smaller, encasement of SMA + celiac trunk)

PANCREATIC LIPOMATOSIS

Etiology:

1. Atherosclerosis of elderly
2. Obesity
3. Steroid therapy
4. Cushing syndrome
5. Main pancreatic duct obstruction
6. Cystic fibrosis
7. Malnutrition
8. Hemochromatosis
9. Viral infection
10. Schwachman-Diamond syndrome

US:

√ increased pancreatic echogenicity

CT:

√ "marbling" of pancreatic parenchyma / total fatty replacement / lipomatous pseudohypertrophy

PANCREATIC PSEUDOCYST

= collection of pancreatic fluid encapsulated by fibrous tissue

Etiology: (1) Acute pancreatitis; pseudocysts mature in 6 – 8 weeks

(2) Chronic pancreatitis

(3) Posttraumatic

(4) Pancreatic cancer

Incidence: 2 – 4% in acute pancreatitis

10 – 15% in chronic pancreatitis

Location: 2/3 within pancreas

Atypical location (may dissect along tissue planes in 1/3):

(a) intraperitoneal: mesentery of small bowel / transverse colon / sigmoid colon

(b) retroperitoneal: along psoas muscle; may present as groin mass / in scrotum

(c) intraparenchymal: liver, spleen, kidney

(d) mediastinal (through esophageal hiatus > aortic hiatus > foramen of Morgagni > erosion through diaphragm): may present as neck mass

Plain film / contrast radiograph:

√ smooth extrinsic indentation of posterior wall of stomach / inner duodenal sweep (80%)

√ indentation / displacement of splenic flexure / transverse colon (40%)

√ downward displacement of duodenojejunal junction

√ gastric outlet obstruction

√ splaying of renal collecting system / ureteral obstruction

US (pseudocyst detectable in 50 – 92%; 92 – 96% accuracy):
√ usually single + unilocular cyst
√ multilocular in 6%
√ fluid-debris level / internal echoes (may contain sequester, blood clot, cellular debris from autolysis)
√ septations (rare; sign of infection / hemorrhage)
√ may increase in size (secondary to hypertonicity of fluid, communication with pancreatic duct, hemorrhage, erosion of vessel)
√ obstruction of pancreatic duct / CBD
CT:
√ fluid in pseudocyst (0 – 30 HU)
√ cyst wall calcification (extremely rare)
Pancreatography:
√ communication with pancreatic duct in 50%

Cx (in 40%):
1. Rupture into abdominal cavity, stomach, colon, duodenum
2. Hemorrhage / formation of pseudoaneurysm
3. Infection
  √ gas bubbles (DDx: fistulous communication to GI tract)
  √ increase in attenuation of fluid contents
4. Intestinal obstruction
Prognosis: spontaneous resolution (in 20 – 50%) secondary to rupture into GI tract / pancreatic / bile duct
DDx: pancreatic cystadenoma, cystadenocarcinoma, necrotic pancreatic carcinoma, fluid-filled bowel loop, fluid-filled stomach, duodenal diverticulum, aneurysm

PANCREATITIS
Etiology:
A. IDIOPATHIC (20%)
B. ALCOHOLISM: acute pancreatitis (15%); chronic pancreatitis (70%)
C. CHOLELITHIASIS: acute pancreatitis (75%); chronic pancreatitis (20%)
D. METABOLIC DISORDERS
  1. Hypercalcemia in hyperparathyroidism (10%), multiple myeloma, amyloidosis, sarcoidosis
  2. Hereditary pancreatitis: autosomal dominant, only Caucasians affected, most common cause of large spherical pancreatic calcifications in childhood, recurrent episodes of pancreatitis, development into pancreatic carcinoma in 20 – 40%; pronounced dilatation of pancreatic duct; pseudocyst formation (50%); associated with type I hypercholesterolemia
  3. Hyperlipidemia Types I and V
  4. Kwashiorkor = Tropical pancreatitis
E. INFECTION / INFESTATION
  1. Viral infection (mumps, hepatitis, mononucleosis)
  2. Parasites (ascariasis, clonorchis)
F. TRAUMA
  1. Penetrating ulcer
  2. Blunt / penetrating trauma

3. Surgery (in 0.8% of Billroth-II resections, 0.8% of splenectomies, 0.7% of choledochal surgery, 0.4% of aortic graft surgery)
G. STRUCTURAL ABNORMALITIES
  1. Pancreas divisum
  2. Choledochocele
H. DRUGS
Azathioprine, thiazide, furosemide, ethacrynic acid, sulfonamides, tetracycline, phenformin, procainamide, steroids (eg, renal transplant)
I. MALIGNANCY
Pancreatic carcinoma (in 1%), metastases, lymphoma

Theories of pathogenesis:
Reflux of bile / pancreatic enzymes / duodenal succus
(a) terminal duct segment shared by common bile duct + pancreatic duct
(b) obstruction at papilla of Vater from inflammatory stenosis, edema / spasm of sphincter of Oddi, tumor, periduodenal diverticulum
(c) incompetent sphincter of Oddi

Acute Pancreatitis
= inflammatory disease of pancreas producing temporary changes with restoration of normal anatomy + function following resolution
Path:
  1. EDEMATOUS PANCREATITIS:
  edema, congestion, leukocytic infiltrates; mortality rate of 4%
  2. NECROTIZING PANCREATITIS:
  proteolytic destruction of pancreatic parenchyma; mortality rate of 80 – 90%
    (a) HEMORRHAGIC PANCREATITIS:
    + fat necrosis and hemorrhage
    (b) SUPPURATIVE PANCREATITIS:
    + bacterial infection
A. Diffuse form (52%)
B. Focal form (48%): location of head:tail = 3:2

Clinical stages:
I = EDEMATOUS PANCREATITIS
  • rapid improvement following conservative therapy
  • gradual decrease of elevated enzymes
  Mortality: 5%
II = PARTIALLY NECROTIZING PANCREATITIS
  • delayed / no response to conservative therapy
  • delayed / no normalization of enzymes
  • leukocytosis of <16,000
  • hyperglycemia of <200 mg/100 ml
  • hypocalcemia of >4 mval/l
  • base deficit of <4 mval/l
  Mortality: 30 – 75%
III = TOTALLY NECROTIZING PANCREATITIS
  • deterioration under conservative therapy
  • leukocytosis of >16,000
  • hyperglycemia of >200 mg/100 ml
  • hypocalcemia of <4 mval/l

- base deficit of >4 mval/l
  Mortality: 100% (40% by 2nd day, 75% by 5th day, 100% by 10th day)

- abdominal pain, nausea, vomiting
- raised pancreatic amylase + lipase in blood + urine
- increased amylase-creatinine clearance ratio

√ NO findings on US / CT in 29%
Abdominal film:
  √ "colon cutoff" sign = dilated transverse colon with abrupt change to a gasless descending colon (inflammation via phrenicocolic ligament causes spasm + obstruction at the splenic flexure impinging on a paralytic colon)
  √ "sentinel loop" (10 – 55%) = localized segment of gas-containing bowel in duodenum (in 20 – 45%) / terminal ileum / cecum
  √ "renal halo" sign = water density of inflammation in anterior pararenal space contrasts with perirenal fat; more common on left side
  √ mottled appearance of peripancreatic area (secondary to fat necrosis in pancreatic bed, mesentery, omentum)
  √ intrapancreatic gas bubbles (from acute gangrene / suppurative pancreatitis)
  √ "gasless abdomen" = fluid-filled bowel associated with vomiting
  √ ascites
CXR (findings in 14 – 71%):
  √ pleural effusion (in 5%), usually left-sided, with elevated amylase levels (in 85%)
  √ diaphragmatic elevation, atelectasis (20%), pulmonary infiltrates, ARDS
UGI:
  √ esophagogastric varices (from splenic vein obstruction)
  √ enlarged tortuous edematous rugal folds along antrum + greater curvature (20%)
  √ widening of retrogastric space (from pancreatic enlargement / inflammation in lesser sac)
  √ diminished duodenal peristalsis + edematous folds
  √ widening of duodenal sweep + downward displacement of ligament of Treitz
  √ Poppel sign = edematous swelling of papilla
  √ Frostberg inverted 3 sign = segmental narrowing with fold thickening of duodenum
  √ jejunal + ileal fold thickening (proteolytic spread along mesentery)
BE:
  √ narrowing, nodularity, fold distortion along inferior haustral row of transverse colon ± descending colon
Cholangiography:
  √ long gently tapered narrowing of CBD
  √ prestenotic biliary dilatation
  √ smooth / irregular mucosal surface
Bone films (findings in 6%):
  secondary to metastatic intramedullary lipolysis + fat necrosis

√ punched out / permeative destruction of cancellous bone + endosteal erosion
√ aseptic necrosis of femoral / humeral heads
√ metaphyseal infarcts, predominantly in distal femur + proximal tibia
US (pancreatic visualization in 62 – 78%):
  √ hypoechoic diffuse / focal enlargement of pancreas
  √ dilatation of pancreatic duct (if head focally involved)
  √ extrapancreatic hypoechoic mass with good acoustic transmission (= phlegmonous pancreatitis)
  √ fluid collection: lesser sac (60%), L > R anterior pararenal space (54%), posterior pararenal space (18%), around left lobe of liver (16%), in spleen (9%), mediastinum (3%), iliac fossa, along transverse mesocolon / mesenteric leaves of small intestine
  Fate of fluid collection:
    (a) complete resolution
    (b) pseudocyst formation
    (c) bacterial infection = abscess
  √ pseudocyst formation (52%): extension into lesser sac, transverse mesocolon, around kidney, mediastinum, lower quadrants of abdomen
CT (pancreatic visualization in 98%):
  √ no detectable change in size / appearance (29%)
  √ hypodense (5 – 20 HU) mass in phlegmonous pancreatitis; may persist long after complete recovery
  √ hyperdense areas (50 – 70 HU) in hemorrhagic pancreatitis for 24 – 48 hours
  √ enlargement with convex margins + indistinctness of gland with parenchymal inhomogeneity
  √ thickening of anterior pararenal fascia
  √ non-contrast-enhancing parenchyma during bolus injection (= pancreatic necrosis)
Angiography:
  √ may be normal
  √ hypovascular areas (15 – 56%)
  √ hypervascularity + increased parenchymal stain (12 – 45%)
  √ venous compression secondary to edema
  √ formation of pseudoaneurysms (in 10% with chronic pancreatitis): splenic artery (50%), pancreatic arcades, gastroduodenal artery
Cx:
  1. Phlegmon (18%) = solid mass characterized by edema, infiltration of inflammatory cells + necrosis: extension into lesser sac, anterior pararenal space, transverse mesocolon, small bowel mesentery, retroperitoneum, pelvis
  2. Pseudocyst formation (10%)
  3. Hemorrhage (3%)
  4. Abscess (2 – 10%): 2 – 4 weeks after severe acute pancreatitis; most commonly due to E. coli
     √ may contain gas within pancreatic bed
     DDx: air secondary to intestinal fistula
  5. Pancreatic ascites
  6. Biliary duct obstruction
  7. Thrombosis of splenic vein / SMV

8. Pseudoaneurysm
   (a) rupture into preexisting pseudocyst
   (b) digestion of arterial wall by enzymes
   Incidence: in up to 10% of severe pancreatitis
   Location: splenic artery (most common), gastroduodenal, pancreatico-duodenal, hepatic artery
   Mortality: 37% for rupture, 16 – 50% for surgery

Rx
1. Conservative (NPO, gastric tube, atropine, analgesics, sedation, prophylactic antibiotics) for stage I
2. Early surgery in stages II and III

Chronic Pancreatitis
= continuing inflammatory disease of pancreas characterized by irreversible damage to anatomy + function

A. CHRONIC CALCIFYING PANCREATITIS:
   √ protein plugs / calculi within ductal system

B. CHRONIC OBSTRUCTIVE PANCREATITIS:
   secondary to slow growing tumor / surgical duct ligation / ampullary stenosis
   √ dilatation of pancreatic duct
   √ normal sized / focally or diffusely enlarged / small atrophic gland
   √ calcifications uncommon
- acute exacerbation of epigastric pain (93%): decreasing with time due to progressive destruction of gland, usually painless after 7 years
- jaundice (42%) from common bile duct obstruction
- steatorrhea (80%)
- diabetes mellitus (58%)
- secretin test with decreased amylase + bicarbonate in duodenal fluid

Plain film:
   √ numerous irregular calcifications (in 20 – 50% of alcoholic pancreatitis) PATHOGNOMONIC
UGI:
   √ displacement of stomach / duodenum by pseudocyst
   √ shrinkage / fold induration of stomach (DDx: linitis plastica)
   √ stricture of duodenum
Cholangiopancreatography (most sensitive imaging modality):
   √ slight ductal ectasia / clubbing of side branches (minimal disease)
   √ "nipping" = narrowing of the origins of side branches
   √ dilatation >2 mm, tortuosity, wall rigidity, main ductal stenosis (moderate disease)
   √ "beading, chain of lakes, string of pearls" = dilatation, stenosis, obstruction of main pancreatic duct + side branches (severe disease)
   √ intraductal protein plugs / calculi

√ prolonged emptying of contrast material
√ may have stenosis / obstruction + prestenotic dilatation of CBD
US / CT:
   √ irregular (73%) / smooth (15%) / beaded (12%) pancreatic ductal dilatation (in 41 – 68%)
   √ small atrophic gland (in 10 – 54%)
   √ pancreatic mostly intraductal calcifications (4 – 68%)
   √ inhomogeneous gland with increased echogenicity (62%)
   √ irregular pancreatic contour (45 – 60%)
   √ focal (12 – 30%) / diffuse (27 – 45%) pancreatic enlargement
   √ mostly mild biliary ductal dilatation (29%)
   √ intra- / peripancreatic pseudocysts (20 – 25%)
   √ segmental portal hypertension (= splenic vein thrombosis + splenomegaly) in 11%
   √ arterial pseudoaneurysm formation
   √ peripancreatic fascial thickening + blurring of organ margins (16%)
   √ ascites / pleural effusion (9%)
Angiography:
   √ increased tortuosity + angulation of pancreatic arcades + intrahepatic arteries (88%)
   √ luminal irregularities / focal fibrotic arterial stenoses (25 – 75%) / smooth beaded appearance
   √ irregular parenchymal stain
   √ venous compression / occlusion (20 – 50%)
   √ portoportal shunting + gastric varices without esophageal varices

Cx: pancreatic carcinoma (2 – 4%), jaundice, pseudocyst formation, pancreatic ascites, thrombosis of splenic / mesenteric / portal vein
Rx: surgery for infected pseudocyst, GI bleeding from portal hypertension, common bile duct obstruction, gastrointestinal obstruction

PAPILLARY STENOSIS
Etiology:
A. PRIMARY PAPILLARY STENOSIS (10%)
   1. Congenital malformation of papilla
   2. Sequelae of acute / chronic inflammation
   3. Adenomyosis
B. SECONDARY PAPILLARY STENOSIS (90%)
   1. Mechanical trauma of stone passage (choledocholithiasis in 64%; cholecystolithiasis in 26%)
   2. Functional stenosis: associated with pancreas divisum, history of pancreatitis
   3. Reflex spasm
   4. Previous surgical manipulation
   5. Periampullary neoplasm

√ prestenotic dilatation of CBD
√ increase in pancreatic duct diameter (83%)
√ long smooth narrowing / beak (fibrotic stenosis)
√ prolonged bile-to-bowel transit time >45 minutes on Tc-IDA scintigraphy

PERICHOLECYSTIC ABSCESS

Cause: subacute perforation of gallbladder wall
subsequent to gangrene + infarction due to
acute cholecystitis

Prevalence: 2 – 20%

Location:
- (a) gallbladder bed (most common)
√ low-level echo area in liver adjacent to
gallbladder
- (b) intramural
√ small low-level echo area within thickened
gallbladder wall
- (c) intraperitoneal
√ low-level echo area within peritoneal cavity
adjacent to gallbladder

Rx: (1) Emergency operation
(2) Antibiotic treatment + elective operation
(3) Percutaneous abscess drainage

PORCELAIN GALLBLADDER

= calcium incrustation of gallbladder wall

Incidence: 0.6 – 0.8% of cholecystectomy patients

M:F = 1:5

Histo:
- (a) flakes of dystrophic calcium within chronically
inflamed + fibrotic muscular wall
- (b) microliths scattered diffusely throughout mucosa,
submucosa, glandular spaces, Rokitansky-Aschoff
sinuses

Associated with   gallstones in 90%
- minimal symptoms
√ curvilinear (muscularis) / granular (mucosal)
calcifications in segment of wall / entire wall
√ nonfunctioning GB on oral cholecystogram
√ highly echogenic shadowing curvilinear structure in GB
fossa (DDx: stone-filled contracted GB)
√ echogenic GB wall with little acoustic shadowing (DDx:
emphysematous cholecystitis)
√ scattered irregular clumps of echoes with posterior
acoustic shadowing

Cx: 10 – 20% develop carcinoma of gallbladder

PORTAL HYPERTENSION

- normal hepatic blood flow of 1.5 l/min (= 25% of cardiac
output) passes through portal system (2/3) + through
hepatic artery (1/3)

Classification:
A. Dynamic / hyperkinetic portal hypertension
congenital / traumatic / neoplastic arterioportal fistula
B. Increased portal venous resistance
@ PREHEPATIC
— portal vein thrombosis (portal phlebitis, oral
contraceptives, coagulopathy, neoplastic
invasion, pancreatitis, neonatal omphalitis)
— portal vein compression (tumor, trauma,
lymphadenopathy, portal phlebosclerosis,
pancreatic pseudocyst)
@ INTRAHEPATIC (= obstruction of portal venules)
— presinusoidal
1. Congenital hepatic fibrosis

2. Idiopathic noncirrhotic fibrosis
3. Primary biliary cirrhosis
4. Wilson disease
5. Sarcoid liver disease
6. Toxic fibrosis (arsenic, copper, PVC)
7. Reticuloendotheliosis
8. Myelofibrosis
9. Felty syndrome
10. Schistosomiasis
11. Chronic malaria
— sinusoidal
1. Hepatitis
2. Sickle cell disease
— postsinusoidal
1. Cirrhosis (most frequent): Laënnec
cirrhosis, postnecrotic cirrhosis from
hepatitis
2. Veno-occlusive disease of liver
@ POSTHEPATIC
1. Budd-Chiari syndrome
2. Constrictive pericarditis
3. CHF (tricuspid incompetence)

- elevated hepatic wedge pressure (HWP) = portal
venous pressure (normal <10 mm Hg); normal values
seen in presinusoidal portal hypertension
- caput medusae
- hemorrhaging esophageal varices (50%)

@ Splanchnic system:
√ portal vein >13 mm (57% sensitivity, 100%
specificity)
√ SMV + splenic vein >10 mm; coronary vein >4 mm;
recanalized umbilical vein >3 mm (size of vessels
not related to degree of portal hypertension or
presence of collaterals)
√ loss of respiratory increase of splanchnic vein
diameters (80% sensitivity, 100% specificity)
√ portal vein aneurysm
√ portal vein thrombosis
√ cavernous transformation of portal vein
√ increased echogenicity + thickening of portal vein
walls
Doppler US:
√ continuous portal vein flow without respiratory
changes
√ may have hepatofugal flow within spontaneous
splenorenal shunts (indicates high incidence of
hepatic encephalopathy)
√ dilated hepatic artery may demonstrate elevated
resistive index >0.78
@ Porto-systemic collaterals:
√ varices = serpentine tubular rounded structures
= esophageal, gastrosplenic, omental, splenorenal,
hemorrhoidal, retroperitoneal shunting veins (in up to
88%)
√ gallbladder wall varices in thickened gallbladder wall
(in 80% associated with portal vein thrombosis)
@ Cruveilhier-Baumgarten syndrome (20 – 30%)
= recanalized paraumbilical vein

√ hypoechoic channel in ligamentum teres
  (a) size <2 mm (in 97% of normal subjects; in 14% of patients with portal hypertension)
  (b) size ≥2 mm (86% sensitivity for portal hypertension)
√ arterial signal on Doppler US in 38%
√ hepatofugal venous flow (82% sensitivity, 100% specificity for portal hypertension)
@ Spleen
  √ splenomegaly (absence does not rule out portal hypertension)
  √ siderotic Gamna-Gandy nodules in 13% (due to perifollicular + trabecular hemorrhage)
    √ multiple 3 – 8 mm low-intensity spots on FLASH / GRASS images
    √ multiple hyperechoic spots on US
    √ multiple faint calcifications on CT
√ ascites
Cx: Acute gastrointestinal bleeding (mortality of 30 – 50% during 1st bleeding)

SEGMENTAL PORTAL HYPERTENSION
= splenic vein occlusion / superior mesenteric vein occlusion

PORTAL VEIN THROMBOSIS
Etiology:
  A. IDIOPATHIC (mostly): ? neonatal sepsis
  B. SECONDARY:
    (1) Tumor invasion by HCC, cholangiocarcinoma, pancreatic carcinoma, gastric carcinoma / extrinsic compression by tumor
    (2) Trauma; blood dyscrasia; clotting disorder; estrogen therapy; Cx of splenectomy for myeloproliferative disease, severe dehydration
    (3) Intraabdominal sepsis with phlebitis; pancreatitis; ascending cholangitis
    (4) Cirrhosis + portal hypertension (5%)

Age: predominantly children, young persons
• abdominal pain
• portal systemic encephalopathy
• hematemesis (esophageal varices)

√ nonvisualization of portal vein
√ calcification within clot / wall of portal vein
√ splenomegaly
√ ascites
Plain film:
  √ hepatosplenomegaly
  √ enlarged azygos vein
  √ paraspinal varices
UGI:
  √ esophageal varices
  √ thickening of bowel wall
US:
  √ echogenic material within vessel lumen (67%)
  √ increase in portal vein diameter (57%)
  √ portosystemic collateral circulation (48%)
  √ enlargement of thrombosed segment >15 mm (38%)

√ cavernous transformation = **cavernoma** (19%)
  = failure to visualize the extrahepatic portal vein + presence of multiple tubular structures with portal venous flow
√ thickening of lesser omentum
CECT:
  √ low-density center in portal vein surrounded by peripheral enhancement
  √ portal vein density 20 – 30 HU less than aortic density after contrast
MR:
  √ areas of flow void in portal area + abnormal signal intensity in main portal vein
Angio:
  √ "thread and streaks" sign of tumor thrombus (streaky contrast opacification of tumor vessels)

Cx: (1) Hepatic infarction
     (2) Bowel infarction

POSTCHOLECYSTECTOMY SYNDROME
= symptoms recurring / persisting after cholecystectomy
Incidence:
  mild recurrent symptoms in 9 – 25%; severe symptoms in 2.6 – 32% (result of 1,930 cholecystectomies):
    — completely cured (61%)
    — satisfactory improvement with
      (a) persistent mild dyspepsia (11%)
      (b) mild attacks of pain (24%)
    — failure with
      (a) occasional attacks of severe pain (3%)
      (b) continuous severe distress (1.7%)
      (c) recurrent cholangitis (0.7%)
Causes:
  A. BILIARY CAUSES
    (a) Incomplete surgery:
      1. Gallbladder / cystic duct remnant
      2. Retained stone in cystic duct remnant
      3. Overlooked CBD stone
    (b) Operative trauma
      1. Bile duct stricture
      2. Bile peritonitis
    (c) Bile duct pathology
      1. Fibrosis of sphincter of Oddi
      2. Biliary dyskinesia
      3. Biliary fistula
    (d) Residual disease in neighboring structures
      1. Pancreatitis
      2. Hepatitis
      3. Cholangitis
    (e) Overlooked bile duct neoplasia
  B. EXTRABILIARY CAUSES (erroneous preoperative diagnosis)
    (a) Other GI tract disease
      1. Inadequate dentition
      2. Hiatus hernia
      3. Peptic ulcer
      4. Spastic colon
    (b) Anxiety state, air swallowing
    (c) Abdominal angina

(d) Carcinoma outside gallbladder
(e) Coronary artery disease

RICHTER SYNDROME

= development of large cell / diffuse histiocytic lymphoma in patients with CLL
Etiology: transformation / dedifferentiation of CLL lymphocytes
Incidence in CLL patients: 3 – 10%
Median age: 59 years
Medium time interval after diagnosis of CLL: 24 months
• fever (65%) without evidence of infection
• increasing lymphadenopathy + hepatosplenomegaly (46%)
• weight loss (26%)
• abdominal pain (26%)
Location: bone marrow, lymph nodes, liver, spleen, bowel, lung, pleura, kidney, dura
Prognosis:
  Median survival time: 4 months from diagnosis of lymphoma; 14% remission rate

SCHISTOSOMIASIS

Worldwide major cause of portal hypertension: 200 million people affected
Types:
  A. SCHISTOSOMA HAEMATOBIUM
     in Africa, Mediterranean, Southwest Asia
  B. SCHISTOSOMA MANSONI
     in parts of Africa, Arabia, West Indies, northern part of South America
  C. SCHISTOSOMA JAPONICUM
     coastal areas of China, Japan, Formosa, Philippines, Celebes
Cycle:
  cercariae enter lymphatics + blood system via thoracic duct; larvae are transported into mesenteric capillaries; mature in portal system + liver into worms; worms live in pairs in copula within portal vein + tributaries for 10 – 15 years; female swims against blood flow to reach venules of urinary bladder (S. haematobium) or intestine + rectum (S. mansoni, S. japonicum); deposits eggs in wall of urinary bladder or intestines, eggs pass with urine + feces; hatch within water to release miracidia which infect snail hosts; cercariae emerge after maturation from snails
Infection: cercaria penetrate human skin / buccal mucosa from contaminated water (slow-moving streams, irrigation canals, paddy fields, lakes)
Histo: granulomatous reaction + fibrosis along portal vein branches
@ Liver
  √ marked diffuse thickening + echogenicity of walls of portal venules
  √ hepatosplenomegaly
  √ portal vein dilatation in 73% (portal hypertension)
  √ normal parenchymal echogenicity
@ GI tract
  √ gastric + esophageal varices
  √ polypoid bowel wall masses (esp. in sigmoid)

  √ granulomatous colitis
  √ strictures with extensive pericolic inflammation
Cx: ileus

SCHWACHMAN-DIAMOND SYNDROME

= rare congenital absence of pancreatic exocrine tissue, 2nd most frequent cause of exocrine pancreatic insufficiency in childhood
• pancreatic insufficiency
• recurrent respiratory and skin infections (secondary to bone marrow hypoplasia)
• dwarfism (metaphyseal dysostosis)
• normal electrolytes in sweat
• tends to improve with time
√ total fatty replacement of pancreas

SOLID AND PAPILLARY NEOPLASM OF PANCREAS

= SOLID AND CYSTIC TUMOR = PAPILLARY-CYSTIC NEOPLASM = SOLID AND PAPILLARY EPITHELIAL NEOPLASM
= rare, low-grade malignant tumor; often misclassified as nonfunctioning islet cell tumor, cystadenoma, cystadenocarcinoma of pancreas
Mean age: 27 (range 10 – 46) years ; M:F = 1:9
Path: large well-encapsulated mass with considerable hemorrhagic necrosis + cystic degeneration
• gradually enlarging abdominal mass

Location: tail of pancreas (most frequently)
√ sharply defined inhomogeneous round / lobulated pancreatic mass with solid + cystic portions
√ may be completely cystic (when complicated by extensive necrosis)
√ mean diameter of 10 cm (range 3 – 15 cm)
√ dystrophic calcification may occur
√ hypovascular with no contrast enhancement / enhancement of solid tissue projecting toward center of mass
US:
  √ echogenic mass with necrotic center
Prognosis: excellent after excision; metastases in 4%
DDx:
  (1) Microcystic adenoma (innumerable tiny cysts, older age group)
  (2) Mucinous cystic neoplasm (large uni- / multilocular cysts, older age group)
  (3) Nonfunctioning islet cell tumor (hypervascular)

SPLENIC INFARCTION

Most common cause of focal defects
Cause:
  1. Bacterial endocarditis (responsible in 50%), valve vegetation, cardiac thrombus, atheromatous plaque
  2. Sickle cell disease (leading to functional asplenia)
  3. Periarteritis nodosa
  4. Postembolization therapy
  5. Focal inflammatory process (eg, pancreatitis)
  6. Myeloproliferative / lymphoproliferative disorders (CML most common), polycythemia vera

7. Myelofibrosis with myeloid metaplasia + splenomegaly
8. Metastatic carcinoma
9. Gaucher disease

mnemonic: "PSALMS"
   Pancreatic carcinoma, **P**ancreatitis
   Sickle cell disease / trait
   Adenocarcinoma of stomach
   Leukemia
   Mitral stenosis with emboli
   Subacute bacterial endocarditis

- LUQ pain, fever
- elevated erythrocyte sedimentation rate, leukocytosis
- abnormal lactate dehydrogenase levels
- √ focal wedge-shaped peripheral defect

SPLENOSIS

= autotransplantation of splenic tissue to other sites following trauma
Age: young men with history of trauma / splenectomy
Time of detection: mean of 10 years (range of 6 months – 32 years) after trauma
Location: diaphragmatic surface, liver, omentum, mesentery, peritoneum, pleura
√ multiple small encapsulated sessile implants (few mm – 3 cm)
√ demonstrated by Tc-99m sulfur colloid; In-111 labeled platelets; Tc-99m heat-damaged RBC (best detection rate)
DDx: accessory spleen

SPONTANEOUS PERFORATION OF COMMON BILE DUCT

Pathogenesis: unknown (? CBD obstruction, localized mural malformation, ischemia, trauma)
Age: 5 weeks – 3 years of age
- vague abdominal distension
- mild persistent hyperbilirubinemia
- varying acholic stools
US:
   √ biliary ascites / loculated subhepatic fluid
   √ localized pseudocholedochal cyst in porta hepatis
Hepatobiliary scintigraphy:
   √ radioisotope diffusion throughout peritoneal cavity

THOROTRASTOSIS

Thorotrast   = 25% colloidal suspension of thorium dioxide; used as contrast agent between late 1920s and mid 1950s, in particular for cerebral angiography and liver spleen imaging; chemically inert with high atomic number of 90; >100,000 people injected
Thorium dioxide   = consists of 11 radioactive isotopes (thorium-232 is major isotope); decay by means of alpha, beta, and gamma emission; biologic half-life of 1.34×10^{10} years; hepatic dose of 1000 – 3000 rads in 20 years
Distribution: phagocytosed by RES + deposited in liver (70%), spleen (30%), bone marrow, abdominal lymph nodes (20%)
√ metallic density contrast material in spleen, lymph nodes, liver
√ spleen may be contracted / nonfunctional
Cx: hepatic fibrosis, angiosarcoma (50%), cholangio-carcinoma, hepatocellular carcinoma (latency period of 3 – 40 years; mean 26 years)

UNDIFFERENTIATED SARCOMA OF LIVER

= EMBRYONAL SARCOMA = 4th most frequent hepatic tumor in childhood
Age: <2 months (in 5%); 6 – 10 years (in 52%); by 15 years (in 90%); up to 30 years
Histo: stellate / spindle-shaped sarcomatous cells arranged in whorls + sheets with foci of hematopoiesis (50%)
- RUQ mass
- mild anemia + leukocytosis (50%)
- elevated liver enzymes (33%)
- fever (5%)
Location: right lobe (75%); left lobe (10%); both lobes (15%)
√ 10 – 20 cm in size
NUC:
   √ photodefect on sulfur colloid scan
US / CT:
   √ large intrahepatic masses with cystic areas (necrosis + hemorrhage)
Angio:
   √ hyper- / hypovascular with stretching of vessels
   √ scattered foci of neovascularity
Prognosis: mostly results in death within 12 months
DDx: mesenchymal hamartoma

DIFFERENTIAL DIAGNOSIS OF GASTROINTESTINAL DISORDERS

ABNORMAL INTRAABDOMINAL AIR

Abnormal air collection

1. Abnormally located bowel
   Chilaiditi syndrome, inguinal hernia
2. Pneumoperitoneum
3. Retropneumoperitoneum
   Perforation of duodenum / rectum / ascending + descending colon, diverticulitis, ulcerative disease, endoscopic procedure
4. Gas in bowel wall
   Gastric pneumatosis, phlegmonous gastritis, endoscopy, rupture of lung bulla
5. Gas within abscess
   Located in subphrenic, renal, perirenal, hepatic, pancreatic space, lesser sac
6. Gas in biliary system
   Hepatobiliary fistula, surgery, duodenal ulcer, duodenal diverticulum, cancer, stone, patulous ampulla, emphysematous cholecystitis
   √   gas outlines choledochus ± gallbladder
   √   peripheral branches of bile ducts not filled
7. Gas in portal venous system
   Generally associated with intestinal necrosis (air leakage) / infection with gas-forming organisms in: vascular accidents, superior mesenteric artery syndrome, diabetes, imperforate anus, duodenal atresia, esophageal atresia, diarrhea, dead fetus
   √   branching air within 2 cm of liver periphery

Pneumoperitoneum
Etiology:
A. DISRUPTION OF WALL OF HOLLOW VISCUS
   (a) blunt / penetrating trauma
      1. Perforated foreign body (eg, thermometer injury to rectum, vaginal stimulator in rectum)
      2. Compressor air directed toward anus
   (b) iatrogenic perforation
      1. Laparoscopy / laparotomy (58%): absorbed in 1 – 24 days dependent on initial amount of air introduced and body habitus (80% in asthenic, 25% in obese patients)
         Δ   After 3 days free air should be followed with suspicion!
      2. Leaking surgical anastomosis
      3. Endoscopic perforation
      4. Enema tip injury
      5. Diagnostic pneumoperitoneum
   (c) diseases of GI tract
      1. Perforated gastric / duodenal ulcer
      2. Perforated appendix
      3. Ingested foreign body perforation
      4. Diverticulitis (ruptured Meckel diverticulum / sigmoid diverticulum, jejunal diverticulosis)
      5. Necrotizing enterocolitis with perforation

6. Inflammatory bowel disease (eg, toxic megacolon)
7. Obstruction[†] (gas traversing intact mucosa): neoplasm, imperforate anus, Hirschsprung disease, meconium ileus
8. Ruptured pneumatosis cystoides intestinalis[†] with "balanced pneumoperitoneum" (= free intraperitoneal air tamponades cysts maintaining a balance between intracystic air + pneumoperitoneum)
9. Idiopathic gastric perforation = spontaneous perforation in premature infants (congenital gastric muscular wall defect)

B. THROUGH PERITONEAL SURFACE
   (a) transperitoneal manipulation
      1. Abdominal needle biopsy / catheter placement
      2. Mistaken thoracentesis / chest tube placement
      3. Endoscopic biopsy
   (b) extension from chest[‡]
      1. Dissection from pneumomediastinum (positive pressure breathing, rupture of bulla / bleb, chest surgery)
      2. Bronchopleural fistula
   (c) rupture of urinary bladder
   (d) penetrating abdominal injury
C. THROUGH FEMALE GENITAL TRACT[†]
   (a) iatrogenic
      1. Perforation of uterus / vagina
      2. Culdocentesis
      3. Rubin test = tubal patency test
      4. Pelvic examination
   (b) spontaneous
      1. Intercourse, orogenital insufflation
      2. Douching
      3. Knee-chest exercise, water skiing, horseback riding
D. INTRAPERITONEAL
   1. Gas-forming peritonitis
   2. Rupture of abscess
Note [†] = asymptomatic spontaneous pneumoperitoneum without peritonitis

√ air in lesser peritoneal sac
√ gas in scrotum (through open processus vaginalis)
Large collection of gas:
   √ abdominal distension, no gastric air-fluid level
   √ "wall sign" = "Rigler sign" = "bas-relief sign" = air on both sides of bowel as intraluminal gas + free air outside (usually requires >1,000 ml of gas)
   √ "football sign" = large pneumoperitoneum outlining entire abdominal cavity
   √ outline of falciform ligament (medial RUQ); most common structure outlined

√ "telltale triangle sign" = triangular air pocket between 3 loops of bowel
√ "inverted V sign" = outline of both lateral umbilical ligaments
√ "urachus sign" = outline of middle umbilical ligament

RUQ gas (best place to look for small collections):
√ single large area of hyperlucency over the liver
√ oblique linear area of hyperlucency outlining the posteroinferior margin of liver
√ doge's cap sign = triangular collection of gas in Morison pouch (posterior hepatorenal space)
√ air outlining fissure of ligamentum teres hepatis (= posterior free edge of falciform ligament) seen as sharply defined slitlike area of hyperlucency between 10th and 12th rib within 2.5 – 4.0 cm of right vertebral border 2 – 7 mm wide and 6 – 20 mm long
√ "saddlebag / mustache / cupola sign" = gas trapped below central tendon of diaphragm
√ parahepatic air = gas bubble lateral to right edge of liver

Pseudopneumoperitoneum
= process mimicking free air
A. ABDOMINAL GAS
  (a) gastrointestinal gas
    1. Pseudo-wall sign = apposition of gas-distended bowel loops
    2. Chilaiditi syndrome
    3. Diaphragmatic hernia
    4. Diverticulum of esophagus / stomach / duodenum
  (b) extraintestinal gas
    1. Retroperitoneal air
    2. Subdiaphragmatic abscess
B. CHEST
  1. Pneumothorax
  2. Empyema
  3. Irregularity of diaphragm
C. FAT
  1. Subdiaphragmatic intraperitoneal fat
  2. Interposition of omental fat between liver + diaphragm

Pneumoretroperitoneum
Causes:
  (1) Traumatic rupture (usually duodenum)
  (2) Perforation of duodenal ulcer
  (3) Gas abscess of pancreas (usually extends into lesser sac)
  (4) Urinary tract gas (trauma, infection)
  (5) Dissected mediastinal air
√ kidney outlined by gas
√ outline of psoas margin ± gas streaks in muscle bundles

Pneumatosis cystoides intestinalis
= multiple thin-walled, noncommunicating, gas-filled cysts of various sizes located in subserosa ± submucosa with a normal mucosa + muscularis
Age: adulthood

Location: predominantly in lower colon

1. PRIMARY PNEUMATOSIS INTESTINALIS (15%)
   Cause: idiopathic
2. SECONDARY PNEUMATOSIS INTESTINALIS (85%)
   Causes:
     (a) intestinal trauma
       1. Ingestion of caustic agents
       2. Gastrointestinal endoscopy + biopsy
       3. Jejunoileal bypass surgery
       4. Postoperative bowel anastomosis
       5. Abdominal trauma
       6. Parenteral nutrition
       7. Barium enema
     (b) intestinal ischemia / infarction
       1. Necrotizing enterocolitis
       2. Mesenteric vascular disease
     (c) intestinal obstruction
       1. Imperforate anus
       2. Hirschsprung disease
       3. Pyloric stenosis
       4. Meconium plug syndrome
       5. Neoplasm
     (d) infection
       1. Primary infection of bowel wall
       2. Intestinal parasites, tuberculosis
       3. Perforated jejunal diverticulum
       4. Peritonitis
       5. Steroid therapy
     (e) inflammation
       1. Pyloric / duodenal ulcer
       2. Inflammatory bowel disease
       3. Collagen vascular disease: scleroderma, systemic lupus erythematosus, periarteritis
       4. Whipple disease
     (f) chronic obstructive bronchopulmonary disease
       1. Emphysema
       2. Bullous disease of lung
       3. Chronic bronchitis
       4. Asthma
       5. Artificial ventilation

• asymptomatic
√ radiolucent clusters of cysts along contour of bowel wall (best demonstrated on CT)
√ segmental mucosal nodularity (DDx: polyposis)
√ ± pneumoperitoneum
Cx: asymptomatic large pneumoperitoneum (may persist for months / years)

Soap bubble appearance in abdomen of neonate
1. Feces in infant fed by mouth
2. Meconium ileus:
   gas mixed with meconium, usually RLQ
3. Meconium plug:
   gas in and around plug, in distribution of colon
4. Necrotizing enterocolitis: submucosal pneumatosis
5. Atresia / severe stenosis: pneumatosis
6. Hirschsprung disease:
   impacted stool, sometimes pneumatosis

ABDOMINAL CALCIFICATIONS

Diffuse abdominal calcifications
1. Cystadenoma of ovary
   - √ granular, sandlike psammomatous calcifications
2. Pseudomyxoma peritonei
   - (a) pseudomucinous adenoma of ovary
   - (b) mucocele of appendix
3. Undifferentiated abdominal malignancy
4. Tuberculous peritonitis
   - √ mottled calcifications, simulating residual barium
5. Meconium peritonitis
6. Oil granuloma
   - √ annular, plaquelike

Focal alimentary tract calcifications
A. ENTEROLITHS
1. Appendicolith: in 10 – 15% of acute appendicitis
2. Stone in Meckel diverticulum
3. Diverticular stone
4. Rectal stone
5. Proximal to partial obstruction
B. MESENTERIC CALCIFICATIONS
1. Dystrophic calcification of omental fat deposits + appendices epiploicae (secondary to infarction / pancreatitis / TB)
2. Cysts: mesenteric cyst, hydatid cyst
C. INGESTED FOREIGN BODIES
   trapped in appendix, diverticula, proximal to stricture
1. Calcified seeds + pits
2. Birdshot
D. TUMOR
1. Mucocele of appendix
   - √ crescent-shaped / circular calcification
2. Mucinous adenocarcinoma of stomach / colon
   = COLLOID CARCINOMA
   - √ small mottled / punctate calcifications in primary site ± in regional lymph node metastases, adjacent omentum, metastatic liver foci
3. Gastric / esophageal leiomyoma: calcifies in 4%
4. Lipoma

Abdominal wall calcifications
A. IN SOFT TISSUES
1. Hypercalcemic states
2. Idiopathic calcinosis
B. IN MUSCLE
   - (a) Parasites:
     1. Cysticercosis = Taenia solium
        - √ round / slightly elongated calcifications
     2. Guinea worm = dracunculiasis
        - √ stringlike calcifications up to 12 cm long
   - (b) Injection sites
     from quinine, bismuth, calcium gluconate, calcium penicillin
   - (c) Myositis ossificans
C. IN SKIN
1. Soft-tissue nodules: papilloma, neurofibroma, melanoma, nevi
2. Scar: √ linear density
3. Colostomy / ileostomy
4. Tattoo markings

Abdominal vascular calcifications
A. ARTERIES
1. Atheromatous plaques
2. Arterial calcifications in diabetes mellitus
B. VEINS
   Phleboliths = calcified thrombus, generally seen below interspinous line
1. normal / varicose veins
2. hemangioma
C. LYMPH NODES
1. Histoplasmosis / tuberculosis
2. Chronic granulomatous disease
3. Residual lymphographic contrast
4. Silicosis

ABNORMAL INTRAABDOMINAL FLUID
Ascites
A. TRANSUDATE:
   (1) Hypoproteinemia (2) CHF (3) Constrictive pericarditis (4) Chronic renal failure (5) Cirrhosis (6) Budd-Chiari syndrome
B. EXUDATE:
   (1) Carcinomatosis (2) Polyserositis (3) TB peritonitis (4) Pancreatitis (5) Meigs syndrome
C. Hemorrhagic / chylous fluid

Early signs (accumulation in pelvis):
- √ round central density in pelvis + ill-defined bladder top
- √ thickening of peritoneal flank stripe
- √ space between properitoneal fat and gut >3 mm

Late signs:
- √ Hellmer sign = medial displacement of lateral liver margins
- √ medial displacement of ascending + descending colon
- √ obliteration of hepatic + splenic angles
- √ bulging flanks
- √ gray abdomen
- √ floating centralized loops
- √ separation of loops

HIGH-DENSITY ASCITES
1. Tuberculosis: 20 – 45 HU; may be lower
2. Ovarian tumor
3. Appendiceal tumor

Neonatal ascites
A. GASTROINTESTINAL
   - (a) perforation of hollow viscus
     Meconium peritonitis
   - (b) inflammatory lesions
     Meckel diverticulum, appendicitis
   - (c) cyst rupture
     Mesenteric / omental / choledochal cyst
   - (d) bile leakage
     Biliary obstruction / perforation

B. PORTOHEPATIC
    (a) <u>extrahepatic portal vein obstruction</u>
       Atresia of veins, compression by mass
    (b) <u>intrahepatic portal vein obstruction</u>
       Portal cirrhosis (neonatal hepatitis), biliary
       cirrhosis (biliary atresia)

C. URINARY TRACT
    Δ Urine ascites (most common cause) from lower
    urinary tract obstruction + upper urinary tract
    rupture:
    Posterior / anterior urethral valves, ureterovesical /
    ureteropelvic junction obstruction, renal / bladder
    rupture, anterior urethral diverticulum, bladder
    diverticula, neurogenic bladder, extrinsic bladder
    mass

D. GENITAL
    Ruptured ovarian cyst, hydrometrocolpos

E. HYDROPS FETALIS
    Immune hydrops, nonimmune hydrops (usually
    cardiac causes)

F. MISCELLANEOUS
    Chylous ascites, lymphangiectasia, congenital
    syphilis, trauma, idiopathic

Chylous ascites

IN ADULTS:	1.	Inflammatory process	(35%)
	2.	Tumor	(30%)
	3.	Idiopathic	(23%)
	4.	Trauma	(11%)
	5.	Congenital	(1%)
IN CHILDREN:	1.	Congenital	(39%)
	2.	Inflammatory process	(15%)
	3.	Trauma	(12%)
	4.	Tumor	(3%)
	5.	Idiopathic	(33%)

Fluid collection

mnemonic: "BLUSCHINGS"
Biloma
Lymphocele, **L**ymphoma (almost anechoic)
Urinoma
Seroma
Cyst (pseudocyst, peritoneal inclusion cyst)
Hematoma (aneurysm, AVM)
Infection, **I**nfestation (empyema, abscess,
    Echinococcus)
Neoplasm (necrotic)
GI tract (dilated loops, ileus, duplication)
Serosa (ascites, pleural fluid, pericardial effusion)

MECHANICAL INTESTINAL OBSTRUCTION
  = occlusion / constriction of bowel lumen

Gastric outlet obstruction
A. CONGENITAL LESION
    1. Antral mucosal diaphragm = antral web
    2. Gastric duplication: usually along greater
       curvature, abdominal mass in infancy
    3. Hypertrophic pyloric stenosis

B. INFLAMMATORY NARROWING
    1. Peptic ulcer disease: cause in adults in 60 – 65%
    2. Corrosive gastritis
    3. Crohn disease, sarcoidosis, syphilis, tuberculosis

C. MALIGNANT NARROWING
    1. Antral carcinoma: cause in adults in 30 – 35%
    2. Scirrhous carcinoma of pyloric channel

D. OTHERS
    1. Prolapsed antral polyp / mucosa
    2. Bezoar
    3. Gastric volvulus
    4. Postoperative stomal edema

Abdominal plain film:
  √ large smoothly marginated homogeneous mass
    displacing transverse colon + small bowel inferiorly
  √ one / two air-fluid levels

Duodenal obstruction
A. CONGENITAL
    1. Annular pancreas
    2. Peritoneal bands = Ladd bands
    3. Aberrant vessel

B. INFLAMMATORY NARROWING
    1. Chronic duodenal ulcer scar
    2. Acute pancreatitis: phlegmon, abscess,
       pseudocyst
    3. Acute cholecystitis: perforated gallstone

C. NTRAMURAL HEMATOMA
    1. Blunt trauma (accident, child abuse)
    2. Anticoagulant therapy
    3. Blood dyscrasia

D. TUMORAL NARROWING
    1. Primary duodenal tumors
    2. Tumor invasion from pancreas, right kidney, lymph
       node enlargement

E. EXTRINSIC COMPRESSION
    1. Aortic aneurysm
    2. Pseudoaneurysm

F. OTHERS
    1. Superior mesenteric artery syndrome from
       extensive burns, body cast, rapid weight loss,
       prolonged bed rest
    2. Bezoar (in gastrectomized patient)

mnemonic: "VA BADD TU BADD"

<u>child</u>	<u>adult</u>
Volvulus	**T**umor
Atresia	**U**lcer
Bands	**B**ands
Annular pancreas	**A**nnular pancreas
Duplication	**D**uplication
Diverticulum	**D**iverticulum

Abdominal plain film:
  √ double bubble sign = air-fluid levels in stomach +
    duodenum

Jejunal and ileal obstruction
A. CONGENITAL
    1. Ileal atresia / stenosis

2. Enteric duplication: located on antimesenteric side, mostly in ileum
3. Mid-gut volvulus from arrest in rotation + fixation of small bowel during fetal life
4. Mesenteric cyst from meconium peritonitis: located on mesenteric side
5. Meckel diverticulum

B. EXTRINSIC BOWEL LESIONS
  1. Fibrous adhesions (in 75%) from previous surgery / peritonitis
  2. Hernias (inguinal, femoral, umbilical, paraduodenal, foramen of Winslow, incisional, Spigelian, obturator)
  3. Volvulus
  4. Masses: neoplasm, abscess

C. LUMINAL OCCLUSION
  1. Swallowed foreign body, bezoar, gallstone, bolus of Ascaris lumbricoides, inspissated milk
  2. Meconium ileus: √ microcolon in cystic fibrosis
  3. Meconium ileus equivalent
  4. Intussusception (tumor, Meckel diverticulum, chronic ulcer, adhesion)
  5. Tumor (rare)

D. INTRINSIC BOWEL WALL LESION
  1. Strictures from neoplasm, Crohn disease, tuberculous enteritis, parasitic disease, potassium chloride tablets, surgical anastomosis, irradiation, massive deposition of amyloid
  2. Intramural hemorrhage: blunt trauma, Henoch-Schönlein purpura
  3. Vascular insufficiency: arterial / venous occlusion

ACQUIRED SMALL BOWEL OBSTRUCTION IN CHILDHOOD
  mnemonic: "AAIIMM"
    Adhesions
    Appendicitis
    Intussusception
    Incarcerated hernia
    Malrotation
    Meckel diverticulum

SMALL BOWEL OBSTRUCTION IN ADULT
  mnemonic: "SHAVIT"
    Stone (gallstone ileus)
    Hernia
    Adhesion
    Volvulus
    Intussusception
    Tumor

Abdominal plain film:
  √ "candy cane" appearance in erect position = >3 distended small bowel loops >3 cm with gas-fluid levels (>3 – 5 hours after onset of obstruction)
  √ disparity in size between obstructed loops and contiguous small bowel loops of normal caliber beyond site of obstruction
  √ small bowel positioned in center of abdomen
  √ little / no gas + stool in colon with complete mechanical obstruction after 12 – 24 hours

√ "stretch sign" = erectile valvulae conniventes completely encircle bowel lumen
√ "stepladder appearance" in low obstruction (the greater the number of dilated bowel loops the more distal the site of obstruction)
√ "string-of-beads" indicate peristaltic hyperactivity to overcome mechanical obstruction
√ hyperactive peristalsis / aperistalsis = fatigued small bowel
CAVE: little / no gas in small bowel from fluid-distended loops may lead one to overlook obstruction
UGI:
  √ "snake head" appearance = active peristalsis forms bulbous head of barium column in an attempt to overcome obstruction
  √ barium appears in colon >12 hours
Enteroclysis for adhesive obstruction:
  √ abrupt change in caliber of bowel with normal caliber / collapsed bowel distal to obstruction
  √ stretched folds of normal pattern
  √ angulated + fixed bowel segment

STRANGULATED OBSTRUCTION
  Cause: adhesion, volvulus, incarcerated hernia
  Strangulation = mechanical obstruction + interruption of segmental blood supply
  √ fixation of bowel loop
    √ "pseudotumor" in unchanged position (from closed loop obstruction)
    √ "coffee bean" appearance
  √ featureless bowel wall with flattening of valvulae (from edema / hemorrhage)
  √ increasing intraluminal fluid
  √ separation of bowel loops (from exudate / free fluid)
  √ free intraperitoneal gas (from frank perforation)

Colonic obstruction
Incidence: 25% of all intestinal obstructions
A. NEONATAL COLONIC OBSTRUCTION
  1. Meconium plug syndrome
  2. Colonic atresia
  3. Anorectal malformation: rectal atresia, imperforate anus
B. LUMINAL OBTURATION
  1. Fecal impaction
    √ bubbly pattern of large mass of stool
  2. Fecaloma
  3. Gallstone (in sigmoid narrowed by diverticulitis)
  4. Intussusception
C. BOWEL WALL LESION
  (a) <u>malignant</u> (60 – 70% of obstructions) Predominantly in sigmoid
  (b) <u>inflammatory</u>
    1. Crohn disease
    2. Ulcerative colitis
    3. Mesenteric ischemia
    4. Sigmoid diverticulitis (15%)
      √ stenotic segment >6 cm
    5. Acute pancreatitis

(c) <u>infectious</u>
   Infectious granulomatous process (actinomycosis,
   tuberculosis, lymphogranuloma venereum),
   parasitic disease (amebiasis, schistosomiasis)
(d) <u>wall hematoma</u>
   Blunt trauma, coagulopathy
D. EXTRINSIC
   (a) <u>mass impression</u>
      1. Endometriosis
      2. Large tumor mass: prostate, bladder, uterus,
         tubes, ovaries
      3. Pelvic abscess
      4. Hugely distended bladder
      5. Mesenteritis
      6. Poorly formed colostomy
   (b) <u>severe constriction</u>
      1. Volvulus (3rd most common cause): sigmoid
         colon, cecum, transverse colon, compound
         volvulus (= ileosigmoid knot)
      2. Hernia: transverse colon in diaphragmatic
         hernia, sigmoid colon in left inguinal hernia
      3. Adhesion

Abdominal plain film patterns:
   (a) dilated colon only = competent ileocecal valve
   (b) dilated small bowel (25%) = incompetent ileocecal
       valve
   (c) dilated colon + dilated small bowel = ileocecal valve
       obstruction secondary to cecal overdistension
   √ gas-fluid levels distal to hepatic flexure (fluid is
      normal in cecum + ascending colon); sign not valid
      with diarrhea / saline catharsis / enema
   √ cecum most dilated portion (in 75% of cases);
      critical at 10 cm diameter (high probability for
      impending perforation)
   Δ The lower the obstruction the more proximal the
      distension!
   BE: emergency barium enema of unprepared colon in
        suspected obstruction!
        <u>contraindicated</u> in toxic megacolon, pneumatosis
        intestinalis, portal vein gas, extraluminal gas

ILEUS
= ADYNAMIC / PARALYTIC / NONOBSTRUCTIVE
  ILEUS
= derangement impairing proper distal propulsion of
  intestinal contents
Cause:
— in neonate:
   1. Hyperbilirubinemia
   2. Intracranial hemorrhage
   3. Aspiration pneumonia
   4. Necrotizing enterocolitis
   5. Aganglionosis
— in child / adult:
   1. Postoperative ileus
      • usually resolves by 4th postoperative day
   2. Visceral pain: obstructing ureteral stone, common
      bile duct stone, twisted ovarian cyst, blunt
      abdominal / chest trauma

3. Intraabdominal inflammation / infection: peritonitis,
   appendicitis, cholecystitis, pancreatitis, salpingitis,
   abdominal abscess, hemolytic-uremic syndrome,
   gastroenteritis
4. Ischemic bowel disease
5. Anticholinergic drugs: atropine, propantheline,
   morphine + derivatives, tricyclic antidepressants,
   dilantin, phenothiazines, hexamethonium bromide
6. Neuromuscular disorder: diabetes, hypothyroidism,
   porphyria, lead poisoning, uremia, hypokalemia,
   amyloidosis, urticaria, sprue, scleroderma, Chagas
   disease, vagotomy, myotonic dystrophy, CNS
   trauma, paraplegia, quadriplegia
7. Systemic disease: septic / hypovolemic shock,
   urticaria
8. Chest disease: lower lobe pneumonia, pleuritis,
   myocardial infarction, acute pericarditis, congestive
   heart failure
9. Retroperitoneal disease: hemorrhage (spine
   trauma), abscess

mnemonic: "Remember the P's"
   Pancreatitis
   Pendicitis
   Peptic ulcer
   Perforation
   Peritonitis
   Pneumonia
   Porphyria
   Postoperative
   Potassium deficiency
   Pregnancy
   Pyelonephritis

• intestinal sounds decreased / absent
• abdominal distension
√ large + small bowel ± gastric distension
√ decreased small bowel distension on serial films
√ delayed but free passage of contrast material
Rx: not amenable to surgical correction

Localized ileus
= isolated distended loop of small / large bowel
  = SENTINEL LOOP
Often associated with an adjacent acute inflammatory
  process
Etiology:
   1. Acute pancreatitis: duodenum, jejunum,
                             transverse colon
   2. Acute cholecystitis: hepatic flexure of colon
   3. Acute appendicitis: terminal ileum, cecum
   4. Acute diverticulitis: descending colon
   5. Acute ureteral colic: GI tract along course of
                             ureter

Pseudoobstruction
A. Transient pseudoobstruction:
   1. Electrolyte imbalance
   2. Renal failure
   3. Congestive heart failure

B. Chronic pseudoobstruction
1. Scleroderma
2. Amyloidosis
C. Idiopathic pseudoobstruction in young women
with no apparent cause

ESOPHAGUS

Esophageal contractions
Δ Esophageal motor acitivity needs to be evaluated in
recumbent position without influence of gravity!
PERISTALTIC EVENT = coordinated contractions of
esophagus
PERISTALTIC SEQUENCE = aboral stripping wave
clearing esophagus

1. PRIMARY PERISTALSIS
= orderly peristaltic sequence with progressive
aboral stripping traversing entire esophagus with
complete clearance of barium; centrally mediated
(medulla) swallow reflex via glossopharyngeal +
vagal nerve; initiated by swallowing
√ rapid wave of inhibition followed by slower wave of
contraction
Δ Normal peristaltic sequence will be interrupted by
repetitive swallowing before peristaltic sequence is
complete!
2. SECONDARY PERISTALSIS
= local peristaltic wave identical to primary
peristalsis but elicited through esophageal
distension = sensorimotor stretch reflex
Δ Esophageal motility can be evaluated with barium
injection through nasoesophageal tube despite
patient's inability to swallow!
3. TERTIARY CONTRACTIONS
= nonpropulsive esophageal motor event without
clearing of esophagus
Δ Presence of tertiary activity does not necessarily
imply a significant motility disturbance!
(a) nonsegmental = partial luminal indentation
(b) segmental = luminal obliteration (rare)
√ "curling" = erratic segmental contractions
√ "rosary-bead" appearance

Abnormal esophageal peristalsis
A. PRIMARY MOTILITY DISORDERS
1. Achalasia
2. **Diffuse esophageal spasm**
• severe intermittent pain while swallowing
√ compartmentalization of esophagus by
numerous tertiary contractions
Dx: extremely high pressures on manometry
3. Presbyesophagus
4. Chalasia
5. Congenital TE fistula
6. Intestinal pseudoobstruction
B. SECONDARY MOTILITY DISORDERS
(a) Connective tissue disease
1. Scleroderma
2. SLE

3. Rheumatoid arthritis
4. Polymyositis
5. Dermatomyositis
6. Muscular dystrophy
(b) Chemical / physical injury
1. Reflux / peptic esophagitis
2. S/P vagotomy
3. Caustic esophagitis
4. Radiotherapy
(c) Infection
Fungal: candidiasis
Parasitic: Chagas disease
Bacterial: TB, diphtheria
Viral: herpes simplex
(d) Metabolic disease
1. Diabetes mellitus
2. Amyloidosis
3. Alcoholism
4. Electrolyte disturbances
(e) Endocrine disease
1. Myxedema
2. Thyrotoxicosis
(f) Neoplasm
(g) Drug-related
atropine, propantheline, curare
(h) Muscle disease
1. Myotonic dystrophy
2. Muscular dystrophy
3. Oculopharyngeal dystrophy
4. Myasthenia gravis (disturbed motility only in
striated muscle of upper 1/3 of esophagus)
√ persistent collection of barium in upper
third of esophagus
√ findings reversed by cholinesterase
inhibitor edrophonium (Tensilon®)
(i) Neurologic disease
1. Parkinsonism
2. Multiple sclerosis
3. CNS neoplasm
4. Amyotrophic lateral sclerosis
5. Bulbar poliomyelitis
6. Cerebrovascular disease
7. Huntington chorea
8. Ganglioneuromatosis
9. Wilson disease
10. Friedreich ataxia
11. Familial dysautonomia (Riley-Day)
12. Stiff-man syndrome

Diffuse esophageal dilatation
= ACHALASIA PATTERN = MEGAESOPHAGUS

A. ESOPHAGEAL MOTILITY DISORDER
1. Idiopathic achalasia
2. Chagas disease: patients commonly from South
America; often associated with megacolon +
cardiomegaly
3. Postvagotomy syndrome
4. Scleroderma
5. Systemic lupus erythematosus

6. Presbyesophagus
7. Ehlers-Danlos syndrome
8. Diabetic / alcoholic neuropathy
9. Anticholinergic drugs
10. Idiopathic intestinal pseudoobstruction
    = degeneration of innervation
11. Amyloidosis: associated with macroglossia, thickened small bowel folds
12. Esophagitis

B. DISTAL OBSTRUCTION
   1. Infiltrating lesion of distal esophagus / gastric cardia (eg, carcinoma) = pseudoachalasia
   2. Benign stricture
   3. Extrinsic compression

mnemonic: "MA'S TACO in an SH"
   Muscular disorder (eg, myasthenia gravis)
   Achalasia
   Scleroderma
   Trypanosomiasis (Chagas disease)
   Amyloidosis
   Carcinoma
   Obstruction
   Stricture (lye, potassium, tetracycline)
   Hiatal hernia

Air esophagram
1. Normal variant
2. Scleroderma
3. Distal obstruction: tumor, stricture, achalasia
4. Thoracic surgery
5. Mediastinal inflammatory disease
6. S/P total laryngectomy (esophageal speech)
7. Endotracheal intubation + PEEP

Tracheobronchoesophageal fistula
A. CONGENITAL
   1. Congenital tracheoesophageal fistula

B. MALIGNANT
   1. Lung cancer
   2. Metastases to mediastinal lymph nodes
   3. Esophageal cancer
   Often following radiation treatment of these tumors!

C. TRAUMATIC
   1. Instrumentation (esophagoscopy, bougienage, pneumatic dilatation)
   2. Blunt ("crush injury") / penetrating chest trauma
   3. Surgery
   4. Foreign body perforation
   5. Corrosives
   6. Postemetic rupture = Boerhaave syndrome

D. INFECTIOUS / INFLAMMATORY
   — TB, syphilis, histoplasmosis, actinomycosis, Crohn disease
   — Perforated diverticulum
   — Pulmonary sequestration / cyst

Esophageal diverticulum
1. ZENKER DIVERTICULUM (pharyngoesophageal)
2. INTERBRONCHIAL DIVERTICULUM
   = traction diverticulum
   Response to pull from fibrous adhesions following lymph node infection (TB), contains all 3 esophageal layers
   Location: usually on right anterolateral wall of interbronchial segment
   √ calcified mediastinal nodes
3. INTERAORTICO-BRONCHIAL DIVERTICULUM
   = thoracic pulsion diverticulum
   Location: on left anterolateral wall between inferior border of aortic arch + upper margin of left main bronchus
4. EPIPHRENIC DIVERTICULUM (rare)
   Location: usually on lateral esophageal wall, right > left, in distal 10 cm
   √ often associated with hiatus hernia
5. INTRAMURAL ESOPHAGEAL PSEUDODIVERTICULOSIS
   √ outpouching from mucosal glands

Esophageal inflammation
A. CONTACT INJURY
   (a) reflux related
       1. Peptic ulcer disease
       2. Barrett esophagus
       3. Scleroderma (patulous LES)
       4. Nasogastric intubation
   (b) caustic
       1. Foreign body
       2. Corrosives
   (c) thermic
       Habitual ingestion of excessively hot meals / liquids
B. RADIATION INJURY
C. INFECTION
   1. Candidiasis
   2. Herpes simplex virus / CMV
   3. Diphtheria
D. SYSTEMIC DISEASE
   (a) dermatologic disorders
       Pemphigoid, epidermolysis bullosa
   (b) others:
       1. Crohn disease
       2. Graft-versus-host disease
       3. Behçet disease
       4. Eosinophilic gastroenteritis

Esophageal ulceration
A. PEPTIC
   1. Reflux esophagitis: scleroderma
      √ shallow / deep ulcers in distal esophagus
   2. Barrett esophagus
   3. Crohn disease
      √ aphthous ulcers in variable location
   4. Dermatologic disorders: benign mucous membrane pemphigoid, epidermolysis bullosa dystrophica, Behçet disease

B. INFECTIOUS
  1. Herpes
     √ discrete superficial ulcers in midesophagus
  2. Cytomegalovirus
     √ large flat ulcer in mid- or distal esophagus
C. CONTACT INJURY / EXTERNAL INJURY
  1. Corrosives: alkali, strictures in 50%
  2. Alcohol-induced esophagitis
  3. Drug-induced: antibiotics, quinidine, potassium chloride
     √ discrete superficial ulcers in midesophagus
  4. Radiotherapy: smooth stricture >4500 rads
     √ shallow / deep ulcers conforming to radiation portal
  5. Nasogastric tube
     √ elongated stricture in middle + distal 1/3
  6. Endoscopic sclerotherapy
D. MALIGNANT
  1. Esophageal carcinoma
Location:
@ Upper esophagus
  1. Barrett ulcer in islets of gastric mucosa
@ Midesophagus
  1. Herpes esophagitis
  2. CMV esophagitis
  3. Drug-induced esophagitis
@ Distal esophagus
  1. Reflux esophagitis
  2. CMV esophagitis
DDx:
  1. Sacculation
     = outpouching in distal esophagus due to asymmetric scarring in reflux esophagitis
  2. Esophageal intramural pseudodiverticula
  3. Artifact
     (a) tiny precipitates of barium
     (b) transient mucosal crinkling in inadequate distension
     (c) irregular Z-line

Focal esophageal narrowing
  1. **Web**
     = 1– 2 mm thick (vertical length) area of complete / incomplete circumferential narrowing
     Location: cervical / thoracic; occasionally multiple
  2. **Ring**
     = 5 – 10 mm thick (vertical length) area of complete / incomplete circumferential narrowing
  3. **Stricture**
     = >10 mm in vertical length

Long smooth esophageal narrowing
  1. Congenital esophageal stenosis
     √ at junction between middle + distal third
     √ web-like / tubular stenosis of 1 cm in length
  2. Surgical repair of esophageal atresia
     √ interruption of primary peristaltic wave at anastomosis
     √ secondary contractions may produce retrograde flow with aspiration

√ impaction of food
  3. Caustic burns = alkaline burns
  4. Gastric acid: reflux, hyperemesis gravidarum
  5. Intubation: reflux + compromise of circulation
  6. Radiotherapy for esophageal carcinoma; tumor of lung, breast, or thymus; lymphoma; metastases to mediastinal lymph nodes
     Onset of stricture: usually 4 – 8 months post Rx
     Dose: 3000 – 5000 rad
  7. Post infection: moniliasis (rare)

LOWER ESOPHAGEAL NARROWING
  mnemonic: "SPADE"
  Scleroderma
  Presbyesophagus
  Achalasia; **A**nticholinergics
  Diffuse esophageal spasm
  Esophagitis

Double-barrel esophagus
  1. Dissecting intramural hematoma from emetogenic injury
  2. Mallory-Weiss tear
     trauma, esophagoscopy (in 0.25%), bougienage (in 0.5%), ingestion of foreign bodies, spontaneous (bleeding diathesis)
  3. Intramural abscess
  4. Intraluminal diverticulum
  5. Esophageal duplication (if communication with esophageal lumen present)

Esophageal filling defect
A. BENIGN TUMORS
   <1% of all esophageal tumors
   (a) <u>Submucosal tumor</u> (75%)
       = nonepithelial, intramural
       1. Leiomyoma (50% of all benign tumors)
       2. Lipoma, fibroma, lipoma, fibrolipoma, myxofibroma, hamartoma, hemangioma, lymphangioma, neurofibroma, schwannoma, granular cell myoblastoma
          √ primary wave stops at level of tumor
          √ proximal esophageal dilatation + hypotonicity
          √ rigid esophageal wall at site of tumoral implant
          √ disorganized / altered / effaced mucosal folds around defect
          √ tumor shadow on tangential view extending beyond esophageal margin
   (b) <u>Mucosal tumor</u> (25%) = epithelial, intraluminal
       1. Fibrovascular / inflammatory polyp; adenomatous polyp
       2. Squamous papilloma, fibropapilloma
       3. Villous adenoma, fibroadenoma
          √ no interruption of primary peristaltic wave
          √ well-circumscribed central radiolucent defect
          √ symmetrical ampullary distension of esophagus around defect
          √ no change of mucosal pattern at periphery of defect

B. MALIGNANT TUMORS
1. Esophageal cancer, varicoid squamous cell carcinoma
2. Gastric cancer
3. Leiomyosarcoma, carcinosarcoma, pseudosarcoma
4. Metastases: malignant melanoma, lymphoma (<1% of gastrointestinal lymphomas), stomach, lung, breast
C. VASCULAR
varices
D. INFECTION / INFLAMMATION
Candida / herpes esophagitis, drug-induced inflammatory reaction
E. CONGENITAL / NORMAL VARIANT
prolapsed gastric folds, esophageal duplication cyst
F. FOREIGN BODIES
chicken bone, fish bone, pins, coins, small toys, meat, air bubble

Esophageal mucosal nodules / plaques
1. Candida esophagitis
   √ diffuse / localized discrete plaques
2. Reflux esophagitis (early stage)
   √ tiny poorly defined nodules in distal esophagus
3. Barrett esophagus
   √ localized reticular pattern often adjacent to distal aspect of high stricture
4. Glycogen acanthosis
   √ diffuse / localized nodules / plaques
5. Superficial spreading carcinoma
   √ localized coalescent nodules / plaques
6. Artifacts (undissolved effervescent agent, air bubbles, debris)

Abnormal esophageal folds
A. TRANSVERSE FOLDS
1. **Feline esophagus**
   frequently seen with gastroesophageal reflux; normally found in cats
   √ transient contraction of longitudinally oriented muscularis mucosae
2. Fixed transverse folds
   due to scarring from reflux esophagitis
   √ stepladder appearance in distal esophagus
B. LONGITUDINAL FOLDS
normally 1 – 2 mm wide in collapsed esophagus; >3 mm with submucosal edema / inflammation
1. Gastroesophageal reflux
2. Opportunistic infection
3. Caustic ingestion
4. Irradiation

DDx:
1. Varices
   √ tortuous / serpentine folds that can be effaced by esophageal distension
2. Varicoid carcinoma
   √ fixed rigid folds with abrupt demarcation due to submucosal spread

Extrinsic esophageal impression
Cervical causes of esophageal impression
A. OSSEOUS LESIONS
1. Anterior marginal osteophyte / DISH
2. Anterior disk herniation
3. Cervical trauma + hematoma
4. Osteomyelitis
5. Bone neoplasm
B. ESOPHAGEAL WALL LESIONS
(a) muscle
   1. Cricopharyngeus
   2. Esophageal web
(b) vessel
   1. Pharyngeal venous plexus
   2. Lymph node enlargement
C. ENDOCRINE ORGANS
1. Thyroid / parathyroid enlargement (benign / malignant)
2. Fibrotic traction after thyroidectomy
D. Retropharyngeal / mediastinal abscess

Thoracic causes of esophageal impression
A. NORMAL INDENTATIONS
Aortic arch, left main stem bronchus, left inferior pulmonary vein, diaphragmatic hiatus
B. ABNORMAL VASCULATURE
Right-sided aortic arch, cervical aortic arch, aortic unfolding, aortic tortuosity, aortic aneurysm, double aortic arch ("reverse S"), coarctation of aorta ("reverse figure 3"), aberrant right subclavian artery = arteria lusoria (semilunar / bayonet-shaped imprint upon posterior wall of esophagus), aberrant left pulmonary artery (between trachea + esophagus), anomalous pulmonary venous return (anterior), persistent truncus arteriosus (posterior)
C. CARDIAC CAUSES
(a) enlargement of chambers
   Left atrial / left ventricular enlargement: mitral disease (esophageal displacement backwards + to the right)
(b) pericardial masses
   Pericardial tumor / cyst / effusion
D. MEDIASTINAL CAUSES
Mediastinal tumor, lymphadenopathy (metastatic, tuberculous), inflammation, cyst
E. PULMONARY CAUSES
Pulmonary tumor, bronchogenic cyst, atypical pulmonary fibrosis (retraction)
F. ESOPHAGEAL ABNORMALITIES
1. Esophageal diverticulum
2. Paraesophageal hernia
3. **Esophageal duplication:** R:L = 2:1, mostly tubular shape, almost never communicating; intramural / paraesophageal, 60% at lower esophagus

STOMACH
Gastric pneumatosis
A. INFECTION
1. Emphysematous gastritis

B. ISCHEMIA
1. Gastric ulcer disease with intramural perforation
2. Severe necrotizing gastroenteritis
3. Gastric carcinoma
4. Volvulus
5. Gastric infarction

C. TRAUMA
(a) Iatrogenic
1. Recent gastroduodenal surgery
2. Endoscopy (1.6%)
(b) Ingested material:
1. Corrosive gastritis
2. Acid ingestion

D. OVERDISTENSION (increased intraluminal pressure)
1. Gastric outlet obstruction
2. Volvulus
3. Overinflation during gastroscopy
4. Profuse vomiting

E. DISSECTING AIR
1. Pulmonary bulla rupturing along esophageal wall / mediastinum

F. IDIOPATHIC
1. Nonbacterial gastric emphysema = intramural gastric emphysema

√ thin discrete sharply defined streaks of gas in submucosa ± subserosa
√ irregular radiolucent band of innumerable small bubbles with constant relationship to each other
√ bulging of mucosa
√ gas within portal venous system

Gastric atony
= gastric retention in the absence of mechanical obstruction
Pathophysiology: reflex paralysis

A. ACUTE GASTRIC ATONY
(may develop within 24 – 48 hours)
1. Acute gastric dilatation: secondary to decreased arterial perfusion (ischemia, congestive heart failure) in old patients, usually fatal
2. Postsurgical atony, ureteral catheterization
3. Immobilization: body cast, paraplegia, postoperative state
4. Abdominal trauma: especially back injury
5. Severe pain: renal / biliary colic, migraine headaches, severe burns
6. Infection: peritonitis, pancreatitis, appendicitis, subphrenic abscess, septicemia

B. CHRONIC GASTRIC ATONY
1. Neurologic abnormalities: brain tumor, bulbar poliomyelitis, vagotomy, tabes
2. Muscular abnormalities: scleroderma, muscular dystrophy
3. Drug-induced atony: atropine, morphine, heroin, ganglionic blocking agents
4. Electrolyte imbalance: diabetic ketoacidosis, hypercalcemia, hypocalcemia, hypokalemia, hepatic coma, uremia, myxedema

5. Diabetes mellitus = gastroparesis diabeticorum (0.08% incidence)
6. Emotional distress
7. Lead poisoning
8. Porphyria

• abdominal distension
• vascular collapse (decreased venous return)
• vomiting
√ large stomach filled with air + fluid (up to 7,500 ml)
√ retention of barium
√ absent / diminished peristaltic activity
√ patulous pylorus
√ frequently dilated duodenum
DDx: gastric volvulus, pyloric stenosis

Narrowing of stomach
= linitis plastica type of stenosis

A. MALIGNANCY
1. Scirrhous gastric carcinoma (involving portion / all of stomach)
2. Hodgkin lymphoma, NHL
3. Metastatic involvement (carcinoma of breast, pancreatic carcinoma, colonic carcinoma)

B. INFLAMMATION
1. Chronic gastric ulcer disease with intense spasm
2. Pseudo-Billroth-I pattern of Crohn disease
3. Sarcoidosis
√ polypoid appearance, pyloric hypertrophy
√ gastric ulcers, duodenal deformity
4. Eosinophilic gastritis
5. Polyarteritis nodosa
6. Stenosing antral gastritis / hypertrophic pyloric stenosis

C. INFECTION
1. Tertiary stage of syphilis
√ absent mucosal folds + peristalsis
√ no change over years
2. Tuberculosis (rare)
√ hyperplastic nodules / ulcerative lesion / annular lesion
√ pyloric obstruction, may cross into duodenum
3. Histoplasmosis
4. Actinomycosis
5. Strongyloidiasis
6. Phlegmonous gastritis
7. Toxoplasmosis

D. TRAUMA
1. Corrosive gastritis
2. Radiation injury
3. Gastric freezing
4. Hepatic arterial chemotherapy infusion

E. OTHERS
1. Perigastric adhesions (normal mucosa, no interval change, normal peristalsis)
2. Amyloidosis
3. Pseudolymphoma
4. Exogastric mass (hepatomegaly, pancreatic pseudocyst)

Antral narrowing
mnemonic: "SPICER"
Sarcoidosis, **S**yphilis
Peptic ulcer disease
Infection (tuberculosis)
Cancer
Eosinophilic granuloma
Radiation

Widened retrogastric space
A. PANCREATIC MASSES (most common cause)
   1. Acute + chronic pancreatitis
   2. Pancreatic pseudocyst
   3. Pancreatic cystadenoma + carcinoma
B. OTHER RETROPERITONEAL MASSES
Sarcoma, renal tumor, adrenal tumor, lymph node enlargement, abscess, hematoma
C. GASTRIC MASSES
   1. Leiomyoma, leiomyosarcoma
D. OTHERS
   1. Aortic aneurysm
   2. Choledochal cyst
   3. Obesity
   4. Postsurgical disruptions + adhesions
   5. Ascites
   6. Gross hepatomegaly + enlarged caudate lobe
   7. Hernia involving omentum

Intramural-extramucosal lesions of stomach
√ sharply delineated marginal / contour defect
√ stretched folds over intact mucosa
√ acute angle at margins
√ may ulcerate centrally
√ may become pedunculated and acquire polypoid appearance over years

A. NEOPLASTIC
   1. Leiomyoma   (48%)
   2. Neurogenic tumors   (14%)
   3. Heterotopic pancreas (12%)
   4. Fibrous tumor   (11%)
   5. Lipoma   (7%)
   6. Hemangioma   (7%)
   7. Glomus tumor   (rare)
   8. Carcinoid
   9. Metastatic tumor
B. INFLAMMATION / INFECTION
   1. Granuloma: (1) Foreign body granuloma (2) Sarcoidosis (3) Crohn disease (4) Tuberculosis (5) Histoplasmosis
   2. Eosinophilic gastritis
   3. Tertiary syphilis: infiltrative / ulcerative / tumorous type
   4. Echinococcal cyst
C. PANCREATIC ABNORMALITIES
   1. Ectopic pancreas
   2. Annular pancreas
   3. Pancreatic pseudocyst
D. DEPOSITS
   1. Amyloid

   2. Endometriosis
   3. Localized hematoma
E. OTHERS
   1. Varices (ie, fundal)
   2. Duplications (4% of all GI tract duplications)

Gastric filling defects
A. INTRINSIC WALL LESIONS
  (a) <u>benign</u> (most common)
   1. Polyps: hyperplastic, adenomatous, villous, hamartomatous (Peutz-Jeghers syndrome, Cowden disease)
   2. Leiomyoma
   3. Granulomatous lesions:
    (a) Eosinophilic granuloma (b) Crohn disease (c) Tuberculosis (d) Sarcoidosis
   4. Pseudolymphoma = benign reactive proliferation of lymphoid tissue
   5. Extramedullary hematopoiesis
   6. Ectopic pancreas
   7. Gastric duplication cyst
   8. Intramural hematoma
   9. Esophagogastric herniation
  (b) <u>malignant</u>
   1. Gastric carcinoma, lymphoma
   2. Gastric sarcoma: leiomyosarcoma, liposarcoma, leiomyoblastoma
   3. Gastric metastases: melanoma, breast, pancreas, colon
B. EXTRINSIC IMPRESSIONS ON STOMACH
in 70% nonneoplastic (extrinsic pseudotumors in 20%)
  (a) <u>normal organs</u>: organomegaly, tortuous aorta, heart, cardiac aneurysm
  (b) <u>benign masses</u>: cysts of pancreas, liver, spleen, adrenal, kidney; gastric duplication, postoperative deformity (eg, Nissen fundoplication)
  (c) <u>malignant masses</u>: enlarged celiac nodes
  (d) <u>inflammatory lesion</u>: left subphrenic abscess / hematoma
  — lateral displacement: enlarged liver, aortic aneurysm, enlarged celiac nodes
  — medial displacement: splenomegaly, mass in colonic splenic flexure, cardiomegaly, subphrenic abscess
C. INTRALUMINAL GASTRIC MASSES
   1. Bezoar
   2. Foreign bodies: food, pills, blood clot, gallstone
D. TUMORS OF ADJACENT ORGANS
Pancreatic carcinoma + cystadenoma, liver carcinoma, carcinoma of gallbladder, colonic carcinoma, renal carcinoma, adrenal carcinoma, lymph node involvement
E. THICKENED GASTRIC FOLDS

Bull's eye lesions
A. PRIMARY NEOPLASMS
   1. Leiomyoma, leiomyosarcoma
   2. Lymphoma
   3. Carcinoid

4. Primary carcinoma
B. HEMATOGENOUS METASTASES
    1. Malignant melanoma
        √ usually spares large bowel
    2. Breast cancer (15%)
        √ scirrhous appearance in stomach
    3. Cancer of lung
    4. Renal cell carcinoma
    5. Kaposi sarcoma
    6. Bladder carcinoma
C. ECTOPIC PANCREAS
    in duodenum / stomach
D. EOSINOPHILIC GRANULOMA
    most frequently in stomach

Lesions involving stomach and duodenum
1. Lymphoma: in <33% of patients with lymphoma
2. Gastric carcinoma: in <5%, but 50 x more common than lymphoma
3. Peptic ulcer disease
4. Tuberculosis: in 10% of gastric TB
5. Crohn disease: pseudo-Billroth-I pattern
6. Strongyloidiasis
7. Eosinophilic gastroenteritis

Thickened gastric folds
A. INFLAMMATION / INFECTION
    1. Inflammatory gastritis:
        alcoholic, hypertrophic, antral, corrosive, postirradiation, gastric cooling
    2. Crohn disease
    3. Sarcoidosis
    4. Infectious gastritis:
        bacterial invasion, bacterial toxins from botulism, diphtheria, dysentery, typhoid fever, anisakiasis, TB, syphilis
    5. Pseudolymphoma
B. MALIGNANCY
    1. Lymphoma
    2. Gastric carcinoma
C. INFILTRATIVE PROCESS
    1. Eosinophilic gastritis
    2. Amyloidosis
D. PANCREATIC DISEASE
    1. Pancreatitis
    2. Direct extension from pancreatic carcinoma
E. OTHERS
    1. Zollinger-Ellison syndrome
    2. Ménétrièr disease
    3. Gastric varices

Gastric ulcer
A. HORMONAL
    1. Zollinger-Ellison syndrome
    2. Hyperparathyroidism (in 1.3 – 24%)
        duodenum:stomach = 4:1; M:F = 3:1
        Δ Duodenal ulcers predominantly in females!
        Δ Gastric ulcers predominantly in males!
        • absence of gastric hypersecretion

3. Steroid-induced ulcer
    Gastric > duodenal location; frequently multiple + deep ulcers
    Commonly associated with erosions
    • bleeding (in 1/3)
4. Curling ulcer (burn) (in 0.09 – 2.6%)
5. Retained gastric antrum
B. INFLAMMATION
    1. Peptic ulcer disease
    2. Gastritis
    3. Radiation-induced ulcer
C. BENIGN MASS
    1. Leiomyoma
    2. Granulomatous disease
    3. Pseudolymphoma (lymphoid hyperplasia)
D. MALIGNANT MASS
    1. Gastric carcinoma
    2. Lymphoma (2% of all gastric neoplasms)
        √ multiple ulcers with aneurysmal appearance
    3. Leiomyosarcoma, neurogenic sarcoma, fibrosarcoma, liposarcoma
    4. Metastases
        (a) hematogenic: malignant melanoma, breast cancer, lung cancer
        (b) per continuum: pancreas, colon, kidney
E. DRUGS
    ASA: greater curvature

Complications of postoperative stomach
1. Filling defect of gastric remnant
2. Retained gastric antrum
3. Dumping syndrome
4. Afferent loop syndrome
5. Stomal obstruction
    (a) temporary reversible: edema of suture line, abscess / hematoma, potassium deficiency, inadequate electrolyte replacement, hypoproteinemia, hypoacidity
    (b) late mechanical: stomal ulcer (75%)

mnemonic: "LOBULATING"
Leaks (early)
Obstruction (early)
Bezoar
Ulcer (especially marginal)
Loop (afferent loop syndrome)
Anemia (macrocytic secondary to decreased intrinsic factor)
Tumor (? increased incidence)
Intussusception
Not feeling well after meals (dumping syndrome)
Gastritis (bile reflux)

Filling defect of gastric remnant
A. IATROGENIC
    Surgical deformity / plication defect, suture granuloma
B. INFLAMMATORY
    Bile reflux gastritis, hyperplastic polyps

C. INTUSSUSCEPTION
1. **Jejunogastric intussusception**
   (efferent loop in 75%, afferent loop in 25%)
   (a) acute form: high intestinal obstruction, left hypochondriac mass, hematemesis
   (b) chronic / intermittent form: may be self-reducing
       √ "coil spring" appearance of gastric filling defect
2. Gastrojejunal / gastroduodenal mucosal prolapse
   • often asymptomatic
   • bleeding, partial obstruction
D. NEOPLASTIC
1. Gastric stump carcinoma = >5 years after resection for benign disease; 15% within 10 years; 20% after 20 years
2. Recurrent carcinoma (10%) secondary to incomplete removal of gastric cancer
3. Malignancy at anastomosis (incomplete resection)
E. INTRALUMINAL MATTER: Bezoar

Gastric surgical procedures

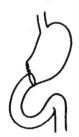

Billroth I

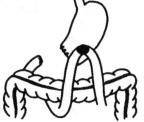

Billroth II

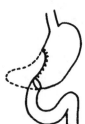

Shoemaker

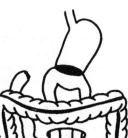

retrocolic (Polya)

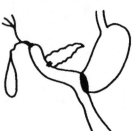

Whipple

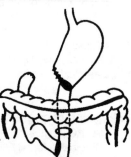

Roux-en-Y

SMALL BOWEL
Enlargement of papilla of Vater
A. Normal variant
   identified in 60% of UGI series; atypical location in 3rd portion of duodenum in 8%; 1.5 cm in diameter in 1% of normals
B. Papillary edema
   1. Impacted stone
   2. Pancreatitis (Poppel sign)
   3. Acute duodenal ulcer disease
   4. Papillitis
C. Perivaterian neoplasms
   = tumor mass + lymphatic obstruction
   1. Adenocarcinoma
   2. Adenomatous polyp (premalignant lesion)
   √ irregular surface + erosions
D. Lesions simulating enlarged papilla
   1. Benign spindle cell tumor
   2. Ectopic pancreatic tissue

Thickened duodenal folds
A. INFLAMMATION
   (a) within bowel wall: peptic ulcer disease, Zollinger-Ellison syndrome, regional enteritis, lymphoid hyperplasia, uremia
   (b) surrounding bowel wall: pancreatitis, cholecystitis
B. INFECTION
   Giardiasis, TB, strongyloidiasis, nontropical sprue
C. NEOPLASIA
   Lymphoma, metastases to peripancreatic nodes
D. DIFFUSE INFILTRATIVE DISORDER
   Whipple disease, amyloidosis, mastocytosis, eosinophilic enteritis, intestinal lymphangiectasia
E. VASCULAR DISORDER
   Duodenal varices, mesenteric arterial collaterals, intramural hemorrhage, chronic duodenal congestion (congestive heart failure, portal venous hypertension)
F. GLANDULAR ENLARGEMENT
   Brunner gland hyperplasia, cystic fibrosis

mnemonic: "BAD HELP"
   Brunner gland hyperplasia
   Amyloidosis
   Duodenitis (Z-E syndrome, peptic)
   Hemorrhage
   Edema, **E**ctopic pancreas
   Lymphoma
   Pancreatitis, **P**arasites

Duodenal filling defect
A. EXTRINSIC
   Gallbladder impression, CBD impression, gas-filled diverticulum
B. INTRINSIC TO WALL
   (a) benign neoplastic mass
       Adenoma, leiomyoma, lipoma, hamartoma (Peutz-Jeghers syndrome), prolapsed antral polyp, Brunner gland adenoma, villous adenoma, islet cell tumor

(b) <u>malignant neoplastic mass</u>
Carcinoid tumor, adenocarcinoma, ampullary carcinoma, lymphoma, sarcoma, metastasis (stomach, pancreas, gallbladder, colon, kidney, melanoma), retroperitoneal lymph node involvement

(c) <u>non-neoplastic mass</u>
Papilla of Vater, choledochocele, duplication cyst, pancreatic pseudocyst, duodenal varix, mesenteric artery collaterals, intramural hematoma, adjacent abscess, stitch abscess, ectopic pancreas, heterotopic gastric mucosa, prolapsed antral mucosa, Brunner gland hyperplasia, benign lymphoid hyperplasia

C. INTRALUMINAL
Blood clot, foreign body (fruit pit, gallstone, feeding tube)

Extrinsic pressure effect on duodenum
A. BILE DUCTS
Normal impression, dilated CBD, choledochal cyst
B. GALLBLADDER
Normal impression, gallbladder hydrops, Courvoisier phenomenon, gallbladder carcinoma, pericholecystic abscess
C. LIVER
Hepatomegaly, hypertrophied caudate lobe, anomalous hepatic lobe, hepatic cyst, hepatic tumor
D. RIGHT KIDNEY
Bifid collecting system, hydronephrosis, multiple renal cysts, polycystic kidney disease, hypernephroma
E. RIGHT ADRENAL
Adrenal carcinoma, enlargement in Addison disease
F. COLON
Duodenocolic apposition due to anomalous peritoneal fixation, carcinoma of hepatic flexure
G. VESSELS
Lymphadenopathy, duodenal varices, dilated arterial collaterals, aortic aneurysm, intramural / mesenteric hematoma

Widened duodenal sweep
A. NORMAL VARIANT

B. PANCREATIC LESION
1. Acute pancreatitis
2. Chronic pancreatitis
3. Pancreatic pseudocyst
4. Pancreatic carcinoma
5. Metastasis to pancreas
6. Pancreatic cystadenoma

C. VASCULAR LESION
1. Lymph node enlargement: lymphoma, metastasis, inflammation
2. Cystic lymphangioma of the mesentery

D. RETROPERITONEAL MASS
1. Aortic aneurysm
2. Choledochal cyst

Duodenal narrowing
A. DEVELOPMENTAL ANOMALIES
1. Duodenal atresia
2. Congenital web / duodenal diaphragm
3. Intraluminal diverticulum
4. Duodenal duplication cyst
5. Annular pancreas
6. Midgut volvulus, peritoneal bands (Ladd bands)
B. INTRINSIC DISORDERS
(a) <u>inflammation / infection</u>
1. Postbulbar ulcer
2. Crohn disease
3. Sprue
4. Tuberculosis
5. Strongyloidiasis
(b) <u>tumor</u>
Duodenal / ampullary malignancy
C. DISEASE IN ADJACENT STRUCTURES
1. Pancreatitis, pseudocyst, pancreatic carcinoma
2. Cholecystitis
3. Contiguous abscess
4. Metastases to pancreaticoduodenal nodes (lymphoma, lung cancer, breast cancer)
D. TRAUMA
1. Duodenal rupture
2. Intramural hematoma
E. VASCULAR
1. Superior mesenteric artery syndrome
2. Aorticoduodenal fistula
3. Preduodenal portal vein (anterior to descending duodenum)

Dilated duodenum
Megaduodenum = marked dilatation of entire C-loop
Megabulbus = dilatation of duodenal bulb only

A. VASCULAR COMPRESSION
Superior mesenteric artery syndrome, abdominal aortic aneurysm, aorticoduodenal fistula
B. PRIMARY DUODENAL ATONY
(a) scleroderma, dermatomyositis, SLE
(b) Chagas disease, aganglionosis, neuropathy, surgical / chemical vagotomy
(c) focal ileus: pancreatitis, cholecystitis, peptic ulcer disease, trauma
(d) altered emotional status, chronic idiopathic intestinal pseudo-obstruction
C. INFLAMMATORY / NEOPLASTIC INDURATION OF MESENTERIC ROOT
Crohn disease, tuberculous enteritis, pancreatitis, peptic ulcer disease, strongyloidiasis, metastatic disease
D. FLUID DISTENSION
Celiac disease, Zollinger-Ellison syndrome

Postbulbar ulceration
1. Benign postbulbar peptic ulcer
√   medial aspect of upper 2nd portion
√   incisura pointing to ulcer
√   occasionally barium reflux into common bile duct

√   ring stricture
√   stress- and drug-induced ulcers heal without
     deformity
2. Zollinger-Ellison syndrome
   √   multiple ulcers distal to duodenal bulb
   √   thickening of folds + hypersecretion
3. Leiomyoma
4. Malignant tumors:
   (a) primaries
       Adenocarcinoma, lymphoma, sarcoma
   (b) contiguous spread
       Pancreas, colon, kidney, gallbladder
   (c) hematogenous spread
       Melanoma, Kaposi sarcoma
   (d) lymphogenic spread
       Metastases to periduodenal lymph nodes
5. Granulomatous disease: Crohn disease, TB
6. Aorticoduodenal fistula
7. Mimickers: ectopic pancreas, diverticulum

Benign duodenal tumors
1. Leiomyoma   (27%)
2. Adenomatous polyp   (21%)
3. Lipoma   (21%)
4. Brunner gland adenoma   (17%)
5. Angiomatous tumor   (6%)
6. Ectopic pancreas   (2%)
7. Duodenal cyst   (2%)
8. Neurofibroma   (2%)
9. Hamartoma   (2%)

Malignant duodenal tumors
1. Adenocarcinoma (73%)
   Location: 40% in duodenum, most often in 2nd + 3rd
               portion = periampullary neoplasm
   (a) suprapapillary: apt to cause obstruction + bleeding
   (b) peripapillary: extrahepatic jaundice
   (c) intrapapillary: GI bleeding
   May be associated with Peutz-Jeghers syndrome
   √   annular / polypoid / ulcerative
   Metastases: regional lymph nodes (2/3)
   DDx: (1) Primary bile duct carcinoma
            (2) Ampullary carcinoma
2. Leiomyosarcoma (14%)
   Most often beyond 1st portion of duodenum
   √   up to 20 cm in size
   √   frequently ulcerated exophytic mass
3. Carcinoid (11%)
4. Lymphoma (2%)
   √   marked wall thickening
   √   bulky periduodenal lymphadenopathy

Small bowel diverticula
A. TRUE DIVERTICULA
   (a) Duodenal diverticula
       1. Racemose diverticula: bizarre, lobulated
       2. Giant diverticula
       3. Intraluminal diverticula: result of congenital
          web / diaphragm

   (b) Jejunal diverticulosis
   (c) Meckel diverticulum
B. PSEUDODIVERTICULA
   1. Scleroderma
   2. Crohn disease
   3. Lymphoma
   4. Mesenteric ischemia
   5. Communicating ileal duplication
   6. Giant duodenal ulcer

Small bowel ulcer
Aphthous ulcers of small bowel
A. INFECTION
   1. Yersinia enterocolitis (25%)
   2. Salmonellosis
   3. Tuberculosis
   4. Rickettsiosis
B. INFLAMMATION
   1. Crohn disease (22%)
   2. Behçet syndrome
   3. Reiter syndrome
   4. Ankylosing spondylitis

Large nonstenotic ulcers of small bowel
1. Primary nonspecific ulcer   47% incidence
2. Yersiniosis   33%
3. Crohn disease   30%
4. Tuberculosis   18%
5. Salmonellosis / shigellosis   7%
6. Meckel diverticulum   5%

Cavitary small bowel lesions
1. Lymphoma (exoenteric form)
2. Leiomyosarcoma (exoenteric form)
3. Primary adenocarcinoma
4. Metastases (especially malignant melanoma)

Separation of bowel loops
A. INFILTRATION OF BOWEL WALL / MESENTERY
   (a) inflammation / infection
       1. Crohn disease
       2. TB
       3. Radiation injury
       4. Retractile mesenteritis
       5. Intraperitoneal abscess
   (b) deposits
       1. Intestinal hemorrhage / mesenteric vascular
          occlusion
       2. Whipple disease
       3. Amyloidosis
   (c) tumor
       1. Carcinoid tumor: local release of serotonin
          responsible for muscular thickening +
          fibroplastic proliferation = desmoplastic
          reaction
       2. Primary carcinoma of small bowel (unusual
          presentation)
       3. Lymphoma
       4. Neurofibromatosis

B. ASCITES
Hepatic cirrhosis (75%), peritonitis, peritoneal carcinomatosis, congestive heart failure, constrictive pericarditis, primary / metastatic lymphatic disease
C. EXTRINSIC MASS
1. Peritoneal mesothelioma, mesenteric tumors (fibroma, lipoma, fibrosarcoma, leiomyosarcoma, malignant mesenteric lymphoid tumor, metastases)
2. Intraperitoneal abscess
3. Retractile mesenteritis (fibrosis, fatty infiltration, panniculitis)

Dilatated small bowel & normal folds
mnemonic: "SOS"
Sprue
Obstruction
Scleroderma

A. EXCESSIVE FLUID
(a) mechanical obstruction
due to adhesion, hernia, neoplasm
√ "string-of-beads sign" = air bubbles between mucosal folds in a fluid-filled small bowel
√ "pseudotumor sign" = closed loop obstruction
(b) malabsorption syndromes
1. Celiac disease, tropical + nontropical sprue
2. Lactase deficiency
B. BOWEL WALL PARALYSIS
= functional ileus = adynamic ileus
1. Surgical vagotomy
2. Chemical vagotomy from drug effects: atropine-like substances, morphine, L-dopa, glucagon
3. Chagas disease
4. Metabolic: hypokalemia, diabetes
5. Intrinsic + extrinsic intraabdominal inflammation
6. Chronic idiopathic pseudo-obstruction
C. VASCULAR COMPROMISE
1. Mesenteric ischemia (atherosclerosis)
2. Acute radiation enteritis
3. Amyloidosis
4. SLE
D. BOWEL WALL DESTRUCTION
1. Lymphoma
2. Scleroderma (smooth muscle atrophy)
3. Dermatomyositis

Normal small bowel folds & diarrhea
1. Pancreatic insufficiency
2. Lactase deficiency
3. Lymphoma / pseudolymphoma

Abnormal small bowel folds
Thickened folds of stomach + small bowel
1. Lymphoma
2. Crohn disease
3. Eosinophilic gastroenteritis
4. Zollinger-Ellison syndrome
5. Ménétrièr disease

6. Cirrhosis = gastric varices + hypoproteinemia
7. Amyloidosis
8. Whipple disease

Thickened smooth folds ± dilatation
A. EDEMA
(a) hypoproteinemia
Cirrhosis, nephrotic syndrome, protein-losing enteropathy (celiac disease, Whipple disease)
(b) increased capillary permeability
Angioneurotic edema, gastroenteritis
(c) increased hydrostatic pressure
Portal venous hypertension
(d) Zollinger-Ellison syndrome
B. HEMORRHAGE
(a) vessel injury
Ischemia, infarction, trauma
(b) vasculitis
Connective tissue disease, Henoch-Schönlein purpura, thrombangiitis obliterans, irradiation
(c) hypocoagulability
Hemophilia, anticoagulant therapy, hypofibrinogemia, circulating anticoagulants, fibrinolytic system activation, idiopathic thrombocytopenic purpura, coagulation defects (leukemia, lymphoma, multiple myeloma, metastatic carcinoma), hypoprothrombinemia
C. LYMPHATIC BLOCKAGE
1. Tumor infiltration: lymphoma, pseudolymphoma
2. Irradiation
3. Mesenteric fibrosis
4. Intestinal lymphangiectasia
5. Whipple disease
D. DEPOSITS
1. Eosinophilic enteritis
2. Pneumatosis intestinalis
3. Amyloidosis
4. Abetalipoproteinemia
5. Crohn disease
6. Graft-versus-host disease
7. Immunologic deficiency: hypo- / dysgammaglobulinemia

Thickened irregular folds ± dilatation
A. INFLAMMATION
1. Crohn disease
B. NEOPLASTIC
1. Lymphoma, pseudolymphoma
C. INFECTION
(a) protozoan
Giardiasis, strongyloidiasis, hookworm
(b) bacterial
Yersinia enterocolitica, typhoid fever, tuberculosis
(c) fungal: histoplasmosis
(d) AIDS-related infection
D. IDIOPATHIC
(a) lymphatic dilatation
1. Lymphangiectasia

2. Inflammatory process, tumor growth, irradiation fibrosis
3. Whipple disease
   (b) <u>cellular infiltration</u>
   1. Eosinophilic enteritis
   2. Mastocytosis
   (c) <u>deposits</u>
   1. Zollinger-Ellison syndrome
   2. Amyloidosis
   3. Alpha chain disease: defective secretory IGA system
   4. A-β-lipoproteinemia: recessive, retinitis pigmentosa, neurologic disease
   5. A-α-lipoproteinemia
   6. Fibrocystic disease of the pancreas
   7. Polyposis syndrome

   mnemonic: "G. WILLIAMS"
   Giardiasis
   Whipple disease, **W**aldenström macroglobulinemia
   Ischemia
   Lymphangiectasia
   Lymphoma
   Inflammation
   Amyloidosis, **A**gammaglobulinemia
   Mastocytosis, **M**alabsorption
   Soft tissue neoplasm (carcinoid, lipoma)

Tethered small bowel folds

= indicative of desmoplastic reaction
√ kinking, angulation, tethering, separation of bowel loops
1. Carcinoid
2. Postoperative in Gardner syndrome
3. Retractile mesenteritis
4. Hodgkin disease
5. Peritoneal implants
6. Endometriosis
7. Tuberculous peritonitis
8. Mesothelioma
9. Postoperative adhesions

Atrophy of small bowel folds

1. Celiac disease
2. Chronic radiation injury

Delayed small bowel transit

= transit time >6 hours
   mnemonic: "SPATS DID"
   Scleroderma
   Potassium (hypokalemia)
   Anxiety
   Thyroid (hypothyroidism)
   Sprue
   Diabetes (poorly controlled)
   Idiopathic
   Drugs (opiates, atropine, phenothiazine)

Multiple stenotic lesions of small bowel

1. Crohn disease

2. End-stage radiation enteritis
3. Metastatic carcinoma
4. Endometritis
5. Eosinophilic gastroenteritis
6. Tuberculosis
7. Drug-induced (eg, potassium chloride tablets)

Small bowel filling defects
Solitary filling defect

A. INTRINSIC TO BOWEL WALL
   (a) <u>benign neoplasm</u>: leiomyoma (97%), adenoma, lipoma, hemangioma, neurofibroma
   (b) <u>malignant primary</u>: adenocarcinoma, lymphoma (desmoplastic response), sarcoma, carcinoid
   (c) <u>metastases</u>: from melanoma, lung, kidney, breast
   (d) <u>inflammation</u>: inflammatory pseudotumor
   (e) <u>infection</u>: parasites
B. EXTRINSIC TO BOWEL WALL
   1. Duplication cyst
   2. Endometrioma
C. INTRALUMINAL
   1. Gallstone ileus
   2. Parasites (ascariasis, strongyloidiasis)
   3. Inverted Meckel diverticulum
   4. Blood clot
   5. Foreign body, bezoar, pills, seeds

Multiple filling defects of small bowel

A. POLYPOSIS SYNDROMES
   1. Peutz-Jeghers syndrome
   2. Gardner syndrome
   3. Disseminated gastrointestinal polyposis
   4. Generalized gastrointestinal juvenile polyposis
   5. Cronkhite-Canada syndrome
B. BENIGN TUMORS
   1. Multiple simple adenomatous polyps
   2. Hemangioma
   3. Leiomyoma, neurofibroma
   4. Nodular lymphoid hyperplasia
      = normal terminal ileum in children + adolescents; may be associated with dysgammaglobulinemia
      √ symmetric fairly sharply demarcated filling defects
   5. Varices (= multiple phlebectasia in jejunum, oral mucosa, tongue, scrotum)
C. MALIGNANT TUMORS
   1. Carcinoid tumor
   2. Lymphoma
      (a) primary lymphoma (rarely multiple)
      (b) secondary lymphoma: gastrointestinal involvement in 63% of disseminated disease; 19% in small intestine
   3. Metastases: melanoma > lung > breast > choriocarcinoma > kidney > stomach, uterus, ovary, pancreas
D. INTRALUMINAL
   1. Gallstones

2. Foreign bodies, food particles, seeds, pills
3. Parasites: ascariasis, strongyloidiasis, hookworm, tapeworm

Sandlike lucencies of small bowel
1. Waldenström macroglobulinemia
2. Mastocytosis
3. Histoplasmosis
4. Nodular lymphoid hyperplasia
5. Intestinal lymphangiectasia
6. Eosinophilic gastroenteritis
7. Lymphoma
8. Crohn disease
9. Whipple disease
10. Yersinia enterocolitis
11. Cronkhite-Canada syndrome
12. Cystic fibrosis
13. Food particles / gas bubbles
14. Strongyloides stercoralis

SMALL BOWEL TUMORS
Incidence: 1:100,000; 1.5 – 6% of all neoplasms in the GI tract;
Malignant:benign = 1:1
Symptomatic malignant:symptomatic benign = 3:1
Location of small bowel primaries:
   ileum (41%), jejunum (36%), duodenum (18%)
ROENTGENOGRAPHIC APPEARANCE:
(1) pedunculated intraluminal tumor, usually originating from mucosa
   √ smooth / irregular surface without visible mucosal pattern
   √ moves within intestinal lumen twice the length of the stalk
(2) sessile intraluminal tumor without stalk, usually from tissues outside mucosa
   √ smooth / irregular surface without visible mucosal pattern
(3) intra- / extramural tumor
   √ base of tumor greater than any part projecting into the lumen
   √ mucosal pattern visible, may be stretched
(4) serosal tumor
   √ displacement of adjacent loops
   √ small bowel obstruction (rare)
   √ coil-spring pattern of intussusceptum

Benign small bowel tumors
*   asymptomatic (80%)
*   melena, pain, weakness
*   palpable abdominal mass (20%)
Types:
   1. Leiomyoma   (36 – 49%)
   2. Adenoma   (15 – 20%)
   3. Lipoma   (14 – 16%)
      Location: duodenum (32%), jejunum (17%), ileum (51%)
   4. Hemangioma   (13 – 16%)
   5. Lymphangioma   (5%)
      Location: duodenum > jejunum > ileum

6. Neurogenic tumor   (1%)

Malignant small bowel tumors
*   asymptomatic (10 – 30%)
*   pain due to intermittent obstruction (80%)
*   weight loss (66%)
*   gastrointestinal blood loss (50%)
*   palpable abdominal mass (50%)

   1. Carcinoid (46 – 48%)
   2. Adenocarcinoma (25 – 26%)
      may arise in villous tumors / de novo
      Location: duodenum (48%), jejunum (44%), ileum (8%)
      √ annular stricture (60%)
      √ lobulated / ovoid polypoid sessile mass (41%)
      √ ulceration (27%)
   3. Lymphoma (16 – 17%)
   4. Leiomyosarcoma (9 – 10%)
   5. Vascular malignancy (1%)
   6. Fibrosarcoma (0.3%)
   7. Metastatic tumor

Ileocecal valve abnormalities
A. Lipomatosis: >40 years of age, female
   √ stellate / rosette pattern
B. NEOPLASM
   1. Lipoma, adenomatous polyp, villous adenoma
   2. Carcinoid tumor
   3. Adenocarcinoma: 2% of all colonic cancers
   4. Lymphoma: often involving terminal ileum
C. INFLAMMATION
   1. Crohn disease
   2. Ulcerative colitis
      √ patulous valve, fixed in open position
   3. Tuberculosis
      √ "Fleischner sign" = wide gaping ileocecal valve associated with narrowing of the immediately adjacent ileum
   4. Amebiasis
      √ terminal ileum not involved (in United States)
   5. Typhoid fever, anisakiasis, schistosomiasis, actinomycosis
   6. Cathartic abuse
D. PROLAPSE
   (a) antegrade: indistinguishable from lipomatosis / prolapsing mucosa / neoplasm
   (b) retrograde
E. INTUSSUSCEPTION
F. LYMPHOID HYPERPLASIA

COLON
Colon cutoff sign
= abrupt cutoff of gas column at splenic flexure
Causes:
   1. Acute pancreatitis (inflammatory exudate along transverse mesocolon)
   2. Colonic obstruction
   3. Mesenteric thrombosis
   4. Ischemic colitis

Coned cecum
A. INFLAMMATION
1. Crohn disease
   √ involvement of ascending colon + terminal ileum
2. Ulcerative colitis
   √ backwash ileitis (in 10%)
   √ gaping ileocecal valve
3. Appendicitis
4. Typhlitis
5. Perforated cecal diverticulum
B. INFECTION
1. Tuberculosis
   √ colonic involvement more prominent than that of terminal ileum
2. Amebiasis
   √ involvement of cecum in 90% of amebiasis
   √ thickened ileocecal valve fixed in open position
   √ reflux into normal terminal ileum
   √ skip lesions in colon
3. Actinomycosis
   • palpable abdominal mass
   • indolent sinus tracts in abdominal wall
4. Blastomycosis
5. **Anisakiasis**
   from ingestion of raw fish with ascaris-like nematode
6. Typhoid, Yersinia
C. TUMOR
1. Carcinoma of the cecum
2. Metastasis to cecum

Colonic thumbprinting
= sharply defined fingerlike marginal indentations at contours of wall
1. ISCHEMIA = Ischemic colitis
   Occlusive vascular disease, hypercoagulability state, hemorrhage into bowel wall (bleeding diathesis, anticoagulants), traumatic intramural hematoma
2. INFLAMMATION
   Ulcerative colitis, Crohn colitis
3. INFECTION
   Acute amebiasis, schistosomiasis, strongyloidiasis, cytomegalovirus (in renal transplant recipients), pseudomembranous colitis
4. MALIGNANT LESIONS
   Localized primary lymphoma, hematogenous metastases
5. MISCELLANEOUS
   Endometriosis, amyloidosis, pneumatosis intestinalis, diverticulosis, diverticulitis, hereditary angioneurotic edema

Colonic urticaria pattern
A. OBSTRUCTION
1. Obstructing carcinoma
2. Cecal volvulus
3. Colonic ileus
B. ISCHEMIA
C. INFECTION / INFLAMMATION
1. Yersinia enterocolitis

2. Herpes
3. Crohn disease
D. URTICARIA

Colonic ulcers
A. IDIOPATHIC
1. Ulcerative colitis
2. Crohn colitis
B. ISCHEMIC
1. Ischemic colitis
C. TRAUMATIC
1. Radiation injury
2. Caustic colitis
D. NEOPLASTIC
1. Primary colonic carcinoma
2. Metastases (prostate, stomach, lymphoma, leukemia)
E. INFLAMMATORY
1. Pseudomembranous colitis
2. Pancreatitis
3. Diverticulitis
4. Behçet syndrome
5. Solitary rectal ulcer syndrome
6. Nonspecific benign ulceration
F. INFECTION
(a) protozoan
   1. Amebiasis
   2. Schistosomiasis
   3. Strongyloidiasis
(b) bacterial
   1. Shigellosis, salmonellosis
   2. Staphylococcal colitis
   3. Tuberculosis
   4. Gonorrheal proctitis
   5. Yersinia colitis
   6. Campylobacter fetus colitis
(c) fungal
   Histoplasmosis, mucormycosis, actinomycosis, candidiasis
(d) viral
   1. Lymphogranuloma venereum
   2. Herpes proctocolitis
   3. Cytomegalovirus (transplants)

APHTHOUS ULCERS
1. Crohn disease
2. Amebic colitis
3. **Yersinia enterocolitis**
   Organism: Gram-negative
   • fever, diarrhea, RLQ pain
   Location: terminal ileum
   √ thickened folds + ulceration
   √ lymphoid nodular hyperplasia
4. Behçet syndrome
5. Lymphoma
6. Ischemia

Double-tracking of colon
= longitudinal extraluminal tracks paralleling the colon
1. Diverticulitis: generally 3 – 6 cm in length

2. Crohn disease: generally >10 cm
3. Primary carcinoma: wider + more irregular

Colonic narrowing
A. CHRONIC STAGE OF ANY ULCERATING COLITIS
   (a) <u>inflammatory</u> : ulcerative colitis, Crohn colitis, solitary rectal ulcer syndrome, nonspecific benign ulcer
   (b) <u>infectious</u>: amebiasis, schistosomiasis, bacillary dysentery, TB, fungal disease, lymphogranuloma venereum, herpes zoster, cytomegalovirus, strongyloides
   (c) <u>ischemic</u>: ischemic colitis
   (d) <u>traumatic</u>: radiation injury, cathartic colon, caustic colitis
B. MALIGNANT LESION
   (a) <u>primary</u>: colonic carcinoma (annular / scirrhous); complication of ulcerative colitis + Crohn colitis
   (b) <u>metastatic</u>: from prostate, cervix, uterus, kidney, stomach, pancreas, primary intraperitoneal sarcoma
      — hematogenous (eg, breast)
      — lymphangitic spread
      — peritoneal seeding
C. EXTRINSIC PROCESS
   (a) <u>inflammation</u>: retractile mesenteritis, diverticulitis, pancreatitis
   (b) <u>deposits</u>: amyloidosis, endometriosis, pelvic lipomatosis
D. POSTSURGICAL
   Adhesive bands, surgical anastomosis
E. NORMAL
   Cannon point

Rectal narrowing
1. Pelvic lipomatosis + fibrolipomatosis
2. Lymphogranuloma venereum
3. Radiation injury of rectum
4. Chronic ulcerative colitis

Enlarged presacral space
Normal width <5 mm in 95%; abnormal width >10 mm
A. RECTAL INFLAMMATION / INFECTION
   Ulcerative colitis, Crohn colitis, idiopathic proctosigmoiditis, radiation therapy
B. RECTAL INFECTION
   1. Proctitis (TB, amebiasis, lymphogranuloma venereum, radiation, ischemia)
   2. Diverticulitis
C. BENIGN RECTAL TUMOR
   1. Developmental cyst (dermoid, enteric cyst, tail gut cyst)
   2. Lipoma, neurofibroma, hemangioendothelioma
D. MALIGNANT RECTAL TUMOR
   1. Adenocarcinoma, cloacogenic carcinoma
   2. Lymphoma, sarcoma, lymph node metastases
   3. Prostatic carcinoma, bladder tumors, cervical cancer, ovarian cancer
E. BODY FLUIDS / DEPOSITS
   1. Hematoma: surgery, sacral fracture
   2. Pus: perforated appendix, presacral abscess
   3. Serum: edema, venous thrombosis
   4. Deposit of fat: pelvic lipomatosis, Cushing disease
   5. Deposit of amyloid: amyloidosis
F. SACRAL TUMOR
   1. Sacrococcygeal teratoma, anterior sacral meningocele
   2. Chordoma, metastasis to sacrum
G. MISCELLANEOUS
   1. Inguinal hernia containing segment of colon
   2. Colitis cystica profunda
   3. Pelvic lipomatosis

Colonic filling defects
Single colonic filling defect
A. BENIGN TUMOR
   1. Polyp (hyperplastic, adenomatous, villous adenoma, villoglandular); most common benign tumor
   2. Lipoma
      Most common intramural tumor, 2nd most common benign tumor; M < F
      Location: ascending colon + cecum > left side of colon
   3. Carcinoid: 10% metastasize
   4. Spindle cell tumor (leiomyoma, fibroma, neurofibroma); 4th most common benign tumor; rectum > cecum
   5. Lymphangioma, hemangioma
B. MALIGNANT TUMOR
   (a) <u>primary tumor</u>: carcinoma, sarcoma
   (b) <u>secondary tumor</u>:
      Metastases (breast, stomach, lung, pancreas, kidney, female genital tract), lymphoma, invasion by adjacent tumors
C. INFECTION
   1. Ameboma
   2. Polypoid granuloma: schistosomiasis, TB
D. INFLAMMATION
   1. Inflammatory pseudopolyp: ulcerative colitis, Crohn disease
   2. Periappendiceal abscess
   3. Diverticulitis
   4. Foreign body perforation
E. NONSESSILE INTRALUMINAL BODY
   1. Fecal impaction
   2. Foreign body
   3. Gallstone
   4. Bolus of Ascaris worms
F. MISCELLANEOUS
   1. Endometriosis
      3rd most common benign tumor
      Location: sigmoid colon, rectosigmoid junction (at level of cul-de-sac)
      • may cause bleeding (after invasion of mucosa)
   2. Localized amyloid deposition
   3. Suture granuloma
   4. Intussusception

5. Pseudotumor (adhesions, fibrous bands)
6. Colitis cystica profunda

Multiple colonic filling defects
A. NEOPLASMS
   (a) <u>polyposis syndrome</u>: familial polyposis, Gardner syndrome, Peutz-Jeghers syndrome, Turcot syndrome, juvenile polyposis syndrome, disseminated gastrointestinal polyps, multiple adenomatous polyps
   (b) <u>hematogenous metastases</u>: from breast, lung, stomach, ovary, pancreas, uterus
   (c) <u>multiple tumors</u>
      1. benign: neurofibromatosis, colonic lipomatosis, multiple hamartoma syndrome (Cowden disease)
      2. malignant: lymphoma, leukemia, adenocarcinoma
B. INFLAMMATORY PSEUDOPOLYPS
   Ulcerative colitis, Crohn colitis, ischemic colitis, amebiasis, schistosomiasis, strongyloidiasis, trichuriasis
C. ARTIFACTS
   Feces, air bubbles, oil bubbles, mucus strands, ingested foreign body (eg, corn kernels)
D. MISCELLANEOUS
   Nodular lymphoid hyperplasia, lymphoid follicular pattern, hemorrhoids, diverticula, pneumatosis intestinalis, colitis cystica profunda, colonic urticaria, submucosal colonic edema secondary to obstruction, cystic fibrosis, amyloidosis, ulcerative pseudopolyps, proximal to obstruction

Cecal filling defect
A. ABNORMALITIES OF THE APPENDIX
   1. Acute appendicitis / appendiceal abscess
   2. Crohn disease
   3. Inverted appendiceal stump / appendiceal intussusception
   4. Mucocele
   5. Myxoglobulosis
   6. Appendiceal neoplasm: carcinoid tumor (90%), leiomyoma, neuroma, lipoma, adenocarcinoma, metastasis
B. COLONIC LESION
   1. Ameboma
   2. Primary cecal neoplasm
   3. Ileocolic intussusception
   4. Lipomatosis of ileocecal valve
C. UNUSUAL ABNORMALITIES
   1. Ileocecal diverticulitis (in 50% < age 30 years)
   2. Solitary benign ulcer of the cecum
   3. Adherent fecolith (eg, in cystic fibrosis)
   4. Endometriosis
   5. Burkitt lymphoma

mnemonic: "CECUM TIPSALE"
Carcinoma
Enteritis
Carcinoid
Ulcerative colitis
Mucocele of appendix
Tuberculosis
Intussusception
Periappendiceal abscess
Stump of the appendix
Ameboma
Lymphoma
Endometriosis

Carpet lesions of colon
= flat lobulated lesions with alteration of surface texture + little / no protrusion into lumen
Location: rectum > cecum > ascending colon
Causes:
A. NEOPLASMS
   1. Tubular / tubulovillous / villous adenoma
   2. Familial polyposis
   3. Adenocarcinoma
   4. Submucosal tumor spread (from adjacent carcinoma)
B. MISCELLANEOUS
   1. Nonspecific follicular proctitis
   2. Biopsy site
   3. Endometriosis
   4. Rectal varices
   5. Colonic urticaria

Colonic polyp
Terminology:
1. **Polyp**
   = mass projecting into the lumen of a hollow viscus above the level of the mucosa; usually arises from mucosa, may derive from submucosa / muscularis propria
   (a) neoplastic: adenoma / carcinoma
   (b) nonneoplastic: hamartoma / inflammatory polyp
2. **Pseudopolyp**
   = scattered island of inflamed edematous mucosa on a background of denuded mucosa
   (a) pseudopolyposis of ulcerative colitis
   (b) "cobblestoning" of Crohn disease
3. **Postinflammatory (filiform) polyp**
   = fingerlike projection of submucosa covered by mucosa on all sides following healing + regeneration of inflammatory (most common in ulcerative colitis) / ischemic / infectious bowel disease

Histologic Classification:
A. ADENOMATOUS POLYPS
   1. Familial polyposis
   2. Gardner syndrome
   3. Peutz-Jeghers syndrome (some in SB + colon)
   4. Turcot syndrome
B. INFLAMMATORY POLYPS
   1. Juvenile polyposis
   2. Cronkhite-Canada syndrome
C. HAMARTOMATOUS POLYPS
   1. Peutz-Jeghers syndrome (most in small bowel)

2. Cowden disease
D. POLYPOSIS LOOK-ALIKES
1. Inflammatory polyposis
2. Lymphoid hyperplasia
3. Lymphoma
4. Metastases
5. Pneumatosis coli

Polyposis syndromes

= more than 100 polyps in number

Mode of transmission:
A. HEREDITARY
(a) <u>autosomal dominant</u>
1. Familial (multiple) polyposis
2. Gardner syndrome
3. Peutz-Jeghers syndrome
(b) <u>autosomal recessive</u>
1. Turcot syndrome
B. NONHEREDITARY
1. Cronkhite-Canada syndrome
2. Juvenile polyposis

<u>MESENTERY</u>
Mesenteric masses
A. ROUND SOLID MASSES
Δ Benign primary tumors are more common than malignant primary tumors!
1. Metastases especially from colon, ovary (most frequent neoplasm of mesentery)
2. Lymphoma
3. Leiomyosarcoma (more frequent than leiomyoma)

4. Neural tumor (neurofibroma, ganglioneuroma)
5. Lipoma (uncommon), lipomatosis, liposarcoma
6. Fibrous histiocytoma
7. Hemangioma
8. Desmoid tumor (most common primary)
B. ILL-DEFINED MASSES
Metastases (ovary), lymphoma, fibromatosis, fibrosing mesenteritis (associated with Gardner syndrome), lipodystrophy, panniculitis
C. LOCULATED CYSTIC MASSES
Lymphangioma (most common), pseudomyxoma peritonei, mesenteric cyst, hematoma
D. OMENTAL CAKE
Lymphoma, tuberculosis, mesothelioma
E. STELLATE MASSES
Mesothelioma, metastases, fibrosing mesenteritis, tuberculous peritonitis, desmoid tumor

Regional patterns of lymphadenopathy
@ Retrocrural nodes
Abnormal size: >6 mm
Common cause: lung carcinoma, mesothelioma, lymphoma
@ Gastrohepatic ligament nodes
= superior portion of lesser omentum suspending stomach from liver
Abnormal size: >8 mm
Common cause: carcinoma of lesser curvature of stomach, distal esophagus, lymphoma, pancreatic cancer, melanoma, colon + breast cancer
DDx: coronary varices

	Single Polyp	**Multiple Polyps**
Neoplastic (10 %) — epithelial	1. Tubular adenoma 2. Tubulovillous adenoma 3. Villous adenoma 4. Turcot syndrome	1. Familial adenomatosis coli 2. Adenomatosis of GI tract 3. Gardner syndrome
— nonepithelial	1. Carcinoid 2. Leiomyoma 3. Lipoma 4. Hem-, lymphangioma 5. Fibroma, neurofibroma	
Nonneoplastic (90 %) — unclassified	1. Hyperplastic polyp	1. Hyperplastic polyposis
— hamartomatous	1. Juvenile polyp 2. Peutz-Jeghers syndrome	1. Juvenile polyposis
— inflammatory	1. Ulcerative colitis 2. Benign lymphoid polyp 3. Fibroid granulation polyp	1. Cronkhite-Canada syndrome 2. Ulcerative colitis

@ Porta hepatis nodes
    = in porta hepatis extending down hepatoduodenal
      ligament, anterior + posterior to portal vein
    Abnormal size: >6 mm
    Common cause: carcinoma of gallbladder + biliary
                        tree, liver, stomach, pancreas,
                        colon, lung, breast
    Cx: high extrahepatic biliary obstruction
@ Pancreaticoduodenal nodes
    = between duodenal sweep + pancreatic head
      anterior to IVC
    Abnormal size: >10 mm
    Common cause: lymphoma, pancreatic head,
                        colon, stomach, lung, breast
                        cancer

@ Perisplenic nodes
    = in splenic hilum
    Abnormal size: >10 mm
    Common cause: NHL, leukemia, small bowel
                        neoplasm, ovarian cancer,
                        carcinoma of right / transverse
                        colon
@ Retroperitoneal nodes
    = periaortic, pericaval, interaortocaval
    Abnormal size: >10 mm
    Common cause: lymphoma, renal cell, testicular,
                        cervical, prostatic carcinomas
@ Celiac and superior mesenteric artery nodes
    = preaortic nodes
    Abnormal size: >10 mm
    Common cause: any intraabdominal neoplasm
@ Pelvic nodes
    = along common, external + internal iliac vessels
    Abnormal size: >15 mm
    Common cause: carcinoma of bladder, prostate,
                        cervix, uterus, rectum

Enlarged lymph node with low-density center
1. Tuberculosis
2. Pyogenic infection
3. Whipple disease
4. Lymphoma
5. Metastatic disease after radiation + chemotherapy

Gastrointestinal hemorrhage
Mortality: approx. 10%
Δ Barium examination should be avoided in acute
bleeders!

Sources:
A. UPPER GASTROINTESTINAL HEMORRHAGE
    = bleeding site proximal to ligament of Treitz
    @ Esophagogastric junction
        1. Esophageal varices (17%): 50% mortality
        2. Mallory-Weiss syndrome (7 – 14%):
           very low mortality
    @ Stomach
        1. Acute hemorrhagic gastritis (17 – 27%)
        2. Gastric ulcer (10%)

3. Pyloroduodenal ulcer (17 – 25%)
    Mortality: <10% if under age 60; >35% if
                  over age 60
@ Other causes (14%): visceral artery aneurysm,
    vascular malformation, neoplasm, vascular-
    enteric fistula
    Average mortality: 8 – 10%

B. LOWER GASTROINTESTINAL HEMORRHAGE
    @ Small intestine
        Tumor (eg, leiomyoma, metastases), ulcers,
        diverticula (eg, Meckel diverticulum),
        inflammatory bowel disease (eg, Crohn
        disease), vascular malformation, visceral artery
        aneurysm, aortoenteric fistula
    @ Colorectal (70%)
        1. Diverticula (most common): hemorrhage in
           25% of patients with diverticulosis;
           spontaneous cessation of bleeding in 80%;
           recurrent bleeding in 25%
        2. Colonic angiodysplasia = dilated submucosal
           arteries + veins overlying mucosal thinning
           (? secondary to mucosal ischemia)
        3. Colitis, tumors, mesenteric varices

INFANTILE GASTROINTESTINAL BLEEDING
(1) Peptic ulcer (2) Varices (3) Ulcerated Meckel
diverticulum

Intramural hemorrhage
Causes:
A. VASCULITIS
    1. Henoch-Schönlein purpura
B. TRAUMA
C. COAGULATION DEFECT
    1. Anticoagulant therapy
    2. Thrombocytopenia
    3. Disseminated intravascular coagulation
D. DISEASES WITH COAGULATION DEFECT
    1. Hemophilia
    2. Leukemia, lymphoma
    3. Multiple myeloma
    4. Metastatic carcinoma
    5. Idiopathic thrombocytopenic purpura
E. ISCHEMIA (often fatal)

• abdominal pain
• melena
Site: submucosal / intramural / mesenteric
√ "stacked coin" / "picket fence" appearance of mucosal
    folds (due to symmetric infiltration of submucosal blood)
√ "thumbprinting" = rounded polypoid filling defect (due to
    focal accumulation of hematoma in bowel wall)
√ separation + uncoiling of bowel loops
√ narrowing of lumen + localized filling defects
    (asymmetric hematoma)
√ no spasm / irritability
√ mechanical obstruction + proximal distension of loops
Prognosis: resolution within 2 – 6 weeks

GI abnormalities in chronic renal failure and renal transplantation

@ Esophagus
  1. Esophagitis
     Cause: Candida, CMV, herpes
@ Stomach & duodenum
  1. Gastritis
     √ thickened gastric folds (38%)
     √ edema + erosions
     Cause:
     (a) imbalance of gastrin levels + gastric acid
         secretion due to (1) reduced removal of
         gastrin from kidney with loss of cortical mass
         (2) impaired acid feedback mechanism (3)
         hypochlorhydria
     (b) opportunistic infection (eg, CMV)
  2. Gastric ulcer (3.5%)
  3. Duodenal ulcer (2.4%)
  4. Duodenitis (47%)
@ Colon
  More severely + frequently affected after renal
  transplantation
  1. Progressive distention + pseudoobstruction
     Contributing factors: dehydration, alteration of diet,
        inactivity, nonabsorbable antacids, high-dose
        steroids
  2. Ischemic colitis
     (a) primary disease responsible for end-stage
         renal disease (eg, diabetes, vasculitis)
     (b) trauma of renal transplantation
  3. Diverticulitis
     Contributing factors: chronic obstipation, steroids,
        autonomic nervous dysfunction
  4. Pseudomembranous colitis
  5. Uremic colitis = nonspecific colitis
  6. Spontaneous colonic perforation
     Cause: nonocclusive ischemia, diverticula,
        duodenal + gastric ulcers
@ Pancreas
  1. Pancreatitis
     Cause: hypercalcemia, steroids, infection,
        immunosuppressive agents, trauma
@ General
  1. GI hemorrhage
     Cause:
        gastritis, ulcers, colonic diverticula, ischemic
        bowel, infectious colitis, pseudomembranous
        colitis, nonspecific cecal ulceration
  2. Bowel perforation (in 1 – 4% of transplant recipients)
  3. Opportunistic infection
     Organisms: Candida, herpes, CMV, strongyloides
  4. Malignancy
     (a) skin tumors
     (b) lymphoma

Protein-losing enteropathy

A. DISEASE WITH MUCOSAL ULCERATION
  1. Carcinoma
  2. Lymphoma
  3. Inflammatory bowel disease
  4. Peptic ulcer disease

B. HYPERTROPHIED GASTRIC RUGAE
  1. Ménétrièr disease

C. NONULCERATIVE MUCOSAL DISEASE
  1. Celiac disease
  2. Tropical sprue
  3. Whipple disease
  4. Allergic gastroenteropathy
  5. Gastrocolic fistula
  6. Villous adenoma of colon

D. LYMPHATIC OBSTRUCTION
  1. Intestinal lymphangiectasia

E. HEART DISEASE
  1. Constrictive pericarditis
  2. Tricuspid insufficiency

Malabsorption

= deficient absorption of any essential food materials
  within small bowel

(1) PRIMARY MALABSORPTION
  = the digestive abnormality is the only abnormality
    present
  1. Celiac disease = nontropical sprue
  2. Tropical sprue
  3. Disaccharidase deficiencies
(2) SECONDARY MALABSORPTION
  = occurring during course of gastrointestinal
    disease
  (a) enteric
    1. Whipple disease
    2. Parasites: hookworm, Giardia, fish tapeworm
    3. Mechanical defects: fistulas, blind loops,
       adhesions, volvulus, short circuits
    4. Neurological: diabetes, functional diarrhea
    5. Inflammatory: enteritis (viral, bacterial,
       fungal, nonspecific)
    6. Endocrine: Zollinger-Ellison syndrome
    7. Drugs: neomycin, phenindione, cathartics
    8. Collagen disease: scleroderma, lupus,
       polyarteritis
    9. Lymphoma
    10. Benign + malignant small bowel tumors
    11. Vascular disease
    12. CHF, agammaglobulinemia, amyloid,
        abetalipoproteinemia, intestinal
        lymphangiectasia
  (b) gastric
    Vagotomy, gastrectomy, pyloroplasty, gastric
    fistula (to jejunum, ileum, colon)
  (c) pancreatic
    Pancreatitis, pancreatectomy, pancreatic cancer,
    cystic fibrosis
  (d) hepatobiliary
    Intra- and extrahepatic biliary obstruction, acute
    + chronic liver disease

ROENTGENOGRAPHIC SIGNS IN MALABSORPTION

√   SMALL BOWEL WITH NORMAL FOLDS + FLUID
1. Maldigestion (deficiency of bile salt / pancreatic enzymes)
2. Gastric surgery
3. Alactasia

√   SMALL BOWEL WITH NORMAL FOLDS + WET
1. Sprue
2. Dermatitis herpetiformis

√   DILATED DRY SMALL BOWEL
1. Scleroderma
2. Dermatomyositis
3. Pseudoobstruction: no peristaltic activity

√   DILATED WET SMALL BOWEL
1. Sprue
2. Obstruction
3. Blind loop

√   THICKENED STRAIGHT FOLDS + DRY SMALL BOWEL
1. Amyloidosis (malabsorption is unusual)
2. Radiation
3. Ischemia
4. Lymphoma (rare)
5. Macroglobulinemia (rare)

√   THICKENED STRAIGHT FOLDS + WET SMALL BOWEL
1. Zollinger-Ellison syndrome
2. Abetalipoproteinemia: rare inherited disease characterized by CNS damage, retinal abnormalities, steatorrhea, acanthocytosis

√   THICKENED NODULAR IRREGULAR FOLDS + DRY SMALL BOWEL
1. Lymphoid hyperplasia
2. Lymphoma
3. Crohn disease
4. Whipple disease
5. Mastocytosis

√   THICKENED NODULAR IRREGULAR FOLDS + WET SMALL BOWEL
1. Lymphangiectasia
2. Giardiasis
3. Whipple disease (rare)

SMALL BOWEL NODULARITY WITH MALABSORPTION
mnemonic: "**W**hat **I**s **H**is **M**ain **A**im? **L**ay **E**ggs, **B**y **G**od"

Whipple disease
Intestinal lymphangiectasia
Histiocytosis
Mastocytosis
Amyloidosis
Lymphoma, **L**ymph node hyperplasia
Edema
Blood
Giardiasis

ANATOMY AND FUNCTION OF GASTROINTESTINAL TRACT

Gastrointestinal hormones

Cholecystokinin

= CCK = 33 amino acid residues (former name: Pancreozymin); the 5 C-terminal amino acids are identical to those of gastrin, causing similar effects as gastrin

Produced in: duodenal + upper intestinal mucosa
Released by: fatty acids, some amino acids (phenylalanine, methionine), hydrogen ions

Effects:
@ Stomach
(1) weakly stimulates HCl secretion
(2) given alone: inhibits gastrin, which leads to decrease in HCl production
(3) stimulates pepsin secretion
(4) stimulates gastric motility
@ Pancreas
(1) stimulates secretion of pancreatic enzymes (= Pancreozymin)
(2) stimulates bicarbonate secretion (weakly by direct effect; strongly through potentiating effect on secretin)
(3) stimulates insulin release
@ Liver
(1) stimulates water + bicarbonate secretion
@ Intestine
(1) stimulates secretion of Brunner glands
(2) increases motility
@ Biliary tract
(1) strong stimulator of gallbladder contraction
(2) relaxation of sphincter of Oddi

Gastrin

= 17 amino acid peptide amide; PENTAGASTRIN = acyl derivative of the biologic active C-terminal tetrapeptide amide

Produced in: antral cells + G-cells of pancreas
Released by: mediated by neuroendocrine cholinergic reflexes
     (a) vagal stimulation, gastric distension
     (b) short-chain alcohol (ethanol, propanol)
     (c) amino acids (glycine, ß-alanine)
     (d) caffeine
     (e) hypercalcemia
Inhibited by: drop in pH of antral mucosa to <3.5

Effects:
@ Stomach:
(1) stimulation of gastric HCl secretion from parietal cells, which in turn:
(2) increases pepsinogen production by chief cells through local reflex
(3) increased antral motility
(4) trophic effect on gastric mucosa (parietal cell hyperplasia)

@ Pancreas
(1) strong increase in enzyme output
(2) weakly stimulates fluid + bicarbonate output
(3) stimulates insulin release
@ Liver
(1) water + bicarbonate secretion
@ Intestine
(1) stimulates secretion of Brunner glands
(2) increases motility
@ Gallbladder
(1) stimulates contraction
@ Esophagus
(1) increases resting pressure of LES

Glucagon

Produced in: α-cells (and β-cells) of pancreas
Released by: low blood glucose levels
Effects:
@ Intestines
(1) hypotonic effect on duodenum > jejunum > stomach > colon
@ Hormones
(1) releases catecholamines from the adrenal gland that paralyse intestinal smooth muscle
(2) increases serum insulin + glucose levels (mobilization of hepatic glycogen)
@ Biliary tract
(1) increases bile flow
(2) relaxes gallbladder + sphincter of Oddi

Dose for radiologic imaging: 1 mg maximum
Δ IV administration causes a quick response + rapid dissipation of action!
Δ IM administration prolongs onset + increases length of action!
Side effects: nausea + vomiting, weakness, dizziness (delayed onset of 11/2 – 4 hours after IM administration)
Contraindication: Diabetes mellitus

Secretin

Produced in: duodenal mucosa
Released by: hydrogen ions providing a pH <4.5
Effects:
@ Stomach
(1) inhibits gastrin activity, which leads to decrease in HCl secretion
(2) stimulates pepsinogen secretion by chief cells (potent pepsigogue)
(3) decreases gastric and duodenal motility + contraction of pyloric sphincter
@ Pancreas
(1) increases alkaline pancreatic secretions ($NaHCO_3$)
(2) weakly stimulates enzyme secretion

(3) stimulates insulin release
@ Liver
  (1) stimulates water + bicarbonate secretion (most potent choleretic)
@ Intestine
  (1) stimulates secretion of Brunner glands
  (2) inhibits motility
@ Esophagus
  (1) opens LES

Gastric cells

1. Chief cells
  = peptic / zymogenic cells
  Location: body + fundus
  produce: pepsinogen
2. Parietal cells
  = oxyntic cells
  Location: body + fundus
  produce: H^+, Cl^-, intrinsic factor, prostaglandins
3. Mucous neck cells
  produce: mucoprotein, mucopolysaccharide, aminopolysaccharide sulfate
4. Argentaffin cells
  = enteroendocrine cells
  Location: body + fundus
  produce: glucagon-like substance (A-cells), somatostatin (D-cells), vasoactive intestinal polypeptide (D_1-cells), 5-hydroxytryptamine (EC-cells)
5. G-cells
  Location: pylorus
  produce: gastrin

Small bowel peristalsis

A. INCREASED
  1. Vagal stimulation
  2. Acetylcholine
  3. Anticholinesterase (eg, neostigmine)
  4. Cholecystokinin
B. DECREASED
  1. Atropine (eg, Pro-Banthine®)
  2. Bilateral vagotomy

Effect of bilateral vagotomy

= cholinergic denervation
(1) decreased MOTILITY of stomach + intestines
(2) decreased GASTRIC SECRETION
(3) decreased TONE OF GALLBLADDER + bile ducts
(4) increased TONE OF SPHINCTERS (Oddi + lower esophageal sphincter)

Lower esophageal anatomy

A. **Esophageal Vestibule**
  = saccular termination of lower esophagus with upper boundary at tubulovestibular junction + lower boundary at esophagogastric junction
  √ collapsed during resting state
  √ assumes bulbous configuration with swallowing
  (a) tubulovestibular junction = A-level = junction between tubular and saccular esophagus

(b) phrenic ampulla = bell-shaped part above diaphragm (term should be discarded because of dynamic changes of configuration)
(c) submerged segment = infrahiatal part of esophagus
  √ widening / disappearance is indicative of GE reflux disease

B. **Gastroesophageal Junction**
  Site: at upper level of gastric sling fibers, straddles cardiac incisura demarcating the left lateral margin of GE junction
C. **Z-line** = B-level = squamocolumnar junction line not acceptable criterion for locating GE junction
  Site: 1 – 2 cm above gastric sling fibers
D. **Lower Esophageal Sphincter**
  = physiologic 2 – 4 cm high pressure zone corresponding to esophageal vestibule
  √ tightly closed during resting state
  √ assumes bulbous configuration with swallowing

Muscular rings of esophagus

A Ring
= contracted / hypertrophied muscles in response to incompetent GE sphincter
• rarely symptomatic / dysphagia
Location: at tubulovestibular junction = superior aspect of vestibule
√ usually 2 cm proximal to GE junction at upper end of vestibule
√ varies in caliber during the same examination, may disappear on maximum distension
√ broad smooth narrowing with thick rounded margins
√ visible only if tubular esophagus above + vestibule below are distended

B Ring
= sling fibers representing a U-shaped thickening of inner muscle layers with open arm of U toward lesser curvature = inferior aspect of vestibule
Location: < 2 cm from hiatal margins
√ only visible when esophagogastric junction is above hiatus
√ thin ledge-like ring just below the mucosal junction (Z-line)

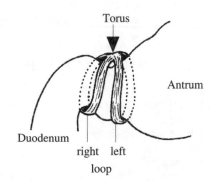

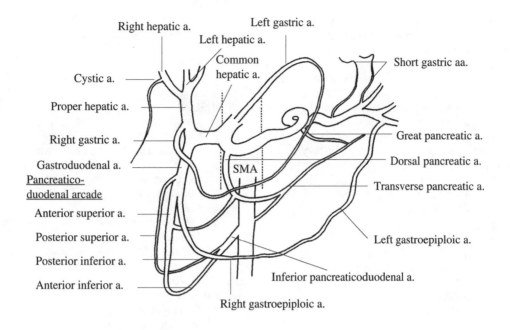

Blood Supply of Stomach, Duodenum, and Pancreas

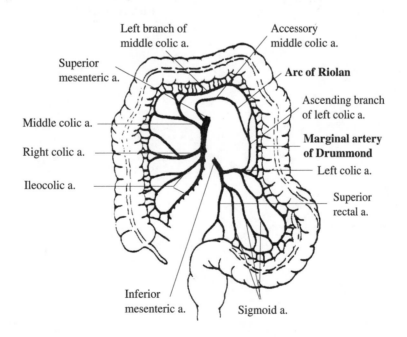

Blood Supply of Large Intestine

Pylorus

= fan-shaped specialized circular muscle fibers with:
- (a) distal sphincteric loop = right canalis loop
  - √ corresponds to radiologic pyloric sphincter
- (b) proximal sphincteric loop = left canalis loop
  - √ 2 cm proximal to distal sphincteric loop on greater curvature (seen during complete relaxation)
- (c) torus = fibers of both sphincters converge on the lesser curvature side to form a muscular prominence; prolapse of mucosa between sphincteric loops produces a niche simulating ulcer

√ pyloric channel 5 –10 mm long, wall thickness of 4 – 8 mm
√ concentric indentation of the base of the duodenal bulb

Small bowel folds

A. NORMAL FOLD THICKNESS
- @   jejunum   1.7 – 2.0 mm   >2.5 mm pathologic
- @   ileum   1.4 – 1.7 mm   >2.0 mm pathologic

B. NORMAL NUMBER OF FOLDS
- @   jejunum   4 – 6 / inch
- @   ileum   3 – 5 / inch

C. NORMAL FOLD HEIGHT
- @   jejunum   3.5 – 7.0 mm
- @   ileum   2.0 – 3.5 mm

D. NORMAL LUMEN DIAMETER
- @   upper jejunum   3.0 – 4.0 cm   >4.5 cm pathologic
- @   lower jejunum   2.5 – 3.5 cm   >4.0 cm pathologic
- @   ileum   2.0 – 2.8 cm   >3.0 cm pathologic

RULE OF 3's:
- Δ wall thickness <3 mm
- Δ valvulae conniventes <3 mm
- Δ diameter <3 cm
- Δ air-fluid levels <3

Intestinal gas

A. INFLUX
1. Aerophagia ....2 l
2. Liberation from intestinal tract
    - (a) neutralization of bicarbonate in secretions (CO_2) ....8 l
    - (b) bacterial fermentation (CO_2, H_2, CH_4, H_2S) ... 15 l
3. Diffusion from blood (N_2, O_2, CO_2)

B. EFFLUX
1. Diffusion from intestines into blood and expulsion from lung ....50 l
2. Expulsion from anus ....2 l

Intestinal fluid

A. INFLUX
1. Oral ingestion ....2.5 l
2. Intestinal secretions ....8.2 l
    - saliva...1.5 l
    - bile ....0.5 l
    - gastric secretions .... 2.5 l
    - pancreatic secretions ....0.7 l
    - intestinal secretions ....3.0 l

B. EFFLUX
1. Peranal ....0.1 l
2. Intestinal resorption (primarily in ileum + ascending colon) ....10.6 l

GASTROINTESTINAL DISORDERS

ACHALASIA
= failure of organized peristalsis + relaxation at level of lower esophageal sphincter
Etiology:
- (a) idiopathic: abnormality of Auerbach plexus / medullary dorsal nucleus; ? neurotropic virus, ? gastrin hypersensitivity
- (b) Chagas disease

√ megaesophagus = dilatation of esophagus beginning in upper 1/3, ultimately entire length
√ small / absent gastric air bubble
√ stasis in thoracic esophagus filled with retained secretions + alimentary residue
√ absence of primary peristalsis below level of cricopharyngeus
√ nonperistaltic contractions
√ "bird beak" / "rat tail" deformity = V-shaped conical + symmetric tapering of stenotic segment with most marked narrowing at GE junction
√ Hurst phenomenon = temporary transit through cardia when hydrostatic pressure of barium column is above tonic LES pressure
√ sudden esophageal emptying after ingestion of carbonated beverage (eg, Coke)
√ "vigorous achalasia" = numerous tertiary contractions in nondilated distal esophagus of early achalasia
√ prompt relaxation of LES upon amyl nitrate inhalation (smooth-muscle relaxant)

Cx: esophageal carcinoma in 7% (usually midesophagus)
Rx: pneumatic dilatation / surgical myotomy
DDx: (1) Neoplasm (separation of gastric fundus from diaphragm; normal peristalsis; asymmetric tapering)
      (2) Peptic stricture of esophagus

ADENOMA OF SMALL BOWEL
Location: duodenum (21%), jejunum (36%), ileum (43%) esp. ileocecal valve
Histo: (1) Hamartomatous polyp (77%), multiple in 47%, 1/3 of multiple lesions associated with Peutz-Jeghers syndrome
      (2) adenomatous polyp (13%), may have malignant potential
      (3) polypoid gastric heterotopic tumor (10%)

ADENOMATOUS COLONIC POLYP
= EPITHELIAL POLYP
Most common benign colonic tumor (68 – 79%)
Predisposed:
previously detected polyp / cancer; family history of polyps / cancer; idiopathic inflammatory bowel disease; Peutz-Jeghers syndrome; Gardner syndrome; familial polyposis

Incidence: 3% in 3rd decade; 10% in 7th decade; 26% in 9th decade
Location: rectum (21 – 34%); sigmoid (26 – 38%); ascending colon (9 – 12%); transverse colon (12 – 13%); descending colon (6 – 18%); multiple in 35 – 50% (usually <5 – 10 in number)
Histo:
1. Tubular adenoma (75%)
   = cylindrical glandular structure lined by stratified columnar epithelium
   malignant potential: <10 mm in 1%; 10 – 20 mm in 10%; >20 mm in 35%
2. Tubulovillous adenoma (15%)
   = mixture between tubular + villous adenoma
   malignant potential: <10 mm in 4%; 10 – 20 mm in 7%; >20 mm in 46%
3. Villous adenoma (10%)
   = infolding of papillary projections of glandular structure ("villous fronds")
   malignant potential: <10 mm in 10%; 10 – 20 mm in 10%; >20 mm in 53%
   - potassium depletion

Size & Malignancy:
<5 mm in 0%; 5 – 9 mm in 1%; 10 – 20 mm in 10%; >20 mm in 46% malignant
Δ All polyps >10 mm should be removed!
Δ Time for adenoma-carcinoma sequence probably averages 10 – 15 years!
- asymptomatic (75%)
- diarrhea, abdominal pain
- peranal hemorrhage (67%)

Colonoscopy (incomplete in 16 – 43%)
BE (rate of detection of polyps <10 mm higher with double than single contrast; false-negative rate of 7%):
√ sessile flat / round polyp
√ pedunculated polyp: stalk >2 cm in length almost always indicative of a benign polyp
√ suggestive of malignancy: irregular lobulated surface, broad base = width of the base greater than height, retraction of colonic wall = dimpling / indentation / puckering at base of tumor, interval growth
√ lacelike / reticular surface pattern CHARACTERISTIC for villous adenoma (occasionally in tubular adenoma)

DDx:
(1) Nonneoplastic: hyperplastic polyp, inflammatory pseudopolyp, lymphoid tissue, ameboma, tuberculoma, foreign body granuloma, malakoplakia, heterotopia, hamartoma
(2) Neoplastic subepithelial: lipoma, leiomyoma, neurofibroma, hemangioma, lymphangioma, endothelioma, myeloblastoma, sarcoma, lymphoma, enteric cyst, duplication, varix, pneumatosis, hematoma, endometriosis

AFFERENT LOOP SYNDROME

= PROXIMAL LOOP SYNDROME = BLIND LOOP SYNDROME

= partial intermittent obstruction of afferent loop leading to overdistension of loop by gastric juices after Billroth II gastrojejunostomy

Cause:

gastrojejunostomy with left-to-right anastomosis (= proximal jejunal loop attached to greater curvature instead of lesser curvature), mechanical factors (intussusception, adhesion, kinking), inflammatory disease, neoplastic infiltration of local mesentery or anastomosis, idiopathic motor dysfunction

• postprandial epigastric fullness relieved by bilious vomiting
• vitamin B_{12} deficiency with megaloblastic anemia
• afferent loop with abnormal bacterial flora (Gram negative, resembling colon in quality + quantity)

UGI:

√ preferential emptying of stomach into proximal loop
√ proximal loop stasis
√ regurgitation

CT:

√ rounded water-density masses adjacent to head + tail of pancreas forming a U-shaped loop
√ oral contrast material may not enter loop
√ may result in biliary obstruction (increased pressure at ampulla)

Rx: antibiotic therapy

AIDS

Δ Gastrointestinal involvement due to Kaposi sarcoma + opportunistic infections!

Opportunistic organisms:

CMV, Mycobacterium avium intracellulare, Cryptosporidium, Candida, Pneumocystis

1. AIDS-related cholangitis

    Organism: CMV, Cryptosporidium
    • RUQ pain, fever, jaundice, abnormal LFT
    √ irregular dilatation of intra- and extrahepatic bile ducts similar to sclerosing cholangitis

2. Liver abscess
3. Splenomegaly (very common)
4. Splenic infarction (septic emboli)
5. CMV esophagitis
6. Cryptosporidium antritis
    √ area of focal gastric thickening + ulceration
7. CMV gastritis
    frequently affects GE junction + prepyloric antrum
8. AIDS enteritis

    (a) **Cryptosporidium enteritis**
        Location: proximal small bowel
        √ small bowel dilatation of proximal jejunal loops
        √ small bowel thickening (mimicking sprue)
        √ thickening + effacement of mucosal folds
        √ "toothpaste" appearance of small bowel
    (b) **Mycobacterium avium intracellulare enteritis**
        = PSEUDO-WHIPPLE DISEASE
        • diarrhea, malabsorption
        √ dilatation of distal small bowel

√ mucosal fold thickening + nodularity
√ mesenteric + retroperitoneal lymphadenopathy
√ splenomegaly

9. AIDS colitis
    — ischemic bowel
    — acute appendicitis
    — neutropenic colitis
    — pseudomembranous colitis
    — infectious colitis / ileitis
        CMV colitis / ileitis
        • hematochezia, crampy abdominal pain, fever
        Path: small vessel vasculitis resulting in hemorrhage, ischemic necrosis, ulceration
        Location: terminal ileum
        √ marked bowel wall thickening
        √ double-ring / target sign (due to increased submucosal edema)
        √ ascites
        √ inflammation of pericolonic fat + fascia

10. Bowel obstruction
    (a) infection
    (b) intussusception (Kaposi sarcoma, lymphoma)

AMEBIASIS

= primary infection of the colon by protozoan Entamoeba histolytica

Countries: worldwide distribution, most common in warm climates; South Africa, Egypt, India, Asia, Central + South America (20%); United States (5%)

Route: contaminated food / water (human cyst carriers); cyst dissolves in small bowel; trophozoites settle in colon; proteolytic enzymes + hyaluronidase lyse intestinal epithelium; may embolize into portal venous + systemic blood system

Histo: amebic invasion of mucosa + submucosa causing tiny ulcers, which spread beneath mucosa + merge into larger areas of necrosis; mucosal sloughing; secondary bacterial infection

• asymptomatic for months / years
• acute attacks of diarrhea (loose mucoid blood-stained stools)
• fever, headache, nausea

Location: (areas of relative stasis) right colon + cecum (90%) > hepatic + splenic flexures > rectosigmoid

√ loss of normal haustral pattern with granular appearance (edema, punctate ulcers)
√ "collarbutton" ulcers
√ cone-shaped cecum
√ several cm long stenosis of bowel lumen in transverse colon, sigmoid colon, flexures (result of healing + fibrosis); in multiple segments
√ ameboma = hyperplastic granuloma with bacterial invasion of amebic abscess; usually annular + constricting / intramural mass / cavity continuous with bowel lumen; shrinkage under therapy in 3 – 4 weeks
√ ileocecal valve thickened + fixed in open position with reflux

√ involvement of distal ileum (10%)
Dx: stool examination / rectal biopsy
Cx: (1) Toxic megacolon with perforation
(2) Amebic abscess in liver (2%), brain, lung
(transdiaphragmatic spread of infection),
pericolic, ischiorectal, subphrenic space
(3) Intussusception in children (due to ameboma)
(4) Fistula formation (colovesical, rectovesical,
rectovaginal, enterocolic)

AMYLOIDOSIS

= deposition of a protein-polysaccharide material in
various organs leads to hypoxia, mucosal edema,
hemorrhage, ulceration, mucosal atrophy, muscle
atrophy
Histo: amorphous eosinophilic hyaline material
deposited around terminal blood vessels, stains
with Congo red + crystal violet
A. PRIMARY AMYLOIDOSIS
probably autosomal dominant inheritance with
immunologically determined dysfunction of plasma
cells
• idiopathic amyloid deposition in liver, spleen,
kidneys, adrenals, bowel
B. SECONDARY AMYLOIDOSIS
(a) following prolonged infectious / inflammatory
process: rheumatoid arthritis (in 20%),
tuberculosis, leprosy, chronic pyelonephritis,
lymphoreticular malignancy, paraplegia, old age
(b) associated with multiple myeloma (in 10%)
Δ GI involvement in primary more common than in
secondary amyloidosis!
• malabsorption (diarrhea, protein loss)
• occult GI bleeding
• obstruction
• macroglossia
@ Esophagus
√ loss of peristalsis
√ megaesophagus
@ Stomach
• postprandial epigastric pain + heartburn
• acute erosive hemorrhagic gastritis
(a) diffuse infiltrative form
√ small-sized stomach with rigidity + loss of
distensibility simulating linitis plastica (from
thickening of gastric wall)
√ effaced rugal pattern
√ diminished / absent peristalsis
√ marked retention of food
(b) localized infiltration (often located in antrum)
√ irregularly narrowed + rigid antrum
√ thickened rugae
√ superficial erosions / ulcerations
(c) amyloidoma = well-defined submucosal mass
@ Small bowel
(a) diffuse form (more common)
√ diffuse uniform thickening of valvulae
conniventes in entire small bowel
√ broadened flat undulated mucosal folds
(mucosal atrophy)

√ "jejunization" of ileum
√ impaired intestinal motility
√ small bowel dilatation
(b) localized form (less common)
√ multiple pea- / marble-sized deposits
√ pseudoobstruction = physical + plain film
findings suggesting mechanical obstruction with
patent large + small bowel on barium
examination
Cx: small bowel infarction
@ Colon: √ pseudopolyps in colon
@ Bone: √ bone cysts
Dx: by rectal / gingival biopsy
DDx: Whipple disease, intestinal lymphangiectasia,
lymphosarcoma

ANGIODYSPLASIA OF COLON

= VASCULAR ECTASIA = ARTERIOVENOUS
MALFORMATION
Acquired lesion
Associated with: aortic stenosis (20%)
Incidence at autopsy: 2%
Age: majority >55 years
Location: (a) cecum + ascending colon (majority)
(b) descending + sigmoid colon (25%)
• chronic intermittent low-grade bleeding
• occasionally massive bleeding
√ "vascular tufts" = cluster of vessels during arterial phase
along antimesenteric border
√ early opacification of ileocolic vein
√ densely opacified dilated tortuous ileocolic vein into late
venous phase
√ contrast extravasation (unusual)

ANORECTAL ATRESIA

= first trimester embryologic event
Incidence: 1:5,000 livebirths
A. LOW ANOMALY: bowel has passed through levator
sling; anal opening in abnormal location (perineal
fistula)
B. HIGH ANOMALY: bowel ends above levator sling;
opening into vagina / posterior urethra (air in bladder
in males; air in vagina in females)
√ distance between rectal air and skin will not accurately
outline the extent of atretic rectum and anus (varying
length during crying with increase in abdominal pressure
+ contraction of levator ani muscle)
US:
√ ≤15 mm distance between anal dimple + distal rectal
pouch on transperineal images indicates low lesion
OB-US (earliest detection by 26 – 28 weeks GA):
√ dilated colon + normal amniotic fluid
Associated with: (part of VACTERL syndrome)
(1) Duodenal atresia / stenosis (20%)
(2) Esophageal atresia (20%)
(3) Spinal anomalies (50%): defective sacral
segmentation
(4) Arrest of descent of urorectal septum (50%)
(most commonly when rectum ends above levator
sling)

(5) GU anomalies (25 – 35%): M > F
    more common in supralevator than infralevator
    termination
(6) Cardiac anomalies
(7) Caudal regression syndrome (anorectal atresia,
    sacral agenesis, renal agenesis / dysplasia, lower
    limb hypoplasia, sirenomelia)

ANTRAL MUCOSAL DIAPHRAGM
  = antral web
Age range: 3 months – 80 years
Associated with: gastric ulcer (30 – 50%)
• symptomatic if opening <1 cm
Location: usually 1.5 cm from pylorus (range 0 – 7 cm)
√ constant symmetrical band of 2 – 3 mm thickness
  traversing the antrum perpendicular to long axis of
  stomach
√ "double bulb" appearance (in profile)
√ concentric / eccentric orifice
√ normal peristaltic activity

APPENDICITIS
Incidence: 7 – 12% in Western world population
Etiology: obstruction of appendiceal lumen by lymphoid
              hyperplasia (60%), fecolith (33%), foreign
              bodies (4%), stricture, tumor, parasite; Crohn
              disease (in 25%)
Peak age: 2nd – 3rd decade
• classic signs + symptoms not present in 20 – 30% (32 –
  45% rate of misdiagnosis in women between ages 20 –
  40)
• fever (56%)
• nausea + vomiting (40%)
• RLQ pain (72%)
• leukocytosis (88%)
Atypical location: within pelvis (30%), extraperitoneal (5%)

Abdominal plain film (abnormalities seen in <50%):
  √ usually laminated calcified appendicolith in RLQ (in 7
    – 15%)
    Δ Appendicolith + abdominal pain = 90% probability
      of acute appendicitis!
    Δ Appendicolith in acute appendicitis means a high
      probability for gangrene / perforation!
  √ paucity of intestinal gas in RLQ
  √ "cecal ileus" = gas-fluid level in cecum in gangrene
    (= local paralysis)
  √ small bowel dilatation with air-fluid level in terminal
    ileum + cecum (infrequent sign of mechanical
    obstruction)
  √ distortion of psoas margin + flank stripes
  √ focal increase in thickness of lateral abdominal wall
    in 32% (= edema between properitoneal fat line +
    cecum)
  √ loss of properitoneal fat line
  √ thickening of cecal wall
  √ loss of definition of right inferior hepatic outline (= free
    peritoneal fluid)
  √ fluid / pus in cul-de-sac
  √ pneumoperitoneum (rare)

BE / UGI (accuracy 50 – 84%):
  √ failure to fill appendix with barium (normal finding in
    up to 35%)
  √ indentation along medial wall of cecum (= edema at
    base of appendix / matted omentum / periappendiceal
    abscess)
US: (75 – 96% sensitivity, 90 – 95% overall accuracy;
    nondiagnostic study in 4% due to inadequate
    compression of RLQ); useful in ovulating women
    (false-negative appendectomy rate in males 15%, in
    females 35%)
  √ visualization of noncompressible appendix as a blind-
    ending tubular aperistaltic structure (seen only in 2%
    of normals)
  √ target appearance of ≥6 mm in total diameter on
    cross-section / mural wall thickness ≥2 mm
  √ diffuse hypoechogenicity (associated with higher
    frequency of perforation)
  √ lumen may be distended with anechoic / hyperechoic
    material
  √ visualization of appendicolith (6%)
  √ localized periappendiceal fluid collection
  √ prominent pericecal fat
CT (appendix rarely visualized):
  √ circumferential symmetrical thickening of wall of
    appendix
  √ linear streaky densities in pericecal / mesenteric /
    pelvic fat
  √ phlegmon = pericecal soft-tissue mass
  √ appendicolith = homogeneous / ringlike calcification
    (25%)
  √ pericecal / mesenteric / pelvic abscess = poorly
    encapsulated single / multiple fluid collection with air /
    extravasated contrast material
DDx: colitis, diverticulitis, small bowel obstruction,
         infectious enteritis, duodenal ulcer, pancreatitis,
         intussusception, Crohn disease, mesenteric
         lymphadenitis, ovarian torsion, pelvic inflammatory
         disease
Rx: finding of appendicolith is sufficient evidence to
         perform prophylactic appendectomy in
         asymptomatic patients (50% have perforation /
         abscess formation at surgery)

ASCARIASIS
= most common parasitic infection in world; cosmopolitan
  occurrence; endemic along Gulf Coast, Ozark
  Mountains, Nigeria, Southeast Asia
Organism: Ascaris lumbricoides = roundworm parasite,
               15 – 35 cm in length; production of 200,000
               eggs daily
Cycle: infection by contaminated soil, eggs hatch in
          duodenum, larvae penetrate into venules /
          lymphatics, carried to lungs, migrate to alveoli
          and up the bronchial tree, swallowed, maturation
          in jejunum within 2.5 months
Age: children age 1 – 10 years
• colic
• eosinophilia
• appendicitis

- hematemesis / pneumonitis
- jaundice (if bile ducts infested)

Location: jejunum > ileum (99%), duodenum, stomach, CBD, pancreatic duct

√ 15 – 35 cm long tubular filling defects
√ barium-filled enteric canal outlined within Ascaris
√ whirled appearance, occasionally in coiled clusters ("bolus of worms")

Cx: (1) Perforation of bowel (2) Mechanical obstruction

BARRETT ESOPHAGUS

= replacement of squamous epithelium with columnar metaplasia in lower esophagus

Cause: gastroesophageal reflux; contributing factors: genetic influence, alcohol, tobacco

Incidence: in 2 – 10% of patients with reflux esophagitis

Distribution: circumferential / focal
√ large deep peptic ulcer
√ stricture in upper / middle esophagus several cm long; occasionally distal stricture (DDx: peptic stricture without Barrett esophagus)
√ fine reticular pattern located distally from stricture
√ gastroesophageal reflux (common)
√ uptake of Tc-99m pertechnetate by columnar epithelium

Cx: adenocarcinoma in 8 – 10%

BEHÇET SYNDROME

= uncommon multisystem inflammatory disorder of unknown etiology with relapsing course

Age at onset: 3rd decade; M:F = 2:1

Major criteria: buccal + genital ulceration, ocular inflammation, skin lesions

Minor criteria: thrombophlebitis, GI + CNS lesions, arthritis, family history

- abdominal pain + diarrhea (50%)

@ Mucocutaneous: aphthous stomatitis, papules, pustules, vesicles, folliculitis, erythema nodosum-like lesions
@ Genital : ulcers on penis + scrotum / vulva + vagina
@ Ocular : relapsing iridocyclitis, hypopyon, chorioditis, papillitis, retinal vasculitis
@ Articular: mild nondestructive arthritis
@ Vascular: migratory thrombophlebitis
@ CNS : chronic meningoencephalitis
@ Esophagus: ulceration, stenosis, perforation
@ Small bowel: ulceration, perforation
@ Colon : multiple discrete deep ulcers in normal mucosa (DDx: granulomatous / ulcerative colitis)

DDx: Reiter syndrome, Steven-Johnson syndrome, SLE, ulcerative colitis, ankylosing spondylitis

BEZOAR

= intraintestinal mass composed of accumulated ingested material

Predisposition:
previous gastric surgery, massive overindulgence of food with high fiber contents

(a) Phytobezoar (55% of all bezoars):
= poorly digested fibers, skin + seeds of fruits and vegetables usually forming in stomach, may become impacted in small bowel
- history of recent ingestion of pulpy foods
Food: oranges, persimmons (most common, unripe persimmons contain the tannin shibuol that forms a gluelike coagulum after contact with dilute acid)
Site of impaction: stomach, jejunum, ileum
√ intraluminal filling defect without constant site of attachment to bowel wall
√ interstices filled with barium
√ coiled-spring appearance (rare)
√ partial / complete obstruction
Cx: decubitus ulceration + pressure necrosis of bowel wall
DDx: lobulated / villous adenoma, leiomyosarcoma, metastatic melanoma, intussusception

(b) Trichobezoar (hair):
80% are < age 30, almost exclusively in females;
Associated with gastric ulcer in 24 – 70%

BOERHAAVE SYNDROME

= complete transmural disruption of esophageal wall with extrusion of gastric content into mediastinum / pleural space secondary to food bolus impaction
- forceful vomiting with sudden onset of pain (substernal, left chest, in neck, pleuritic, abdominal)
- dyspnea
- NO hematemesis (blood escapes outside esophageal lumen)
√ rent of 2 – 5 cm in length, 2 – 3 cm above GE junction, predominantly on anterior right side
√ pleural effusion on left >> right side / hydropneumothorax
√ mediastinal emphysema (single most important plain film finding)
√ "V-sign of Naclerio" = air between lower thoracic aorta + diaphragm
√ extravasation of contrast medium into mediastinum / pleura

BRUNNER GLAND HYPERPLASIA

Etiology: hyperplasia secondary to hyperacidity
Physiology: secrete a clear viscous alkaline substance into crypts of Lieberkühn
MORPHOLOGIC TYPES:
1. Diffuse nodular hyperplasia
2. Circumscribed nodular hyperplasia: in suprapapillary portion
3. Single adenomatous hyperplastic polyp: in duodenal bulb
Location: duodenal glands begin in vicinity of pylorus extending distally within proximal 2/3 of duodenum
√ multiple nodular filling defects (usually limited to 1st portion of duodenum
√ "cobblestoning" (most common finding)

√ occasionally single large mass ± central ulceration

BURKITT LYMPHOMA
= most common type of non-Hodgkin lymphoma in children; initially described in Africa

Etiology: tumor from undifferentiated B-cell-derived lymphocytes; associated with Epstein-Barr virus
Age: children + young adults
Histo: characteristic "starry sky" plattern
Location: salivary glands, thyroid, ovary, small bowel, bone marrow; often multicentric in origin; rarely in lymph nodes

• jaw mass
• abdominal mass
• paraplegia
• NO peripheral leukemia
√ usually intraabdominal extranodal involvement with sparing of spleen

A. ENDEMIC FORM (Africa, New Guinea)
    50% of all childhood cancers in central Africa
    Age: 6 – 8 years
    Location: mandible, maxilla
B. NONENDEMIC FORM
    Age: 10 – 12 years
    Location: abdominal involvement (69%): tumors of small bowel (terminal ileum), mesentery, retroperitoneum, ovaries, uterus
    √ well-defined sharply marginated homogeneous tumors (75%)
    √ ascites (13%)
    √ renal masses / enlargement (5%)
    √ hydronephrosis (28%)
    √ conspicuous absence of lymph node disease
    √ pleural effusion (most common chest abnormality)
Rx: dramatic response to chemotherapy

CARCINOID
= most common primary tumor of small bowel + appendix; belongs to APUDomas; M:F = 2:1
Path: firm yellow submucosal nodule arising from argentophil Kulchitsky cells in the crypts of Lieberkühn (= argentaffinoma); invasion into mesentery incites an intense fibrotic reaction
Histo: resemble adenocarcinomas but do not have their aggressive behavior; malignant with invasion through muscularis
Biochemistry:
tumor elaborates (1) ACTH (2) histamine (3) bradykinin (4) kallikrein (5) serotonin = 5-hydroxytryptamine (from tryptophan over 5-hydroxytryptophan), which is metabolized in liver by monamine oxidase into 5-hydroxyindole acetic acid (5-HIAA) and excreted in urine; 5-hydroxytryptophan is destroyed in pulmonary circulation
• asymptomatic (66%)
• pain / obstruction (19%)
• weight loss (16%)
• palpable mass (14%)

• **Carcinoid syndrome** (7% of small bowel carcinoids) caused by excess serotonin levels, requires that serotonin metabolism (to 5-HIAA in liver) is bypassed
  (a) with liver metastases
  (b) with primary pulmonary / ovarian carcinoids
  • recurrent diarrhea (70%)
  • right-sided endocardial fibroelastosis (35%) resulting in tricuspid regurgitation + pulmonary valve stenosis + right heart failure
  • attacks precipitated by ingestion of food / alcohol
  • asthmatic wheezing (15%)
  • desquamative skin lesions (5%)
  • cutaneous flushing (rare)

Metastases:
to lymph nodes, liver (in 90% of patients with carcinoid syndrome), lung, bone (osteoblastic)
(a) incidence versus tumor size
    tumor of   <1 cm   (in 75%)   metastasizes in   2%
    tumor of   1 – 2 cm (in 20%)   metastasizes in 50%
    tumor of   >2 cm   (in 5%)   metastasizes in 85%
(b) incidence versus location
    tumor in ileum   (in 28%)   metastasizes in 35%
    tumor in appendix   (in 46%)   metastasizes in   3%
    tumor in rectum   (in 17%)   metastasizes in   1%
RULE OF 1/3:   Δ 1/3 have metastases
                Δ 1/3 are multiple
                Δ 1/3 have another malignancy
Location:
@ GI tract (>95%): between gastric cardia and anus
    (a) appendix (30 – 90%): commonly benign; surgical incidence of 0.03 – 0.7%
    (b) small bowel (25 – 35%): 91% in ileum (in 1/3 multiple); 7% in jejunum, 2% in duodenum
    (c) rectum (10%): metastasize in 10%
    (d) colon (5%): ascending colon, often malignant
    (e) rare in stomach
@ Others: bronchus, thyroid, pancreas, biliary tract, teratomas (ovarian, sacrococcygeal, testicular)
@ may be multicentric

UGI:
√ small smooth submucosal mass impinging eccentrically on lumen
√ angulation + kinking of loops leading to obstruction (DIAGNOSTIC)
√ spiculated / tethered appearance of mucosal folds (desmoplastic reaction)
√ separation of loops due to large mesenteric metastases
CT:
√ stellate radiating pattern + beading of mesenteric neurovascular bundles (desmoplastic reaction)
√ retraction + shortening of mesentery
√ displacement + kinking + separation of adjacent bowel loops
√ segmental thickening of adjacent bowel loops (encasement of mesenteric vessels leads to chronic ischemia)
√ low-density lymphadenopathy (due to necrosis)

√ liver metastases may become isodense following slow contrast infusion

Angio:
√ thickening + foreshortening of mesenteric vessels
√ kinking of small- and medium-sized vessels with stellate configuration
√ venous occlusion / mesenteric varices
√ encasement of medium-sized vessels
√ simulated hypervascularity secondary to fibrotic retraction of mesenteric vessels

NUC (I-123 MIBG imaging):
√ uptake in 44 – 63% (higher frequency of radiotracer uptake in midgut carcinoids + with elevated serotonin levels)

Cx: second primary malignant neoplasm in other location (36% at necropsy)
Rx: Somatostatin / SMS 201-995
DDx: oat-cell carcinoma, pancreatic carcinoma, medullary thyroid carcinoma, retractile mesenteritis, desmoplastic carcinoma / lymphoma

CATHARTIC COLON

= prolonged use of stimulant-irritant cathartics (>15 years) resulting in neuromuscular incoordination from chronically increased muscular activity + tonus
Agents: castor oil, senna, phenolphthalein, cascara, podophyllum, aloin
Location: involvement of colon proximal to splenic flexure
√ effaced mucosa with flattened smooth surface
√ diminished / absent haustrations
√ "pseudostrictures" = smoothly tapered areas of narrowing are typical (sustained tonus of circular muscles)
√ poor evacuation of barium
√ flattened + gaping ileocecal valve
√ shortened but distensible ascending colon
DDx: "burned out" ulcerative colitis with right-sided predominance (very similar)

CHAGAS DISEASE

= damage of ganglion cells by neurotoxin liberated from protozoa Trypanosoma cruzi resulting in aperistalsis of GI tract + dilatation
Endemic to Central + South America (esp. eastern Brazil)
Histo: decreased number of cells in medullary dorsal motor nucleus + Wallerian degeneration of vagus + decrease / loss of argyrophilic cells in myenteric plexus of Auerbach
Peak age: 30 – 50 years; M:F = 1:1
• intermittent / persistent dysphagia
• odynophagia (= fear of swallowing)
• foul breath, regurgitation
• aspiration
• Mecholyl test: abnormal response indicative of deficient innervation; 2.5 – 10 mg methacholine subcutaneously followed by severe tetanic nonperistaltic contraction 2 – 5 minutes after injection, commonly in distal half of esophagus, accompanied by severe pain
@ Dilatative cardiomyopathy (myocarditis)

@ Megacolon (bowels move at intervals of 8 days to 5 months)
   Cx: impacted feces, sigmoid volvulus
@ Esophagus: changes as in achalasia

CHALASIA

= continuously relaxed sphincter with free reflux in the absence of a sliding hernia
Etiology: elevated submerged segment
Causes: (1) Delayed development of esophagogastric region in newborns
           (2) Scleroderma, Raynaud disease
           (3) S/P forceful dilatation / myotomy for achalasia
√ free / easily induced reflux

CHRONIC IDIOPATHIC INTESTINAL PSEUDOOBSTRUCTION

= nonpropulsive intestine characterized by impaired response to intestinal dilatation without definable cause; ? autosomal dominant
Age: all ages, M:F = 1:1
• recurrent attacks of abdominal distension, periumbilical pain, nausea, vomiting, constipation
√ mild to marked gaseous distension of duodenum + proximal small bowel
√ esophageal dilation + hypoperistalsis (lower third)
√ excessive duodenal dilation (DDx: megaduodenum, superior mesenteric artery syndrome)
√ ligament of Treitz may be placed lower than usual
√ delayed transit of barium through affected segments
√ disordered motor activity (fluoroscopy)

COLITIS CYSTICA PROFUNDA

= rare benign condition characterized by submucosal mucus-containing cysts lined by normal colonic epithelium
Etiology: probably related to chronic inflammation
Age: primarily disease of young adults
• brief periods of bright red rectal bleeding
• mucous / bloody discharge
• intermittent diarrhea
Location: (a) localized to rectum (most commonly) / sigmoid
           (b) generalized colonic process (less common)
√ nodular polypoid / cauliflower-like lesions <2 cm in size, containing no gas
√ spiculations mimicking ulcers (barium-filled clefts between nodules)
DDx: pneumatosis (rarely affects rectum)

COLORECTAL CARCINOMA

Most common cancer of GI tract; 2nd most common cause of death from malignancy after lung cancer (in men) + breast cancer (in women)
Predisposed: socioeconomic status, diet low in fiber + high in fat, obesity (in men), asbestos worker, familial polyposis, Gardner syndrome, Turcot syndrome, Peutz-Jeghers syndrome

Incidence: 15% of all newly diagnosed cancers; 13% of all cancer deaths; 151,000 new cases / year with 61,300 deaths; 6.5% lifetime probability of any white person to develop colorectal cancer; 3/100,000 in 30 – 34-year-olds; 532/100,00 for >85-year-olds

Risk factors:
1. Colonic adenoma
    — malignancy in 5% of tubular adenomas
    — malignancy in 40% of villous adenomas
    Δ 93% of colorectal carcinomas arise from adenomatous polyp!
    Δ A patient with one adenoma has a 9% chance of having a colorectal carcinoma in next 15 years!
    Δ 5% of adenomas 5 mm in size develop into invasive cancers (5 mm is considered critical mass of intraepithelial neoplasia)!
2. Family history of benign / malignant colorectal tumors, 3 – 5 x risk in first-degree relatives
3. Chronic ulcerative colitis (3 – 5% incidence; cumulative incidence of 26% after 25 years of colitic symptoms)
4. Prominent lymphoid follicular pattern
5. History of endometrial / breast cancer
6. Crohn disease (particularly in bypassed loops / in vicinity of chronic fistula)
7. Pelvic irradiation
8. Ureterosigmoidostomy

Age: peak age 50 – 70 years;
          median age of 71 years for colon cancer;
          median age of 69 years for rectal cancer
Histo: (1) Adenocarcinoma with varied degrees of differentiation
            (2) Mucinous carcinoma (uncommon)
            (3) Squamous cell carcinoma + adenoacanthoma (rare)

Staging:
    Duke   A: limited to bowel wall (15%)
    Duke   B: extension through bowel wall into serosa / mesenteric fat (35%)
    Duke   C : lymph node metastases (50%)
            C_1: + growth limited to bowel wall
            C_2: + growth extending into adipose tissue
    Duke   D : distant metastases

Metastases:
1. liver (15 – 20% at time of surgery)
2. retroperitoneal + mesenteric nodes (15%)
3. hydronephrosis (13%)
4. adrenal (10%)
5. lung
6. ovarian metastases
7. psoas muscle tumor deposit
8. malignant ascites
9. bone (extremely infrequent)
• rectal bleeding
• positive fecal occult blood testing (2 – 6% positive-result rate ; 5 – 10% positive predictive value):
  Hemoccult (hematein) , Hemoquant (porphyrins), Haemselect (hemoglobin)

• progressive elevation of carcinoembryonic antigen (CEA) >10 µg/l indicative of recurrent / metastatic disease

Location:
    rectum (15 – 41%), sigmoid (20 – 37%), descending colon (10 – 11%), transverse colon (12%), ascending colon (8 – 16%), cecum (8 – 10%); "aging gut" = right-sided lesions increasing with age
Colonoscopy: successful examination to cecum in 57– 84%; fails to detect 12% of colonic polyps (10% in areas never reached by colonoscope)
BE (sensitivities for polyps >1 cm: single contrast 77 – 94%, double contrast 82 – 98%; for polyps <1 cm: single contrast 18 – 72%, double contrast 61 – 83%):
√ fungating polypoid carcinoma
√ annular ulcerating carcinoma = "saddle lesion" / "apple-core lesion"
√ scirrhous carcinoma: rare variant with circumferential + longitudinal spread; often seen in ulcerative colitis
√ curvilinear / mottled calcifications (rare)
CT: staging accuracy of 48 – 90%, for lymph node metastases of 25 – 73%
CT staging (poor accuracy compared with Duke classification):
Stage 1   intramural polypoid mass
Stage 2   thickening of bowel wall
Stage 3   slight invasion of surrounding tissues
Stage 4   massive invasion of surrounding tissue + adjacent organs / distant metastases
√ low density mass + low density lymph nodes in mucinous adenocarcinoma
√ psammomatous calcifications in mucinous adenocarcinoma
MR (staging accuracy of 73%, 40% sensitivity for lymph node metastases)

Prognosis:
    40 – 50% overall 5-year survival rate; 80 – 90% with Duke A; 70% with Duke B; 33% with Duke C; 5% with Duke D; recurrence at line of anastomosis (11 – 50%) within 1 year after resection in 50%, within 2 years after resection in 80%
    Risk:
        of   5% for synchronous colon cancer
        of   14% for synchronous cancer with "sentinel polyp"
        of   35% for additional adenomatous polyp
        of   3% for metachronous colon cancer
        of 3.8% for extracolonic malignancy

Cx: (1) Obstruction (frequently in descending + sigmoid colon)
         (2) Perforation
         (3) Intussusception
         (4) Pneumatosis cystoides intestinalis
DDx: (1) Prolapsing ileocecal valve (change on palpation)
         (2) Spasm (intact mucosa, released by propantheline bromide)
         (3) Diverticulitis

COLONIC VOLVULUS
= most common form of volvulus
A. VOLVULUS OF CECUM
Associated with malrotation + long mesentery
Age peak: 20 – 40 years; M > F
√ "kidney-shaped" distended cecum, usually positioned in LUQ
√ tapered end of barium column points toward torsion
B. VOLVULUS OF SIGMOID
= sigmoid twists on mesenteric axis
Usually in elderly / psychiatrically disturbed
Degree of torsion: 360° (50%), 180° (35%), 540° (10%)
√ greatly distended paralyzed loop with fluid-fluid levels, mainly on left side, extending toward diaphragm (erect film)
√ "coffee bean sign" = distinct midline crease corresponding to mesenteric root in largely gas-distended loop (supine)
√ "bird-of-prey sign" = tapered hooklike end of barium column
CT:
√ "whirl sign" = tightly torsioned mesentery formed by twisted afferent + efferent loop

CONGENITAL INTESTINAL ATRESIA
Incidence: 1:300 livebirths
Location: jejunum + ileum (70%), duodenum (25%), colon (5%)
√ "triple bubble sign" = intraluminal gas in stomach + duodenal bulb + proximal jejunum as pathognomonic sign for jejunal atresia
√ gasless lower abdomen (gut usually air-filled by 4 hours after birth)
√ meconium peritonitis
√ polyhydramnios (in 50% with duodenal / proximal jejunal atresia; rarely in ileal / colonic atresia)

CRICOPHARYNGEAL ACHALASIA
= hypertrophy of cricopharyngeus muscle (= upper esophageal sphincter) with failure of complete relaxation
Etiology:
1. Normal variant without symptoms: seen in 5 – 10% of adults
2. Compensatory mechanism to gastroesophageal reflux
3. Neuromuscular dysfunction of deglutition
   (a) primary neural disorders:
       Brainstem disorder (bulbar poliomyelitis, syringomyelia, multiple sclerosis, amyotrophic lateral sclerosis); central / peripheral nerve palsy; cerebrovascular occlusive disease; Huntington chorea
   (b) primary muscle disorder:
       Myotonic dystrophy; polymyositis; dermatomyositis; sarcoidosis; myopathies secondary to steroids / thyroid dysfunction; oculopharyngeal myopathy
   (c) myoneural junction disorder:
       Myasthenia gravis; diphtheria; tetanus

- mostly asymptomatic
- dysphagia
Δ Cineradiography / videotape recording required for demonstration !
√ distension of proximal esophagus + pharynx
√ smoothly outlined shelf- / liplike projection posteriorly at level of cricoid (= pharyngoesophageal junction) = level of C5/6
√ barium may overflow into larynx + trachea
Cx: Zenker diverticula
Rx: cricopharyngeal myotomy

CROHN DISEASE
= REGIONAL ENTERITIS = disease of unknown etiology with prolonged + unpredictable course characterized by discontinuous + asymmetric involvement of entire GI tract
Path: transmural inflammation (noncaseating granuloma with Langhans giant cells and epitheloid cells, edema, fibrosis); obstructive lymphedema + enlargement of submucosal lymphoid follicles; ulceration of mucosa overlying lymphoid follicles
Age: onset between 15 – 30 years; M:F = 1:1
- recurrent episodes of diarrhea
- colicky / steady abdominal pain
- low-grade fever
- weight loss, anorexia
- occult blood + anemia
- perianal abscess / fistula (40%)
- malabsorption (30%)
Associated with erythema nodosum, pyoderma gangrenosum
INTESTINAL MANIFESTATIONS
@ Esophagus (rare)
@ Stomach (1 – 2%) = granulomatous gastritis
  √ pseudo-post Billroth-I appearance
  √ "rams horn sign" = poorly distensible smooth tubular narrowed antrum + widened pylorus + narrow duodenal bulb
  √ aphthous ulcers (= pinpoint erosions)
  √ cobblestone mucosa
  √ antral-duodenal fistula
@ Duodenum (4 – 10%)
  almost always associated with gastric involvement
  Location: duodenal bulb + proximal half of duodenum
  √ superficial erosions / aphthoid ulcers (early lesion)
  √ thickened duodenal folds
@ Small bowel (80%) = regional enteritis
  terminal ileum (alone / in combination in 95%); jejunum / ileum (15 – 55%)
  √ thickening + slight nodularity of circular folds
  √ aphthous ulcers
  √ cobblestone mucosa / ulceration
  √ commonly associated with medial cecal defect
@ Colon (22 – 55%) = granulomatous colitis
  particularly on right side with rectum + sigmoid frequently spared

√ tiny 1 – 2 mm nodular filling defects (lymphoid follicular pattern)

√ aphthous ulcers with "target / bull's-eye" appearance

√ "transverse stripe sign" = 1 cm long straight stripes representing contrast medium within deep grooves of coarse mucosal folds

√ long fistulous tracts parallel to bowel lumen

@ Rectum (14 – 50%)

√ deep / collar-button ulcers

√ rectal sinus tracts

Phases:

(a) Earliest changes

√ nodular enlargement of lymphoid follicles

√ blunting / flattening / distortion / straightening / thickening of valvulae conniventes (obstructive lymphedema, usually first seen in terminal ileum)

√ aphthoid ulcers = nodules with shallow central barium collection

(b) Advanced nonstenotic phase

√ skip lesions (90%) = discontinuous involvement with intervening normal areas

√ cobblestone appearance = serpiginous longitudinal + transverse ulcers separated by areas of edema

√ thick + blunted small bowel folds (inflammatory infiltration of lamina propria + submucosa)

√ straightening + rigidity of small bowel loops with luminal narrowing (spasm + submucosal edema)

√ separation + displacement of small bowel loops (from lymphedematous wall thickening / increase in mesenteric fat / enlarged mesenteric lymph nodes / perforation with abscess formation)

√ pseudopolyps = islands of hyperplastic mucosa between denuded mucosa

√ inflammatory polypoid masses

√ sessile / pedunculated / filiform postinflammatory polyps

√ diffuse mucosal granularity due to 0.5 – 1 mm round lucencies (= blunted + fused villi seen en face)

√ pseudodiverticula = pseudosacculations = bulging area of normal wall opposite affected scarred wall on antimesenteric side

(c) Stenotic phase

√ "string sign" = strictures (most frequently in terminal ileum) / marked narrowing of rigid loops

√ normal proximal loops may be dilated with stasis ulcers + fecoliths

CT:

√ homogeneous density of thickened bowel wall (DDx: ulcerative colitis with inhomogeneous attenuation)

√ "double halo configuration" (50%) = intestinal lumen surrounded by inner ring of low attenuation (= edematous mucosa) + outer ring of soft-tissue density (= thickened fibrotic muscularis + serosa) (DDx: radiation enteritis, ischemia, mesenteric venous thrombosis, acute pancreatitis)

√ luminal narrowing + proximal dilatation

√ skip areas of asymmetrical bowel wall thickening of 10 – 20 mm in 82% (DDx: ulcerative colitis with a mean thickness of 8 mm)

√ "creeping fat" = massive proliferation of mesenteric fat (40%) with mass effect separating small bowel loops

√ mesenteric adenopathy (18%)

√ abscess (DDx: postoperative blind loop)

US:

√ thickening of bowel wall (65%) about 8 mm (DDx: ulcerative colitis)

√ inflammatory mass (14%), abscess (4%)

√ distended fluid-filled loops (12%)

Prognosis: recurrence rate of up to 39% after resection (commonly at the site of the new terminal ileum, most frequently during first 2 years after resection); mortality rate of 7% at 5 years, 12% at 10 years after 1st resection

Cx:

(1) Fistula (33%):

(a) enterocolic: most frequently between ileum and cecum

(b) enterocutaneous: rectum-to-skin; rectum-to-vagina

(c) perineal fistula + sinus tracts

Δ Crohn disease is 3rd most common cause of fistula / sinus tracts (*DDx:* iatrogenic [most common cause], diverticula [2nd most common cause])!

(2) Intramural sinus tracts

(3) Abscess (DDx: acute appendicitis)

(4) Free perforation (rare)

(5) Toxic megacolon

(6) Small bowel obstruction (15%)

(7) Hydronephrosis (from ureteric compression, generally on right side)

(8) Adenocarcinoma in ileum / colon (particularly in bypassed loops / in vicinity of chronic fistula)

Δ 4 – 20 x increased risk of colonic adenocarcinoma compared to general population with a latency period of 25 – 30 years!

(9) Lymphoma in large + small bowel

DDx:

(1) Yersinia (in terminal ileum, resolution within 3 – 4 months)

(2) Tuberculosis (more severe involvement of cecum, pulmonary TB)

(3) Actinomycosis, histoplasmosis, blastomycosis, anisakiasis

(4) Segmental infarction (acute onset, elderly patient)

(5) Radiation ileitis (appropriate history)

(6) Lymphoma (no spasm, luminal narrowing is uncommon, tumor nodules)

(7) Carcinoid tumor (tumor nodules)

(8) Eosinophilic gastroenteritis

(9) Potassium stricture

EXTRAINTESTINAL MANIFESTATIONS

@ Hepatobiliary

1. Fatty infiltration of liver (steroid therapy, hyperalimentation)

2. Hepatic abscess
3. Gallstones (28 – 34%)
   3 – 5 x higher risk than expected; stone formation caused by interrupted enterohepatic circulation with malabsorption of bile salts in terminal ileum; risk correlates with length of diseased ileum / resected ileum / duration of disease
4. Acute cholecystitis
5. Sclerosing cholangitis (10%) + hepatoma
6. Bile duct + gallbladder carcinoma
@ Genitourinary
1. Urolithiasis: oxalate / uric acid stones
2. Hydronephrosis
3. Renal amyloidosis
4. Cystitis
5. Ileoureteral / ileovesical fistula (5 – 20%)
@ Musculoskeletal
   • clubbing of fingers
   • seronegative peripheral migratory arthritis (5 – 20%); may precede bowel disease in 10%; increased with colonic disease; resection of diseased bowel leads to regression of symptoms
1. Periostitis
2. Hypertrophic osteoarthropathy
3. Sacroiliitis
4. Ankylosing spondylitis
5. Avascular necrosis of femoral head (steroid Rx)
6. Pelvic osteomyelitis (contiguous involvement)
7. Muscle abscess
@ Erythema nodosum, uveitis

CRONKHITE-CANADA SYNDROME
= non-neoplastic nonhereditary inflammatory polyps (as in juvenile polyposis) associated with ectodermal abnormalities
Histo: inflammatory polyps resembling juvenile / retention polyps = multiple cystic spaces filled with mucin secondary to degenerative changes
Age: 62 years (range 42 – 75 years); M < F
• exudative protein-losing enteropathy
• diarrhea (disaccharidase deficiency, bacterial overgrowth in small intestine)
• severe weight loss
• abdominal pain
• nail atrophy
• brownish hyperpigmentation of skin
• alopecia
√ multiple polyps
Location: stomach (100%); small bowel (>50%); colon (100%)
Prognosis: rapidly fatal in women within 6 – 18 months (cachexia); tendency toward remission in men

CYSTIC FIBROSIS
= MUCOVISCIDOSIS = FIBROCYSTIC DISEASE
= autosomal disorder characterized by mucous plugging of exocrine glands secondary to increased viscosity of secreted mucus; heterozygous in 5%; more common in Caucasians

• high sweat chlorides
• chronic obstipation
• infertility
• decreased urinary PABA excretion
• sinusitis
• exocrine pancreatic insufficiency (endocrine function not affected)
√ large distended colon with mottled appearance (retained bulky dry stool)
√ rectal prolapse
√ meconium ileus (10 – 15%)
√ microcolon
√ thickened folds in duodenum, small bowel, colon
√ calcific chronic pancreatitis
√ increased pancreatic echogenicity
√ cirrhosis
√ bronchiectasis

DESMOID TUMOR
= uncommon benign tumor consisting of fibrous tissue with insidious growth = desmos = "band / tendon" = subgroup of fibromatoses
Types:
   1. ABDOMINAL DESMOID
      Location: mesentery (most common mesenteric primary), musculoaponeurosis of rectus, internal oblique muscle; occasionally external oblique muscle
   2. EXTRAABDOMINAL DESMOID
      = musculoaponeurotic fibromatosis
      Location: pelvis, chest wall, mediastinum

Age: peak age in 3rd decade, 70% between 20 and 40 years of age; M:F = 1:3
Path: poorly circumscribed coarsely trabeculated tumor resembling scar tissue, confined to musculature + overlying aponeurosis
Histo: elongated spindle-shaped cells of uniform appearance, septated by dense bands of collagen, infiltration of adjacent tissue (DDx: low-grade fibrosarcoma, reactive fibrosis)
Associated with Gardner syndrome, multiple pregnancies, prior trauma
• firm slowly growing deep-seated mass

Size: 5 – 20 cm in diameter
MR:
   √ hypointense to muscle on T1WI + variable intensity on T2WI
CT:
   √ ill-defined / well-circumscribed mass
   √ usually higher attenuation than muscle
   √ ± enhancement
   √ retraction, angulation, distortion of small / large bowel with mesenteric infiltration
US:
   √ sharply defined + smoothly marginated mass of low / medium / high echogenicity
Cx: compression / displacement of bowel / ureter, intestinal perforation

Prognosis: locally aggressive growth; 25 – 65% recurrence rate
Rx: local resection + radiotherapy, antiestrogen therapy
DDx:
(1) Malignant tumor: fibrosarcoma, rhabdomyosarcoma, synoviosarcoma, liposarcoma, fibrous histiocytoma, lymphoma, metastasis
(2) Benign tumor: neurofibroma, neuroma, leiomyoma
(3) Acute hematoma

DISACCHARIDASE DEFICIENCY
= enzyme deficiencies for any of the disaccharides (maltose, lactose, etc.)
A. PRIMARY
B. SECONDARY to other diseases (eg, Crohn disease)
Pathophysiology:
(a) unabsorbed disaccharides produce osmotic diarrhea
(b) bacterial fermentation produces short chain volatile fatty acids causing further osmotic + irritant diarrhea
√ normal small bowel series without added lactose
√ abnormal small bowel series done with lactose (50 g added to 600 cm³ of barium suspension)
√ small + large bowel distension
√ dilution of barium
√ shortening of transit time

DIVERTICULAR DISEASE OF COLON
= overactivity of smooth muscle causing herniation of mucosa + submucosa through muscle layers
Incidence:
5 – 10% in 5th decade; 33 – 48% over age 50; 50% past 7th decade; M:F = 1:1; most common affliction of colon in developed countries
Cause: decreased fecal bulk (diet high in refined fiber + low in roughage)
Location:
in 80% in sigmoid (= narrowest colonic segment with highest pressure); in 17% distributed over entire colon; in 4 – 12% isolated to cecum / ascending colon

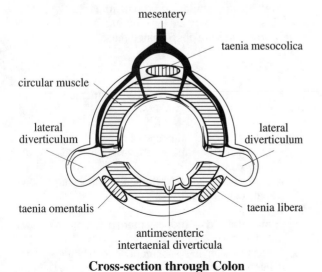

mesentery
taenia mesocolica
circular muscle
lateral diverticulum
lateral diverticulum
taenia omentalis
taenia libera
antimesenteric intertaenial diverticula

Cross-section through Colon

Prediverticular Disease of Colon
= longitudinal + circular smooth muscle thickening with redundancy of folds secondary to myostatic contracture
√ "saw-tooth sign" = crowding + thickening of haustral folds (shortening of colonic segment)
√ plump marginal indentations
√ superimposed muscle spasm (relieved by antispasmodics)
DDx: hemorrhage; ischemia; radiation changes; pseudomembranous colitis

Colonic Diverticulosis
= acquired herniations of mucosa + muscularis mucosae through the muscularis propria with wall components of mucosa, submucosa, serosa = false diverticula of pulsion type
Site:
(a) lateral diverticula arise between mesenteric + antimesenteric teniae on opposite sides
(b) antimesenteric intertaenial diverticula opposite of mesenteric side
Intramural type vasa recta (= nutrient arteries) pass through the circular muscle (weakness in muscular wall) and are carried over the fundus of the diverticula as it enlarges
√ Size: initially tiny (3 – 10 mm) V-shaped protrusion increasing up to several cm in diameter
√ bubbly appearance of air-containing diverticula
√ residual barium within diverticula from previous study
√ spiky irregular outline (antimesenteric intertaenial ridge is typical site for intramural diverticula)
√ smooth dome-shaped appendages with a short neck
√ may be pointed, attenuated, irregular with variable filling
√ circular line with sharp outer edge + fuzzy blurred inner edge (en face view in double contrast BE)
√ **Giant Sigmoid Diverticulum** = large gas-containing cyst (air entrapment secondary to ball-valve mechanism) arising in left iliac fossa
CT:
√ diverticula
√ distorted luminal contour + muscular hypertrophy

Colonic Diverticulitis
= perforation of diverticulum with intramural / localized pericolic abscess
Incidence: in 10 – 25% of diverticular disease
Pathogenesis: mucosal abrasion from inspissated fecal material leads to perforation of thin wall
• pain + local tenderness + mass in LLQ
• fever, leukocytosis

Location: sigmoid colon (most commonly)
√ localized ileus / bowel obstruction (kinking / edema)
√ gas in abscess / fistula
√ pneumoperitoneum (rare)
√ focal area of eccentric luminal narrowing caused by pericolic / intramural inflammatory mass
√ marked thickening + distortion of mucosal folds

√ extraluminal contrast = PERIDIVERTICULITIS
  √ "double-tracking" = pericolonic longitudinal sinus tract
  √ pericolonic collection = peridiverticular abscess
  √ fistula to bladder / small bowel / vagina
√ ± pattern of small bowel obstruction (if small bowel adheres to abscess)
CT:
  √ fine linear strands within pericolic fat (98%)
  √ diverticula (84%)
  √ circumferential bowel wall thickening of 4 – 12 mm (70%)
  √ frank abscess (47%)
  √ fluid ± air of peritonitis (16%)
  √ fistula formation (14%):
    most commonly colovesical, also colovaginal, coloenteric, colocutaneous
  √ colonic obstruction (12%)
  √ intramural sinus tracts (9%)
  √ ureteral obstruction (7%)
Prognosis:
  (a) self-limiting (usually)
  (b) transmural perforation
  (c) superficial ulceration
  (d) chronic abscess
DDx:
  (1) Colonic neoplasm (shorter segment, heaped-up margins, ulcerated mucosa)
  (2) Crohn colitis (double-tracking longer than 10 cm)
Rx: antibiotics, surgery (in 25%), percutaneous abscess drainage

Colonic Diverticular Hemorrhage

Not related to diverticulitis
Incidence: in 3 – 47% of diverticulosis
Location: 75% located in ascending colon (larger neck + dome of diverticula)
• massive rectal hemorrhage without pain
√ extravasation of radionuclide tracers
√ angiographic contrast pooling in bowel lumen
Rx: (1) transcatheter infusion of vasoconstrictive agents (Pitressin®)
    (2) embolization with Gelfoam®

DUMPING SYNDROME

= early postprandial vascular symptomatology of sweating, flushing, palpitation, feeling of weakness and dizziness
Pathophysiology:
rapid entering of hypertonic solution into jejunum resulting in fluid shift from blood compartment into small bowel
Incidence: 1 – 5% ; M:F = 2:1
Δ Roentgenologic findings not diagnostic!

√ rapid emptying of barium into small bowel (= loss of gastric reservoir function)
Rx: lying down, diet
DDx: late postprandial hypoglycemia (90 – 120 minutes after eating)

DUODENAL ATRESIA

= most common cause of congenital duodenal obstruction; second most common site of gastrointestinal atresias after ileum
Incidence: 1:10,000; M:F = 1:1
Etiology: defective vacuolization of duodenum between 6th – 11th weeks of fetal life; rarely from vascular insult (extent of obstruction usually involves larger regions with vascular insult)
Age at presentation: first few days of life
• persistent bilious vomiting a few hours after birth / following 1st feeding
• rapid deterioration secondary to loss of fluids + electrolytes
Isolated sporadic anomaly (30 – 52%)
Associated anomalies (in 60%):
  (1) Down syndrome (20 – 33%);
    Δ 25% of fetuses with duodenal atresia have Down syndrome!
    Δ <5% of fetuses with Down syndrome have duodenal atresia!
  (2) CHD (8 – 50%): endocardial cushion defect, VSD
  (3) Gastrointestinal anomalies (26%): esophageal atresia, biliary atresia, duodenal duplication, imperforate anus, small bowel atresia, intestinal malrotation, Meckel diverticulum, transposed liver, annular pancreas (20%)
  (4) Urinary tract anomalies (8%)
  (5) Vertebral + rib anomalies (37%)

Location: (a) usually distal to ampulla of Vater (80%)
        (b) proximal duodenum (20%)
√ "double bubble sign" = gas-fluid levels in duodenal bulb + gastric fundus
√ total absence of intestinal gas in small / large bowel
√ colon of normal caliber
OB-US (usually not identified prior to 24 weeks GA):
  √ "double bubble sign" = simultaneous distension of stomach + 1st portion of duodenum, continuity of fluid between stomach + duodenum must be demonstrated
  √ increased gastric peristalsis
  √ polyhydramnios (100%)
DDx: (1) Prominent incisura angularis causing bidissection of stomach
    (2) Choledochal cyst
Cx: prematurity (40%) secondary to preterm labor related to polyhydramnios

DUODENAL DIVERTICULUM

Incidence: 1 – 5% of GI studies; 22% of autopsies
A. PRIMARY DIVERTICULUM
  = mucosal prolapse through muscularis propria
  Location: 2nd portion (62%), 3rd portion (30%), 4th portion (8%)
  Site: medial wall in region of papilla (88%), posteriorly (8%), lateral wall (4%)
B. SECONDARY DIVERTICULUM
  = all layers of duodenal wall = true diverticulum as complication of duodenal / periduodenal inflammation

Location: almost invariably in 1st portion of
                duodenum
• mostly asymptomatic
Cx: (1) Perforation + peritonitis (2) Bowel obstruction
        (3) Biliary obstruction (4) Bleeding (5) Diverticulitis

DUODENAL ULCER
Incidence: 200,000 cases/year; 2 – 3 x more frequent
                than gastric ulcers; M:F = 3:1
Pathophysiology:
    too much acid in duodenum from (a) abnormally high
    gastric secretion (b) inadequate neutralization
Predisposed: cortisone therapy, severe cerebral injury,
                after surgery, chronic obstructive
                pulmonary disease
Location:
    (a)   bulbar (95%):
            anterior wall (50%), posterior wall (23%), inferior
            wall (22%), superior wall (5%)
    (b)   postbulbar (3 – 5%):
            majority on medial wall of supraampullary region;
            tendency for hemorrhage in 66%, M:F = 7:1
√ frequently small round / ovoid / linear ulcer niche
√ "kissing ulcers" = ulcers opposite from each other on
    anterior + posterior wall
√ giant duodenal ulcer >3 cm (rare) with higher morbidity
    + mortality; may be overlooked by simulating a normal /
    deformed duodenal bulb
√ "cloverleaf deformity, hourglass stenosis" (healed stage)
    with prestenotic dilatation of recesses

Cx: (1)   Obstruction (5%)
        (2)   Perforation (<10%): anterior > posterior wall;
                fistula to gallbladder
        (3)   Penetration (<5%) = sealed perforation
        (4)   Hemorrhage (15%): melena > hematemesis

DUODENAL VARICES
= dilated collateral veins secondary to portal hypertension
    (posterior superior pancreaticoduodenal vein)
√ lobulated filling defects (best demonstrated in prone
    position, maximal luminal distension will obliterate them)
√ commonly associated with fundal + esophageal varices

DUPLICATION CYST
Incidence: 15% of pediatric abdominal masses are
                gastrointestinal
Location: mesenteric surface of ileum > ileocecal
                junction > duodenum > greater curvature of
                stomach
√ elongated tubular / spherical cystic mass with inner
    echogenic mucosal lining paralleling outer wall of cyst
√ cyst paralleling normal bowel lumen
Cx: bowel obstruction
DDx:
    (1)   Omental cyst (greater omentum / lesser sac,
            multilocular)
    (2)   Mesenteric cyst (between leaves of small bowel
            mesentery)
    (3)   Meckel diverticulum (communicates with GI tract)

ECTOPIC PANCREAS
= PANCREATIC REST
Incidence: 2 – 10% of autopsies; M:F = 2:1
• asymptomatic
Location: distal greater curvature of antrum / pylorus
                (80%), duodenal bulb, jejunum, ileum, Meckel
                diverticulum; lesions may be multiple
√ smooth cone- / nipple-shaped submucosal nodule 1 – 5
    cm in size
√ central umbilication representing orifice of filiform duct

EOSINOPHILIC GASTROENTERITIS
= uncommon self-limited form of gastroenteritis with
    remissions + exacerbations characterized by infiltration
    of eosinophilic leukocytes into stomach / small bowel
    wall + usually marked peripheral eosinophilia
Cause: unknown
Histo: fibrous tissue + eosinophilic infiltrate of
            gastrointestinal mucosa
Age: in children + young adults with allergy +
            eosinophilia

A. EOSINOPHILIC GRANULOMA
    = FIBROUS POLYPOID LESION
    = INFLAMMATORY PSEUDOTUMOR
    = localized form / circumscribed type
    Location: almost exclusively in stomach (most
                    common in antrum + pylorus)
    √ submucosal polypoid mass / pedunculated polyp

B. EOSINOPHILIC GASTROENTERITIS
    = diffuse type
    = eosinophilic infiltration of mucosa, submucosa, and
        muscular layers of small intestine ± stomach by
        mature eosinophils (? gastric pendant to Löffler
        syndrome)

• recurrent episodes of abdominal pain, diarrhea, vomiting
• weight loss
• hematemesis (from ulceration)
• peripheral eosinophilia, anemia
• history of systemic allergy / food allergy
Location: entire small bowel (particularly jejunum),
                distal stomach, omentum, mesentery
Site: (a) mucosal (b) muscular (c) serosal (rare)

@ Stomach (almost always limited to antrum)
    √ "wet stomach"
    √ ulcers are rare
    (a) mucosal type
        √ enlarged gastric rugae / cobblestone nodules /
            polyps
    (b) muscular type
        √ thickened + rigid wall with narrowed gastric
            antrum / pylorus
        √ bulky intraluminal mass up to 9 cm in size
        Cx: pyloric obstruction
    DDx: hypertrophic gastritis, lymphoma, carcinoma
@ Small bowel (involved in 50%)
    √ separation of small bowel loops

(a) mucosal type
- malabsorption + hypoproteinemia
- √ thickening + distortion of folds predominantly in jejunum

(b) submucosal / muscular type
- √ motility disturbance
- √ small-bowel obstruction
- √ effacement of mucosal pattern + narrowing of lumen

(c) serosal type
- √ ascites

Prognosis: tendency toward spontaneous remission
Rx: steroids / removal of sensitizing agent

ESOPHAGEAL ATRESIA + TRACHEOESOPHAGEAL FISTULA

= incomplete division of primitive foregut into respiratory + digestive tracts characterized by failure of formation of tubular esophagus + abnormal communication between esophagus + trachea; occuring at 3rd – 5th week of intrauterine life

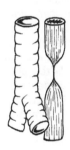

Esophageal atresia **9%**

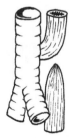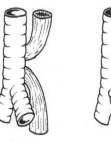

1%   **2%**   **82%**
Esophageal atresia + TE fistula

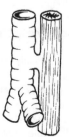

TE fistula without esophageal atresia **6%**

Incidence: 1:2,000 – 4,000 livebirths; most common sporadic congenital anomaly diagnosed in childhood

Associated anomalies (17 – 70%):
1. Cardiac (15 – 39%): patent ductus arteriosus, ASD, VSD, right-sided aortic arch (5%)
2. Musculoskeletal (24%): radial ray hypoplasia, vertebral anomalies
3. Gastrointestinal (20%): anorectal anomalies, duodenal atresia
4. Genitourinary (12%): unilateral renal agenesis
5. Chromosomal (10 – 19%): trisomy 18, 21, 13

mnemonic: "ARTICLES"
Anal atresia
Renal anomalies
TE fistula
Intestinal atresia / malrotation
Cardiac anomaly (PDA, VSD)
Limb anomalies (radial ray hypoplasia, polydactyly)
Esophageal atresia
Spinal anomalies

mnemonic: "VACTERL"
Vertebral anomalies
Anorectal anomaly
Cardiovascular anomalies
Tracheo-
Esophageal fistula
Renal anomalies
Limb anomalies

- drooling from excessive accumulation of pharyngeal secretions (esophageal atresia = EA)
- obligatory regurgitation of ingested fluids (EA)
- coughing + choking during feeding (TEF)
- recurrent pneumonia + progressive respiratory distress of variable severity (tracheo-esophageal fistula = TEF)

Location: between upper 1/3 + lower 1/3 of esophagus just above carina

Esophageal *atresia without fistula* (8 – 9%)
Associated anomalies in 17% (mostly Down syndrome + other atresias of GI tract)

Esophageal *atresia with fistula*
1. Proximal TE fistula (1%)
2. Distal TE fistula (82 – 86%)
3. Proximal + distal TE fistula (1 – 2%)
Associated anomalies in 30% (mostly cardiovascular)

Tracheoesophageal *fistula without atresia* (6%)
Associated anomalies in 23% (mostly cardiovascular)

√ "coiled tube" = inability to pass feeding tube into stomach (esophageal atresia)
√ retrotracheal air-filled pouch causing compression / displacement of esophagus
√ gasless abdomen (esophageal atresia ± proximal TE fistula)

√ bowel gas present in 90% (distal TE fistula / H-type fistula)

√ non- / hypoperistaltic esophageal segment (6 – 15 cm) in midesophagus

√ aspiration pneumonia, esp. in dependent upper lobes

OB-US (anomalies not identified before 24 weeks GA):

  √ polyhydramnios in 33 – 60% (= obstruction to flow of amniotic fluid)

    Δ TE-fistula with esophageal atresia is cause of polyhydramnios in only 3%!

  √ absence of fluid-distended stomach (in 10 – 40%; in remaining cases TE-fistula / gastric secretions allow some gastric distention)

  √ small abdomen (low birth weight in 40%)

  √ distended proximal pouch of atretic esophagus

Cx after repair:
  (1) Anastomotic leak
  (2) Recurrent TE fistula
  (3) Aspiration pneumonia secondary to
      (a) esophageal stricture
      (b) disordered esophageal motility distal to TE fistula
      (c) gastroesophageal reflux
DDx: pharyngeal pseudodiverticulum (traumatic perforation of posterior pharynx from finger insertion into oropharynx during delivery / tube insertion)

ESOPHAGEAL CANCER

Incidence: <1% of all cancers; 4 – 10% of all GI malignancies; 9,000 cases/year (United States); M:F = 4:1; blacks:whites = 2:1

High-risk regions: Iran, parts of Africa, Italy, China

Predisposing factors:
  achalasia (risk factor of 1000 x), asbestosis, Barrett esophagus, celiac disease, ionizing radiation, caustic stricture (risk factor of 1000 x), Plummer-Vinson syndrome, tannins, alcohol, tobacco, history of oral / pharyngeal cancer, tylosis palmaris et plantaris

  mnemonic: "BELCH SPAT"
    Barrett esophagus
    EtOH abuse
    Lye stricture
    Celiac disease
    Head and neck tumor
    Smoking
    Plummer-Vinson syndrome
    Achalasia
    Tylosis

Histo:
  (1) Squamous cell carcinoma (95%)
  (2) Adenocarcinoma (4%) arising from mucosal / submucosal glands or heterotopic gastric mucosa or columnar-lined epithelium (Barrett)
      (a) in 70% from Barrett esophagus
      (b) at gastroesophageal junction
  (3) Mucoepidermoid carcinoma, adenoid cystic carcinoma

  (4) Carcinosarcoma = pseudosarcoma = spindle-cell squamous carcinoma
      Age: in men >45 years
      Location: usually middle third of esophagus
      √ large bulky polypoid smooth, lobulated, scalloped intraluminal mass, may be pedunculated
  (5) Leiomyosarcoma, rhabdomyosarcoma, fibrosarcoma, malignant lymphoma

Cancer Staging:
  TNM system:
    T_1 tumor <5 cm in length without circumferential involvement
    T_2 tumor >5 cm in length / circumferential or obstructive lesion
    T_3 extra-esophageal spread
  CT staging (Moss):
    Stage 1 intraluminal tumor / localized wall thickening of 3 – 5 mm
    Stage 2 localized / circumferential wall thickening >5 mm
    Stage 3 contiguous spread into adjacent mediastinum (trachea, main stem bronchi, aorta, pericardium)
      √ loss of fat planes (nonspecific, often still resectable)
      √ mass in contact with aorta >90° (in 20 – 70% still resectable)
      √ displacement / compression of airway (50 – 100% accuracy for invasion)
      √ esophagotracheal / -bronchial fistula (unresectable)
    Stage 4 distant metastases
      √ enlarged abdominal lymph nodes >10 mm (12 – 85% accuracy)
      √ hepatic, pulmonary, adrenal metastases
      √ direct erosion of vertebral body

• dysphagia (87 – 95%) of <6 months duration
• weight loss (71%)
• retrosternal pain (46%)
• regurgitation (29%)
Location: upper 1/3 (15 – 20%); middle 1/3 (37 – 44%); lower 1/3 (38 – 43%)
RADIOLOGIC TYPES:
  (1) Polypoid / fungating form (most common)
      √ sessile / pedunculated tumor with lobulated surface
      √ protruding, irregular, polycyclic, overhanging, steplike "apple core" lesion
  (2) Ulcerating form
      √ large ulcer niche within bulging mass
  (3) Infiltrating form
      √ gradual narrowing with smooth transition (DDx: benign stricture)
  (4) Varicoid form = superficial spreading carcinoma
      Histo: longitudinal extension within wall without invasion beyond mucosa / submucosa
      √ tiny confluent nodules / plaques
      DDx: Candida esophagitis

Metastases:
- (a) lymphogenic: anterior jugular chain + supraclavicular nodes (primary in upper 1/3); paraesophageal + subdiaphragmatic nodes (primary in middle 1/3); mediastinal + paracardial + celiac trunk nodes (primary in lower 1/3)
- (b) hematogenous: lung, liver, adrenal gland

Cx: fistula formation to trachea / bronchi / mediastinum
Prognosis: 3 – 20% 5-year survival rate

ESOPHAGEAL INTRAMURAL PSEUDODIVERTICULOSIS
= dilated excretory ducts of deep esophageal adnexal mucous glands
Etiology: uncertain
Incidence: about 100 cases in world literature
Site: diffuse / segmental involvement
In 90% associated with:
   any severe esophagitis (most often reflux / Candida), esophageal stricture
√ multiple tiny rounded / flask-shaped barium collections in longitudinal rows parallel to long axis of esophagus
√ appear to "float" outside esophagus without apparent communication with lumen
√ commonly associated with strictures in distal esophagus

ESOPHAGEAL PERFORATION
Cause:
- (1) Emetogenic injury of the esophagus from sudden increase in intraabdominal pressure + relaxation of distal esophageal sphincter in the presence of a moderate to large amount of gastric contents
- (2) Closed chest trauma
- (3) Complication of endoscopy, dilatation of stricture, bougie, disruption of suture line following surgical anastomosis, attempted intubation
- (4) Esophageal carcinoma
- (5) Retained foreign body (coin, aluminum pop-tops, metallic button, safety pin, invisible plastic toy) leading to perforation (in pediatric age group)
- • rapid onset of overwhelming sepsis

Plain film (norma in 12%):
√ pneumomediastinum
√ subcutaneous emphysema of the neck
√ delayed widening of the mediastinum (secondary to mediastinitis)
√ hydrothorax (after rupture into pleural cavty), usually unilateral
√ hydropneumothorax (often not initially seen)
√ confirmation with contrast study

A. UPPER ESOPHAGEAL LACERATION
   √ widening of upper mediastinum
   √ right-sided hydrothorax
B. DISTAL ESOPHAGEAL LACERATION
   √ left-sided hydrothorax
   √ little mediastinal changes
Cx: (1) Acute mediastinitis (2) Obstruction of SVC (3) Mediastinal abscess

ESOPHAGEAL VARICES
= dilated submucosal veins due to increased collateral blood flow from portal venous system to azygos system
A. UPHILL VARICES
   = collateral blood flow from portal vein via azgos vein into SVC (usually lower esophagus dains via left gastric vein into portal vein)
   Cause:
   - (a) intrahepatic obstruction from cirrhosis
   - (b) splenic vein thrombosis (usually gastric varices)
   - (c) obstruction of hepatic veins
   - (d) IVC obstruction below hepatic veins
   - (e) IVC obstruction above hepatic vein entrance / CHF
   - (f) marked splenomegaly / splenic hemangiomatosis (rare)
   √ varices in lower half of esophagus
B. DOWNHILL VARICES
   = collateral blood flow from SVC via azygos vein into IVC / portal venous system (upper esophagus usually drains via azygos vein into SVC)
   Cause: obstruction of superior vena cava distal to entry of azygos vein most commonly due to lung cancer, lymphoma, retrosternal goiter, thymoma, mediastinal fibrosis
   √ varices in upper 1/3 of esophagus

EXAMINATION TECHNIQUE
- (a) small amount of barium (not to obscure varices)
- (b) relaxation of esophagus (not to compress varices): refrain from swallowing because succeeding swallow initiates a primary peristaltic wave that lasts for 10 – 30 seconds; sustained Valsalva maneuver precludes from swallowing
- (c) in LAO projection with patient recumbent / in Trendelenburg position ± Valsalva maneuver / deep inspiration

Plain film:
√ paraspinal widening (in 5% of patients with portal hypertension)
UGI:
√ thickened sinuous interrupted mucosal folds (earliest sign)
√ tortuous radiolucencies of variable size + location
√ "worm-eaten" smooth lobulated filling defects
CT:
√ thickened esophageal wall + lobulated outer contour
√ scalloped esophageal luminal masses
√ right- / left-sided soft-tissue masses (= paraesophageal varices)
√ marked enhancement following dynamic CT
Cx: bleeding in 28% within 3 years; exsanguination in 10 – 15%
DDx: varicoid carcinoma of esophagus

ESOPHAGEAL WEB
= ringlike constriction covered by squamous epithelium on superior + inferior surfaces
Age: middle-aged females

? association with:
Plummer-Vinson syndrome = Paterson-Kelly syndrome (iron deficiency anemia, stomatitis, glossitis, dysphagia, spoon-shaped nails)
Location: in cervical esophagus near cricopharyngeus (most common); webs may be multiple
√ visualized during maximal distension (in one tenth of a second)
√ arises at right angles from anterior esophageal wall
√ thin delicate membrane of uniform thickness of <3 mm

Cx: high risk of upper esophageal + hypopharyngeal carcinoma
DDx: stricture (circumfeential + thicker)

ESOPHAGITIS

Acute Esophagitis
√ thickened >3 mm wide folds with irregular lobulated contour
√ mucosal nodularity (= multiple ulcerations + intervening edema)
√ erosions
√ vertically oriented ulcers usually 3 – 10 mm in length
√ inflammatory esophagogastric polyp = proximal gastric fold extending across esophagogastric junction (rare)
√ abnormal motility

Candida Esophagitis
= MONILIASIS = CANDIDIASIS
Predisposed:
individuals with depressed immunity (hematologic disease, renal transplant, leukemia, chronic debilitating disease, diabetes mellitus, steroids, chemotherapy, radiotherapy, AIDS), antibiotics, scleroderma, strictures, achalasia, S/P fundoplication
Path: patchy, creamy-white plaques covering a friable erythematous mucosa
• dysphagia (= difficult swallowing)
• severe odynophagia (= painful swallowing from segmental spasm)
• intense retro- / substernal pain
• associated with thrush (= oral moniliasis) in 20 – 80%

Location: predilection for lower 1/2 of esophagus
√ involvement of long esophageal segments
√ longitudinal plaques = grouping of tiny 1 – 2 mm nodular filling defects with linear orientation
√ "cobblestone" appearance = mucosal nodularity in early stage (from growth of colonies on surface)
√ shaggy / fuzzy / serrated contour (from coalescent plaques, pseudomembranes, erosions, ulcerations, intramural hemorrhage) in fulminant candidiasis
√ narrowed lumen (rom spasm, pseudomembranes, marked edema)
√ "intramural diverticulosis" = multiple tiny indentations + protrusions
√ sluggish / absent primary peristalsis
√ strictures (rare)
√ mycetoma resembling large intraluminal tumor (rare)

Diagnostic sensitivity:
endoscopy (97%), double contrast (88%), single contrast (55%)
Cx: systemic candidiasis
Rx: Mycostatin®
DDx:
reflux esophagitis, herpes esophagitis, acute caustic ingestion, intramural pseudodiverticulosis, squamous papillomatosis, glycogen acanthosis, Barrett esophagus, superficial spreading carcinoma, epidermolysis bullosa, varices

Caustic Esophagitis
= CORROSIVE ESOPHAGITIS
Corrosive agents:
lye (sodium hydroxide), washing soda (sodium carbonate), household cleaners, iodine, silver nitrate, household bleaches, Clinitest® tablets (tend to be neutralized by gastric acid)
Δ Severity of injury dependent on contact time + concentration of corrosive material!
Associated with   injury to pharynx + stomach (7 – 8%): antral burns more common with acid (buffering effect of gastric acid on alkali)
Location: middle + lower thirds of esophagus
Stage I :   acute necrosis from protein coagulation
√ mucosal blurring (edema)
√ diffusely atonic + dilated esophagus
√ tertiary contractions
Stage II :   frank ulceration in 3 – 5 days
√ ulceration + pseudomembranes
Stage III :   scarring + stricture from fibroblastic activity
√ long segmental stricture aft 10 days when acute edema subsides (7 – 30%)
Cx:
(1) Esophageal / gastric perforation during ulcerative stage
(2) Squamous cell carcinoma in injured segment

Chronic Esophagitis
√ luminal narrowing with tapered transition to normal + proximal dilatation
√ circumferential / eccentric stricture
√ sacculations = pseudodiverticula

Cytomegalovirus Esophagitis
√ discrete superficial ulcers indistinguishable from herpes esophagitis
√ one / more large ovoid flat ulcers (up to several cm in size)

Drug-induced Esophagitis
Agents: tetracycline, doxycycline, potassium chloride, quinidine, aspirin, ascorbic acid, alprenolol chloride, emepronium bromide
• severe odynophagia
• history of taking medication with little / no water immediately before going to bed
Location: midesophagus at site of compression by aortic arch / left mainstem bronchus

√ superficial solitary / several discrete / localized clusters of tiny ulcers distributed circumferentially

√ dramatic healing of lesion 7 – 10 days after withdrawal of offending agent

DDx: herpes esophagitis

Herpes Esophagitis

Organism: Herpes simplex virus type I (DNA core virus) secreted in saliva of 2% of healthy population

Age: 15 – 30 years; usually males

- history of recent exposure to sexual partners with herpetic lesions on lips / buccal mucosa
- flulike prodrome of 3 – 10 days (fever, sore throat, upper respiratory infection, myalgia)
- acute odynophagia

Location: mid-esophagus

√ discrete superficial punctate / linear / stellate ulcers on normal mucosa (without plaques)

Dx: rising serum titer for HSV type 1, viral culture, immunofluorescent staining for HSV antigen, demonstration of intranuclear inclusions

Reflux Esophagitis

= esophageal inflammation secondary to reflux of acid-peptic contents of the stomach; reflux occurs if resting pressure of LES <5 mmHg (may be normal event if followed by rapid clearing)

Histo: basal cell hyperplasia with wall thickening + thinning of epithelium, mucosal edema + erosions, inflammatory infiltrate

Determinants:
 (1) Frequency of reflux
 (2) Adequacy of clearing mechanism
 (3) Volume of refluxed material
 (4) Potency of refluxed material
 (5) Tissue resistance

Reflux preventing features:
 (1) Lower esophageal sphincter
 (2) Phrenoesophageal membrane
 (3) Length of subdiaphragmatic esophagus
 (4) Gastroesophageal angle of His (70 – 110°)

May be associated with:
 sliding hiatal hernia (in most patients), scleroderma, nasogastric intubation

- heartburn, epigastric discomfort
- choking, globus hystericus
- retrosternal pain
- thoracic / cervical dysphagia

Site: usually lower 1/3 / lower 1/2 with continuous disease extending proximally from GE junction

√ segmental esophageal narrowing (edema / spasm / stricture)

√ granular / finely nodular appearance of thickened longitudinal mucosal folds with poorly defined borders (mucosal edema + inflammation) in early stages

√ single marginal ulcer / erosion at or adjacent to gastroesophageal junction

√ multiple areas of superficial ulceration in distal esophagus

√ prominent mucosal fold ending in polypoid protuberance within hiatal hernia / cardia

√ interruption of primary peristalsis at inflamed segment

√ nonperistaltic waves in distal esophagus following deglutition (85%)

√ incomplete relaxation of LES (75%), incompetent sphincter (33%)

√ acid test = abnormal motility elicited by acid barium (pH 1.7)

√ "felinization" = transverse ridges of esophagus secondary to contraction of muscularis mucosae (similar to cat esophagus)

NUC (pertechnetate):
 √ esophageal activity (Barrett esophagus similar to ectopic gastric mucosa)

REFLUX TESTS
 1. Reflux of barium in RPO position, may be elicited by coughing / deep respiratory movements / swallowing of saliva + water / anteflexion in erect position: only in 50% accurate
 2. Water-siphon test: in 5% false negative; large number of false positives
 3. Tuttle test = measurement of esophageal pH: 96% accurate
 4. Radionuclide gastroesophageal reflux test (typically combined with gastric emptying test):
 Technique: ROI drawn over distal esophagus + compared with time-activity curve over stomach, scaled to 4%
 √ esophageal activity >4% stomach activity

Cx of reflux:
 (a) from acid + pepsin acting on esophageal mucosa:
  1. Motility disturbance
  2. Stricture
  3. Schatzki ring
  4. Barrett esophagus
  5. Iron-deficiency anemia
  6. Reflux / peptic esophagitis
 (b) from aspiration of gastric contents
  1. Acute aspiration pneumonia
  2. Mendelson syndrome
  3. Pulmonary fibrosis

Viral Esophagitis

Predisposed: immunocompromised, eg, underlying malignancy, debilitating illness, radiation treatment, steroids, chemotherapy, AIDS

FAMILIAL ADENOMATOUS POLYPOSIS

= FAMILIAL MULTIPLE POLYPOSIS = autosomal dominant disease with 80% penetrance (gene for familial polyposis localized on chromosome 5); sporadic occurrence in 1/3

Incidence: 1:7,000 to 1:24,000 livebirths

Histo: tubular / villotubular adenomatous polyps; usually about 1,000 adenomas

Age: polyps appear around puberty

- family history of colonic polyps (66%)
  Δ Screening of family members after puberty!
- clinical symptoms begin during 3rd – 4th decade (range 5 – 55 years)
- vague abdominal pain, weight loss
- diarrhea, bloody stools
- protein-losing enteropathy (occasionally)

Associated with:
(1) Hamartomas of stomach in 49%
(2) Adenomas of duodenum in 25%
(3) Periampullary carcinoma
√ "carpet of polyps" = myriads of 2 – 3 mm (up to 2 cm) polypoid lesions
@ Colon (100%):   more numerous in distal colon; always affecting rectum
   √ normal haustral pattern
@ Stomach (5%)
@ Small bowel (<5%)

Cx: malignant transformation: colon > stomach > small bowel (in 12% by 5 years; in 30% by 10 years; in 100% by 20 years after diagnosis; age at carcinomatous development usually 20 – 40 years; multiple carcinomas in 48%)
Rx: prophylactic total colectomy in late teens / early twenties before symptoms develop +
(1) Permanent ileostomy
(2) Continent endorectal pull-through pouch
(3) Kock pouch (= distal ileum formed into a one-way valve by invaginating the bowel at skin site)
DDx: other polyposes, lymphoid hyperplasia, lymphosarcoma, ulcerative colitis with inflammatory pseudopolyps

GALLSTONE ILEUS

0.4 – 5% of all small bowel obstructions in elderly; M:F = 1:4
- previous history of gallbladder disease
- intermittent episodes of abdominal cramps, nausea, vomiting

TRIAD:
√ mechanical small bowel obstruction (in 86%)
√ gas within biliary tree (in 69%)
√ ectopic gallstone (in 25%)

GARDNER SYNDROME

= autosomal dominant disease (? variant of familial polyposis) characterized by a triad of (1) colonic polyposis (2) osteomas (3) soft tissue tumors
Histo: adenomatous polyps
Age: 15 – 30 years
Associated with: ? MEA complex
(1) periampullary / duodenal carcinoma (12%)
(2) thyroid carcinoma
(3) adrenal adenoma / carcinoma
(4) parathyroid adenoma
(5) pituitary chromophobe adenoma
(6) carcinoid, adenoma of small bowel
(7) retroperitoneal leiomyoma

- skin pigmentation
Δ Familial polyposis + Gardner syndrome may occur in the same family!
Δ Extraintestinal manifestations occur usually earlier than in intestinal polyposis!
@ Polyposis
   Location: colon (100%), stomach (5 – 68%), duodenum (90%), small bowel (<5%)
   √ multiple colonic polyps appearing during puberty, increasing in number during 3rd – 4th decade
   √ lymphoid hyperplasia of terminal ileum
   √ hamartomas of stomach
@ Soft tissue tumors
   (a) sebaceous / epidermoid inclusion cysts (scalp, back, face, extremities)
   (b) fibroma, lipoma, leiomyoma, neurofibroma
   (c) desmoid tumors (3 – 29%); peritoneal adhesions (desmoplastic tendency); mesenteric fibrosis, retroperitoneal fibrosis, mammary fibromatosis, marked keloid formation, hypertrophied scars (anterior abdominal wall) arise 1 – 3 years after surgery
     - GI / urinary tract obstruction
@ Osteomatosis of membranous bone (50%)
   Location: calvarium, mandible (81%), maxilla, ribs, long bones
@ Long bones
   √ localized wavy cortical thickening / exostoses
   √ slight shortening + bowing
@ Teeth
   √ odontoma, unerupted supernumerary teeth, hypercementosis
   √ tendency toward numerous caries (dental prosthesis at early age)

Cx: malignant transformation in 100% (average age at death is 41 years if untreated)
Rx: prophylactic total colectomy at about 20 years of age

GASTRIC CARCINOMA

3rd most common GI malignancy after colorectal + pancreatic cancer, 6th leading cause of cancer deaths
Prevalence: declining; 24,000 cases/year in USA

Predisposed:
pernicious anemia (risk factor of 2), chronic atrophic gastritis, adenomatous + villous polyp (7 – 27% are malignant), gastrojejunostomy, Billroth II > Billroth I
Histo: adenocarcinoma (95%); rarely squamous cell carcinoma / adenoacanthoma
Staging:
T_1 tumor limited to mucosa / submucosa
T_2 tumor involves muscle / serosa
T_3 tumor penetrates through serosa
T_{4a} invasion of adjacent contiguous tissues
T_{4b} invasion of adjacent organs, diaphragm, abdominal wall
N_1 involvement of perigastric nodes within 3 cm of primary along greater / lesser curvature

N$_2$ involvement of regional nodes >3 cm from primary along branches of celiac axis

N$_3$ paraaortic, hepatoduodenal, retropancreatic, mesenteric nodes

M$_1$ distant metastases

Location: mostly distal third of stomach + cardia; 60% on lesser curvature, 10% on greater curvature; esophagogastric junction in 30%

Probability of malignancy of an ulcer: at lesser curvature 10 – 15%, at greater curvature 70%, in fundus 90%

MORPHOLOGY

1. Polypoid / fungating carcinoma
2. Ulcerating / penetrating carcinoma (70%)
3. Infiltrating / scirrhous carcinoma (5 – 15%)
   = linitis plastica
   Histo: frequently signet ring cell type + increase in fibrous tissue
   Location: antrum, fundus + body (38%)
   √ firmness, rigidity, reduced capacity of stomach, aperistalsis in involved area
   √ granular / polypoid folds with encircling growth
4. Superficial spreading carcinoma
   = confined to mucosa / submucosa; 5-year survival of 90%
   √ patch of nodularity
   √ little loss of elasticity
5. Advanced carcinoma

EARLY GASTRIC CANCER (20%)
= invasion limited to mucosa + submucosa (T$_1$ lesion)
Classification of Japan Research Society for Gastric Cancer:

Type I Protruded type = >0.5 cm height with protrusion into gastric lumen (10 – 20%)

Type II Superficial type = <0.5 cm height

IIa slightly elevated surface (10 – 20%)

IIb flat / almost unrecognizable (2%)

IIc slightly depressed surface (50 – 60%)

Type III Excavated type (5 – 10%)

ADVANCED GASTRIC CANCER (T$_2$ lesion and higher)
Bormann classification:

Type 1 broad-based elevated polypoid lesion

Type 2 elevated lesion + ulceration + well-demarcated margin

Type 3 elevated lesion + ulceration + ill-defined margin

Type 4 ill-defined flat lesion

Type 5 unclassified, no apparent elevation

UGI:
√ rigidity
√ filling defect
√ amputation of folds ± ulceration ± stenosis
√ calcifications (mucinous adenocarcinoma)

CT:
√ irregular nodular luminal surface
√ asymmetric thickening of folds
√ mass of uniform density / varying attenuation
√ wall thickness >6 mm with gas distension + 13 mm with positive contrast material distension
√ increased density in perigastric fat
√ enhancement exclusively in linitis plastica type
√ nodules of serosal surface (= dilated surface lymphatics)
√ diameter of esophagus at gastroesophageal junction larger than adjacent aorta (DDx: hiatal hernia)
√ lymphadenopathy below level of renal pedicle (3%)

Metastases:
1. along peritoneal ligaments
   (a) gastrocolic lig.: transverse colon, pancreas
   (b) gastrohepatic + hepatoduodenal lig.: liver
2. local lymph nodes
3. hematogenous: liver (most common), adrenals, ovaries, bone (1.8%), lymphangitic carcinomatosis of lung (rare)
4. peritoneal seeding:
   rectal wall = Blumer shelf
5. left supraclavicular lymph node = Virchow node

Prognosis:
overall 5-year survival rate of 5 – 18%, mean survival time of 7 – 8 months;
— 85% 5-year survival in stage T$_1$
— 52% 5-year survival in stage T$_2$
— 47% 5-year survival in stage T$_3$
— 17% 5-year survival in stage N$_{1-2}$
— 5% 5-year survival in stage N$_3$

GASTRIC DIVERTICULUM
stomach is least common site of diverticula
Incidence: 1:600 – 2,400 of UGI studies
Etiology: (a) traction secondary to scarring / periantral inflammation = true diverticulum
(b) pulsion (less common) = false diverticulum

Prognostic Parameters of Gastric Carcinoma			
Tumor size	Metastases	Limited to Submucosa	5-year Survival Rate
1 cm	11%		87%
2 cm	25%	70%	67%
3 cm	45%		35%
4 cm	59%	60%	33%
>4 cm	72%	33%	

Age: beyond 40 years
Location: juxtacardia on posterior wall (75%), prepyloric
                    (15 – 22%), greater curve (3%)
Often associated with aberrant pancreas in antral location
√ pliability + varying degrees of distension
√ NO mass, edema or rigidity of adjacent folds
DDx: small ulcer in intramural-extramucosal mass

GASTRIC DUPLICATION CYST
= intramural cyst lined with secretory epithelium (may
  grow)
Age: in 75% detected before age 12

Location: frequently on greater curvature (65%)
√ seldom communicates with main gastric lumen at one /
  both ends
√ may ulcerate
√ up to 12 cm in size

GASTRIC EMPHYSEMA
= relatively benign condition of mucosal disruption
Cause:
   (1) Severe vomiting
   (2) Gastroscopic manipulation
   (3) Increased intraluminal pressure in gastric outlet
        obstruction
   (4) Rupture + dissection of subpleural blebs in bullous
        emphysema
   (5) Cystic pneumatosis = benign idiopathic round
        submucosal air lucencies

GASTRIC POLYP
Incidence: 1.5 – 5%, most common benign gastric
                    tumor
Associated with: hyperacidity + ulcers, chronic atrophic
                         gastritis, gastric carcinoma
Prognosis: low incidence of malignant transformation

1. INFLAMMATORY POLYP (75 – 90%)
   = HYPERPLASTIC POLYP = REGENERATIVE
     POLYP
   Histo: proliferated gastric mucosa + acute and
                   chronic inflammatory infiltrates in lamina
                   propria; no malignant potential
   Associated with: chronic atrophic gastritis, pernicious
                              anemia
   Location: random distribution within stomach, often in
                   antrum + body
   √ sharply delineated polyp with smooth circular border
   √ "Mexican hat sign" = stalk seen en face overlying the
     head of polyp
   √ sessile / pedunculated, usually multiple polyps
   √ usually <1 cm in diameter without progression
   √ no contour defect of stomach
2. ADENOMATOUS POLYP (10 – 20%)
   = true neoplasm with malignant potential (as high as
     51%, increasing with size)
   Associated with: Gardner syndrome, coexistent
                              gastric carcinoma
   Location: more commonly in antrum (antrum spared in

      Gardner syndrome)
   √ elliptical / mushroom-shaped; often single
   √ usually >1.5 cm in diameter
   √ smooth / irregular lobulated contour
3. HAMARTOMATOUS POLYP (rare)
   Histo: densely packed gastric glands
   Associated with: Peutz-Jeghers syndrome
   √ usually <2 cm in diameter
4. RETENTION POLYP (rare)
   Histo: dilated cystic glands + stroma
   Associated with: Cronkhite-Canada syndrome
5. VILLOUS POLYP (rare)
   √ trabeculated / lobulated slightly irregular contour
   Cx: malignant transformation
DDx:
   (1) Ménétrièr disease (antrum spared)
   (2) Eosinophilic polyp (peripheral eosinophilia, linitis
        plastica appearance, small bowel changes)
   (3) Lymphoma
   (4) Carcinoma

GASTRIC ULCER
Benign Gastric Ulcer
95% of all gastric ulcers
Causes:
   (1) Stress
   (2) Burns = curling ulcer
   (3) Cerebral disease = Cushing ulcer
   (4) Uremia
   (5) Severe prolonged illness
   (6) Gastritis
   (7) Steroid therapy
   (8) Intubation
   (9) Stasis ulcer proximal to pyloric / duodenal
        obstruction
   (10) HPT (25% with ulcer disease)
Pathophysiology:
   disrupted mucosal barrier with vulnerability to acid +
   secretion of large volume of gastric juice containing
   little acid
Incidence: 5:10,000; 100,000/year (United States)
Age peak: 55 – 65 years; M:F = 1:1
Multiplicity:
   (a) multiple in 2 – 8% (17 – 24% at autopsy),
        especially in patients on Aspirin®
   (b) coexistent duodenal ulcer in 5 – 64%;
        gastric:duodenal = 1:3 (adults) = 1:7 (children)
• abdominal pain: in 30% at night, in 25% precipitated
  by food

Location: lesser curvature at junction of corpus +
                antrum within 7 cm from pylorus; proximal
                half of stomach in older patients (geriatric
                ulcer); adjacent to GE junction within hiatal
                hernia
√ ulcer size usually <2 cm (range 1 – 250 mm);
  in 4% >40 mm
√ Haudek niche = conical / collar button-shaped barium
  collection projecting outside gastric contour (profile
  view)

√ Hampton line = 1 mm thin straight lucent line traversing the orifice of the ulcer niche (seen on profile view + with little gastric distension) = ledge of touching overhanging gastric mucosa of undermined benign ulcer

√ ulcer collar = smooth thick lucent band interposed between the niche and gastric lumen (thickened rim of edematous gastric wall) in well distended stomach

√ ulcer mound = smooth, sharply delineated, gently sloping extensive tissue mass surrounding a benign ulcer (edema + lack of wall distensibility) in well distended stomach

√ ulcer crater = round / oval barium collection with smooth border on dependent side (en face view)

√ halo defect = wide lucent band symmetrically surrounding ulcer resembling extensive ulcer mound (viewed en face)

√ ring shadow: ulcer on nondependent side (en face view)

√ radiating thick folds extending directly to crater edge fusing with the effaced marginal fold of the ulcer collar / halo of ulcer mound

√ incisura defect = smooth, deep, narrow, sharp indentation on greater curvature opposite a niche on lesser curvature at / slightly below the level of the ulcer (spastic contraction of circular muscle fibers)

Prognosis:
    healing in 50% by 3 weeks, in 100% by 6 – 8 weeks; slower healing in older patients; only complete healing proves benignancy
Cx: bleeding, perforation

Malignant Gastric Ulcer

Incidence: 5% of ulcers are malignant
Prognosis: partial healing may occur
Location: anywhere within stomach; fundal ulcers above level of cardia are usually malignant

√ ulcer location within gastric lumen, ie, not projecting beyond expected margin of stomach (profile view)

√ eccentrically located ulcer within the tumor

√ irregularly shaped ulcer

√ shallow ulcer with width greater than depth

√ nodular ulcer floor

√ abrupt transition between normal mucosa + abnormal tissue at some distance (usually 2 – 4 cm) from ulcer edge

√ rolled / rounded / shouldered edges surrounding ulcer

√ nodular irregular folds approaching ulcer with fused / clubbed / amputated tips

√ rigidity / lack of distensibility

√ associated large irregular mass

√ **Carman meniscus sign** = curvilinear lens-shaped intraluminal form of crater with convexity of crescent toward gastric wall and concavity toward gastric lumen (profile view, usually under compression) found in specific type of ulcerating carcinoma, seen only infrequently; wall aspect can also be concave / flat

√ **Kirklin meniscus complex** = Carman sign (appearance of crater) + radiolucent slightly elevated rolled border

GASTRIC VOLVULUS

= abnormal degree of rotation of one part of stomach around another part, usually requires >180° twisting to produce complete obstruction

Etiology: (a) abnormality of suspensory ligaments (hepatic, splenic, colic, phrenic)
            (b) unusually long gastrohepatic + gastrocolic mesenteries

Usually associated with diaphragmatic abnormality:
(1) Paraesophageal hiatus hernia in 33%
(2) Eventration

Types:
(a) ORGANOAXIAL VOLVULUS
    rotation around a line extending from cardia to pylorus
(b) MESENTEROAXIAL VOLVULUS
    rotation around an axis extending from lesser to greater curvature

• severe epigastric pain
• vigorous attempts to vomit without results
• inability to pass tube into stomach
√ massively distended stomach in LUQ extending into chest
√ incomplete / absent entrance of barium into stomach
√ barium demonstrates area of twist
Cx: intramural emphysema, perforation
DDx: gastric atony, acute gastric dilatation, pyloric obstruction

GASTRITIS

Corrosive Gastritis

Agents:
(a) <u>acid, formaldehyde</u>
    • clinically usually silent
    Location: esophagus usually unharmed, severe gastric damage, duodenum may be involved (newer potent materials cause atypical distribution)

(b) <u>alkaline</u>
    Location: pylorus + antrum most frequently involved

A. ACUTE CHANGES (edema + mucosal sloughing)
    √ marked enlargement of gastric rugae + erosions / ulceration
    √ complete cessation of motor activity
    √ gas in portal venous system
    Cx: perforation

B. CHRONIC CHANGES
    √ firm thick non-pliable wall
    √ stenotic / incontinent pylorus (if involved)
    √ gastric outlet obstruction (cicatrization) after 3 – 10 weeks

Emphysematous Gastritis

= rare but severe form of widespread phlegmonous gastritis subsequent to mucosal disruption characterized by gas in wall of stomach

Cause of mucosal disruption:
  ingestion of toxic / corrosive substances (most
  common), alcohol abuse, trauma, gastric infarction,
  necrotizing enterocolitis, ulcer

Histo: bacterial invasion of submucosa + subserosa
Organism: Hemolytic streptococcus, Clostridia
            welchii, E. coli, S. aureus
• explosive onset of abdominal pain, nausea, chills,
  fever, leukocytosis
• bloody foul smelling emesis

√ linear small gas bubbles within grossly thickened
  gastric wall
√ may be associated with gas in portal vein
Cx: cicatricial stenosis / sinus tract formation
Prognosis: 60 – 80% mortality

Erosive Gastritis
= HEMORRHAGIC GASTRITIS
Incidence: 0.5 – 10% of GI studies
Etiology   (in 50% without causative factors):
  (1) Peptic disease: emotional stress, alcohol, acid,
      corrosives, severe burns, antiinflammatory
      agents (aspirin, steroids, phenylbutazone,
      indomethacin)
  (2) Infection: Herpes simplex virus, CMV, Candida
  (3) Crohn disease: aphthoid ulcers identical in
      appearance to varioliform erosions
Histo: epithelial defect not penetrating beyond
            muscularis mucosae
• 10 – 20% of all GI hemorrhages (usually without
  significant blood loss)
• vague dyspepsia, ulcerlike symptoms

Location: antrum, rarely extending into fundus;
            aligned on surface of gastric rugal folds
√ varioliform erosion = tiny fleck of barium surrounded
  by radiolucent halo ("target lesion") <5 mm, usually
  multiple
√ incomplete erosion = linear streaks / dots of barium
  without surrounding mound of edema / inflammation
√ nodularity / scalloping of prominent antral folds
√ contiguous duodenal disease may be present
√ limited distensibility, poor peristalsis / atony, delayed
  gastric emptying

Phlegmonous Gastritis
Etiology: septicemia, local abscess, postoperative
            stomach, complication of gastric ulcer /
            cancer
Organism: Streptococcus
Path: multiple gastric wall abscesses, which may
            communicate with lumen
• severe fulminating illness
• patient may vomit pus
Location: usually limited to stomach not extending
            beyond pylorus; submucosa is the most
            severely affected gastric layer
√ barium dissection into submucosa + serosa

GIARDIASIS
= overgrowth of commensal parasite Giardia lamblia
Organism:
  Giardia lamblia (flagellated protozoan); often harmless
  contaminant of duodenum + jejunum in motile form
  (= trophozoite) attached to mucosa by suction disk,
  nonmotile form (= cyst) shed in feces; capable of
  pathogenic behavior with invasion of gut wall
Incidence: 1.5 – 2% of population in United States,
            infests 4 – 16% of inhabitants of tropical
            countries, found in 3 – 20% of children in
            parts of Southern United States
Predisposed: altered immune mechanism
            (dysgammaglobulinemia, nodular lymphoid
            hyperplasia of ileum)
Histo: blunted villi (may be misdiagnosed as celiac
            disease especially in children), cellular infiltrate of
            acute + chronic inflammation in lamina propria
• abdominal pain, weight loss, failure to thrive (especially
  in children)
• spectrum from asymptomatic to severe debilitating
  diarrhea, steatorrhea (related to number of organisms)
• reduced fat absorption (simulating celiac disease)

Location: most pronounced in duodenum + jejunum
√ thickened distorted mucosal folds in duodenum +
  jejunum (mucosal edema) with normal ileum
√ marked spasm + irritability with rapid change in direction
  + configuration of folds
√ hypersecretion with blurring + indistinctness of folds
√ hyperperistalsis with rapid transit time
√ segmentation of barium (from motility disturbance +
  excess intraluminal fluid)
√ ± lymphoid hyperplasia (associated with immunoglobulin
  deficiency state)

Dx: (1) Detection of Giardia lamblia cysts in formed
            feces or trophozoites in diarrheal stools
        (2) Trophozoites in duodenal aspirate / jejunal
            biopsy
DDx: Strongyloides / hookworm infection
Rx: quinacrine (Atabrine®)

GLYCOGEN ACANTHOSIS
= benign degenerative condition with accumulation of
  cellular glycogen within squamous epithelial lining of
  esophagus; etiology unknown
Incidence: in up to 15% of endoscoped patients
Histo: hyperplasia + hypertrophy of squamous mucosal
            cells secondary to increased glycogen; no
            malignant potential
• asymptomatic
• white oval mucosal plaques of 2 – 15 mm in diameter on
  otherwise normal appearing mucosa

Location: middle (common) / distal esophagus
√ multiple 1 – 3 mm rounded nodules / plaques
Dx: biopsy
DDx: Candida esophagitis (lesions disappear under
            treatment in contrast to glycogen acanthosis)

GRAFT-VERSUS-HOST DISEASE

= immunocompetent cells from donor bone marrow react against recipient tissues following bone marrow transplant for treatment of leukemia / lymphoma / aplastic anemia

Incidence: 30 – 70% of patients with allogeneic (= donor genetically different from host) transplant

Target organs: GI tract, skin, liver

@ Skin
- macular erythematous rash on face, trunk, extremities

@ Liver
- elevation of hepatic enzymes ± liver failure

@ GI tract
- profuse secretory diarrhea
- abdominal cramping, nausea, vomiting

Path: severe mucosal atrophy / destruction
√ "ribbon bowel" = small bowel fold thickening + effacement (DDx: viral enteritis, ischemia, celiac disease, radiation, soybean allergy)
√ loss of haustration, spasm, edema, ulceration, granular mucosal pattern of colon
√ prolonged coating of abnormal bowel for days
√ severely decreased transit time

Prognosis: fatal in up to 15% (due to opportunistic infections)
Rx: steroids + cyclosporine
DDx: superinfection with enteroviruses

HEMANGIOMA OF SMALL BOWEL

Increased incidence in: Turner syndrome, tuberous sclerosis, Osler-Weber-Rendu disease

Location: duodenum (2%), jejunum (55%), ileum (42%)
√ multiple sessile compressible intraluminal filling defects
√ nodular segmental mucosal abnormality
√ phleboliths in intestinal wall

HENOCH-SCHÖNLEIN PURPURA

= allergic vasculitis precipitated by allergies, insect sting, bacterial + viral infections, drugs (eg, penicillin, sulfonamides, aspirin)

Age: children + adults
- purpuric skin rash on legs + extensor surfaces on arms
- microscopic hematuria (from proliferative glomerulo-nephritis with IgA deposits demonstrated by immunofluorescence)
- arthralgias
- abdominal pain + GI bleeding
√ thickened valvulae conniventes (due to hemorrhage + edema)
Rx: high doses of corticosteroids

HIATAL HERNIA

Associated with: diverticulosis (25%), reflux esophagitis (25%), duodenal ulcer (20%), gallstones (18%)

A. SLIDING HIATAL HERNIA (99%)
= AXIAL HERNIA = CONCENTRIC HERNIA
= esophagogastric junction remains in chest with portion of peritoneal sac forming part of wall of hernia

Etiology: rupture of phrenicoesophageal membrane due to repetitive stretching with swallowing
Incidence: increasing with age
√ reducible in erect position
√ epiphrenic bulge = entire vestibule + sleeve of stomach are intrathoracic
√ distance between B ring (if visible) and hiatal margin >2 cm
√ peristalsis ceases above hiatus (end of peristaltic wave delineates esophagogastric junction)
√ tortuous esophagus having an eccentric junction with hernia
√ numerous coarse thick gastric folds within suprahiatal pouch (>6 longitudinal folds)
√ ± gastroesophageal reflux
CT:
√ dehiscence of diaphragmatic crura >15 mm
√ pseudomass within / above esophageal hiatus
√ increase in fat surrounding distal esophagus (= herniation of omentum through phrenicoesophageal ligament)
DDx: normal temporary cephalad motion of esophagogastric junction by 1 – 2 cm into chest due to contraction of longitudinal muscle during esophageal peristalsis

B. PARAESOPHAGEAL HERNIA (1%)
= ROLLING HIATAL HERNIA = PARAHIATAL HERNIA = portion of stomach superiorly displaced into thorax with esophagogastric junction remaining in subdiaphragmatic position
√ cardia in normal position
√ herniation of portion of stomach anterior to esophagus
√ frequently nonreducible
√ may be associated with gastric ulcer of lesser curvature at level of diaphragmatic hiatus

C. TOTALLY INTRATHORACIC STOMACH
= defect in central tendon of diaphragm in combination with slight volvulus in transverse axis of stomach behind heart
√ cardia may be intrathoracic (usually) / subdiaphragmatic
√ great gastric curvature either on right / left side

D. CONGENITALLY SHORT ESOPHAGUS
(not true hernia, very rare)
= gastric ectopy by lack of lengthening of esophagus
√ nonreducible intrathoracic gastric segment (in erect / supine position)
√ cylindrical / round intrathoracic segment with large sinuous folds
√ short straight esophagus
√ circular narrowing at gastroesophageal junction, frequently with ulcer
√ gastroesophageal reflux

HERNIA
External Hernia
= bowel extending outside the abdominal cavity
Incidence: 95% of all hernias

Location:
1. Inguinal hernia
2. Femoral hernia
3. Spigelian hernia = hernia through internal oblique muscle, beneath external oblique muscle at lateral margin of rectus sheath (linea semilunaris)
4. Petit lumbar triangle
5. Obturator foramen
6. Sciatic notch
7. Diaphragmatic hernia (foramen of Bochdalek + Morgagni)
8. Richter hernia = entrapment of one wall of the bowel in hernia orifice, usually seen in older women with femoral hernias

Internal Hernia

Incidence: 5% of all hernias, responsible for <1% of mechanical small bowel obstruction

Classification of hernias:
(a) retroperitoneal: usually congenital containing a hernial sac
   1. paraduodenal (Treitz ligament)
   2. foramen of Winslow
   3. intersigmoid
   4. pericecal / ileocolic
   5. supravesical
(b) anteperitoneal:
   small group of hernias without a peritoneal sac
   1. transmesenteric (transverse / sigmoid mesocolon)
   2. transomental
   3. pelvic (including broad ligament)

A. PARADUODENAL HERNIA (53%)
   (a) through fossa of Landzert on left side (3/4)
      √   lateral to 4th portion of duodenum and behind descending + transverse mesocolon
   (b) through fossa of Waldeyer on right side (1/4)
      √   caudal to SMA and inferior to 3rd portion of duodenum
B. LESSER SAC HERNIA (<10%)
   through foramen of Winslow in retrogastric location
   Invaginated gut:
      ileum > jejunum, cecum, appendix, ascending colon, Meckel diverticulum, gallbladder, greater omentum
C. HERNIA THROUGH BROAD LIGAMENT (very rare) after laceration / fenestration from surgery or during pregnancy

HIRSCHSPRUNG DISEASE
= AGANGLIONOSIS OF THE COLON = AGANGLIONIC MEGACOLON
= absence of parasympathetic ganglia in muscle (Meissner plexus) + submucosal layers (Auerbach plexus) secondary to an arrest of craniocaudal migration of neuroblasts before 12th week leading to relaxation failure of the aganglionic segment
Incidence: 1:5,000 – 8,000 livebirths; usually sporadic; familial in 4%

Age: full-term infant during first 6 weeks of life (70 – 80%); M:F = 4 – 9:1; extremely rare in premature infants
Associated with: Trisomy 21 (2%)
Location:
   at varying distances proximal to anus, usually rectosigmoid
   (a)   short segment disease   (80%)
   (b)   long segment disease   (15%)
   (c)   total colonic aganglionosis (5%)
   (d)   skip aganglionosis = sparing of rectum (very rare)
• failure to pass meconium within first 24 hours of life
• intermittent constipation + paradoxical diarrhea (25%)
• rectal manometry with absence of spike activity
√ "transition zone" = aganglionic segment appears normal in size
√ dilatation of large + small bowel aborally from transition zone
√ marked retention of barium on delayed films after 24 hours
√ normal appearing rectum in 33%
√ 10 – 15 cm segment of persistent corrugated / convoluted rectum (= abnormal uncoordinated contractions of the aganglionic portion of colon) in 31% (DDx: colitis, milk allergy, normal intermittent spasm of rectum)
N.B.: avoid digital exam / cleansing enema prior to radiographic studies!
OB-US:
   √ dilated small bowel / dilated colon

Cx: (1)   Necrotizing enterocolitis
      (2)   Cecal perforation (secondary to stasis, distension, ischemia)
      (3)   Obstructive uropathy
Dx: suction mucosal biopsy of rectum (increased acetylcholinesterase activity)
Rx: (1)   Swenson pull-through procedure
      (2)   Duhamel operation
      (3)   Soave procedure

HODGKIN DISEASE
Incidence: 0.75% of all cancers diagnosed each year
Age: bimodal peaks at age 25 – 30 years and 75 – 80 years
Histo: Reed-Sternberg cell = binucleate cell with prominent centrally located nucleolus
   (1)   Lymphocyte predominance (5%)
      = abundance of normal-appearing lymphocytes + relative paucity of abnormal cells; often diagnosed in younger people; frequently early stage; systemic symptoms are uncommon; most favorable natural history
   (2)   Nodular sclerosis (78%)
      = lymph nodes traversed by broad bands of birefringent collagen separating nodules, which consist of normal lymphocytes, eosinophils, plasma cells, and histiocytes; most common subtype; typically mediastinal involvement; 1/3 with systemic symptoms

(3) <u>Mixed cellularity</u> (17%)
= diffuse effacement of lymph nodes with lymphocytes, eosinophils, plasma cells + relative abundance of atypical mononuclear and Reed-Sternberg cells; more commonly advanced stage at presentation and older age

(4) <u>Lymphocyte depletion</u> (1%)
= paucity of normal appearing lymphocytes + abundance of abnormal mononuclear and Reed-Sternberg cells; least common subtype with worst prognosis; associated with advanced stage and systemic symptoms

STAGE
I involvement of single lymph node region
II involvement of ≥ 2 lymph node regions on same side of diaphragm
III lymph node involvement on both sides of diaphragm
IV diffuse / disseminated involvement of ≥ 1 extralymphatic organs / tissues ± associated lymph node involvement
E = extralymphatic site
S = splenic involvement
A = absence of fever, night sweats, >10% weight loss in past 6 months
B = presence of fever, night sweats, >10% weight loss in past 6 months
• painless lymphadenopathy
• alcohol-induced pain
• unexplained fevers, night sweat, weight loss
• generalized pruritus
Location: intestinal involvement uncommon (10 – 15%); duodenum + jejunum (67%); terminal ileum (20%)
√ narrow rigid obstructive lesion
√ abundance of desmoplastic reaction (DDx from NHL)
√ infiltrating (60%); polypoid (26%); ulcerated (14%)
Prognosis: excellent for isolated / localized disease

HYPERPLASTIC POLYP OF COLON
= intestinal metaplasia consisting of mucous glands lined by a single layer of columnar epithelium; NO malignant potential
Path: infolding of epithelium into the glandular lumen
Location: rectum
√ usually <5 mm in diameter

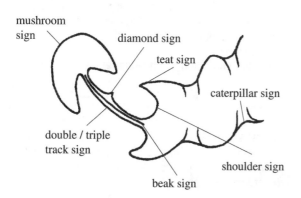

HYPERTROPHIC PYLORIC STENOSIS
= idiopathic hypertrophy and hyperplasia of circular muscle fibers of pylorus with proximal extension into gastric antrum
Incidence: 3:1,000; M:F = 4 – 5:1
Etiology: inherited as a dominant polygenic trait; increased incidence in firstborn boys; acquired rather than congenital condition

A. INFANTILE FORM
Age: manifestation at 2 – 8 weeks of life
• nonbilious projectile vomiting (sour formula / clear gastric contents) with progression over a period of several weeks after birth (15 – 20%)
• positive family history
• olive-shaped mass
• nasogastric aspirate >10 ml (92% sensitive, 86% specific)
UGI:
Precautions: (1) empty stomach via nasogastric tube before study
              (2) remove contrast at end of study
√ pyloric wall thickness >10 mm
√ elongation + narrowing of pyloric canal (2 – 4 cm in length)
√ "double / triple track sign" = crowding of mucosal folds in pyloric channel
√ "string sign" = passing of small barium streak through pyloric channel
√ Twining recess = "diamond sign" = transient triangular tentlike cleft / niche in midportion of pyloric canal with apex pointing inferiorly secondary to mucosal bulging between two separated hypertrophied muscle bundles on the greater curvature side within pyloric channel
√ "pyloric teat" = outpouching along lesser curvature due to disruption of antral peristalsis
√ "antral beaking" = mass impression upon antrum with streak of barium pointing toward pyloric channel
√ Kirklin sign = "mushroom sign" = indentation of base of bulb (in 50%)
√ gastric distension with fluid
√ active gastric hyperperistalsis
√ "caterpillar sign" = gastric hyperperistaltic waves
US:
√ "target sign" = hypoechoic ring of hypertrophied pyloric muscle around echogenic mucosa centrally on cross-section
√ "cervix sign" = indentation of muscle mass on fluid-filled antrum on longitudinal section
√ pyloric volume >1.4 cm³ (= 1/4 $\prod$ x [maximum pyloric diameter]² x pyloric length); most accurate criteria independent of contracted or relaxed state
√ pyloric muscle wall thickness ≥3 mm
√ pyloric transverse diameter ≥13 mm with pyloric channel closed
√ elongated pyloric canal ≥17 mm in length
√ exaggerated peristaltic waves
√ delayed gastric emptying of fluid into duodenum

Cx: hypochloremic metabolic alkalosis
DDx:
1. Infantile pylorospasm (variable caliber of antral narrowing, antral peristalsis, resolves in several days, effective treatment with metoclopramide hydrochloride)
2. Milk allergy
3. Eosinophilic gastroenteritis

B. ADULT FORM (secondary to mild infantile form)
- acute obstructive symptoms uncommon
- nausea, intermittent vomiting
- postprandial distress, heartburn
Associated with:
   (1) peptic ulcer disease (in 50 – 74%) (prolonged gastrin production secondary to stasis of food)
   (2) chronic gastritis (54%)
- √ persistent elongation (2 – 4 cm) + concentric narrowing of pyloric channel
- √ parallel + preserved mucosal folds
- √ antispasmodics show no effect on narrowing
- √ proximal benign ulcer (74%), usually near incisura

TORUS HYPERPLASIA = FOCAL PYLORIC HYPERTROPHY
- = localized muscle hypertrophy on the lesser curvature
- = milder atypical form of HPS
- √ flattening of distal lesser curvature

INTESTINAL LYMPHANGIECTASIA
A. CONGENITAL LYMPHANGIECTASIA = PRIMARY PROTEIN-LOSING ENTEROPATHY
   = generalized congenital malformation of lymphatic system with atresia of the thoracic duct + gross dilatation of small bowel lymphatics; usually sporadic; may be inherited
   Age: presentation before 30 years
   - asymmetric generalized lymphedema (due to protein-losing enteropathy with hypoproteinemia)
   - chylous pleural effusions (45%)
   - diarrhea (60%), steatorrhea (20%)
   - vomiting (15%)
   - abdominal pain (15%) + distension
   - decreased albumin + globulin
   - lymphocytopenia (90%)
   - decreased serum fibrinogen, transferrin, ceruloplasmin

B. ACQUIRED LYMPHANGIECTASIA
   Causes leading to dilatation of intestinal lymphatics:
   1. Mesenteric adenitis
   2. Retroperitoneal fibrosis
   3. Diffuse small bowel lymphoma
   4. Pancreatitis
   5. Pericardial effusion with obstruction of thoracic duct
   - peripheral edema / anasarca (KEY SYMPTOM)
   - chylous + serous effusion
   - diarrhea, vomiting, abdominal pain, malabsorption, steatorrhea

- hypoproteinemia secondary to protein loss into intestinal lumen

Path: dilatation of lymph vessels in mucosa + submucosa + abundance of foamy fat-staining macrophages (negative for PAS)
- √ diffuse symmetric marked enlargement of folds in jejunum + ileum (due to dilated intestinal lymphatics + hypoproteinemic edema)
- √ slight separation + rigidity of folds
- √ dilution of barium column (considerable increase in intestinal secretions from malabsorption)
- √ no / mild dilatation of bowel
- Lymphangiogram (not always diagnostic):
  - √ hypoplasia of lower extremity lymphatics
  - √ occlusion of thoracic duct / large tortuous thoracic duct
  - √ obstruction of cisterna chyli with backflow into mesenteric + intestinal lymphatics
  - √ hypoplastic lymph nodes
- *Dx:*   small bowel biopsy (dilated lymphatics in lamina propria + vascular core)
- *Rx:*   low-fat diet with medium-chain triglycerides (direct absorption into portal venous system)
- *DDx:* (1) Whipple disease (more segmentation + fragmentation, wild folds)
         (2) Amyloidosis (edema + secretions usually absent)
         (3) Hypoalbuminemia (less pronounced symmetrical thickening of folds, less prominent secretions)

INTRALUMINAL DUODENAL DIVERTICULUM
- = congenital lesion secondary to elongation of an incomplete duodenal diaphragm
- *Age at presentation:*   in young adult
- easy satiety
- vomiting
- upper abdominal cramping pain
- Location: 2nd – 3rd portion of duodenum
- √ barium-filled sac within duodenal lumen (pathognomonic picture) = "windsock, comma, teardrop" appearance
- √ anchored to the lateral wall of the duodenum
- √ "halo" sign = duodenal mucosa covers outer + inner wall of diverticulum

INTRAMURAL ESOPHAGEAL RUPTURE
- = DISSECTING INTRAMURAL HEMATOMA = mucosal tear with dissecting hemorrhage into submucosa and involvement of venous plexus
- hematemesis
- √ intramural hematoma simulates retained solid material within lumen
- √ "mucosal stripe sign" = dissected mucosa floating within lumen

INTUSSUSCEPTION
- = invagination or prolapse of a segment of intestinal tract (= intussusceptum) into the lumen of adjacent intestine (= intussuscipiens)

A. IN CHILDREN (94%)

Most common abdominal emergency of early childhood, leading cause of acquired bowel obstruction in childhood

Etiology:

(1) idiopathic (over 95%): mucosal edema + lymphoid hyperplasia following viral gastroenteritis; predominantly at ileocecal valve

(2) lead point (5%): Meckel diverticulum (most common), lymphosarcoma, polyp, enterogenous cyst, duplication cyst, suture granuloma, appendiceal inflammation, Henoch-Schönlein purpura, inspissated meconium; usually >6 years of age

Age: peak incidence between 6 months and 2 years; 3 – 9 months (40%); <1 year (50%); <2 years (75%); >3 years (<10%); M:F = 2:1

- abrupt onset of violent crampy pain (90%), vomiting (85%)
- abdominal mass (60%)
- "currant jelly" bloody stools (60%)

Location: ileocolic (75 – 95%) > ileoileal (4%) > colocolic

Cx: vascular compromise secondary to incorporation of mesentery (hemorrhage, infarction, acute inflammation)

B. IN ADULTS (6%)

Etiology:

(1) specific cause (80%): benign tumor (1/3), malignant tumor (1/5), lipoma, Meckel diverticulum, prolapsed gastric mucosa, aberrant pancreas, adhesions, foreign body, feeding tube, chronic ulcer (TB, typhoid), prior gastroenteritis, gastroenterostomy, trauma without anatomic lead point:
celiac disease, scleroderma, Whipple disease, fasting, anxiety, agonal state

(2) idiopathic (20%)

- recurrent episodes of colicky pain, nausea, vomiting

Location: ileoileal (40%) > ileocolic (13%)

Plain film (no abnormality in 25%):

√ soft-tissue mass

√ small bowel obstruction (50 – 60%) with nipplelike termination of gas shadow

Antegrade barium study:

√ "coil spring" appearance

√ beaklike abrupt narrowing of barium column demonstrating a central channel

Retrograde barium study:

√ convex intracolic mass + "coiled spring" pattern

CT:

√ "multiple concentric rings" = 3 concentric cylinders (central cylinder = canal + wall of intussusceptum; middle cylinder = crescent of mesenteric fat; outer cylinder = returning intussusceptum + intussuscipiens)

√ proximal obstruction

US:

√ "doughnut / target / bull's eye sign" (on transverse sections) = concentric rings of alternating hypoechoic + hyperechoic layers with central hyperechoic portion

√ "pseudokidney / hayfork sign" on longitudinal sections

HYDROSTATIC / PNEUMATIC REDUCTION

Δ <1% mortality if reduction occurs <24 hours after onset!

Overall success rate: 18 – 90%

Contraindications: pneumoperitoneum, peritonitis, hypovolemic shock

Technique:

(1) Sedation with morphine sulfate (0.2 mg/kg IM) / fentanyl citrate IV

(2) 60% wt/vol barium enema with container between 24 – 36 inches above level of anus

(3) Maximally 3 attempts for 3 minutes each

(4) Reduction should be accomplished within 10 minutes

(5) Extensive reflux into small bowel desirable to exclude residual ileoileal intussusception

"RULE OF THREES" = (1) 3 feet above table
(2) no more than 3 attempts
(3) 3 minutes per attempt

Alternative medium: 1:4 Gastrografin-water solution raised to a height of 5 feet

Cx: perforation (0.4%); reduction of nonviable bowel; incomplete reduction; missed lead point

Prognosis: 3.5 – 10% rate of recurrence

ISCHEMIC COLITIS

= nonocclusive vascular disease within the territory of the inferior mesenteric artery characterized by acute onset + rapid clinical and radiographic evolutionary changes

Etiology: diminished blood flow within bowel wall (mucosa + submucosa most sensitive to ischemia); major mesenteric vessels usually patent

Precipitating factors:

(a) bowel obstruction: volvulus, carcinoma (proximal bowel segment affected)

(b) thrombosis: cardiovascular disease, collagen vascular disease, sickle cell disease, hemolytic-uremic syndrome, oral contraceptives

(c) trauma: history of aortoiliac reconstruction (2%) with ligation of IMA

Age: >50 years

- abrupt onset of lower abdominal pain + rectal bleeding
- abdominal tenderness, diarrhea

Location: left colon (90%), splenic flexure (80%) + sigmoid ("watershed areas"), rectum spared

Plain film (usually normal):

√ segmental thumbprinting = marginal indentations on mesenteric side (rare finding on plain film)

BE (in 90% abnormal):

Δ Single contrast may efface thumbprinting, but double contrast overall is more sensitive!

√ thumbprinting (75%) due to submucosal hemorrhage + edema

√ transverse ridging = markedly enlarged mucosal folds (spasm), some wall pliability is preserved

√ serrated mucosa = inflammatory edema + superficial longitudinal / circumferential ulceration

√ deep penetrating ulcers (late)

CT:

√ symmetrical / lobulated segmental thickening of colonic wall

√ irregular narrowed atonic lumen (= thumbprinting)

√ curvilinear collection of intramural gas

√ portal + mesenteric venous air

√ blood clot in SMA / SMV

Angio (findings similar to inflammatory disease):

√ normal / slightly attenuated arterial supply

√ mild acceleration of arteriovenous transit time

√ small tortuous ectatic draining veins

Prognosis:

(1) Transient ischemia = complete resolution within 1 – 3 months

(2) Stricturing ischemia = incomplete delayed healing
    √ narrowed foldless segment of several cm in length with smooth tapering margins

(3) Gangrene with necrosis + perforation (extremely uncommon)

JEJUNAL DIVERTICULUM

= acquired mucosal herniation;
frequently multiple (= jejunal diverticulosis)

Incidence: 0.1% on UGI, 1% of autopsy series; M > F

Site: on mesenteric border near entrance of blood vessels

• upper abdominal pain

Plain film:

√ slight dilatation of jejunal loops

BE:

√ may not fill (narrow neck / stagnant secretions)

√ trapped barium on delayed film after 24 hours

Cx:

(1) Blind loop syndrome with bacterial overgrowth
    • steatorrhea, diarrhea, malabsorption, weight loss
    • macro- / microcytic anemia

(2) Free perforation = leading cause of pneumoperitoneum without peritonitis

(3) Hemorrhage

(4) Diverticulitis

(5) Intestinal obstruction

JUVENILE POLYPOSIS

= retention / inflammatory polyp = polyp with inflammatory changes secondary to chronic irritation

Δ Most common familial / nonfamilial colonic polyp in children (75%)!

Histo: hyperplasia of mucous glands; retention cysts develop with obstruction of gland orifices (multiple mucin-filled spaces)

Peak age: 4 – 6 years (range 1 – 10 years); M:F = 3:2

• rectal bleeding (95%) most commonly as intermittent bright red hematochezia

• anemia, pain

• diarrhea, constipation

• abdominal pain (from intussusception)

• rectal prolapse (rare)

Location: rectosigmoid (80%); rare in small bowel + stomach

√ solitary polyp (75%); multiple polyps (1/3) of smooth round contour

√ lesion of pinpoint size / up to several cm in diameter

√ invariably on stalk of variable length

√ autoamputation / regression with time

KAPOSI SARCOMA

Incidence: 11 – 34%; 95% in homosexual men

Location:

@   GI tract (40%):
     anywhere within GI tract; often multifocal
     Δ GI tract is the only site of involvement in <5%!

@   Lymph nodes + skin:
     associated with high frequency of GI tract involvement

√ thickened nodular folds

√ submucosal nodules ± central umbilication

√ polypoidal mass

√ infiltrating lesion

LADD BANDS

= congenital peritoneal bands extending from cecum / hepatic flexure over anterior surface of 2nd / 3rd portion of duodenum causing duodenal obstruction at its 2nd portion (even without volvulus)

Associated with   malrotation

LEIOMYOMA

2/3 occur in stomach

Leiomyoma of Esophagus

Most common benign tumor of esophagus; 50% of all esophageal benign tumors

Incidence: 1:1,119 (autopsy study)

Age: young adults, 3% in children (associated with Alport syndrome in 22%); M>F

• asymptomatic

• dysphagia, odynophagia, dyspepsia

• hematemesis if large (rare)

Site: frequently lower + mid 1/3 of esophagus; intramural; multiple leiomyomas in 3%

√ 2 – 15 cm large smooth well-defined intramural mass causing eccentric thickening of wall + deformity of lumen

√ may have coarse calcifications
    Δ Leiomyoma is the only calcifying esophageal tumor!

√ ulceration uncommon

√ diffuse leiomyomatosis / multiple leiomyomas in children

CT:

√ uniform soft-tissue density

√ diffuse contrast enhancement

CAVE: high percentage misdiagnosed as extrinsic lesion!

Leiomyoma of Small Bowel
Most common benign tumor of small bowel
Location: duodenum (21%), jejunum (48%),
            ileum (31%); single in 97%
Site: mainly serosal (50%), mainly intraluminal (20%),
        intramural (10%)
Size: <5 cm (50%), 5 – 10 cm (25%), >10 cm (25%)
√ small ulcer + large barium-filled cavity (central
  necrosis + communication with lumen)
√ hypervascular

Leiomyoma of Stomach
2nd most common benign gastric tumor (after gastric
polyp), most common of calcified benign tumors
Location: pars media (39%), antrum (26%),
            pylorus (12%), fundus (12%), cardia (10%)
Site: intraluminal submucosal (60%), exophytic
        subserosal (35%), combined intramural-
        extramural dumbbell type mass (5%)
√ average size of 4.5 cm
√ ovoid mass with smooth margin + smooth surface
  (most frequently)
√ forms right angle with gastric wall
√ ulcerated in 50%
√ pedunculated intraluminal tumor in submucosal
  growth (rare)
√ "iceberg phenomenon" = large extraluminal
  component in subserosal growth
√ calcifies in 4%
Cx: (1) Hemorrhage (acute / chronic)
     (2) Obstruction (tumor bulk / intussusception)
     (3) Infection
     (4) Fistulization / perforation
     (5) Malignant degeneration (benign:malignant =
         3:1)

LEIOMYOSARCOMA
Leiomyosarcoma of Small Bowel
Location: duodenum (26%), jejunum (34%),
            ileum (40%)
√ usually >6 cm in size
√ nodular mass: intraluminal (10%), intraluminal
  pedunculated (5%), intramural (15%), chiefly extrinsic
  (66%)
√ mucosa may be stretched + ulcerated (50%)
√ may show central ulcer pit / fistula communicating
  with a large necrotic center
√ intussusception

Leiomyosarcoma of Stomach
Incidence: 0.1 – 3% of all gastric malignancies
Age: 10 – 73 years; M > F
Histo: pleomorphism, hypercellularity, mitotic figures,
        cystic degeneration, necrosis
• GI bleeding (from ulceration)
• obstruction
Location: anterior / posterior wall of body of stomach
Metastases:
  (a) hematogenous to liver, lung, peritoneum; rarely
      to bone + soft tissue

  (b) direct extension into omentum, retroperitoneum
  (c) lymph nodes (rare)

√ average size of 12 cm
√ intramural mass
√ may be pedunculated
√ large masses tend to be exogastric
√ very frequently ulcerated
CT:
  √ lobulated irregular outline
  √ central zones of low density (necrosis with
    liquefaction)
  √ air / positive contrast within tumor (= ulceration)
  √ dystrophic calcifications

Carney Syndrome
Triad of (1) Gastric leiomyosarcoma
          (2) Functioning extraadrenal paraganglioma
          (3) Pulmonary chondromas
Incidence: 24 patients reported; M:F = 1:11

LIPOMA
Most common submucosal tumor in colon
Incidence: in colon in 0.25% (autopsy)
Location: colon (particularly cecum + ascending colon)
            > duodenum > ileum > stomach > jejunum >
            esophagus
• asymptomatic
• crampy pain, hemorrhage (rare)

√ smooth, sharply outlined, round / ovoid globular mass
  of 1 – 3 cm in diameter
√ short thick pedicle in 1/3 caused by repeated peristaltic
  activity (prone to intussuscept)
√ marked radiolucency
√ change in shape + size on compression due to softness
√ "squeeze sign" = sausage-shaped mass on
  postevacuation radiographs
CT:
  √ sharply defined intramural mass of fat density
Cx: intussusception (rare) / ulceration (rare)
Prognosis: NO liposarcomatous degeneration

LYMPHOGRANULOMA VENEREUM
= LGV = sexually transmitted disease caused by virus
Chlamydia trachomatis producing a nonspecific
granulomatous inflammatory response in infected
mucosa (mononuclear cells + macrophages), perirectal
lymphatic invasion
Location: rectum, may extend to sigmoid + descending
            colon
M:F = 3.4:1

√ narrowing + shortening + straightening of rectosigmoid
√ widening of retrorectal space
√ irregularity of mucosa + ulcerations
√ paracolic abscess
√ fistula to pericolic area, rectum, vagina (common)
Rx: tetracyclines effective in acute phase before
      scarring has occurred

LYMPHOID HYPERPLASIA

Incidence: normal variant in 13% of BE examinations
Histo: hyperplastic lymph follicles in lamina propria
(Peyer patches), probably compensatory attempt
for immunoglobulin deficiency
Etiology:
(1) Normal in child / young adult
(2) Self-limiting local / systemic inflammation / infection
/ allergy
(3) May be related to immunodeficiency / dysgammaglobulinemia with small bowel involvement
Age: (a) generally in children <2 years
(b) in adults invariably associated with late onset
immunoglobulin deficiency (IgA, IgM)
Associated with: splenomegaly, large tonsils,
eczematous dermatitis, achlorhydria,
pernicious anemia, acute pancreatitis,
colonic carcinoma
At risk for:
(1) **Good syndrome** (10%)
= gastric carcinoma + benign thymoma +
lymphoid hyperplasia
(2) Respiratory infections
(3) Giardia lamblia infection (90%)
(4) Functional thyroid abnormalities
Location: primarily jejunum, may involve entire small
bowel, ascending colon + hepatic flexure,
seldom in sigmoid / rectum
• malabsorption (diarrhea + steatorrhea)
• low serum concentrations of IgA, IgG, IgM
√ mucosa studded with innumerable 1 – 3 mm small
uniform polypoid lesions
√ lesions may be umbilicated (uncommon)

LYMPHOMA

Classification:
A. PRIMARY LYMPHOMA OF BOWEL
(a) localized (b) diffuse
Predisposed: Arabs + Middle Eastern Jews
Associated with   celiac disease
B. SECONDARY INTESTINAL LYMPHOMA
as part of generalized systemic process

Incidence: 10% of patients with abdominal lymphoma
have bowel involvement
Median age: 60 years
Histo: predominantly NHL (lymphosarcoma, reticulum
cell sarcoma); in 15% Hodgkin disease
May be associated with   enlargement of extraabdominal
lymph nodes, malabsorption
Radiographic types:
(a) polypoid / nodular (47%)
√ enlarged nodular folds
(b) ulcerative (42%)
√ ulcerative lesions, may be complicated by
perforation
√ aneurysmal configuration
(c) diffusely infiltrating (11%)
√ diffuse hoselike thickening of bowel wall
√ decreased / absent peristalsis

CT staging:
Stage I   tumor confined to bowel wall
Stage II   limited to local nodes
Stage III   widespread nodal disease
Stage IV   disseminated to bone marrow, liver, other
organs

Location: 10 – 25% of NHL are extranodal; stomach >
small bowel > colon > esophagus;
multicentric in 10 – 50%
√ enlargement of spleen
√ enlargement of regional lymph nodes

@ Esophagus
least common site of GI involvement (in <1%)
@ Stomach
1 – 5% of all gastric malignancies; most common site
of extranodal Hodgkin disease; 25% of extranodal
lymphoma; mostly NHL with histiocytic cell type;
isolated primary gastric malignancy in 10%
Site: arises in lymphoid tissue of lamina propria; no
predilection for any particular region of
stomach
Direct extension into: pancreas, spleen, transverse
colon, liver
√ flexibility of gastric wall preserved
√ duodenum often affected when antrum involved
√ circumscribed mass with endogastric / exogastric
(25%) growth
√ broad tortuous mucosal folds over large portions of
stomach (diffuse form)
√ large irregular ulcers
CT:
√ diffuse involvement of entire stomach (50%),
typically more than half of gastric circumference
√ segmental involvement (15%)
√ ulcerated mass (8%)
√ average wall thickness of 4 – 5 cm
√ luminal irregularity (66%)
√ hyperrugosity (58%)
Prognosis: 55% 5-year survival rate after resection
@ Small bowel
1/5 of all small bowel malignancies; most common
malignant small bowel tumor; multiple sites of
involvement in 1/5; most common cause of
intussusception in children >6 years
Location: ileum (51%), jejunum (47%),
duodenum (2%),
Site: arising from lymphoid patches of Peyer
Types:
(a) infiltrating lymphoma with plaquelike
involvement of wall >5 cm in length (80%) /
>10 cm in length (20%) (DDx: Crohn disease)
√ ± ulceration (considerable excavation)
√ desmoplastic response
√ thickened valvulae with corrugated
appearance
√ aneurysmal dilatation (secondary to
destruction of autonomic nerve plexus +
muscle / tumor necrosis)

(b) single / multiple polypoid mucosal / submucosal masses
  √ cobblestone defects due to lymphomatous polyps
  √ nodules may ulcerate
  √ may cause intussusception
  √ sprue pattern
(c) endoexoenteric mass
  √ large mass with only small intramural component
  √ ± ulcer + fistulae + aneurysmatic dilatation
(d) mesenteric / retroperitoneal adenopathy
  √ single / multiple extraluminal masses displacing bowel
  √ ill-defined confluent mass engulfing + encasing multiple loops of adjacent bowel
  √ "sandwich configuration" = mass surrounding mesenteric vessels that are separated by perivascular fat
  √ conglomerate mantle of retroperitoneal + mesenteric mass

@ Colon
  Less commonly involved than stomach / small bowel; 1.5% of all abdominal lymphomas
  Location: cecum most commonly involved (85%)
  √ single mass > diffuse infiltration > polypoid lesion
  √ paradoxical dilatation
  √ gross mural circumferential / focal soft-tissue thickening (average size of 5 cm)
  √ slight enhancement
  √ massive regional + distant mesenteric + retroperitoneal adenopathy
  DDx: frequently resembles inflammatory disease / polyposis

Prognosis:
  (a) 71 – 82% 2-year survival rate in isolated bowel lymphoma
  (b) 0% 2-year survival rate in stage IV disease with bowel involvement
Cx during chemotherapy: perforation (9 – 40%), hemorrhage

MALIGNANT MELANOMA
= develops from melanocytes derived from neural crest cells, arising in preexisting benign nevi
Incidence: 1% of all cancers
@ Skin primary
  Clark Staging:
    Level I   all tumor cells above basement membrane (in situ lesion)
    Level II tumor extends to papillary dermis
    Level III tumor extends to interface between papillary + reticular dermis
    Level IV tumor extends between bundles of collagen of reticular dermis
    Level V   tumor invasion of subcutaneous tissue (in 87% metastatic)
  Breslow staging:
    thin   <0.75 mm depth of invasion

    intermediate 0.76 – 3.99 mm depth of invasion
    thick   >4 mm depth of invasion

METASTASES:
  latent period of 2 – 20 years after initial diagnosis (most commonly 2 – 5 years)
  Primary site: head + neck (79%), eye (77%), GU system (67%), GI tract (in up to 60%)
  @ Lymphadenopathy
    — in 23% with level II + IV
    — in 75% with level V
  @ Bone (11 – 17%)
    • often initial manifestation of recurrence
    • poor prognosis
    Location: axial skeleton (80%), ribs (38%)
  @ Lung (70% at autopsy)
    most common site of relapse;
    respiratory failure most common cause of death
  @ Liver (17 – 23%; 58 – 66% at autopsy)
    √ single / multiple lesions 0.5 – 15 cm in size
    √ larger lesion often necrotic
    √ may be partially calcified
  @ Spleen (1 – 5%; 33% at autopsy)
    √ single / multiple lesions of variable size
    √ solid / cystic
  @ GI tract + mesentery (4 – 8%)
    • abdominal pain, GI bleeding
    Location: small intestine (35 – 50%), colon (14 – 20%), stomach (7 – 20%)
    √ multiple submucosal nodules ± "bull's-eye / target" appearance = central ulceration
    √ irregular amorphous cavity (exoenteric growth)
    √ intussusception (10 – 20%)
  @ Kidney (up to 35% at autopsy)
  @ Adrenal (11%, up to 50% at autopsy)
  @ Subcutis
Prognosis: 30 – 40% eventually die from this tumor

MALLORY-WEISS SYNDROME
= mucosal + submucosal tear with involvement of venous plexus
Pathophysiology: violent projection of gastric contents against lower esophagus
Age: 30 – 60 years; M > F
Predisposed: alcoholics
• history of repeated vomiting prior to hematemesis
• massive painless hematemesis

Location: at / above / below (76%) esophagogastric junction
√ longitudinal single tear in 77%, in 23% multiple tears
√ extravasation of barium
Angio:
  √ bleeding site at gastric cardia
DDx: peptic ulcer / ulcerative gastritis

MASTOCYTOSIS
= systemic disease with mast cell proliferation in skin + RES (lamina propria of small bowel; bone; lymph nodes; liver; spleen) associated with eosinophils + lymphocytes

Age: <6 months old (in 50%)
- nausea, vomiting, diarrhea, steatorrhea
- urticaria pigmentosa
- abdominal pain, anorexia
- alcohol intolerance
- tachycardia, asthma, flushing, headaches, pruritus (histamine liberation)
@ Small bowel
  √   generalized irregular distorted thickened folds ± wall thickening
  √   diffuse pattern of 2 – 3 mm sandlike mucosal nodules
  √   urticaria-like lesions of gastric + intestinal mucosa
@ Liver & spleen
  √   hepatosplenomegaly
@ Bone
  √   sclerotic bone lesions
Dx: jejunal biopsy demonstrates an excess of mast cells
Cx: (1) Peptic ulcer disease (histamine-mediated acid secretion)
       (2) Leukemia
Rx: antihistamines, histamine decarboxylase inhibitors, sodium chromoglycase

MECKEL DIVERTICULUM
= persistence of the omphalomesenteric duct (= vitelline duct), which usually obliterates by 5th embryonic week; most commonanomaly of the GI tract
Incidence: 2 – 3% of population
Age: majority in children <10 years of age; M:F = 3:1
Histo: contains heterotopic tissue in 12 – 16%: gastric / pancreatic / colonic mucsa;
       Δ Frequency of ectopic gastric mucosa:
       30% overall; 60% in symptomatic children; in >95% with GI hemorrhage

Location: within terinal 6 feet of ileum; in 94% on antimesenteric border
RULE OF 2's: (1) in 2% of population
              (2) symptomatic usually before age 2
              (3) located within 2 feet of ileocecal valve
              (4) length of 2 inches

NUC (>85% sensitivity, >95% specificity, >88% accuracy):
  N.B.:   sensitivity drops after adolescence, because patients asymptomatic throughout childhood are less likely to have ectopic gastric mucosa
  Δ Tc-99m pertechnetate is excreted by mucoid cells of gastric mucosa, excretion is not deendent on presence of parietal cells
  Preparation:
    (1) No irritative measures for 48 hours (contrast studies, endoscopy, cathartics, enemas, drugs irritating GI tract)
    (2) Fasting for 3 – 6 hours (results in decreased gastric secretion + diminished bowel peristalsis)
    (3) Evacuation of bowel + bladder prior to study
  Dose: 5 – 20 mCi (100 µCi/kg) Tc-99m pertechnetate

Radiation dose: 0.54 rad/2 mCi for thyroid;
                   0.3 rad/2 mCi for large intestine;
                   0.2 rad/2 mCi for stomach
Imaging: serial images in 5 – 10 minute-intervals for 1 hour
√ improved visualization through
  (a) pentagastrin = stimulates uptake (6 µg/kg SC 20 min prior to pertechnetate)
  (b) cimetidine = inhibits secretion (maximum 300 mg/dose IV 1 hour prior)
  (c) glucagon = decreases peristalsis (50 µg/kg IM 5 – 10 minutes prior)
√ poor visualization with use of perchlorate + atropine (= depressed uptake)
False-positive results:
  (1) Ectopic gastric mucosa in gastrogenic cyst, enteric duplication, normal small bowel, Barrett esophagus
  (2) Increased blood pool in AVM, hemangioma, hypervascular tumor, aneurysm
  (3) Duodenal ulcer, ulcerative colitis, Crohn disease, appendicitis, laxative abuse
  (4) Intussusception, intestinal obstruction, volvulus
  (5) Urinary tract obstruction,calyceal diverticulum
  (6) Anterior meningomyelocele
  (7) Poor technique
False-negative results:
  (1) Insufficient mass of ectopic gastric mucosa
  (2) Dilution of intraluminal activity (hemorrhage / hypersecretion)
Cx (in 20%):
  (1) GI bleeding secondary to ulceration
  (2) Acute diverticulitis
  (3) Intestinal obstruction secondary to intussusception / fibrous bands / volvulus (when attached to umbilicus)
  (4) Malignant tumor (rare): carcinoma, sarcoma, carcinoid
  (5) Chronic abdominal pain

MECONIUM ILEUS
= low sall bowel obstruction secondary to inspissated meconium, which impacts in distal ileum
Age: may develop in utero (in 15%)
Associated with:
  mucoviscidosis (= cystic fibrosis) with thick + sticky meconium due to deficiency of pancreatic secretions (in almost 100%)
  Δ 10 – 15% of infants with cystic fibrosis present with meconium ileus!
√ numerous dilated small bowel loops with paucity of air-fluid levels
√ "bubbly" / "frothy" appearance of intestinal contents
√ "soap bubble" / "applesauce" in RLQ
√ multiple round / oval filling defects in distal ileum
√ microcolon (unused colon)
OB-US:
  √ unusual echogenic intraluminal areas in small bowel (DDx: normal transient inspissated meconium)
  √ usually polyhydramnios

√ small bowel dilatation
Cx (in 40 – 50%): volvulus, ischemia, necrosis, perforation, meconium peritonitis, atresia
Rx: (1) Gastrografin enema (attention to fluid + ectrolyte balance)
(2) Acetylcysteine eema

MECONIUM ILEUS EQUIVALENT
DISTAL INTESTINAL OBSTRUCTION SYNDROME
= clinical condition characterized by abdominal pain + palpable mass in RLQ + partial / complete obstruction at level of terminal ileum / cecum / ascending colon in patients with cystic fibrosis
Incidence: 7 – 41% of patients with cystic fibrosis; higher prevalence in adult patients
Cause: undigested food residues, motility disturbance, dilatation of bowel leading to fecal stasis
√ bubbly granular fecal mass in RLQ
√ partial / complete small bowel obstruction
√ thickening of mucosal folds
√ cystic fibrosis of lung
Cx: intussusception, volvulus
Rx: increasing dose of pancreatic enzyme supplements, mucolytic agents orally / with enema

MECONIUM PERITONITIS
sterile chemical peritonitis secondary to perforation of bowel proximal to high-grade / complete obstruction that seals in utero due to inflammatory response
Incidence: 1:35,000 livebirths
Age: antenatal perforation after 3rd month of gestation
Cause:
(1) Atresia (secondary to ischemic event) (50%)
    (a) of small bowel (usually ileum or jejunum)
    (b) of colon (uncommon)
(2) Bowel obstruction (46%)
    (a) meconium ileus
    (b) volvulus, internal hernia
    (c) intussusception,congenital bands, Meckel diverticulum
(3) Hydrometrocolpos
Δ Meconium peritonitis due to cystic fibrosis diagnosed in utero in 8% + at birth in 15 – 40%!
Types:
(a) fibroadhesive type:
    = intense chemical reaction of peritoneum, which seals off the perforation
    √ dense mass with calcium deposits
(b) cystic type:
    = cystic cavity formed by fixation of bowel loops surrounding the perforation site, which continues to leak meconium
    √ cyst outlined by calcific rim
√ intra-abdominal calcifications (conspicuously absent in cystic fibrosis)
    √ small flecks of calcifications scattered throughout abdomen
    √ larger aggregates of calcifications along inferior surface of liver / flank / processus vaginalis / scrotum

√ obstructive roentgen signs following birth
√ microcolon = "unused colon"
OB-US:
√ polyhydramnios (64 – 71%)
√ fetal ascites (54 – 57%)
√ bowel dilatation (27 – 29%)
√ intraabdominal bright echogenic mass
√ multiple linear / clumped foci of calcifications (84%); may develop within 12 hours after perforation
√ meconium pseudocyst = well-defined hypoechoic mass surrounded by an echogenic calcified wall (= contained perforation)
DDx: (1) Intraabdominal teratoma
(2) Fetal gallstones
(3) Isolated liver calcifications
Mortality: up to 62%

MECONIUM PLUG SYNDROME
= local inspissation of meconium leading to low colonic obstruction secondary to colonic inertia (functional); not related to meconium ileus
Age: newborn infant, many of diabetic mothers
• abdominal distension
• vomiting
• failure to pass meconium

√ distended transverse + ascending colon + dilated small bowel (proximal to obstruction)
√ occasionally bubbly appearance in colon
√ presacral pseudotumor (no gas in rectum)
√ double-contrast effect = barium between meconium plug + colonic wall

Rx: water-soluble enema
DDx: Hirschsprung disease

MELANOSIS COLI
= benign brown-black discoloration of colonic mucosa
Incidence: 10% of autopsies
Cause: ? chronic anthracene cathartic usage
• asymptomatic
Prognosis: no malignant potential

MÉNÉTRIÈR DISEASE
= GIANT HYPERTROPHIC GASTRITIS
= HYPERPLASTIC GASTROPATHY caracterized by excessive mucus production and TRIAD of (1) Giant mucosal hypertrophy (2) Hypoproteinemia (3) Hypochlorhydria
Histo: hyperplasia of glandular tissue + microcyst formation, mucosal thickness up to 6 mm (normal range: 0.6 – 1.0 mm)
Age: 20 – 70 years; M:F = 2:1
Associated with benign gastric ulcer (13 – 72%)
• protein-losing enteropathy with hypoproteinemia + peripheral edema
• weight loss
• gastrointestinal bleeding
• absent / decreased acid secretion (>50%) epigastric pain vomiting

Location: throughout fundus + body, particularly
             prominent along greater curvature, antrum
             usually spared (DDx to lymphoma: usually in
             antrum)
√ markedly enlarged + tortuous gastric folds in spite of
  adequate gastric distension
√ relatively abrupt demarcation between normal +
  abnormal areas
√ marked hypersecretion (mucus)
√ preserved pliability
CT:
   √ wall thickening of proximal stomach
   √ nodular symmetric folds
DDx: lymphoma, polypoid variety of gastric carcinoma,
       acute gastritis, chronic gastritis, gastric varices

MESENTERIC / OMENTAL CYST

= lymphatic hamartoma lined by mesothelial cells with
  serous, chylous, (occasionally) hemorrhagic fluid
  contents
Location: small bowel mesentery (78%)
• asymptomatic
√ single multilocular cyst up to several cm in size
√ omental cysts may be pedunculated
CT:
   √ near-water density / soft-tissue density
   √ ± fluid levels related to fat + water components

Cx: torsion, hemorrhage, intestinal obstruction

MESENTERIC ISCHEMIA

Etiology:
   (a) arterial: atheromatous disease, embolic disease,
       dissecting aortic aneurysm, fibromuscular
       hyperplasia, vasculitis, endotoxin shock,
       hypoperfusion (shock, hypovolemia), disseminated
       intravascular coagulation, direct trauma
       — **"abdominal angina"** = intermittent mesenteric
          ischemia in severe arterial stenosis with
          inadequate collateralization provoked by food
          ingestion
       — **occlusive mesenteric infarction** = thrombosis
          at atherosclerotic site / embolus; 90% mortality
          rate
       — **nonocclusive mesenteric ischemia**
          = preexisting atherosclerosis with systemic low-
          flow state (cardiac failure / intraoperative
          hypotension)
   (b) venous: young patient, often following abdominal
       surgery
   (c) incarceration of hernia, volvulus, constriction by
       adhesive bands, intussusception

Pathophysiology: mucosa is most sensitive area to
anoxia from arterial / venous occlusion with early
ulcerations leading to formation of strictures

Consequences:
dependent on magnitude of insult, duration of process,
adequacy of collaterals

   (a) reversible ischemia
       1. Complete restitution of bowel wall secondary to
          abundant collaterals
       2. Healing with fibrosis + stricture formation
   (b) irreversible ischemia
       1. Transmural infarction with bowel perforation

• first crampy, then continuous abdominal pain with acute
  event
• gross rectal bleeding
• malabsorption with chronic vascular disease + strictures
Signs of mesenteric embolization:
   • acute abdominal pain
   • cardiac disease predisposing to embolization
   • gut emptying (vomiting / diarrhea)
   • WBC >12,000/µl with left shift (80%)
Location: (a) any segment of small bowel
             (b) distal transverse colon, splenic flexure,
                  cecum (most common)
Plain film:
   √ gasless abdomen (= fluid-filled loops from exudation)
     (21%)
   √ bowel distension to splenic flexure (= perfusion
     territory of SMA) in 43%
   √ "thumbprinting" (36%) = thickening of bowel wall +
     valvulae (edema)
   √ small bowel pseudoobstruction (most frequently in
     thrombosis)
   √ pneumatosis (= dissection of luminal gas into bowel
     wall) (28%)
   √ mesenteric + portal vein gas (14%)
   √ ascites (14%)
Barium:
   (a) Acute:
        √ "scalloping / thumbprinting" = thickening of wall +
          valvulae
        √ "picket fencing"
        √ separation + uncoiling of loops
        √ narrowed lumen
        √ circumferential ulcer
   (b) Subacute:
        √ flattening of one border
        √ pseudosacculation / pseudodiverticula on
          antimesenteric border
   (c) Chronic:
        √ 7 – 10 cm long smooth pliable strictures
        √ dilatation of gut between strictures
        √ thinned + atrophic valvulae
        Cx: obstruction
CT:
   (a) Specific findings in only 26%:
        √ pneumatosis intestinalis (22 – 57%)
        √ portal venous gas (13 – 36%) / mesenteric vein
          gas (28%)
        √ thumbprinting (26%)
   (b) Nonspecific findings
        √ focal / diffuse bowel dilatation (56 – 71%) with
          gas (43%) / fluid (29%)
        √ thickening of intestinal wall (64%)
        √ thrombosis of SMA (7%)

√ pneumoperitoneum (7%)
√ ascites (43%)
Angio:
√ occlusion / vasoconstriction / vascular beading
√ embolus lodged at major branching points distal to first 3 cm of SMA
NUC:
(a) IV / IA Tc-99m sulfur colloid / labeled leukocytes, Ga-citrate, Tc-99m pyrophosphate:
√ tracer accumulation 5 hours after onset of ischemia (more intense uptake with transmural infarcts)
(b) intraperitoneal injection of Xe-133 in saline is absorbed by intestine:
√ decreased washout with abnormal perfusion of strangulated bowel
Prognosis:
(1) Massive infarction of small + large bowel if mesenteric embolization occurs proximal to middle colic artery (= limited collateral flow)
(2) Focal segments of intestinal ischemia if mesenteric embolization occurs distal to middle colic artery (= good collateral flow)
Mortality: 80 – 92% for intestinal infarction

MESOTHELIOMA
= only primary tumor of peritoneum
Age: 55 – 66 years; M >>F
Associated with: asbestos disease

Location: pleura (67%), peritoneum (30%), pericardium (2.5%), processus vaginalis (0.5%)
√ thickening of mesentery, omentum, peritoneum, bowel wall
√ nodular masses in anterior parietal peritoneum
√ disproportionately small amount of ascites
CT:
√ nodular irregular thickening of peritoneal surfaces
√ localized masses
√ infiltrating sheets of tissue
√ foci of calcifications
√ ascites of near-water density
√ stellate configuration of neurovascular bundles
√ pleated thickening of mesenteric leaves
NUC:
√ diffuse uptake of gallium-67

METASTASES TO SMALL BOWEL
Origin: colon > stomach > breast > ovary > uterine cervix > melanoma > lung > pancreas
Spread:
(1) Intraperitoneal seeding: ovary, breast, GI tract
(2) Hematogenous dissemination with submucosal deposits: melanoma, breast, lung, Kaposi sarcoma
(3) Direct extension from adjacent neoplasm: ovary, uterus, prostate, pancreas, colon, kidney

√ fixation + tenting + transverse stretching (= across long axis) of folds secondary to mesenteric + peritoneal infiltration (most common form)

UGI:
√ single mass protruding into lumen resembling annular carcinoma
√ "bull's-eye" lesions = multiple polypoid masses with sizable ulcer craters
√ obstruction from kinking / annular constriction / large intraluminal mass
√ compression by direct extension of primary tumor / involved nodes
CT:
√ soft-tissue density nodules / masses
√ sheets of tissue causing thickening of bowel wall + mesenteric leaves
√ fixation + angulation of bowel loops (in tumors with desmoplastic response)
√ ascites

METASTASES TO STOMACH
Organ of origin: malignant melanoma, breast, lung, colon, prostate, leukemia, secondary lymphoma
• GI bleeding + anemia (40%)
• epigastric pain

√ solitary mass (50%)
√ multiple nodules (30%)
√ linitis plastica (20%): especially breast
√ multiple umbilicated nodules: melanoma

MIDGUT VOLVULUS
= torsion of entire gut around SMA due to a short mesenteric attachment of small intestine in incomplete rotation (normally 270° counterclockwise rotation); nonrotation = 90° or less; malrotation = 90 – 270°
In 20% associated with:
(1) Duodenal atresia
(2) Duodenal diaphragm
(3) Duodenal stenosis
(4) Annular pancreas

• acute symptoms in newborn (medical emergency): bile-stained vomiting (intermittent, postprandial, projectile); abdominal distension; shock
• intermittent obstructive symptoms in older child: recurring attacks of nausea, vomiting and abdominal pain

Plain film:
√ dilated air-filled duodenal bulb + paucity of gas distally
√ "double bubble sign" = air-fluid levels in stomach + duodenum
Barium studies:
√ duodenojejunal junction (ligament of Treitz) located lower than duodenal bulb + to the right of expected position
√ spiral course of midgut loops = "apple peel / corkscrew" appearance
√ duodenal fold-thickening + thumbprinting (mucosal edema + hemorrhage)
√ abnormally high position of cecum

CT:
- √ whirllike pattern of small bowel loops + adjacent mesenteric fat converging to the point of torsion (during volvulus)
- √ SMV to the left of SMA (NO volvulus)
- √ chylous mesenteric cyst (from interference with lymphatic drainage)

US:
- √ distended proximal duodenum with arrowhead-type compression over spine
- √ superior mesenteric vein to the left of SMA
- √ thick-walled bowel loops below duodenum + to the right of spine associated with peritoneal fluid

Angio:
- √ "barber pole sign" = spiraling of SMA
- √ tapering / abrupt termination of mesenteric vessels
- √ marked vasoconstriction + prolonged contrast transit time
- √ absent venous opacification / dilated tortuous superior mesenteric vein

Cx: intestinal ischemia + necrosis in distribution of SMA (bloody diarrhea, ileus, abdominal distension)

MUCOCELE OF APPENDIX

A. MUCOCELE
  = distension of appendix with sterile mucus
  Etiology:
    luminal obstruction by fecolith, foreign body, carcinoid, endometriosis, adhesions, volvulus; mucinous cystadenoma / cystadenocarcinoma of appendix (occasionally)
  Incidence: 0.07 – 0.24%
  - √ globular, smooth-walled, broad-based mass invaginating into cecum
  - √ peripheral rimlike calcifications frequent
  CT:
    - √ round sharply defined mass with homogeneous low attenuation content
  US:
    - √ ovoid, complex cystic mass with internal echoes
  Cx: pseudomyxoma peritonei

B. MYXOGLOBULOSIS
  = rare variant of mucocele of the appendix characterized by clusters of pearly white mucous balls intermixed with mucus
  - usually asymptomatic
  - may appear as acute appendicitis
  - √ multiple 1 – 10 mm small rounded annular, nonlaminated calcified spherules (PATHOGNOMONIC)
  DDx: inverted appendiceal stump, acute appendicitis, carcinoma of the cecum

NECROTIZING ENTEROCOLITIS

= NEC = ischemic bowel disease secondary to hypoxia, perinatal stress, infection (endotoxin), congenital heart disease
Incidence: most common GI emergency in premature infants

Age: develops >48 – 72 hours after birth; in 90% within first 10 days of life
Path: acute inflammation + mucosal ulceration + widespread transmural necrosis
Organism: not yet isolated; often occurs in miniepidemics within nursery
Predisposed:
    premature infant (50 – 80%), Hirschsprung disease, bowel obstruction (small bowel atresia, pyloric stenosis, meconium ileus, meconium plug syndrome)

Location: usually in terminal ileum (most commonly involved), cecum, right colon; rarely in stomach, upper bowel
- blood-streaked stools (in 50%); explosive diarrhea
- bile emesis
- mild respiratory distress
- generalized sepsis
- √ disarrayed bowel gas pattern (no longer normal array of polygons)
- √ distension of small bowel and colon (loops wider than vertebral body L1) ± air-fluid levels, commonly in RLQ (1st sign)
- √ tubular loops of bowel
- √ bowel wall thickening + "thumbprinting"
- √ persistent abnormal loop of bowel without change for >24 hours
- √ pneumatosis intestinalis (80%) in curvilinear shape (= subserosal) or bubbly / cystic (= submucosal gas collection from gas-forming organisms / dissection of intraluminal gas)
- √ "bubbly" appearance of bowel due to gas in wall / intraluminal gas / fecal matter (intraluminal contents are composed of blood, sloughed colonic mucosa, intraluminal gas, some fecal material)
- √ gas in portal venous system (frequently transient, does not imply hopeless outcome)
- √ ascites
- √ pneumoperitoneum (immediate surgery required)
- N.B.: Barium enema is contraindicated! May be used judiciously in selected cases with radiologic + clinical doubt!
- *Cx:*   (1) Inflammatory stricture after healing (BE follow-up in survivors)
            (2) Bowel perforation in 12 – 32%

PELVIC LIPOMATOSIS + FIBROLIPOMATOSIS

= nonmalignant overgrowth of adipose tissue with minimal fibrotic + inflammatory components compressing soft tissue structures within pelvis
Age: 9 – 80 years (peak 25 – 60 years); M:F = 10:1; NO racial predominance for blacks; obesity NOT contributing factor
- often incidental finding
- urinary frequency, flank pain, suprapubic tenderness
- recurrent urinary tract infections
- low back pain, fever
- √ elongation + narrowing of rectum
- √ elevation of rectosigmoid + sigmoid colon out of pelvis
- √ increase in sacrorectal space >10 mm

√ stretching of sigmoid colon
√ elongation + elevation of urinary bladder with symmetrical inverted pear shape
√ elongation of posterior urethra
√ pelvic lucency; CT confirmatory
√ medial / lateral displacement of ureters
Cx of fibrolipomatosis:
  (1) Ureteral obstruction (40% within 5 years)
  (2) IVC obstruction

PERITONEAL METASTASES
= intraabdominal spread of tumor
Origin: ovary, stomach, colon, pancreas
√ massive ascites
√ desmoplastic reaction at (a) anterior border of rectum (Blumer shelf) (b) mesenteric side of terminal ileum
CT:
  √ increased density of linear network in mesenteric fat
  √ loculated fluid collections in peritoneal cavity
  √ apparent thickening of mesenteric vessels (= fluid within leaves of mesentery)
  √ adnexal mass of cystic / soft-tissue density (= Krukenberg tumor)
  √ small nodular densities on peritoneal surface
  √ "omental cake" = thickening of greater omentum
  √ lobulated mass in pouch of Douglas

PEUTZ-JEGHERS SYNDROME
= autosomal dominant disease with incomplete penetrance characterized by intestinal polyposis + mucocutaneous pigmentation (= hamartomatosis); often spontaneous mutation
Incidence: 1:7,000 livebirths; in 50% familial, in 50% sporadic; most frequent of polyposis syndromes to involve small intestines
Age: 25 years at presentation (range 10 – 30 years)
Path: multiple small sessile / large pedunculated polyps
Histo:
  benign hamartomatous polyp with smooth muscle core arising from muscularis mucosae + extending into polyp; misplaced epithelium in submucosa, muscularis propria, subserosa frequently surrounding mucin-filled spaces
  Location: small bowel (jejunum + ileum > duodenum) > colon > stomach; esophagus spared
Associated with: carcinoma of GI tract (2 – 3%), pancreas, breast, ovary; adenoma of bronchus + bladder
• mucocutaneous pigmentation (similar to freckles) = 1 – 5 mm small elongated melanin spots on mucous membranes (lower lips, gums, palate) + facial skin (nose, cheeks, around eyes) + volar aspects of toes and fingers (100%)
• cramping abdominal pain (small bowel intussusception in 47%)
• rectal bleeding, melena (30%)
• prolapse of polyp through anus
• chronic hypochromic anemia
@ Small bowel (>95%)
  √ multiple polyps separated by wide areas of intervening flat mucosa

√ multilobulated surface of larger polyps
√ myriads of 1 – 2 mm nodules = carpet of polyps
√ intussusception usually confined to small bowel
@ Colon + rectum (30%)
  √ multiple scattered 1 – 30 mm polyps; NO carpeting
@ Stomach + duodenum (25%)
  √ diffuse involvement with multiple polyps
@ Respiratory + urinary tract

Cx: (1) Transient intussusception (pedunculated polyp)
     (2) Carcinoma of breast, pancreas (13%), reproductive organs [endometrium, malignant adenoma of cervix, ovary (in 5%), testis], GI tract (2 – 3%)
Rx: (1) Endoscopic removal of all polyps
     (2) Surgery is reserved for obstruction, severe bleeding, malignancy
Prognosis: decreased life expectancy due to development of cancer
DDx: familial adenomatous polyposis, juvenile polyposis (similar age), Cowden syndrome, Cronkhite-Canada syndrome

POSTCRICOID DEFECT
= variable defect seen commonly in the fully distended cervical esophagus; no pathologic value
Etiology: redundancy of mucosa over rich postcricoid submucosal venous plexus
Incidence: in 80% of normal adults
Location: anterior aspect of esophagus at level of cricoid cartilage
√ tumor- / weblike lesion with variable configuration during swallowing

DDx: submucosal tumor, esophageal web (persistent configuration)

POSTINFLAMMATORY POLYPOSIS
= PSEUDOPOLYPOSIS
= re-epithelialized inflammatory polyps as sequelae of mucosal ulceration
Etiology: ulcerative colitis (10 – 20%); granulomatous colitis (less frequent); schistosomiasis (endemic); amebic colitis (occasionally); toxic megacolon
Location: most common in left hemicolon, may occur in stomach / small intestine
√ sessile + frondlike appearance (often)
√ filiform polyposis = multiple wormlike projections only attached at their bases (CHARACTERISTIC)
  Pathogenesis: ulcerative undermining of strips of mucosa with re-epithelialization of denuded surfaces of tags + bowel wall
Prognosis: NO malignant potential
DDx: familial polyposis (polyps terminate in bulbous heads)

PRESBYESOPHAGUS
= defect in primary peristalsis + LES relaxation associated with aging

Incidence: 15% in 7th decade; 50% in 8th decade;
                85% in 9th decade
Associated with: hiatus hernia, reflux
• usually asymptomatic

√ impaired / no primary peristalsis
√ often repetitive nonperistaltic tertiary contractions in
   distal esophagus
√ mild / moderate esophageal dilatation
√ poor LES relaxation
DDx: diabetes, diffuse esophageal spasm, scleroderma,
        esophagitis, achalasia, benign stricture, carcinoma

PROLAPSED ANTRAL MUCOSA

= prolapse of hypertrophic + inflammatory mucosa of
  gastric antrum into duodenum resulting in pyloric
  obstruction
√ mushroom- / umbrella- / cauliflower-shaped filling defect
   at duodenal base
√ filling defect varies in size + shape
√ redundant gastric rugae can be traced from pyloric
   antrum through pyloric channel
√ gastric hyperperistalsis

PSEUDOMEMBRANOUS COLITIS

Etiologic agent: cytotoxin produced by Gram-negative
                     Clostridium difficile
Predisposed:
  (a) complication of antibiotic therapy with tetracycline,
      penicillin, ampicillin, clindamycin, lincomycin,
      amoxicillin, chloramphenicol, cephalosporins
  (b) following surgery / renal transplantation /
      irradiation; intestinal vascular insufficiency
  (c) shock, uremia
  (d) proximal to large bowel obstruction
  (e) debilitating diseases: lymphosarcoma, leukemia
Histo: pseudomembranes (exudate composed of
           leukocytes, fibrin, mucin, sloughed necrotic
           epithelium) on a partially denuded colonic
           edematous mucosa (mucosa generally intact)
• profuse watery diarrhea, abdominal cramps, tenderness
• confluent pseudomembranes seen on endoscopy
Plain film:
  √ adynamic ileus pattern = moderate gaseous
     distension of small bowel + colon
  √ edematous, distorted haustral markings
  √ transverse bands = marked thickening + distortion of
     haustra
  √ diffusely shaggy + irregular surface (confluent
     pseudomembranes)
  √ "thumbprinting" most prominent in transverse colon
BE (CONTRAINDICATED in severe cases):
  √ pseudoulcerations = barium filling clefts between
     pseudomembranes
  √ irregular ragged polypoid contour of colonic wall
  √ discrete multiple filling defects of 2 – 4 mm in size
     (DDx: polyposis, nodular form of lymphoma)
CT:
  √ irregular colonic wall with circumferential thickening
  √ homogeneous enhancement due to hyperemia

Dx: (1) Stool assay for Clostridium difficile cytotoxin
        (2) Pseudomembranes on proctosigmoidoscopy
Cx: Peritonitis
Prognosis: 15% mortality; most patients recover within 2
               weeks
Rx: discontinuation of suspected antibiotic +
        administration of vancomycin / metronidazole with
        attention to fluid and electrolyte balance

PSEUDOMYXOMA PERITONEI

= "jelly belly" = "gelatinous ascites" = slow insidious
  accumulation of large amounts of intraperitoneal
  gelatinous material secondary to peritoneal
  carcinomatosis from mucinous cystadenocarcinoma
Etiology:
  ruptured mucinous adenocarcinoma of appendix / ovary;
  rarely associated with malignancy of colon, stomach,
  uterus, pancreas, common bile duct, urachal duct,
  omphalomesenteric duct
• slowly progressive massive abdominal distension
• recurrent abdominal pain
√ thickening of peritoneal + omental surfaces
√ omental cake
√ posterior displacement of bowel loops + mesentery
√ voluminous septated / loculated pseudoascites
√ several thin-walled cystic masses of different size
   throughout abdominal cavity
√ scalloped contour of liver margins
√ annular / semicircular calcifications (rare but highly
   suggestive)
DDx: peritoneal metastases, pancreatitis with
        pseudocysts, pyogenic peritonitis, widespread
        echinococcal disease
Prognosis: 50% 5-year survival rate

RADIATION INJURY

= obliterative endarteritis with irradiation in excess of
  4,000 – 4,500 rads
Incidence: 5%; increased risk after pelvic surgery
√ radiographic changes within field of radiation only

Radiation Gastritis

Permanent radiographic findings of radiation injury
   appear 1 month to 2 years after therapy
√ gastric ulceration + deformity (pylorus)
√ enlargement + effacement of gastric folds
√ antral narrowing + rigidity (similar to linitis plastica)

Radiation Enteritis

Permanent radiographic findings of radiation injury
   appear >1 – 2 years following irradiation
Predisposed: women (cancer of cervix, endometrium,
                 ovary), patients with bladder cancer
• crampy abdominal pain (from intermittent obstruction)
• persistent diarrhea
• occult intestinal hemorrhage
Location: ileum; concomitant radiation damage to
               colon / rectum
√ irregular nodular thickening of folds with straight
   transverse course ± ulcerations

√ serrated bowel margin
√ thickened bowel wall with luminal narrowing
√ multiple strictures + partial mechanical obstruction
√ separation of adjacent bowel loops by >2 mm
√ shortening of small bowel
√ fixation + immobilization of bowel loops with similar radiographic appearance between examinations (from dense desmoplastic response to irradiation)
CT:
√ increased attenuation of mesentery
DDx: Crohn disease, lymphoma, ischemia, hemorrhage

Radiation Injury of Rectum
Manifestation of radiation colitis can occur up to 15 years following irradiation
Predisposed: 90% in women (carcinoma of cervix)
• tenesmus, diarrhea, bleeding, constipation
√ ridgelike appearance of mucosa (submucosal fibrosis)
√ irregularly outlined ulcerations (rare)
CT:
√ narrowed partially distensible rectum
√ thick homogeneous rectal wall
√ "target sign" = submucosal circumferential lucency
√ proliferation of perirectal fat >10 mm
√ thickening of perirectal fascia
√ "halo effect" = increase in pararectal fibrosis
Cx: (1) Obstruction
(2) Colovaginal / coloenteric fistula formation

RECTAL CANCER
Staging accuracy:
(1) Digital rectal examination: 68 – 83%; limited to lesions within 10 cm of anal verge
(2) CT: 66 – 92%, better for more extensive regional spread
(3) MR: 74 – 93%
(4) Transrectal ultrasound: 67 – 94%; limited to lesions <14 cm from anal verge + nonstenotic lesions

Pathologic staging of rectal cancer:			
Astler-Coller	TNM	Description	5-year survival
A	$T_1N_0M_0$	limited to submucosa	80%
B1	$T_2N_0M_0$	limited to muscularis	70%
B2	$T_3N_0M_0$	transmural extension	60–65%
C1	$T_2N_1M_0$	nodes (+), into muscularis	35–45%
C2	$T_3N_1M_0$	nodes (+), transmural	25%
D	M_1	distant metastasis	<25%

Transrectal US:
Normal layers: (a) hyperechoic interface of balloon + mucosa (b) hypoechoic mucosa + muscularis mucosa (c) hyperechoic submucosa (d) hypoechoic muscularis propria (e) hyperechoic serosa
√ hypoechoic mass disrupting rectal wall
√ no interruption of hyperechoic submucosa = tumor confined to mucosa + submucosa
√ no interruption of hyperechoic serosa = tumor confined to rectal wall
√ break in outermost hyperechoic layer = tumor penetrates into perirectal fat
√ hypoechoic perirectal lymph nodes (= tumor involvement)

RETAINED GASTRIC ANTRUM
Cause: retention of endocrinologically active gastric antrum in continuity with pylorus + duodenum
Pathophysiology:
bathing of antrum in alkaline duodenal juice stimulates secretion of gastrin
Associated with gastric ulcers in 30 – 50%

√ duodenogastric reflux of barium through pylorus (diagnostic)
√ giant marginal ulcer / several marginal ulcers usually on jejunal side of anastomosis (large false-negative + false-positive rate; correct positive rate of 28 – 60%)
√ large amount of secretions
√ edematous mucosa of jejunal anastomotic segment
√ lacy / cobweblike small bowel pattern (hypersecretion)
Cx: gastrojejunocolic fistula

RETRACTILE MESENTERITIS
= CHRONIC FIBROSING MESENTERITIS = CHRONIC SUBPERITONEAL SCLEROSIS = MESENTERIC PANNICULITIS = LIPOSCLEROTIC MESENTERITIS = MESENTERIC LIPODYSTROPHY = MESENTERIC WEBER-CHRISTIAN DISEASE
= rare disorder of unknown etiology characterized by fibro-fatty thickening of small bowel mesentery

Etiology: ? trauma, previous surgery, ischemia
Path: spectrum ranging from mesenteric lipodystrophy through mesenteric panniculitis to mesenteric fibrosis
Histo: chronic inflammation with a dense collection of lymphocytes + plasma cells + lipid-laden macrophages; desmoplastic reaction; fat necrosis; calcifications
Associated with:
(1) Gardner syndrome, familial polyposis
(2) Fibrosing mediastinitis, retroperitoneal fibrosis
(3) Lymphoma, lymphosarcoma
(4) Carcinoid tumor
(5) Metastatic gastric / colonic carcinoma
(6) Whipple lipodystrophy
(7) Weber-Christian disease
Age: most common in 6th decade; M:F = 2:1
• crampy abdominal pain
• nausea + vomiting; mild weight loss
• low-grade fever

Location: root of mesentery extending toward mesenteric border of bowel
Plain film:
√ soft tissue mass with calcifications
√ ± thumbprinting (from vascular congestion)

UGI:
- √ compression / distortion of duodenum near ligament of Treitz
- √ separation of small bowel loops with fixation, kinking + angulation

CT:
- √ mass of fat density interspersed with soft tissue density (fibrous tissue) + calcifications
- √ mesenteric thickening with fine stellate pattern extending to bowel border
- √ retraction of small bowel loops
- √ single mesenteric soft tissue mass (fibroma)
- √ multiple nodules throughout mesentery (fibromatosis)

Prognosis: usually benign course

DDx: metastatic gastric / colonic adenocarcinoma; carcinoid tumor; mesenteric lymphoma; liposarcoma of mesentery

SCHATZKI RING

= LOWER ESOPHAGEAL MUCOSAL RING = constant lower esophageal ring (mucosal thickening) presumed to result from reflux esophagitis = thin annular peptic stricture

Incidence: 6 – 14% of population; old age > young age; M > F

Histo: usually squamous epithelium on upper surface + columnar epithelium on undersurface; may be covered totally by squamous epithelium or columnar epithelium

- asymptomatic (if ring >20 mm)
- dysphagia (if ring <12 mm)

Location: near the squamo-columnar junction; in region of B ring at inferior margin of lower esophageal sphincter

- √ permanently present nondistensible transverse ring with constant shape + size (range of 3 – 18 mm)
- √ 2 – 4 mm thick shelflike projection into lumen with smooth symmetric margins
- √ visible only with adequate distension of esophagogastric region and when located above the esophageal hiatus of the diaphragm
- √ best demonstrated in prone position during arrested deep inspiration with Valsalva maneuver while barium column passes through esophagogastric region
- √ short esophagus + intrahiatal / intrathoracic gastric segment = sliding hiatal hernia if Schatzki ring located 1 – 2 cm above diaphragmatic hiatus

Prognosis: decrease in caliber over 5 years (in 25 – 33%)

Cx: impaction of food bolus (associated with severe chest pain)

Rx: (1) Proper mastication of food
         (2) Endoscopic rupture
         (3) Esophageal dilatation (radiographically often lack of caliber change after successful dilatation)

DDx: annular peptic stricture (usually thicker, asymmetric, irregular surface, associated with thickened esophageal folds, serration of esophageal margins)

SCLERODERMA

= PROGRESSIVE SYSTEMIC SCLEROSIS = PSS

Age: 30 – 50 years; M:F = 1:3

Histo: vasculitis + submucosal fibrosis extending into muscularis, smooth muscle atrophy

- skin changes, Raynaud phenomenon, arthritis
- abdominal pain, diarrhea, occasional malabsorption
- multiple episodes of pseudoobstruction

Intestinal involvement in 40 – 45% (may precede other manifestations)

@ Esophagus (in 42 – 95%)
- Δ First GI tract location to be involved!
- dysphagia (50%)
- heartburn (30%)
- √ normal peristalsis above aortic arch (striated muscle in proximal 1/3 of esophagus)
- √ hypotonia / atony + hypokinesia in distal 2/3 of esophagus
- √ deficient emptying in recumbent position
- √ thin / vanished longitudinal folds
- √ mild to moderate dilatation of esophagus
- √ chalasia (= patulous lower esophageal sphincter)
- √ gastroesophageal reflux (70%)
- √ erosions + superficial ulcers (from asymptomatic reflux esophagitis: NO protective esophageal contraction)
- √ fusiform stricture usually 4 – 5 cm above gastroesophageal junction (from reflux esophagitis)
- √ esophageal shortening + sliding hiatal hernia

Cx: peptic stricture, Barrett esophagus, adenocarcinoma

@ Stomach (less frequent involvement)
- √ gastric dilatation
- √ decreased motor activity + delayed emptying

@ Small bowel (up to 45%)
- rapidly progressing disease once small intestine is involved
- malabsorption (delayed intestinal transit time + bacterial overgrowth)
- √ marked dilatation of small bowel (in particular duodenum = megaduodenum, jejunum) simulating small bowel obstruction
  CAVE: misdiagnosis of obstruction may lead to exploratory surgery!
- √ abrupt cutoff at SMA level (atrophy of neural cells with hypoperistalsis)
- √ prolonged transit time with barium retention in duodenum up to 24 hours
- √ "hidebound / accordion" pattern (60%) = sharply defined folds of normal thickness with decreased intervalvular distance (tightly packed folds) within dilated segment (due to predominant involvement of circular muscle)
- √ pseudodiverticula (10 – 40%) = asymmetric sacculations with squared tops + broad bases on mesenteric side (due to eccentric smooth muscle atrophy)
- √ pneumatosis cystoides intestinalis + pneumoperitoneum (occasionally)

√ excess fluid with bacterial overgrowth (="pseudo-blind loop syndrome")
√ normal mucosal fold pattern
Cx: intussusception without anatomic lead point
@ Colon (up to 40 – 50%)
- constipation (common), may alternate with diarrhea
√ pseudosacculations + wide-mouthed "diverticula" on antimesenteric side (formed by repetitive bulging through atrophic areas) in transverse + descending colon
√ eventually complete loss of haustrations (simulating cathartic colon)
√ marked dilatation (may simulate Hirschsprung disease)
√ stercoral ulceration (from retained fecal material)
Cx: life-threatening barium impaction
@ Chest
√ bibasilar interstitial fibrosis
@ Bones
√ acroosteolysis (Raynaud phenomenon)
√ soft tissue calcifications

DDx:
(1) Dermatomyositis (similar radiographic findings)
(2) Sprue (increased secretions, segmentation, fragmentation, dilatation most significant in midjejunum, normal motility)
(3) Obstruction (no esophageal changes, no pseudodiverticula)
(4) Idiopathic intestinal pseudoobstruction (usually in young people)

SOLITARY RECTAL ULCER SYNDROME
= benign condition with misleading name
Cause:
? congenital malformation of colonic mucosal glands, inflammation as a result of rectal infection, mucosal ischemia, ergotamine tartrate therapy, prolapse of anterior rectal wall with traumatization of rectal mucosa by anal sphincter during defecation
Path:
small / large, single / multiple shallow ulcers; 25% broad-based, 18% patchy granular / velvety hyperemic mucosa; rectal stenosis through confluent circumferential lesion
Histo:
obliteration of lamina propria by fibromuscular proliferation of muscularis mucosae, streaming of fibroblasts + muscle fibers between crypts, misplaced mucosal glands deep to muscularis mucosae; diffuse increase in mucosal collagen

- chronic rectal bleeding
- passage of mucus
- disordered defecation
- tenesmus
BE:
√ ulcer
√ polypoid lesion / nodules
√ stricture

Evacuation proctography:
√ failure of anorectal angle to open while straining
√ excessive perineal descent

Prognosis:
(1) Little change over time
(2) Considerable change in appearance of lesion
(3) Transfusions necessitated by massive blood loss

SPRUE
= classic disease of malabsorption
Path: villous atrophy (truncation) + elongation of crypts of Lieberkühn + round cell infiltration of lamina propria (plasma cells + lymphocytes)

A. TROPICAL SPRUE
Etiology: infectious agent cured with antibiotics; geographic distribution (India, Far East, Puerto Rico)
Age: any age group
- glossitis
- hepatosplenomegaly
- macrocytic anemia + leukopenia
Prognosis: spontaneous resolution after months / years
Rx: responds well to folic acid + broad-spectrum antibiotics

B. NONTROPICAL SPRUE
= CELIAC DISEASE = GLUTEN-SENSITIVE ENTEROPATHY
= characterized by malabsorption resulting from atrophy of small intestinal villi
May be hereditary: detected in 15% of 1st degree relatives
Age: childhood and 30 – 40 years
Rx: gluten-free diet

- diarrhea, steatorrhea (CLASSIC but found only in minority of patients)
- crampy abdominal pain (from intussusception)
- lassitude, weight loss
- stomatitis, anemia (iron / folate / vitamin B_{12} deficiency)• neuropathy, depression
- infertility
- osteomalacia with bone pain
Location: duodenum + jejunum > remainder of small bowel
Small bowel follow-through:
√ small bowel dilatation is HALLMARK in untreated celiac disease (70 – 95%), best seen in mid + distal jejunum (due to intestinal hypomotility); degree of dilatation related to severity of disease
√ hypersecretion-related artifacts:
√ air-fluid levels in small bowel (rare)
√ segmentation = breakup of normal continual column of barium creating large masses of barium in dilated segments separated by stringlike strands from adjacent clumps due to excessive fluid; best seen on delayed films

√ flocculation = coarse granular appearance of small clumps of disintegrated barium due to excess fluid best seen at periphery of intestinal segment; occurs especially with steatorrhea

√ fragmentation = scattering = faint irregular stippling of residual barium resembling snowflakes associated with segmentation due to excessive fluid

√ "moulage sign" (50%) = smooth contour with effaced featureless folds resembling tubular wax mold (due to atrophy of the folds of Kerckring); CHARACTERISTIC of sprue if seen in duodenum + jejunum

√ "jejunization" of ileal loops (= adaptive response to decreased jejunal mucosal surface) = SPECIFIC

√ long / normal / short transit time

√ nonpropulsive peristalsis (flaccid + poorly contracting loops)

√ normal / thickened / effaced mucosal folds (depending on hypoproteinemia)

√ colonlike haustrations in well-filled jejunum (secondary to spasm + cicatrization from transverse ulcers)

√ transient nonobstructive intussusception (20%) without anatomic lead point

√ "bubbly bulb" = peptic duodenitis = mucosal inflammation, gastric metaplasia, Brunner gland hyperplasia

Enteroclysis:
√ decreased number of folds in proximal jejunum (≤3 folds per inch)

√ increased number of folds in distal ileum (>5 folds per inch)

√ tubular featureless lumen

√ mosaic pattern = 1 – 2 mm polygonal islands of mucosa surrounded by barium-filled distinct grooves (10%)

CT:
√ small bowel dilatation + increased fluid content ± mucosal fold thickening

√ mild to moderate lymphadenopathy in mesentery / retroperitoneum (up to 12%)

Cx:
(1) Ulcerative jejunoileitis
= multiple chronic benign ulcers (sausage appearance of small bowel) with hemorrhage, perforation + obstruction
Age: 5th – 6th decade
Location: jejunum > ileum > colon
Prognosis: frequently fatal
Rx: small bowel resection
(2) Hyposplenism (30 – 50%)
√ small atrophic spleen
(3) Cavitary mesenteric lymph node syndrome characterized by:
(a) mesenteric lymph node cavitation
(b) splenic atrophy
(c) villous atrophy of small intestinal mucosa
√ enlarged lymph nodes of low attenuation ± fat-fluid levels (filled with lipid-rich hyaline material) within jejunoileal mesentery
Prognosis: usually fatal disorder

(4) Malignant tumors
(a) lymphoma (in 8%): commonly diffuse + nodular
√ enlarged nodular folds, ulcers, extrinsic mass effect
(b) adenocarcinoma of small bowel (6%)
(c) squamous cell carcinoma of pharynx / esophagus (in 6%) during 6th – 7th decade
(5) Generalized lymphadenopathy with lymphocytosis (mimicking lymphoma)
(6) Sigmoid volvulus (rare)

Dx: (1) Jejunal / duodenal biopsy
(2) Improvement of small bowel abnormalities after a few months on a gluten-free diet
Cause for relapse:
hidden dietary gluten, diabetes, bacterial overgrowth, intestinal ulceration, development of lymphoma

DDx:
(1) Esophageal hypoperistalsis: scleroderma, idiopathic pseudoobstruction
(2) Gastric abnormalities: Zollinger-Ellison syndrome, chronic granulomatous disease, eosinophilic enteritis, amyloidosis, malignancy
(3) Tiny nodular defects on thickened folds: Whipple disease, intestinal lymphangiectasia, Waldenström macroglobulinemia
(4) Small 1 – 3 mm nodules: lymphoid hyperplasia associated with giardiasis and immunoglobulin deficiency disease, diffuse lymphoma
(5) Small nodules of varying sizes: systemic mastocytosis, amyloidosis, eosinophilic enteritis, Cronkhite-Canada syndrome
(6) Bowel wall narrowing, kinking, scarring, ulceration: regional enteritis, bacterial / parasitic infection, carcinoid, vasculitis, ischemia, irradiation

STRONGYLOIDIASIS
= parasitic infection in tropics + subtropics
Organism: helminthic parasite Strongyloides stercoralis
Cycle: enters body through skin, passes through lung, settles in duodenum + upper jejunum
Path: edema + inflammation of intestinal wall secondary to invasion by larvae; flattening of villi; ova in mucosal crypts
• asymptomatic (in majority)
• pneumonitis
• severe malnutrition (malabsorption, steatorrhea)
• persistent vomiting
• worms, larvae, eggs in stool

√ paralytic ileus (massive invasion)
√ edematous folds, spasm, dilatation of proximal 2/3 of duodenum
√ ulceration
√ stenosis in 3rd + 4th part of duodenum
√ rigid pipe stem appearance + irregular narrowing of duodenum (in advanced cases)
Prognosis: high mortality in undernourished patients

SUPERIOR MESENTERIC ARTERY SYNDROME
= VASCULAR COMPRESSION OF DUODENUM
= WILKIE SYNDROME = CHRONIC DUODENAL ILEUS
= BODY CAST SYNDROME
= vascular compression of 3rd portion of duodenum within aortomesenteric compartment; probably representing a functional reflex dilatation
Etiology:
narrowing of angle between SMA + aorta to 10 – 22° (normal 45 – 65°):
congenital, weight loss, visceroptosis due to loss of abdominal muscle tone (as in pregnancy), asthenic built, exaggerated lumbar lordosis, prolonged bed rest in supine position (body cast, whole-body burns, surgery)
- repetitive vomiting
- abdominal cramping

√ megaduodenum = pronounced dilatation of 1st + 2nd portion of duodenum + frequently stomach, best seen in supine position
√ vertical linear compression defect in transverse portion of duodenum overlying spine
√ abrupt change in caliber distal to compression defect
√ relief of compression by postural change into prone knee-elbow position

TERTIARY ESOPHAGEAL CONTRACTIONS
= disordered up-and-down movement of bolus
Cause:
1. Presbyesophagus
2. Diffuse esophageal spasm
3. Hyperactive achalasia
4. Neuromuscular disease:
   diabetes mellitus, Parkinsonism, amyotrophic lateral sclerosis, multiple sclerosis, thyrotoxic myopathy, myotonic dystrophy
5. Obstruction of cardia:
   neoplasm, distal esophageal stricture, benign lesion, S/P repair of hiatal hernia
Age: in 5 – 10% of normal adults during 4th – 6th decade
Location: in lower 2/3 of esophagus
√ spontaneous repetitive nonpropulsive contraction
√ "yo-yo" motion of barium
√ "corkscrew" appearance = scalloped configuration of barium column
√ "rosary bead" / "shish kebab" configuration = compartmentalization of barium column
√ no lumen-obliterating contractions

TOXIC MEGACOLON
= acute transmural fulminant colitis with neurogenic loss of motor tone + rapid development of extensive colonic dilatation >5.5 cm in transverse colon (damage to entire colonic wall + neuromuscular degeneration)
Etiology:
1. Ulcerative colitis (most common)
2. Crohn disease
3. Amebiasis, salmonellosis
4. Pseudomembranous colitis
5. Ischemic colitis

Histo: widespread sloughing of mucosa + thinning of frequently necrotic muscle layers
- systemic toxicity
- profuse bloody diarrhea

√ colonic ileus with marked dilatation of transverse colon
√ few air-fluid levels
√ increasing caliber of colon on serial radiographs without redundancy
√ loss of normal colonic haustra + interhaustral folds
√ coarsely irregular mucosal surface
√ pseudopolyposis = mucosal islands in denuded ulcerated colonic wall
√ pneumatosis coli ± pneumoperitoneum
CT:
  √ distended colon filled with large amounts of fluid + air
  √ distorted haustral pattern
  √ irregular nodular contour of thin wall
  √ intramural air / small collections
BE: CONTRAINDICATED due to risk of perforation
Prognosis: 20% mortality

TUBERCULOSIS
Rarely encountered in Western hemisphere, increased incidence in AIDS; usually associated with pulmonary tuberculosis (in 6 – 38%)
Etiology:
(1) Ingestion of tuberculous sputum
(2) Hematogenous spread from tuberculous focus in lung to submucosal lymph nodes, associated with radiographic evidence of pulmonary TB in <50%
(3) Primary infection by cow milk (Mycobacterium bovis)
Path:
(a) ulcerative form (most frequent): ulcers with their long axis perpendicular to axis of intestine, undermining + pseudopolyps
(b) hypertrophic form: thickening of bowel wall (transmural granulomatous process)
Organisms: M. tuberculosis, M. bovis, M. avium-intracellulare
Age: 20 – 40 years
- weight loss, abdominal pain (80 – 90%)
- nausea, vomiting
- tuberculin skin test negative in most patients with primary intestinal TB

Location: ileocecal area > ascending colon > jejunum > appendix > duodenum > stomach > sigmoid > rectum
@ Tuberculous peritonitis (in 1/3)
  Δ Most common presentation
  Cause: hematogenous spread / rupture of mesenteric node
  (a) wet type = exudative ascites with high protein contents + leukocytes
  (b) dry type = caseous adenopathy + adhesions
  (c) fibrotic type = omental cakelike mass with separation + fixation of bowel loops

CT:
- √ high-density ascites (20 – 45 HU)
- √ enlarged lymph nodes (90%) with low-density centers in 40% (due to caseous necrosis)
  Location: peripancreatic + mesentery, retroperitoneum
- √ irregular masses of soft-tissue density in omentum + mesentery (common)
Cx: small bowel obstruction (adhesions from serosal tubercles)

@ Ileocecal area (80 – 90%)
  Δ Most commonly affected bowel
  Cause: relative stagnation of intestinal contents + abundance of lymphoid tissue (Peyer patches)
- √ Stierlin sign = rapid emptying of narrowed terminal ileum (due to persistent irritability) on BE
- √ thickened ileocecal valve (mass effect)
- √ Fleischner sign = "inverted umbrella" defect = wide gap of patulous ileocecal valve + narrowed rigid cecum
- √ deep fissures + ulcers with sinus tracts / enterocutaneous fistulas / perforation
  DDx: Crohn disease, cecal carcinoma

@ Colon
  Site: segmental colonic involvement, esp. on right side
- √ rigid contracted cone-shaped cecum (spasm / transmural fibrosis)
- √ spiculations + wall thickening
- √ diffuse ulcerating colitis + pseudopolyps
- √ shortening + short hourglass strictures
  DDx: ulcerative colitis, Crohn disease, amebiasis (spares terminal ileum), colitis of bacillary dysentery, ischemic colitis, pseudomembranous colitis

@ Gastroduodenal
  Site: simultaneous involvement of pylorus + duodenum
- √ stenotic pylorus with gastric outlet obstruction
- √ narrowed antrum (linitis plastica appearance)
- √ antral fistula
- √ multiple large and deep ulcerations on lesser curvature
- √ thickened duodenal folds with irregular contour / dilatation
  DDx: carcinoma, lymphoma, syphilis

@ Esophagus
  Least common GI tract manifestation
- √ ulceration
- √ stricture
- √ mass
- √ sinus tract formation

TURCOT SYNDROME
= autosomal recessive disease with
  (a) colonic polyposis
  (b) CNS tumors (especially supratentorial glioblastoma, occasionally medulloblastoma)
Age: symptomatic during 2nd decade

Histo: adenomatous polyps
- diarrhea
- seizures
- √ multiple 1 – 30 mm polyps in colon + rectum
Cx: malignant transformation of colonic polyps in 100%
Prognosis: death from brain tumor in 2nd + 3rd decade

TYPHLITIS
= transmural necrotizing inflammatory process of cecum in neutropenic patients; typhlos = cecum
Histo: edema + ulceration of entire bowel wall; necrosis + perforation possible
Organisms: Pseudomonas, Candida, CMV, Klebsiella, E. coli, B. fragilis, Enterobacter
Predisposed: common in childhood leukemia, aplastic anemia, lymphoma, immunosuppressive therapy (eg, renal transplant), AIDS
Location: cecum + ascending colon, appendix + distal ileum may become secondarily involved
- abdominal pain, may be localized to RLQ
- watery diarrhea
- fullness / palpable mass in RLQ
- fever, neutropenia
- hematochezia / occult blood

- √ fluid-filled masslike density in RLQ
- √ distension of nearby small bowel loops
- √ thumbprinting of ascending colon
- √ circumferential thickening of cecal wall >4 mm
- √ occasionally pneumatosis
CT:
- √ circumferential cecal wall thickening (>1 – 3 mm)
- √ may have intramural pneumatosis
- √ pericolonic inflammation

Cx: (1) Perforation (BE is a risky procedure)
      (2) Abscess formation
DDx: (1) Leukemic / lymphomatous deposits (more eccentric thickening)
      (2) Appendicitis with periappendicular abscess (normal cecal wall thickness)
      (3) Diverticulitis
      (4) Inflammatory bowel disease

ULCERATIVE COLITIS
= common idiopathic inflammatory bowel disease with continuous concentric + symmetric colonic involvement
Etiology: ? hypersensitivity / autoimmune disease
Path: predominantly mucosal disease with exudate + edema + crypt abscesses (HALLMARK) resulting in shallow ulceration
Age peak: 20 – 40 years + 60 – 70 years; M:F = 1:1
- alternating periods of remission + exacerbation
- bloody diarrhea
- electrolyte depletion, fever, systemic toxicity
- abdominal cramps
Extracolonic manifestations:
  - iritis, erythema nodosum, pyoderma gangrenosum
  - pericholangitis, chronic active hepatitis, primary sclerosing cholangitis, fatty liver

- spondylitis, peripheral arthritis, coincidental rheumatoid arthritis (10 – 20%)
- thrombotic complications

Location: begins in rectum with proximal progression (rectum spared in 4%)
(a) rectosigmoid in 95% (diagnosed by rectal biopsy); continuous circumferential involvement often limited to left side of colon
(b) terminal ileum in 10 – 25% ("backwash ileitis")

Plain film:
√ hyperplastic mucosa, polypoid mucosa, deep ulcers
√ diffuse dilatation with loss of haustral markings
√ toxic megacolon
√ free intraperitoneal gas
√ complete absence of fecal residue (due to inflammation)

BE:
(a) acute stage
√ narrowing + incomplete filling (spasm + irritability)
√ fine mucosal granularity = stippling of barium coat (from diffuse mucosal edema + hyperemia + superficial erosions)
√ spicules + serrated bowel margins (tiny superficial ulcers)
√ "collar button" ulcers (= undermining of ulcers)
√ "double-tracking" = longitudinal submucosal ulceration over several cm
√ hazy / fuzzy quality of bowel contour (excessive secretions)
√ "thumbprinting" = symmetric thickening of colonic folds
√ pseudopolyps = scattered islands of edematous mucosa + reepithelialized granulation tissue within areas of denuded mucosa
√ widening of presacral space
√ obliterated rectal folds = valves of Houston (43%)
(b) subacute stage
√ distorted irregular haustra
√ inflammatory polyps = sessile frondlike / rarely pedunculated lesions (= localized mucosal inflammation resulting in polypoid protuberance)
√ coarse granular mucosa (= mucosal replacement by granulation tissue)
(c) chronic stage
√ shortening of colon (= reversible spasm of longitudinal muscle) with depression of flexures
√ "leadpipe" colon = rigidity + symmetric narrowing of lumen
√ widening of haustral clefts / complete loss of haustrations (DDx: cathartic colon)
√ "burnt-out colon" = fairly distensible colon without haustral markings + without mucosal pattern
√ hazy / fuzzy quality of bowel contour (excessive secretions)
√ postinflammatory polyps (12 – 19%) = small sessile nodules / long wormlike branching + bridging outgrowths (= filiform polyposis)

√ "backwash ileitis" (5 – 30%) involving 4 – 25 cm of terminal ileum with patulous ileocecal valve + absent peristalsis + granularity
CT:
√ wall thickening <10 mm

Cx:
(1) Toxic megacolon ± perforation in 5 – 10% (DDx: granulomatous / ischemic / amebic colitis)
Δ Most common cause of death in ulcerative colitis!
(2) Colonic adenocarcinoma (3 – 5%):
25 x increased risk after 7 – 8 years; higher incidence of multiple carcinomas particularly with pancolitis + onset of disease in childhood
Location: distal transverse colon, descending colon, rectum
√ narrowed segment of 2 – 6 cm in length with eccentric lumen + irregular contour + flattened rigid tapered margins = scirrhous carcinoma
√ annular / polypoid carcinoma
(3) Colonic strictures (10%)
smooth contour with fusiform pliable tapering margins, usually short + single stricture; commonly in sigmoid / rectum / transverse colon; usually after minimum of 5 years of disease; rarely cause for obstruction (DDx: colonic carcinoma)

DDx: (1) Familial polyposis (no inflammatory changes)
(2) Cathartic colon (more extensive in right colon)

DDx between CROHN DISEASE and ULCERATIVE COLITIS
mnemonic: "LUCIFER M"

	Crohn Disease	Ulcerative Colitis
Location	right side	left side
Ulcers	deep	shallow
Contraction	no	yes
Ileocecal valve	thickened	gaping
Fistulae	yes	no
Eccentricity	yes	no
Rate of carcinoma	slight increase	marked increase
Megacolon	unusual	yes

VILLOUS ADENOMA
Villous Adenoma of Colon
Incidence: 7% of all colonic tumors
Age: presentation late in life; M = F
Location: rectum + sigmoid (75%), cecum, ileocecal valve; 2% of all tumors in rectum + colon
Associated with: other GI tumors (25%)
- sensation of incomplete evacuation
- rectal bleeding
- excretion of copious amounts of thick mucus
- fatiguability, weakness
- electrolyte depletion syndrome in 4% (dehydration, hyponatremia, hypokalemia)
√ may completely encircle the colon

√ bulky tumor with spongelike corrugated appearance (arium within interstices)

√ striated "brushlike" surface

√ soft pliable tumor with change in shape

√ innumerable mucosal projections (= fronds) with reticular / granular surface pattern (if villous elements constitute >75% of tumor, diagnosis can be made on BE)

√ apparent decrease in size on postevacuation films

Cx: malignant transformation / invasion (in 36%) related to size of tumor <5 cm (9%); >5 cm (55%); >10 cm (100%)

Villous Adenoma of Duodenum

More common in colon + rectum; fewer than 50 cases in world literature

√ sessile, soft nonobstructive mass

√ "lace" / "soap bubble" pattern

√ preservation of peristaltic activity + bowel distensibility

WALDENSTRÖM MACROGLOBULINEMIA

= malignant neoplasm of plasma cells with production of abnormal IgM proteins

Histo: macroglobulin proteinaceous hyaline material fills lacteals in lamina propria of small bowel villi with secondary lymphatic distension + edema

Age: late-life onset

• lymphadenopathy

• hepatosplenomegaly

• diarrhea, steatorrhea, malabsorption

• anemia, bleeding diathesis

• IgM elevation

• hyperviscosity

@   Small bowel (rarely involved)

√ small bowel dilatation

√ uniform diffuse thickening of valvulae conniventes with spike-like configuration (jejunum + proximal ileum)

√ granular surface of punctate filling defects (distended villi)

Dx: characteristic M-spike in serum electrophoresis

WHIPPLE DISEASE

= INTESTINAL LIPODYSTROPHY

= chronic multisystem disease thought to be caused by infection with an as yet unidentified bacterium

Path:

PAS-positive material (periodic acid Schiff) = glyco-protein within foamy macrophages in the submucosa of the jejunum (bacterial cell wall) + fat deposits within intestinal submucosa and lymph nodes causing lymphatic obstruction + dilatation

Age: 40 – 49; M:F = 9:1; Caucasians

• recurrent and migratory arthralgias / nondeforming arthritis (65 – 95%); arthritis may precede Whipple disease in 10% up to 10 years

• malabsorption, steatorrhea, abdominal pain

• weight loss, fever

• polyserositis

• generalized lymphadenopathy

• skin pigmentation similar to Addison disease

Organ involvement: virtually every organ system, small bowel, joints, heart, CNS, eyes, skin

√ moderate thickening of jejunal + duodenal folds (from mucosal + submucosal infiltration by PAS-positive macrophages combined with lymphatic obstruction)

√ micronodularity (= swollen villi) and wild mucosal pattern

√ hypersecretion, segmentation, fragmentation (occasionally if accompanied by hyperproteinemia)

√ NO / minimal dilatation of small bowel

√ NO rigidity of folds

√ NO ulcerations

√ normal transit time (approximately 3 hours)

√ hepatosplenomegaly

CT:

√ bulky 3 – 4 cm large low-density lymph nodes in mesenteric root + retroperitoneum (due to extracellular neutral fat + fatty acids)

√ thickening of bowel wall

√ splenomegaly

√ ascites

√ pleuropericarditis

√ sacroiliitis

Dx: jejunal biopsy, abdominal / peripheral lymph node biopsy

Rx: long-term broad-spectrum antibiotics (tetracycline)

DDx: (1)   Sprue (marked dilatation, no fold thickening, pronounced segmentation + fragmentation)

(2)   Intestinal lymphangiectasia (thickened folds throughout small bowel)

(3)   Amyloidosis

(4)   Lymphoma

PSEUDO-WHIPPLE DISEASE IN AIDS

similar clinical picture caused by Mycobacterium avium intracellulare

√ wall + fold thickening of small bowel loops

√ mesenteric lymphadenopathy

ZENKER DIVERTICULUM

= posterior hypopharyngeal pouch = pharyngoesophageal diverticulum = pulsion diverticulum with herniation of mucosa + submucosa through oblique + transverse muscle bundles (pseudodiverticulum) of the cricopharyngeal muscle

Etiology: cricopharyngeal dysfunction (cricopharyngeal achalasia / premature closure) results in increased intraluminal pressure

• compressible neck mass

• dysphagia, regurgitation of food

• foul breath

Location: at pharyngoesophageal junction in midline of Killian dehiscence / triangle of Laimer, at level of C5/6

√ posterior barium extension in upper half of semilunar depression on the posterior wall of esophagus (cricopharyngeal muscle)

√ barium-filled sac extending caudally behind + usually to left of esophagus

√ partial obstruction of esophagus from external pressure of sac contents

√ partial barium reflux from diverticulum into hypopharynx

ZOLLINGER-ELLISON SYNDROME

= peptic ulcer diathesis associated with marked hypersecretion of gastric acid + gastrin-producing non-β islet cell tumor of pancreas

Causes:

A. GASTRINOMA (90%) = non-β islet cell tumor with continuous gastrin production

Location: 87% in pancreas, 13% in medial wall of duodenum (gastrinoma triangle), stomach, jejunum, spleen, retroperitoneum, ovary

60% malignant, 40% benign, solitary in 50%

Associated with MEN-Type I (in 10 – 40%)

Sensitivity of preoperative localization:

25% for US, 35% for CT, 20% for MRI, 68% for selective angiography, 63% for portal venous sampling

B. PSEUDO Z-E SYNDROME = COWLEY SYNDROME = antral G-cell hyperplasia (10%) (increase in number of G-cells in gastric antrum)

• lack of gastrin elevation after secretin injection

• exaggerated gastrin elevation after protein meal

Age: middle age; M>F

• Clinical tetrad:

(1) Gastric hypersecretion: refractory response to histamine stimulation test concerning HCl concentration; increased basal secretion (>60% of augmented secretion is diagnostic)

(2) Hypergastrinemia >180 pg/ml

(3) Hyperacidity with basal acid output >15 mEq/h

(4) Diarrhea (30%), steatorrhea (40%): may be sole complaint in 10%, frequently nocturnal; secondary to inactivation of pancreatic enzymes by large volumes of HCl

• severe intractable pain (90%)

• ulcer perforation (30%)

√ ulcers (atypical location + course should suggest diagnosis):

Location: duodenal bulb (65%) + stomach (20%), near ligament of Treitz (25%), duodenal C-loop (5%), distal esophagus (5%)

Multiplicity: solitary ulcer (90%), multiple ulcers (10%)

√ recurrent / intractable ulcers

√ marginal ulcers in postgastrectomy patient

(a) on gastric side of anastomosis

(b) on mesenteric border of efferent loop

√ prominence of area gastricae (hyperplasia of parietal cell mass)

√ enlargement of rugal folds

√ sluggish gastric peristalsis (? hypokalemia)

√ "wet stomach" = dilution of barium by excess secretions in nondilated nonobstructed stomach

√ gastroesophageal reflux (common) + esophagitis

√ dilatation of duodenum + upper small bowel (fluid overload)

√ thickened folds in duodenum + jejunum (edema)

√ rapid small-bowel transit time

mnemonic: "FUSED"

Folds (thickened, gastric folds)

Ulcers (often multiple, postbulbar)

Secretions increased (refractory to histamine)

Edema (of proximal small bowel)

Diarrhea

Cx: (1) Malignant islet cell tumor (in 60%)

(2) Liver metastases will continue to stimulate gastric secretion

Rx:

(1) Control of gastric hypersecretion:

(a) H2-receptor antagonist: cimetidine, ranitidine, famotidine

(b) Hydrogen-potassium adenosine triphosphatase inhibitor (omeprazole)

(2) Resection of gastrinoma if found (because of malignant potential)

(3) Total gastrectomy

DIFFERENTIAL DIAGNOSIS OF UROGENITAL DISORDERS

RENAL FAILURE
= reduction in renal function
- rise in serum creatinine >2.5 mg/dl

Acute renal failure
= clinical condition associated with rapid steadily increasing azotemia ± oliguria (<500 ml urine per day) over days / weeks

Etiology
- A. PRERENAL
  = renal hypoperfusion secondary to systemic illness
  1. Fluid + electrolyte depletion
  2. Hemorrhage
  3. Hepatic failure + hepatorenal syndrome
     √ abnormally elevated resistive index
  4. Cardiac failure
  5. Sepsis
  √ normal resistive index <0.70
- B. RENAL (most common)
  1. Acute tubular necrosis:
     ischemia, nephrotoxins, radiographic contrast, hemoglobulinuria, myoglobulinuria, myocardial infarction, burns
     √ resistive index ≥ 0.75
  2. Acute glomerulonephritis + small vessel disease:
     acute poststrep glomerulonephritis, rapidly progressive glomerulonephritis, lupus, polyarteritis nodosa, Schönlein-Henoch purpura, subacute bacterial endocarditis, serum sickness, Goodpasture syndrome, malignant hypertension, hemolytic uremic syndrome, drug-related vasculitis, abruptio placentae
     √ normal resistive index <0.70
  3. Acute tubulointerstitial nephritis:
     drug reaction, pyelonephritis, papillary necrosis
     √ abnormal resistive index
  4. Intrarenal precipitation (hypercalcemia, urate, myeloma protein)
  5. Arterial / venous obstruction
  6. Cortical necrosis
- C. POSTRENAL (5%)
  = result of outflow obstruction (rare)
  1. Prostatism
  2. Tumors of bladder, retroperitoneum, pelvis
  3. Calculus
  √ hydronephrosis
- D. CONGENITAL
  Bilateral renal agenesis / dysplasia / infantile polycystic kidney disease, congenital nephrotic syndrome, congenital nephritis, perinatal hypoxia

Incidence: ATN + prerenal disease account for 75% of acute renal failure

Chronic renal failure
= decrease in renal function over months / years

Etiology:
- A. INFLAMMATION / INFECTION
  1. Glomerulonephritis
  2. Chronic pyelonephritis
  3. Tuberculosis
  4. Sarcoidosis
- B. VASCULAR
  1. Renal vascular disease
  2. Bilateral renal vein thrombosis
- C. DYSPROTEINEMIA
  1. Myeloma
  2. Amyloid
  3. Cryoglobulinemia
  4. Waldenström macroglobulinemia
- D. METABOLIC
  1. Diabetes
  2. Gout
  3. Hypercalcemia
  4. Hyperoxaluria
  5. Cystinosis
  6. Fabry disease
- E. CONGENITAL
  1. Polycystic kidney disease
  2. Multicystic dysplastic kidney
  3. Medullary cystic disease
  4. Alport syndrome
  5. Infantile nephrotic syndrome
- F. MISCELLANEOUS
  1. Hepatorenal syndrome
  2. Radiation

Abnormal tubular function
- A. PROXIMAL TUBULE
  reabsorbs almost all of glucose, amino acids, phosphate
  - glycosuria (Toni-Fanconi syndrome)
  - aminoaciduria (cysteinuria)
  - phosphaturia (phosphate diabetes, thiazides)
- B. DISTAL TUBULE
  absorbs most of water
  - diabetes insipidus

Renal tubular acidosis
= inability of kidney to excrete an acid urine, resulting in systemic metabolic acidosis

Functional types:
- A. TYPE I = DISTAL TYPE
  = impaired ability to secrete H^+ in distal tubule
  Higher incidence of nephrocalcinosis, nephrolithiasis, osteomalacia
  - acid load test with NH_4Cl

B. <u>TYPE II</u> =   <u>PROXIMAL TYPE</u>
= impaired capacity to absorb HCO_3^- in proximal tubule
Most common in renal insufficiency, hyperparathyroidism
- bicarbonate titration test

Pathophysiology:
(a) loss of phosphate = osteomalacia / rickets
(b) loss of calcium   = nephrocalcinosis + renal calculi
(c) loss of potassium   = muscle weakness
(d) loss of bicarbonate = hyperchloremic acidosis
- alkaline urine
- potassium wasting, loss of sodium
- hypercalciuria (continued mobilization of bone calcium)
- hyperchloremic acidosis (low plasma bicarbonate)

Consequences:
- chronic renal failure (damage from nephrocalcinosis + secondary pyelonephritis)
- muscle weakness, hyporeflexia, paralysis (due to hypokalemia)
- bone pain (due to osteomalacia)
√ rickets / osteomalacia
√ nephrocalcinosis / stone formation (marked reduction of urinary citrate)

Categories:
1. INFANTILE RTA = PRIMARY RTA TYPE II
   = LIGHTWOOD SYNDROME
   Cause: late development of enzyme carbonic anhydrase; male patients
   Prognosis: spontaneous remission by age 2 in majority of patients
   √ nephrocalcinosis in 25%

2. PRIMARY RTA TYPE I
   autosomal dominant; female patients
   Age: presents in early adult life
   √ nephrocalcinosis in 75%
   √ osteomalacia in 50%
3. ACQUIRED RTA
   (a) TYPE I:
       Sjögren syndrome, cryoglobulinemia, light chain proteinuria, amphotericin B toxicity, toluene toxicity, outdated tetracyclines, lithium toxicity, heavy metal intoxication, renal transplant, radiation therapy, chronic renal disease
   (b) TYPE II
       cystinuria, Wilson disease, primary + secondary hyperparathyroidism, Fanconi syndrome, glycogen storage disease

Arterial hypotension
Cause: intrarenal hypovolemia, primary vasoconstriction, reduced glomerular filtration, depletion of intratubular urine volume

Δ May occur as a contrast reaction!
Urogram reverts to normal after reversion of hypotension!
√ bilateral small smooth kidneys (compared with size on preliminary films)
√ increasingly dense nephrogram
√ usually NO opacification of collecting system
√ initially opacification of collecting system if hypotension occurs during contrast injection

Diabetes insipidus
1. <u>Hypothalamic diabetes insipidus</u>
   = vasopressin production is reduced to <10%
   Cause:
   (a) rare autosomal dominant X-linked genetic disorder
   (b) pituitary destruction: craniopharyngioma, surgery, head trauma, complication of meningitis, eosinophilic granuloma
2. <u>Psychogenic water intoxication</u>
   = compulsive intake of large amounts of fluid, which leads to inhibition of normal vasopressin production
   - water deprivation test
3. <u>Primary nephrogenic diabetes insipidus</u>
   = rare sex-linked recessive genetic disorder with unresponsiveness of tubules + collecting system to vasopressin (in infants + young males)
4. <u>Secondary nephrogenic diabetes insipidus</u>
   Cause:
   drug toxicity, analgesic nephropathy, sickle cell anemia, hypokalemia, hypercalcemia, chronic uremic nephropathy, postobstructive uropathy, reflux nephropathy, amyloidosis, sarcoidosis

Hypercalcemia
mnemonic: "SHAMPOO DIRT"
Sarcoidosis
Hyperparathyroidism, **H**yperthyroidism
Alkali-milk syndrome
Metastases, **M**yeloma
Paget disease
Osteogenesis imperfecta
Osteopetrosis
D vitamin intoxication
Immobility
Renal tubular acidosis
Thyazides

Polycythemia
Cause: increased level of erythropoietin (acting on erythroid stem cells) secondary to a decrease in pO_2; erythropoietin precursor is produced in juxtaglomerular epitheloid cells of kidney + converted in blood
RENAL
A. INTRARENAL
   1. Vascular impairment
   2. Renal cell carcinoma (5%)
   3. Wilms tumor
   4. Benign fibroma
   5. Simple cyst (14%)
   6. Polycystic kidney disease

B. POSTRENAL
1. Obstructive uropathy (14%)
EXTRARENAL
A. LIVER DISEASE
1. Hepatoma
2. Regenerating hepatic cells
B. ADRENAL DISEASE
1. Pheochromocytoma
2. Aldosteronoma
3. Cushing disease
C. CNS DISEASE
1. Cerebellar hemangioblastoma
D. Large uterine myomas

NOT in: renal vein thrombosis, multicystic dysplastic
kidney, medullary sponge kidney

Wetting

1. **Enuresis**
= manifestation of neuromuscular vesicourethral
immaturity; M:F = 3:2
• intermittent wetting, usually at night during sleep
• often positive history of enuresis from one parent
• normal physical examination
√ no structural abnormality; urography NOT indicated
2. **Epispadia**
= incomplete fusion of infravesical portion of urinary
tract
• urinary incontinence from incompetent bladder neck /
urethral sphincter
√ abnormally wide symphysis pubis (>1 cm)
3. Sacral agenesis
= segmental defect (below S2) with deficiency of
nerves that innervate bladder, urethra, rectum, feet
Δ Children of diabetic mothers are affected in 17%!
4. **Extravesical infrasphincteric ectopic ureter**
only affects girls as boys do NOT have infrasphincteric
ureteral orifices
(a) ureter draining upper pole of duplex system exits
below urethral sphincter (90%)
(b) ureter draining single system with ectopic
extravesical orifice (10%)
5. **Synechia vulvae**
= adhesive fusion of minor labia directs urine primarily
into vagina from where it dribbles out post micturition
6. **Vaginal reflux**
in obese older girls with fat thighs and fat labia
7. Miscellaneous
Posterior urethral valves, urethral stricture, urethral
diverticula

KIDNEY

Absent renal outline on plain film

A. ABSENT KIDNEY
1. Congenital absence
2. S/P nephrectomy
B. SMALL KIDNEY
1. Renal hypoplasia
2. Renal atrophy

C. RENAL ECTOPIA
1. Pelvic kidney
2. Crossed fused ectopia
3. Intrathoracic kidney
D. OBLITERATION OF PERIRENAL FAT
1. Perirenal abscess
2. Perirenal hematoma
3. Renal tumors

Unilateral large smooth kidney

A. PRERENAL:
(a) arterial: acute arterial infarction
(b) venous: acute renal vein thrombosis
B. INTRARENAL:
(a) congenital: duplicated pelvocalyceal system,
crossed fused ectopia,
multicystic dysplastic kidney,
adult polycystic kidney (in 8%
unilateral)
(b) infectious: acute bacterial nephritis
(c) adaptation: compensatory hypertrophy
C. POSTRENAL:
(a) collecting system: obstructive uropathy

mnemonic: "AROMA"
Acute pyelonephritis
Renal vein thrombosis
Obstructive uropathy
Miscellaneous (compensatory hypertrophy, duplication)
Arterial obstruction (infarction)

Bilateral large kidneys

Average renal length by X-ray: M = 13 cm; F = 12.5 cm
1. PROTEIN DEPOSITION
Amyloidosis, multiple myeloma
2. INTERSTITIAL FLUID ACCUMULATION
Acute tubular necrosis, acute cortical necrosis, acute
arterial infarction, renal vein thrombosis
3. CELLULAR INFILTRATION
(a) Inflammatory cells: acute interstitial nephritis,
acute bacterial nephritis
(b) Malignant cells   : leukemia / lymphoma
4. PROLIFERATIVE / NECROTIZING DISORDERS
(a) Glomerulonephritis (GN)
Acute (poststreptococcal) GN, rapidly progressive
GN, idiopathic membranous GN,
membranoproliferative GN, lobular GN, IgA
nephropathy, glomerulosclerosis,
glomerulosclerosis related to heroin abuse
(b) Multisystem disease
Polyarteritis nodosa, systemic lupus
erythematosus, Wegener granulomatosis, allergic
angitis, diabetic glomerulosclerosis, Goodpasture
syndrome (lung hemorrhage + glomerulonephritis),
Schönlein-Henoch syndrome (anaphylactoid
purpura), thrombotic thrombocytopenic purpura,
focal glomerulonephritis associated with subacute
bacterial endocarditis
5. URINE OUTFLOW OBSTRUCTION
Bilateral hydronephrosis: congenital / acquired

6. HORMONAL STIMULUS
Acromegaly, compensatory hypertrophy, nephromegaly associated with cirrhosis / hyperalimentation / diabetes mellitus
7. DEVELOPMENTAL
Bilateral duplication system, horseshoe kidney, polycystic kidney disease
8. MISCELLANEOUS
Acute urate nephropathy, glycogen storage disease, hemophilia, sickle cell disease, Fabry disease, physiologic response to contrast material and diuretics

Unilateral small kidney

A. PRERENAL = VASCULAR
1. Lobar infarction
2. Chronic infarction
3. Renal artery stenosis
4. Radiation nephritis
B. INTRARENAL = PARENCHYMAL
1. Congenital hypoplasia
2. Multicystic dysplastic kidney (in adult)
3. Postinflammatory atrophy
C. POSTRENAL = COLLECTING SYSTEM
1. Reflux nephropathy = chronic atrophic pyelonephritis
2. Postobstructive atrophy

Bilateral small kidneys

A. PRERENAL = VASCULAR
1. Arterial hypotension (acute)
2. Generalized arteriosclerosis
3. Atheroembolic disease
4. Benign & malignant nephrosclerosis
B. INTRARENAL
1. Hereditary nephropathies: medullary cystic disease, hereditary chronic nephritis (Alport syndrome)
2. Chronic glomerulonephritis
3. Amyloidosis (late)
C. POSTRENAL
1. Papillary necrosis
D. CAUSES OF UNILATERAL SMALL KIDNEY occurring bilaterally

Depression of renal margins

1. Fetal lobation
   √ notching between normal calices
2. Splenic impression
   √ flattened upper outer margin of left kidney
3. Chronic atrophic pyelonephritis
   √ indentation over clubbed calices
4. Renal infarct
   √ normal calices
5. Chronic renal ischemia
   √ normal calices

Increased echogenicity of renal cortex

= RENAL MEDICAL DISEASE = diffuse increase in cortical echogenicity with preservation of corticomedullary junction

Path: deposition of collagen / calcium
√ echointensity of cortex equal to or greater than liver / spleen + equal to renal sinus
1. Acute / chronic glomerulonephritis
2. Renal transplant rejection
3. Lupus nephritis
4. Hypertensive nephrosclerosis
5. Renal cortical necrosis
6. Methemoglobulinuric renal failure
7. Alport syndrome
8. Amyloidosis
9. Diabetic nephrosclerosis
10. End-stage renal disease

Hyperechoic renal pyramids in children

A. Nephrocalcinosis
   (a) iatrogenic (most common cause): furosemide (Rx for BPD), vitamin D (Rx for hypophosphatemic rickets)
   (b) noniatrogenic:
      1. Idiopathic hypercalcemia
      2. Williams syndrome
      3. Absorptive hypercalcemia
      4. Hyperparathyroidism
      5. Milk-alkali syndrome
      6. Kenny-Caffey syndrome
      7. Distal renal tubular acidosis
      8. Malignant tumors
      9. Chronic glomerulonephritis
      10. Sjögren syndrome (distal RTA)
      11. Sarcoidosis
B. Metabolic disease
   1. Gout
   2. Lesch-Nyhan syndrome (urate)
   3. Fanconi syndrome
   4. Glycogen storage disease (distal RTA)
   5. Wilson disease (distal RTA)
   6. Alpha 1-antitrypsin deficiency
   7. Tyrosinemia
   8. Cystinosis
   9. Oxalosis
   10. Crohn disease
C. Hypokalemia
   1. Primary aldosteronism
   2. Pseudo-Bartter syndrome
D. Protein deposits
   1. Infant dehydration with presumed Tamm-Horsfall proteinuria
   2. Toxic shock syndrome
E. Vascular congestion
   1. Sickle cell anemia
F. Infection
   1. Candida / CMV nephritis
   2. AIDS-associated Mycobacterium avium-intracellulare
G. Fibrosis of renal pyramids
H. Cystic medullary disease
   1. Medullary sponge kidney
   2. Congenital hepatic fibrosis with tubular ectasia
I. Intrarenal reflux
   1. Chronic pyelonephritis

Enlargement of iliopsoas compartment
A. INFECTION
- (a) from retroperitoneal organs
    1. Renal infection
    2. Complicated pancreatitis
    3. Postoperative aortic graft infection
- (b) from spine
    1. Osteomyelitis / postoperative complication of bone surgery
    2. Discitis / postoperative complication from disc surgery
- (c) from GI tract
    1. Crohn disease
    2. Appendicitis
- (d) others
    1. Pelvic inflammatory disease / postpartum infection
    2. Sepsis

B. HEMORRHAGE
1. Coagulopathy and anticoagulant therapy
2. Ruptured aortic aneurysm
3. Postoperative aneurysm repair / other surgery / trauma

C. NEOPLASTIC DISEASE
- (a) Extrinsic
    1. Lymphoma
    2. Metastatic lymphadenopathy
    3. Bone metastases with soft tissue involvement
    4. Retroperitoneal sarcoma
- (b) Intrinsic
    1. Muscle tumors
    2. Nervous system tumors
    3. Lipoma / liposarcoma

D. MISCELLANEOUS
1. Pseudoenlargement of psoas muscle compared to de facto atrophy of contralateral side in neuromuscular disease
2. Fluid collections
   urinoma, lymphocele, pancreatic pseudocyst, enlargement of iliopsoas bursa
3. Pelvic venous thrombosis
   √ diffuse swelling of all muscles (edema)

RENAL MASS

Unilateral renal masses
SOLID MASSES
A. TUMORS
- (a) <u>malignant</u>: adenocarcinoma, malignant lymphoma / Hodgkin disease, adult nephroblastoma, metastases, Wilms tumor, sarcoma, oncocytoma, invasive transitional cell carcinoma
- (b) <u>benign</u>: adenoma, hamartoma (angiomyolipoma), mesenchymal tumor (lipoma, fibroma, myoma, hemangioma)

B. INFLAMMATORY MASSES
acute focal bacterial nephritis, renal abscess, xanthogranulomatous pyelonephritis, malakoplakia, tuberculoma

FLUID-FILLED MASSES
A. CYSTS
- (a) Simple renal cyst
- (b) Inherited cystic disease:
    multicystic dysplastic kidney disease (Potter Type II), multilocular cystic nephroma
- (c) Focal hydronephrosis

B. ARTERIOVENOUS MALFORMATION

Δ Lesions <1 cm often cannot be clearly characterized

Δ Lesions 1 – 1.5 cm can often be ignored, particularly in elderly / patients with significant other disease

Bilateral renal masses
A. MALIGNANT TUMORS
1. Malignant lymphoma / Hodgkin disease
2. Metastases
3. Renal cell carcinoma
4. Wilms tumor

B. BENIGN TUMORS
1. Angiomyolipoma
2. Nephroblastomatosis

C. CYSTS
1. Adult polycystic kidney disease
2. Acquired cystic kidney disease

Renal mass in neonate
A. UNILATERAL
1. Multicystic kidney (15%)
2. Hydronephrosis (25%)
   - (a) UPJ obstruction
   - (b) upper moiety of duplication
3. Renal vein thrombosis
4. Mesoblastic nephroma
5. Rare: Wilms tumor, teratoma

B. BILATERAL
1. Hydronephrosis
2. Polycystic kidney disease
3. Multicystic kidney + contralateral hydronephrosis
4. Nephroblastomatosis
5. Bilateral multicystic kidney

Renal mass in older child
A. SINGLE MASS
1. Wilms tumor
2. Multilocular cystic nephroma
3. Focal hydronephrosis
4. Traumatic cyst, abscess
5. Renal cell carcinoma
6. Malignant rhabdoid tumor
7. Teratoma
8. Clear cell sarcoma of kidney
9. Intrarenal neuroblastoma

B. MULTIPLE MASSES
1. Nephroblastomatosis
2. Multiple Wilms tumors
3. Angiomyolipoma
4. Lymphoma
5. Leukemia
6. Adult polycystic kidney disease
7. Abscesses

Avascular mass in kidney

mnemonic: "CHEAT"
Cyst
Hematoma
Edema
Abscess
Tumor

Low-density retroperitoneal mass

1. Lipoma
   √ sharply marginated, homogeneously fatty mass
2. Lymphangioma
   √ similar to lipoma if enough fat content
3. Adrenal myelolipoma
   √ density between fat + water
   √ usually nonhomogeneous, occasionally with hemorrhage ± calcifications
4. Renal angiomyolipoma
   √ intrarenal component
   √ hypervascular with large feeding arteries, multiple aneurysms, laking without shunting, tortuous circumferential vessels, whorled parenchymal + venous phase
5. Xanthogranulomatous pyelonephritis
   √ nonfunctioning kidney replaced by low-density material + central staghorn calculus
6. Metastatic retroperitoneal tumors
7. Renal cell carcinoma
8. Fibrosarcoma, fibrous histiocytoma, mesenchymal sarcoma, malignant teratoma
   √ density close to muscle
9. Liposarcoma

Growth pattern of renal tumors in adults

A. EXPANSILE GROWTH
   1. Renal cell carcinoma
   2. Oncocytoma
   3. Angiomyolipoma
   4. Juxtaglomerular tumor
   5. Metastatic tumor (eg, lymphoma)
   6. Mesenchymal tumor
B. INFILTRATIVE GROWTH
   1. Lymphoma / leukemia
   2. Invasive transitional cell carcinoma
   3. Metastatic tumor
   4. Renal cell carcinoma

Local bulge in renal contour

A. CYST
   1. Simple renal cyst
B. TUMOR
   1. Adenocarcinoma
   2. Angiomyolipoma
   3. Pseudotumor
C. INFECTION
   1. Subcapsular abscess
   2. XGP
D. TRAUMA
   1. Subcapsular hematoma
E. DILATED COLLECTING SYSTEM

Multiloculated renal mass

A. NEOPLASTIC DISEASE
   1. Multiloculated renal cell carcinoma
   2. Multilocular cystic nephroma
   3. Cystic Wilms tumor
   4. Necrotic tumors
      (a) mesoblastic nephroma
      (b) clear cell sarcoma
B. RENAL CYSTIC DISEASE
   1. Localized renal cystic disease
   2. Septated cyst
   3. Segmental multicystic kidney
   4. Complicated cyst
C. INFLAMMATORY DISEASE
   1. Echinococcus
   2. Segmental XGP
   3. Abscess
   4. Malakoplakia
D. VASCULAR LESIONS
   1. AV fistula
   2. Organizing hematoma

Focal area of increased renal echogenicity

1. Chronic renal infarction
2. Angiomyolipoma
3. Cavernous renal hemangioma
4. Renal cell carcinoma
5. Angiosarcoma
6. Undifferentiated sarcoma
7. Oncocytoma
8. Metastasis
9. Acute focal bacterial nephritis

Renal sinus mass

A. TUMORS
   1. Transitional cell carcinoma
   2. Lymphoma
   3. Metastasis to sinus lymph nodes
   4. Mesenchymal tumor: lipoma, fibroma, myoma, hemangioma
   5. Plasmacytoma
   6. Myeloid metaplasia
B. MISCELLANEOUS
   1. Sinus lipomatosis
   2. Parapelvic cyst
   3. Saccular aneurysm
   4. Urinoma

Hypoechoic renal sinus

A. SOLID
   1. Fibrolipomatosis
   2. Column of Bertin
   3. Duplex kidney
   4. TCC / RCC
B. CYSTIC
   1. Multiple parapelvic cysts
   2. Caliectasis
   3. Dilated veins

Renal pseudotumor

= anomalies of lobar anatomy that may simulate a tumor

A. PRIMARY

1. **Large column of Bertin**

   = large septum / cloison of Bertin = large cloison
   = focal cortical hyperplasia = benign cortical rest
   = focal renal hypertrophy

   = persistence of normal septal cortex / excessive infolding of cortex usually in the presence of partial or complete duplication

   Location: between upper and interpolar portion

   √ mass <3 cm in largest diameter

   √ lateral indentation of renal sinus

   √ deformation of adjacent calices + infundibula

   √ mass continuous with renal cortex

   √ enhancement pattern like renal cortex

   √ echogenicity similar to cortex

2. **Dromedary hump**

   = subcapsular nodule = splenic bump

   = secondary to prolonged pressure by spleen during fetal development

   Location: in mid portion of lateral border of left kidney

   √ triangular contour + elongation of middle calyx

   √ enhancement pattern like renal cortex

3. **Hilar lip**

   = supra- / infrahilar bulge = medial part of kidney above / below sinus

   Location: most frequently medial to left kidney just above renal pelvis (on transaxial scan)

   √ enhancement pattern like cortex with medulla

4. **Fetal lobation**

   = persistent cortical lobation

   14 individual lobes with centrilobar cortex located around calices

5. **Lobar dysmorphism**

   complete diminutive lobe situated deep within renal substance with its own diminutive calyx in its central portion

B. ACQUIRED

1. **Nodular compensatory hypertrophy**

   areas of unaffected tissue in the presence of focal renal scarring from chronic atrophic pyelonephritis (= reflux nephropathy), surgery, trauma, infarction;

   √ hypertrophy usually evident within 2 months; less likely to occur > age 50

   DDx: accessory spleen, medial lobule of spleen, splenosis, normal / abnormal bowel, pancreatic disease, gallbladder, adrenal abnormalities

   Dx: static radionuclide imaging / renal arteriography / CT

ABNORMAL NEPHROGRAM

Nonvisualized kidney on excretory urography

A. ABSENCE OF KIDNEY

1. Agenesis
2. Ectopia

B. LOSS OF PERFUSION

1. Chronic infarction
2. Unilateral renal vein thrombosis

3. Fractured kidney

C. URINARY OBSTRUCTION

1. Hydronephrosis
2. Ureteropelvic junction obstruction

D. REPLACED NORMAL RENAL PARENCHYMA

1. Multicystic dysplastic kidney
2. Unilateral polycystic kidney disease
3. Renal tumor (RCC, TCC, Wilms tumor)
4. Xanthogranulomatous pyelonephritis

Abnormal nephrogram due to Impaired Perfusion

1. Systemic hypotensive reaction as reaction to contrast material / cardiac failure / dehydration

   Pathophysiology: drop in perfusion pressure after contrast reaches kidney leads to increased salt + water reabsorption and slowed tubular transit

   √ prolonged bilateral dense nephrograms
   = persistent increasing nephrogram

   √ decrease in renal size

   √ loss of pyelogram after initial opacification

   NUC (use of glomerular filtration agent [eg, Tc-99m DTPA] preferred):

   √ prolonged cortical transit + reduced excretion

2. Impaired perfusion of renal artery

   (a) in renal artery stenosis

   √ decreased nephrographic opacity + rim nephrogram

   √ hyperconcentration in collecting system

   √ ureteral notching

   NUC (glomerular filtration agent [eg, Tc-99m DTPA] preferred):

   √ decreased perfusion with prolonged excretory phase

   (b) in renal artery occlusion (thrombosis, embolism)

   √ absent nephrogram

3. Impaired perfusion of small arteries

   Trueta shunting = transient rerouting of blood flow from cortex to medulla

   Causes:

   (a) reflex spasm during arterial angiography secondary to catheter trauma / pressure injection of highly concentrated contrast medium

   (b) chronic renal disorders (collagen vascular disease, malignant nephrosclerosis, chronic glomerulonephritis

   (c) necrotizing vasculitis (polyarteritis nodosa, scleroderma, hypertensive nephrosclerosis)

   CT, Angio:

   √ inhomogeneous opacification of cortex

   IVP:

   √ irregular cortical nephrogram = spotted nephrogram

4. Acute venous outflow obstruction in renal vein thrombosis

   √ obstructive nephrogram

   √ progressive increase in opacity of entire kidney

Abnormal nephrogram due to <u>Impaired Tubular Transit</u>

Causes:
- A. EXTRARENAL: ureteric obstruction (eg, stone)
  - √ obstructive nephrogram
    NUC:
    before decrease in renal function use of glomerular filtration agent (eg, Tc-99m DTPA); with decrease in renal function use of plasma flow agents (eg, Tc-99m MAG3 / I-123 Hippuran) preferred
    - √ continuous increase in renal activity
    - √ dilatation of collecting system
- B. INTRARENAL
  - (a) segmental: limb of duplication system, calyceal obstruction, interstitial edema
    - √ segmental nephrogram
  - (b) protein precipitation: Tamm-Horsfall protein (a normal mucoprotein product of proximal nephrons), Bence Jones protein (multiple myeloma), uric acid precipitation (acute urate nephropathy), myoglobulinuria, hyperproteinuric state
    - √ striated nephrogram
    NUC:
    before decrease in renal function use of glomerular filtration agent (eg, Tc-99m DTPA); with decrease in renal function use of plasma flow agents (eg, Tc-99m MAG3 / I-123 Hippuran) preferred
    - √ prolonged cortical transit time + prolonged excretory phase

Abnormal nephrogram due to <u>Abnormal Tubular Function</u>

1. Acute tubular necrosis
   - √ immediate persistent nephrogram (common)
   - √ progressive increasing opacity (rare)
2. Contrast-induced renal failure

Cortical rim nephrogram

= rim of cortex continues to receive flow from capsular vessels

Cause:
1. Acute total main renal artery occlusion
2. Renal vein thrombosis
3. Acute tubular necrosis
4. Severe chronic urinary obstruction

Increasingly dense nephrogram

= initially faint nephrogram becoming increasingly dense over hours to days

Mechanism:
- (a) diminished plasma clearance of contrast material
- (b) leakage of contrast material into renal interstitial spaces
- (c) increase in tubular transit time

Cause:
- A. VASCULAR = diminished perfusion
  1. Systemic arterial hypotension (bilateral)

  2. Severe main renal artery stenosis (unilateral)
  3. Acute tubular necrosis (in 33%): due to contrast material nephrotoxicity
  4. Acute renal vein thrombosis

- B. INTRARENAL
  1. Acute glomerular disease

- C. COLLECTING SYSTEM
  1. Intratubular obstruction
     - (a) uric acid crystals (acute urate nephropathy)
     - (b) precipitation of Bence Jones protein (myeloma nephropathy)
     - (c) Tamm-Horsfall protein (severely dehydrated infants / children)
  2. Acute extrarenal obstruction: ureteral calculus

Striated urographic nephrogram

= fine linear bands of alternating lucency + density in area of tubules and collecting ducts
1. Systemic hypotension
2. Intratubular obstruction (Tamm-Horsfall proteinuria)
3. Acute bacterial nephritis / pyelonephritis
4. Renal contusion
5. Medullary sponge kidney
6. Medullary cystic disease
7. Infantile polycystic kidney disease
8. Renal vein thrombosis
9. Acute extrarenal obstruction

Striated angiographic nephrogram

= random patchy densities reflecting redistribution of blood flow from the cortical vasculature to the vasa recta of the medulla
1. Obliterative diseases of the renal microvasculature: polyarteritis nodosa, scleroderma, necrotizing angiitis, catheter-induced vasospasm
2. Acute bacterial nephritis
3. Renal vein thrombosis

Vicarious contrast material excretion during IVP

= biliary contrast material detected radiographically following intravenous administration of contrast material

Normal contrast excretion:
<2% of urographic dose of diatrizoates + iothalamates are handled by hepatobiliary excretion

Pathophysiology:
increase in protein binding due to prolonged intravascular contact + acidosis

Cause:
1. Uremia (reduction in glomerular filtration + uremia-associated acidosis)
2. Acute unilateral obstruction (increase in circulation time + transient intracellular acidosis)
3. Spontaneous urinary extravasation (prolonged vascular contact of contrast material)

Spontaneous urinary contrast extravasation

= SPONTANEOUS PYELORENAL BACKFLOW

Etiology:

physiologic "safety valve" for obstructed urinary tract with pressures of 80 – 100 mm Hg in collecting system due to ipsilateral ureteral obstruction from distal stone impaction; pressure is proportional to degree + duration of acute obstruction + dose of contrast material

Incidence: 0.1 – 18%; M>F (male ureter less compliant)

Criteria:

(a) absence of recent ureteral instrumentation
(b) absence of previous renal / ureteral surgery
(c) absence of destructive urinary tract lesion
(d) absence of external trauma
(e) absence of external compression
(f) absence of pressure necrosis due to stone

Types:

1. Pyelotubular backflow
   = opacification of terminal portions of collecting ducts (= papillary ducts = ducts of Bellini) as a physiologic phenomenon (in 13% with low osmolality + in 0.4% with high osmolality contrast media), wrongly termed "backflow"
   √ wedge-shaped brushlike lines from calyx towards periphery
2. Pyelosinus backflow
   = contrast extravasation from ruptured fornices along infundibula, renal pelvis, proximal ureter; most common form
   Cx: urinoma, retroperitoneal fibrosis
3. Pyelointerstitial backflow
   = contrast flow from pyramids into subcapsular tubules
4. Pyelolymphatic backflow
   = contrast extravasation into periforniceal + peripelvic lymphatics
   √ visualization of small lymphatics draining medially
5. Pyelovenous backflow
   = forniceal rupture into interlobar / arcuate veins; very rare

COLLECTING SYSTEM

Caliceal abnormalities

A. OPACIFICATION OF COLLECTING TUBULES
   1. Pyelorenal backflow
   2. Medullary sponge kidney
B. PAPILLARY CAVITY
   1. Papillary necrosis
   2. Caliceal diverticulum
   3. Tuberculosis / brucellosis
C. LOCALIZED CALIECTASIS
   1. Reflux nephropathy = chronic atrophic pyelonephritis
   2. Compound calyx
   3. Hydrocalyx
   4. Congenital megacalyx
   5. Localized postobstructive caliectasis
   6. Localized tuberculosis / papillary necrosis
D. GENERALIZED CALIECTASIS
   1. Postobstructive atrophy
   2. Congenital megacalices
   3. Obstructive uropathy (hydronephrosis)

4. Nonobstructive hydronephrosis
5. Diabetes insipidus

Widened collecting system

A. OBSTRUCTIVE UROPATHY
   1. Acute obstruction
   2. Chronic obstruction
   3. Obstructed upper pole moiety of duplicated collecting system
B. NONOBSTRUCTIVE WIDENING
   (a) Congenital
      1. Megacalicosis
         underdevelopment of papillae, usually unilateral
      2. Congenital primary megaureter
         widened ureter with normally tapered distal end
      3. Megacystis-megaureter syndrome
      4. Prune-belly syndrome
   (b) Increased urine volume
      1. High-flow states: diabetes insipidus, osmotic diuresis, dehydrated patient undergoing rehydration, unilateral kidney
      2. Vesicoureteral reflux
   (c) Atony of renal collecting system
      1. Infection: ie, acute pyelonephritis
      2. Pregnancy
         Etiology: ? obstruction by enlarged ovarian veins / uterus; progesterone induced decrease in ureteral tone
         Incidence: 3 – 4% of pregnant women
         Time: at end of 1st trimester, maximal in 3rd trimester
         Location: right (90%), left (67%); ureter widened only to pelvic brim
         Prognosis: resolution within a few weeks to 6 months after delivery
      3. Retroperitoneal fibrosis
   (d) Distended urinary bladder
   (e) Previous obstruction: dilatation remains in spite of relief of obstruction

Filling defect in collecting system

mnemonic: "6 C's & 2 P's"
   Clot
   Cancer
   Cyst
   Calculus
   Candida + other fungi
   Cystitis cystica
   Polyp
   Papilla (sloughed)

Nonopaque intraluminal mass in collecting system

A. NONOPAQUE CALCULUS
   uric acid, xanthine, matrix
   √ smooth, rounded, not attached
B. TISSUE SLOUGH
   1. Papillary necrosis

2. Cholesteatoma
3. Fungus ball
4. Inspissated debris ("mucopus")
C. VASCULAR
   1. Blood clot: history of hematuria
      √ change in appearance over time
D. FOREIGN MATERIAL
   1. Air
      from bladder via reverse peristalsis, direct
      trauma, renoalimentary fistula
   2. Foreign matter

Mucosal mass in collecting system
NEOPLASTIC
A. BENIGN TUMOR
   1. Aberrant papilla = papilla without calyx
      protruding into major infundibulum
   2. Endometriosis
   3. **Fibroepithelial polyp** = fibrous polyp
      = fibroepithelioma = vascular fibrous polyp
      = polypoid fibroma
      = mesodermal tumor with fibrovascular
      stroma + normal transitional cell epithelium
      Age: 20 – 40 years
      • intermittent abdominal / flank pain
      • gross hematuria (rare)
      √ elongated cylindrical filling defect with
        smooth margins
      √ mobile on thin pedicle
B. MALIGNANT TUMOR
   (a) Uroepithelial tumors
       1. Transitional cell carcinoma (85 – 91%)
       2. Squamous cell carcinoma (10 – 15%)
          Predisposing factors:
             calculi (50 – 60%), chronic infection,
             leukoplakia, phenacetin abuse
          √ infiltrating / superficially spreading
       3. Mucinous adenocarcinoma
          = metaplastic transformation
       4. Sarcoma (extremely rare)
   (b) Metastases: breast (most common),
       melanoma, stomach, lung, cervix, colon,
       prostate

INFLAMMATION / INFECTION
   1. Tuberculosis
   2. Candidiasis
   3. Schistosomiasis
   4. Pyeloureteritis cystica
   5. Leukoplakia
   6. Malakoplakia
   7. Xanthogranulomatous pyelonephritis

VASCULAR
   1. Submucosal hemorrhage:
      trauma, anticoagulant therapy, acquired
      circulating anticoagulants, complication of
      crystalluria / microlithiasis
      √ thumbprinting with progressive improvement

2. Vascular notching:
   ureteropelvic varices, renal vein occlusion, IVC
   occlusion, vascular malformation, retroaortic left
   renal vein, "nutcracker" effect on left renal vein
   between aorta and SMA
3. Polyarteritis nodosa

PROMINENT MUCOSAL FOLDS
   1. Redundant longitudinal mucosal folds of
      intermittent hydronephrosis (UPJ obstruction,
      vesicoureteral reflux) or after relief of obstruction
   2. Chemical / mechanical irritation
   3. Urticaria (Stevens-Johnson syndrome
      = erythema multiforme bullosa)
   4. Leukoplakia (= squamous metaplasia)
   5. Ureteral diverticulosis
      = rupture of the roofs of cysts in ureteritis cystica

Effaced collecting system
A. EXTRINSIC COMPRESSION
   (1) Unilateral / bilateral global enlargement of renal
       parenchyma
   (2) Renal sinus masses: hemorrhage; parapelvic cyst;
       sinus lipomatosis
B. SPASM / INFLAMMATION
   (1) Infection: acute pyelonephritis, acute bacterial
       nephritis, acute tuberculosis
   (2) Hematuria
C. INFILTRATION
   Malignant uroepithelial tumors
D. OLIGURIA
   1. Antidiuretic state
   2. Renal ischemia
   3. Oliguric renal failure

RENAL CYSTIC DISEASE
Potter classification
POTTER SYNDROME
   = any renal condition associated with severe
     oligohydramnios
   • peculiar facies with wide-set eyes, parrot beak nose,
     pliable low-set ears, receding chin
Type   I   : infantile PCKD
Type   II   : multicystic dysplastic kidney disease,
               multilocular cystic nephroma
       IIa : kidneys of normal / increased size
       IIb : kidneys reduced in size
Type   III : adult PCKD, tuberous sclerosis, medullary
               sponge kidney
Type   IV   : ureteropelvic junction obstruction with
               development of small cortical cysts / cystic
               dysplasia

Renal cystic disease
A. SIMPLE RENAL CYST
   1. Intrarenal
   2. Parapelvic
B. POLYCYSTIC RENAL DISEASE
   1. Adult PCKD
   2. Infantile PCKD

C. CYSTIC MEDULLARY DISEASE
1. Uremic medullary cystic disease
2. Juvenile nephronophthysis
3. Medullary sponge kidney
D. RENAL DYSPLASIA
1. Multicystic dysplastic kidney
2. Segmental / focal renal dysplasia
3. Familial renal dysplasia
E. NEUROCUTANEOUS DYSPLASIA
1. Tuberous sclerosis
2. Von Hippel-Lindau syndrome
F. CYSTIC TUMORS
1. Multilocular cystic nephroma
2. Cystic Wilms tumor
3. Cystic renal cell carcinoma
G. ACQUIRED RENAL CYSTIC DISEASE
1. Acquired cystic disease of uremia
2. Infectious cysts (TB, Echinococcus, abscess)
3. Medullary necrosis
4. Pyelogenic cyst

Syndromes with multiple cortical cysts
1. Von Hippel-Lindau syndrome
2. Tuberous sclerosis
3. Meckel-Gruber syndrome
4. Zellweger syndrome = cerebrohepatorenal syndrome
5. Jeune syndrome
6. Conradi syndrome = chondrodysplasia punctata
7. Oro-facial-digital syndrome
8. Trisomy 13
9. Turner syndrome

RENAL CALCIFICATION

Calcified renal mass
Δ A calcified renal mass is malignant in 75% of cases!
A. TUMOR
1. Renal cell carcinoma (calcifies in 10%)
   √ calcifications generally nonperipheral, sometimes along fibrous capsule
2. Wilms tumor
B. INFECTION
1. Abscess
   Δ Tuberculous abscess frequently calcifies!
   Δ Pyogenic abscess rarely calcifies!
2. Echinococcal cyst
   Renal involvement in 3% of hydatid disease; 50% of echinococcal cysts calcify
3. Xanthogranulomatous pyelonephritis
   √ large obstructive calculus in >70%
C. CYSTS
Calcification related to prior hemorrhage and infection
1. Simple renal cyst (calcifies in 1%)
2. Multicystic dysplastic kidney (in adult)
3. Adult polycystic kidney disease
4. Milk of calcium (cyst, caliceal diverticulum, obstructed hydrocalyx)
DDx: residual pantopaque used in cyst puncture
D. VASCULAR
1. Subcapsular / perirenal hematoma

2. Renal artery aneurysm
   √ circular cracked eggshell appearance
3. Congenital / posttraumatic arteriovenous fistula

Nephrocalcinosis
= NEPHROLITHIASIS
= calcium salts in renal parenchyma
Incidence: 0.1 – 6%; M>F

mnemonic: "MARCH"
Medullary sponge kidney
Alkali excess
Renal medullary / cortical necrosis, **R**TA
Chronic glomerulonephritis
Hyperoxaluria, **H**ypercalcemia, **H**ypercalciuria

Medullary Nephrocalcinosis
= calcifications involving the distal convoluted tubules in the loops of Henle
Incidence: 95% of all nephrocalcinoses
Causes:
A. HYPERCALCIURIA
(a) endocrine
1. Hyperparathyroidism in 5% (primary >> secondary)
2. Paraneoplastic syndrome of lung + kidney primary (ectopic parathormone production)
3. Cushing syndrome
4. Diabetes insipidus
5. Hyperthyroidism
(b) alimentary
1. Milk-alkali syndrome (excess calcium + alkali = milk + antacids)
2. Hypervitaminosis D
3. Beryllium poisoning
(c) osseous
1. Osseous metastases, multiple myeloma
2. Prolonged immobilization
3. Progressive senile osteoporosis
(d) renal
1. Renal tubular acidosis (in 73% of primary RTA)
2. Medullary sponge kidney
3. **Bartter syndrome**
   tubular disorder with potassium + sodium wasting, hyperplasia of juxtaglomerular apparatus, hyperaldosteronism, hypokalemic alkalosis, and normal blood pressure
(e) drug therapy
1. Furosemide (in infants)
2. Prolonged ACTH therapy
3. Vitamin E (orally)
4. Calcium (orally)
(f) miscellaneous
1. Sarcoidosis
2. Idiopathic hypercalcuria
3. Idiopathic hypercalcemia

B. HYPEROXALURIA = OXALOSIS
   1. **Primary hyperoxaluria**
      = Hereditary hyperoxaluria (more common)
      = rare autosomal recessive inherited enzyme deficiency of carboligase with diffuse oxalate deposition in kidneys, heart, blood vessels, lung, spleen, bone marrow
      Type I = glyoxalate metabolism
      Type II = hydroxypyruvate metabolism
      Age: usually <5 years
      Prognosis: early death in childhood
   2. **Secondary hyperoxaluria**
      = Enteric hyperoxaluria (rare)
      Cause: disturbance of bile acid metabolism after jejunoileal bypass, ileal resection, blind loop syndrome, Crohn disease, increased ingestion (green leafy vegetables), pyridoxine deficiency, ethylene glycol poisoning, methoxyflurane anesthesia
C. HYPERURICOSURIA
   1. Gouty kidney
   2. Lesch-Nyhan syndrome
D. URINARY STASIS
   1. Milk-of-calcium in pyelocaliceal diverticulum
   2. Medullary sponge kidney
E. DYSTROPHIC CALCIFICATION
   1. Renal papillary necrosis

√ normal-sized / occasionally enlarged kidneys (medullary sponge kidney)
√ grouped rounded / linear calcifications
√ small poorly defined / large coarse granular calcifications in renal pyramids
US:
   √ absence of hypoechoic papillary structures (earliest sign)
   √ hyperechoic rim at corticomedullary junction + around tip and sides of pyramids
   √ solitary focus of hyperechogenicity at tip of pyramid near fornix
   √ increased echogenicity of renal pyramids ± shadowing (no acoustic shadowing with small + light calcifications)
DDx of hyperechoic medulla in newborns:
   Oliguria with transient tubular blockage by Tamm-Horsfall proteinuria
Cx: often followed by urolithiasis

Cortical Nephrocalcinosis
Incidence: 5% of all nephrocalcinoses
Causes:
   1. Acute cortical necrosis
   2. Chronic glomerulonephritis
   3. Alport syndrome = hereditary nephritis + deafness
   4. Congenital oxalosis, primary hyperoxaluria
   5. Chronic paraneoplastic hypercalcemia
   6. Rejected renal transplant
US:
   √ homogeneously increased echogenicity of renal parenchyma > liver echogenicity

Retroperitoneal calcification
A. NEOPLASM
   1. Wilms tumor (in 10%)
   2. Neuroblastoma (in 50%): fine granular / stippled / amorphous
   3. Teratoma: cartilage / bone / teeth, pseudodigits, pseudolimbs
   4. Cavernous hemangioma: phleboliths
B. INFECTION
   1. Tuberculous psoas abscess
   2. Hydatid cyst
C. TRAUMA
   1. Old hematoma

RENOVASCULAR DISEASE
Renal aneurysm
A. EXTRARENAL ANEURYSM (2/3)
   1. Congenital
   2. Atherosclerotic
   3. Fibromuscular dysplasia
   4. Mycotic
      2.5% of all aneurysms
      Cause: bacteremia, SBE, perivascular extension of inflammation
      Organism: Streptococcus, Staphylococcus, Pneumococcus, Salmonella
      Locations: thoracic aorta, SMA, peripheral branches of middle cerebral artery, large arteries of extremities, intrarenal (rare), in areas of preexisting vascular disease
   5. Neurofibromatosis
   6. Trauma + renal artery angioplasty

B. INTRARENAL ANEURYSM (1/3)
   in interlobar and more peripheral branches
   1. Congenital
      Age at Dx: 30 years; M:F = 1:1
      • hypertension in 25% (from segmental renal ischemia)
      √ aneurysm close to vascular bifurcations, may calcify
   2. Atherosclerotic (may calcify)
   3. Polyarteritis nodosa
   4. SLE
   5. Drug abuse vasculitis
      Kidney most commonly affected organ
      Cause:
         (a) immunologic injury from circulating hepatitis antigen-antibody complexes producing a necrotizing angiitis
         (b) bacterial endocarditis
         (c) drug-related
         (d) impurity-related
      Drugs: metamphetamine, heroin, LSD
      √ multiple small aneurysms in interlobar branches near corticomedullary junction
      √ inhomogeneous spotty nephrogram
   6. Allergic vasculitis
   7. Neoplasm (renal cell carcinoma in 14%; adult Wilms tumor)

8. Hamartoma (angiomyolipoma in 50%)
9. Wegener granulomatosis
10. Metastatic arterial myxoma
11. Transplant rejection
12. Neurofibromatosis

Cx: (1) Hypertension (unusual) (2) Perinephric / retroperitoneal hemorrhage (3) Formation of AV fistula (4) Peripheral renal embolization (5) Thrombosis

Spontaneous renal hemorrhage
A. RENAL TUMOR (57 – 63%)
  (a) malignant (30 – 33%):
    RCC, TCC of renal pelvis, Wilms tumor, lipo-, fibro-, angiosarcoma
  (b) benign (24 – 33%):
    angiomyolipoma, lipoma, adenoma, fibromyoma, ruptured hemorrhagic cyst
B. VASCULAR DISEASE (18 – 26%)
  Vasculitis (eg, polyarteritis nodosa in 13%), arteriovenous malformation, ruptured aneurysm, segmental renal infarction
C. INFLAMMATION / INFECTION (7 – 10%)
  1/2 with + 1/2 without abscess
D. COAGULOPATHY
  Anticoagulation therapy, bleeding diathesis, long-term hemodialysis

Subcapsular hematoma
√ subcapsular mass with flattening of renal parenchyma
√ total resorption / formation of pseudocapsule with calcification
Angio: √ avascular mass
Cx: Page kidney (ischemia, release of renin, hypertension)

Renovascular hypertension
1. Atherosclerosis (60%)
2. Fibromuscular dysplasia (35%)
3. Neurofibromatosis
4. Pheochromocytoma
5. Fibrous bands (congenital stenosis)
6. Arteritis (Takayasu disease)
7. Emboli
8. Thrombosis
9. Aneurysm
10. Renal cyst
11. Neoplasm
12. Perirenal hematoma

URETER

Ureteral deviation
A. LUMBAR URETER
  (a) Lateral deviation (common):
    1. Hypertrophy of psoas muscle
    2. Enlargement of paracaval / para-aortic lymph nodes
    3. Aneurysmal dilatation of aorta
    4. Neurogenic tumors
    5. Fluid collections (abscess, urinoma, lymphocele, hematoma)
  (b) Medial deviation:
    1. Retrocaval ureter (on right side only)
    2. Retroperitoneal fibrosis
B. PELVIC URETER
  (a) Medial deviation:
    1. Hypertrophy of iliopsoas muscle
    2. Enlargement of iliac lymph nodes
    3. Aneurysmal dilatation of iliac vessels
    4. Bladder diverticulum at UVJ (Hutch)
    5. Following abdominoperineal surgery + retroperitoneal lymph node dissection
    6. Pelvic lipomatosis
  (b) Lateral deviation with extrinsic compression
    1. Pelvic mass (eg, fibroids, ovarian tumor)

Ureteral stricture
A. INTRINSIC CAUSE
  (a) mucosal
    1. Primary ureteral tumors
  (b) mural
    1. **Endometriosis**
      common disorder in menstruating women (15%);
      ureteral involvement is rare and indicates widespread pelvic disease
      √ abrupt smooth stricture of 0.5 – 2.5 cm length
      √ rectosigmoid involvement on BE
    2. Tuberculosis, schistosomiasis
    3. Traumatic
      ureterolithotomy, endoscopic stone extraction, hysterectomy
    4. Amyloidosis
      √ distal stricture with submucosal calcification
    5. Nonspecific (rare)
B. EXTRINSIC CAUSE
  1. Endometriosis
    extrinsic form:intrinsic form = 4:1
  2. Abscess
    tuboovarian, appendiceal, perisigmoidal
  3. Inflammatory bowel disease
    (eg, Crohn disease, diverticulitis)
  4. Radiation fibrosis
  5. Metastases
    cervix, endometrium, ovary, rectum, prostate, breast, lymphoma
  6. Iliac artery aneurysm (with perianeurysmal fibrosis)

Megaureter
A. VESICOURETERAL REFLUX
  (a) Primary vesicoureteral reflux
    1. Primary reflux megaureter
      abnormal ureteral tunnel at UVJ
    2. Prune belly syndrome
  (b) Secondary vesicoureteral reflux
    1. Hypertonic neurogenic bladder
    2. Bladder outlet obstruction
    3. Posterior urethral valves

B. OBSTRUCTION
  (a) Primary obstruction
      1. Intrinsic ureteral obstruction (stone, stricture, tumor)
      2. Ectopic ureter
      3. Ureterocele
      4. Ureteral duplication: tortuous dilated ureter of upper moiety
  (b) Secondary obstruction
      1. Retroperitoneal obstruction: tumor, fibrosis, aortic aneurysm
      2. Bladder wall mass
      3. Bladder outlet obstruction: eg, prostatic enlargement
C. NONREFLUX-NONOBSTRUCTED MEGAURETER
      1. Congenital primary megaureter = megaloureter
      2. Polyuria: eg, diabetes insipidus, acute diuresis
      3. Infection
      4. Ureter remaining wide after relief of obstruction

ADRENAL GLAND
Adrenocortical hyperfunction
  1. Cushing syndrome = hypercortisolism
  2. Conn syndrome = hyperaldosteronism
  3. Adrenogenital syndrome

Adrenal medullary disease
  1. Neuroblastoma
  2. Ganglioneuroblastoma
  3. Ganglioneuroma
  4. Pheochromocytoma

Adrenal cortical disease
  1. Adrenal hyperplasia
  2. Adrenocortical adenoma
  3. Adrenocortical carcinoma
  4. Cushing syndrome
  5. Conn syndrome
  6. Adrenogenital syndrome

Small unilateral adrenal tumor
  Δ Incidental discovery of adrenal mass in 1% of CT!
      (a) mass <3 cm in diameter is likely benign
      (b) mass >5 cm in diameter is likely malignant
      (c) CT attenuation values <0 HU indicate nonhyperfunctioning adenomas

  1. Cortical adenoma (in 1 – 9% of autopsies)
  2. Metastasis (27% of all tumors): lung (40%), breast (20%), renal cell carcinoma, gastrointestinal tumors, melanoma
      Δ 50% of adrenal masses in oncologic patients represent benign nonhyperfunctioning adenomas!
  3. Pheochromocytoma
  4. Asymmetric hyperplasia
  5. Granulomatous disease (TB, histoplasmosis)
      √ diffuse enlargement / discrete mass
      √ ± cystic changes ± calcification
  6. Myelolipoma: rare benign tumor composed of hematopoietic cells + fat similar to bone marrow

Large solid adrenal mass
  1. Cortical carcinoma
  2. Pheochromocytoma
  3. Neuroblastoma / ganglioneuroma
  4. Myelolipoma
  5. Metastasis
  6. Hemorrhage
  7. Inflammation
  8. Abscess (eg, histoplasmosis, tuberculosis)

Bilateral large adrenals
  1. Hyperplasia
  2. Inflammation
  3. Hemorrhage
  4. Metastases

Cystic adrenal mass
  1. Old hemorrhage
  2. Cyst: pancreatic pseudocyst, degenerated adenoma, hydatid cyst, endothelial lined vascular cystic space
  3. Neuroblastoma (rare)
  4. Cystic adenoma

Adrenal calcification
  A. TUMOR
      1. Neuroblastoma
      2. Pheochromocytoma
      3. Adrenal adenoma
      4. Adrenal carcinoma
      5. Dermoid
  B. VASCULAR
      1. Hemorrhage (neonatal, sepsis)
  C. INFECTION
      1. Tuberculosis
      2. Histoplasmosis
      3. Waterhouse-Friderichsen syndrome
  D. ENDOCRINE
      1. Addison disease (TB)
  E. OTHERS
      1. Wolman disease

URINARY BLADDER
Bilateral narrowing of urinary bladder
  A. WITH ELEVATION OF BLADDER FLOOR
      1. Pelvic lipomatosis
      2. Pelvic hematoma
         Cause: trauma, anticoagulant therapy, spontaneous rupture of blood vessels, blood dyscrasia (rare), bleeding neoplasm (rare)
      3. Chronic cystitis
  B. WITH SUPERIOR COMPRESSION OF BLADDER
      1. Thrombosis of IVC
         Cause: trauma, hypercoagulability state (oral contraceptives), extension of thrombi from lower extremity, abdominal sepsis, Budd-Chiari syndrome, compression of IVC by neoplasm
         √ collaterals through gonadal veins, ascending lumbar veins, vertebral plexus, retroperitoneal veins, portal vein (via hemorrhoidal veins)
         √ notching of distal ureter by ureteral veins

2. Pelvic lymphadenopathy
   Cause: lymphoma (most often)
   √ polycyclic asymmetric compression of bladder
   √ medial displacement of pelvic segment of
       ureters
   √ lateral displacement of upper ureters
3. Hypertrophy of iliopsoas muscles
4. Bilateral pelvic masses
   (a) bilateral lymphocysts (following radical pelvic
       surgery)
   (b) bilateral urinomas
   (c) bilateral pelvic abscesses

Small bladder capacity
Cause: thickened / fibrotic bladder wall; bladder
            resection; disuse of bladder
• urinary frequency
• progressive rise in bladder pressure during filling
√ reduced bladder compliance
√ thickened bladder wall + decreased bladder volume
√ vesicoureteral reflux

1. **Interstitial cystitis**
   Age: postmenopausal female
   • pink pseudoulceration of bladder mucosa
      characteristically at vertex of bladder (= Hunner
      ulcer)
2. **Hemorrhagic cystitis**
   (a) nonspecific: negative culture
   (b) viral (adenovirus): negative culture, viral exanthem
   (c) cytotoxic: cyclophosphamide (Cytoxan®), in 15%
       of patients within 1st year of treatment
3. **Tuberculous cystitis**
   √ irritable hypertonic bladder with decreased capacity
   √ disease process usually starts at trigone spreading
       upwards and laterally
   √ calcification of bladder wall (rare)
4. **Cystitis cystica**
   = bacterial infection; more common in females
   √ cystogram insensitive
5. Schistosomiasis infection of bladder
   √ calcifications of bladder wall (common)
6. Radiation cystitis

Bladder wall thickening
Normal bladder wall thickness (regardless of age +
gender):
   <5 mm   in nondistended bladders
   <3 mm   in well distended bladders

A. TUMOR
   1. Neurofibromatosis
B. INFECTION / INFLAMMATION
   1. Cystitis
C. MUSCULAR HYPERTROPHY
   1. Neurogenic bladder
   2. Bladder outlet obstruction (eg, posterior urethral
       valves)
D. UNDERDISTENDED BLADDER

Bladder wall calcification
A. INFLAMMATION
   1. Schistosomiasis (50%)
      √ relatively normal distensibility
   2. Tuberculosis
      √ bladder markedly contracted
   3. Postirradiation cystitis
   4. Bacillary UTI (extremely uncommon)
B. NEOPLASM
   TCC, squamous cell carcinoma, leiomyosarcoma,
   hemangioma, neuroblastoma, osteogenic sarcoma

mnemonic: "SCRITT"
   Schistosomiasis
   Cytoxan
   Radiation
   Interstitial cystitis
   Tuberculosis
   Transitional cell carcinoma

Masses extrinsic to urinary bladder
A. NORMAL / ENLARGED ORGANS
   1. Uterus, leiomyomatous uterus, pregnant uterus
   2. Distended rectosigmoid
   3. Ectopic pelvic kidney
   4. Prostate cancer / BPH
B. SOLID PELVIC TUMORS
   1. Lymphadenopathy
   2. Bone tumor from sacrum / coccyx
   3. Rectosigmoid mass
   4. Hip arthroplasty
   5. Neurogenic neoplasm, meningomyelocele
   6. Pelvic lipomatosis / liposarcoma
C. CYSTIC PELVIC LESIONS
   (a) congenital / developmental
      1. Urachal cyst
      2. Müllerian duct cyst
      3. Gartner duct cyst
      4. Anterior meningocele
      5. Hydrometrocolpos
   (b) related to trauma
      1. Hematoma (eg, rectus sheath hematoma)
      2. Urinoma
      3. Lymphocele
      4. Abscess
      5. Aneurysm
      6. Mesenteric cyst
   (c) cyst of genitalia
      1. Prostatic cyst
      2. Cyst of seminal vesicle
      3. Cyst of vas deferens
      4. Ovarian cyst
      5. Hydrosalpinx
      6. Vaginal cyst
   (d) cyst of urinary bladder
      1. Bladder diverticulum
   (e) cyst of GI tract
      1. Peritoneal inclusion cyst
      2. Fluid-filled bowel

Urinary bladder wall masses
A. CONGENITAL
1. Congenital septum
2. Simple ureterocele
3. Ectopic ureterocele
B. BLADDER TUMORS
C. INFLAMMATION / INFECTION
1. Cystitis: hemorrhagic ~, abacterial ~, bullous ~, edematous ~, interstitial ~, eosinophilic ~, granulomatous ~, emphysematous ~, cystitis cystica, cyclophosphamide cystitis, cystitis glandularis (premalignant lesion with villous lesions in bladder dome from proliferation of "intestine-like" glands in submucosa)
2. Tuberculosis
3. Schistosomiasis
4. Malakoplakia
D. HEMATOMA
after instrumentation, surgery, trauma

VOIDING DYSFUNCTION
A. FAILURE TO STORE URINE
  • urinary frequency, urgency, incontinence
  Bladder causes:
1. Involuntary detrusor contractions
    (a) detrusor instability (idiopathic / neurogenic)
    (b) detrusor hyperreflexia (upper cord lesion)
2. Poor bladder compliance
    (a) detrusor hyperreflexia
    (b) bladder wall fibrosis
3. Sensory urgency
    (a) infection, inflammation, irritation
    (b) neoplasia
4. Vesicovaginal fistula
5. Psychogenic condition
  Sphincter causes:
1. Stress incontinence
2. Sphincteric incontinence
  Extravesical ectopic insertion of ureter in females
B. FAILURE TO EMPTY BLADDER
  • poor flow, straining, hesitancy
  • inability to completely empty bladder
  Bladder causes:
1. Detrusor areflexia (sacral arc lesion)
2. Impaired detrusor contractility (myogenic)
3. Psychogenic condition
  Bladder outlet obstruction:
1. Bladder neck contracture
2. Prostatic enlargement
3. Detrusor-external sphincter dyssynergia
4. Scarring from surgery / radiation therapy
5. Ectopic ureterocele
6. Urethral stenosis
7. Urethral kinking (eg, due to cystocele)

Detrusor instability
= MOTOR URGE INCONTINENCE = UNSTABLE BLADDER
Condition resembles that of immature bladder before toilet training

Patient groups:
(1) symptoms of nocturnal enuresis + frequency / incontinence dating back to childhood
(2) idiopathic instability occurring in middle age
(3) outflow obstruction commonly in men
(4) degenerative instability secondary to cardiovascular + neurologic disease later in life
  • frequency, urgency, urge incontinence, occasionally nocturia
  • hesitancy + difficulty in voiding may occur in men without significant prostatic hypertrophy
  √ involuntary bladder contractions with no relationship to bladder distension
  √ progressively vigorous contractions during bladder filling
  √ postural instability limited to upright position
  √ impaired milk-back due to high bladder pressure
  √ strong aftercontractions following bladder emptying
  Cx: thickening of bladder wall, bladder diverticula
  Rx: treatment of obstruction, anticholinergic drug (oxybutynin), operative increase in bladder capacity

Sensitive bladder (sensory urgency)
Cause:
  cystitis (reduced compliance), some cases of stress incontinence (filling of bladder neck induces urgency)
  • frequency, urgency, sometimes nocturia
  √ patient uncomfortable with low bladder filling
  √ no abnormal rise in bladder pressure
  √ normal voiding function

Stress incontinence
= SPHINCTER WEAKNESS INCONTINENCE
Cause:
(a) female: congenital bladder neck weakness, pregnancy, childbirth, aging (secondary to changes in anatomic relationship of urethra + bladder base)
(b) male: S/P prostatectomy with damage to distal sphincter
  • frequency, urgency (involuntary filling of bladder neck)
  √ opening of bladder neck during coughing
  √ impairment of milk-back mechanism (= retrograde emptying of urethra during interruption of voiding phase does not occur)
  √ urethrovesical descent (in type I + II)
  Chain cystography:
  √ posterior urethrovesical angle (= angle between posterior urethra + bladder base) increased >100°
  √ upper urethral axis (= angle between upper urethra + vertical line) increased >35°

Prostatic obstruction
= urethral compression by hypertrophic prostatic tissue
  • difficulty in voiding
  • reduction in flow rate
  √ high-pressure bladder
  √ slow + prolonged flow
  √ increase in bladder capacity with reduced contractility (late)

Detrusor-sphincter dyssynergia
= overactivity of bladder neck muscle with failure to relax at beginning of voiding
Cause: spinal cord lesion / trauma above level of sacral outflow
- difficulty in voiding ± frequency
- lifelong history of poor stream
- √ collarlike indentation of bladder neck during voiding (= persistent / intermittent narrowing of membranous urethra)
- √ may have high voiding pressure + reduced flow
- √ trapping of contrast in urethra during interruption of flow
- √ massive reflux into prostatic ducts during voiding (due to high pressure within prostatic urethra)
- √ severely trabeculated "Christmas-tree" bladder + bilateral hydroureteronephrosis
Rx: bladder neck incision

Incontinence
1. Stress incontinence
2. Vesicovaginal / ureterovaginal fistula
3. Overflow incontinence
   (secondary to lesions of sacral spinal cord / sacral reflex arc or severe outlet obstruction)
4. Reflex voiding
   (a) hyperreflexive lesion (lesion of upper spinal cord)
   (b) uninhibited / unstable bladder
5. Urge incontinence
6. Continual dribbling
   (extravesical ectopic termination of ureter)
7. Psychogenic incontinence

MALE GENITAL TRACT

Calcifications of male genital tract
A. VAS DEFERENS
   1. Diabetes mellitus: in muscular outer layer
   2. Degenerative changes
   3. TB, syphilis, nonspecific UTI: intraluminal
B. SEMINAL VESICLES
   Gonorrhea, TB, schistosomiasis, bilharziosis
C. PROSTATE
   Calcified corpora amylacea, TB

Acutely symptomatic scrotum
= acute unilateral scrotal swelling ± pain
Cause:
   epididymitis:torsion = 3:2   <20 years of age
   epididymitis:torsion = 9:1   >20 years of age
A. Torsion
   1. Torsion of testis
   2. Torsion of testicular appendages
      accounts for 5% of scrotal pathology; both located near upper pole of testes
      Frequency:
         appendix testis:appendix epididymis = 9:1
   3. Scrotal fat necrosis
   4. Strangulated hernia

B. Infection / inflammation
   1. Acute epididymitis
   2. **Orchitis**
      Etiology:
         (1) bacterial infection
         (2) complication of mumps in 20%:
            in adolescents + young adults; usually developing 4 – 5 days later; unilateral involvement in >90%; parotitis precedes orchitis in 84%, simultaneous in 3%, later in 4%, without parotitis in 10%
   3. Intrascrotal abscess
C. Hemorrhage
   1. Testicular trauma
   2. Hemorrhage into testicular tumor

Scrotal mass
1. Inflammation   (48%)
2. Hydrocele   (24%)
3. Torsion   (9%)
4. Varicocele   (7%)
5. Spermatocele   (4%)
6. Cysts   (4%)
7. Malignant tumor (2%)
8. Benign tumor   (0.7%)

Cystic lesions of testis
Incidence: 4 – 10%
A. NON-NEOPLASTIC
   1. **Testicular cyst**
      - nonpalpable
      Often associated with spermatocele
      Location: related to rete testis (in 92%)
   2. **Tunica albuginea cyst**
      - palpable
      - √ solitary small marginally located cyst
   3. **Tubular ectasia of rete testis**
      Age: middle-aged to elderly
      Often associated with spermatocele
      - nonpalpable
      Location: mediastinum testis
      - √ elliptical hypoechoic mass with branching tubular structures ± cysts
   4. Congenital cystic dysplasia of testis (extremely rare)
B. NEOPLASTIC
   Δ 24% of all testicular tumors have cystic component!
   - palpable
   - √ in combination with solid element

DDx: hematoma, inflammation, seminoma, Leydig cell tumor

Prostatic cysts
1. **Müllerian duct cyst**
   from remnants of paramesonephric (= müllerian) duct which has regressed by 3rd fetal month
   Age: 3rd – 4th decade
   - obstructive / irritative urinary tract symptoms
   - suprapubic / rectal pain
   - hematuria

Location: arise from region of verumontanum slightly lateral to midline
√ large cyst usually with cephalad extension above prostate
√ aspirate contains serous / mucous clear brown / green fluid, NEVER spermatozoa
√ rarely contains calculi
Cx: infection, hemorrhage, carcinomatous transformation

2. **Utricle cyst**
Secondary to dilatation of prostatic utricle (sometimes believed to be a remnant of the müllerian duct)
Age: 1st – 2nd decade
• postvoid dribbling
• obstructive / irritative urinary tract symptoms
• suprapubic / rectal pain
• hematuria
May be associated with hypospadia, incomplete testicular descent, unilateral renal agenesis
Location: arise in midline from verumontanum
√ 8 – 10 mm long cyst usually without extension above prostate
Dx: endoscopic catheterization with aspiration of white / brown fluid occasionally containing spermatozoa
Cx: infection, hemorrhage, carcinomatous transformation

3. **Ejaculatory duct cyst**
Cause: congenital / acquired obstruction of ejaculatory duct
• perineal pain, dysuria, ejaculatory pain
• hematospermia
Location: along expected course of ejaculatory duct
√ intraprostatic cyst within central zone
√ aspirate contains spermatozoa with normal testicular function
√ cyst commonly contains calculi
√ cystic dilatation of ipsilateral seminal vesicle
√ contrast injection into cyst outlines seminal vesicle

4. **Cystic degeneration of BPH**
Most common cystic lesion of prostate
Location: transition zone
√ usually small cyst within nodules of benign prostatic hyperplasia

5. **Retention cyst**
= dilatation of glandular acini
Cause: acquired obstruction of glandular ductule
Age: 5 – 6th decade
Location: transition / central / peripheral zone
√ 1 – 2 cm smooth-walled unilocular cyst

6. **Cavitary / diverticular prostatitis**
Cause: fibrosis of chronic prostatitis constricts ducts leading to stagnation of exudate + breakdown of intraacinar septa with cavity formation

• history of long-standing inflammatory condition
√ "Swiss cheese" prostate

7. **Prostatic abscess**
Age: 5 – 6th decade
• fever, chills
• urinary frequency, urgency, dysuria, hematuria
• perineal / lower back pain
• focally enlarged tender prostate
√ hypo- / anechoic mass with irregular wall + septations

8. Parasitic cyst (Echinococcus, bilharziosis)

9. Cystic carcinoma

Hypoechoic lesion of prostate
1. Adenocarcinoma (35%)
2. Benign prostatic hyperplasia (18%)
3. "Normal" prostatic tissue (18%)
4. Prostatitis: eg, granulomatous prostatitis (14%)
5. Atrophy: eg, fibrosis following TURP (10%)
6. Prostatic dysplasia (6%)

Ambiguous genitalia
• cryptorchidism   • labial fusion
• clitoromegaly   • epi- / hypospadia
Sex assignment based on
(1) karyotype (2) gonadal biopsy (3) genital anatomy

FEMALE PSEUDOHERMAPHRODITISM
Cause: exposure to excessive androgens in 1st trimester, often associated with adrenogenital syndrome
Karyotype: 46,XX
• masculinized external genitalia
√ normal ovarian, uterine, vaginal anatomy

MALE PSEUDOHERMAPHRODITISM
Cause: deficiency of testicular secretions / abnormal response by target organs
Karyotype: 46,XY
• feminized / ambiguous external genitalia
√ undescended male testes

TRUE HERMAPHRODITISM
Karyotype: 46,XX / 46,XY
√ ovarian + testicular tissue present together = ovary / ovotestis / testis

MIXED GONADAL DYSGENESIS
= testis + gonadal streak with XO/XY karyotype
√ uterus usually present

ANATOMY AND FUNCTION OF UROGENITAL TRACT

Urogenital Embryology

Renal Vascular Anatomy

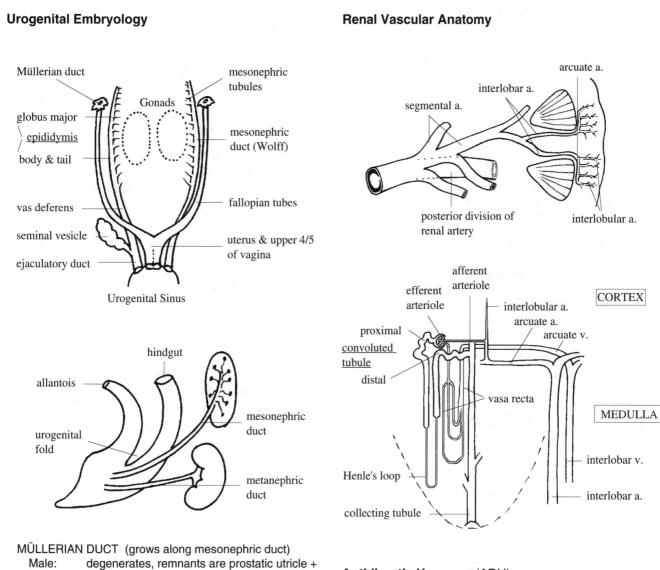

MÜLLERIAN DUCT (grows along mesonephric duct)
Male: degenerates, remnants are prostatic utricle + appendix testis
Female: uterus, fallopian tubes
PRONEPHROS
vestigial remnant / completely absent
MESONEPHROS   degenerates
mesonephric tubules: efferent ductules (M);
                         epinephron (F)
mesonephric duct: vas deferens, ejaculatory duct, seminal vesicles (M); vanishes (F)

METANEPHROS (kidney)
(1) metanephric duct buds from mesonephric duct at 4th week to form ureter, pelvis, calices, collecting ducts (10 – 12 generations)
(2) metanephric vesicles form around terminal branches of collecting ducts
    Δ Polycystic kidney disease is believed to be a failure of linkage!

Antidiuretic Hormone (ADH)
Production site: supraoptic nuclei of hypothalamus, transported to neurohypophysis
Stimulus: fluid loss with increase in osmolality
Effects: (1) 10 x increase in permeability of collecting ducts (= concentrated urine)
        (2) decreased blood flow through vasa recta leads to increased hypertonicity of interstitium (= countercurrent multiplier mechanism)

Renal physiology
GLOMERULAR FILTRATION RATE (GFR)
$[P] \times GFR = [U] \times U_{vol}$

$$GFR = \{[U] \times U_{vol}\} / [P] = 125 \text{ ml/min} = 20\% \text{ of RPF}$$

Substrate: inulin; Tc-99m DTPA

TUBULAR SECRETION (Tm)

$$[U] \times U_{vol} = [P] \times GFR + Tm$$

Tm = { [U] × U$_{vol}$} - {[P] × GFR}

Substrate: p-aminohippurate (PAH); I-131 Hippuran

RENAL PLASMA FLOW (RPF)

$$[P] \times RPF = [U] \times U_{vol}$$

RPF = {[U] × U$_{vol}$} / [P]

Substrate: p-aminohippurate

[P]	= concentration in plasma
GFR	= glomerular filtration rate
[U]	= concentration in urine
U$_{vol}$	= urine volume
Tm	= transport maximum (across tubular cells)
RPF	= renal plasma flow

Renal imaging in newborn infant

Δ low glomerular filtration rate (GFR):
— on first day of life: 21% of adult values
— by 2 weeks of age: 44% of adult values
— at end of 1st year: close to adult values
Δ limited capacity to concentrate urine
IVP: √ occasional failure of renal visualization
NUC: √ improved visualization on radionuclide studies

Contrast excretion

UROGRAPHIC DENSITY depends on

$$[U] = \{[P] \times GFR\} / U_{vol}$$

1. Concentration of contrast material in plasma [P] is a function of
   (a)   total iodine dose
   (b)   contrast injection rate
   (c)   volume distribution
   Rapid decline of concentration of contrast material in vessels is due to:
   (1)   rapid mixing within vascular compartment
   (2)   diffusion into extravascular extracellular fluid space (capillary permeation)
   (3)   renal excretion
2. Glomerular filtration rate (GFR): 99% filtered
3. Urine volume (U$_{vol}$) ie, activity of ADH:
   (a)   in dehydrated state with increased ADH activity concentrations of contrast material are higher
   Dehydration is considered a risk-potentiating factor for nephrotoxicity!
   (b)   in volume-expanded state with decreased ADH activity concentrations of contrast material are lower
   Patients with CHF require higher doses of contrast material!

MEGLUMINE: no metabolization, excreted by glomerular filtration alone
Meglumine effect of osmotic diuresis:
   (a) lower concentration of urinary iodine per ml urine
   (b) greater distension of collecting system
   N.B.: Avoid meglumine in "at risk" patients (higher incidence of contrast reactions than sodium!)

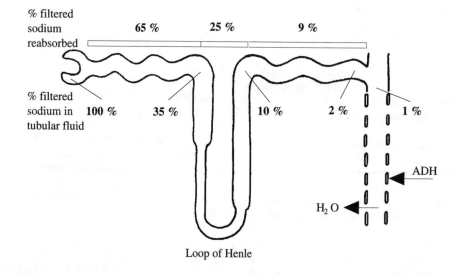

Sodium Reabsorption

hypertonicity is maintained within the medullary interstitium by the countercurrent multiplier system of the loop of Henle and the vasa recta; ADH increases permeability of collecting ducts for water

SODIUM: extensive reabsorption by tubules with delayed excretion
Sodium effect of reabsorption:
  (a) increased concentration of urinary iodine (improved visualization)
  (b) less distension of collecting system (ureteral compression necessary)

DEVELOPMENTAL RENAL ANOMALIES

A. NUMERARY RENAL ANOMALY
  1. Supernumerary kidney
  2. Complete / partial duplication
  3. Abortive calyx
  4. Unicalyceal (unipapillary) kidney

B. RENAL UNDERDEVELOPMENT
  1. Congenital renal hypoplasia
  2. Renal agenesis
  3. Renal dysgenesis

C. RENAL ECTOPIA
  Normal location of kidneys: 1st – 3rd lumbar vertebra

  1. Longitudinal ectopia
     Location: pelvic, sacral, lower lumbar level, intrathoracic; L > R
     √ must demonstrate aberrant arteries
     DDx: displacement through diaphragmatic hernia (nonaberrant); hypermobile kidney
     Pelvic kidney
        Incidence: 1:725 births
        May be associated with:
           (1) vesicoureteral reflux
           (2) hydronephrosis due to abnormally high insertion of ureter into renal pelvis
           (3) hypospadia (common)

  2. Crossed ectopia
     (a) fused (common)
     (b) separate (rare)
     √ invariably aberrant renal arteries
     √ distal ureter inserts into trigone on the side of origin

  3. Renal fusion
     = "lump, cake, disc, horseshoe"
     Cx: aberrant arteries may cross and obstruct ureter
     Horseshoe kidney
        Incidence: 0.2 – 1% (at autopsy)
        Associated with (in 50%):
           (1) Caudal ectopia
           (2) Vesicoureteral reflux
           (3) Hydronephrosis
        √ fusion of R + L kidney at lower (90%) / upper (10%) pole
        √ renal long axis medially oriented
        √ preaortic renal isthmus at L4/5
        √ ureters passing anteriorly
        Cx: renal calculi

  4. Renal malrotation
     √ collecting structures may be positioned ventrally (most common), lateral (rare), dorsal (rarer), transverse (along AP axis)
     √ "funny looking calices" = developmental usually nonobstructive ectasia

ADRENAL ANATOMY
from periphery to centrum:
  (a) renin-angiotensin-dependent outer adrenal cortex:
     zona **g**lomerulosa = mineralocorticoid (aldosterone)
  (b) corticotropin-dependent inner adrenal cortex:
     zona **f**asciculata = cortisol
     zona **r**eticularis = sex hormones (androgen, estrogen)
  (c) medulla = norepinephrine, epinephrine

Normal size	:	3 – 5 x 3 x 1 cm
Normal weight	:	3 – 5 g
Visualization by CT	:	Left side 100%, Right side 99%
by US	:	Left side 45%, Right side 80%

ANATOMY OF SCROTAL CONTENTS

Average size of testis	:	3.8 x 3.0 x 2.5 cm (decreasing with age)
Size of globus major	:	11 x 7 x 6 mm (decreasing with age)
Scrotal wall thickness	:	2 – 8 mm (3 – 6 mm in 89%)
Hydrocele	:	small to moderate in 14% of normals
Testicular cysts	:	in 8% of normals (average size 2 – 3 mm), numbers increasing with age
Epididymal cysts	:	in 30% of normals (average size 4 mm)
Epididymal calcification	:	in 3%

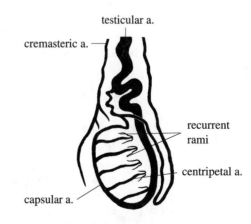

Arterial supply to scrotum

ZONAL ANATOMY OF PROSTATE
Normal weight: 20 ± 6 g
Normal size: 2.8 cm (craniocaudad), 2.8 cm
   (anteroposterior), 4.8 cm (width)
A. Outer gland
   1. Central zone: surrounds ejaculatory ducts from
      their entrance at prostatic base to
      verumontanum;
      25% of glandular tissue

   2. Peripheral zone: extends from base of prostate to
      apex along rectal surface;
      70% of glandular tissue
B. Inner gland
   1. Transition zone: on each side of internal sphincter;
      4% of glandular tissue;
      enlarges with BPH
   2. Periurethral zone: surrounding urethra; 1% of
      glandular tissue

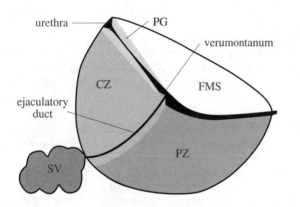

Midsagittal Section through Normal Prostate

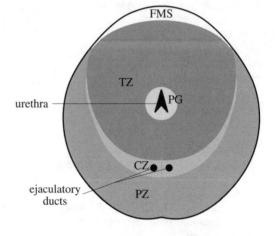

Transverse Section through Prostate with BPH
= enlargement of transition zone

CZ	=	central zone	PZ	=	peripheral zone
TZ	=	transition zone	SV	=	seminal vesicles

PG	=	periurethral glands
FMS	=	fibromuscular stroma

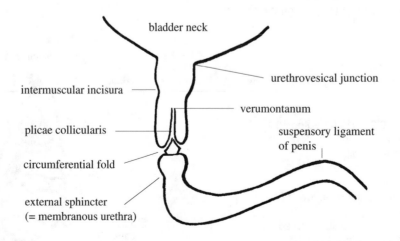

Urethrogram: normal urethral folds in LPO

RENAL, ADRENAL, URETERAL, VESICAL, AND SCROTAL DISORDERS

ABORTIVE CALYX
= developmental anomaly with short blind-ending
outpouching of pyramid without papillary invagination
Location: (a) renal pelvis
(b) infundibulum (mostly upper pole)

ACQUIRED CYSTIC KIDNEY DISEASE
= ACQUIRED CYSTIC DISEASE OF UREMIA
= renal cysts in patients on long-term hemodialysis (in
17% <5 cysts per kidney, in 40% no cysts
Δ Successful transplant prevents occurrence of cysts /
tumor!
Incidence: in 27 – 47% after approximately 3 years; in
80% after 4 years; approaching 100% after
>5 years
Proposed etiologies:
(a) altered compliance of tubular basement membrane
(b) obstruction due to focal proliferation of tubular
epithelium
(c) obstruction of ducts by interstitial fibrosis / oxalate
crystals
(d) toxicity from circulating metabolites
(e) vascular insufficiency
Histo: cysts lined by flattened cuboidal / papillary
epithelium

√ small end-stage kidneys (<280 g)
√ multiple 0.5 – 2 cm cysts bilaterally (early = small,
late = large)
In 13 – 20% associated with:
(a) small papillary / tubular / solid clear-cell adenomas
1 cm in diameter
(b) renal cell carcinoma

Cx: spontaneous hemorrhage into cyst
(macrohematuria / retroperitoneal hemorrhage from
cyst rupture)

AIDS
• azotemia, proteinuria, hematuria, pyuria (in 38 – 68%
sometime during illness)
• progressive renal failure (10%)
1. **HIV nephropathy** (40%)
= characterized by nephrotic-range proteinuria +
rapidly progressive renal failure
Histo: focal segmental glomerulosclerosis,
microcystic dilatation of tubules, intratubular
casts
√ global enlargement of both kidneys
CT:
√ medullary hyperattenuation (14%)
US:
√ increased cortical echogenicity
MRI:
√ loss of corticomedullary differentiation
Prognosis: death within 6 months

2. Renal infection with Pneumocystis carinii (8%)
√ punctate renal calcifications confined to cortex
√ associated calcifications in spleen, liver, lymph
nodes, adrenal glands
3. Renal lymphoma (3 – 11%)
AIDS-related lymphoma: NHL > Burkitt lymphoma,
Hodgkin disease

√ multiple renal masses
√ direct extension of retroperitoneal lymphadenopathy
engulfing kidney, renal sinus, ureter
4. Cystitis (22%)
Organisms: routine Gram-negative species, Candida,
Beta-hemolytic streptococci, Salmonella,
CMV
√ bladder wall thickening

ACUTE CORTICAL NECROSIS
= rare disorder with patchy / universal necrosis of renal
cortex + proximal convoluted structures secondary to
distension of glomerular capillaries with
dehemoglobulinized RBCs; medulla and 1 – 2 mm of
peripheral cortex are spared

Etiology:
(a) Obstetric patient (most often): abruptio placentae
= premature separation of placenta with concealed
hemorrhage (50%), septic abortion, placenta previa
(b) Children: severe dehydration + fever, infection,
hemolytic uremic syndrome, transfusion reaction
(c) Adults: sepsis, dehydration, shock, myocardial
failure, burns, snakebite, abdominal aortic surgery,
hyperacute renal transplant rejection
• protracted + severe oliguria / anuria

EARLY SIGNS
√ diffusely enlarged smooth kidneys
√ absent / faint nephrogram
US: √ loss of normal corticomedullary region with
hypoechoic outer rim of cortex
NUC: √ severely impaired renal perfusion

LATE SIGNS
√ small kidney (after a few months)
√ "tramline" / punctate calcifications along margins of
viable and necrotic tissue (as early as 6 days)
US:
√ hyperechoic cortex with acoustic shadowing
Prognosis: poor chance of recovery

ACUTE DIFFUSE BACTERIAL NEPHRITIS
= ACUTE SUPPURATIVE PYELONEPHRITIS
= more severe and extensive form of acute pyelonephritis,
which may lead to diffuse necrosis (phlegmon)

Organisms: Proteus, Klebsiella > E. coli
Predisposed: diabetics (60%)

ACUTE INTERSTITIAL NEPHRITIS
= infiltration of interstitium by lymphocytes, plasma cells, eosinophils, few PMNs + edema

Causes: allergic / idiosyncratic reaction to drug exposure (methicillin, sulfonamides, ampicillin, cephalothin, penicillin, anticoagulants, phenindione, diphenylhydantoin)
• eosinophilia (develops 5 days to 5 weeks after exposure)
√ large smooth kidneys with thick parenchyma
√ normal / diminished contrast density
US: √ normal / increased echogenicity

ACUTE TUBULAR NECROSIS
= temporary reversible marked reduction in tubular flow rate

Etiology:
(a) DRUGS: bichloride of mercury, ethylene glycol (antifreeze), carbon tetrachloride, bismuth, arsenic, uranium, urographic contrast material (especially when associated with glomerulosclerosis in diabetes mellitus), aminoglycosides (gentamicin, kanamycin)
(b) ISCHEMIA: major trauma, massive hemorrhage, postpartum hemorrhage, crush injury, myoglobulinuria, compartmental syndrome, septic shock, cardiogenic shock, burns, transfusion reaction, severe dehydration, pancreatitis, gastroenteritis, renal transplantation, cardiac surgery, biliary surgery, aortic resection
Pathophysiology: profound reduction in renal blood flow due to elevated arteriolar resistance

√ smooth large kidneys, especially increase in AP diameter >4.63 cm (due to interstitial edema)
√ diminished / absent opacification of collecting system
√ immediate persistent dense nephrogram (75%)
√ increasingly dense persistent nephrogram (25%)
√ diffuse calcifications (rare)
US:
    √ normal to diminished echogenicity of medulla
    √ sharp delineation of swollen pyramids
    √ normal (89%) / increased (11%) echogenicity of cortex
    √ elevated resistive index ≥ 0.75 (in 91% excluding patients with hepatorenal syndrome); unusual in prerenal azotemia
Angio:
    √ normal arterial tree with delayed emptying of intrarenal vessels
    √ slightly delayed / normal venous opacification
NUC:
    √ poor concentration of Tc-99m glucoheptonate / Tc-99m DTPA
    √ well maintained renal perfusion
    √ better renal visualization on immediate postinjection images than on delayed images
    √ progressive parenchymal accumulation of I-131 Hippuran / Tc-99m MAG3
    √ no excretion

ADDISON DISEASE
= PRIMARY ADRENAL INSUFFICIENCY
Δ 90% of adrenal cortex must be destroyed!
Cause:
1. Idiopathic adrenal atrophy (60 – 70%): likely autoimmune disorder
2. Granulomatous disease: tuberculosis, sarcoidosis
3. Fungal infection: histoplasmosis, blastomycosis, coccidioidomycosis
4. Adrenal hemorrhage: anticoagulation therapy, bleeding, coagulation disorders, sepsis, shock
5. Bilateral metastatic disease (rare)
√ diminutive glands (in idiopathic atrophy + chronic inflammation)
√ enlarged glands (acute inflammation, acute hemorrhage, metastasis)

ADRENAL HEMORRHAGE
Cause:
(a) NEWBORN
    Associated with birth trauma (forceps / breech delivery), hypoxia (prematurity), infants of diabetic mothers, septicemia, hemorrhagic disorders
    Age: 1st week of life
    Site: R > L; bilateral in 10%
(b) ADULT
    Following anticoagulant therapy, stress caused by sepsis (Waterhouse-Friderichsen syndrome), surgery, trauma (mostly right side), tumor
√ mass displacing renal axis
√ gradual decrease in size
√ peripheral calcification after 1 week
US:
    √ initially echogenic becoming progressively hypoechoic (degeneration, lysis)
CT:
    √ high-attenuation mass (50 – 90 HU) in acute / subacute stage

ADRENOCORTICAL ADENOMA
A. NONHYPERFUNCTIONING
    characterized by
    (a) normal lab values of adrenal hormones
    (b) NO pituitary shut-down of the contralateral gland
    (c) activity on NP-59 radionuclide scans
    Incidence: incidental finding in 1% at CT, 3% at autopsy
√ surveillance CT to confirm lack of growth
Rx: surgical removal for masses 3 – 5 cm as indeterminate potentially malignant neoplasms

B. HYPERFUNCTIONING
    1. Primary hyperaldosteronism
    2. Cushing syndrome (10%)
    3. Virilization
√ contralateral atrophic gland (secondary to ACTH suppression with autonomous adenoma)
√ unilateral focus of I-131 NP-59 radioactivity + contralateral absence of iodocholesterol accumulation (DDx: hyperplasia [bilateral activity])

√ well-defined sharply marginated mass <5 cm in size (average size 2.0 – 2.5 cm)
√ mild homogeneous enhancement
√ adenoma may calcify
CT:
  √ soft-tissue density / cystic density (mimicked by high cholesterol content) with poor correlation between functional status and HU number
  √ small adenomas <1 cm often go undetected
  √ contralateral gland often normal / atrophic
Angio:
  √ tumor blush + neovascularity; occasionally hypovascular
  √ pooling of contrast material
  √ enlarged central vein with high flow
  √ arcuate displacement of intraadrenal veins
  √ bilateral adrenal venous sampling in up to 40% unsuccessful in localizing
MR:
  √ mass iso- / hypointense (rarely hyperintense) to liver on T2WI
  √ mild enhancement + quick washout on Gd-dimeglumine enhanced study
  (DDx: metastases tend to have higher signal intensities [however 20 – 30% overlap])

ADRENOCORTICAL CARCINOMA
- 20% nonfunctioning
- 50% hyperfunctioning (in 10 – 15% Cushing syndrome)

Size: usually >5 cm (median size 12 cm; in 16% <6 cm)
√ frequently heterogeneous mass with irregular margins
√ occasionally calcified
√ invasion of IVC
√ metastases to regional lymph nodes, liver, lung, bone
CT:
  √ central areas of low attenuation (tumor necrosis)
  √ inhomogeneous enhancement (foci of hemorrhage + central necrosis)
MRI:
  √ hyperintense to liver on T2WI
Angio:
  √ enlarged adrenal arteries
  √ neovascularity, occasionally with parasitization
  √ AV shunting; multiple draining veins
NUC:
  √ usually bilateral nonvisualization with I-131 NP-59 (carcinomatous side does not visualize because amount of uptake is small for size of lesion; contralateral side does not visualize because carcinoma is releasing sufficient hormone to cause pituitary feedback shutdown of contralateral gland)
Biopsy: may appear histologically benign in well-differentiated adenocarcinoma

Prognosis: 0% 5-year survival rate

ADRENOCORTICAL HYPERPLASIA
Responsible for 8% of Cushing syndrome and 10 – 20% of hyperaldosteronism

Cause:
1. Corticotropin-dependent (85%): pituitary causes, ectopic corticotropin production, production of corticotropin-releasing factor
2. Primary pigmented nodular adrenocortical hyperplasia
3. Primary aldosteronism (rare)
Incidence: 4 x increased in patients with malignancy
Age: 70 – 80% in adults; 19% in children
Types:
(1) Smooth hyperplasia (common)
  √ bilateral normal sized glands
  √ thickened + elongated glands
(2) Cortical nodular hyperplasia (less common)
  √ normal glands ± appreciable micronodular configuration
  √ thickened gland with macronodular configuration (nodules up to 2.5 cm)
Angio:
  √ normal venogram: may show enlarged gland
  √ minimally increased hypervascularity
  √ focal accumulation of contrast medium
NUC:
  √ asymmetric bilateral NP-59 uptake (related to urinary cortisol excretion) without dexamethasone suppression in Cushing syndrome
  √ bilateral foci of NP-59 uptake with dexamethasone suppression (nondiagnostic ≥5 days)

ADRENOGENITAL SYNDROMES
A. CONGENITAL TYPE
  = impaired cortisol + aldosterone synthesis secondary to enzyme defect (22-hydroxylase / 11-β-hydroxylase) with increased ACTH stimulation by pituitary gland (negative feedback mechanism)
  M < F
  - virilization of female fetus
  - precocious puberty in male
  - pseudohermaphroditism (clitoral hypertrophy, ambiguous external genitalia, urogenital sinus)
  √ symmetrically enlarged + thickened adrenal glands

B. ACQUIRED TYPE
  M < F
  (a) adrenal hyperplasia / adenoma / carcinoma
  (b) ovarian / testicular tumor
  (c) gonadotropin-producing tumor: pineal, hypothalamic, choriocarcinoma
  - virilization
  - Cushing syndrome

AMYLOIDOSIS
= accumulation of extracellular eosinophilic protein substances

1. PRIMARY AMYLOIDOSIS
  kidneys involved in 35%

2. SECONDARY AMYLOIDOSIS
  kidneys involved in >80%, also affected are breast, tongue, alimentary tract, spleen, connective tissue

Causes: tuberculosis, osteomyelitis, bronchiectasis, ulcerative colitis, rheumatoid arthritis, Still disease, multiple myeloma, Waldenström macroglobulinemia, familial Mediterranean fever

√ smooth normal to large kidneys with increase in parenchymal thickness (early stage)
√ small kidneys = renal atrophy (late stage)
√ occasionally attenuated collecting system
√ increase in cortical echogenicity (deposition of amyloid in glomeruli and interstitium) + prominence of corticomedullary junction + obscuration of arcuate aa.
√ nephrographic density normal to diminished
US:
    √ normal to increased echogenicity
Cx: renal vein thrombosis

ANALGESIC NEPHROPATHY
= renal damage from ingestion of salicylates in combination with phenacetin / acetaminophen in a cumulative dose of 1 kg
Incidence: United States (2 – 10%), Australia (20%)
Age: middle-aged; M:F = 1:4
- gross hematuria
- hypertension
- renal colic (passage of renal tissue)
- renal insufficiency (2 – 10% of all end-stage renal failures)
- ANALGESIC SYNDROME: history of psychiatric therapy, abuse of alcohol + laxatives, headaches, pain in cervical + lumbar spine, peptic ulcer, anemia, splenomegaly, arteriosclerosis, premature aging
√ papillary necrosis
√ scarring of renal parenchyma ("wavy outline"); bilateral in 66%, unilateral in 5%
√ renal atrophy
√ papillary urothelial tumors in calices / pelvis (mostly TCC / squamous cell carcinoma), in 5% bilateral

ANGIOMYOLIPOMA
= RENAL HAMARTOMA = benign mesenchymal tumor
Histo: tumor composed of fat, smooth muscle, aggregates of thick-walled blood vessels
Types:
(1) Isolated AML (80%) = sporadic AML
    solitary + unilateral (in 80% on R side), NO stigmata of tuberous sclerosis; M:F = 1:2.3 – 12.5; commonly in women between 40 – 60 years of age
(2) AML associated with tuberous sclerosis (in 20%)
    in 80% of patients with tuberous sclerosis; commonly bilateral + multiple
- small lesions are asymptomatic
- acute flank / abdominal pain (due to hemorrhage)
- shock (due to massive retroperitoneal hemorrhage)
- hematuria
√ often large component of extrarenal tumor
√ calcifications (6%)
Plain film:
    √ fat lucency (in <10%)

CT:
    √ fat density (diagnostic)
US:
    √ intensely echogenic tumor (due to high fat content)
    √ less echogenic areas due to hemorrhage, necrosis, dilated calyces
MRI:
    √ variable areas of high signal intensity on T1WI (DDx: hemorrhagic cyst, solid tumor)
Angio:
    √ hypervascular mass (95%) with enlarged interlobar + interlobular feeding arteries, tortuous irregular aneurysmally dilated vessels (1/3), venous pooling, "sunburst" / "whorled" / "onion peel" appearance, no AV shunting
Cx: hemorrhagic shock from bleeding into angiomyolipoma or into retroperitoneum
DDx: renal / perirenal lipoma

ARTERIOVENOUS MALFORMATION
(1) Congenital AVM
(2) Acquired AVM: trauma, spontaneous rupture of aneurysm, very vascular malignant neoplasm
Histo:
(a) cirsoid = multiple coiled vascular channels grouped in cluster; supplied by one / more arteries; draining into one / more veins
(b) cavernous = single well-defined artery feeding into a single vein (rare)
√ large unifocal mass
√ focally attenuated and displaced collecting system
√ homogeneously enhancing mass
√ curvilinear calcification
US:
    √ tubular anechoic structure (DDx: hydronephrosis, hydrocalix)

BENIGN PROSTATIC HYPERTROPHY
Incidence: 50% between ages 51 + 60 years; 75 – 80% of all men >80 years of age
Histo: fibromyoadenomatous nodule (most common), muscular + fibromuscular + fibroadenomatous + stromal nodules
Age: initial growth onset <30 years of age; onset of clinical symptoms at 60 ± 9 years
- sensation of full bladder, nocturia
- trouble initiating micturition
- decreased urine caliber + force
- dribbling at termination of micturition

Location: transition + periurethral zone proximal to verumontanum forming "lateral lobes" (82%), "median lobe" (12%)
√ oval (61%) / round (22%) / pear-shaped (17%) enlargement of central gland
√ posterior + lateral displacement of outer gland (= prostate proper) creating cleavage plane of fibrous tissue between hyperplastic tissue + compressed prostatic tissue (= surgical capsule) often demarcated by displaced intraductal calcifications

Rx: open prostatectomy (glands >80 g), transurethral resection of prostate = TURP (glands <80 g); Δ Only 4 – 5% of patients need surgical treatment!

BLADDER CALCULI

Etiology:
1. FOREIGN BODY NIDUS CALCULI
   from self-introduced objects, bladder wall-penetrating bone fragments, prostatic chips, nonabsorbable suture material, fragments of Foley balloon catheter, pubic hair, presence of intestinal mucosa (in bladder augmentation, ileal conduit, repaired bladder exstrophy)
2. STASIS CALCULI
   in bladder outflow obstruction, vesical diverticula, lower urinary tract infection (in particular Proteus), cystocele, neuropathic bladder dysfunction
3. MIGRANT CALCULI
   = renal calculi spontaneously passing into bladder
4. IDIOPATHIC / PRIMARY / ENDEMIC CALCULI
   in North Africa, India, Indonesia; in young boys of low socioeconomic class (nutritional deficiency?)
√ single stone in 86%
Rate of recurrence after removal: 41%

BLADDER CONTUSION

= intramural hematoma
√ no extravasation
√ lack of normal distensibility
√ crescent-shaped filling defect in contrast-distended bladder

BLADDER DIVERTICULUM

= cavity formed by herniation of bladder mucosa through muscular wall, joined to the bladder cavity by a constricted neck
Etiology: (a) persistent lower urinary tract obstruction (enlarged prostate, bladder neck stenosis)
(b) congenital
Average age: 57 years; M:F = 9:1
Sites: areas of congenital weakness of muscular wall at
(a) ureteral meatus
(b) posterolateral wall (Hutch diverticulum = paraureteral)
Cx: (1) Vesical carcinoma in 0.8 – 7% secondary to chronic inflammation (average age 66 years)
(2) Ureteral obstruction
(3) Ureteral reflux

BLADDER RUPTURE

Extraperitoneal Rupture of Bladder (80%)

Cause: pelvic fracture (sharp bony spicule) or avulsion tear at fixation points of puboprostatic ligaments
Location: usually close to base of bladder anterolaterally
Plain film:
√ "pear-shaped" bladder
√ loss of obturator fat planes
√ paralytic ileus

√ upward displacement of ileal loops
Contrast examination:
√ flame-shaped contrast extravasation into perivesical fat, best seen on postvoid films, may extend into thigh / anterior abdominal wall
US:
√ "bladder within a bladder" = bladder surrounded by fluid collection

Intraperitoneal Rupture of Bladder (20%)

Causes:
(a) usually as a result of invasive procedure (cystoscopy), stab wound, surgery
(b) blunt trauma with sudden rise in intravesical pressure (requires distended bladder)
Location: usually at dome of bladder
√ contrast extravasation into paracolic gutters
√ contrast outlining small bowel loops
√ uriniferous ascites

BLADDER TUMORS

Incidence: 3% of all neoplasms; most common tumor of genitourinary tract
• painless hematuria (60%)
IVP: 70% accuracy rate

STAGING

T 1	= A	= lesions involving mucosa + submucosa
T 2	= B_1	= invasion of superficial muscle layer
T 3a	= B_2	= invasion of deep muscular wall
T 3b	= C	= invasion of perivesical fat
T 4	= D	= extension to perivesical organs (seminal vesicles, prostate, rectum)

Staging accuracy: 50% clinically; 32 – 80% for CT; 73% for MRI

Overstaging due to: edema following endoscopy / endoscopic resection, fibrosis from radiation therapy

A. EPITHELIAL TUMORS (95%)
1. Transitional cell carcinoma (95%)
   multicentric, aniline dyes
2. Squamous cell carcinoma (4%)
   worst prognosis; secondary to chronic disorders (infection, stricture, calculi), schistosomiasis, bladder diverticula
3. Adenocarcinoma (1%)
   most common in bladder exstrophy, less common in cystitis glandularis + urachal carcinoma (at dome of bladder in urachal remnant)

B. NONEPITHELIAL TUMORS
(a) <u>primary benign tumors</u>
1. Leiomyoma (most common)
   • hematuria secondary to ulceration
   Site: submucosal / intramural / subserosal
2. Rhabdomyoma (rare)
3. **Hemangioma of the bladder** (0.6%)
   Age: <20 years (in >50%), M:F = 1:1
   May be associated with   Klippel-Trénaunay syndrome

- gross painless hematuria
- cutaneous hemangiomas over abdomen, perineum, thighs in 25 – 30%
- √ compressible solitary (2/3) / multiple (1/3) masses ± phleboliths
4. Neurofibroma
   generalized neurofibromatosis in 60%
5. Nephrogenic adenoma
   Associated with   cystitis cystica / cystitis glandularis
6. Endometriosis
   on posterior wall, urinary symptoms in 80%
7. Pheochromocytoma (0.5%)
   from paraganglia of bladder wall; 7% are malignant
   - postmicturitional adrenergic attack
(b) primary malignant tumors
   1. Rhabdomyosarcoma
   2. Leiomyosarcoma
      rarely at trigone; mainly >40 years of age
   3. Primary lymphoma
      2nd most common nonepithelial tumor of urinary bladder
      Age: 40 years; M:F = 1:3
      Location: submucosal; at bladder base + trigone
(c) secondary tumors
   1. Lymphoma
      at autopsy in NHL (15%); Hodgkin disease (5%)
   2. Leukemia
      at autopsy in 22%; microscopic involvement
   3. Metastases
      1.5% of bladder malignancies; solitary / multiple nodules
      melanoma > stomach > breast > kidney > lung
   4. Direct extension (common)
      from prostate, rectum, sigmoid, cervix, ovary

CHOLESTEATOMA

= keratin ball = keratinized squamous epithelium shed into lumen
- history of UTIs
- repeated episodes of renal colic
Location: renal pelvis > upper ureter
√ mottled / stringy filling defects in collecting system
√ dilatation of pelvicaliceal system (with obstruction)
√ calcification of keratinized material possible
Δ Not a premalignant condition!

CHRONIC GLOMERULONEPHRITIS

Cause: after acute poststreptococcal glomerulonephritis
- late presentation without prior clinically apparent acute phase
- hypertension
- renal failure
√ small smooth kidneys with wasted parenchyma
√ normal papillae + calices
√ patchy nephrogram with diminished density of contrast material

√ cortical calcification (uncommon)
US:
   √ increased echogenicity
   √ small kidneys with vicarious sinus lipomatosis
Angio:
   √ marked reduction in renal blood flow + reflux of contrast material into aorta
   √ severely pruned + tortuous interlobar and arcuate arteries
   √ nonvisualization of interlobular arteries
   √ delayed contrast clearance from interlobar arteries

CLEAR CELL SARCOMA OF KIDNEY

= rare highly malignant renal tumor of childhood with predilection for bone metastasis
Incidence: up to 6% of renal tumors in children
Histo: composed of well-defined polygonal to stellate cells with vacuolization, ovoid to rounded nuclei, prominent capillary pattern + tendency toward cyst formation separated by slightly thickened septa
Age: 1 – 6 years; M:F = 1:1
- increasing abdominal girth + palpable abdominal mass
- lethargy, weight loss
- hematuria
√ expansile mass (8 – 16 cm) with dominant soft-tissue component
√ cystic component of varying size (few mm – 5 cm) + multiplicity (58%)
√ amorphous / linear calcifications (25%)
√ renal mass crossing midline (58%)
US:
   √ inhomogeneous renal mass of soft-tissue density
   √ well-defined hypoechoic central area (= necrosis)
   √ mass of fluid-filled cystic spaces
CT:
   √ inhomogeneous enhancement less than that of normal renal parenchyma
   √ low-attenuation areas (= necrosis)
   √ water-density areas (= cysts)
Prognosis: worse than Wilms tumor
DDx: cystic form of Wilms tumor, multilocular cystic nephroma, cystic dysplasia

CONGENITAL RENAL HYPOPLASIA

= miniaturization with reduction in number of renal lobes, number of calices and papillae, amount of nephrons (+ smallness of cells)
VARIANT: **Ask-Upmark kidney** = aglomerular focal hypoplasia
√ unilateral small kidney
√ decreased number of papillae + calices (5 or less)
√ hypertrophied contralateral kidney
√ absent renal artery
√ hypoplastic disorganized renal veins

CONN SYNDROME

= PRIMARY HYPERALDOSTERONISM = excess mineralocorticoid production (sodium resorption, potassium excretion)

M:F = 1:2
- hypertension (secondary to hypernatremia); responsible for 2% of all systemic hypertension
- hypokalemia + hyperkaliuria
- metabolic alkalosis
- depressed renin levels

Path:
  (a) adenoma (89%): solitary aldosteronoma (70%); multiple (13%); microadenomatosis (6%)
  (b) bilateral hyperplasia (11%): diffuse / nodular
  (c) adrenocortical carcinoma (<1%)

√ small aldosteronoma of 1.7 cm average size (range 0.5 – 3.5 cm); bilateral in 6%
√ soft-tissue density / low attenuation
√ usually hypervascular, rarely hypovascular

Adrenal venography : 76% accuracy
Adrenal venous blood sampling: 91% accuracy, 75% sensitivity
CT : 60 – 80% sensitivity

NUC:
√ I-131 NP-59 uptake following dexamethasone suppression
  √ bilateral early visualization (<5 days) implies adrenal hyperplasia
  √ unilateral early visualization implies adenoma
  √ late bilateral visualization (>5 days) may be normal

Rx: adrenalectomy for neoplasms; medical treatment for hyperplasia

CUSHING SYNDROME
= HYPERCORTISOLISM = excessive cortisol secretion
Etiology:
  A. ACTH-INDEPENDENT
    1. Exogenous cortisol
    2. Primary adrenal abnormality (20%):
      (a) primary pigmented nodular adrenocortical hyperplasia (children, young adults)
      (b) adrenocortical adenoma (10 – 20% of cases; 10% in adults, 15% in children)
      (c) adrenocortical carcinoma (5 – 10% of cases; 10% in adults, 66% in children)
  B. ACTH-DEPENDENT
    = overproduction of corticotropin with adrenal hyperplasia (in up to 85%)
    1. Exogenous ACTH
    2. Paraneoplastic ectopic ACTH production (20%): oat cell carcinoma of lung (8%), liver cancer, prostate cancer, ovarian cancer, breast cancer, carcinoid, bronchial adenoma, pancreatic islet cell tumor, medullary carcinoma of thyroid, thymoma, pheochromocytoma
    3. Cushing disease
      = CNS disease due to basophilic / chromophobe adenoma / overactive pituitary
    4. Hypothalamic dysfunction
    5. Production of corticotropin-releasing factor (rare)

Incidence: 1:1,000 autopsies; M:F = 1:4
Age: 3rd – 4th decade (highest incidence); more often following pregnancy

- central obesity, buffalo hump, moon face
- striae, acne
- impaired glucose tolerance / diabetes mellitus
- hypertension
- elevated plasma cortisol levels
- excessive excretion of urinary 17-hydroxy-corticosteroids
- dexamethasone suppression test / metyrapone test
√ retarded bone maturation
√ osteoporosis
√ excess callus formation

EPIDIDYMITIS
Acute Epididymitis
= ACUTE EPIDIDYMO-ORCHITIS
most common acute pathologic process in postpubertal age secondary to ascending infection (usually beginning as prostatitis)

Incidence: 634,000 cases/year; <10 years in 0%; 20 – 30 years in 72%
Organism: E. coli + S. aureus (85%), Gonococcus (12%), TB (2%); <35 years of age Chlamydia trachomatis + Neisseria gonorrheae; >35 years of age Escherichia coli + Proteus mirabilis; nonspecific epididymitis in 20%

- fever
- increasing pain over 1 – 2 days
- epididymal swelling + tenderness
- pyuria (95%)
- positive urine culture
- leukocytosis (50%)
- dysuria + frequency (25%)
- prostatic tenderness (infrequent)

Location: may have focal involvement as in focal epididymitis (25%), focal orchitis (10%)

US:
√ enlarged epididymis with decreased echogenicity
√ hydrocele + skin thickening

Color Duplex:
√ increased number + concentration of identifiable vessels in affected region (= hyperemia)
√ peak systolic velocity (PSV) >15 cm/s with PSV ratio >1.9 compared to normal side
√ detection of venous flow

NUC (true positive rate of 99%):
√ symmetrical perfusion of iliac + femoral vessels
√ markedly increased perfusion through spermatic cord vessels (testicular + deferential arteries)
√ curvilinear increased activity laterally in hemiscrotum on static images (also centrally if testis involved)
√ increased activity of scrotal contents on static images (hyperemia + increased capillary permeability)

Cx: (1) Focal / diffuse orchitis (20 – 40%)
    (2) Epididymal abscess (6%) / testicular abscess (6%)
    (3) Infarction (3%) from extrinsic compression of testicular blood flow
    (4) Late testicular atrophy (21%)

DDx: (1) Testicular abscess (increased perfusion with centrally decreased uptake)
(2) Hydrocele (normal perfusion, no uptake)
(3) Testicular tumor (slightly increased perfusion; in- / decreased uptake)

Chronic Epididymitis
US:
√ enlarged hyperechoic epididymis

GANGLIONEUROBLASTOMA
= tumor of sympathetic nervous system that is intermediate in cellular maturity between neuroblastoma and ganglioneuroma; metastatic potential
Incidence: less common than neuroblastoma / ganglioneuroma
Age: early childhood; M:F = 1:1
Location: posterior mediastinum, abdomen
√ extension through neural foramen into epidural space
√ nerve root / spinal cord compression

GANGLIONEUROMA
= may represent end-stage of maturation of a neuroblastoma; without metastatic potential
Histo: mature ganglion cell
Age: 2nd + 3rd decade; 60% <20 years; M:F = 1:1
Location: posterior mediastinum (43%); adrenal gland (20%)
• rarely hormone-active
√ dumbbell-shaped large mass extending from paraspinous region through neural foramen into epidural space
√ frequently calcified
DDx: neurofibroma (no calcification), schwannoma (no calcification), neuroblastoma (calcified)

HEMOLYTIC-UREMIC SYNDROME
= most common cause of acute renal failure in children requiring dialysis; characterized by thrombotic microangiopathy with typical features of DIC
Cause:
(1) Infection: enterotoxic E. coli, Shigella dysenteriea I, Streptococcus pneumoniae, Salmonella typhi, Coxsackie virus, ECHO virus, adenovirus
(2) Associated medical condition: pregnancy, SLE + other collagen vascular disease, malignancy, malignant hypertension
(3) Drugs: oral contraceptives, cyclosporine, mitomycin, 5-fluorouracil
Age: usually children <2 years
Histo: microangiopathy including endothelial swelling + thrombus formation in glomerulus + renal arterioles
CLASSIC TRIAD:
• hemolytic anemia
• thrombocytopenia
• acute renal failure
• recent bout of gastroenteritis (commonly with E. coli)
• sudden palor, irritability
• bloody diarrhea

• dyspnea (due to fluid retention, heart failure, pleural effusion)
• convulsions
• rapid rise in blood urea nitrogen level out of proportion to plasma creatinine level (= result of cell lysis)

@ Kidney (sometimes only organ involved):
√ kidneys of normal / slightly increased size
√ hyperechoic cortex
Doppler-US:
√ diastolic flow absent / reversed / reduced (= increase in resistance to flow)
√ return to normal waveforms predates return of urine output
Scintigraphy:
√ lack of renal perfusion
@ Liver: hepatomegaly, hepatitis
@ Heart: myocarditis
@ Intestines: perforation, intussusception, pseudomembranous colitis
@ Brain (up to 50%): drowsiness, personality changes, coma, hemiparesis, seizures (up to 40%)
Prognosis: complete spontaneous recovery (in 85%)

HEREDITARY CHRONIC NEPHRITIS
= ALPORT SYNDROME = probably autosomal dominant trait with presence of fat-filled macrophages ("foam cells") in the corticomedullary junction and medulla
(a) males: progressive renal insufficiency, death usually < age 50
(b) females: nonprogressive
• polyuria
• anemia
• salt wasting
• hyposthenuria
• nerve deafness
• ocular abnormalities (congenital cataracts, nystagmus, myopia, spherophakia)
• NO hypertension
√ small smooth kidneys
√ diminished density of contrast material
√ cortical calcifications

HERMAPHRODITISM
= TRUE HERMAPHRODITISM = TRUE INTERSEX
= condition characterized by presence of ovotestis
Incidence: rare (500 cases in world literature); <10% of all intersex conditions
Age: diagnosed within first 2 decades (75%)

Classification:
Class I : normal female genitalia (80%)
Class II : enlarged clitoris
Class III: partially fused labioscrotal folds
Class IV: fused labioscrotal folds
Class V : hypoplastic scrotum + penoscrotal hypospadia
Class VI: normal male genitalia

Genotype: 46,XX (>50%) / 46,XY

- inguinal hernia
- lower abdominal pain (due to endometriosis)
- lower abdominal tumor (dysgerminoma, myomatous uterus)

Reared as boy:
- cryptorchidism
- short penis
- slight degree of hypospadia
- urogenital sinus at base of penis
- penile urethra (extremely rare)
- effective spermatogenesis (rare)

Reared as girl:
- development of breasts
- hematuria (= menstruation via urogenital sinus opening)
- internal female organs + female fertility
- amenorrhea
- separate urethral + vaginal openings (uncommon)

Gonads:
ovotestis (64%): bilateral ovotestes in 20% / ovary on one side and testis on other / testis or ovary on one side and ovotestis on other

Location: in pelvis (predominantly ovarian tissue); in scrotum / inguinal region (predominantly testicular tissue)

√ ovotestis with heterogeneous appearance due to combination of testicular tissue + ovarian follicles
√ hypoplastic uterus

HYDROCELE

= collection of fluid between parietal and visceral layers of tunica vaginalis; most common type of fluid collection in scrotum

(A) PRIMARY = IDIOPATHIC HYDROCELE
without predisposing lesion as congenital defect of lymphatic drainage
(B) SECONDARY HYDROCELE
(a) inflammation (epididymitis, epididymo-orchitis)
(b) testicular tumor (in 10 – 40%)
(c) trauma / postsurgical
(d) torsion, infarction
(C) CONGENITAL HYDROCELE
= ascites in scrotum through communication with peritoneal cavity (= open processus vaginalis); may be associated with inguinal hernia
(D) INFANTILE HYDROCELE
= hydrocele with fingerlike extension into funicular process but without communication with peritoneal cavity

US:
√ anechoic, good back wall, through transmission
√ with low level echoes ± septations: hematocele / pyocele / cholesterol crystals

HYDRONEPHROSIS

A. OBSTRUCTIVE UROPATHY = HYDRONEPHROSIS
= dilatation of collecting structures without functional deficit
B. OBSTRUCTIVE NEPHROPATHY = dilatation of collecting system with renal functional impairment

US:
Grading system of hydronephrosis:
Grade 0 = homogeneous central renal sinus complex without separation
Grade 1 = separation of central sinus echoes of ovoid configuration; continuous echogenic sinus periphery; 52% predictive value for obstruction
Grade 2 = separation of central sinus echoes of rounded configuration; dilated calices connecting with renal pelvis; continuity of echogenic sinus periphery
Grade 3 = replacement of major portions of renal sinus; discontinuity of echogenic sinus periphery

False-negatives: staghorn calculus filling entire collecting system, hyperacute renal obstruction (system not yet dilated), spontaneous decompression of obstruction, fluid-depleted patient with partial obstruction
False-positives: full bladder, increased urine flow (overhydration, medications, following urography, diabetes insipidus, diuresis in nonoliguric azotemia), acute pyelonephritis, postobstructive / postsurgical dilatation, vesicoureteral reflux

Amount of collecting system dilatation depends on:
(a) duration of obstruction
(b) renal output
(c) presence of spontaneous decompression

Δ Amount of residual renal cortex is of prognostic significance!

Acute Hydronephrosis
Cause:
(1) Passage of calculus with sites of stone impaction at points of ureteral narrowing:
(a) ureterovesicle junction (70%)
(b) ureteropelvic junction
(c) crossing of iliac vessels
(2) Passage of blood clot (from carcinoma, AV malformation, trauma, anticoagulant therapy), sloughed necrotic papilla
(3) Suture on ureter
(4) Ureteral edema following instrumentation
(5) Sulfonamide crystallization in nonalkalinized urine
(6) Normal pregnancy
- pain (50%)
- urinary tract infection (36%)
- nausea + vomiting (33%)
√ normal-sized kidney with normal parenchymal thickness
√ increasingly dense nephrogram
√ delayed appearance of contrast (decreased glomerular filtration)
√ increasingly dense nephrogram over time ("obstructed nephrogram")

√ minimally dilated collecting system + ureter
√ widening of forniceal angles
√ delayed images demonstrate site of obstruction
√ vicarious contrast excretion through gallbladder (uncommon)

Cx: spontaneous urinary extravasation (0.1 – 18%) from forniceal / pelvic tear (= pyelosinus reflux)

Chronic Hydronephrosis
= most frequent cause of abdominal mass in first 6 months of life (25% of all neonatal abdominal masses)
Causes:
(a) acquired: benign + malignant tumors of the ureter; ureteral strictures; benign prostatic hyperplasia; retroperitoneal tumor / fibrosis; neurogenic bladder; cervical / prostatic carcinoma; pelvic mass (lymphoma, abscess, ovarian), urethral polyps; urethral neoplasm, acquired urethral strictures
(b) congenital

• insidious course
√ large kidney with wasted parenchyma
√ diminished nephrographic density (decreased clearance)
√ early "rim" sign (thin band of radiodensity surrounding calices)
√ delayed opacification of collecting system
√ moderate to marked widening of collecting system
√ tortuous dilated ureter
NUC:
√ photopenic area during vascular phase
√ accumulation of radionuclide tracer within hydronephrotic collecting system on delayed images
Cx: superimposed infection (= pyonephrosis)

Congenital Hydronephrosis
Mostly isolated malformation
Incidence: 1:100 – 300 births
Risk of recurrence: 2 – 3% for siblings
Age at presentation: 25% by age 1 year, 55% by age 5 years
Causes:
1. UPJ obstruction (22 – 67%)
2. Posterior urethral valves (18%)
3. Ectopic ureterocele (14%)
4. Prune belly syndrome (12%)
5. Ureteral + UVJ obstruction (8%)
6. Others: severe vesicoureteral reflux, bladder neck obstruction, hypertrophy of verumontanum, urethral diverticulum, congenital urethral strictures, anterior urethral valves, meatal stenosis
May be associated with: Down syndrome (17 – 25%)
• palpable abdominal mass
• intermittent flank + periumbilical pain
• failure to thrive
• vomiting
• hematuria, infection

Location: 70% unilateral
OB-US:
√ AP diameter of renal pelvis ≥4 mm between 14 – 32 weeks, ≥7 mm after 32 weeks
√ caliceal distension communicating with renal pelvis
Δ Postnatal evaluation after 4 – 7 days of age!

Prognosis: parenchymal atrophy + renal impairment (dependent on severity + duration)

Focal Hydronephrosis
= HYDROCALICOSIS = HYDROCALYX = obstructed drainage of one portion of kidney
Causes: (1) Congenital: partial / complete duplication
(2) Infectious stricture: eg, TB
(3) Infundibular calculus
(4) Tumor
(5) Trauma
√ unifocal mass, commonly in upper pole
√ absent polar group of calices (early)
√ dilated polar group (late) with displacement of adjacent calices
√ delayed opacification in obstructed group
√ focally replaced nephrogram
US:
√ anechoic cystic lesion with smooth margins
CT:
√ focal area of water density with smooth margin and thick wall

JUXTAGLOMERULAR TUMOR
= RENINOMA = rare tumor arising from renin-producing juxtaglomerular cells
Age: mean age of 31 years; M<F
Path: small foci of hemorrhage + pseudocapsule
• hypertension
• moderate to severe headaches
• polydypsia, polyuria, enuresis

Location: just beneath renal capsule
√ renal mass of usually 2 – 3 cm in size
US:
√ echogenic mass ± areas of necrosis / hemorrhage
CT:
√ isodense tumor on NECT, hypodense on CECT
Angio:
√ angiographically hypovascular tumor
√ renal venous blood sampling yields high renin level
Dx: combination of elevated renin without renal arterial lesion + hypovascular solid renal mass

LEUKEMIA
Δ Most common malignant cause of bilateral global renal enlargement!
Incidence: renal involvement in 63% of autopsies
(a) Diffuse involvement:
leukemic cells infiltrate the interstitial tissue; tubules are replaced (more common in lymphocytic than in granulocytic forms); no relationship to peripheral white blood cell count

(b) Focal involvement:
   rarely cause for unifocal renal mass: chloroma, myeloblastoma, myeloblastic sarcoma
- renal impairment (from leukemic infiltrate, hyperuricemia, septicemia, hemorrhage)
- hypertension
- √ large smooth kidneys bilaterally
- √ normal or diminished density on nephrogram
- √ occasionally attenuated collecting system with nonopaque filling defects (clot, uric acid)
- √ retroperitoneal lymphadenopathy

US:
   √ loss of definition + distortion of central sinus complex
   √ normal to increased coarse echoes throughout renal cortex + preservation of renal medullae
   √ single / multiple focal anechoic masses

DDx: Hodgkin disease, malignant lymphoma, multiple myeloma

LEUKOPLAKIA
= KERATINIZING SQUAMOUS METAPLASIA / DYSPLASIA = DYSKERATOSIS
Cause: chronic infection (80%) / stones (40%)
Histo: large confluent areas / scattered patches of squamous metaplasia of transitional cell epithelium with keratinization + cellular atypia in deeper layers
Peak age: 4th – 5th decade;
   M:F = 1:1 (with involvement of renal pelvis)
   M:F = 4:1 (with involvement of bladder)
Location: bladder > renal pelvis > ureter; bilateral in 10%
- hematuria (30%)
- recurrent UTIs
- pathognomonic passage of gritty flakes, soft tissue stones, white chunks of tissue (desquamated keratinized epithelial layers) leading to colic, fever, chills
- √ corrugated / striated irregularities of pelvocalyceal walls, localized / generalized
- √ plaquelike intraluminal mass with "onion skin" pattern of contrast material in interstices
- √ caliectasis + pyelectasis common (with obstruction)
- √ ridging / filling defects of ureter
- √ associated with calculi in 25 – 50%

Cx: premalignant condition for epidermoid carcinoma in 12% (controversial!)

LOBAR NEPHRONIA
= ACUTE FOCAL BACTERIAL NEPHRITIS = focal variant of acute pyelonephritis with single / multiple areas of suppuration + necrosis
Organisms: E. coli > Proteus > Klebsiella
Predisposed:
   patients with altered host resistance (diabetes [60%], immunosuppression), chronic catheterization, mechanical / functional obstruction, trauma
- fever, flank pain, pyuria
- √ focal area of absent nephrogram / distorted pyelogram
- √ renal arteries displaced, renal veins compressed
- √ hypoechoic mass with ill-defined margins and disruption of corticomedullary border, NO fluid collection

√ low attenuation zone with poorly defined transition to surrounding parenchyma
√ Ga-67 uptake
√ vesicoureteral reflux often present
Cx: scarring, abscess

LOCALIZED CYSTIC DISEASE
= multiple simple cysts involving only one portion of the kidney
- no family history
Histo: dilated ducts and tubules varying in size from mm to several cm
Prognosis: not progressive

LYMPHOMA
Incidence: in 2.7 – 6% renal involvement
Types:
   (1) NON-HODGKIN LYMPHOMA
       renal involvement detected in 5% of abdominal CT, in 33 – 65% of autopsies; occurs usually late in disease
   (2) HODGKIN LYMPHOMA
       renal involvement in 13% of autopsies
Patterns of involvement:
   (a) primary renal lymphoma (very rare)
   (b) hematogenous dissemination: uni- / bilateral
       — single / multiple foci
       — diffuse infiltration
   (c) direct extension from adjacent pararenal lymphomatous disease, usually extranodal
- clinically silent (50%)
- flank pain, mass, weight loss
- hematuria
- compromise of renal function (urinary tract obstruction, renal vein compression, diffuse infiltration of kidney, superimposed infarct)
- √ unilateral:bilateral = 3:1
- √ multiple nodular masses (29 – 61%)
- √ invasion from retroperitoneal disease (11%)
- √ single bulky tumor (7%), small solitary tumor (7 – 48%)
- √ diffuse infiltration (6 – 19%), microscopic infiltration (7%)
- √ neovascularity, encasement, vascular displacement (occasionally palisade-like configuration)

US:
   √ single / multiple anechoic / hypoechoic masses
   √ renal enlargement + decreased parenchymal echoes

MALAKOPLAKIA
= uncommon chronic inflammatory response to Gram-negative infection
Organism: E. coli (in 94%); diabetes mellitus predisposes
Histo: submucosal histiocytic granulomas containing large foamy mononuclear cells (Hansemann macrophages) with intracytoplasmatic basophilic PAS-positive inclusion bodies (Michaelis-Gutmann bodies) consisting of incompletely destroyed E. coli bacterium surrounded by lipoprotein membranes
Peak age: 5th – 7th decade; M:F = 1:4

- hematuria
- raised yellow lesion <3 cm in diameter

Location: bladder > lower 2/3 of ureter > upper ureter > renal pelvis; multifocal in 75%; bilateral in 50%

√ multiple dome-shaped smooth mural filling defects
√ scalloped appearance if lesions confluent
√ generalized pelviureteral dilatation (if obstructive)
√ displacement of pelvocaliceal system + distorted central sinus complex
√ multifocal parenchymal masses may cause diminished / absent nephrogram

DDx: pyeloureteritis cystica

MALPOSITIONED TESTIS

= MALDESCENDED TESTIS

testes are normally within scrotum by 28 – 32 weeks MA

Incidence: at birth in 10% (in babies >2,500 g in 3.4%; in premature babies in 30%); by 3 – 4 months in 0.8%; at puberty in 0.2 – 0.8%

1. **Pseudocryptorchidism**

= RETRACTILE TESTIS = unusually spastic cremasteric muscle

2. **Cryptorchidism**

= arrested descent of testis along its normal course bilateral in 10%, anorchia in 3 – 5%

Location: high scrotal, inguinal canal, abdomen (20%)

3. **Ectopia testis**

= deviation from the usual pathway

Location: interstitial (on oblique muscle), pubopenile, perineal, femoral triangle

Cx: (1) Sterility
         (2) Malignancy: most commonly seminoma, 48 x risk, 4 – 11% of all testicular tumors found in cryptorchidism
         (3) Torsion: 10 x risk in cryptorchidism

Test sensitivity:
US   : 20 – 88% (DDx: lymph node)
CT   : 95%
Venography : 50 – 90%

MECKEL-GRUBER SYNDROME

= autosomal recessive disease characterized by occipital encephalocele, polycystic kidneys, polydactyly

Incidence: 1:12,000 – 50,000; more common among Yemenite Jews

Risk of recurrence: 25%; carrier frequency of 1:56

- history of affected siblings

OB-US:
√ large polycystic kidneys containing 2 – 10 mm cysts
√ occipital encephalocele
√ postaxial polydactyly
√ microcephaly
√ cleft lip and palate
√ moderate-to-severe oligohydramnios (onset midtrimester)
√ inability to visualize urine within fetal bladder

OB management:
1. Chromosomal analysis to exclude trisomy 13 (if no prior family history)
2. Option of pregnancy termination <24 weeks GA
3. Nonintervention for fetal distress >24 weeks GA

Prognosis: invariably fatal at birth due to pulmonary hypoplasia + renal failure

DDx: trisomy 13

MEDULLARY CYSTIC DISEASE

= NEPHRONOPHTHISIS

Histo:
variable number of medullary cysts (100 µ to 2 cm) + progressive periglomerular and interstitial fibrosis + tubular atrophy with dilatation of some proximal tubules

Types:
(1) <u>MEDULLARY CYSTIC DISEASE</u> = ADULT ONSET
autosomal dominant, in young adults, rapidly progressive course with uremia + death in 2 years
(2) <u>JUVENILE NEPHRONOPHTHISIS</u> = JUVENILE ONSET
autosomal recessive, in children 3 – 5 years, average duration of 10 years before uremia and death occurs

- salt-wasting, polyuria, hyposthenuria, polydypsia
- failure to thrive, growth retardation (in early teens)
- uremia, severe anemia, normal sediment, hypertension (only in late phase)

√ bilateral normal / small kidneys with smooth contour + thin cortex

IVP:
√ poor opacification of renal collecting system
√ "medullary nephrogram" = medullary striations persistent for up to 2 hours; occasionally replaced by sharply defined multiple thin-walled lucencies

Retrograde pyelogram:
√ communication between collecting system + cysts

US / CT:
√ increased parenchymal echogenicity + loss of corticomedullary junction
√ multiple small medullary / corticomedullary cysts

MEDULLARY SPONGE KIDNEY

= dysplastic cystic dilatation of papillary + medullary portions of collecting ducts (first few generations of metanephric duct branchings)

Incidence: 0.5%

Age: young to middle-aged adults; sporadic

May be associated with: Ehlers-Danlos syndrome, parathyroid adenoma, Caroli disease

- often asymptomatic

√ medullary nephrocalcinosis (40 – 80%) with one / more calculi up to 5 mm
√ "bunch of flowers" = thick dense streaks of contrast material radiating from pyramids peripherally representing papillary cysts / ectatic ducts (DDx: dense papillary blush in normals)
√ may be unilateral in 25%
√ may involve only one pyramid / all pyramids (25%)

Cx: urolithiasis, hematuria, infection

DDx:
(1) Normal variant ("papillary blush" without distinct streaks / nephrocalcinosis / pyramidal enlargement)
(2) Renal tuberculosis (larger more irregular calcifications + cavitations + strictures + ulcerations)
(3) Papillary necrosis (sloughed papilla + caliceal ring sign)
(4) Medullary nephrocalcinosis (no ectatic ducts / cysts, calcifications beyond pyramids)
(5) Juvenile polycystic kidney disease (bilateral renal enlargement + hepatic periportal fibrosis)
(6) Caliceal diverticulum (small, solitary, located between pyramid)

MEGACALICOSIS

= CONGENITAL MEGACALICES = nonprogressive caliceal dilatation caused by hypoplastic medullary pyramids
Age: any age;   M >> F
May be associated with   primary megaureter
• normal glomerular filtration rate
Site: entire kidney / part of kidney; unilateral / bilateral
√ kidney usually enlarged with prominent fetal lobation
√ reduced parenchymal thickness (medulla affected, NOT cortex)
√ mosaic-like arrangement of dilated calices (polygonal + faceted appearance, NOT globular as in obstruction)
√ increased number of calices
√ ABSENT caliceal cupping (semilunar instead of pyramidal configuration of papillae)
√ NO dilatation of pelvis / ureters, NORMAL contrast excretion
Cx: (1) Hematuria (2) Stone formation

MEGACYSTIS-MICROCOLON SYNDROME

= MEGACYSTIS-MICROCOLON-INTESTINAL HYPOPERISTALSIS SYNDROME (MMIH)
= functional obstruction of bladder + colon characterized by
(1) Enlarged urinary bladder
(2) Small colon
(3) Strikingly short small intestine suspended on a primitive dorsal mesentery
(4) Markedly enlarged hydronephrotic kidneys with little remaining parenchyma
Incidence: 26 cases reported;   predominantly in females
May be associated with: diaphragmatic hernia, PDA, teeth at birth
• distended abdomen (large bladder + dilated small bowel loops)
• intestinal pseudo-obstruction (NO peristaltic activity)

OB-US:
√ polyhydramnios (in spite of dilated bladder) / normal amount of amniotic fluid
√ megacystis
√ bilateral hydroureteronephrosis
√ female sex

BE:
√ microcolon (transient feature of narrow rectum + sigmoid)
√ malrotation / malfixation or foreshortening of small bowel
VCUG
√ distended unobstructed bladder
Prognosis: lethal in most cases

MEGALOURETER

= CONGENITAL PRIMARY MEGAURETER = TERMINAL URETERECTASIS = ACHALASIA OF URETER
= intrinsic congenital dilatation of lower juxtavesical orthotopic ureter
Cause: aperistaltic juxtavesical (1.5 cm long) segment secondary to faulty development of muscle layers of ureter (functional, NOT mechanical obstruction)
Incidence: all ages; M:F = 2:1
Associated disorders (in 40%):
(a) contralateral: UPJ obstruction, reflux, ureterocele, ureteral duplication, renal ectopia, renal agenesis
(b) ipsilateral: caliceal diverticulum, megacalicosis, papillary necrosis
• asymptomatic (mostly)
• pain
• abdominal mass
• hematuria
• infection

Location: L:R = 3:1, bilateral in 20 – 40%
√ prominent localized dilatation of pelvic ureter (up to 5 cm in diameter) usually not progressive, but may involve entire ureter + collecting system
√ vigorous non-propulsive to-and-fro motion in dilated segment
√ functional smoothly tapered narrowing of intravesical ureter
√ NO reflux, NO stenosis

MESOBLASTIC NEPHROMA

= FETAL RENAL HAMARTOMA = BENIGN CONGENITAL WILMS TUMOR = BENIGN FETAL HAMARTOMA = FETAL MESENCHYMAL TUMOR = LEIOMYOMATOUS HAMARTOMA = CONGENITAL FIBROSARCOMA = FIBROMYXOMA
= nonfamilial benign fibromyomatoid mass arising from renal connective tissue
Incidence: most common renal neoplasm in neonate; 3% of all renal neoplasms in children
Age: 3 months mean age at presentation; may occasionally go undetected until adulthood; M > F
Histo: smooth muscle cells + immature fibroblasts + islands of embryonic glomeruli, tubules, vessels, hematopoietic cells, cartilage
In 14% associated with   prematurity, polyhydramnios, GI + GU tract malformations, neuroblastoma
• large flank mass
• hematuria (20%) / hypertension (4%), anemia

√ usually replaces 60 – 90% of renal parenchyma
√ may produce multiple cystic spaces
√ NO sharp cleavage plane towards normal parenchyma, may extend beyond capsule
√ calcifications (rare)
√ NO venous extension (DDx from Wilms tumor)
IVP:
  √ large noncalcified renal mass with distortion of collecting system
  √ usually NO herniation into renal pelvis (DDx from MLCN)
US:
  √ evenly echogenic tumor with concentric echogenic + hypoechoic rings resembling uterine fibroids
  √ complex mass with hemorrhage + cyst formation + necrosis
Angio:
  √ hypervascular mass with neovascularity + displacement of adjacent vessels
Cx: transformation to metastasizing spindle cell sarcoma (rare)
Rx: complete resection
Prognosis: excellent

METASTASES TO KIDNEY

Δ Most common malignant tumor of the kidney (2 x as frequent as primaries)!
most common primaries: bronchus, breast, non-Hodgkin lymphoma, stomach
less common primaries: chloroma, myeloblastoma, myeloblastic sarcoma, melanoma, osteogenic sarcoma, choriocarcinoma (10 – 50% incidence), Hodgkin lymphoma, rhabdomyosarcoma

MULTICYSTIC DYSPLASTIC KIDNEY

= MULTICYSTIC DYSGENETIC KIDNEY (MCDK)
= MULTICYSTIC KIDNEY (MCK) = Potter Type II
Δ Second most common cause of an abdominal mass in neonate (after hydronephrosis)!
Δ Most common form of cystic disease in infants!
Incidence: 1:10,000 (for bilateral MCDK); M:F = 2:1 (for unilateral MCDK); more common among infants of diabetic mothers
Risk of recurrence: 2 – 3%
Etiology: (sporadic)
extrarenal obstruction / atresia <8 – 10 weeks of fetal life leads to aberrant development of collecting ducts and tubules + failure of development of nephrons + cystic expansion of abnormal tubules (after 20 weeks of MA)
Histo: immature glomeruli + tubules reduced in number + whorling mesenchymal tissue, cartilage (33%), cysts
Associated with renal anomalies of contralateral side in 30 – 50%:
  (1) Ureteropelvic junction obstruction (7 – 27%)
  (2) Horseshoe kidney (5 – 9%)
  (3) Ureteral anomalies (5%)
  (4) Renal hypoplasia (4%)
  (5) Vesicoureteral reflux

  (6) Malrotation
Fatal form: bilateral MCDK (4.5 – 21%), contralateral renal agenesis (0 – 11%)

• abdominal mass
• asymptomatic if unilateral (may go undetected until adulthood)
• recurrent urinary tract infections, intermittent abdominal pain, nausea + vomiting, hematuria, failure to thrive
• fatal due to pulmonary hypoplasia if bilateral

Location:
  1. UNILATERAL multicystic dysplastic kidney
    most common form (80 – 90%); L:R = 2:1 secondary to pelvoinfundibular atresia
  2. SEGMENTAL / focal renal dysplasia
    = "multilocular cyst" secondary to
      (a) high-grade obstruction of upper pole moiety in duplex kidney from ectopic ureterocele
      (b) single obstructed infundibulum
  3. BILATERAL cystic dysplasia
    in the presence of severe obstruction in utero from posterior urethral valves / urethral atresia with oligohydramnios + pulmonary hypoplasia

Types:
  (1) MULTICYSTIC KIDNEY (Potter IIa)
    √ large kidney with multiple large cysts + little visible renal parenchyma
  (2) HYPOPLASTIC / DIMINUTIVE FORM (Potter IIb)
    √ echogenic small kidney

APPEARANCE RELATED TO SITE OF OBSTRUCTION
  @ ureteropelvic junction
    √ single / several large / multiple medium-sized cysts in large kidney
  @ distal ureter / urethra
    √ small / no cysts in small kidney

APPEARANCE RELATED TO TIME OF INSULT
  (a) early onset between 8th – 11th week
    √ small / atretic renal pelvis + calices
    √ 10 – 20 cysts + loss of reniform appearance
  (b) late onset = HYDRONEPHROTIC FORM
    √ large central cyst (= dilated pelvis) often communicating with cysts
    √ some renal function may be demonstrated

√ large kidney with lobulated contour in infancy
√ incidental finding of small kidney in adults (secondary to arrested growth)
√ ipsilateral atretic ureter
√ contralateral renal hypertrophy
√ calcification: curvilinear / ringlike in wall of cysts in 30% of adults, rarely in children
IVP + NUC:
  Δ NUC preferred over IVP in first month of life as concentrating ability of even normal neonatal kidneys is suboptimal!
  √ no function (rarely faint contrast accumulation)

US:
- √ normal renal architecture replaced
- √ random cysts of varying shape + size ("cluster of grapes") with largest cyst in peripheral nonmedial location (100% accurate)
- √ cysts separated by septa (100% accurate)
- √ central sinus complex absent (100% accurate)
- √ no communication between multiple cysts (93% accurate)
- √ no identification of parenchymal rim or corticomedullary differentiation (74% accurate)
- √ cysts begin to disappear in infancy
- √ kidney may be small + atrophic (as little as 1 g) / normal / large
- √ oligohydramnios in bilateral MCDK / unilateral MCKD + contralateral urinary obstruction

Angio:
- √ absent / hypoplastic renal artery; angiography unnecessary since a DDx to long-standing functionless kidney is not possible

OB-management:
- (1) Routine antenatal care + evaluation by pediatric urologist following delivery if unilateral
- (2) Option of pregnancy termination if ≤24 weeks GA
- (3) Nonintervention for fetal distress if >24 weeks GA

Cx: (1) Renin-dependent hypertension (rare)
            (2) Malignancy in <1:330
DDx: hydronephrosis

MULTILOCULAR CYSTIC NEPHROMA

= MLCN = PERLMANN TUMOR = MULTILOCULAR RENAL CYST = CYSTIC NEPHROMA = CYSTIC ADENOMA / HAMARTOMA / LYMPHANGIOMA = CYSTIC / POLYCYSTIC NEPHROBLASTOMA = PARTIALLY POLYCYSTIC KIDNEY = WELL-DIFFERENTIATED POLYCYSTIC WILMS TUMOR

= rare nonhereditary benign neoplasm originating from metanephric blastema with malignant potential (same common ancestor cell line as nephroblastoma)

Histo: undifferentiated mesenchymal and primitive glomerulotubular elements

Age: biphasic age + sex distribution: <4 years in 73% male, >4 years in 89% female; boys 3 months to 4 years (peak 3 – 24 months) + women 4 – 8th decade (peak 50 – 60 years)

- commonly asymptomatic
- hematuria

- √ unilateral unifocal well-circumscribed mass (characteristic) usually in lower pole
- √ cluster of noncommunicating cysts of various sizes separated by thick septa
- √ tortuous fine vessels coursing through septa
- √ thick fibrous capsule
- √ calcifications (uncommon): peripheral / nonperipheral; curvilinear to flocculent
- √ gelatinous fluid

IVP:
- √ distortion of calices / hydronephrosis secondary to nonfunctional mass

- √ often herniation into renal pelvis

US:
- √ cluster of cysts separated by thick septa (SUGGESTIVE PATTERN)
- √ occasionally solid character (finely cystic structure with jelly-like contents + solid components)

Cx: development into nephroblastoma (in infants) / sarcoma (in older patients)
Rx: nephrectomy

MULTIPLE MYELOMA

Δ Administration of contrast material poses potential hazards!

Δ It is essential that dehydration is avoided!

Impairment of renal function:
- (1) Precipitation of abnormal proteins into tubule lumen (30 – 50%)
- (2) Toxicity of Bence-Jones proteins on tubules
- (3) Impaired renal blood flow secondary to increased blood viscosity
- (4) Amyloidosis
- (5) Nephrocalcinosis from hypercalcemia

- Tamm-Horsfall proteinuria (tubular cell secretion)
- √ smooth normal to large kidneys (initially), become small with time
- √ occasionally attenuated pelvo-infundibulo-caliceal system
- √ normal to diminished contrast material density; increasingly dense in acute oliguric failure

US:
- √ normal to increased echogenicity

NUC in bone scintigraphy:
- √ non-specific increased parenchymal activity

MYCETOMA

= FUNGUS BALL

Organism: typically Candida, Aspergillus, Mucor, Cryptococcus, Phycomycetes, Actinomycetes mostly mycelial (M-form) or occasionally yeast cells (Y-form)

Predisposed: diabetics, debilitating illness, prolonged antibiotic therapy, leukemia, lymphoma, thymoma, immunosuppression

- flank pain, passing of tissue, hematuria (extremely rare)
- renal candidiasis associated with candidemia
- Candida cystitis preceded by vaginal candidiasis

- √ unilateral nonvisualization of kidney (most frequent)
- √ large irregular filling defect extending into dilated calices (retrograde contrast study)
- √ necrotizing papillitis from Candida nephritis (common)
- √ lacelike pattern (on antegrade contrast study)

NEPHROBLASTOMATOSIS

= persistent metanephrogenic blastema as a potential precursor of Wilms tumor; primitive renal tissue normally present up to 36 weeks gestational age

Incidence: in 12 – 33% of kidneys with single and 100% of kidneys with bilateral Wilms tumor

Age: neonatal period, infancy, childhood

Associated with:
    hemihypertrophy, sporadic aniridia, Klippel-Trenaunay
    syndrome, Beckwith-Wiedemann syndrome,
    pseudohermaphroditism, splenic agenesis with hepatic
    malformation
√ kidneys may be enlarged
√ deformity of pelvocaliceal system
US:
    √ subtle subcapsular hypoechoic nodules / cysts
    √ nephromegaly with decreased parenchymal echoes
CT:
    √ hypodense subcapsular nodules after contrast
      enhancement

NEPHROGENIC ADENOMA

= uncommon benign metaplastic response to urothelial
    injury / prolonged irritation
Cause: (a) trauma: accident, surgery, instrumentation,
               renal transplantation
           (b) irritation: calculi, chronic infection
Age: 3 weeks – 83 years; M:F = 3:1 (more common in
           females <20 years of age)
Path: discrete raised papillary / polypoid areas
           projecting from epithelial surface
Histo: variable number of small tubules + cysts +
           papillae lined with a single layer of cuboidal / low
           columnar cells
• hematuria, dysuria
• asymptomatic
Location: bladder (72%), renal pelvis, ureter, urethra;
           strong correlation between location + site of
           insult to urothelium
√ filling defect
Rx: resection / fulguration
DDx: inflammatory / malignant urothelial lesions

NEUROBLASTOMA

Most common solid abdominal mass of infancy (12.3% of
all perinatal neoplasms), 3rd most common malignant
tumor in infancy (after leukemia + CNS tumors), 2nd most
common tumor in childhood (Wilms tumor more common
in older children), 7% of all childhood cancers; 15% of
cancer deaths in children
Incidence: 1:7,100 to 1:10,000 livebirths; 500 cases per
               year in USA; 20% hereditary
Origin: neural crest
Path: round irregular lobulated mass of 50 – 150 g with
              areas of hemorrhage + necrosis
Histo: small round cells slightly larger than lymphocytes
              with scant cytoplasm; Horner-Wright rosettes
              = one / two layers of neuroblasts surrounding a
              central zone of tangled neurofibrillary processes
Age: 25% during 1st year; 50% <2 years; 75% in <4
              years; 90% in <8 years; occasionally present at
              birth; M:F = 1:1
May be associated with aganglionosis of bowel, CHD
• pain + fever (30%)
• palpable abdominal mass (45 – 54%)
• bone pain, limp, inability to walk (20%)
• myoclonus of trunk + extremities

• cerebellar ataxia, nystagmus (20%)
• opsoclonus = spontaneous conjugate + chaotic eye
  movements (sign of cerebellar disease)
• orbital ecchymosis / proptosis (12%)
• intractable diarrhea (9%) due to increase in vasoactive
  intestinal polypeptides (VIP)
• increased catecholamine production (75 – 90%):
  in 95% excreted in urine as vanillylmandelic acid (VMA)
  / homovanillic acid (HVA)
• hypertension (up to 30%)
• acute cerebellar encephalopathy
• paroxysmal episodes of flushing, tachycardia,
  headaches, sweating
• rise in body temperature
• hyperglycemia

Stages
I   limited to organ of origin
II   regional spread not crossing midline
III   extension across midline
IV   metastatic to distant lymph nodes, liver, bone,
       brain, lung
IVs   stages I + II with disease confined to liver, skin,
       bone marrow WITHOUT radiographic evidence
       of skeletal metastases
Metastases:
    bone (60%), regional lymph nodes (42%), orbit (20%),
    liver (15%), intracranial (14%), lung (10%)
    Δ Metastases are first manifestation in up to 60%!
    Hutchinson syndrome
        (1) primary adrenal neuroblastoma (2) extensive
        skeletal metastases, particularly skull (3) proptosis
        (4) bone pain
    Pepper syndrome
        (1) primary adrenal neuroblastoma (2) massive
        hepatomegaly from metastases
    Blueberry muffin syndrome
        (1) primary adrenal neuroblastoma (2) multiple
        metastatic skin lesions
    Δ Bone marrow aspirate positive in 50 – 70% at time of
    initial diagnosis!
    Δ 2/3 of patients >2 years have disseminated disease!

@ Skeletal metastases:
    √ periosteal reaction
    √ osteolytic focus / multicentric lytic lesions
    √ lucent horizontal metaphyseal line
    √ vertical linear radiolucent streaks in
      metadiaphysis of long bones
    √ pathologic fracture
    √ vertebral collapse
    √ widened cranial sutures (subjacent dural
      metastases)
    √ sclerotic lesions with healing
    DDx: Ewing sarcoma, rhabdomyosarcoma,
            leukemia, lymphoma
@ Intracranial + maxillofacial metastases:
    Site: dura, brain substance
@ Pulmonary metastases:
    √ nodular infiltrates

√ rib erosion
√ mediastinal + retrocrural lymphadenopathy (common)
Location: anywhere within sympathetic neural chain
@ abdomen
  (a) adrenal (36%): almost always unilateral
  (b) both adrenals (7 – 10%)
  (c) extraadrenal in sympathetic chain (18%)
@ thorax + posterior mediastinum (14%): aortic bodies
@ neck (5%): carotid ganglia
@ pelvis (5%): organ of Zuckerkandl
@ skull / esthesioneuroblastoma of olfactory bulb, cerebellum, cerebrum (2%)
@ other sites (10%): eg, intrarenal (very rare)
@ unknown (10%)
√ large suprarenal mass with irregular shape + margins (82%)
√ heterogeneous texture with low density areas from hemorrhage + necrosis (55%)
√ stippled / coarse calcifications (36 – 70%)
√ "drooping lily" sign = displacement of kidney inferolaterally without distortion of collecting system
√ hydronephrosis (24%)
√ inseparable from kidney ± invasion of kidney (32%)
√ propensity for extension into spinal canal through neural foramen with erosion of pedicles (15%)
√ extension across midline (55%) (DDx: Wilms tumor)
√ retroperitoneal adenopathy / contiguous extension (73%)
√ retrocrural adenopathy (27%)
√ encasement of IVC + aorta, celiac axis, SMA (32%)
√ caval involvement = indicator of unresectability
√ liver metastases (18 – 66%); invasion of liver (5%)
Angio:
  √ hypo- / hypervascular mass
US:
  √ hyper- / hypoechoic mass with acoustic shadows
NUC:
  √ focal uptake of I-131 / I-123 MIBG radioactivity (82% sensitivity; 88% specificity)
  √ tracer uptake on bone scan (60%)
OB-US:
  • maternal symptoms of catecholamine excess
  √ mixed cystic + solid mass in adrenal region
  √ may exhibit acoustic shadowing (calcifications)
  √ hydrops fetalis (severe anemia secondary to metastases to bone marrow, mechanical compression of IVC, hypersecretion of aldosterone)

2-year survival rate versus age at presentation:
  60% if patient's age   <1 year
  20% if patient's age   1 – 2 years
  10% if patient's age   >2 years
  Δ May revert to benign ganglioneuroma in 0.2%!
Survival rate versus stage:
  80% for stage I
  60% for stage II
  30% for stage III
  7% for stage IV
  75 – 87% for stage IVs

DDx: exophytic Wilms tumor, mesoblastic nephroma, multicystic kidney, retroperitoneal teratoma, adrenal hemorrhage, hepatic hamartoma / hemangioma, infradiaphragmatic sequestration

NEUROGENIC BLADDER
Neuroanatomy: bladder innervation of detrusor muscle by parasympathetic nerves S2 – S4
Etiology: congenital (myelomeningocele); trauma; neoplasm (spinal, CNS); infection (herpes, polio); inflammation (multiple sclerosis, syrinx); systemic disorder (diabetes, pernicious anemia)
A. SPASTIC BLADDER
  "upper motor neuron" lesion above conus
B. ATONIC BLADDER
  "lower motor neuron lesion" below conus

ONCOCYTOMA
= PROXIMAL TUBULAR ADENOMA = BENIGN OXYPHILIC ADENOMA
Incidence: 2 – 14% of renal tumors
Age: middle- to old-aged subjects; M:F = 1.7:1
Path:
  well-encapsulated tan-colored tumor of well-differentiated proximal tubular cells (benign adenoma) + oncocytes = large eosinophilic / oxophilic cells (granular eosinophilic cytoplasm with large number of mitochondria); similar tumors seen in thyroid, parathyroid, salivary glands, adrenals; pathologic diagnosis requires entire tumor because well-differentiated renal cell carcinoma may have oncocytic features
√ renal mass of 6 cm average size (0.3 – 26 cm)
√ tumor of homogeneous low attenuation / hypoechogenicity (>50%)
√ well-demarcated with pseudocapsule
√ central stellate scar in 30% (in lesions >3 cm only due to organization of central infarction + hemorrhage after tumor growth has outstripped blood supply)
Angio:
  √ spoke-wheel configuration (80%), homogeneous parenchymal phase (71%)
Tc-99m DMSA:
  √ photopenic area (tubular cells do not function normally)
Rx: local resection / heminephrectomy

PAGE KIDNEY
= renin-angiotensin mediated hypertension caused by renal compression in a perinephric / subcapsular location
Etiology: (1) Spontaneous hematoma (most common) (2) Blunt trauma (3) Cyst (4) Tumor

√ stretching + splaying of intrarenal vessels
√ slow arterial washout
√ distortion of renal contour + thinning of renal parenchyma
√ enlarged + displaced capsular artery

PAPILLARY NECROSIS

= NECROTIZING PAPILLITIS = ischemic necrobiosis of medulla (loops of Henle + vasa recta) secondary to interstitial nephritis (interstitial edema) or intrinsic vascular obstruction

Cause:

mnemonic: "POSTCARD"

Pyelonephritis
Obstructive uropathy
Sickle cell disease
Tuberculosis, **T**rauma
Cirrhosis = alcoholism, **C**oagulopathy
Analgesic nephropathy
Renal vein thrombosis
Diabetes mellitus

also: dehydration, severe infantile diarrhea, hemophilia, Christmas disease, acute tubular necrosis, transplant rejection, postpartum state, high-dose urography, intravesical instillation of formalin, thyroid cancer

Types:
1. Necrosis in situ = necrotic papilla detaches but remains unextruded within its bed
2. Medullary type (partial papillary slough) = single irregular cavity located concentric / eccentric in papilla with long axis paralleling the long axis of the papilla + communicating with calyx
3. Papillary type (total papillary slough)

Phases:
(1) Enlargement of papilla (papillary swelling)
(2) Fine projections of contrast material alongside papilla (tract formation)
(3) Medullary cavitation / complete slough of papilla
- flank pain, dysuria, fever, chills
- ureteral colic, hematuria
- acute oliguric renal failure
- hypertension
- proteinuria, pyuria, hematuria, leukocytosis

Location:
(a) localized / diffuse
(b) bilateral distribution (systemic cause)
(c) unilateral (obstruction, renal vein thrombosis, acute bacterial nephritis)
√ normal or small kidney (analgesic nephropathy) / large kidney (acute fulminant)
√ smooth / wavy renal contour (analgesic nephropathy)
√ diminished density of contrast material in nephrogram; rarely increasingly dense
√ wasted parenchymal thickness
√ widened fornix (necrotic shrinkage)
√ club-shaped calyx (detached papilla)
√ displaced collecting system (enlarged septal cortex from edema)
√ intraluminal filling defect (sloughed papilla)
√ calcifications: papillary / curvilinear / ringlike (attached papilla)
US: √ multiple round / triangular cystic spaces in medulla with echo reflections of arcuate arteries at periphery of cystic spaces

Cx: higher incidence of transitional cell carcinoma in analgesic abusers (8 x); higher incidence of squamous cell carcinoma
DDx: (1) Postobstructive renal atrophy
        (2) Congenital megacalices (normal renal function)

PARAGANGLIOMA

= rare neuroendocrine tumor arising from paraganglionic tissue found between base of skull and floor of pelvis; belong to amine-precursor-uptake decarboxylation (APUD) system characterized by cytoplasmic vesicles containing catecholamines

Types:
(1) Adrenal paraganglioma arising from adrenal medulla = **pheochromocytoma**
(2) Aorticosympathetic paraganglioma associated with sympathetic chain + retroperitoneal ganglia
(3) Parasympathetic paraganglioma including branchiomeric **chemodectoma**, vagal + visceral autonomic paraganglioma
- paroxysmal / permanent hypertension (due to secretion of vasopressor amines) with headache, pallor, perspiration, palpitations
- tumor may secrete catecholamine (= **functional paraganglioma**); proportion of hormonally active tumors high for pheochromocytomas, intermediate for aorticosympathetic paragangliomas, low for parasympathetic paragangliomas
- pheochromocytomas secrete norepinephrine + epinephrine, extraadrenal paragangliomas secrete only norepinephrine, some paragangliomas produce dopamine
- determination of free norepinephrine most sensitive with gas chromatography / high-pressure liquid chromatography (HPLC) performed on 24-hour urine specimens

Location of functioning paragangliomas:
(a) adrenal medulla (>80%)
(b) extraadrenal intraabdominal (8 – 16%)
(c) extraadrenal in head, neck, chest (2 – 4%)
(d) multiple paragangliomas in up to 20%, particularly in hereditary disorders (multiple endocrine neoplasia syndromes, neuroectodermal syndromes)
Cx: malignant transformation in 2 – 10%

PARATESTICULAR TUMORS

Only 4% of all scrotal tumors
A. BENIGN TUMOR
   1. **Adenomatoid tumor** (30%)
      = benign slow-growing neoplasm within epididymis (particularly in globus minor)
      Age: 2nd – 4th decade
      √ well-marginated mass with echogenicity equal to / greater than testis
   2. Polyorchidism
   3. Others: carcinoid, papillary cystadenoma of epididymis, leiomyoma, fibroma, adrenal rest, cholesteatoma, lipoma

B. MALIGNANT TUMOR
  1. Sarcomas: rhabdomyo-, leiomyo-, lipo-, fibro-, embryonal sarcoma
  2. Metastases

PHEOCHROMOCYTOMA

= ADRENAL PARAGANGLIOMA
= rare tumor of chromaffin tissue; responsible for 0.1% of hypertensions

Incidence: 0.13% in autopsy series; sporadic occurrence in 94%

Histo: chromaffin tumor cells contain chromagranin within secretory granules, tumor tends to form "Zellballen" (cell balls)

Age: 5% in childhood

Symptomatology secondary to excess catecholamine production:
- asymptomatic (9%)
- headaches, sweating, flushing, palpitations, anxiety, tremor
- nausea, vomiting, abdominal pain, chest pain
- paroxysmal (47%) / sustained (37%) hypertension
  (a) elevated catecholamine
  (b) functional renal vasoconstriction
  (c) renal artery stenosis (fibrosis, intimal proliferation, tumor encasement)
- hypoglycemia during hypertensive crisis
- elevated urine vanillylmandelic acid (VMA) in 54%; in up to 22% false-negative result because VMA not excreted

Associated with:
(1) Multiple endocrine neoplasia (MEN) in 6%:
  - pheochromocytoma asymptomatic in 50%
  (a) Sipple syndrome = MEN type II (= type 2A)
    = medullary carcinoma of thyroid + parathyroid adenoma + pheochromocytoma
  (b) **Mucosal neuroma syndrome** = MEN type III (= type 2B)
    = medullary carcinoma of thyroid + intestinal ganglioneuromatosis + pheochromocytoma
    - long slender extremities (Marfanoid)
    - prominent lips
    - nodular deformity of tongue (mucosal neuromas of tongue often initially diagnosed by dentists)
    - corneal limbus thickening
    √ thickened colonic folds + abnormal haustral pattern + diverticula
    √ multiple submucosal neuromas throughout small bowel, may act as lead point for intussusception
(2) Neuroectodermal disorder
  (a) tuberous sclerosis
  (b) von Hippel-Lindau disease
  (c) neurofibromatosis
(3) Familial pheochromocytosis
(4) **Carney syndrome** = paraganglioma + gastric epitheloid leiomyosarcoma + pulmonary chondroma

Location: anywhere in sympathetic nervous system from neck to sacrum; subdiaphragmatic in 98%
  (a) adrenal medulla (85 – 90%)
  (b) extraadrenal (10 – 15% in adults, 31% in children): para-aortic sympathetic chain (8%), organ of Zuckerkandl at origin of inferior mesenteric artery (2 – 5%), gonads, urinary bladder (1%)

Multiplicity:
  10% in nonfamilial adult cases
  32% in nonfamilial childhood cases
  65% in familial syndromes

RULE OF TENS:
  10% bilateral / multiple   **10**% extraadrenal
  10% malignant   **10**% familial

CT: localization accurate in 91% with tumor >2 cm in size; up to 40% in extraadrenal location are missed by CT; 93 – 100% sensitivity
  √ discrete round / oval mass with a mean size of 5 cm (range 3 – 12 cm)
  √ solid / cystic / complex mass with low-density areas secondary to hemorrhage / necrosis
  √ calcifications may be present
  Δ IV injection of iodinated contrast material may precipitate hypertensive crisis in patients not on alpha-blockers!

NUC: I-131 / I-123 MIBG (metaiodobenzylguanidine) scan (80 – 90% sensitivity; 98% specificity)
  Useful:
  (a) with clear clinical / laboratory evidence of tumor but no adrenal abnormality on CT / MRI
  (b) in detecting extra-adrenal pheochromocytomas by whole-body scintigraphy

MRI:
  √ iso- / slightly hypointense to liver on T1WI
  √ extremely hyperintense on T2WI
  √ marked homo- / inhomogeneous enhancement

Angio: intraarterial injection CONTRAINDICATED (induces hypertensive crisis)
  √ venous blood sampling (at different levels in IVC)
  √ localization by aortography in >91%
  √ usually hypervascular lesion with intense tumor blush
  √ slow washout of contrast material
  √ enlarged feeding arteries + neovascularity ("spoke-wheel" pattern)
  √ parasitization from intrarenal perforating branches

Cx: malignancy in 2 – 14%; metastases (may be hormonally active) to bone, lymph nodes, liver, lung

Rx:
(1) Surgical removal curative
(2) Alpha-adrenergic blocker (phenoxybenzamine / phentolamine)
(3) Beta-adrenergic blocker (propranolol)
(4) I-131 MIBG used to treat metastases

DDx: nonfunctioning adrenal adenoma, adrenocortical carcinoma, adrenal cyst

POLYARTERITIS NODOSA

= PERIARTERITIS NODOSA = systemic vascular disease with focal necrotizing inflammation of vessel walls affecting medium + small arteries; mucoid degeneration + fibrinoid necrosis begins within media; main vessels spared (DDx: necrotizing angiitis, mycotic aneurysm)

M > F
- malaise, low-grade fever, weight loss
- renal failure

@ Kidney is most frequently affected organ (85%)
  √ multiple small intrarenal aneurysms (interlobar, arcuate, interlobular arteries)
  √ aneurysms may disappear (thrombosis) or appear in new locations
  √ arterial narrowing + thrombosis (chronic stage / healing stage)
  √ multiple small cortical infarcts
  Cx: perinephric / subcapsular hemorrhage (rupture of aneurysm)
@ Liver (66%)
@ Mesenteric vessels (50%)
  - abdominal pain, ulcer formation, GI bleeding, intestinal infarction
@ Skeletal muscle (39%)
@ Skin (20%)

POLYCYSTIC KIDNEY DISEASE

Autosomal Dominant Polycystic Kidney Disease

= ADULT POLYCYSTIC KIDNEY DISEASE
= slowly progressive disease with nearly 100% penetrance and great variation in expressivity
Incidence: 1:1,000 people carry the mutant gene; 3rd most prevalent cause of chronic renal failure
Risk of recurrence: 50%

Histo:
    abnormal rate of tubule divisions (Potter Type III) with hypoplasia of portions of tubules left behind as the ureteral bud advances; cystic dilatation of Bowman capsule, loop of Henle, proximal convoluted tubule, coexisting with normal tissue

Mean age at diagnosis:
    43 years (neonatal / infantile onset has been reported); M:F = 1:1
    Onset of cyst formation:
    — 54% in 1st decade
    — 72% in 2nd decade
    — 86% in 3rd decade
    morphologic evidence in all patients by age 80

Associated with:
  (1) Cysts in: liver (25 – 50%), pancreas (9%); rare in lung, spleen, thyroid, ovaries, uterus, testis, seminal vesicles, epididymis, bladder
  (2) Aneurysm: saccular "berry" aneurysm of cerebral arteries (10 – 30%)
  (3) Mitral valve prolapse

- symptomatic at mean age of 35 years (cysts are growing with age)
- hypertension (50 – 70%)
- azotemia
- hematuria, proteinuria
- lumbar / abdominal pain

√ bilaterally large kidneys with multifocal round lesions; unilateral enlargement may be the first manifestation of the disease
√ cysts may calcify in curvilinear rim- / ring-like irregular amorphous fashion
√ elongated + distorted + attenuated collecting system
√ nodular puddling of contrast material on delayed images
√ "Swiss cheese" nephrogram = multiple lesions of varying size with smooth margins
√ polycystic kidneys shrink after beginning of renal failure, after renal transplantation, or on chronic hemodialysis
NUC: poor renal function on Tc-99m DTPA scan
  √ multiple areas of diminished activity, cortical activity only in areas of functioning cortex
US:
  √ multiple cysts in cortical region (adults)
  √ diffusely echogenic when cysts small (children)
  √ renal contour poorly demarcated
OB-US:
  √ enlarged kidneys with increased echogenicity / multiple cysts (usually in 3rd trimester), earliest sonographic diagnosis at 14 weeks, may appear unilateral
  √ oligohydramnios / normal amount of amniotic fluid

Atypical rare presentation:
  (a) unilateral adult PCKD
  (b) segmental adult PCKD
  (c) adult PCKD in utero / neonatal period (simulating infantile PCKD in appearance but without impaired renal function)
Cx:
  (1) Death from uremia (59%) / cerebral hemorrhage (secondary to hypertension or ruptured aneurysm [13%]) / cardiac complications (mean age 50 years)
  (2) Renal calculi
  (3) Urinary tract infection
  (4) Cyst rupture
  (5) Hemorrhage

DDx:
  (1) Multiple simple cysts (less diffuse, no family history)
  (2) von Hippel-Lindau disease (cerebellar hemangioblastoma, retinal hemangiomas, occasionally pheochromocytomas)
  (3) Acquired uremic cystic disease (kidneys small, no renal function, transplant)
  (4) Infantile PCKD (usually microscopic cysts)

Autosomal Recessive Polycystic Kidney Disease
= INFANTILE POLYCYSTIC KIDNEY DISEASE
= POLYCYSTIC DISEASE OF CHILDHOOD
= Potter Type I

Incidence: 1: 6,000 to 1:50,000 livebirths; F > M;
carrier frequency of 1:112

Path:
@   kidney: abnormal proliferation + dilatation of
collecting tubules resulting in multiple 1 – 2 mm
cysts
@   liver: periportal fibrosis often with abnormal
proliferation + dilatation of bile ducts
@   pancreas: pancreatic fibrosis

A.   ANTENATAL FORM (most common)
90% of tubules show cystic changes
•   onset of renal failure in utero
√   oligohydramnios and dystocia (large abdominal
mass)
Prognosis:
death from renal failure / respiratory insufficiency
(pulmonary hypoplasia) within 24 hours in 75%,
within 1 year in 93%; uniformly fatal

B.   NEONATAL FORM
60% of tubules show ectasia + minimal hepatic
fibrosis + bile duct proliferation
•   onset of renal failure within 1st month of life
Prognosis:
death from renal failure / hypertension /
left ventricular failure within 1st year of life

C.   INFANTILE FORM
20% of renal tubules involved + mild / moderate
periportal fibrosis
•   disease appears by 3 – 6 months of age
Prognosis:
death from chronic renal failure / systemic arterial
hypertension / portal hypertension

D.   JUVENILE FORM
10% of tubules involved + gross hepatic fibrosis +
bile duct proliferation
•   disease appears at 1 – 5 years of age
Prognosis: death from portal hypertension

Δ The less severe the renal findings the more severe
the hepatic findings!

@   Lung
√   severe pulmonary hypoplasia
√   pneumothorax / pneumomediastinum
@   Liver
•   portal venous hypertension
√   tubular cystic dilatation of small intrahepatic bile
ducts
√   increase in liver echogenicity (from congenital
hepatic fibrosis)
@   Kidneys
√   bilateral gross renal enlargement
√   faint nephrogram + blotchy opacification on initial
images
√   increasingly dense nephrogram
√   poor visualization of collecting system

√   "sunburst nephrogram" = striated nephrogram
with persistent radiating opaque streaks
(collecting ducts) on delayed images
√   prominent fetal lobation
CT:
√   prolonged corticomedullary phase
US:
√   hyperechoic enlarged kidneys (unresolved 1 –
2 mm cystic / ectatic dilatation of renal tubules
increase number of acoustic interfaces)
√   loss of corticomedullary differentiation, poor
visualization of renal sinus + renal borders
√   occasionally discrete macroscopic cysts
√   compressed / minimally dilated collecting
system
OB-US (as early as 17 weeks GA):
√   progressive renal enlargement with renal
circumference:abdominal circumference ratio
>0.30
√   hyperechoic renal parenchyma
√   nonvisualization of urine in fetal bladder
√   oligohydramnios (33%)
OB management:
(1)   Chromosome studies to determine if other
malformations present (eg, trisomy 13 / 18)
(2)   Option of pregnancy termination <24 weeks
(3)   Nonintervention for fetal distress >24 weeks
if severe oligohydramnios present
Risk of recurrence: 25%
DDx: Meckel-Gruber syndrome

POSTERIOR URETHRAL VALVES
= congenital thick folds of mucous membrane located in
posterior urethra (prostatic + membranous portion) distal
to verumontanum

Type I :   (most common) mucosal folds (vestiges of
Wolffian duct) extend anteroinferiorly from the
caudal aspect of the verumontanum, often fusing
anteriorly at a lower level
Type II: (rare) mucosal folds extend anterosuperiorly from
the verumontanum toward the bladder neck
(nonobstructive normal variant, probably a
consequence of bladder outlet obstruction)
Type III: diaphragmlike membrane located below the
verumontanum (= abnormal canalization of
urogenital membrane)
Time of discovery: prenatal (8%), neonatal (34%), 1st
year (32%), 2nd – 16th year (23%),
adult (3%)
•   urinary tract infection (fever, vomiting) in 36%
•   obstructive symptoms in 32% (hesitancy, straining,
dribbling [20%], enuresis [20%])
•   palpable kidneys / bladder in neonate (21%)
•   failure to thrive (13%)
•   hematuria (5%)

VCUG:
√   vesicoureteral reflux, mainly on left side (<50%)
√   fusiform distension + elongation of proximal posterior
urethra persisting throughout voiding

√ transverse / curvilinear filling defect in posterior urethra
√ diminution of urethral caliber distal to severe obstruction
√ hypertrophy of bladder neck
√ trabeculation + sacculation of bladder wall
√ large postvoid bladder residual

OB-US:
√ male gender
√ oligohydramnios (related to severity + duration of obstruction)
√ hypoplastic / multicystic dysplastic kidney (if early occurrence)
√ overdistended urinary bladder (megacystis) in 30%
√ thick-walled urinary bladder + trabeculations (best seen after decompression)
√ bilateral hydroureteronephrosis (+ pulmonary hypoplasia)
√ dilated renal pelvis may be absent in renal dysplasia / rupture of bladder / pelviureteric atresia
√ urine leak: urinoma, urine ascites, urothorax

OB management:
(1) Induction of labor as soon as fetal lung maturity established if diagnosed during last 10 weeks of pregnancy
(2) Vesicoamniotic shunting may be contemplated if diagnosed remote from term (68% survivors)

Cx: (1) Neonatal urine leak (ascites, urothorax, urinoma) in 13%
(2) Neonatal pneumothorax / pneumomediastinum in 9%
(3) Prune belly syndrome
(4) Renal dysplasia (if obstruction occurs early during gestation)

Prognosis: depends upon duration of obstruction prior to corrective surgery; nephrectomy for irreversible damage (13%)

DDx: (1) UPJ obstruction (2) UVJ obstruction (3) Primary megaureter (4) Massive vesicoureteral reflux (5) Megacystis-microcolon-intestinal hypoperistalsis syndrome

POSTINFLAMMATORY RENAL ATROPHY

= acute bacterial nephritis with irreversible ischemia as an unusual form of severe Gram-negative bacterial infection in patients with altered host resistance in spite of proper antibiotic treatment

Histo: occlusion of interlobar arteries / vasospasm

√ small smooth kidney
√ papillary necrosis in acute phase

POSTOBSTRUCTIVE RENAL ATROPHY

= generalized papillary atrophy usually following successful surgical correction of urinary tract obstruction and progressing in spite of relief of obstruction
√ small smooth kidney, usually unilateral
√ dilated calices with effaced papillae
√ thinned cortex

PROSTATE CANCER

Incidence: 8.7% in white males, 9.4% in black males, increasing with age; 132,000 new cases in U.S. (1992); 2nd most common malignancy in males (after lung cancer)
Δ One out of 11 males will develop prostate cancer!

Risk factors: advancing age, presence of testes, cadmium exposure, animal fat intake

Histo:
(a) nodular pattern
(b) nodular-infiltrating pattern
(c) infiltrating pattern

• prostate specific antigen (PSA) may be elevated
(a) enzyme-linked immunosorbent assay
(b) polyclonal radioimmunoassay (Proscheck®, Abbott PSA®)
(c) monoclonal radioimmunoassay (Hibratech®): normal value of 0.1 – 4 ng/ml

Adjustment of normal values in reference to prostate volume (height x width x length x 0.52):
x 0.2 for Hibratech®, x 0.11 for Proscheck®, x 0.12 for Abbott PSA®

Staging (American Joint Committee on Cancer):
A   nonpalpable tumor
A_1 focal well-differentiated tumor <1.5 cm in diameter
A_2 diffuse poorly differentiated tumor; >5% of chips from transurethral resection contain cancer
B   palpable tumor confined to prostate
B_1 lesion <1.5 cm in diameter
B_2 tumor >1.5 cm / involving more than one lobe
C   tumor with capsular involvement
C_1 capsular invasion
C_2 capsular penetration
C_3 seminal vesicle involvement
D   distant metastasis
D_1 involvement of pelvic lymph nodes
D_2 distant metastases to bone / lymph nodes
Δ At initial presentation >75% have stage C + D!

Grading (Gleason score 2 – 10):
low numbers refer to well-differentiated, high numbers to anaplastic tumors; primary predominant grade (1 – 5) is added to secondary less representative area with highest degree of dedifferentiation (1 – 5)

Metastases to lymph nodes:
0% in stage A_1, 34% in stage A_2, 18% in stage B_1, 34% in stage B_2, 57% in stage C; 10% with Gleason grade ≤5; 70% with Gleason grade 9 / 10

Location: peripheral zone (70%), transition zone (20%), central zone (10%)
US (21% positive predictive value):
√ hypoechoic (61%) / mixed (2%) / hyperechoic (2%) lesion; not detectable isoechoic lesion (35%)
√ asymmetric enlargement of gland

√ deformed contour of prostate
√ heterogeneous texture
Size versus rate of detection:
  ≤5 mm (36%), 6 – 10 mm (65%), 11 – 15 mm (53%),
  16 – 20 mm (84%), 21 – 25 mm (92%), ≥26 mm
  (75%)
DDx of hypoechoic lesion: external sphincter, veins,
  neurovascular bundle, seminal vesicle, dilated duct,
  small prostatic cyst, acute prostatitis, benign prostatic
  hyperplasia, dysplasia, sonographic artifact
Prognosis: increase in tumor volume increases
  probability of capsular penetration,
  metastasis, histologic dedifferentiation
Mortality: 2.6% for white males, 4.5% for black males;
  34,000 deaths/1992

PRUNE BELLY SYNDROME

= EAGLE-BARRETT SYNDROME
= congenital nonhereditary multisystem disorder; almost
  exclusively in males
TRIAD: 1. Absent abdominal wall musculature
         2. Urinary tract obstruction
         3. Cryptorchidism
Etiology:
  massive abdominal distension secondary to urethral
  obstruction / transient ascites / intestinal duplication cyst
  / megacystis-microcolon syndrome causes pressure
  atrophy of abdominal wall muscles; bladder distension
  interferes with descent of testes
Incidence: 1:35,000 to 1:50,000 livebirths; almost
  exclusively in males
Groups:
  (1) Obstruction of urethra (most commonly urethral
    atresia)
    Associated with: malrotation, intestinal atresia,
      imperforate anus, skeletal abnormalities, CHD,
      Hirschsprung disease, congenital cystic
      adenomatoid malformation
    √   bladder wall hypertrophy
    Prognosis: death shortly after birth
  (2) Functional abnormality of bladder emptying (more
    common)
    no associated abnormalities
    √   large floppy urinary bladder
    √   large urachal remnant
    Prognosis: chronic urinary tract problems

• wrinkled flaccid appearance of hypotonic abdominal wall
  with bulging flanks (agenesis / hypoplasia of muscles in
  lower + medial parts of abdominal wall)
• bilateral cryptorchidism
√ impaired renal function
√ no / mild hydronephrosis
√ dilated tortuous laterally placed ureters
√ large distended urinary bladder
√ persistence of urachal remnant
√ dilated prostatic urethra (absence of prostate)
√ urethral obstruction (occasionally posterior urethral
  valves), renal dysplasia, oligohydramnios, pulmonary
  hypoplasia (in severe cases)

VCUG:
  √ reflux into utriculus / seminal vesicles
  √ ± reflux into ureters
  √ diverticula of urethra (megalourethra)
Cx: respiratory infections (ineffective cough)

PYELOCALICEAL DIVERTICULUM

= PYELOGENIC CYST = PERICALICEAL CYST
= CALICEAL DIVERTICULUM
= uroepithelium-lined pouch extending from a peripheral
  point of the collecting system into adjacent renal
  parenchyma
TYPE I (calyx):
  more common; connected to caliceal cup, usually at
  fornix; bulbous shape; narrow connecting infundibulum
  of varying length; few millimeters in diameter; in polar
  region especially upper pole
TYPE II (pelvis):
  interpolar region; communicates directly with pelvis;
  usually larger and rounder; neck short and not easily
  identified

Cause:
  (1) Developmental origin from ureteral bud remnant
    (obstruction of peripheral aberrant "minicalyx")
  (2) Acquired: reflux, infection, rupture of simple cyst /
    abscess, infundibular achalasia / spasm,
    hydrocalyx secondary to inflammatory fibrosis of an
    infundibulum
√ formation of single / multiple stones (50%) or milk of
  calcium (fluid-calcium level)
√ opacification may be delayed and remain so for
  prolonged period
√ mass effect on adjacent pelvocaliceal system if large
  enough
Cx: recurrent infection
DDx: ruptured simple nephrogenic cyst, evacuated
  abscess / hematoma, renal papillary necrosis,
  medullary sponge kidney, hydrocalyx due to
  infundibular narrowing from TB / crossing vessel /
  stone / infiltrating carcinoma

PYELONEPHRITIS

= upper urinary tract infection with pelvic + caliceal +
  parenchymal inflammation

Acute Pyelonephritis

= episodic urinary tract infection
Etiology:
  infected urine from lower tract during adulthood; in
  5% anatomic abnormality (obstruction, stone, stasis);
  (DDx: chronic atrophic pyelonephritis secondary to
  vesicoureteral reflux in infancy)
Pathway of infection:
  (a) ascending bacterial infection usually due to P-
    fimbriated E. coli (fimbriae facilitate adherence to
    mucosal surface): initial colonization of ureter in
    areas of turbulent flow leads to paralysis of
    ureteral smooth muscle function with dilatation +
    obstruction of collecting system

(b) vesicoureteral reflux + pyelotubular backflow: P-fimbriated E. coli not necessary for infection

(c) hematogenous spread (12 – 20%) with Gram-positive cocci

Organism: E. coli > Proteus > Klebsiella, Enterobacter, Pseudomonas

Age: any; M << F

• fever + chills + flank pain
• leukocytosis
• microscopic hematuria
• pyuria

Indication for imaging:
   (1) diabetes (2) analgesic abuse (3) neuropathic bladder (4) history of urinary tract stones (5) atypical organism (6) poor response to antibiotics (7) frequent recurrences
√ normal urogram in 75%!
√ smooth normal / enlarged kidney(s), focal >> diffuse involvement of kidney
√ delayed opacification of collecting system
√ compression of collecting system (edema)
√ nonobstructive ureteral dilatation (rare, effect of endotoxins)
√ immediate persistent dense nephrogram, rarely striated
√ diminished nephrographic density (global / wedge-shaped / patchy)
√ nonvisualization of kidney (in severe pyelonephritis, rare)
√ "tree-barking" = mucosal striations (rare)
US:
   √ swollen kidney with decreased echogenicity
   √ thickened sonolucent corticomedullary bands
   √ loss of corticomedullary junction demarcation
   √ loss of central sinus echoes
   √ wedge-shaped zones of decreased attenuation
CT:
   √ small foci of low attenuation (= microabscesses 1 – 5 mm) without mass defect
   √ delayed / decreased enhancement

Prognosis:
   (1) Quick response to antibiotic treatment will leave no scars
   (2) Delayed treatment of acute pyelonephritis during first 3 years of life can severely affect renal function later in life: decreased renal function, hypertension (33%), end-stage renal disease (10%)

Emphysematous Pyelonephritis
= fulminant infection of kidney + perirenal tissues with gas in and around enlarged nonfunctioning kidney + formation of abscess

Organism: E. coli > Proteus >> Clostridia (rare)
Mechanism: pyelonephritis leads to ischemia + low O_2 tension with anaerobic metabolism; facultative anaerobe organisms form CO_2

Predisposed: immunocompromised patients, esp. diabetics (in 90% of cases); obstructed kidney (in 40%); F > M
√ gas within collecting system
√ streaks / bubbles of gas in interstitium of renal parenchyma radiating from medulla to cortex
√ subcapsular / perinephric gas
Mortality: 40 – 50% (71% for antibiotic Rx, 30% for nephrectomy)
Rx: prompt surgical drainage

Xanthogranulomatous Pyelonephritis
= chronic suppurative granulomatous infection in chronic obstruction (calculus, stricture, carcinoma) originating in medulla
Incidence: 681,000 surgically proven cases of chronic pyelonephritis
Organisms: Proteus mirabilis, E. coli
Path: replacement of corticomedullary junction with soft yellow nodules; calices filled with pus and debris
Histo: diffuse infiltration by plasma cells + lipid-laden macrophages (xanthoma cells)
Peak age: 5th – 7th decade; all ages affected, may occur in infants; M:F = 1:3

• pyuria   (95%)
• flank pain   (80%)
• fever   (70%)
• palpable mass   (50%)
• weight loss   (50%)
• microscopic hematuria   (50%)
• reversible hepatic dysfunction with elevated liver function tests (50%)

A. DIFFUSE XGP   (83 – 90%)
B. SEGMENTAL / FOCAL XGP   (10 – 17%)
   = tumefactive form due to obstructed single infundibulum / one moiety of duplex system
   DDx: renal cell carcinoma

√ kidney globally enlarged (smooth contour uncommon) / focal renal mass
√ contracted pelvis with dilated calices
√ totally absent / focally absent nephrogram
√ central obstructing calculus: staghorn calculus in 75%
√ extension of inflammation into perirenal space, pararenal space, ipsilateral psoas muscle, colon, spleen, diaphragm, posterior abdominal wall, skin
Retrograde:
   √ complete obstruction at ureteropelvic junction / infundibulum / proximal ureter
   √ contracted renal pelvis, dilated deformed calices + nodular filling defects
   √ irregular parenchymal masses with cavitation
CT:
   √ low attenuation masses replacing renal parenchyma
US:
   √ hypoechoic dilated calices with echogenic rim

√ hypoechoic masses frequently with low-level internal echoes replacing renal parenchyma
√ loss of corticomedullary junction
√ parenchymal calcifications are uncommon
Angio:
  √ stretching of segmental / interlobar arteries around large avascular masses
  √ hypervascularity / blush around periphery of masses in late arterial phase (= granulation tissue)
  √ venous encasement + occlusion
  DDx: hydronephrosis, avascular tumor

PYELOURETERITIS CYSTICA
Cause: chronic urinary tract irritant (stone / infection)
Histo: numerous small submucosal epithelial-lined cysts representing cystic degeneration of epithelial cell nests within lamina propria (cell nests of von Brunn) formed by downward proliferation of buds of surface epithelium that have become detached from the mucosa
Organisms: E. coli > M. tuberculosis, Enterococcus, Proteus, schistosomiasis
Predisposed: diabetics
Age: 6th decade; more prevalent in women

Location: bladder >> proximal 1/3 of ureter > ureteropelvic junction; unilateral >> bilateral
√ multiple small round smooth lucent defects of 1 – 3 mm in size; scattered discrete / clustered
√ persist unchanged for years in spite of antibiotic therapy

DDx: (1) Spreading / multifocal TCC
     (2) Vascular ureteral notching

PYONEPHROSIS
= presence of pus in dilated collecting system secondary to infected hydronephrosis
Path: purulent exudate composed of sloughed urothelium + inflammatory cells from early formation of microabscesses + necrotizing papillitis
Organism: most commonly E. coli
US:
  √ dispersed / dependent internal echoes within dilated pelvocalyceal system
  √ shifting urine-debris level
  √ dense peripheral echoes in nondependent location + shadowing (gas from infection)
Cx: 1. XGP
    2. Renal abscess
    3. Perinephric abscess
    4. Fistula to duodenum, colon, pleura

RADIATION NEPHRITIS
Histo: interstitial fibrosis, tubule atrophy, glomerular sclerosis, sclerosis of arteries of all sizes, hyalinization of afferent arterioles, thickening of renal capsule
Threshold dose: 2300 rads over 5 weeks
• clinically resembling chronic glomerulonephritis

√ normal / small smooth kidney consistent with radiation field
√ parenchymal thickness diminished (globally / focally; related to radiation field)
√ diminished nephrographic density

REFLUX ATROPHY
Cause: increased hydrostatic pressure of pelvocaliceal urine with atrophy of nephrons secondary to long-standing vesicoureteral reflux
√ small smooth kidney with loss of parenchymal thickness
√ widened collecting system with effaced papillae
√ longitudinal striations from redundant mucosa when collecting system is collapsed
NOT to confuse with reflux nephropathy !

REFLUX NEPHROPATHY
= CHRONIC ATROPHIC PYELONEPHRITIS = ascending bacterial urinary tract infection secondary to reflux of infected urine from lower tract + tubulointerstitial inflammation in childhood (hardly ever endangers adult kidney); most common cause of small scarred kidney
Etiology:
3 essential elements: (1) Infected urine
                  (2) Vesicoureteral reflux
                  (3) Intrarenal reflux
Age: usually young adults (subclinical diagnosis starting in childhood); M < F
• fever, flank pain, frequency, dysuria
• hypertension, renal failure
• may have no history of significant symptoms

Site: predominantly affecting poles of kidneys secondary to presence of compound calyces having distorted papillary ducts of Bellini (= papillae with gaping openings instead of slitlike openings of interpolar papillae)
√ normal / small kidney; uni- / bilateral; uni- / multifocal
√ focal parenchymal thinning with contour depression in upper / lower pole (more compound papillae in upper pole), scar formation only up to age 4
√ retracted papilla with clubbed calyx subjacent to scar
√ contralateral / focal compensatory hypertrophy (= pseudotumor)
√ dilated ureters (secondary to reflux) sometimes with linear striations (redundant / edematous mucosa)
US:
  √ focally increased echogenicity within cortex (scar)
Angio:
  √ small tortuous intrarenal arteries, pruning of intrarenal vessels
  √ vascular stenoses, occlusion, aneurysms
  √ inhomogeneous nephrographic phase
NUC (Tc-99m glucoheptonate / DMSA with SPECT most sensitive method):
  √ focal / multifocal photon deficient areas

RENAL / PERIRENAL ABSCESS
= usually complication of renal inflammation with liquefaction; 2% of all renal masses

Pathway of infection:
  (a) ascending (80%): associated with obstruction
      (UPJ, ureter, calculus)
  (b) hematogenous (20%): infection from skin, teeth,
      lung, tonsils (S. aureus), endocarditis,
      intravenous drug abuse
Organisms: E. coli, Proteus
• urine culture often negative

Renal Abscess

  • negative urine analysis / culture (in up to 20%)
  IVP:
    √ focal mass displacing collecting system
  CT:
    √ focal renal mass with thick enhancing wall +
      thickened Gerota fascia
    √ centrally diminished attenuation
  US:
    √ slightly hypoechoic (early), hypo- to anechoic (late)
      mass with irregular margins + increased through-
      transmission ± septations ± microbubbles of gas
  NUC (Ga-67 citrate / In-111 leukocytes):
    √ hot spot
  DDx: cystic renal cell carcinoma

Carbuncle

= collection of many small abscesses

Perinephric Abscess

= extension of renal abscess through capsule
Predisposed: diabetics (in 30%), urolithiasis

  √ loss of psoas margin / obscuration of renal contour
  √ renal displacement
  √ focal renal mass
  √ scoliosis concave to involved side
  √ respiratory immobility of kidney
  √ gas in renal fossa
  √ unilateral impaired excretion
  √ pleural effusion

RENAL ADENOMA

Most common cortical lesion; increased frequency in
tobacco users
Incidence: in 1% of individuals (autopsy statistic)
Age: usually >30 years; M > F

Types:
  (1) Papillary / cystadenoma (38%)
  (2) Tubular adenoma (38%)
  (3) Mixed type adenoma (21%)
  (4) Alveolar adenoma (3%) = precursor of
      hypernephroma

  √ usually <3 cm in size
  √ impossible to differentiate from renal cell carcinoma
  Cx: premalignant / potentially malignant

  Δ Small adenoma <3 cm should be considered a renal cell
  carcinoma of low metastatic potential!

RENAL AGENESIS

Mechanism:
  (a) formation failure
      = failure of ureteral bud to form
      • absence of ipsilateral hemitrigone and ureteral
        orifice
  (b) induction failure
      = failure of growing ureteral bud to induce
        metanephric tissue
      • blind ending ureter

A. UNILATERAL RENAL AGENESIS
  Incidence: 1:600 – 1,000 pregnancies
  Risk of recurrence: 4.5%
  Often coexisting with other anomalies:
      genital tract anomalies (40% of females, 12% of
      males); Turner syndrome, trisomy, Fanconi anemia,
      Laurence-Moon-Biedl syndrome
  Δ 70% incidence of genital abnormalities if only one
    kidney visualized!
  √ absent adrenal gland (11%)
  √ absent / rudimentary renal vessels
  √ colon occupies renal fossa
  √ compensatory contralateral renal hypertrophy (50%)

B. BILATERAL RENAL AGENESIS (= Potter syndrome)
  Incidence: 1:3,000 to 1:10,000 pregnancies;
                  M:F = 2.5:1
  Risk of recurrence: <1%
  • Potter's facies = low set ears, redundant skin,
    parrot-beaked nose, receding chin
  √ severe oligohydramnios (after 14 weeks MA)
  √ bilateral absence of renal outline (after 12 weeks)
  √ flat discoid adrenals (simulating kidneys with
    hypoechoic rim + thin central sinus)
  √ inability to visualize urine in fetal bladder (after 13
    weeks); negative furosemide test (20 – 60 mg IV)
    not diagnostic (fetuses with severe IUGR may not
    be capable of diuresis)
  √ bell-shaped thorax (pulmonary hypoplasia)
  √ compression deformities of extremities = clubfoot,
    flexion contractures, joint dislocations
  Prognosis: stillbirths (24 – 38%); invariably fatal in the
              first days of life (pulmonary hypoplasia)
  DDx: functional cause of in utero renal failure

RENAL ARTERY STENOSIS

Responsible for 2 – 10% of systemic arterial hypertension
Hemodynamic significance determined by:
  (a) elevated renin levels in renal vein of affected kidney
      ≥1.5:1
  (b) collateral vessels
  (c) greater than 70% stenosis with poststenotic
      dilatation
  (d) transstenotic intraarterial pressure gradient ≥40
      mm Hg
  (e) decrease in renal size
Causes:
  1. Atheromatous lesion (mostly in proximal 2 cm)
  2. Fibromuscular dysplasia

3. Uncommon: renal artery aneurysm, arteriovenous malformation / fistula, Takayasu disease, thrombangitis obliterans, syphilitic arteritis, dissecting aortic aneurysm, postradiation artery stenosis, neurofibromatosis, thrombosis, embolus (atrial fibrillation, prosthetic valve thrombi, cardiac myxoma, paradoxical emboli, atheromatous emboli), trauma, aortic dissection

Histo: tubular atrophy and shrinkage of glomeruli
- abdominal / flank pain
- hematuria
- hypertension
- oliguria, anuria
- low urine sodium concentration

√ normal / decreased renal size (R 2 cm < L; L 1.5 cm < R) with smooth contour
√ vascular calcifications (aneurysm / atherosclerosis)
IVP (60% true-positive rate, 22% false-negative rate):
  √ delayed appearance of contrast material (decreased glomerular filtration)
  √ increased density of contrast material (increased water reabsorption)
  √ delayed washout of contrast material (prolonged urine transit time)
  √ lack of distension of collecting system
  √ global attenuation of contrast density, urogram may be normal with adequate collateral circulation
  √ notching of proximal ureter (enlargement of collateral vessels)
NUC (88% sensitivity):
  Captopril radionuclide renography used for screening in renovascular hypertension!
  √ reduced / absent perfusion of kidney
  √ poor visualization / nonvisualization on delayed images
Duplex US:
  √ increased peak systolic frequency shift at stenosis
  √ poststenotic spectral broadening ± flow reversal
  √ peak velocity >100 cm/sec (for >50% stenosis; 0 – 42% sensitive, 79 – 92% specific)
  √ absence of blood flow during diastole (for >50% stenosis)
  √ ratio of peak renal artery velocity to peak aortic velocity >3.5 (for >60% stenosis; 0 – 91% sensitive, 37 – 97% specific)
Problems:
  (a) technically inadequate examinations in 6 – 49%; usually limited to children + thin adults
  (b) multiple renal arteries in 20 – 28%
  (c) "false" tracings from large collateral vessels / reconstituted segments of main renal artery

Arteriosclerosis of Kidney
Age: >50 years; M > F
Path: lesion primarily involving intima
Location: main renal artery (93%) + additional stenosis of renal artery branch (7%); bilateral in 31%
Associated with   arteriosclerosis of aorta

√ eccentric stenosis in proximal 2 cm of renal artery, frequently involving orifice

Fibromuscular Dysplasia of Renal Artery
Incidence:
  35% of renal artery stenoses; 1,100 patients reported (by 1982) with involvement of renal artery in 60% + extracranial carotid artery in 30%
Age: most common cause of renovascular hypertension in children + young adults <40 years; M:F = 1:3
Associated with   fibromuscular dysplasia of other aortic branches in 1 – 2%: celiac a., hepatic a., splenic a., mesenteric a., iliac a., internal carotid a.

- hypertension
- progressive renal insufficiency

Sites: mid- and distal main renal artery (79%), renal artery branches (4%), combination (17%); proximal third of main renal artery spared in 98%; bilateral in 2/3; R:L = 4:1

1. INTIMAL FIBROPLASIA (1 – 2%)
   Path: circumferential / eccentric fibrous tissue between intima + internal elastic lamina
   Age: children + young adults
   Site: main renal artery + major segmental branches; often bilateral
   √ narrow annular radiolucent band
   √ poststenotic fusiform dilatation
2. MEDIAL FIBROPLASIA (60 – 70%)
   Path: multiple fibromuscular ridges + severe mural thinning with loss of smooth muscle + internal elastic lamina
   Site: mid + distal renal artery + branches
   √ "string of beads" = alternating areas of stenoses + aneurysms
3. MEDIAL HYPERPLASIA (5 – 15%)
   Path: smooth muscle hyperplasia within arterial media
   Site: main renal artery and branches
   √ long smooth tubular narrowing
4. PERIMEDIAL FIBROPLASIA (20%)
   Path: fibroplasia of outer 1/2 of media replacing external elastic lamina
   Site: distal main renal artery
   √ long irregular stenosis, beading
   √ NO aneurysm formation (not wider than unaffected segment)
5. MEDIAL DISSECTION (5 – 10%)
   Path: new channel in outer 1/3 of media within external elastic lamina
   Site: main renal artery + branches
   √ false channel, aneurysm
6. ADVENTITIAL FIBROPLASIA (<1%)
   Path: adventitial + periarterial proliferation in fibrofatty tissue
   Site: main renal artery, large branches
   √ long segmental stenosis

Cx: (1) Giant aneurysm
     (2) AV fistula between renal artery + vein (in medial fibroplasia)

Rx: (1) Resection of diseased segment with end-to-end anastomosis
     (2) Replacement by autogenous vein graft, excision + repair by patch angioplasty
     (3) Transluminal balloon angioplasty

Neurofibromatosis

Hypertension in neurofibromatosis due to:
(1) Pheochromocytoma
(2) Renal artery stenosis
Δ Renal artery involvement mainly seen in children!

Types:
(a) mesodermal dysplasia of arterial wall with fibrous transformation (common)
(b) narrowing of main renal artery by periarterial neurofibroma (rare)

√ saccular funnel-shaped aneurysm involving aorta / main renal artery
√ smooth / nodular stenosis (mural / adventitial neurofibroma) in proximal renal artery
√ intrarenal aneurysm (rare)
DDx: fibromuscular dysplasia; congenital renal artery stenosis

RENAL CELL CARCINOMA
= RCC = RENAL ADENOCARCINOMA
= HYPERNEPHROMA
Incidence: 80 – 90% of all renal malignant primaries in adults; 1 – 3% of all visceral cancers
Age: 6th – 7th decade (generally >40 years); peak age of 55 years; may occur in children; M:F = 2–3:1
Path:
arises from proximal tubular cells; 30% found incidentally with imaging
(a) clear cell carcinoma (95%): hypervascular, >50 years
(b) papillary adenocarcinoma (5%): hypovascular, 40 – 50 years, slow growing, well encapsulated, metastasize late

Predisposed:
(1) Tobacco; phenacetin abuse
(2) von Hippel-Lindau syndrome (10 – 25%): often small intracystic tumors (hemangioblastoma, retinal angioma, renal cysts)
(3) Acquired cystic disease of uremia (7 x increased risk)

Multiple RCC: commonly in von Hippel-Lindau syndrome; bilateral in 1 – 3%

Stage I : tumor confined to renal capsule
          √ sharply defined convex interface with perirenal fat

II : confined to Gerota fascia = perirenal fascia
     √ irregular interface between tumor + fat
III : extension into renal vein or IVC ± positive lymph nodes; extension into perirenal fat
IV: extension into adjacent organs; distant metastases
Regional extension: into lymph nodes (9 – 20%); into IVC (4 – 10%)

Metastases:
  Spread to:
    lung (55%); lymph nodes (34%); liver (33%); bone (32%); adrenals (19%); contralateral kidney (11%); brain (6%); heart (5%); spleen (5%); bowel (4%); skin (3%); ureter (rare)
  Incidence:
    (a) tumors <4 cm: 8.5% for grade II tumors
    (b) tumors 4 – 8 cm in size: 18% for grade II tumors, 50% for grade III tumors

• hematuria (56%), flank pain (36%), weight loss (27%), fever (11%)
• varicocele (2%)
• anemia (40%)
• Stauffer syndrome (15%) = abnormal liver function in absence of hepatic metastases
• Paraneoplastic syndromes: polycythemia (4%), hypercalcemia

√ mass, bulge, discontinuity of renal contour
√ calcification (10 – 20%): usually central + amorphous
√ extrinsic compression + displacement of pelvis + calices
√ cysts: (a) cystic necrotic tumor (40%)
         (b) cystadenocarcinoma (2 – 5%)
         (c) renal cell carcinoma in wall of cyst (3%)
√ tumor growth into renal vein / IVC (30%)
IVP:
  √ diminished function (parenchymal replacement, hydronephrosis)
US:
  √ isoechoic (44%) / hypoechoic (35%) / hyperechoic (21%) mass (DDx: complicated cyst, angiomyolipoma)
  √ inhomogeneity due to hemorrhage, necrosis, cystic degeneration
MRI (best modality to assess stage III + IV disease):
  √ low to medium signal intensity on T1WI; hyperintense areas are usually due to hemorrhage
  √ heterogeneous signal intensity on T2WI
Angio:
  √ typically hypervascular (95%) with puddling of contrast + occasional AV shunting
  √ enlarged tortuous poorly tapering feeding vessels
  √ coarse neovascularity + formation of small aneurysms
  √ parasitization of lumbar, adrenal, subcostal, mesenteric artery branches
  √ poorly defined tumor margins

Prognosis: 10-year survival rate for stage I + II 60 – 70%, for stage III 40%, for stage IV 0%
Recurrence: in 11% after 10 years

RENAL CYST

Simple Cortical Renal Cyst

Acquired lesion possibly secondary to tubular obstruction; accounts for 62% of all renal masses

Incidence: in 1 – 2% of all urograms; in 3 – 5% of all autopsies

Age: peak incidence after age 30 years; increasing frequency with age (in 0.22% in pediatric age group, in 50% over age 50)

May be associated with: tuberous sclerosis, von Hippel-Lindau disease, Caroli disease, neurofibromatosis

√ large and unifocal when peripheral
√ focal attenuation + displacement of collecting system
√ focally replaced nephrogram with smooth margin, thin wall and "beak sign"
US (90 – 100% accuracy of US & CT):
  √ spherical / ovoid in shape
  √ anechoic without internal echoes
  √ smooth clearly demarcated walls
  √ acoustic enhancement beyond cyst
CT:
  √ near water density lesion (<20 HU), thin wall, smooth interface with renal parenchyma, no enhancement
Cystography:
  √ smooth wall, clear aspirate with low lactic dehydrogenase, no fat content
Cx: (1) Hemorrhage in 1 – 11.5%
      (2) Infection
      (3) Tumor within cyst in <1%

Atypical Renal Cyst

Cause: hemorrhage / infection
√ delicate septa (10 – 15%)
√ peripheral + curvilinear calcification (1%)

Complicated Renal Cyst

(a) hemorrhagic cyst
(b) infected cyst
√ round sharply marginated lesion
US:
  √ thick-walled with internal echoes
CT:
  √ increased density secondary to hemorrhage / high protein contents (= hyperattenuating cyst with approximately 50 – 80 HU)
  √ no contrast enhancement
DDx: abscess, hematoma, renal artery aneurysm, cystic tumor

Parapelvic Cyst

= spherical fluid-filled masses intimately attached to renal pelvis without connection to pelvocaliceal system

Incidence: 4 – 6% of all renal cysts
Etiology: probably ectatic lymphatic channels / ? from urine extravasation
• serous fluid

√ soft tissue density in renal sinus
√ focal displacement + smooth effacement of collecting system
√ stretching of collecting system when generalized
√ rarely curvilinear calcification of cyst wall (4%)
US:
  √ anechoic mass with acoustic enhancement, irregular shape
Cx: obstructive caliectasis
DDx: hydronephrosis

RENAL DYSGENESIS

= undifferentiated tissue of renal anlage
Pathologic NOT radiologic diagnosis
√ renal vessels usually absent; occasionally small vascular channels

RENAL INFARCTION

Causes:
  1. Trauma: blunt abdominal trauma, traumatic avulsion of renal artery, surgery
  2. Embolism:
     (a) Cardiac: rheumatic heart disease with arrhythmia (atrial fibrillation), myocardial infarction, prosthetic valves, myocardial trauma, left atrial / mural thrombus, myocardial tumors, subacute bacterial endocarditis
     (b) Catheters: angiographic catheter manipulation, umbilical artery catheter above level of renal arteries
  3. Thrombosis:
     arteriosclerosis, thrombangitis obliterans, polyarteritis nodosa, syphilitic cardiovascular disease, aneurysm (aorta / renal artery), sickle cell disease
  4. Sudden complete renal vein thrombosis

Acute Renal Infarction

√ normal / large kidney with smooth contour
√ normal / expanded parenchymal thickness
√ normal / attenuated collecting system, often only opacified by retrograde pyelography
√ absent / diminished nephrogram with cortical rim enhancement, rarely striations
US:
  √ diminished echogenicity (within <24 hours)
  √ normal echogenicity (echoes appear within 7 days)
NUC (SPECT imaging with Tc-99m DMSA):
  √ photon-deficient area

Lobar Renal Infarction

Early signs:
  √ focal attenuation of collecting system (tissue swelling)
  √ focally absent nephrogram (triangular with base at cortex)
Late signs:
  √ normal / small kidney(s)
  √ focally wasted parenchyma with NORMAL interpapillary line (portion of lobe / whole lobe / several adjacent lobes)

CT:
√ nonperfused area corresponding to vascular division, cortical rim sign
US:
√ focally increased echogenicity

Chronic Renal Infarction
Path: all elements of kidney atrophied with replacement by interstitial fibrosis
√ normal / small kidney with smooth contour
√ globally wasted parenchyma
√ diminished / absent contrast material density
US:
√ increased echogenicity (by 17 days)
Angio:
√ normal intrarenal venous architecture
√ late visualization of renal arteries on abdominal aortogram

Atheroembolic Renal Disease
= dislodgement of multiple atheromatous emboli from the aorta into renal circulation (below level of arcuate arteries)
√ normal / small kidneys with smooth contour or shallow depressions
√ wasted parenchymal thickness
√ diminished density of contrast material
CT:
√ patchy nephrographic distribution
Angio:
√ embolic occlusion

Arteriosclerotic Renal Disease
= disseminated process involving most of the interlobar + arcuate arteries causing uniform shrinkage of kidney
Age: generally over 60 years
Accelerated development in: scleroderma, polyarteritis nodosa, chronic tophaceous gout
• often associated with hypertension (NEPHROSCLEROSIS)

√ normal / small kidneys
√ smooth contour with random shallow contour depressions (infarctions)
√ uniform loss of cortical thickness
√ normal / effaced collecting system (fat proliferation)
√ increased pelvic radiolucency (vicarious sinus fat proliferation)
√ calcification of medium-sized intrarenal arteries
US:
√ increased echogenicity possible
√ increased size of renal sinus echoes (fatty replacement)

Nephrosclerosis
Histo: thickening + hyalinization of afferent arterioles, proliferative endarteritis, necrotizing arteriolitis, necrotizing glomerulitis
• arterial hypertension

(a) BENIGN NEPHROSCLEROSIS
(b) MALIGNANT NEPHROSCLEROSIS (rapid deterioration of renal function)
√ radiographic appearance similar to arteriosclerotic kidney

RENAL TRANSPLANT
Complications in 10%
Δ Problematic period between 4 days and 3 weeks after surgery!
• hypertension in 50% (from rejection / arterial stenosis)

Prognosis: 7 – 8 years half-life of cadaver kidneys; 13 – 24 years half-life of transplant from living-related donor

Acute Tubular Necrosis in Renal Transplant
= primary nonfunctioning with improvement over time (few days – 1 month) secondary to ischemic insult
— ATN more frequent in cadaveric than living-related donor transplant
— ATN greater in transplants with more than one renal artery
— ATN related to length of ischemic interval
• no constitutional symptoms
• elevated urine sodium
• oliguria may begin immediately after transplantation / may be delayed for several days

US:
√ transient enlargement of transplant
√ transient increase in resistive index
Scintigram:
√ normal / slightly decreased transplant perfusion
√ decreased + delayed radiopharmaceutical uptake
√ delayed / decreased / absent excretion of Tc-99m
DDx: acute rejection (serial renal studies help to differentiate)

Rejection of Renal Transplant
Δ Most common cause of parenchymal failure!

1. **Hyperacute rejection**
   = humeral rejection with circulating antibodies present in recipient at time of transplantation, usually following retransplantation
   Path: thrombosed arterioles + cortical necrosis
   Time of onset: within minutes after transplantation
   √ complete absence of renal perfusion + renal function on Tc-99m DTPA scan (DDx: complete arterial / venous occlusion)
   Rx: requires immediate reoperation

2. **Accelerated acute rejection**
   = combination of antibody + cell-mediated rejection
   Time of onset: 2 – 5 days after transplantation

3. **Acute rejection**
   = cellular rejection predominantly dependent on cellular immunity

Time of onset: after 1st week; peak incidence at 2nd – 5th week

Path:
- (a) acute interstitial rejection
  = edema of interstitium with lymphocytic infiltration of capillaries + lymphatics
- (b) acute vascular rejection (rare)
  = proliferative endovasculitis + vessel thrombosis
- low urine sodium, increase in serum creatinine
- hypertension
- oliguria
- fever
- tenderness of transplant
- weight gain

US (30 – 50% negative predictive value):
- √ mild transplant enlargement (most reliable)
- √ increased cortical thickness
- √ increased cortical echogenicity
- √ medullary enlargement with prominence of pyramids
- √ indistinct corticomedullary boundaries

Doppler:
- √ initially <u>decrease</u> in resistive index (? autoregulatory mechanism)
- √ increase in resistive index with increasing severity of rejection

NUC:
- √ may show decreased renal perfusion + renal function
- √ initally perfusion may be normal with only function decreased (DDx to ATN may not be possible on single study)
- √ subsequent exams (1 – 3 day intervals) demonstrate decreasing renal perfusion
- √ prolonged excretory phase
- √ poor and inhomogeneous nephrogram

Angio:
- √ rapid tapering + pruning of interlobar arteries
- √ multiple stenoses + occlusions
- √ nonvisualization of interlobular arteries
- √ prolonged arterial opacification (normally <2 seconds)

4. **Chronic rejection**
   = slow relentless progressive process resulting in interstitial scarring + fibrosis
   Path: endothelial proliferation in small arteries + arterioles; glomerular lesions (? recurrence of patient's original glomerulonephritis)
   Time of onset: months to years after transplantation
   - √ small kidney
   - √ diminished number of intrarenal vessels
   - √ vascular pruning / stenoses / occlusions

Cyclosporin Nephrotoxicity
Action: impedes rejection process with narrow therapeutic window

Histo:
- (a) acutely: damage to tubules, microthrombosis of kidney (secondary to activation of coagulation cascade)
- (b) chronically: hyaline deposition within arterial walls
- √ NO change in renal size / resistive index

Urologic Problems with Renal Transplant

1. **Ureteral obstruction** (1 – 10%)
   - (a) acute: secondary to technical problems
   - (b) late: secondary to ischemia or previous extravasation
   Causes:
   stricture (most commonly at ureterovesicle junction), ureteral kinking, edema at ureteroneo-cystostomy, ureteropelvic fibrosis, crossing vessels, blood clot, lymphocele, fungus ball, calculus
   - √ pyelocaliectasis
   - √ normal resistive index strongly argues against obstruction unless ureteral leak is present
   DDx: low-pressure dilatation secondary to denervation (confirmed by Whitaker test)

2. **Urine extravasation** (3 – 10%)
   Causes:
   - (1) Distal ureteral necrosis secondary to interruption of blood supply (early) / vascular insufficiency due to rejection (late)
   - (2) Leakage from ureteroneocystostomy site
   - (3) Leakage from anterior cystostomy closure site
   - (4) Segmental renal infarction
   - high creatinine level in fluid collection
   Prognosis: high morbidity + mortality (death from transplant infection + septicemia)

3. **Pararenal fluid collection**
   Incidence: in up to 50% of transplantations
   - (1) Lymphocele (10%)
     arises within 1 month after transplantation
     - does not contain creatinine
     - √ mean diameter of 11 cm
     - √ thick septae (50%) + internal debris
     - *Rx:* long-term catheter drainage / surgical marsupialization
   - (2) Urinoma
     - √ rarely septated + smaller than lymphoceles
   - (3) Abscess, hematoma
     - √ photopenic region with displacement / impression on kidney / urinary bladder

Vascular Problems with Renal Transplant
A. PRERENAL
   1. **Renal artery stenosis** (1 – 12%)
      Time of onset:
      within 3 years; cadaver kidney > young donor kidney > living-related donor kidney

(a) short-segment stenosis at anastomosis: technical (75%), use of clamp / cannula, trauma, ischemia of donor vessel

(b) long-segment stenosis: trauma during allograft harvesting, faulty operative technique, chronic rejection, atherosclerosis, kinking, scar formation

- recent onset of hypertension
- renal dysfunction
- bruit over graft site (occasionally)
- √ increase in maximum frequency shift at stenotic site >7.5 kHz (3 MHz transducer) or >12.5 kHz (5 MHz transducer): 94% sensitivity + 86% specificity
- √ gross poststenotic turbulence (supportive evidence)
- √ dampened signals distal to stenosis

2. **Renal artery thrombosis** (1 – 5%)
   Cause: rejection, faulty surgical technique
   Time of onset: within 1st month
   Predisposed: allografts with disparate vessel size, multiple anastomoses, intramural vessel injury due to faulty handling, rejection
   - early sudden onset of anuria

   - √ global absence of perfusion, uptake, excretion
   - √ segmental infarction due to occlusion of polar artery
   - √ hypo- / hyperechoic area ± cortical thickening
   - √ no flow in affected area

3. **Pseudoaneurysm**
   Cause: percutaneous biopsy with vascular injury, faulty surgical technique, perivascular infection
   Location:
   (a) at anastomotic site: due to suture rupture, anastomotic leakage, vessel wall ischemia
   (b) mostly of arcuate arteries within allograft: following needle biopsy, mycotic infection
   - √ hypoechoic mass
   - √ mixed arterial + venous pulsations within mass
   Prognosis: mostly spontaneous regression

4. **Arteriovenous fistula**
   Cause: percutaneous biopsy with vascular injury, faulty surgical technique, perivascular infection
   - hypertension, hematuria, high-output cardiac failure
   - √ high-velocity low-resistance flow in feeding artery
   - √ arterialization of waveform in draining vein
   - √ turbulence + high frequency velocity shift
   - √ exaggerated focal color around lesion (= perivascular soft-tissue vibration)

5. **Renal allograft necrosis**
   = total lack of perfusion in an area of renal cortex associated with variable degrees of medullary necrosis
   Cause: rejection, surgical ligature, preexistent arterial lesion, severe ATN, prolonged time of warm ischemia
   Pattern:
   1. Small focal necrosis
   2. Large isolated area of infarction (segmental arterial occlusion)
   3. Outer cortical necrosis
   4. Cortical necrosis with large patches
   5. Diffuse cortical necrosis
   6. Cortical + medullary necrosis
   7. Necrosis of whole kidney (occlusion of main renal artery)
   MR:
   - √ slightly hyperintense (ischemic necrosis) / hypointense (hemorrhagic necrosis) / isointense area on T2WI
   - √ hypointense areas on Gd-DTPA images
   US:
   - √ hypoechoic (ischemic necrosis) / iso- or hyperechoic (hemorrhagic necrosis) areas
   - √ swollen area (probably cortical edema)
   - √ absence of arterial perfusion by color duplex (not sensitive for small infarcts / superficial cortical necrosis)
   - √ elevated resistive indexes + no / reversed diastolic flow

B. POSTRENAL
   Renal / iliac vein thrombosis (4.2 – 5%)
   - abrupt onset of renal dysfunction
   - graft tenderness
   - hematuria, proteinuria
   - √ enlargement of transplant
   - √ prolonged arterial transit time without arterial occlusions + arterial spasms
   - √ diminished cortical perfusion
   - √ absent venous flow
   - √ reversed diastolic arterial flow
   - √ decreased systolic rise time

HIGH VASCULAR IMPEDANCE OF RENAL TRANSPLANT
   = Pulsatility index (A-B/mean) or resistive index (A-B/B) of Doppler signals greater than 1.8 or 0.75 indicate a reduction in diastolic flow velocity
   Causes:
   (a) intrinsic vascular obstruction
      1. Acute vascular rejection (later stage)
      2. Renal vein obstruction
   (b) increased intraparenchymal pressure
      1. Severe ATN
      2. Severe pyelonephritis: CMV, herpes, E. coli, C. albicans
      3. Extrarenal compression: large collection, hematoma

4. Urinary obstruction (doubted!)
5. Excessive pressure by transducer

Gastrointestinal Problems with Renal Transplant
Incidence: 40%

1. Gastrointestinal hemorrhage
   (a) Upper GI tract bleeding
   gastric erosions, gastric / duodenal ulcers
   Mortality rate: 2 – 3 x of normal
   (b) Lower GI tract bleeding
   hemorrhoids, pseudomembranous colitis, cecal ulcers, colonic polyps

2. GI tract perforation (3%)
   Causes: spontaneous, antacid impaction, perinephric abscess, diverticular disease
   Location: colon > small bowel > gastroduodenal
   Mortality rate: approaches 75% (because of delayed diagnosis)

Aseptic Necrosis with Renal Transplant
Most common long-term disabling complication; femoral head most common site, bilateral in 59 – 80%
Frequency: 5 – 29%
Time of onset: symptoms develop 5 – 126 (mean 9 – 19) months after transplantation
Risk factors:
   dose + method of glucocorticoid administration, duration + quality of dialysis before transplantation, secondary hyperparathyroidism, allograft dysfunction, liver disease, previous transplantation, iron overload, increased protein catabolism during dialysis
Pathophysiology of corticosteroid therapy:
   (1) Fat embolism (fat globules occlude subchondral end arteries)
   (2) Increase in fat cell volume in closed marrow space (increase in intramedullary pressure leads to diminished perfusion)
   (3) Osteopenia (increased bone fragility)
   (4) Reduced sensibility to pain (loss of protection against excessive stress)
Histo: fragmentation, compression, resorption of dead bone, proliferation of granulation tissue, revascularization, production of new bone
• 40% asymptomatic
• joint pain
• restriction of movement

Sites: femoral head, femoral condyles (lateral > medial condyle), humeral head
√ subchondral bone resorption
√ patchy osteosclerosis
√ collapse / fragmentation of bone
Bone scan:
   √ decreased uptake (early) = interruption of blood supply
   √ increased uptake (late) secondary to
   (a) revascularization + bone reparation
   (b) degenerative osteoarthritis

Posttransplant Lymphoproliferative Disorder
= abnormal proliferation of B-cell lymphocytes strongly associated with Epstein-Barr virus infection (in 80%); up to 11% may arise from T-cell lymphocytes
Incidence: 2% of organ transplant recipients
   Δ De novo malignancy affects 6% of renal transplant recipients, in 20% NHL (especially affecting CNS)
   Δ Prevalence of NHL is 35 x greater than in general population!
Cause: sequela of chronic immunosuppression with limited ability to suppress neoplastic activity
Types:
   1. Polyclonal B-cell hyperplasia (nearly identical to infectious mononucleosis)
   2. Monoclonal non-Hodgkin lymphoma
Time of onset: as early as 1 month after transplantation
Location:
@ Lymph nodes: tonsils, cervical neck nodes
@ Gastrointestinal tract
@ Thorax
   √ multiple / solitary well-circumscribed pulmonary nodules ± mediastinal lymphadenopathy (DDx: cryptococcosis, fungus, Kaposi sarcoma)
   √ patchy air-space consolidation (DDx: edema, infection, rejection)
Rx: (1) Antiviral agents
   (2) Reduction / cessation of immunosuppressive agents
   (3) Surgical resection of tumor mass (complete resolution in 63%)

RENAL VEIN THROMBOSIS
Causes:
A. Intrinsic
   (a) children: dehydration from vomiting, diarrhea, glycosuria in infants of diabetic mothers, sepsis, umbilical vein catheterization, enterocolitis
   (b) adults: membranous GN, pyelonephritis, amyloidosis, polyarteritis nodosa, sickle cell anemia, thrombosis of IVC, renal neoplasia (50%), low flow states (CHF, constrictive pericarditis), diabetic nephropathy, lupus nephropathy, sarcoidosis, hypercoagulable states, trauma
B. Extrinsic
   carcinoma of pancreatic tail invading renal vein (in 75%), lymphoma, metastases to retroperitoneum (bronchogenic carcinoma)
Radiographic appearance varies with:
(1) rapidity of venous occlusion (2) extent of occlusion (3) availability of collateral circulation (4) site of occlusion in relation to collateral pathways

Acute Renal Vein Thrombosis
= no time for effective development of collaterals; hemorrhage from ruptured venules + capillaries
• gross hematuria
• flank mass
• consumptive thrombocytopenia
• anuria

√ smooth enlargement of kidney
√ diminished radiographic density
√ little / no pyelocaliceal visualization
√ focal hemorrhagic infarction + capsular rupture
US:
√ diminished echogenicity
√ dilated renal vein / IVC with thrombus
CT: √ exaggerated + prolonged corticomedullary differentiation
√ retroperitoneal hemorrhage
Angio:
√ absent inflow from renal vein into IVC
√ thrombus extending into IVC
NUC:
√ no characteristic pattern on sequential functional study
Cx: (1)   Pulmonary emboli (50%)
(2)   Severe renal atrophy (may show complete recovery)

Subacute Renal Vein Thrombosis
= good collateral drainage; impaired function with steady state or recanalization
√ enlarged edematous boggy kidney
√ slightly diminished / normal nephrographic density (may increase over time)
√ compression of collecting system ("spidery calices")

Chronic Renal Vein Thrombosis
= indolent stage
• 80 – 90% asymptomatic
• nephrotic syndrome (proteinuria, hypercholesterolemia, anasarca)
√ normal excretory urogram in 25% (with good collateral circulation especially if left side affected)
√ notching of proximal ureter
√ retroperitoneal dilated collaterals
US:
√ increased echogenicity
CT:
√ renal vein + IVC thrombus (24%); perirenal collaterals
√ prolonged corticomedullary differentiation
√ delayed / absent pyelocaliceal opacification + attenuated collecting system
√ thickening of Gerota fascia

RETROCAVAL URETER
= CIRCUMCAVAL URETER = abnormality in embryogenesis of IVC with abnormal persistence of right subcardinal vein ventral to ureter (instead of right supracardinal vein, which is dorsal to right ureter)
Incidence: 0.07%;   M:F = 3:1
• symptoms of right ureteral obstruction

√ ureteral course swings medially over pedicle of L3/4, passing behind IVC, and then exiting anteriorly between IVC and aorta returning to its normal position
√ varying degrees of hydronephrosis + proximal hydroureteronephrosis

RETROPERITONEAL FIBROSIS
= ORMOND DISEASE = CHRONIC PERIAORTITIS
Path: dense hard fibrous tissue enveloping the retroperitoneum with effects on ureter, lymphatics, great vessels
Causes:
A. PRIMARY RETROPERITONEAL FIBROSIS (2/3)
Probably autoimmune disease with antibodies to ceroid (by-product of aortic plaque, which has penetrated into media) leading to systemic vasculitis;
Associated with   fibrosis outside retroperitoneum in 8 – 15%
Age: 31 – 60 years (in 70%); M:F = 2:1
Rx: responsive to corticoids
B. SECONDARY RETROPERITONEAL FIBROSIS (1/3)
(1) Drugs (12%): methysergide, phenacetin, hydralazine, ergotamine, methyldopa, amphetamines, LSD
(2) Tumor (8%): lymphoma, carcinoid, retroperitoneal metastases, Hodgkin disease
(3) Retroperitoneal trauma, surgery, infection
(4) Aneurysm of aorta / iliac arteries (desmoplastic response)
(5) Connective tissue disease: eg, polyarteritis nodosa

Peak age: 40 – 60 years;   M:F = 2:1
• renal insufficiency (50 – 60%)
• dull pain in flank, back, abdomen (90%)
• hypertension
• edema, fever, hydrocele (10%)

Location: around aorta + beyond common iliac bifurcation, rarely extends below pelvic rim, may extend into mediastinum
√ medial deviation of ureters in middle third, typically bilateral
√ hydroureteronephrosis
√ ureterectasis at L4/5 (interference with peristalsis)
√ gradual tapering of ureter (extrinsic compression)
US:
√ hypoechoic homogeneous mass
CT:
√ periaortic mass of attenuation similar to muscle
√ may show contrast enhancement (active inflammation)
NUC:
√ gallium uptake during active inflammation

Rx: (1)   Withdrawal of possible causative agent
(2)   Surgical relief of obstruction
(3)   Corticosteroids

RETROPERITONEAL LIPOSARCOMA
= slow-growing tumor that displaces rather than infiltrates surrounding tissue and rarely metastasizes
Incidence: 2nd most common primary retroperitoneal tumor (after malignant fibrous histiocytoma), 95% of all fatty retroperitoneal tumors

Histo:
rarely arising from lipoma
(a) myxoid form (most common): varying degrees of mucinous + fibrous tissue + relatively little lipid = intermediate differentiation
√ radiodensity between water + muscle
(b) lipogenic form: malignant lipoblasts with large amounts of lipid + scanty myxoid matrix = well-differentiated
√ radiodensity of fat
(c) pleomorphic type (least common): marked cellular pleomorphism, paucity of lipid + mucin = highly undifferentiated
√ radiodensity of muscle

Age: most commonly 40 – 60 years; M > F
Sites: lower extremity (45%), abdominal cavity + retroperitoneum (14%), trunk (14%), upper extremity (7.6%), head & neck (6.5%), miscellaneous (13.5%)

CT:
√ solid pattern: inhomogeneous poorly marginated infiltrating mass with contrast enhancement
√ mixed pattern: focal fatty areas (-40 to -20 HU) + areas of higher density (+ 20 HU)
√ pseudocystic pattern: water-density mass (averaging of fatty + solid connective tissue elements)
√ calcifications in up to 12%

Angio:
√ hypovascular without vessel dilatation / capillary staining / laking

Prognosis: most radiosensitive of soft tissue sarcomas; 32% overall 5-year survival

DDx: malignant fibrous histiocytoma, leiomyosarcoma, desmoid tumor

RHABDOMYOSARCOMA

Most common soft tissue tumor in childhood
Incidence: 4 – 8% of all malignant tumors in children <15 years of age; 10 – 25% of all sarcomas
Age: 75% <5 years of age; peak age 2 – 6 years; M:F = 2:1
Histo:
(a) embryonal rhabdomyosarcoma (>50%)
subtype: polyploidal form = sarcoma botryoides = grapelike
(b) alveolar rhabdomyosarcoma (worst prognosis)
(c) pleomorphic rhabdomyosarcoma (mostly in adults)

Location: head + neck (28 – 36%), trigone + bladder neck (18 – 21%), orbit (10%), extremities (18 – 23%), trunk (7 – 8%), retroperitoneum (6 – 7%), perineum + anus (2%), other sites (7%)
Points of origin in genitourinary rhabdomyosarcoma: trigone, prostate, seminal vesicles, spermatic cord, vulva, vagina, cervix, uterus (arising from the mesenchyme of urogenital ridge)
• urinary frequency
• dysuria
• palpable bladder
• hematuria (late manifestation)

• strangury (= painful urge to void without success)
• vaginal discharge / protruding grapelike mass
√ obstruction of bladder neck with large postvoid residual
√ lobulated grapelike tumor mass with elevation of bladder floor
√ homogeneous echogenicity similar to muscle ± hypoechoic areas (hemorrhage / necrosis)
√ retroperitoneal lymph node enlargement
Angio:
√ diffuse tumor vascularity
Prognosis: (a) 14 – 35% 5-year survival with radical surgery
(b) 60 – 90% 3-year survival with chemotherapy

SCHISTOSOMIASIS
= BILHARZIASIS
Organism: S. haematobium (GU tract) >95%; S. mansoni (GI tract) <5%
Lifecycle: female parasite discharges eggs into urine + feces; hatch within fresh water into miracidia; penetrate snail (intermediate host); develop into cercaria; penetrate human skin (usually foot) + pass into lymphatics; settle in portal veins + migrate into pelvic venous plexus; eggs erode bladder mucosa
• frequency, urgency, dysuria
• dull flank pain (from hydronephrosis)
• hematuria

√ calcifications: linear continuous bladder wall calcification (in 4 – 56%), vesical calculi (in 39%), distal ureteral calcification (in 34%), honey-combed calcification of seminal vesicles
√ multiple inflammatory pseudopolyps in bladder + ureter secondary to granulomas (= bilharziomas)
√ ureteral dilatation (atony secondary to fibrosis / perineuritis)
√ ureteritis cystica / ureteritis calcinosa (= punctate calcifications)
√ ureteral strictures in distal third (in 8%) (most commonly in intravesical portion with cobra-head configuration = pseudoureterocele); Makar stricture = focal stricture at L3
√ vesicoureteral reflux
√ thick-walled fibrotic "flat-topped" bladder with high insertion of ureters
√ reduced bladder capacity with significant postvoid residual (fibrotic stage)
√ urethral stricture with perineal fistulas
Cx: (1) Portal hypertension
(2) Squamous cell carcinoma of bladder (discontinuous calcifications, irregular filling defect)

SCLERODERMA
= PROGRESSIVE SYSTEMIC SCLEROSIS (PSS)
Renal disease common within 3 years of onset
Histo: fibrinoid necrosis of afferent arterioles (also seen in malignant hypertension)

√ renal cortical necrosis
√ spotty inhomogeneous nephrogram (constriction + occlusion of arteries)
√ concomitant arterial ectasia

SCROTAL ABSCESS
Etiology:
(1) Complication of epididymo-orchitis (often in diabetics), missed testicular torsion, gangrenous tumor, infected hematoma, primary pyogenic orchitis
(2) Systemic infection: mumps, smallpox, scarlet fever, influenza, typhoid, syphilis, TB
(3) Septic dissemination from: sinusitis, osteomyelitis, cholecystitis, appendicitis
NUC:
√ marked increase in perfusion, hot hemiscrotum with photon-deficient area representing the abscess on Tc-99m pertechnetate scan (DDx: chronic torsion)
√ increased scrotal uptake with leukocyte imaging
US:
√ hypoechoic / complex fluid collection with low-level echoes (differentiation of intra- from extratesticular abscess location possible)

Cx: (1) Pyocele
(2) Fistulous tract to skin

SEMINAL VESICLE CYST
1. ACQUIRED SEMINAL VESICLE CYST
2. CONGENITAL SEMINAL VESICLE CYST
Associated with anomalies of ipsilateral mesonephric duct:
(1) Ectopic insertion of ipsilateral ureter (92%) into bladder neck / posterior prostatic urethra / ejaculatory duct / seminal vesicle
(2) Ipsilateral renal dysgenesis (80%)
(3) Duplication of collecting system (8%)
Symptomatic age: 21 – 41 years
• abdominal / flank / pelvic / perineal pain exacerbated by ejaculation
• dysuria, frequent urination
• epididymitis in prepubertal boy
• recurrent urinary tract infection

√ cystic mass posterior to urinary bladder (DDx: müllerian duct cyst)
√ dilated ejaculatory duct

SINUS LIPOMATOSIS
= PERIPELVIC LIPOMATOSIS
= PELVIC FIBROLIPOMATOSIS
= PERIPELVIC FAT PROLIFERATION
Etiology:
(1) Normal increase with aging and obesity
(2) Vicarious proliferation of sinus fat with destruction / atrophy of kidney (= replacement lipomatosis)
(3) Extravasation of urine leading to proliferation of fatty granulation tissue
(4) Normal variant

Age: 6th – 7th decade
√ kidney may be enlarged
√ elongated "spiderlike / trumpetlike" pelvocaliceal system
√ infundibula arranged in "spoke-wheel" pattern
√ parenchymal thickness diminished with underlying disease
√ occasionally focal fat deposit with localized deformity of collecting system
Plain film:
√ diminished sinus density
CT:
√ unequivocal fat values
US:
√ echodense / patchy hypoechoic sinus complex

SUPERNUMERARY KIDNEY
= aberrant division of nephrogenic cord into two metanephric tails (rare)
Associated with: horseshoe kidney, vaginal atresia, duplicated female urethra, duplicated penis
Location: most commonly on left side of abdomen caudal to normal kidney
√ supernumerary ureter may insert into ipsilateral kidney / directly into bladder / ectopic site

Cx: hydronephrosis, pyonephrosis, pyelonephritis, cysts, calculi, carcinoma, papillary cystadenoma, Wilms tumor

SYSTEMIC LUPUS ERYTHEMATOSUS
Kidneys involved in 100%, renal disease develops in 50%
Histo: focal membranous glomerulonephritis
Incidence: blacks:caucasians = 3:1; M < F; increased risk in relatives
√ nonerosive arthritis of hands (characteristic)
√ aneurysms in interlobular + arcuate arteries (similar to polyarteritis nodosa)
√ normal / decreased renal size
US:
√ increased parenchymal echogenicity

Cx: (1) Nephrotic syndrome (common)
(2) Renal vein thrombosis (rare)
Prognosis: end-stage renal disease is common cause of death

TESTICULAR INFARCTION
Etiology: torsion, trauma, leukemia, bacterial endocarditis, polyarteritis nodosa, Henoch-Schönlein purpura
√ diffusely hypoechoic small testis
√ hyperechoic regions (hemorrhage / fibrosis)

TESTICULAR TORSION
= SPERMATIC CORD TORSION
Most common scrotal disorder in children, 20% of acute scrotal pathology
Incidence: 1:160, 10-fold risk in undescended testis compared with normal annual incidence of 1:4,000 males

Etiology:
(1) "Bell and clapper" deformity = high insertion of tunica vaginalis on spermatic cord
(2) Abnormally loose mesorchium between testis + epididymis
(3) Extravaginal torsion involving testis + tunica vaginalis due to loose attachment of testicular tunics to scrotum during in utero + perinatal period

Peak age: newborn period + puberty (13 – 16 years); <20 years in 74 – 85%; >21 years in 26%; >30 years in 9%

- sudden severe pain in 100% (frequently at night)
- negative urine analysis (98%)
- history of similar episode in same / contralateral testis (42%)
- nausea + vomiting (50%)
- scrotal swelling + tenderness (42%)
- leukocytosis (32%)
- low-grade fever (20%)
- history of trauma / extreme exertion (13%)

Location:
in 5% bilateral (anomalous suspension of contralateral testis found in 50 – 80%)

Salvage rate:
versus time interval between onset of pain and surgery
80 – 100% .... <6 hours
76% .... 6 – 12 hours
20% .... 12 – 24 hours
near 0% .... >24 hours
spontaneous detorsion in 7%
Δ Testis viable for only 3 – 6 hours!

Cx: testicular atrophy (in 33 – 45%)

Acute Testicular Torsion
70% of patients present within first 6 hours from onset of pain
US (80 – 90% sensitivity):
√ testicular + epididymal enlargement with decreased echogenicity
√ increase in size of spermatic cord
√ scrotal skin thickening
√ hydrocele (occasionally)
√ loss of spermatic cord Doppler signal (sensitivity 44%, specificity 67%)
Color duplex (highly accurate):
√ absence of testicular + epididymal flow
NUC (98% accuracy):
Dose: 5 – 15 mCi Tc-99m pertechnetate
Imaging: at 2 – 5 second intervals for 1 minute (vascular phase); at 5 minute intervals for 20 minutes (tissue phase)
√ decreased perfusion / occasionally normal
√ nubbin sign = bump of activity extending medially from iliac artery denoting reactive increased blood flow in spermatic cord with abrupt termination
√ rounded cold area replacing testis (requires knowledge of side + location of painful testis)

Subacute Testicular Torsion
= MISSED TESTICULAR TORSION
- symptoms present for >24 hours
√ enlarged / normal-sized testis with heterogeneous texture
√ normal NUC angiogram / nubbin sign
√ "doughnut" sign = decreased testicular activity with rim hyperemia of dartos perfusion
MRI:
√ enlarged spermatic cord without increase in vascularity
√ whirlpool pattern (twisting of spermatic cord)
√ torsion knot = low-signal-intensity focus at point of twist (displacement of free protons from epicenter of twist)

TESTICULAR TRAUMA
Δ Testicular rupture is indication for immediate surgical intervention!
Salvageability:
90% if surgical repair occurs <72 hours after trauma;
55% if surgical repair occurs >72 hours after trauma

√ areas of decreased / increased echogenicity (hemorrhage ± necrosis)
√ thickened scrotal wall
√ visualization of fracture plane
√ hematocele, may show thickening + calcification of tunica vaginalis if chronic
√ uriniferous hydrocele from perforated bulbous urethra
√ avascular region on color duplex

TESTICULAR TUMOR
Most common neoplasm in males between ages 25 – 34 years; 1 – 2% of all cancers in males; 1.5% of all childhood malignancies; 4th most common cause of death from malignancy between ages 15 – 34 years (12%)
Incidence per year: 3 – 5:100,000
Peak age: 25 – 35 years
Risk factors:
(a) Caucasian race, Jewish religion
(b) family history of testicular cancer, previous testicular neoplasm
(c) testicular maldescent / atrophy (10 x risk); abdominal site affected in 5%, inguinal site affected in 1.25%
- chronic pain, "heaviness," acute scrotal pain (10%)
- enlarging testis, mass
- gynecomastia, virilization

STAGING
Stage I limited to testis + spermatic cord
Stage II metastases to lymph nodes below diaphragm
   II A nonpalpable
   II B bulky mass
Stage III metastases to lymph nodes above diaphragm
   III A confined to lymphatic system
   III B extranodal metastases

Metastases: at presentation in 4 – 14% to lung, liver, bones, brain, lymph nodes

Tumor activity: monitored by levels of α-fetoprotein + β-HCG

Color duplex:
  √ tumor <1.5 cm is hypovascular, >1.5 cm hypervascular (DDx: orchitis)
  √ distortion of vessels

Prognosis:
  >93% 5-year survival rate for stage I;
  85 – 90% 5-year survival rate for stage II;
  complete remission under chemotherapy in 65 – 75%;
  relapse in 10 – 20% within 18 months

Germ Cell Tumors (95%)
  (a) one histologic type in 65%
  (b) mixed lesion in 35%
      1. Teratocarcinoma (= teratoma + embryonal cell carcinoma)
         2nd most common after seminoma, may occasionally undergo spontaneous regression
      2. Embryonal cell carcinoma + seminoma
      3. Seminoma + teratoma

A. **SEMINOMA** (40 – 50%)
    Most common tumor in undescended testis
    Peak age: 30 – 40 years
    Spread: in 25% metastasized on initial presentation, pulmonary metastases develop in 19%
    • serum α-fetoprotein usually normal
    • β-HCG elevation in 10 – 15%
    √ usually uniformly hypoechoic + confined within tunica albuginea
    Rx: sensitive to radiation + chemotherapy
    Prognosis: 10-year survival rate of 75 – 85%

B. NONSEMINOMA
    1. **Embryonal Cell Carcinoma** (20 – 25%)
       Most common component of mixed testicular tumors
       Peak age: 2nd – 3rd decade and <2 years
       Spread: most aggressive testicular tumor, visceral metastases
       • ± α-fetoprotein elevation
       √ hypoechoic mass with areas of increased echogenicity + cystic areas (hemorrhage / necrosis)
       √ may show invasion of tunica albuginea
       Prognosis: 30 – 35% 5-year survival rate

    2. **Teratoma** (4 – 10%)
       2nd most common testicular tumor in young boys
       Histo: consists of elements from more than one germ cell layer
       Age: benign in children; may transform into malignancy in adulthood

       • serum α-fetoprotein may be elevated
       √ mixed echotexture with sonolucent + highly echogenic components (markedly heterogeneous)
       Prognosis: metastases to lymph nodes, bone, liver in 30% within 5 years

    3. **Choriocarcinoma** (1 – 3%)
       Peak age: 20 – 30 years
       Spread: may rapidly metastasize without evidence of choriocarcinoma in primary lesion, pulmonary metastases develop in 81%
       • serum β-HCG always elevated
       √ mixed echotexture (hemorrhage, necrosis, calcifications)
       Prognosis: nearly 0% 5-year survival rate

    4. **Yolk sac tumor**
       Equivalent to endodermal sinus tumor of ovary
       Age: childhood
       • serum α-fetoprotein always elevated

    5. **Epidermoid cyst of testicle** (<1%)
       = KERATIN CYST = benign teratoma with only ectodermal components
       Age: 20 – 40 years; primarily in whites
       Histo: cyst contains keratin, wall composed of fibrous tissue + lined by squamous epithelium
       √ sharply circumscribed encapsulated round lesion of 0.5 – 10.5 cm in diameter
       √ hyperechoic fibrous cyst wall ± shadowing from calcifications
       √ hypoechoic cyst contents (= laminated keratin debris)
       √ may have echogenic center (= calcification of intraluminal content)
       MRI:
          √ target appearance with fibrous capsule of low signal intensity on T1WI + T2WI , cyst content of high signal intensity on T1WI + T2WI, central calcification with center of low signal intensity

Stromal Cell Tumors = Interstitial Cell Tumors (3%)
  • gynecomastia
  • loss of libido
  • precocious virilism (children)
  • impotence (adults)

1. **Leydig Cell Tumor**
   benign:malignant = 9:1
   • may secrete androgens / estrogens
   √ usually hypoechoic nodule

2. **Sertoli Cell Tumor**
   generally benign with 10% malignant; may secrete estrogens

3. Primitive gonadal stroma tumor (exceedingly rare)

Metastases to Testis (0.06%)
(a) in adults: prostate > lung > kidney > GI tract,
     bladder, thyroid, melanoma
(b) in children: neuroblastoma
√ often multiple and bilateral, mostly hypoechoic,
   occasionally echogenic masses

Lymphoma / Leukemia of Testis
Incidence: 6.7% of all testicular tumors
Lymphoma: most common testicular tumor in men >
         age 50; bilateral in 40%
Leukemia: 92% incidence of testicular involvement on
         autopsy, 8 – 16% on clinical examination
         during therapy, up to 41% on clinical
         examination after therapy
Δ Occult testicular tumor often found in patients in bone
  marrow remission ("gonadal barrier" to chemotherapy)
√ diffuse / focal process of decreased echogenicity

Burned Out Tumor
= AZZOPARDI TUMOR
= spontaneous regression of testicular malignancy
  (teratocarcinoma)
√ highly echogenic focal lesion ± shadowing

SECOND TESTICULAR TUMOR
Risk for second tumor in cryptorchidism:
  15% for inguinal, 30% for abdominal location

Risk for second contralateral tumor:
  500 – 1,000 x ; bilaterality in 1.1 – 4.4%;
  Δ Development interval between 1st + 2nd tumor:
  4 months – 25 years
  Δ Detected in 47% by 2 years; in 60% by 5 years,
  in 75% by 10 years
  Δ Synchronous contralateral tumor in 8 – 10%

  US: a testicular abnormality is malignant in only
      50%!

TUBERCULOSIS
Urogenital tract is the second most common site after
lung; almost always affects the kidney first as a
hematogenous focus from lung / bone / GI tract; evidence
of previous TB on CXR in 10 – 15%; <5% have active
pulmonary disease
Age: usually before age 50; M > F

• gross / microscopic hematuria
• "sterile" pyuria
• frequency, urgency, dysuria
• history of previous clinical TB (25%)

@ EXTRARENAL SIGNS ON ABDOMINAL PLAIN FILM
  √ osseous / paraspinous changes of TB (discitis +
     psoas abscess)
  √ calcified granulomas in liver, spleen, lymph nodes,
     adrenals

@ RENAL MANIFESTATIONS
Unilateral involvement in 75% with hematogenous
spread
√ displacement of collecting system secondary to
   tuberculoma (initial infection)
√ dystrophic amorphous calcifications in
   tuberculomas of renal parenchyma (in 25%)
√ kidney enlarged (early) / small (late) / normal
√ "smudged" papillae = irregularities of surface of
   papillae
√ "moth-eaten" calyx = caliceal erosion (early change)
√ irregular tract formations from calyx into papilla
√ large irregular cavities with extensive destruction =
   papillary necrosis
√ dilated calices (hydrocalicosis) often with sharply
   defined circumferential narrowings (infundibular
   strictures) at one / several sites (most common
   finding)
√ renal calculi (in 10%)
√ "putty kidney" = tuberculous pyonephrosis from
   ureteral stricture
√ autonephrectomy = small shrunken scarred
   nonfunctioning kidney ± dystrophic calcifications
√ infection may extend into peri- / pararenal space +
   psoas

@ URETERAL MANIFESTATIONS
Always with evidence of renal involvement as it
spreads from kidney
Location: either end of ureter (most commonly distal
         1/3), usually asymmetric, may be unilateral

√ ureteral filling defects (= mucosal granulomas)
√ "saw tooth ureter" = irregular jagged contour
   secondary to dilatation + multiple small mucosal
   ulcerations + wall edema (early changes)
√ strictures (late changes):
   "beaded ureter"   = alternating areas of strictures
                    + dilatations
   "corkscrew ureter" = marked tortuosity with
                    strictures + dilatations
   "pipe stem ureter" = rigid aperistaltic short thick
                    and straight ureter
√ vesicoureteral reflux through "fixed" patulous orifice
√ ureteral calcifications uncommon (usually in distal
   portion)

@ BLADDER MANIFESTATIONS
Infection from renal source causing interstitial cystitis
√ thickened bladder wall (= muscle hypertrophy +
   inflammatory tuberculomas)
√ bladder wall ulcerations
√ "shrunken bladder" = scarred bladder with
   diminished capacity
√ bladder wall calcifications (rare)
Cx: fistula / sinus tract

@ SEMINAL VESICULAR + EPIDIDYMAL
  MANIFESTATIONS
Hematogenous infection (NOT ascending)

√ calcifications in 10% (diabetes more common cause)

DDx: brucellosis, fungal infections (identical picture)

UNICALICEAL (UNIPAPILLARY) KIDNEY

Path: OLIGOMEGANEPHRONIA = reduced number of nephrons and enlargement of glomeruli

Associated with: absence of contralateral kidney, other anomalies

- hypertension
- proteinuria
- azotemia

URACHAL CARCINOMA

= rare tumor arising from the urachus (vestigial remnant of cloaca + allantois) within space of Retzius

Incidence: 0.2 – 0.34% of all bladder cancers; 20 – 40% of all primary bladder adenocarcinomas

Histo: (a)   adenocarcinoma (90%) from malignant transformation of columnar metaplasia, in 75% mucin producing
  (b)   TCC, sarcoma, squamous cell carcinoma

Age: 41 – 70 years;   M:F = 3:1

- suprapubic mass, abdominal pain
- hematuria (71%)
- discharge of blood, pus, mucus from umbilicus
- irritative voiding symptoms
- mucous micturition (25%)

Location: supravesical, midline, anterior (80%), in space of Retzius (bounded by transversalis fascia ventrally + peritoneum dorsally)

√ mass anterosuperior to vesical dome with predominantly muscular / extravesical involvement
√ invasion of bladder dome (88%)
√ low attenuation mass in 60% (mucin)
√ often peripheral psammomatous calcifications (70%)
√ markedly increased signal intensity on T2WI

Prognosis: 16% 5-year survival rate

URETERAL DUPLICATION

Complete Duplication

Incidence: 0.5 – 10% of livebirths; in 6% of urograms;   M:F = 1:2;   in 15 – 40% bilateral

Risk of recurrence: 12% in 1st degree relatives

Embryology: ureters develop from separate ureteric buds originating from a single Wolffian duct

(1)   Upper pole moiety
  Ectopic ureter inserts below and medial to orthotopic ureter
  Subject to OBSTRUCTION

(2)   Lower pole moiety
  Orthotopic ureter drains lower pole and interpolar portion + enters bladder at trigone
  Subject to VESICOURETERAL REFLUX

√ two separate echodense renal sinuses + pelves separated by parenchymal bridge

√ atrophic system may simulate a renal mass = nubbin sign
√ obstructed upper pole moiety with tortuous dilated ureter
√ faintly visualized diminutive collecting system
√ paucity of cranial calices
√ flattening of lower pole
√ vesicoureteral reflux into atrophied lower pole

Partial Duplication

√ bifid ureter (in early branching)
√ bifid pelvis (in late branching)
√ "yo-yo" peristalsis = urine moves down the cephalad ureter + refluxes up the lower pole ureter
√ upper pole ureter may end blindly (seen on retrograde injection only)

URETEROCELE

= cystic ectasia of subepithelial segment of intravesical ureter

Simple Ureterocele

= ORTHOTOPIC URETEROCELE = congenital prolapse of dilated distal ureter + orifice into bladder lumen at the usual location of the trigone, typically seen with single ureter

Presentation: incidental finding in adults; M:F = 2:3; bilateral in 33%

√ early filling of bulbous terminal ureter ("cobra head")
√ radiolucent halo (= ureteral wall + adjacent bladder urothelium)
√ round / oval lucent defect near trigone

Cx: (1)   Pyelocaliceal dilatation
  (2)   Prolapse into bladder neck / urethra causing obstruction (rare)
  (3)   Wall thickening secondary to edema from impacted stone / infection

Ectopic Ureterocele

= ureteral bud arising in an abnormal cephalad position from the mesonephric duct and moving caudally resulting in an ureteral orifice distal to trigone within / outside bladder

Incidence: in 10% bilateral

(a)   in single non-duplicated system (20%)
  M:F = 1:1
  • hypoplastic / absent ipsilateral trigone
  √ poor / non-visualized kidney
  √ small / poorly functioning kidney
(b)   in upper moiety ureter of duplex kidney (80%)
  M:F = 1:4

Weigert-Meyer rule = upper moiety ureter passes through the bladder wall to insert inferior + medial to lower moiety ureter below the level of trigone

SITE OF ECTOPIC INSERTION:
  M: proximal to external sphincter:
    low in bladder, bladder neck, prostatic urethra, vas deferens, seminal vesicle (seminal vesical cyst), ejaculatory duct

- NO WETTING in males as insertion is always above external sphincter
- epididymitis in preadolescent male
- urge incontinence (insertion into posterior urethra)

F: infrasphincteric insertion:
distal urethra, vaginal vestibule, vagina, cervix, uterus, fallopian tube, rectum
- WETTING in females only if insertion is below external sphincter
- intermittent / constant dribbling

UPPER MOIETY URETER
= subject to ureteral obstruction from ectopic insertion / aberrant artery crossing
√ hydroureteronephrosis of upper pole of duplex kidney + poor function
√ poor / nonvisualization of upper pole collecting system (delayed films)
√ "drooping lily" appearance = displacement of lower pole collecting system
√ lateral displacement of lower pole collecting system + ureter
√ tortuous dilated lower pole ureter
Cx:
(1) Bladder outlet obstruction (if ureterocele prolapses into bladder neck / urethra)
(2) Contralateral ureteral obstruction (if ectopic ureter large)
(3) Multicystic dysplastic kidney (the further the orifice from normal site of insertion, the more dysplastic the kidney!)

LOWER MOIETY URETER
= subject to vesicoureteral reflux with reflux atrophy / chronic pyelonephritis
√ displacement of proximal orifice upward (shortened course results in reflux)
√ voiding cystogram may show reflux (rare)
Cx: lower pole of duplex kidney may atrophy (in 50%) secondary to chronic pyelonephritis
= reflux nephropathy (from reflux ± infection)
√ clubbed calices underneath focal scars

Pseudoureterocele
= obstruction of an otherwise normal intramural ureter mimicking ureterocele
Causes:
(a) Tumor: bladder tumor (most common in adults), invasion by cervical cancer, pheochromocytoma of intravesical ureter
(b) Edema: from impacted ureteral calculus (most common in children), radiation cystitis, following ureteral instrumentation

√ thick, irregular halo in urinary bladder
√ "cobra head" / "spring onion" appearance of distal ureter
√ NO protrusion of ureter into bladder lumen (oblique views + cystocopy normal)

URETEROPELVIC JUNCTION OBSTRUCTION
M:F = 5:1
Intrinsic causes: primarily functional with impaired formation of urine bolus
(1) partial replacement of UPJ muscle by collagen
(2) abnormal arrangement of junction muscles causing dysmotility (69%) (3) mucosal folds in upper ureter
(4) eosinophilic ureteritis (5) ischemia

Extrinsic causes:
(1) aberrant vessels to lower pole (2) adventitial bands
(3) renal cyst (4) XGP (5) aortic aneurysm

Associated anomalies (27%):
vesicoureteral reflux, bilateral ureteral duplication, bilateral obstructed megaureter, contralateral nonfunctioning kidney, contralateral renal agenesis, meatal stenosis, hypospadia

Location: left > right side; bilateral (30%)
√ large dilated anechoic renal pelvis communicating with calices, but without dilated ureter
IVP:
√ sharply defined narrowing at UPJ
√ widening of the pelvocaliceal system
√ anterior rotation of pelvis
√ broad tangential sharply defined extrinsic compression (in arterial crossing)
√ longitudinal striae of redundant mucosa (in dehydrated state)
√ late changes: unilateral renal enlargement, diminished opacification, wasting of kidney substance
OB-US:
√ enlargement of renal pelvis + branching infundibula + calices
√ anteroposterior diameter of renal pelvis ≥10 mm
√ large unilocular fluid collection (severely dilated collecting system)
DDx: multicystic dysplastic kidney, perinephric urinoma

ADDITIONAL TESTS:
(1) Diuresis excretory urography (Whitfield): accurate in 85%
(2) Diuresis renography (Iodine-131-iodohippurate sodium / Tc-99m-DTPA)
(3) Pressure flow urodynamic study (Whitaker)

URETHRAL TUMORS
BENIGN LESIONS
1. **Fibroepithelial polyp**
in child / young adult; transitional cell epithelium
√ solitary, pedunculated fingerlike filling defect attached near verumontanum
Cx: bladder outlet obstruction
2. **Transitional cell papilloma**
older patient; in prostatic / bulbomembranous urethra; frequently associated with concomitant bladder papillomas
3. **Adenomatous polyp**
young men; adjacent to verumontanum

Histo: columnar epithelium from aberrant prostatic epithelium
- hematuria

4. **Penile squamous papilloma / condyloma acuminata**

in 5% of patients with cutaneous disease (glans penis)
√ verrucous lesion in distal urethra, rarely extension into bladder

5. Others: caruncle, urethral mucosal prolapse, inflammatory tags (in female)

<u>MALIGNANT NEOPLASMS</u>

Incidence: 6th – 7th decade, M:F = 1:5
(a) female
- urethral bleeding
- obstructive symptoms
- dysuria
- mass at introitus
1. Squamous cell carcinoma (70%):
   distal 2/3 of urethra
2. Transitional cell carcinoma (8 – 24%):
   posterior 1/3 of urethra
3. Adenocarcinoma (18 – 28%):
   from periurethral glands of Skene
(b) males
- palpable urethral mass
- periurethral abscess
- obstructive symptoms
- cutaneous fistula
- bloody discharge
Site: bulbomembranous urethra (60%); penile urethra (30%); prostatic urethra (10%)
1. Squamous cell carcinoma (70%)
   secondary to chronic urethritis from venereal disease (44%) + urethral strictures (88%)
2. Transitional cell carcinoma (16%)
   part of multifocal urothelial neoplasia, in 10% after cystectomy for bladder tumor
3. Adenocarcinoma (6%)
   in bulbous urethra originating in glands of Cowper / Littre
4. Melanoma, rhabdomyosarcoma, fibrosarcoma (rare)
5. Metastases from bladder / prostatic carcinoma (rare)

URINOMA

= uriniferous perirenal pseudocyst secondary to tear in collecting system with continuing renal function
Etiology:
(a) nonobstructive: blunt / penetrating trauma, surgery, infection, calculus erosion
(b) obstructive:
   (1) ureteral obstruction (calculus, surgical ligature, neoplasm)
   (2) bladder outlet obstruction (posterior urethral valves)
Δ Augmented by sudden diuretic load of urographic contrast material!

Path: fibroblastic cavity (in 5 – 12 days), dense connective tissue encapsulation (in 3 – 6 weeks)
√ extravasation of contrast material
√ smooth thin-walled cavity (-10 to +30 HU)
  √ sickle-shaped collection = SUBCAPSULAR urinoma
  √ cystic mass in perirenal space = LOCALIZED PERIRENAL urinoma (most common)
  √ cystic mass filling entire perirenal space = DIFFUSE PERIRENAL urinoma
  √ encapsulated expanding intrarenal cystic mass separating renal tissue fragments = INTRARENAL urinoma
√ frequently associated with urine ascites
Cx: retroperitoneal fibrosis, stricture of upper ureter, perinephric abscess
Dx: aspirated fluid with high urea concentration
DDx: lymphocele, hematoma, abscess, renal cyst, pancreatic pseudocyst, ascites

UROEPITHELIAL TUMORS

Incidence: 6 – 10% of all malignant renal tumors
Age: 6th decade; M:F = 2:1

Transitional Cell Carcinoma

Incidence: 85% of all urothelial tumors; 7% of all renal neoplasms; 85% of primary renal pelvic tumors
High-risk group to develop TCC of upper tract:
   (1) high-grade high-stage bladder TCC (2) cystectomy for carcinoma in situ (3) analgesic abuser (8 x increase) (4) employee in aniline dye factory (5) patient from Balkan (6) bladder tumor + vesicoureteral reflux (7) exposure to urothelial carcinogens (cyclophosphamide, tobacco smoke)
Ureteral site: lower 1/3 (70%), mid 1/3 (15%), upper 1/3 (15%)
√ intraluminal mass (60 – 70%): single / multiple, papillary / broad based
√ hydronephrosis
√ parenchymal mass (invasive TCC)
√ stippled appearance (contrast material trapped in interstices)
√ coarse punctate calcific deposits (0.7 – 6.7%)
IVP:
  √ nonopacification of kidney (in advanced tumor with loss of function)
  √ "goblet sign" = "Bergman sign" = ureter dilated distal to obstructing mass (probably secondary to to-and-fro peristalsis of mass)
  √ "catheter-coiling sign" = coiling of catheter on retrograde catheterization
US:
  √ splitting / separation of central renal sinus complex
  √ bulky hypoechoic (similar to renal parenchyma) mass lesion

<u>SYNCHRONOUS TCC</u>
(a) in 39% with primary ureteral TCC
(b) in 24% with primary renal TCC
(c) in 2% with primary bladder TCC

METACHRONOUS TCC IN UPPER TRACT
- (a) in 12% with primary renal + ureteral TCC after 25 months
- (b) in 4% with primary bladder TCC (2/3 within 2 years, up to 20 years)

METACHRONOUS TCC OF BLADDER
- (a) in 23 – 40% after primary renal TCC after 15 – 48 months
- (b) in 20 – 50% after primary ureteral TCC after 10 – 24 months

Squamous Cell Carcinoma
Incidence: 15% of all urothelial tumors
Path: flat ulcerating mass + extensive induration
Associated with: previous chronic renal infection + calculi (25 – 60%)
√ stricture that may simulate extrinsic cause
√ ureteropelvic junction obstruction (common)
√ presence of faceted calculi
√ thickening of pelvocaliceal wall (with superficial spread over large areas)
√ arterial encasement + occlusion + neovascularity
√ enlarged pelvic + ureteric arteries
√ occlusion of renal vein / branches (41%)
Prognosis: poor due to early metastases

UROLITHIASIS
Anderson-Carr-Randall theory of renal stone formation: in the presence of abnormally high calcium excretion exceeding lymphatic capacity, microaggregates of calcium (present in the normal kidney) occur in medulla, increase in size, migrate toward caliceal epithelium, and rupture into calices to form calculi
Formation theory:
- (a) nucleation theory
  = crystal / foreign body initiates formation in urine supersaturated with crystallizing salt
- (b) stone matrix theory
  = organic matrix of urinary proteins + serum serves as framework for deposition of crystals
- (c) inhibitor theory
  = little / no concentration of urinary stone inhibitors results in crystal formation

Incidence: 1:1,000; M > F
Δ 12% of population develop renal stones by age 70
Δ 2 – 3% of population experience an attack of acute renal colic during their lifetime
Δ patients with acute flank pain have ureteral calculi in 67 – 95%

Causes:
Δ 70 – 80% of patients with first-time stones have a specific metabolic disorder

1. Idiopathic urolithiasis
2. Calcium stones
   - (a) with hypercalcemia (50%): hyperparathyroidism, milk-alkali syndrome, hypervitaminosis D, neoplastic disorders, sarcoidosis, Cushing syndrome
   - (b) with normocalcemia (30 – 60%): obstruction, urinary tract infection, vesical diverticulum, horseshoe kidney, medullary sponge kidney, prolonged immobilization, renal tubular acidosis, idiopathic hypercalcuria
3. Hyperoxaluria
   - (a) congenital = deficiency of an enzyme leading to accumulation of glycolate + oxylate
   - (b) acquired = inceased intake of oxalate / oxalate precursors, excess oxalate absorption from large bowel
4. Uric acid lithiasis
   - hyperuricosuria (15 – 20%); stones form in acid urine

	Mineral composition	Opacity
A.	CALCIUM STONES (90%)	
	1. Calcium oxalate monohydrate (= whewellite) + dihydrate (wedellite) (34%)	+++
	√ small, densely opaque, mamillated (stippled appearance)	
	2. Calcium oxalate plus apatite (34%)	+++
	3. Calcium phosphate (= apatite) (5 – 10%)	+++
	rarely pure (= laminated), occasionally forms in infected alkaline urine	
	4. Calcium hydrogen phosphate (= brushite)	+++
	5. Magnesium ammonium phosphate (= struvite) (1%)	++
	laminated, result of urea-splitting organisms (usually Proteus), most common constituent of staghorn calculus	
	6. Struvite plus calcium phosphate (5 – 10%)	++
	associated with infection	
B.	Cystine (3%): mildly opaque	+
C.	Uric acid (5 – 10%): radiolucent	-
D.	Xanthine (extremely rare): nonopaque	-
E.	Matrix (mucoprotein / mucopolysaccharide) (rare): nonopaque	-

(a) with hyperuricemia:
   gout (25%) from excessive intake of meat, fish, poultry, myeloproliferative diseases, antimitotic drugs, chemo- / radiation therapy, uricosuric agents, Lesch-Nyhan syndrome
(b) with normouricemia:
   idiopathic; occurrence in acid concentrated urine (hot climate, ileostomy)
   Rx: raising urinary pH (potassium citrate / sodium bicarbonate)
5. Cystinuria (stones form in acid urine)
   = autosomal recessive disorder in renal tubular reabsorption of cystine, ornithine, lysine, arginine
   Age of onset: after 10 years
   Rx: (1) decreased intake of methionine
        (2) alkalinization of urine
6. Xanthinuria
   = inherited autosomal recessive deficiency of xanthine oxidase (failure of normal oxidation of purines)
7. Urinary tract infection
   Cause: urea-splitting organisms + alkaline environment
   may lead to magnesium ammonium phosphate = struvite stones
8. Any condition causing nephrocalcinosis

Cx: xanthogranulomatous pyelonephritis
Prognosis:
(1) Spontaneous passage of ureteral calculi in 93%
(2) Patient with a first-time calculus has a 50% risk of a new stone forming within 5 years

VARICOCELE

= dilatation + tortuosity of plexus pampiniformis
Components of pampiniform plexus:
(a) internal spermatic vein (ventral location) draining testis
(b) vein of vas deferens (mediodorsal location) draining epididymis
(c) cremasteric vein (laterodorsal location) draining scrotal wall
Etiology:
(1) Retrograde flow into internal spermatic vein secondary to incompetent / absent valve at level of left renal vein / IVC on right side
(2) Compression of left renal vein by tumor, aberrant renal artery, obstructed renal vein
Incidence:
(a) clinical varicocele: in 10 – 15% of adult males, in 21 – 39% of infertile men
(b) subclinical varicocele: in 40 – 75% of infertile men
Theoretical causes for infertility:
(1) increase in local temperature (2) reflux of toxic substances from adrenal gland (3) alteration in Leydig cell function (4) hypoxia of germinative tissue
• scrotal pain
• scrotal swelling
• abnormal spermatogram (impaired motility, immature sperm, oligospermia)

Location: left side (78%), bilateral (16%), right side (6%)

Bidirectional Doppler sonography (erect with quiet breathing):
(1) SHUNT TYPE: insufficent distal valves allow spontaneous + continuous reflux from internal spermatic vein (retrograde flow) into cremasteric vein + vein of vas deferens (orthograde flow) via collaterals
   • sperm quality diminished
   • clinically plexus type (Grade II + III)
     = medium-sized + large varicoceles
(2) STOP TYPE / PRESSURE TYPE: intact distal valves allow only brief period of reflux from spermatic vein into pampiniform plexus under Valsalva maneuver
   • sperm quality normal
   • clinically central type (Grade 0 + I)
     = subclinical + small varicocele
US: diameter of dominant vein in upright position at inguinal canal

	relaxed	during Valsalva
normal	2.2 mm	2.7 mm
small varicocele	2.5 – 4.0	increase of 1.0 mm
moderate varicocele	4.0 – 5.0	increase of 1.2 – 1.5 mm
large varicocele	>5.0	increase of >1.5 mm

VESICOURETERIC REFLUX

A. CONGENITAL REFLUX = PRIMARY REFLUX
   = incompetence of ureterovesical junction unassociated with morphologic abnormalities
   Prevalence: in 1.4% of school girls; in 30% of children with a first episode of UTI
   • short submucosal ureteral tunnel (normally has a length/width ratio of 4:1)
   • large laterally located ureteral orifice
   √ renal scars in 22 – 50%
   Prognosis: disappears in 80%
   Cx: reflux atrophy / nephropathy in 22 – 50%; end-stage renal disease in 5 – 15% of adults

B. ACQUIRED REFLUX = SECONDARY REFLUX
   1. Paraureteric diverticulum = Hutch diverticulum
   2. Duplication with ureterocele
   3. Cystitis (in 29 – 50%)
   4. Urethral obstruction (urethral valves)
   5. Neurogenic bladder
   6. Absence of abdominal musculature (prune belly syndrome)
Cx: renal scarring with UTI (30 – 60%)

GRADES OF REFLUX (VCUG):
   Grade I : √ reflux into distal ureters
   Grade II : √ reflux into collecting system (without caliceal dilatation / blunting)
   Grade III: √ all of the above + mild dilatation of pelvis and calices

Grade IV: √ all of the above + moderate dilatation (clubbing of calices)

Grade V : √ all of the above + severe tortuosity of ureter

Prognosis: (a) grade I – III resolve with maturation of the ureterovesical junction
(b) grade IV – V require surgery to avoid renal scarring + renal impairment + hypertension

Radionuclide cystography:
Δ Lower radiation dose to gonads than fluoroscopic cystography (5 mrad)!
Evaluation of bladder volume at reflux, volume of refluxed urine, residual urine volume, ureteral reflux drainage time
(a) indirect: IV injection of Tc-99m DTPA
(b) direct: instillation of 1 mCi Tc-99m pertechnetate (more sensitive for reflux during filling phase, which occurs in 20%)

US:
√ midline-to-orifice distance >7 – 9 mm has high probability of vesicoureteric reflux

VON HIPPEL-LINDAU SYNDROME
= inherited neurocutaneous dysplasia complex; autosomal dominant (gene located on chromosome 3p) with variable penetrance (80 – 90%) and delayed expression
Age at onset: 2nd – 3rd decade
• visual disturbances (hemorrhage, retinal detachment, glaucoma, uveitis)
• neurologic disorders (from hemangioblastomas)
• polycythemia
@ CNS
1. Hemangioblastomas
most frequent cause of morbidity and mortality
(a) cerebellar (most common)
√ large cystic lesion in posterior fossa with enhancing mural nodule
(b) medullary
(c) spinal
2. Retinal angiomatosis (in 45%)
@ KIDNEYS
1. Cortical renal cysts (75%)
multiple + bilateral (may be confused with adult polycystic kidney disease)
2. Renal cell carcinoma (28 – 45%)
second most frequent cause of mortality
√ multicentric in 87%, bilateral in 75%, may arise from cyst wall
Δ Sensitivity: 35% for angiography, 37% for US, 45% for CT (due to inability to reliably distinguish between cystic RCC, cancer within cyst, atypical cyst)
Δ 50% metastatic at time of discovery
Δ RCC is cause of death in 30 – 50%
3. Renal adenoma
4. Renal hemangioma
@ EPIDIDYMIS
1. Cydstadenoma of epididymis

@ ADRENAL
1. Pheochromocytoma (in 17%): confined to certain families
@ PANCREAS
1. Pancreatic cystadenoma / cystadenocarcinoma
2. Pancreatic islet cell tumor
3. Pancreatic hemangioblastoma
4. Pancreatic cysts (in 30%); incidence in autopsies up to 72%
√ usually multiple and multilocular cysts
@ LIVER
1. Liver hemangioma
2. Adenoma
@ OTHERS
1. Paraganglioma
2. Cysts in virtually any organ: liver, spleen, adrenal, epididymis, omentum, mesentery, lung, bone

WILMS TUMOR
= NEPHROBLASTOMA
Δ Most common malignant abdominal neoplasm in children 1 – 8 years old (10%)!
Δ 3rd most common malignancy in childhood (after leukemia + brain tumors; neuroblastoma more common in infancy)!
Δ 3rd most common of all renal masses in childhood (after hydronephrosis + multicystic dysplastic kidney)!

Incidence: 1:10,000 livebirths; rare during first year; 50% before 3 years, 75% before 5 years; 90% before 8 years; rare in adults; multifocal in 10%; bilateral in 5 – 9%
Age: peak age at 2.5 – 3 years (range of 3 months – 8 years); M:F = 1:1
Histo: arises from undifferentiated metanephric blastema as nephroblastomatosis, recapitulates the developing embryonic kidney
(a) aggregates of small blastemal cells
(b) neoplastic nodules
(c) elongated mesenchymal cells

In 14% associated with:
(1) Beckwith-Wiedemann syndrome (exophthalmos, macrosomia, macroglossia, hepatomegaly, omphalocele, hyperglycemia from islet cell hyperplasia)
(2} Sporadic aniridia
(3) Hemihypertrophy: total / segmental / crossed (2.5%)
(4) Drash syndrome (pseudohermaphroditism, glomerulonephritis, nephrotic syndrome)
(5) Renal anomalies (horseshoe kidney, duplex / solitary / fused kidney)
(6) Genital anomalies (cryptorchidism, hypospadia, ambiguous genitalia)

STAGE:
I tumor limited to kidney
II local extension into perirenal tissue / renal vessels outside kidney / lymph nodes

III not totally resectable (peritoneal implants, other than paraaortic nodes involved, invasion of vital structures)
IV hematogenous metastases (lung, liver, bone [rare], brain)
V bilateral renal involvement (5 – 10%)

- palpable abdominal mass (90%)
- hypertension (47 – 90%)
- abdominal pain (25%)
- fever (15%)
- gross hematuria (7%)
- microscopic hematuria (15 – 20%)

√ large tumor (average size 12 cm)
√ sharply marginated with compressed renal tissue = pseudocapsule
√ partially cystic = focal hemorrhage and necrosis (71%)
√ curvilinear / phlebolithic calcifications (15%); (not stippled as in neuroblastoma)
√ distorted "clobbered" calices
√ tumor may invade IVC / right atrium (4 – 10%)
√ tumor may cross midline
√ hypervascular tumor: enlarged tortuous vessels, coarse neovascularity; small arterial aneurysms, vascular lakes
√ parasitization of vascular supply

US:
√ fairly evenly echogenic mass
√ ± irregular anechoic areas due to central necrosis + hemorrhage
NUC:
√ nonfunctioning kidney (10%)
√ hypo- / iso- / hyperperfusion on radionuclide angiogram
√ absent tracer accumulation on delayed static images

√ displacement of kidney + distortion of collecting system

VARIANT: **Cystic Partially Differentiated Nephroblastoma**
= combination of MLCN + Wilms tumor elements
Incidence: M < F
√ multiple noncommunicating locules
√ polypoid masses within locules

WOLMAN DISEASE
= FAMILIAL XANTHOMATOSIS
= rare autosomal recessive lipidosis with accumulation of cholesteryl esters and triglycerides in visceral foam cells + various tissues
Etiology: deficiency of lysosomal acid lipase
- poor development in neonatal period: failure to gain weight
√ hepatosplenomegaly
√ extensive bilateral punctate calcifications throughout enlarged adrenals (retaining normal shape)
√ generalized osteoporosis
Prognosis: death occurs within first few months of life

ZELLWEGER SYNDROME
= CEREBROHEPATORENAL SYNDROME
autosomal recessive
- muscular hypotonia
- hepatomegaly + jaundice
- craniofacial dysmorphism
- seizures, mental retardation
√ brain dysgenesis (lissencephaly, macrogyria, polymicrogyria)
√ renal cortical cysts
Prognosis: death in early infancy

DIFFERENTIAL DIAGNOSIS OF OBSTETRICAL AND GYNECOLOGICAL DISORDERS

OBSTETRICS
Level I obstetrical ultrasound
Indication: MS-AFP >2 multiples of mean (MOM) on 2 occasions between 14 and 18 weeks MA
Scope of examination:
1. Fetal number
2. Fetal lie
3. Documentation of fetal life
4. Placental location
5. Amniotic fluid volume
6. Gestational dating
7. Detection + evaluation of maternal pelvic masses
8. Survey of fetal anatomy (2nd + 3rd trimester)

Level II obstetrical ultrasound
Indication: AF-AFP >3 standard deviations above mean
Scope of examination:
1. Spina bifida
2. Ventral wall defect (gastroschisis, omphalocele)
3. Upper GI obstruction
4. Cystic hygroma
5. Renal anomalies (obstructive uropathy, renal agenesis)

Elevated alpha-fetoprotein
Origin: formed by yolk sac (4 – 8 weeks) + by fetal liver; levels peak at about 32nd week and decline to low levels at end of pregnancy (a) detectable in amniotic fluid secondary to leakage of fetal serum (transudation, proteinuria) (b) detectable in maternal circulation secondary to leakage from placenta / amniotic fluid
• screening at 14 – 18 weeks
(a) Elevation in MATERNAL SERUM (MS-AFP)
= defined as 2.5 multiples of the median / equivalent to the 5th percentile or 4.5 multiples of mean for multiple gestations
Incidence: 1:500 – 600 infants; 1:100 for infants of diabetic mothers

Multiples of mean MS-AFP	NTD risk General population	Diabetics
1.2	1:4641	1:1202
1.4	1:2578	1:650
1.5	1:1955	1:484
2.0	1:566	1:141
2.1	1:453	1:113
2.8	1:110	
4.0	1:16	

(b) Elevation in AMNIOTIC FLUID (AF-AFP)
Δ elevation of 3 – 5 multiples of the median in 2 – 3:1,000; 1/4 deliver normal babies
Δ elevation >5 multiples of the median in 1 – 2:1,000

Associated with:
A. FETAL ANOMALIES (61%)
1. Neural tube defects: anencephaly, meningocele, myelomeningocele, encephalocele, holoprosencephaly, ventriculomegaly (in 2 – 5% missed by US)
Risk of recurrence: 3% after one affected child; 6% after 2 affected children
2. Ventral wall defects (gastroschisis, omphalocele): sensitivity of 50%
3. Upper GI obstruction (esophageal / duodenal atresia)
4. Cystic hygroma, teratoma
5. Placental anomalies (eg, chorioangioma) + peri- and intraplacental hemorrhage
6. Congenital Finnish nephrosis
7. Feto-maternal hemorrhage
8. Amniotic band syndrome
B. ERRONEOUS DATES (18%): fetus actually older
C. MULTIPLE GESTATIONS (14%)
D. FETAL DEATH IN UTERO (7%) / fetal distress / threatened abortion
E. LOW BIRTH WEIGHT / premature labor
F. MATERNAL DISORDER
1. Hepatitis
2. Hepatoma

Low alpha-fetoprotein
= MS-AFP ≤ 0.5 / AF-AFP ≤ 0.72 multiples of the median
Trisomy syndromes (trisomy 21 & 18)

Use of chromosome analysis
Frequency: 11 – 35% of fetuses with sonographically identified abnormalities have chromosomal abnormalities
1. CNS anomalies: holoprosencephaly (43 – 59%), Dandy-Walker malformation (29 – 50%), cerebellar hypoplasia, agenesis of corpus callosum, myelomeningocele (33 – 50%)
2. Cystic hygroma
3. Omphalocele (30 – 40%)
4. Cardiac malformations
5. Nonimmune hydrops
6. Duodenal atresia
7. Severe IUGR

Uterus large for dates
1. Multiple gestation pregnancy
2. Inaccurate menstrual history
3. Fibroids
4. Polyhydramnios
5. Hydatidiform mole
6. Fetal macrosomia

[handwritten margin notes:]
V. MOLE
Polyhydramnios
Fibroids
Inaccurate history
Large fetus / Macrosomia
Multiple gestation

First trimester bleeding

Δ Affects 25% of all pregnancies, of which 50% terminate in abortion!

A. INTRAUTERINE CONCEPTUS IDENTIFIED
1. Blighted ovum / blighted twin
2. Threatened abortion
3. Implantation bleed
4. Gestational trophoblastic disease

B. NORMAL ENDOMETRIAL CAVITY
(a) with β-hCG level >1,800 mIU/ml
1. Recent spontaneous abortion
2. Ectopic pregnancy
(b) with β-hCG level <1,800 mIU/ml
1. Very early IUP
2. Ectopic pregnancy

Empty gestational sac

1. Normal early IUP between 5 – 7 weeks MA
2. Blighted ovum
DDx: Pseudosac of ectopic pregnancy

AMNIOTIC FLUID VOLUME

Production:
(a) 1st trimester: dialysate of maternal + fetal serum
(b) 2nd + 3rd trimester: fetal urine (600 – 800 cm³/ day near term), fetal lungs (600 – 800 cm³/day near term), amniotic membrane

Assessment of amniotic fluid volume by:
(1) "Gestalt" method: considered the most accurate if performed by experienced operator
(2) Depth of largest vertical pocket: used in BPP but too stringent + flawed
(3) Amniotic Fluid Index (AFI)
(4) Dye / para-amino hippurate dilution technique: 800 cm³ at 34 weeks, 500 cm³ >34 weeks

Polyhydramnios

= amniotic fluid volume >1500 – 2000 cm³ at term
Incidence: 2%
√ fetus does not fill the AP diameter of uterus
√ single largest pocket devoid of fetal parts / cord >8 cm in vertical direction
√ AFI ≥20 – 24 cm
Prognosis: 64% perinatal mortality with severe polyhydramnios

Etiology:
A. IDIOPATHIC (60%)
B. MATERNAL CAUSES (20%)
1. Diabetes (5%)
2. Rh incompatibility
3. Placental tumors: chorioangioma
C. FETAL ANOMALIES (20 - 63%)
(a) gastrointestinal anomalies (6 - 16%)
Impairment of fetal swallowing (esophageal atresia in 3%); high intestinal atresias (1.2 – 1.8%), omphalocele, meconium peritonitis
(b) non-immune hydrops (16%)

(c) neural tube defects (9 – 16%)
Holoprosencephaly, myelomeningocele, ventriculomegaly, agenesis of corpus callosum, encephalocele, microcephaly
(d) chest anomalies (12%)
Diaphragmatic hernia, cystic adenomatoid malformation, tracheal atresia, mediastinal teratoma, primary pulmonary hypoplasia, extralobar sequestration, congenital chylothorax
(e) skeletal dysplasias (11%)
Dwarfism (thanatophoric dysplasia, achondroplasia), kyphoscoliosis, platyspondyly
(f) chromosomal abnormalities (9%)
Trisomy 21, 18, 13
(g) cardiac anomalies (5%)
VSD, truncus arteriosus, ectopia cordis, septal rhabdomyoma, arrhythmia
(h) genitourinary malformations
Cause: ? hormonally mediated polyuria
Unilateral UPJ obstruction, unilateral multicystic dysplastic kidney, mesoblastic nephroma
(i) miscellaneous (8%)
Cystic hygroma, teratoma, amniotic band syndrome, congenital pancreatic cyst

mnemonic: "TARDI"
Twins
Anomalies, fetal
Rh incompatibility
Diabetes
Idiopathic

Oligohydramnios

= amniotic fluid volume <500 cm³ at term
√ single largest pocket devoid of fetal parts / cord ≤1 – 2 cm in vertical direction
√ AFI ≤5 – 7 cm

Etiology:
mnemonic: "DRIPP"
Demise of fetus
Renal anomalies, bilateral (inadequate urine production): renal agenesis / dysgenesis, infantile polycystic kidney disease, prune belly syndrome, posterior urethral valves, urethral atresia, cloacal anomalies
Δ 20-fold increase in incidence of fetal anomalies with oligohydramnios!
IUGR (reduced renal perfusion)
Premature rupture of membranes (most common)
Postmaturity
N.B.: bilateral renal obstruction, if combined with intestinal obstruction, may be associated with polyhydramnios

Cx: pulmonary hypoplasia, cord compression
Prognosis: 77 – 100% perinatal mortality with 2nd trimester oligohydramnios

Dilated cervix

1. Inevitable abortion

2. Incompetent cervix
   = gaping cervix usually develops during 2nd trimester
   Predisposed: cervical trauma (D & C, cauterization), DES exposure in utero with cervical hypoplasia, estrogen medication
   √ visualization of fetal parts / amniotic fluid within dilated endocervical canal (stress test: patient standing with bladder empty)
   Prognosis: 14th – 18th week best time for Rx prior to significant cervical dilatation

3. Premature labor
   = spontaneous onset of palpable, regularly occurring uterine contractions between 20 and 37 weeks MA

Umbilical cord lesions

Δ Persisting 2nd + 3rd trimester umbilical cord cysts are frequently accompanied by fetal anomalies!

A. DEVELOPMENTAL   UOAAM   UFOA² c̄ False cyst

1. **Umbilical hernia**
   = protrusion from anterior abdominal wall with normal insertion of umbilical vessels
   Predisposed:
   blacks, low-birth-weight infants, trisomy 21, congenital hypothyroidism, Beckwith-Wiedemann syndrome, mucopolysaccharidoses
   Prognosis: spontaneous closure in first 3 years of life

2. Omphalomesenteric duct cyst

3. **Allantoic cyst**
   = remnant of umbilical vesicle / allantois located close to fetus
   Histo: lined by single layer of flattened epithelium

4. **Amniotic inclusion cyst**
   = amniotic epithelium entrapped within umbilical cord

5. **Mucoid degeneration of umbilical cord**
   = liquefaction of Wharton jelly / edema = false cyst √

B. ACQUIRED   HUNT for False knot
   1. **False knot**
      = varix of umbilical vessel
      √ irregular protrusions from the cord

   2. **True knot**
      Incidence: 1% of pregnancies
      Cause: excessive fetal movements
      Predisposed: long cord, male fetus, multiparity
      √ localized distension of umbilical vein
      √ tortuosity of cord at level of knot
      Cx: vascular occlusion + fetal death in utero

3. **Umbilical cord hematoma**
   = rupture of the wall of the umbilical vein secondary to mechanical trauma (torsion, loops, knots, traction) / congenital weakness of vessel wall
   Incidence: 1:5,505 to 1:12,699 deliveries
   Location: near fetal insertion of umbilical cord (most common)
   √ hyper- / hypoechoic mass 1 – 2 cm in size, multiple (in 18%)
   Cx: rupture into amniotic cavity with exsanguination
   Prognosis: 52% overall perinatal fetal mortality

4. Neoplasm
   (a) **Angiomyxoma / hemangioma**
      Histo: multiple channels lined by benign endothelium surrounded by edema + myxomatous degeneration of Wharton jelly
      Location: more frequently toward placental end of umbilical cord
      √ hyperechoic mass within cord
      √ may be associated with pseudocyst (= localized collection of edema)
      Cx: nonimmune hydrops
   (b) Other tumors: myxosarcoma, dermoid, teratoma

5. **Umbilical vein varix**
   Incidence: <4% of all umbilical cord abnormalities
   Site: intraamniotic, intraabdominal
   √ fusiform dilatation of umbilical vein
   Cx: (1) Thrombosis with subsequent fetal death
         (2) Partial thrombosis with IUGR

Hematoma, U vein varix, Neoplasm True knot for False knot.

PLACENTA

Abnormal placental size

A. ENLARGEMENT
   = >5 cm in sections obtained at right angles to long axis of placenta
   (a) maternal disease
      1. Maternal diabetes (= villous edema)
      2. Chronic intrauterine infections
      3. Maternal anemia (= normal histology)
      4. Alpha-thalassemia
   (b) fetal disease
      1. Hemolytic disease of the newborn (= villous edema + hyperplasia)
      2. Umbilical vein obstruction
      3. Fetal high-output failure: large chorioangioma, arteriovenous fistula
      4. Fetal malformation: Beckwith-Wiedemann syndrome, sacrococcygeal teratoma, chromosomal abnormality, fetal hydrops
      5. Twin-twin transfusion syndrome

V. mole, Placental Infarct
Massive subchorial thrombus, Intervillous thrombosis, Teratoma
Septal cyst, Perivillous fibrin deposition, ChorioAngioma, Subchorionic fibrin dep. mets

    (c) fetomaternal hemorrhage

B. DECREASE IN SIZE
1. Preeclampsia
   associated with placental infarcts in 33 – 60%
2. IUGR
3. Intrauterine infection
4. Chromosomal abnormality

Vascular spaces of the placenta
1. "Placental cysts"
= large fetal veins located between amnion + chorion anastomosing with umbilical vein
√ sluggish blood flow (detectable by real-time observation)

2. **Basal veins**
= decidual + uterine veins
√ lacy appearing network of veins underneath placenta
DDx: placental abruption

3. **Intraplacental venous lakes**
√ intraplacental sonolucent spaces
√ whirlpool motion pattern of flowing blood

Macroscopic lesions of the placenta   *VP MIT SPASM*
1. **Intervillous thrombosis** (36%)
= intraplacental areas of hemorrhage
Etiology: breaks in villous capillaries with bleeding from fetal vessels
√ sonolucent intraplacental lesions (mm – cm range)
Significance: fetal-maternal hemorrhage (Rh sensitization, elevated AFP levels)

2. **Perivillous fibrin deposition** (22%)
= nonlaminated collection of fibrin deposition
Etiology: thrombosis of intervillous space
Significance: none

3. **Septal cyst** (19%)
Etiology: obstruction of septal venous drainage by edematous villi
√ 5 – 10 mm cyst within septum
Significance: none

4. **Placental infarct** (25%)
= coagulation necrosis of villi
Etiology: disorder of maternal vessels, retroplacental hemorrhage
√ not visualized unless hemorrhagic
Significance: dependent on extent + associated maternal condition

5. **Subchorionic fibrin deposition** (20%)
= laminated collection of fibrin deposition
Etiology: thrombosis of maternal blood in subchorionic space
√ subchorionic sonolucent area
Significance: none

6. Massive subchorial thrombus
= BREUS MOLE = PREPLACENTAL HEMORRHAGE
7. Chorioangioma (1%)
8. Hydatidiform mole
9. Teratoma (rare)
10. Metastatic lesion (rare):
    Melanoma, breast carcinoma, bronchial carcinoma

FETAL CNS ANOMALIES
A. HYDROCEPHALUS
1. Aqueductal stenosis
2. Communicating hydrocephalus
3. Dandy-Walker malformation
4. Choroid plexus papilloma
B. NEURAL TUBE DEFECT
Incidence: 1:500 – 600 livebirths
Risk of recurrence: 3 – 4%
1. Spina bifida
2. Anencephaly
3. Acrania
4. Encephalocele (8 – 15%)
5. Porencephaly
6. Hydranencephaly
7. Holoprosencephaly
8. Iniencephaly
9. Microcephaly
10. Agenesis of corpus callosum
11. Lissencephaly
12. Arachnoid cyst
13. Choroid plexus cyst
14. Vein of Galen aneurysm

FETAL CHEST ANOMALIES
1. Cystic adenomatoid malformation
2. Lung sequestration
3. Bronchogenic cyst
4. Diaphragmatic hernia

Cystic chest mass
1. Bronchogenic cyst
2. Enteric cyst
3. Neurenteric cyst
4. Cystic adenomatoid malformation (Type I)
5. Diaphragmatic abnormalities
6. Pericardial cyst

Complex chest mass
1. Diaphragmatic abnormalities
2. Cystic adenomatoid malformation (Type I, II, III)
3. Pulmonary sequestration
4. Complex enteric cyst

Solid chest mass
1. Diaphragmatic abnormalities
2. Cystic adenomatoid malformation (Type III)
3. Pulmonary sequestration
4. Bronchial atresia
5. Pericardial tumor

Nuchal skin thickening
= skin thickening of posterior neck ≥6 mm
Causes:
A. Normal variant (0.06%)
B. Chromosomal disorders: trisomy 21 (in 45 – 80%), Turner syndrome, trisomy 18, XXX syndrome, XYY syndrome, XXXX syndrome, XXXXY syndrome, 18p-syndrome, 13q-syndrome
C. Nonchromosomal disorders:
　1. Multiple pterygium syndrome = Escobar syndrome
　2. Klippel-Feil syndrome (fusion of cervical vertebrae, CHD, deafness (30%), cleft palate
　3. Zellweger syndrome = cerebrohepatorenal syndrome (large forehead, flat facies, macrogyria, hepatomegaly, cystic kidney disease, contractures of extremities)

FETAL CARDIAC ANOMALIES

Incidence:　1:125 births; most common congenital malformation
Δ 90% occur as isolated multifactorial traits with a recurrence risk of 2 – 4%
Δ 10% are associated with multiple birth defects
Antenatal sonographic diagnosis to prompt cardiac evaluation:
A. ABNORMALITIES IN CARDIAC POSITION
B. CNS
　1. Hydrocephalus
　2. Microcephaly
　3. Agenesis of corpus callosum
　4. Encephalocele (Meckel-Gruber syndrome)
C. GASTROINTESTINAL
　1. Esophageal atresia
　2. Duodenal atresia
　3. Situs abnormalities
　4. Diaphragmatic hernia
D. VENTRAL WALL DEFECT
　1. Omphalocele
　2. Ectopia cordis
E. RENAL
　1. Bilateral renal agenesis
　2. Dysplastic kidneys
F. TWINS
　1. Conjoined twins

Risk factors for congenital heart disease
Prenatal risk factors for congenital heart disease:
A. FETAL RISK FACTORS
　1. Symmetrical IUGR
　2. Fetal bradycardia
　3. Abnormal karyotype (CHD in Down syndrome in 40%; in Trisomy 18 / 13 in >90%; in Turner syndrome in 35%)
　4. Somatic anomalies by US (omphaloceles in 20%, fetal hydrops in 35%)
　5. Oligo- / polyhydramnios

B. MATERNAL RISK FACTORS
　1. Insulin-dependent diabetes mellitus
　2. Collagen vascular disease: SLE
　3. Maternal heart disease
　4. Infection: rubella
　5. Drugs
　　(a) phenytoin (in 2% PS, AS, coarctation, PDA)
　　(b) trimethadione (in 20% transposition, tetralogy, hypoplastic left heart)
　　(c) sex hormones (in 3%)
　　(d) lithium (Ebstein anomaly, tricuspid atresia)
　　(e) alcohol (VSD, ASD)
　　(f) retinoic acid
C. FAMILIAL RISK FACTORS FOR RECURRENCE OF HEART DISEASE
　— overall incidence　: 6 – 8:1,000 livebirths
　— affected sibling　: 1 – 4% (risk doubled)
　— affected parent　: 2.5 – 4%

POOR PROGNOSTIC FEATURES:
　(1) Intrauterine cardiac failure (hydrops)
　(2) Extracardiac anomalies
　(3) Delivery in center without pediatric cardiology

In utero detection of cardiac anomalies
A. ABNORMAL FOUR-CHAMBER VIEW
　1. Septal rhabdomyoma
　2. Endocardial cushion defect
　3. Ventricular septal defect
　4. Epstein anomaly
　5. Single ventricle
B. VENTRICULAR DISPROPORTION
　1. Hypoplastic right / left ventricle
　2. Hypoplastic aortic arch
　3. Aortic / subaortic stenosis
　4. Coarctation of aorta
　5. Ostium primum defect
C. INCREASED AORTIC ROOT DIMENSION
　1. Tetralogy of Fallot
　2. Truncus arteriosus
　3. Hypoplastic left ventricle with transposition
D. DECREASED AORTIC ROOT DIMENSION
　1. Coarctation of aorta
　2. Hypoplastic left ventricle

Structural cardiac abnormalities + fetal hydrops
　1. Atrioventricular septal defect + complete heart block
　2. Hypoplastic left heart　　*ASD, VSD　AVSD*
　3. Critical aortic stenosis　　*C³ – CHB, critical AS,*
　4. Cardiac tumor　　　　　　*cardiac Tumor*
　5. Ectopia cordis　　　　　*P – PA　　　Pe hd*
　6. Dilated cardiomyopathy　*E – Ectopia cordis*
　7. Ebstein anomaly　　　　*H – Hypoplastic Lt. ht.*
　8. Pulmonary atresia　　　*D – Dilated cardiomyopathy*

Fetal echocardiographic views
A. FOUR-CHAMBER VIEW
　1. Position of heart within thorax – *Ectopia cordis, Levo/Dextro*
　2. Number of cardiac chambers *{4, 3 (SV), AV CANAL,*
　3. Ventricular proportion　　　　*Endo cush. defect*
　　↳ hypo Lt. > Rt. ht. synd. / Cardiomyopathy - dilated
　　atria - Ebstein's TS, MS. TR > TS > MR > MS.

[handwritten: ASD, VSD]

4. Integrity of atrial + ventricular septa
5. Position + size + excursion of AV valves *[handwritten: ✓ Ebsteins]*
B. PARASTERNAL LONG-AXIS VIEW
1. Continuity between ventricular septum + anterior aortic wall *[handwritten: TRUNCUS + TRANSPOSITION]*
2. Caliber of aortic outflow tract *[handwritten: – AS, AR.]*
3. Excursion of aortic valve leaflets *[handwritten: –]*
C. SHORT-AXIS VIEW OF OUTFLOW TRACTS
1. Spatial relationship between aorta + pulmonary artery *[handwritten: PA, PS, AS, TRANSPOSITION.]*
2. Caliber of aortic + pulmonary outflow tracts
D. AORTIC ARCH VIEW *[handwritten: – Coarctation]*

FETAL GASTROINTESTINAL ANOMALIES

1. Esophageal atresia ± TE fistula
2. Duodenal atresia
3. Meconium peritonitis
4. Hirschsprung disease
5. Choledochal cyst
6. Mesenteric cyst

Abdominal wall defect *[handwritten: BCG FOR LEO]*
1. Gastroschisis *[handwritten: Bladder exstrophy]*
2. Omphalocele *[handwritten: Cloacal "]*
3. Ectopia cordis *[handwritten: Gastroschisis.]*
4. Cloacal exstrophy *[handwritten: LBW complex]*
5. Bladder exstrophy *[handwritten: Ectopia Cordis]*
6. Limb-body wall complex *[handwritten: Omphalocele.]*

Nonvisualization of fetal stomach
Incidence: 2% (stomach is visualized in almost all normal fetuses by 14 weeks + in all normal fetuses by 19 weeks)
1. Physiologic gastric emptying / intermittent swallowing (repeat scan after 30 minutes)
2. Decreased amniotic fluid volume
3. CNS abnormalities
4. GI tract abnormalities: congenital diaphragmatic hernia, TE fistula with esophageal atresia
5. Cleft palate

Double bubble sign
= fluid filled stomach + proximal duodenum
1. Duodenal atresia (in 30% due to trisomy 21)
2. Duodenal stenosis
3. Duodenal web
4. Annular pancreas
5. Preduodenal portal vein
6. Ladd bands
7. Malrotation

Dilated bowel in fetus *[handwritten: Chief Minister Joins American Medical Association]*
1. Meconium ileus
   Δ All newborns with meconium ileus have cystic fibrosis!
   Δ 10 – 15% of newborns with cystic fibrosis present with meconium ileus!
2. "Apple peel" atresia of small bowel

[handwritten left margin: V. Imp ‖]

3. Jejunal atresia
4. Megacystic-microcolon-intestinal hypoperistalsis syndrome *[handwritten: MMIHS]*
5. Colonic aganglionosis = Hirschsprung disease (may be associated with Down syndrome)
6. Anorectal atresia (associated with CNS abnormalities, part of VACTERL complex)

Bowel obstruction in fetus
Etiology: Intestinal atresia / stenosis secondary to vascular accident, volvulus, meconium ileus, intussusception after organogenesis
Incidence: imperforate anus 1:3,000; small bowel 1:5,000; colon 1:20,000
Pathologic types:
I   one / more transverse diaphragms
II blind-ending loops connected by fibrous string
III complete separation of blind-ending loops
IV apple-peel atresia of small bowel (occlusion of SMA branch)
Associated with: GI anomalies in 45% (malrotation, duplication, microcolon, esophageal atresia)
√ multiple distended bowel loops >7 mm in diameter
√ increased peristalsis
√ polyhydramnios (not seen in distal intestinal obstruction)
Cx: Meconium peritonitis (50%)
DDx: (1) Other cystic masses: duodenal atresia, hydronephrosis, ovarian cyst, mesenteric cyst
(2) Chronic chloride diarrhea

Intraabdominal calcifications in fetus *[handwritten: PTC]*
A. PERITONEAL
1. Meconium peritonitis
2. Plastic peritonitis associated with hydrometrocolpos
B. TUMORS
1. Hemangioma / hemangioendothelioma
2. Hepatoblastoma
3. Metastatic neuroblastoma
4. Teratoma
5. Ovarian dermoid
C. CONGENITAL INFECTION
1. Toxoplasmosis
2. Cytomegalovirus

Cystic mass in fetal abdomen
A. POSTERIOR MID ABDOMEN
1. Cysts of renal origin
2. Hydroureteronephrosis
3. Multicystic dysplastic kidney
4. Paranephric collection
B. RIGHT UPPER QUADRANT
1. Liver cyst
2. Choledochal cyst
C. LEFT UPPER QUADRANT
1. Splenic cyst

D. ANTERIOR MID ABDOMEN
1. Duplication cyst
2. Mesenteric cyst
3. Meconium pseudocyst
4. Dilated bowel
5. Urachal cyst
E. LOWER ABDOMEN
1. Adnexal cyst
2. Hydrometrocolpos
3. Meningocele
4. Sacrococcygeal teratoma

Fetal ascites
A. ASCITES + FETAL HYDROPS
1. Immune hydrops
2. Non-immune hydrops
B. ISOLATED ASCITES
1. Urinary ascites
2. Meconium peritonitis
3. Bowel rupture
4. Ruptured ovarian cyst
5. Hydrometrocolpos
6. Glycogen storage disease

FETAL URINARY TRACT ANOMALIES

1. Bilateral renal agenesis
2. Infantile polycystic kidney disease
3. Adult polycystic kidney disease
4. Multicystic dysplastic kidney
5. Ureteropelvic junction obstruction
6. Megaureter
7. Posterior urethral valves
8. Prune belly syndrome
9. Megacystis-microcolon-intestinal hypoperistalsis syndrome
10. Mesoblastic nephroma
11. Wilms tumor
12. Neuroblastoma

FETAL SKELETAL DYSPLASIA
= heterogeneous group of bone growth disorders resulting in abnormal shape + size of the skeleton
Birth prevalence: 2.4:10,000 births
Prognosis: 23% stillbirths, 32% death in 1st week of life

	Birth prevalence	Perinatal deaths
Thanatophoric dysplasia	0.69:10,000	1:246
Achondroplasia	0.37:10,000	none
Achondrogenesis	0.23:10,000	1:639
Osteogenesis imperf. type II	0.18:10,000	1:799
Osteogenesis imperf., others	0.18:10,000	none
Asphyxiating thoracic dysplasia	0.14:10,000	1:3,196
Chondrodysplasia punctata	0.09:10,000	none
Campomelic dysplasia	0.05:10,000	1:3,196
Chondroectodermal dysplasia	0.05:10,000	1:3,196

CLASSIFICATION
(1) Osteochondrodysplasia
= abnormalities of cartilage / bone growth and development
(2) Dysostosis
= malformation of individual bones singly / in combination
(3) Idiopathic osteolysis
= disorders associated with multifocal resorption of bone
(4) Chromosomal aberration
(5) Primary metabolic disorder

TERMINOLOGY
Micromelia = shortening involves entire limb (eg, humerus, radius + ulna, hand)
Rhizomelia = shortening involves proximal segment (eg, humerus)
Mesomelia = shortening involves intermediate segment (eg, radius + ulna)
Acromelia = shortening involves distal segment (eg, hand)

Lethal bone dysplasia
in order of frequency
1. Thanatophoric dysplasia
2. Osteogenesis imperfecta type II
3. Achondrogenesis type I + II
4. Jeune syndrome (may be nonlethal)
5. Hypophosphatasia, congenital lethal form
6. Chondroectodermal dysplasia (usually nonlethal)
7. Chondrodysplasia punctata, rhizomelic type
8. Camptomelic dysplasia
9. Short-rib polydactyly syndrome
10. Homozygous achondroplasia

Narrow chest
1. Short-rib polydactyly syndrome
2. Asphyxiating thoracic dysplasia
3. Chondroectodermal dysplasia
4. Campomelic dysplasia
5. Thanatophoric dwarfism
6. Homozygous achondroplasia
7. Achondrogenesis
8. Hypophosphatasia

Spine demineralization
1. Achondrogenesis

Large head
1. Achondroplasia
2. Thanatophoric dysplasia

Bowed long bones
1. Campomelic syndrome
2. Osteogenesis imperfecta
3. Thanatophoric dysplasia
4. Hypophosphatasia

Bone fractures
1. Osteogenesis imperfecta
2. Hypophosphatasia
3. Achondrogenesis

Extreme micromelia
1. Achondrogenesis
2. Thanatophoric dysplasia
3. Fibrochondrogenesis
4. Short-rib polydactyly syndrome
5. Diastrophic dysplasia

GYNECOLOGY
Precocious puberty
= early onset of puberty

1. **True precocious puberty**
   = complete precocious puberty
   = early development of gonads + secondary sex characteristics with ovulation before 8 years of age
   Cause:
   (1) Idiopathic activation of hypothalamic-pituitary-gonadal axis (80%)
   (2) Lesion of pituitary gland / hypothalamus
   • increased levels of estrogen + gonadotropin
   √ adult-sized ovaries
   √ dominance of corpus over cervix length

2. **Pseudoprecocious puberty**
   = incomplete precocious puberty
   = early development of secondary sex characteristics without ovulation
   Cause:
   ovarian tumor (eg, granulosa theca-cell tumor, thecoma, choriocarcinoma), ovarian cyst, estrogen-producing adrenal tumor, hypothyroidism, neurofibromatosis, estrogen ingestion
   • low gonadotropin levels
   • increased estradiol levels
   √ prepubertal uterus + ovaries
   √ large ovarian cysts (with McCune-Albright syndrome, neurofibromatosis, isolated autonomous ovarian cyst, cystic neoplasm)

3. **Isolated premature thelarche**
   = breast enlargement
   may occur without endocrine abnormalities
   √ prepubertal uterus + ovaries

4. **Isolated premature adrenarche**
   = pubic hair development
   • increased levels of adrenal androgens
   √ prepubertal uterus + ovaries

Primary amenorrhea
= failure to menstruate by 16 years of age
√ absent / small ovaries:
1. Turner syndrome
2. CNS lesion with decreased gonadotropin release

√ absent uterus:
1. Testicular feminization (endorgan insensitivity to testosterone)
2. Müllerian dysgenesis (= Mayer-Rokitansky-Küster-Hauser syndrome)
√ small uterus:
1. Primary pituitary / hypothalamic lesion
2. Ovarian lesion
3. Turner syndrome
4. In-utero exposure to diethylstilbestrol
√ hydrometrocolpos:
1. Vaginal membrane / septum
√ ovarian enlargement:
1. Polycystic ovarian disease (= Stein-Leventhal syndrome)

Free fluid in cul-de-sac
1. Follicular rupture
2. Ovulation
3. Ectopic pregnancy
4. S/P culdocentesis
5. Ovarian neoplasm
6. Pelvic inflammatory disease

Calcifications of female genital tract
A. UTERUS
   1. Uterine fibroid
B. OVARIES
   1. Dermoid cyst (50%)
   2. Papillary cystadenoma (psammomatous bodies)
   3. Cystadenocarcinoma
   4. Hemangiopericytoma
   5. Gonadoblastoma
   6. Chronic ovarian torsion
   7. Pseudomyxoma peritonei
C. FALLOPIAN TUBES
   1. Tuberculous salpingitis
D. PLACENTA
E. LITHOPEDION

Frequency of pelvic masses
1.	Benign adnexal cyst	34%
2.	Leiomyoma	14%
3.	Cancers	14%
4.	Dermoid	13%
5.	Endometriosis	10%
6.	Pelvic inflammatory disease	8%

Cystic pelvic masses
A. CYSTIC ADNEXAL MASS
B. EXTRAADNEXAL CYSTIC MASS
   1. Peritoneal inclusion cyst
   2. Mesenteric cyst
   3. Lymphocele
   4. Bladder diverticulum
   5. Ectopic gestation
   6. Fluid-distended bowel
   7. Loculated pelvic abscess: appendiceal, diverticular, postoperative

Extrauterine pelvic masses
1. Solid adnexal mass
2. Metastatic disease
3. Lymphoma
4. Pelvic kidney
5. Rectosigmoid carcinoma
6. Prostate carcinoma
7. Benign prostatic enlargement
8. Bladder carcinoma
9. Retroperitoneal tumor
10. Intraperitoneal fat
11. Vascular mass / malformation
12. Hematoma
13. Bowel

ADNEXA

Adnexal masses
A. CYSTIC
1. **Physiologic ovarian cyst**:
   — Graafian follicle: at midcycle <25 mm
   — Corpus luteum: after midcycle <15 mm
2. **Functional / retention cyst**:
   mature follicle fails to involute + continues to enlarge secondary to hormonal imbalance
   - may cause pain (from pressure / hemorrhage)
   √ 4 – 10 cm in diameter
   — <u>Follicular cyst</u> (from preovalutory follicle): may elaborate estrogen, extremely common
   — <u>Corpus luteum cyst</u> (from postovulatory follicle) elaborates progesterone causing delayed menstruation / persistent bleeding
   — <u>Corpus albicans cyst</u> = from corpus luteum following regression of luteal tissue; no hormone production
   — <u>Theca lutein cyst</u>: in hyperstimulated ovary from ovary-stimulating drugs, twins, molar pregnancy, hydrops; elaborates estrogen
   — <u>Serous inclusion cyst</u>: common in postmenopausal women
3. Endometrioma
4. Tuboovarian abscess
5. Dermoid cyst
6. Serous / mucinous cystadenoma
7. Hydrosalpinx
8. Ectopic pregnancy
9. Paraovarian cyst
10. Hydatid cyst of Morgagni
11. Serous / mucinous cystadenocarcinoma
12. Hyperstimulation cysts
13. Peritoneal inclusion cyst

B. SOLID
1. Ovarian tumor
2. Ovarian torsion
3. Fallopian tube carcinoma
4. Polycystic ovaries
   (DDx: pedunculated leiomyoma)

Management of ovarian cyst
A. PREMENOPAUSAL
1. Unilocular cyst ≤2.5 cm ± hemorrhage
   - no follow-up unless on birth control pills
2. Unilocular thin-walled cyst 2.5 – 6 cm without hemorrhage
   - clinical / sonographic follow-up in 1 – 2 months
   - ± addition of hormones
3. Unilocular cyst 2.5 – 6 cm with hemorrhage
   - sonographic follow-up in 1 month
   - ± addition of hormones
4. Unilocular cyst >6 cm
   - consider benign neoplasm

B. POSTMENOPAUSAL
1. Unilocular nonseptated thin-walled cyst <3 cm
   Incidence: 15%
   √ high resistive index (RI) of >0.7
   - serial follow-up
2. Septated cyst / cyst >3 cm / cyst with low RI
   - CA 125 determination
   - surgical exploration

Ovarian tumors
- pressure symptoms: abdominal discomfort, vomiting, flatulence, dyspnea
- pain from adhesions, impaction, torsion
- menstrual irregularity

Cx: (1) Torsion (in 10 – 20%)
       (2) Rupture (rare)
       (3) Infection

CLASSIFICATION
A. <u>Estrogen-producing tumors</u>
   1. Granulosa cell tumor
   2. Theca cell tumor = thecoma
B. <u>Tumors of surface epithelium</u>
   70 – 75% of all ovarian tumors; 90 – 95% of all ovarian cancers
   1. Serous ovarian tumor
   2. Mucinous ovarian tumor
   3. Endometrioid tumor
   4. Cystadenofibroma
   5. Clear cell adenocarcinoma
   6. Brenner tumor
C. <u>Germ cell tumors</u>
   40% of germ cell tumors are malignant
   (a) benign
       1. Dermoid cyst = mature teratoma (most common)
   (b) malignant
       account for 2/3 of ovarian cancers in 1st – 2nd decade of life; <5% of all ovarian neoplasms
       in order of frequency:
       1. Dysgerminoma
       2. Immature teratoma
       3. Endodermal sinus tumor
       4. Embryonal carcinoma
       5. Choriocarcinoma

D. Sex cord-mesenchyme tumors
1. Granulosa cell tumor
2. Theca cell tumor
3. Luteal cell tumor
4. Arrhenoblastoma
E. Connective tissue tumor
1. Fibroma
2. Fibrosarcoma
F. Secondary ovarian tumors
Metastases from: pelvic organs, upper GI tract, breast, bronchus, reticuloendothelial tumors, leukemia
G. Androgen-producing tumors
1. Arrhenoblastoma
2. Sertoli-Leydig cell tumor
3. Clear cell tumor

Solid ovarian tumor
1. Fibroma
2. Thecoma
3. Granulosa cell tumor
4. Sertoli-Leydig cell tumor
5. Brenner tumor
6. Sarcoma
7. Dysgerminoma
8. Endodermal sinus tumor
9. Teratoma
10. Metastasis
11. Endometrioma

UTERUS
Thickened irregular endometrium
Normal endometrial thickness: <1 cm
1. **Endometrial polyps**
Age: mainly 30 – 60 years
Histo: projections of endometrial glands + stroma into uterine cavity
Malignant transformation: in 0.4 – 3.7%

2. **Endometrial hyperplasia**
secondary to prolonged endogenous / exogenous estrogen stimulation
(a) glandular-cystic hyperplasia
(b) adenomatous hyperplasia
√ endometrial thickening >6 mm
Cx: precursor of endometrial cancer
3. Endometritis
4. Primary carcinoma of the endometrium
Location: predominantly in uterine fundus; 24% in isthmic portion)
5. Metastatic carcinoma:
Ovary, cervix, fallopian tube, leukemia
6. Hydatidiform mole
√ echogenic mass with irregular sonolucent areas
7. Incomplete abortion

Diffuse uterine enlargement
1. Diffuse leiomyomatosis
2. Adenomyosis
3. Endometrial carcinoma (15%)

Uterine masses
A. BENIGN
1. Uterine fibroids (99%)
2. Pyometra
3. Hemato- / hydrocolpos
4. Transient uterine contraction (during pregnancy)
5. Bicornuate uterus
6. Adenomyosis
7. Intrauterine pregnancy
B. MALIGNANT
1. Cervical carcinoma
2. Endometrial carcinoma
3. Leiomyosarcoma
4. Invasive trophoblastic disease

ANATOMY AND PHYSIOLOGY OF FEMALE REPRODUCTIVE SYSTEM

Human Chorionic Gonadotropin

= hCG = glycoprotein elaborated by placental trophoblastic cells beginning the 8th day after conception

A. Immunologic Pregnancy Test
= indirect agglutination test for hCG in urine; cross reaction with other hormones / medications possible

Becomes positive at 5 weeks MA

Advantages: readily available, easily + rapidly performed

Disadvantages: frequently false-positive + false-negative results

Sensitivity:
(a) slide: 400 – 15,000 mIU/ml (2 min test time)
(b) test tube: 1,000 – 3,000 mIU/ml (2 hours test time)

B. Radioimmunoassay Pregnancy Test
= measures beta subunit of hCG in serum with a sensitivity as low as 1 – 2 mIU/ml

Becomes positive at 3 weeks MA - *menstrual age.*

Standards:
(1) Second International Standard (2nd IS)
(2) International Reference Preparation (IRP)
100 mIU/ml (2nd IS) = 200 mIU/ml (IRP)
1 ng/ml = 5 – 6 mIU/ml (2nd IS)
         = 10 – 12 mIU/ml (IRP)

Advantages: specific for hCG, sensitive
Disadvantages: requires specialized lab + 3 – 24 hours for completion

Sensitivity:
(a) qualitative: 25 – 30 mIU/ml (3 hours test time)
(b) quantitative: 3 – 4 mIU/ml (24 hours test time)

Rise:
>66% increase of initial β-hCG level over 48 hours in 86% of normal pregnancies
<66% increase of initial β-hCG level over 48 hours in 87% of ectopic pregnancies

Choriodecidua

Chorion = trophoblast + fetal mesenchyme with villous stems protruding into decidua; provides nutrition for developing embryo
(a) chorion frondosum = part adjacent to decidua basalis, forms primordial placenta
(b) chorion laeve = smooth portion of chorion with atrophied villi
(c) "chorionic plate" = amnionic membrane covering the chorionic plate of the placenta

Decidua
(a) decidua basalis = between chorion frondosum + myometrium
(b) decidua capsularis = portion protruding into uterine cavity
(c) decidua parietalis = decidua vera = portion lining the uterine cavity elsewhere

Gestational Sac

Arises from blastocyst which implants into secretory endometrium 6 – 7 days after ovulation, surrounded by echogenic trophoblast

Earliest visualization: mean sac diameter of 3 mm

SAC SIZE: 17 mm by 6th week MA
24 mm by 7th week MA
31 mm by 8th week MA

mean sac diameter grows 1.13 (range 0.71 – 1.75) mm/day; fills chorionic cavity by 11 – 12 weeks MA

VISUALIZATION OF GESTATIONAL SAC

A. in relation to BETA-HCG LEVELS (2nd International Standard):
(serum β-hCG becomes positive 7 – 10 days following conception)
β-hCG levels double every 2 – 3 days during first 60 days of pregnancy
(a) on transabdominal scan:
in 100% with β-hCG levels of >1,800 IU/l
(b) on transvaginal scan:
in 20% with β-hCG levels of <500 IU/l
in 80% with β-hCG levels of 500 – 1,000 IU/l
in 100% with β-hCG levels of >1,000 IU/l

B. in relation to MENSTRUAL AGE
(a) on transabdominal scan:
earliest by 5.5 weeks (diameter of 10 – 12 mm)
(b) on transvaginal scan:
routinely seen by 4.8 – 5.5 weeks MA

√ double decidual sac (DDS) = decidua parietalis adjacent to decidua capsularis: visualization correlates with presence of pregnancy in 98%

Embryo

Developmental stages:
PREEMBRYONIC PERIOD: 2nd – 4th week MA
TRILAMINAR EMBRYONIC DISC: during 5th week MA
EMBRYONIC PERIOD: 6th – 10th week MA
FETAL PERIOD: 11th week MA – term

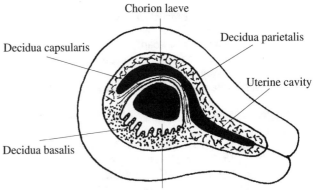

Chorion laeve

Decidua parietalis

Decidua capsularis

Uterine cavity

Decidua basalis

Chorion frondosum

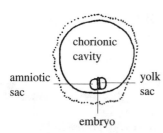

Simple double bleb stage
(earliest detection at 5.5 weeks GA, embryo 2 mm in length

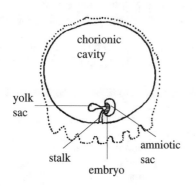

Double bleb + separated yolk sac

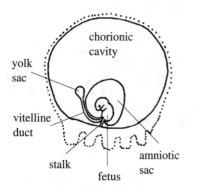

Double bleb + vitelline duct

Average growth rate:
0.7 mm per day / 1.5 mm every 2 days
Earliest visualization: 5.4 weeks MA at CRL of 1.2 mm

VISUALIZATION OF EMBRYO in relation to
GESTATIONAL SAC in 100%:
(a) by transabdominal scan:
with average gestational sac size ≥27 mm
(b) by endovaginal scan:
with average gestational sac size ≥16 mm

VISUALIZATION OF CARDIAC ACTIVITY in 100%:
A. in relation to CRL:
(a) by transabdominal scan : ≥ 9 mm CRL
(b) by transvaginal scan   : ≥ 5 mm CRL
B. in relation to MENSTRUAL AGE:
(a) by transabdominal scan : 7 weeks
(b) by endovaginal scan   : 5 – 6 weeks

CARDIAC ACTIVITY
in 65% of embryos with a CRL of 2 – 4.9 mm
Heart begins to contract at a CRL of 1.5 – 3 mm = 6th
week MA
Δ Cardiac activity predicts a favorable outcome in
90 – 97% of gestations!
Δ Nonvisualization of cardiac activity with CRL of
2 – 12 mm means embryonic demise in 94%!

Yolk sac
= rounded sonolucent structure (outside amniotic cavity)
within chorionic sac (= extracoelomic cavity) connected
to umbilicus via a narrow stalk; formed by proliferation of
endodermal cells at around 4 weeks MA; part of yolk
sac is incorporated into fetal gut, the rest persists as a
sac connected to the fetus by the vitelline duct
Function:
(a) transfer of nutrients from trophoblast to embryo
prior to functioning placental circulation
(b) early formation of blood vessels + blood precursors
on sac wall
(c) formation of primitive gut
(d) source of primordial germ cells

Mean size:
1.0 mm by 4.7 weeks MA; 2.0 mm by 5.6 weeks MA;
3.0 mm by 7.1 weeks MA; 4.0 (2.2 – 5.3) mm by 10
weeks MA; disappears around 12 weeks MA
Earliest visualization:
on endovaginal scan at 4 – 5 weeks MA; in 100% with
GS size of ≥8 mm

Prognosis:
In general abnormal pregnancy outcome (using
endovaginal technique) if
(a) yolk sac absent with GS diameter of ≥8 mm
(b) yolk sac diameter >5.6 mm at <10 weeks MA
(c) embryo visualized without demonstrable yolk sac
(d) yolk sac shape persistently abnormal

Amnionic membrane
= curvilinear echogenic line within chorionic sac; fills
chorionic cavity by 11 – 12 weeks MA; fuses with
chorionic membrane at approximately 16 weeks MA
to form the chorionic plate
Incomplete fusion with chorion frequent
(DDx: subchorionic hemorrhage, twin abortion)

Fetal mensuration
US is more reliable than LMP / physical examination

FETAL AGE
= GESTATIONAL AGE (GA) = "MENSTRUAL AGE" (MA)
= age of pregnancy based on woman's regular last
menstrual period (LMP) projecting the estimated date
of confinement (EDC) at 40 weeks
Δ Note the inaccurate clinical usage of "gestational
age", which strictly speaking refers to the true age of
the pregnancy counting from the day of conception,

whereas "menstrual age" refers to the true age of the pregnancy + approximately 2 weeks counting from the first day of the last menstruation!
Accuracy: 1 – 2 weeks

GESTATIONAL SAC
= average of 3 diameters (craniocaudad, AP, TRV) of anechoic space within sac walls
Δ used for dating between 6 – 12 weeks MA
Accuracy: ± 1 week
Identified as early as 5 weeks MA (on transabdominal scan)

CROWN-RUMP LENGTH (CRL)
= length of embryo; useful up to 12 weeks MA
Accuracy: ± 5 to 7 days
Rule of thumb: MA (in weeks) = CRL (in cm) + 6
Usually identified by 7 weeks MA (transabdominal scan)

BIPARIETAL DIAMETER (BPD)
= measured from leading edge to leading edge of calvarial table at widest transaxial plane of skull
= level of thalami + cavum septi pellucidi + sylvian fissures
Δ Excellent means of estimating GA in 2nd trimester >12 weeks MA
Accuracy of BPD measurement (= "between occasion error"): 2 mm
(a) in 2nd trimester (<24 weeks):± 5 to 7 days (± 9%)
(b) in 3rd trimester: 2 – 4 weeks
less reliable for dating in 3rd trimester because of increasing biologic variability
Δ Diameter of cisterna magna measured from inner margin of occiput to vermis cerebelli: 2 – 10 mm

CEPHALIC INDEX (CI)
= BPD / OFD; measurements of BPD and occipitofrontal diameter (OFD) are both taken from outer to outer edge of calvarium
Δ Confirms appropriate use of BPD if ratio is between 0.70 - 0.86 (2 SD)

HEAD CIRCUMFERENCE (HC)
Used if ratio of BPD/OFD outside 0.70 – 0.86
HC = ([BPD + OFD]/2) X π
Accuracy: slightly less than for BPD

ABDOMINAL CIRCUMFERENCE (AC)
= measured at level of vascular junction of umbilical vein with left portal vein ("hockey stick" appearance) where it is equidistant from the lateral walls in a plane perpendicular to long axis of fetus; measured from outer edge to outer edge of soft tissues
Δ Allows evaluation of head-to-body disproportion
Δ Better predictor of fetal weight than BPD

FEMUR LENGTH (FL)
Δ FL >5 mm below 2 standard deviations suggest skeletal dysplasia!

APPEARANCE OF EPIPHYSEAL BONE CENTERS
in 95% of all cases
— distal femoral epiphysis (DFE): >33 weeks GA
— distal femoral epiphysis (DFE) >5 mm: >35 weeks GA
— proximal tibial epiphysis (PTE): >35 weeks GA
— proximal humeral epiphysis (PHE): >38 weeks GA

DISCORDANT ESTIMATED DATE OF CONFINEMENT (EDC) BY LMP AND BPD:
1. Methodological error in measurement
   (a) wrong axial section
   (b) cranial compression (multiple gestation, breech presentation, oligohydramnios, dolichocephaly)
2. Erroneous LMP
   other measurements (AC, FL) correlate with BPD
3. Abnormal head growth
   (a) BPD less than AC: microcephaly, fetal macrosomia
   (b) BPD more than AC: intracranial abnormality, asymmetrical IUGR

Biophysical Profile (Platt and Manning) = BPP
= in utero Apgar score
Normal parameters (30-minute observation period):
1. NST: reactive *Non-stress test*
   Not included in most BPP evaluations thus decreasing the maximal score to 8!
2. Fetal breathing movement (FBM):
   √ ≥1 breathing period for 60 (30) seconds
   FBM has a circadian rhythm occuring in periods shortly after maternal food intake
   stimulated by: glucose, catecholamine, caffeine, prostaglandin synthetase inhibitor
   suppressed by: barbiturates, benzodiazepine, labor, hypoxia, asphyxia, prostaglandin E2
3. Fetal body movement:
   √ ≥3 discrete movements of limbs / trunk
   influenced by: glucose, gestational age, time of day, maternal drugs, intrinsic rhythm, labor
4. Fetal tone
   upper + lower limbs usually fully flexed with head on chest; least sensitive test parameter
   √ ≥1 episode of extension with return to flexion of limb (focus on hands)
5. Amniotic fluid volume
   √ at least one pocket ≥2 cm (original stringent 1 cm criteria replaced) in vertical diameter in two perpendicular planes without containing loops of cord
Score: 2 points if normal; 0 points if abnormal
Results:
   8 – 10   maximal score
   6   equivocal
   0 – 4   severe fetal compromise, delivery indicated

Amniotic Fluid Index
= sum of vertical depths of largest clear amniotic fluid pockets in the 4 uterine quadrants measured in mm

Method: patient supine, uterus viewed as 4 equal
quadrants, transducer perpendicular to plane
of floor + aligned longitudinally with patient's
spine

Variation: 3.1% intraobserver, 6.7% interobserver
Result:
— 95th percentile: 185 mm at 16 weeks GA, rising to
280 mm at 35 weeks, declining to 190 at 42 weeks
GA
— 5th percentile: 80 mm at 16 weeks, rising to 100 mm
at 23 weeks GA, declining to 70 mm at 42 weeks GA

Stress Tests

1. NON-STRESS TEST (NST)
External monitoring over 20 minutes;
√ at least 4 fetal heart accelerations (>15 bpm over
baseline lasting >15 seconds) following fetal
movement >34 weeks GA
√ no heart accelerations in immaturity, during sleep
cycle, with maternal sedative use
Accuracy:
False-negative rate of 3.2/1000 (if done weekly)
or 1.6/1000 (if done biweekly); 50% false-positive
rate for neonatal morbidity + 80% for neonatal
mortality
2. CONTRACTION STRESS TEST (CST)
External monitoring after injection of oxytocin / maternal
breast stimulation
√ >3 uterine contractions in 10-minute period
Accuracy: False-negative rate of 0.4/1000; 50%
false-positive rate

Placental grading

according to echo appearance of basal zone, chorionic
plate, placental substance
Δ Premature placental calcification is associated with
cigarette smoking, hypertension, IUGR!
Δ Not considered useful because placental grading is
imprecise for fetal dating + for fetal lung maturity!

GRADE 0
√ homogeneous placenta + straight line of chorionic
plate
Time: <30 weeks MA
GRADE 1
√ undulated chorionic plate + scattered bright placental
echoes
Time: seen at any time during pregnancy; in 40% at
term
Δ in 68% L/S ratio >2.0
GRADE 2
√ linear bright echoes parallel to basal plate
√ confluent stippled echoes within placenta
± indentations of chorionic plate
Time: rarely seen in gestations <32 weeks MA;
seen in 40% at term
Δ in 87% L/S ratio >2.0
GRADE 3
√ calcified intercotylidonary septa, often surrounding
sonolucent center

Time: rarely seen in gestations <34 weeks MA;
in 15 – 20% at term
Δ in 100% L/S ratio >2.0 (= strongly correlated with
lung maturity)

PREMATURE PLACENTAL SENESCENCE
= grade 3 placenta seen in gestation <34 weeks MA
Δ in 50% suggestive of maternal hypertension / IUGR

CERVICAL LENGTH

		transabdominal	transvaginal
1st trimester	(<14 wks)	53 ± 17	40 ± 8 mm
2nd trimester	(14 – 28 wks)	44 ± 14	42 ± 10 mm
3rd trimester	(≥ 28 wks)	40 ± 10	32 ± 12 mm

Δ Distended bladder improves visualization but distorts
cervical length on transabdominal US!
Δ Difference between nulli- and multiparous women 10%!

MULTIPLE GESTATION

Incidence: 1% of all births; in 5 – 50% clinically
undiagnosed at term
Occurrence:
twins   in 1:85   pregnancies (= 85[1])
triplets   in 1:7,600   pregnancies (= 85[2])
quadruplets in 1:70,000   pregnancies (= 85[3])
At risk for IUGR: monochorionic-monoamniotic >
monochorionic-diamniotic >
dichorionic-diamniotic
• uterus large for dates
• may have elevated hCG, hPL (human placental
lactogen), AFP levels
√ 2 placentas indicate dichorionic diamniotic pregnancy
√ 1 placenta indicates (a) monochorionic pregnancy (b)
dichorionic pregnancy with fused placenta
√ separating membrane confirms diamniotic pregnancy,
but does not distinguish between mono- / dichorionic
pregnancy

Twin Pregnancy

zygote = fertilized egg
Δ Monozygotic (20 – 30%) and dizygotic (70 – 80%)
twins are sonographically indistinguishable!

1. **Monozygotic twins** (1/3)
= "identical twins"
= division of a single fertilized ovum during earliest
stages of embryogenesis (chorion differentiates 4
days and amnion 8 days after fertilization)
Incidence: 1:250 birth (constant around the world)
√ same sex + identical genotype

(a) DICHORIONIC DIAMNIOTIC (30%)
= separation at two cell stage (= blastomere)
approximately 60 hours after fertilization
√ 2 separate fused / unfused placentas
√ membrane >2 mm due to 2 separate chorionic
sacs + 2 separate amniotic sacs (92% accurate
for dichorionic diamniotic twins)

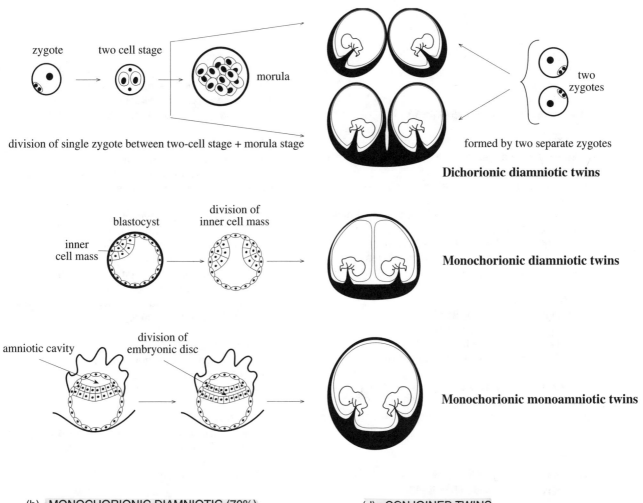

Dichorionic diamniotic twins

Monochorionic diamniotic twins

Monochorionic monoamniotic twins

division of single zygote between two-cell stage + morula stage

formed by two separate zygotes

(b) MONOCHORIONIC DIAMNIOTIC (70%)
    (most common)
    = separation in blastocyst stage between 4th and
      8th day after fertilization (chorion already
      developed and separated from embryo)
    √ 2 separate amniotic sacs within single
      chorionic sac
    Δ Common monochorionic placenta has vascular
      communications in100%!
    Cx: (1) Twin-twin transfusion syndrome
         (2) DIC in surviving twin from transfer of
             thromboplastin; 17% morbidity /
             mortality of survivor after fetal death of
             twin
(c) MONOCHORIONIC MONOAMNIOTIC (1%)
    = division of embryonic disk between 8th and
      13th day after fertilization (amniotic cavity
      already developed)
    √ common amniotic + chorionic sac, no
      separating membrane
    Cx: perinatal mortality up to 50%
         (1) Entangled umbilical cord (70%)
         (2) Conjoined twins (umbilical cord with >
             3 vessels, shared fetal organs,
             continuous fetal skin contour)
Prognosis: 40% survival rate

(d) CONJOINED TWINS
    = division more than 13 days after fertilization is
      usually incomplete; M:F = 3:7
    √ no separating membrane demonstrable
      (monochorionic, monoamniotic)
    √ fetuses commonly face each other
    Cx: perinatal mortality 2.5 times greater than for
        dizygotic twins

2. **Dizygotic twins** (2/3)
    = "fraternal twins"
    (a) fertilization of two ova by two separate
        spermatozoa during two simultaneous ovulations
        (occurring either in both ovaries or in one ovary)
    (b) superfetation = fertilization of two ova by two
        separate spermatozoa during two subsequent
        ovulations (frequency unknown)
    (c) superfecundation = two ova fertilized by two
        different fathers (very rare)
      √ different phenotype; may have different sexes
    Incidence: 1:80 to 1:90 births
    √ different phenotypes; same / opposite sex
    √ always dichorionic diamniotic
    Predisposing factors:
        (1) Advanced maternal age (increased up to age
          35)

(2) Ovulation-inducing agents (multiple pregnancies in 5% with clomiphene, in 30% with Pergonal)

(3) Maternal history of twinning (3 times as frequent compared with normal population)

(4) Increased parity

(5) Maternal obesity

(6) Race (more common in blacks)

GROWTH RATES

Twins should be scanned every 3 – 4 weeks >26 – 28 weeks GA

√ normal individual twins grow at same rate as singletons up to 30 – 32 weeks GA

√ combined weight gain of both twins equals that of a singleton pregnancy

√ body length + head size are little affected

√ BDP growth rates similar to singleton fetuses up to 30 – 32 weeks GA

DISCORDANT GROWTH

= weight difference at birth >25%

Cause: (1) Twin-twin transfusion syndrome
      (2) IUGR of one fetus

√ BPD difference >5 mm (discordant growth in 20 – 30%)

√ discordant HC increases probability of IUGR

√ AC is single most sensitive parameter for IUGR

√ EFW is most sensitive set of combined parameters for IUGR

"FETUS PAPYRACEUS"

= resorption of fluid resulting in paperlike fetal body + compression into adjacent membranes

"VANISHING TWIN"

= disappearance of one twin in utero due to resorption / anembryonic pregnancy

Incidence: 13 – 78% (mean 21%) before 14 weeks GA

Cx:
(1) DIC in response to release of thromboplastin from degenerating fetus
    (a) into maternal circulation
    (b) into monozygotic twin fetus through shared circulation
(2) Velamentous cord insertion (7-fold increase compared with singleton pregnancy)

Prognosis:
(1) Perinatal mortality 5 – 10 times that of singleton pregnancy (91 – 124:1,000 births)
    (a) preterm delivery with birthweight <2500 g
    (b) IUGR (2nd most common cause of perinatal mortality + morbidity)
    (c) amniotic fluid infection (60%)
    (d) premature rupture of membranes (11%)
    (e) twin-twin transfusion syndrome (8%)
    (f) large placental infarct (8%)
    (g) placenta previa
    (h) abruptio placentae
    (i) preeclampsia
    (j) cord accidents
    (k) malpresentations
(2) Fetal death in utero (0.5 – 6.8%; 3 times as often in monochorionic than in dichorionic gestations)
(3) Increased risk of congenital anomalies (23:1,000 births = twice as frequent as in singletons)

Uteroplacental circulation

By 20 weeks MA trophoblast invades maternal vessels and transforms spiral arteries into distended tortuous vessels = uteroplacental arteries

Histo:
(a) in the decidual portion of spiral arteries: proliferating trophoblast from anchoring villi invades lumen of spiral arteries + partially replaces endothelium
(b) in the myometrial portion of spiral arteries: disintegration of smooth muscle elements (loss of elastic lamina) leads to easily distensible vascular system of low resistance

Uterine blood volume flow:
— 50 ml/min shortly after conception
— 500 – 900 ml/min by term

Intervillous blood flow: 140 ± 53 ml/min (by Xe-133 washout)

Doppler waveform:
√ high velocities in diastole similar to those in systole
√ degree of diastolic flow increases as gestation progresses
√ highly turbulent flow

IUGR lesions:
= narrowing of vascular lumen through
(a) thrombosis of decidual segments of uteroplacental arteries
(b) failure of development of myometrial segments of uteroplacental arteries

ANATOMY & FUNCTION OF FEMALE GENITAL ORGANS

Uterine size

1. Neonatal uterus:
tubular structure; length of 2.3 – 4.6 cm (mean 3.4 cm), fundal width of 0.8 – 2.1 cm (mean 1.2 cm), cervical width of 0.8 – 2.2 cm (mean 1.4 cm)
√ echogenic endometrium + endometrial fluid (in 25%) secondary to maternal hormonal stimulation

2. Infantile uterus (infancy to 7 years of age):
length of 2.5 – 3.3 cm, fundal width of 0.4 – 1.0 cm, cervical width of 0.6 – 1.0 cm
√ cervix occupies 2/3 of uterine length

3. Postpubertal uterus:
— nulliparous: 5 – 8 cm (L); 1.6 – 3.0 cm (W); 3 cm (D)
— multiparous: add 2 cm for multiparous dimensions
√ cervix occupies 1/3 of uterine length
√ mean uterine volume of 90 cm³

4. Postmenopausal uterus:
cervix occupies 1/3 of uterine length;
3.5 – 6.5 cm (L); 1.2 – 1.8 cm (W); 2 cm (D)

Uterine zonal anatomy (on T2WI)
Thickness of zones depends on menstrual cycle + hormonal medication
A. Endometrium
√ high signal intensity similar to fat
B. Junctional zone = innermost layer of myometrium
Histo: compact smooth muscle fibers with 3-fold increase in number + size of nuclei compared to outer myometrium
√ low signal intensity (lower water content); seen in 40 – 60%, may not be visible in premenarchal + postmenopausal women
C. Myometrium
√ intermediate signal intensity, increases during secretory phase
CERVICAL ZONES
(a) endocervical canal
√ central zone of high signal intensity on T2WI
(b) myometrium
√ outer zone of low signal intensity similar to junctional zone

Endometrium
(measurements refer to AP diameter of both apposed endometrial layers = double thickness)
1. Menstrual phase (usually 5 days):   2 – 3 mm thick
√ thin interrupted central interphase
2. Proliferative phase (days 6 – 14):   4 – 6 mm thick
√ mildly echogenic interphase surrounded by thin hypoechoic band (= inner layer of myometrium)
3. Periovulatory phase: 6 – 8 mm thick
√ moderately echogenic endometrium
√ "halo sign" = inner hypoechoic layer (= high fluid content of inner functional endometrial layer)
√ 1 – 2 cm of fluid within endometrial lumen
4. Secretory phase (days 15 – 28):   3 – 6 mm thick
√ very echogenic endometrial texture (= tortuous glands + mucin)
5. Postmenopausal: <8 mm thick in 81%
thickness may increase to 15 mm with hormonal replacement (unopposed estrogen, continuous estrogen + progestogen)
Rx: biopsy / D&C if endometrial thickness >8 mm

Ovarian size
Ovarian volume = length x height x width x 0.523
at birth: 1.5 cm (L), 0.25 cm (H), 0.3 cm (W)
<2 years: <0.7 cm³
childhood: 0.75 – 0.86 cm³
6 – 11 years: 1.19 – 2.52 cm³
post puberty: 2.5 – 5 cm (L), 0.6 – 1.5 cm (H), 1.5 – 3 cm (W); 1.8 – 5.7 cm³
MORPHOLOGY
neonate: √ follicles occasionally fail to involute + undergo growth

<8 years: √ solid ovoid structures with homogeneous / finely heterogeneous texture
√ ovaries may contain follicles <9 mm

VISUALIZATION OF OVARIES
after menopause (average onset at age 50):
<5 years post menopause: in 78%
>10 years post menopause: in 64%
following hysterectomy: in 43%

Follicles
During follicular phase (= first 14 days of menstrual cycle) a number of immature primordial follicles begin to mature in response to FSH; by day 5 – 7 the dominant follicle = graafian follicle emerges
√ multiple small cysts = stimulated / unstimulated follicles
√ dominant follicle sonographically detectable by day 8 – 12

Graafian follicle
Size of mature graafian follicle: 17 – 29 mm
√ growth rate 3 mm/day until the last preovulatory 24 hours followed by a sudden increase in diameter
√ cumulus oophorus = 1 mm mural echogenic focus projecting into antrum of follicle + containing oocyte, followed by ovulation within next 36 hours
√ sudden decrease in follicular size (= follicular rupture with extrusion of ovum)
√ corpus luteum of menstruation = 16 – 24 mm cyst with blurred margin + scattered internal echoes representing follicular fluid + blood
√ corpus luteum atreticum = involution + atrophy of corpus luteum on about 24th day of cycle

SIGNS OF OVULATION:
√ development of solid echoes within graafian follicle
√ decrease in diameter / sudden collapse of dominant follicle 28 – 35 hours after LH peak
√ "ring" structure within uterine fundus
√ free fluid appearing in pouch of Douglas

SIGNS OF OVULATORY FAILURE:
√ development of internal echoes prior to 18 mm size
√ continuous cystic enlargement up to 30 – 40 mm

Ovarian Doppler signals
A. NONFUNCTIONING OVARY
√ high-impedance waveform
B. FUNCTIONING OVARY
— days 1 – 6:
√ high-impedance waveform with RI close to 1.0
— days 7 – 22 = mid-follicular to mid-luteal phase = developing dominant follicle + ovulation + corpus luteal phase:
√ continuous diastolic flow with RI close to 0.5
— days 23 – 28 = late luteal phase:
√ high-impedance waveform with RI close to 1.0

OBSTETRICAL AND GYNECOLOGICAL DISORDERS

ABORTION
Rate of spontaneous abortions (= miscarriage)
— >50% of all fertilized ova (estimate)
— 31 – 43% of all implantations (estimate)
— 10 – 25% of clinically diagnosed pregnancies
— 2 – 4% with normal cardiac activity
— decreases with increasing gestational age
Δ Majority of pregnancies lost before 7th week MA!
Etiology: usually due to abnormal karyotype: autosomal trisomy (52%), triploidy (20%), monosomy (15%)

Incomplete Spontaneous Abortion
= retained products of conception, ie, a portion of chorionic villi (placental tissue) / trophoblastic tissue (fetal tissue) remains within uterus
• prolonged bleeding
• infection
US: overall accuracy 96%
√ gestational sac / collection(64%): retained products in 100%
√ sac with dead fetus (19%): retained products in 100%
√ endometrial thickness   >5 mm (3%): retained products in 100%
√ endometrial thickness 2 – 5 mm (7%): retained products in 43%
√ endometrial thickness   <2 mm (7%): retained products in 14%
Cx: endometritis, myometritis, peritonitis, septic shock, diffuse intravascular coagulation (with retention >1 month)

Inevitable Abortion
= gestational sac with fetus having become detached from implantation site; leading to spontaneous abortion within next few hours
Clinical triad:
• severe pain
• uterine contractions
• dilated cervix
√ sac located low within uterus
√ sac surrounded by anechoic zone of blood
√ dilated cervix

Missed Abortion
= dead conceptus within uterine cavity, occurring between 8 – 14 weeks
√ no cardiac activity in a well-defined embryo with CRL >9 mm (on abdominal scans) / CRL >5 mm (on transvaginal scans)
√ gestation not in correspondence with menstrual age
√ sac >25 mm in diameter without an embryo
√ distorted angular sac configuration
√ stringlike debris within gestational sac (in 25%)
√ discontinuous / irregular / thin (2 mm) choriodecidual reaction

√ no double decidual sac
√ low sac position
√ subchorionic collection

Threatened Abortion
= 1st trimester bleeding with a live fetus
Incidence: 20 – 25% of all pregnancies
Clinical triad:
• mild bleeding
• cramping
• closed cervix
Prognosis: 50% develop normally; 50% miscarry
Factors with a poor prognosis:
√ early bradycardia
√ large subchorionic hematoma (DDx: implantation bleed)
√ relative fetal inactivity

Early Embryonic Demise
on endovaginal scan
• beta-hCG level <2 – 3 standard deviations below the mean for given MA / GS size / CRL
√ mean gestational sac size too small for good clinical dates
√ disproportion between embryonic size and mean gestational sac size (difference between mean sac size and CRL <5 mm predictive of miscarriage in 94%)
√ mean gestational sac size of ≥16 mm without embryo
√ gestational sac growth ≤ 0.7 mm/day (normal growth rate of 1.13 mm/day determines appropriate time interval for follow-up scan, ie, when sac is expected to be 27 mm)
√ absence of yolk sac in mean gestational sac size of ≥8 mm (repeat scan in 3 days for confirmation)
√ absence of cardiac activity with CRL of ≥5 mm (repeat scan in 3 days for confirmation)
√ sac position in lower uterine segment / cervix
√ stringlike / granular debris / fluid-fluid level within gestational sac (= intrasac bleeding)

Late Embryonic Demise
on endovaginal scan
√ wrinkled collapsing amniotic membrane
√ irregular distorted shape of gestational sac (DDx: compression by bladder, myoma, contraction)
√ absence of double decidual sac = thin (<2 mm) weakly hyperechoic / irregular choriodecidual reaction

ACARDIA
= ACARDIAC MONSTER = TWIN REVERSED ARTERIAL PERFUSION SEQUENCE (TRAP)
Incidence: 1:30,000 – 35,000 births

Spectrum:
  (1) Holoacardia = no heart at all
  (2) Pseudoacardia = rudimentary cardiac tissue
√ fused placentas
√ polyhydramnios

A. PUMP TWIN
   at increased risk for fetal demise + preterm labor
   √ morphologically normal
   √ cardiac overload signs: hydrops, IUGR,
     hypertrophy of right ventricle, hepatosplenomegaly,
     ascites

B. PERFUSED TWIN
   monochorial placenta (same gender) with vascular
   anastomosis sustains life of acardiac monster;
   wide range of associated abnormalities
   √ absent / rudimentary heart ("acardius")
   √ unidentifiable head / trunk / extremities
Prognosis: mortality of 100% for perfused twin, 50% for
   pump twin

ADENOMYOSIS
= focal / diffuse benign invasion of myometrium by
  endometrium ("endometrial islands")
Incidence: 15 – 27% in hysterectomy specimens
Histo: endometrial glands (resistant to hormonal
  stimulation unlike endometriosis) + stroma within
  myometrium surrounded by hypertrophic smooth
  muscle
Age: multiparous women >30 years during menstrual
  life
Associated with endometriosis (in 36 – 40%)
• hypermenorrhagia, dysmenorrhea
√ smooth uterine enlargement (DDx: diffuse
  leiomyomatosis)
√ occasionally "Swiss cheese" appearance of myometrium
MRI:
  √ no abnormality on T1WI
  √ low intensity lesions on T2WI subjacent to
    endometrium, often isointense to band of junctional
    zone
  √ occasionally central high-intensity spots on T1WI +
    T2WI corresponding to hemorrhagic areas
Cx: infertility
Rx: hysterectomy

AMNIOTIC BAND SYNDROME
= rupture of the amnion exposing the fetus to the injurious
  environment of fibrous mesodermic bands that emanate
  from the chorionic side of the amnion
Incidence: 1:1,200 to 1:15,000 livebirths
√ very thin membrane that flaps with fetal movement or
  attaches to fetus
√ abnormal sheet / bands of tissue that attach to the fetus
  (DDx: uterine synechiae, incomplete amniochorionic
  fusion, amniochorionic separation due to subchorionic
  hemorrhage, fibrin deposits, venous lakes, residual sac
  of blighted twin pregnancy, wisps of umbilical cord)
√ restriction of fetal motion secondary to entrapment of

fetal parts by bands
Associated with FETAL DEFORMITIES (77%):
  1. Limb defects (multiple + asymmetric)
     √ amputation / constriction rings of limbs / digits
     √ distal syndactyly
     √ clubbed feet (30%)
  2. Craniofacial defects
     √ anencephaly
     √ asymmetric lateral encephalocele
     √ facial clefting of lip / palate
     √ asymmetric microphthalmia
     √ incomplete / absent cranial calcification
  3. Visceral defects
     √ gastroschisis ± exteriorization of liver
     √ omphalocele
     √ gibbus deformity of spine

DDx: (1) Chorioamniotic separation
       (2) Intrauterine synechiae

ARRHENOBLASTOMA
Age peak: 25 – 45 years (range 15 – 66 years)
√ solid mass with cystic components (hemorrhage
  ± necrosis)
√ unilateral (95%), up to 27 cm in diameter
Cx: malignant transformation in 22%

BECKWITH-WIEDEMANN SYNDROME
= EMG SYNDROME (**E**xomphalos = omphalocele,
  Macroglossia, **G**igantism); autosomal dominant
Incidence: 1:13,700 livebirths
Constellation:
  (1) Macroglossia
  (2) Visceromegaly
  (3) Omphalocele (10 – 15%)
  (4) Natal / postnatal gigantism
  (5) Nephromegaly
  (6) Facial flame nevus
  (7) Hepatomegaly
  (8) Ear lobe abnormalities
  (9) Hemihypertrophy
  (10) Cardiac anomalies
  (11) Pancreatic hyperplasia
@ Kidney
  √ renal enlargement
  √ increased cortical echogenicity (due to
    glomeruloneogenesis)
  √ accentuation of corticomedullary definition
• neonatal polycythemia
• neonatal hypoglycemia (50%)

Cx: development of malignant tumors (in 10%):
  nephroblastoma, hepatoblastoma, adrenal tumor

BLIGHTED OVUM
= ANEMBRYONIC PREGNANCY; may occur as a
  blighted twin
= gestational sac of >2.5 ml with no identifiable embryo
√ yolk sac identified without embryo
√ empty gestational sac (>6 – 8 weeks MA)

√ gestational sac too small for dates
(a) by transabdominal scan:
    GS usually not visualized before 5 – 5.5 weeks MA;
    yolk sac forms at 4 weeks MA when GS is 3 mm;
    embryo usually visualized by 6 weeks MA
    √ GS size >20 mm of mean diameter without yolk
       sac
    √ GS size >25 mm of mean diameter without
       embryo
    √ absence of GS growth documented on repeat
       scan 7 – 14 days later
(b) by transvaginal scan
    √ GS size >8 mm of mean diameter without yolk
       sac
    √ GS size >16 mm of mean diameter without
       embryo / cardiac activity
Cx: first trimester bleeding

BRENNER TUMOR
Incidence: 1.5 – 2.5%
Associated with: mucinous cystadenoma in 30%
Peak age: 40 – 70 years
• may have estrogenic activity
√ usually hypoechoic solid tumor with well-defined back
  wall, up to 30 cm in diameter
√ bilateral in 5 – 7%

CERVICAL CANCER
6th most common cancer in women, approximately 13,000
new cases/year with 7,000 deaths/year; 3rd most common
gynecological malignancy
Incidence: 12:100,000 women per year
Histo: squamous cell carcinoma (95%),
           adenocarcinoma (5%), unusual clear cell
           adenocarcinoma in women exposed to DES in
           utero
Risk factors: lower socioeconomic class, black race,
           early marriage, increased parity, young
           onset of sexual relations, multiple sexual
           partners, positive herpes virus type II titers

FIGO stage:
0   carcinoma in situ (before invasion)
I   confined to cervix
  Ia   microinvasion of stroma
  Ib   invasion confined to cervix
II   extension beyond cervix but not to pelvic wall /
     lower third of vagina
  IIa   vaginal invasion excluding lower 1/3
  IIb   parametrial involvement excepting pelvic sidewall
III extension to pelvic wall / lower third of vagina
  IIIa invasion of lower 1/3 of vagina
  IIIb parametrial involvement to pelvic wall
IVa mucosal involvement of bladder / rectum
IVb spread to distant organs (paraaortic / inguinal
     nodes, intraperitoneal metastasis)

Significance of tumor size:
  >4 cm: nodal metastases (80%), local recurrence
          (40%), distant metastases (28%)

<4 cm: nodal metastases (16%), local recurrence
        (5%), distant metastases (0%)
Incidence of nodal metastases (77% accuracy for CT,
  78% for MRI):
              0.3% for stage 0, I a
              16%   for stage I b
              33%   for stage II a
              37%   for stage II b
Peak age: 45 – 55 years
• leukorrhea ± vaginal bleeding (<30%)
• postcoital bleeding / metrorrhagia
√ bulky enlargement of cervix (DDx: cervical fibroid)
√ fluid-filled uterus (secondary to obstruction)
√ signs of parametrial invasion: >4 mm soft-tissue strands
  extending from cervix into parametria, cardinal /
  sacrouterine ligaments, irregularity of cervical margins,
  eccentric parametrial enlargement, obliteration of fat
  planes
MRI (76 – 83% accuracy for staging, 82 – 92% accuracy
     for parametrial involvement):
  √ isointense mass on T1WI
  √ hyperintense focal bulge / mass on T2WI (DDx:
     postbiopsy changes, inflammation, nabothian cysts)
  √ blurring + widening of junctional zone secondary to
     obstruction of cervical os (retained secretions in
     uterine cavity)

CHORIOAMNIONIC SEPARATION
(a) normally seen <16 weeks
    = incomplete fusion of amniotic membrane with
      chorionic plate
(b) abnormal >17 weeks MA
    = secondary to hemorrhage
√ membrane extends over fetal surface + stops at origin of
  umbilical cord
√ elevated membrane thinner than chorionic membrane
Cx: rupture of amniotic membrane may lead to amniotic
        band syndrome

CHORIOANGIOMA
= benign vascular malformation of proliferating capillaries
  (= hamartoma)
Incidence: 1:3,500 to 1:20,000 births
Location: usually near the umbilical cord insertion site
√ well-circumscribed intraplacental mass with complex
  echo pattern protruding from the fetal surface of the
  placenta
√ polyhydramnios (in 1/3)
√ arterial signal on Doppler ultrasound in angiomatous
  chorioangioma
Cx: hemorrhage, fetal hydrops, cardiomegaly,
        congestive heart failure, IUGR, premature labor,
        fetal demise (with large lesion)

CHORIOCARCINOMA
5% of gestational trophoblastic diseases
Age: child-bearing age
Histo: excessive trophoblastic proliferation without
           villous structures
• continued vaginal bleeding

- continued elevation of hCG after expulsion of molar / normal pregnancy (25%)
√ mixed hyperechoic pattern (hemorrhage, necrosis)
Spread:
  (a) hematogenous (usually)
  (b) lymphatic + direct extension (occasionally)
Hemorrhagic + necrotic metastases to lung, vagina, kidney (10 – 50%), brain
√ radiodense pulmonary masses with hazy borders due to hemorrhage
√ hyperechoic hepatic foci
Prognosis: fatal with spread to kidneys + brain

CONJOINED TWINS
= incomplete division of embryonic cell mass in monozygotic twins occurring at 13 – 16 days GA
Incidence: 1:30,000 to 1:100,000 livebirths;
             1:600 twin births; M:F = 3:7

Types:
  A. Inferior conjunction:

1.	Diprosopus	two faces + one head and body
2.	Dicephalus	two heads + one body
3.	Ischiopagus	joined by inferior sacrum and coccyx
4.	Pygopagus (20%)	joined by posterolateral sacrum and coccyx

  B. Superior conjunction:

1.	Dipygus	single head, thorax, abdomen + two pelves and four legs
2.	Syncephalus	facial fusion ± thoracic fusion
3.	Craniopagus (6%)	joined between homologous portions of cranial vault

  C. Middle conjunction:

1.	Thoracopagus (18%)	between thoracic walls; conjoined hearts (75%)
2.	Omphalopagus (10%)	joined between umbilicus + xiphoid
3.	Xiphopagus	joined at xiphoid
4.	Thoracoomphalopagus (28%)	

  D. Incomplete duplication (10%): duplication of only one part of body

OB-US (diagnosed as early as 12 weeks GA):
√ single placenta without amniotic membrane (monochorionic, monoamniotic = hallmark of monozygotic twinning)
√ inseparable fetal bodies + skin contours
√ no change in relative position of fetuses
√ both fetal heads persistently at same level (fetuses commonly face each other)
√ bibreech (more common) / bicephalic presentation (cephalic-breech presentation is most common presentation for omphalopagus)
√ polyhydramnios (in almost 50%)
√ single umbilical cord with >3 vessels

√ backward flexion of cervical spine (in anterior fusion)
√ single cardiac motion (shared heart)
Associated malformations:
√ omphalocele
√ congenital heart disease
Prognosis: 39% stillborn; 34% die within first days of life

CORPUS LUTEUM CYST
Types:
  1. Corpus luteum of menstruation
      formed after rupture of follicle + increasing in size until 22nd day of menstrual cycle
      √ usually >12 – 17 mm in size
  2. Corpus luteum of pregnancy
      caused by hCG stimulation during pregnancy
      √ usual size 30 – 40 mm, may grow up to 15 cm in diameter
      √ reaches maximum size after 8 – 10 weeks
      √ usually resolves before 20 weeks GA (12 – 15 weeks), but occasionally persists past 1st trimester
√ thin-walled usually unilateral cyst
√ echogenic (organized clot) / sonolucent (resorbed blood)
√ low-level internal echoes frequent (= hemorrhage)
Cx: rupture with intraperitoneal hemorrhage

CYSTADENOFIBROMA
= variant of serous cystadenoma, rarely malignant
- may produce estrogen excess
√ small multilocular tumor with papillary processes

DERMOID
= DERMOID CYST = MATURE CYSTIC TERATOMA
= congenital tumor containing mature ectodermal elements
Incidence: 11 – 25% of all ovarian neoplasms; 66% of pediatric ovarian tumors; most common ovarian neoplasm
Histo: may contain struma ovarii, carcinoid tumor
Age: reproductive life (80%); age peak 6 – 11 years
- abdominal mass (2/3)
- pain due to torsion / hemorrhage
Site: usually unilateral, bilateral in 12 – 25%
√ cystic mass with average diameter of 10 cm
√ "dermoid plug" = Rokitansky nodule / protuberance = oval / round solid tissue mass (sebaceous material) of 10 – 65 mm projecting into cyst lumen
Plain film (diagnostic in 40%):
√ tooth / bone
√ fat density (SPECIFIC)
CT:
√ round mass of fat floating in interface between two water-density components (93%)
√ Rokitansky nodule = dermoid plug (81%), usually single, may be multiple
√ fat-fluid level (12%)
√ globular calcifications (tooth) / rim of calcification (56%)

US (sensitivity 77 – 87%):
- √ complex mass containing echogenic components (66%)
- √ echogenic focus with acoustic shadowing (due to calcification / mixture of sebum + hair) in a predominantly cystic mass (25 – 44%) (DDx: bowel)
- √ predominantly solid mass (10 – 31%)
- √ purely cystic tumor (9 – 15%)

MR:
- √ hyperintense fat within fluid of low signal intensity on T1WI
- √ hyperintense mass (fat + serous fluid both with high signal intensity) on T2WI

Cx: (1) Malignant degeneration in 1 – 2% (usually within dermoid plug)
(2) Torsion (4 – 16%)
(3) Hydronephrosis

DYSGERMINOMA *highly radiosensitive*

= homologue of testicular seminoma, highly radiosensitive √
Incidence: 1 – 2%
Peak age: 2nd – 3rd decade
- no elevation of AFP / hCG (in 5% syncytiotrophoblastic giant cells present, which can elevate hCG levels)
- √ hyperechoic solid mass, may have areas of hemorrhage + necrosis
- √ bilateral in 15 – 17%
- √ speckled pattern of calcifications (rare)

ECTOPIA CORDIS

= fusion defect of anterior thoracic wall / sternum / septum transversum prior to 9th week of gestation
- A. Thoracic type (60%) = heart outside thoracic cavity protruding through defect in sternum
- B. Abdominal type (30%) = heart protruding into abdomen through gap in diaphragm
- C. Thoracoabdominal type (7%) = in pentalogy of Cantrell
- D. Cervical type (3%) = displacement of heart into cervical region

Associated with:
(1) Facial deformities
(2) Skeletal deformities
(3) Ventral wall defects
(4) CNS malformations: meningocele, encephalocele
(5) Intracardiac anomalies: tetralogy of Fallot, TGA
(6) Amniotic band syndrome
Prognosis: stillbirth / death within first hours / death within first days of life in most cases

ECTOPIC PREGNANCY

= implantation outside the endometrial cavity
Incidence:
1:100 – 400 pregnancies; 9.9:10,000 women annually; 73,700 cases in 1986 in United States; 1.4% of all reported pregnancies; 15% of maternal deaths; coexistent with intrauterine pregnancy in 1:6,800 – 30,000 pregnancies (higher number of coexisting ectopic with ovulation induction)
Risk of recurrence: 10%

Cause: delayed transit of the fertilized zygote secondary to abnormal angulation of oviduct / adhesions from inflammation / slowed tubal transit
Risk factors:
(1) Previous tubal surgery / ligation
(2) Previous PID (30 – 50%)
(3) Ovulation induction
(4) Endometriosis
(5) Previous ectopic pregnancy (25% chance of recurrence)
(6) IUD in place
Δ If the pregnancy cannot be documented as intrauterine the patient should be considered at risk!
Time of manifestation: usually by 7th week of MA

CLASSIC TRIAD (<50%):
- abnormal vaginal bleeding (75 – 86%)
- pelvic pain (97%)
- palpable adnexal mass (30 – 41%)
- secondary amenorrhea (61%)
- cervical tenderness
- positive urinary pregnancy test (50%)
- positive β-hCG does not rise >66% within 48 hours (lower levels + lower rise compared with intrauterine pregnancy)
Δ 0.5% false negative rate with hCG <10 mIU/ml (IRP)!
Location:
(a) tubal (95%): (1) Ampullary ectopic
(2) Isthmic ectopic (92%)
(3) Interstitial ectopic (3%)
(b) other (5%): (1) Abdominal ectopic
(2) Ovarian ectopic
(3) Interligamentary ectopic
(4) Cervical ectopic (exceedingly rare)

Spectrum:
Type 1:   unruptured live ectopic + heartbeat
Type 2:   early embryonic demise without rupture / embryonic structures / heartbeat
Type 3:   ruptured ectopic with blood in pelvis
Type 4:   no sonographic signs of ectopic
Transvesical US:
- √ absence of intrauterine pregnancy (beyond 6 weeks MA / with β-hCG level >1,000 – 2,000 mIU/ml [IRP])
  (a) no IUP by transvesical US = ectopic pregnancy in 43 – 46%
  (b) no IUP by endovaginal US = ectopic pregnancy in 67%
- √ decidual cast = hyperechoic endometrial thickening (50%)
- √ pseudogestational sac = parietal decidual reaction + anechoic fluid center from bleeding (10 – 20%)
- √ echogenic adnexal mass (42%) with small anechoic center = gestational sac ± embryo ± heartbeat
- √ live embryo in adnexa (6 – 17%) = only specific sonographic finding
- √ free abdominal fluid / hyperechoic clot in cul-de-sac
- √ hydro-/ hematosalpinx
- √ corpus luteum within ovary in >50% on side of ectopic pregnancy

Transvaginal US:
- √ extrauterine gestational sac ± live embryo (46 – 71%)
- √ embryonic heartbeat (14 – 28%)
- √ extrauterine gestational sac without live embryo / yolk sac (DDx: hemorrhagic corpus luteum cyst, simple ovarian cyst)
- √ free fluid (40 – 83%): echogenic / particulate fluid (= hemoperitoneum) has 93% positive predictive value for ectopic pregnancy (small amount of anechoic fluid found in 10 – 27% of IUP)
- √ solid / complex adnexal mass (= clotted blood free in peritoneal cavity / hematosalpinx)

Doppler-US:
- √ high-velocity low-impedance flow around extrauterine gestation in 54% (up to 4 kHz shift with 3 MHz transducer, 0.38 ± 0.2 Pourcelot index)
- √ absence of peritrophoblastic flow after 36 days (<0.8 kHz shift with 3 MHz transducer or <1.3 kHz shift with 5 MHz transducer)

INTERSTITIAL ECTOPIC (3 – 4%)
- √ eccentrically placed gestational sac with incomplete / thinned myometrial mantle
- *Prognosis:* massive bleeding from erosion of uterine arteries + veins (pregnancy survives only 12 – 16 weeks GA)
- *DDx:* pregnancy within horn of bicornuate uterus

ABDOMINAL ECTOPIC
- bloating, abdominal pain (fetal movement / peritoneal irritation due to adhesions)
- √ extrauterine location of fetus + placenta
- √ uterus compressed with visible endometrial cavity line
- √ absence of uterine wall between gestation + bladder / abdominal wall
- *Cx:* bowel obstruction / perforation; erosion of pregnancy through abdominal wall

Lithopedion
= "stone child" = very rare obstetrical complication consisting of a dehydrated + calcified demised fetus in an extrauterine pregnancy existing for >3 months without infection

Types:
- (1) Lithokelyphosis = fetal membranes calcified
- (2) Lithokelyphopedion = fetus + membranes calcified
- (3) True lithopedion = only fetus calcified

Maternal age at discovery: 23 – 100 years of age; within 4 – 20 years of fetal demise
Location: most common in adnexae
- √ large densely calcified mass in lower abdomen / upper pelvis
- √ CT scan reveals fetal skeleton
- *DDx:* uterine fibroid, calcified ovarian malignancy / cyst, sarcoma

Dx:
- (1) Laparoscopy (almost 100% accurate)
- (2) Culdocentesis (high probability for ectopic with aspiration of nonclotting blood with a hematocrit >15)

Cx: maternal death in 1:1,000; tubal rupture (10 – 15%)
DDx:
- (1) Hemorrhagic corpus luteum / hematoma
- (2) Adnexal mass: hydrosalpinx, endometrioma
- (3) Fluid-containing small bowel loops
- (4) Eccentrically placed GS in bicornuate / retroflexed / fibroid uterus

ENDODERMAL SINUS TUMOR OF OVARY
= YOLK SAC TUMOR
= rare but highly malignant tumor ~ v. imp.
Histo: resembles endodermal sinuses of the rat yolk sac
Incidence: <1% of all ovarian carcinomas v. imp.
Age: usually adolescence
May be associated with teratoma, dermoid cyst, choriocarcinoma
- frequently abdominal enlargement + pain
- elevated serum AFP (common) imp.

- √ predominantly echogenic solid tumor
- √ cystic areas (epithelial-lined cysts / cysts of coexisting mature teratoma / hemorrhage / necrosis)
- √ bilateral in 1%
- *Rx:* surgery + combination chemotherapy
- *Prognosis:* poor

ENDOMETRIAL CANCER
Most common invasive gynecologic malignancy; v. imp
4th most prevalent female cancer in U.S. women;
34,000 new cases per year with 3,000 deaths
Histo: adenocarcinoma (90 – 95%), sarcoma (1 – 3%)
Peak age: 55 – 62 years; 74% > age 50
Risk factors: nulliparity, late menopause, hormonal replacement therapy, polycystic ovaries, obesity, hypertension, diabetes mellitus

FIGO stage:
- 0 in situ
- I a tumor limited to endometrium
- I b invasion to less than half of myometrium
- I c invasion to more than half of myometrium
- II a endocervical glandular involvement only
- II b cervical stromal invasion
- III a invasion of serosa / adnexa / peritoneal metastases
- III b vaginal metastases
- III c metastases to pelvic / paraortic lymph nodes
- IV a invasion of bladder / bowel mucosa
- IV b distant metastases (lung, brain, bone) including intraabdominal / inguinal lymph nodes
- Δ Clinical staging with dilatation & curettage inaccurate in up to 51%!

Lymph node metastases: 3% with superficial invasion; 40% with deep invasion

- postmenopausal bleeding without hormonal therapy

US:
- √ normal sized / enlarged uterus
- √ echogenic endometrium >5 mm AP thickness (100% negative predictive value, not very specific)

MRI (82 – 92% accuracy for staging, 74 – 87% accuracy for depth of invasion):

√ endometrial cancer has slightly lower signal intensity than endometrium but higher than myometrium on T2WI

v. imp → √ endometrial thickness abnormal if >3 mm (postmenopausal woman) / >10 mm (under estrogen replacement)

v. imp →   *DDx:*   blood clot, uterine secretions, adenomatous hyperplasia

v. imp { √ disruption / absence of junctional zone (myometrial invasion)

v. imp { √ hyperintense areas penetrating into myometrium (deep muscle invasion; 74 – 87% accuracy)

ENDOMETRIOSIS

= encysted functional endometrial tissue outside uterine cavity

Incidence: 5 – 15% of premenopausal women
Etiology:
(1) Peritoneal seeding by retrograde travel of endometrial cells through fallopian tubes
(2) Metaplastic transformation of peritoneal epithelium into endometrial tissue
(3) Traumatic spread (uterine surgery, amniocentesis)
Age: 3rd – 4th decade; dependent on normal hormonal stimulation
• severe dysmenorrhea
• chronic pelvic pain (peritoneal adhesions, bleeding)
• dyspareunia
Location:
(a) internal endometriosis (within uterus)
= ADENOMYOSIS
(b) external endometriosis
typical in: pouch of Douglas, surface of ovary + fallopian tube + uterus, broad ligament, rectovaginal septum
rare in : umbilicus, laparotomy scar, bladder wall, bowel wall (20%), lungs, pleural space, limbs
Morphologic types:
1. Discrete pelvic mass
√ typically cystic space = endometrioma = "chocolate cyst" up to 20 cm in diameter (usually 2 – 5 cm)
√ anechoic / hypoechoic cyst (homogeneous low level echoes = hemorrhagic debris)
√ may contain echogenic material (= clot) appearing as a solid tumor
√ may show layering of debris
√ acoustic enhancement
2. Diffuse form (much more common)
√ often NO detectable abnormality (when lesions small + scattered)
√ frequently multiple cysts bilaterally
√ thickened wall + loss of definition of borders with pelvic organs
MRI (64 – 71% sensitivity; 60 – 82% specificity):
√ hyperintense lesions on all pulse sequences in 47%, hypointense on all pulse sequences in 27%
BE:
• change in bowel habits, rectal pain / bleeding

Path: muscular hypertrophy + fibrosis related to endometriotic deposits in bowel wall
Location: inferior margin of sigmoid colon + anterior wall of rectosigmoid (80%); occasionally multiple lesions
√ single extramucosal mass with crenulated mucosal pattern
√ polypoid intraluminal mass / annular constricting lesion (rare appearance)
CXR:
√ catamenial pneumothorax = spontaneous pneumothorax due to endometriosis of diaphragm
Cx: infertility with involvement of tubes + ovaries (30% of infertility patients show endometriosis)
Dx: laparoscopy

ENDOMETROID TUMOR

Incidence: 15% of all ovarian cancers
Associated with endometrial cancer in 1/3
Histo: resembles endometrial epithelium
√ solid / complex tumor, bilateral in 1/3

FACIAL CLEFTING

= lack of fusion of facial grooves; second most common congenital malformation
Incidence: 1.2 – 1.6:1,000 livebirths
Associated with 72 abnormalities
1. Cleft lip (25%): F > M
associated anomalies: most frequently clubfoot
√ linear defect extending from one side of lip into nostril
√ bilateral in 20%
2. Cleft palate (25%)
associated anomalies in 50%: most frequently clubfoot
3. Cleft lip + palate (50%)
associated anomalies in 13%: most frequently polydactyly
Location: L > R side; in 25% bilateral
√ linear defect extends through alveolar ridge + hard palate reaching the floor of the nasal cavity / orbit

FETAL CARDIAC DYSRHYTHMIAS

normal heart rate: 120 – 160 bpm

Premature Atrial Contractions

= PAC = most common benign rhythm abnormality
√ transient tachycardia / bradycardia
Rx   discontinue smoking, alcohol, caffeine
Follow-up: biweekly auscultation to exclude supraventricular tachycardia

Supraventricular Tachyarrhythmia

Incidence: 1:25,000; most frequent tachyarrhythmia in children
Etiology: viral infection, hypoplasia of sinoatrial tract
Pathogenesis:
(1) Automaticity = irritable ectopic focus discharges at high frequency
(2) Reentry = electric pulse reentering the atria inciting new discharges

Types:
1. Supraventricular tachyarrhythmia (SVT)
   - (a) paroxysmal supraventricular tachycardia
   - (b) paroxysmal atrial tachycardia
   - √ atrial rate of 180 – 300 bpm + ventricular response of 1:1
2. Atrial flutter
   - √ atrial rate of 300 – 460 bpm + ventricular rate of 60 – 200 bpm
3. Atrial fibrillation
   - √ atrial rate of 400 – 700 bpm + ventricular rate of 120 – 200 bpm

Hemodynamics:
fast ventricular rate results in suboptimal filling of heart chambers + decreased cardiac output, overload of RA, CHF

Associated with cardiac anomalies (5 – 10%):
ASD, congenital mitral valve disease, cardiac tumors, WPW syndrome, cardiomyopathy, thyrotoxicosis

OB-US:
- √ M-mode echocardiography with simultaneous visualization of atrial + ventricular contractions allows inference of atrioventricular activation sequence

Cx: congestive heart failure + nonimmune hydrops
Rx: Intrauterine pharmacologic cardioversion (digoxin, verapamil, propranolol, procainamide, quinidine)

Atrioventricular Block
Incidence: 1:20,000 livebirths; in 4 – 9% of all infants with CHD
Etiology:
   (1) Immaturity of conduction system
   (2) Absent connection to AV node
   (3) Abnormal anatomic position of AV node
Associated with:
   (1) Cardiac structural anomalies (45 – 50%): corrected transposition, univentricular heart, cardiac tumor, cardiomyopathy
   (2) Maternal connective tissue disease: lupus erythematosus
Types:
1. First-degree heart block = simple conduction delay
   - √ normal heart rate + rhythm (not reportedly diagnosed in utero)
2. Second-degree heart block
   - (a) Mobitz type I
     - = progressive prolongation of PR interval finally leading to the block of one atrial impulse (Luciani-Wenckebach phenomenon)
     - √ a few atrial contractions are not followed by a ventricular contraction
   - (b) Mobitz type II
     - = intermittent conduction with a ventricular rate as a submultiple of the atrial rate (eg, 2:1 / 3:1 block)
     - √ atrial contraction not followed by ventricular contraction in a constant relationship

3. Third-degree heart block = complete heart block
   - = complete dissociation of atria + ventricles
   - √ slow atrial + ventricular contractions independent from each other
   - *Cx:* decreased cardiac output + CHF

FETAL DEATH IN UTERO
= fetal death during 2nd + 3rd trimesters
Specific signs:
   √ absent cardiac / somatic motion
Nonspecific signs seen not before 48 hours after death:
   √ same / decreased BPD measurement compared to prior exam
   √ development of dolichocephaly
   √ "spalding sign" = overlapping fetal skull bones
   √ distorted fetus without recognizable structures
   √ skin edema (epidermolysis)
   √ increased amount of echoes in amniotic fluid (= fetal tissue fragments)
   √ gas in fetal vascular system

FETAL HYDROPS
Nonimmune Hydrops
= excess of total body water evident as extracellular accumulation of fluid in tissues + serous cavities without antibodies against RBC

Incidence: 1:1,500 to 1:4,000 deliveries
Causes:
1. Cardiac anomalies (40%):
   - (a) structural heart disease (25%): AV septal defect, hypoplastic left heart, rhabdomyoma
   - (b) tachyarrhythmia (15%)
2. Hematologic causes: thalassemia, hemolysis, fetal blood loss
3. Idiopathic (25 – 44%)
4. Twin-twin transfusion (20%)
5. Chromosomal abnormalities (6%): Turner syndrome
6. Skeletal dysplasias: achondroplasia, achondrogenesis, osteogenesis imperfecta, thanatophoric dwarfism, asphyxiating thoracic dysplasia
7. Renal disease (4%): congenital nephrotic syndrome
8. Infections: toxoplasmosis, CMV, syphilis, Coxsackie virus, parvovirus
9. Cervical tumors: teratoma
10. Chest masses: cystic adenomatoid malformation, extralobar sequestration, mediastinal tumor, rhabdomyoma of heart, diaphragmatic hernia
11. Abdominal masses: neuroblastoma, hemangioendothelioma of liver
12. Placental tumors: chorioangioma
Prognosis: 46% death in utero; 17% neonatal death

Immune Hydrops
= ERYTHROBLASTOSIS FETALIS
= lysis of fetal RBCs by maternal IgG antibodies

Pathophysiology:
    rh-negative women (= no D antigen) may become isoimmunized if exposed to Rh-positive blood (= D allotype present); maternal IgM antibodies develop initially, later IgG antibodies with ability to cross placenta (= transplacental passage)
Cause of isoimmunization:
    feto-maternal hemorrhage during pregnancy / delivery / spontaneous or elective abortion

At risk:
    caucasians (15%), blacks (6%), orientals (1%); absence of D antigen originates in Basques
Determination of extent of disease by:
    (1) Optical density shift at 450 nm (= delta OD 450) reflects amount of bilirubin in amniotic fluid
    (2) Percutaneous umbilical cord sampling (PUBS)

√ anasarca (= skin edema)
√ fetal ascites
√ pleural effusion
√ increased diameter of umbilical vein
√ subcutaneous edema (skin thickness >5 mm)
√ polyhydramnios (75%)
√ placentomegaly >6 cm
√ pericardial effusion
√ hepatosplenomegaly

Prophylaxis:
    Rh immune globulin (RhoGAM® = antibody against D antigen) blocks antigen sites on Rh-positive cells in maternal circulation to prevent initiation of maternal antibody production; Rh immune globulin given at 28 weeks to all rh-negative women

FOLLICULAR CYST
= unruptured follicle / ruptured follicle that sealed immediately (after continued stimulation) = failure to ovulate / involute; sign of anovulatory cycle
Predisposed: patients during puberty + menopause; S/P salpingectomy
√ thin-walled, unilocular cyst
√ size usually >2.5 cm / occasionally up to 10 cm in size
√ usually multiple / may be single
√ low-level internal echoes / fluid-debris level / septations / predominantly hyperechoic = hemorrhagic cyst (DDx: teratoma, abscess, torsion, malignancy, ectopic pregnancy)
Prognosis: usually disappears after 1 – 2 menstrual cycles

GASTROSCHISIS
= paraumbilical fusion defect usually on right side secondary to premature interruption of right omphalomesenteric artery (normally persists proximally as superior mesenteric artery) / abnormal involution of right umbilical vein at 5 weeks gestational age; may involve thorax; bowel is nonrotated and lacks secondary fixation to dorsal abdominal wall
Incidence: 1:10,000 to 1:20,000 livebirths, sporadic

Age of occurrence: 37 days of embryonic life
Associated anomalies (5%):
    intestinal atresia / stenosis (25%), IUGR (up to 77%), ectopia cordis
• elevated maternal serum AFP in 75%

√ normal insertion of umbilical cord
√ thickened freely floating bowel loops outside fetal abdomen (lack of peritoneal covering)
√ <3 – 5 cm defect usually on right side of cord insertion
√ no fetal ascites
√ polyhydramnios may be present
Cx: (1) Bowel obstruction / perforation
         (2) Immaturity (65%)
Mortality rate: 7.6 – 28%

GESTATIONAL TROPHOBLASTIC DISEASE
= group of disorders as a result of a combination of male + female gametes arising from trophoblastic elements of the developing blastocyst with invasive tendency + hCG synthesis
1. Benign hydatidiform mole (90%)
2. Invasive mole (5 – 8%)
3. Choriocarcinoma (1 – 2%)

GRANULOSA CELL TUMOR
Most common hormone-active estrogenic tumor of ovary
Incidence: 1 – 3% of all ovarian neoplasms
Age: puberty (5%), reproductive age (45%), postmenopausal (50%)
• precocious puberty
• vaginal bleeding + full breasts

√ multilocular cyst containing fluid / blood (most frequently)
√ size up to 40 cm in diameter, mostly unilateral
√ predominantly hypoechoic mass simulating fibroid
√ endometrial glandular hyperplasia
Cx: malignant transformation is rare

HYDATIDIFORM MOLE
= MOLAR PREGNANCY
Histo: marked edema + enlargement of chorionic villi; disappearance of villous blood vessels + proliferation of trophoblasts
Types:
    1. COMPLETE / CLASSICAL MOLE
        = fertilization of an "empty egg" (= ovum with no active chromosomal material)
        Histo: generalized hydatidiform swelling of all villi + trophoblastic proliferation
        • diploid karyotypem, almost always paternal XX chromosomes
        √ no fetal parts / no chorionic membrane
        Prognosis: in 80% benign, in 20% malignant (choriocarcinoma)
    2. COMPLETE MOLE + COEXISTENT FETUS (2%)
        = molar degeneration of one conceptus of an identical twin pregnancy with same risk of malignant degeneration as in classical mole

3. PARTIAL MOLE
   = areas of molar change alternating with normal villi + fetus with significant congenital anomalies
   Histo: mild to moderate swelling of some villi
   - triploid karyotype (66% XXY; 33% XXX)
   - early onset of preeclampsia
   √ fetal structures present (eg, placenta)
   Prognosis: not associated with malignant transformation

- severe eclampsia prior to 24 weeks
- uterus too large for dates
- 1st trimester bleeding
- abnormal elevation of β-HCG
- passing of grapelike vesicles per vagina
√ uterus larger than dates (in 50%)
√ hyperechoic intrauterine tissue interspersed with numerous punctate hypoechoic areas = hydropic villi
√ in 25% atypical appearance: large hyperechoic areas (blood clot) + areas of cystic degeneration resembling incomplete abortion
√ thick hyperechoic rim around central anechoic zone
√ bilateral theca lutein cysts (18 – 37%), which may take 4 months to regress after evacuation of a molar pregnancy

DDx:
(1) Hydropic degeneration of the placenta (associated with incomplete / missed abortions)
(2) Degenerated uterine leiomyoma
(3) Incomplete abortion = retained products with hemorrhage
(4) Choriocarcinoma

HYDRO- / HEMATOMETROCOLPOS
= accumulation of sterile fluid (hydro~) / blood (hemato~) / pus (pyo~) within uterus (~metria) + vagina (~colpos)
Incidence: 1:16,000 female births
Etiology:
1. Congenital obstruction:
   (a) persistent urogenital sinus = single exit chamber for bladder + vagina; separate orifice for anus; caused by virilization of female fetus / intersex anomaly / arrest of normal vaginal development
      Frequently associated with ambiguous genitalia
      Age: newborn period
   (b) cloacal malformation = single perineal orifice for bladder + vagina + rectum; caused by early embryologic arrest
      Frequently associated with duplex genital tract
      Age: newborn period
   (c) imperforate hymen, transverse vaginal septum, segmental vaginal atresia, imperforate cervix, blind horn of bicornuate uterus, Mayer-Rokitansky-Küster-Hauser syndrome (= agenesis of uterus + vagina with active uterine anlage)
      - primary amenorrhea = "delayed menarche"
      - cyclical abdominal pain
      - interlabial mass
      Age: puberty

Δ Hematometrocolpos / hematocolpos are due to imperforate hymen / transverse vaginal septum
Δ Hematometra is due to cervical dysgenesis + vaginal agenesis / Mayer-Rokitansky-Küster-Hauser syndrome / obstructed uterine horn
May be associated with:
   imperforate anus, hydronephrosis, renal agenesis / dysplasia, polycystic kidneys, duplication of vagina + uterus, sacral hypoplasia, esophageal atresia
2. Acquired obstruction: neoplastic obstruction of endocervical canal / vagina, postpartum infection, attempted abortion, cervical stenosis after radiotherapy, postsurgical scarring, senile contraction

- vague pelvic discomfort
- pain during defecation / urination
- asymptomatic
√ pear-shaped distended uterus ± vagina
√ anechoic / echogenic uterine ± vaginal contents
√ hematosalpinx ± endometriosis
OB-US:
   √ cystic / midlevel echogenic retrovesical mass (mucous secretions secondary to stimulation by maternal estrogens during fetal life)
   √ cystic mass ± fluid-debris level (distended vagina)
   √ bladder often not identified (compression by distended vagina)
DDx: ovarian cyst, duplication cyst, meconium cyst, mesenteric cyst, rectovesical fistula, anterior meningocele, cystic tumor
Cx: endometritis, myometritis, parametritis (= pelvic lymphangitis), pelvic abscess, septic pelvic thrombophlebitis, urinary tract infection

IMMATURE TERATOMA OF OVARY
= EMBRYONAL TERATOMA = MALIGNANT TERATOMA = SOLID TERATOMA
Histo: immature tissue resembling those of the embryo; grade 0 – 3 reflect amount of immature neuroectodermal tissue
May be associated with gliomatosis peritonei = multiple peritoneal implants of mature glial tissue
- elevated AFP levels (50%)
- no elevation of serum hCG levels
√ predominantly solid tumor with numerous cysts of varying size
√ scattered calcifications (due to invariable association with mature teratoma)

INTRAUTERINE CONTRACEPTIVE DEVICE
√ double echogenic line with plastic IUD
√ reverberation echoes with metal IUD

Types of IUD:
1. Lippes loop
   √ 4 – 5 echogenic dots on SAG view
   √ horizontal line / dot on TRV view
2. Saf-T-coil
   √ echogenic solid line on SAG view

√ series of echoes / dot on TRV view
3. Copper 7 / Copper T / Progestasert
   √ dot in fundus + solid line in corpus on SAG view
   √ solid line in fundus + dot in corpus on TRV view
4. Dalkon shield (no longer produced)

"LOST IUD":
= locater device not palpated
Cause: 1. expulsion of IUD
            2. migration of thread
            3. detachment of thread
            4. uterine perforation of IUD
Δ Abdominal plain film indicated if IUD not identified by US!
Cx: pelvic inflammatory disease (2 – 3-fold risk compared to that of non-IUD users)

IUD + PREGNANCY
   √ IUD may not be visualized after 1st trimester (as uterus grows IUD is drawn into cavity)
Prognosis: high risk of septic abortion
Rx: early removal of IUD if string remained in vagina

INTRAUTERINE GROWTH RETARDATION
= process resulting in birth of a neonate with weight below the 10th percentile for gestational age; usually not detectable before 32 – 34 weeks GA (time of maximal fetal growth)
Incidence: 3 – 7% of all deliveries; in 12 – 47% of all twin pregnancies
Etiology:
A. UTEROPLACENTAL INSUFFICIENCY (80%)
   1. Maternal causes
      √ asymmetric IUGR / symmetric IUGR (in severe cases)
      (a) deficient supply of nutrients:
          smoking, maternal malnutrition, multiple gestations, anemia, life in high altitudes
      (b) maternal vascular disease (more common):
          severe diabetes, chronic hypertension, chronic renal disease, collagen disease (eg, SLE) (inadequate placental perfusion)
   2. Primary placental causes
      Extensive placental infarctions, chronic partial separation, placenta previa
B. PRIMARY FETAL CAUSES (20%)
   = decreased intrinsic growth
   √ symmetric IUGR
   Congenital heart disease, genitourinary anomalies, CNS anomalies, chromosomal abnormalities (trisomy 13, 18, 21), viral infection (rubella, CMV)

PHENOTYPES
   1. **Pure symmetrical IUGR** = low profile IUGR
      = proportionate reduction of all fetal measurements due to
      (a) intrinsic alteration in growth potential
      (b) severe nutritional deprivation overwhelming protective brain-sparing mechanism occurring prior to 26 weeks MA + persisting until delivery

   2. **Asymmetrical IUGR** = late flattening IUGR (75%)
      = disproportionate reduction of fetal measurements due to uteroplacental insufficiency with preferential shunting of blood to fetal brain occurring after 26 weeks GA
      √ small body (AC)
      √ high HC/AC and FL/AC ratios (head size + femur length less affected)

MORPHOLOGIC GROWTH PARAMETERS
   AC + EFW have highest sensitivity
   √ BPD growth rate <5th percentile (82% chance of IUGR; 18% false positive; 17% false negative)
   √ HC:AC ratio >95th percentile (71% chance of asymmetrical IUGR)
   √ reduced amniotic fluid volume <1 cm in its broadest dimension anywhere (90% chance of IUGR)
   √ abdominal circumference (AC) <10th percentile (84% chance for IUGR)
   √ grade III placenta

PHYSIOLOGIC FETAL PARAMETERS
   Sequence of events in fetal hypoxia:
      nonreactive CST > absence of fetal breathing > nonreactive NST > diminished fetal movements > absence of fetal movements > absence of fetal tone

Biophysical profile
   Accuracy: False-negative rate of 0.9/1000 pregnancies; 33% sensitivity, 17% positive predictive value

Doppler studies
   1. NON-STRESS TEST (NST)
      Accuracy:
         false-negative rate of 3.2/1000 (if done weekly) or 1.6/1000 (if done biweekly); 50% false-positive rate for neonatal morbidity + 80% for neonatal mortality
   2. CONTRACTION STRESS TEST (CST)
      Accuracy: false-negative rate of 0.4/1000; 50% false-positive rate
   3. UTERINE + UMBILICAL ARTERY WAVEFORM
      √ elevated systolic:diastolic ratio (indicating increased vascular resistance)
   4. FETAL AORTIC FLOW VOLUME
      √ decrease in blood flow <185 – 246 ml/kg/min

Cx: increased risk for perinatal asphyxia, meconium aspiration, electrolyte imbalance from metabolic acidosis, polycythemia, chromosomal / genetic disorder (5 – 15%)
Prognosis: 6 – 8-fold increase in risk for intrapartum + neonatal death

DDx of SGA (fetus small for gestational age):
   (1) Constitutionally small fetus
   (2) Primary growth failure associated with congenital anomalies
   (3) IUGR

INVASIVE MOLE

= CHORIOADENOMA DESTRUENS

Histo: excessive trophoblastic proliferation with presence of villous structure + invasion of myometrium

- history of previous molar gestation / missed abortion (75%)
- continued uterine bleeding
- persistently elevated β-hCG levels
- √ hyperechoic tissue with punctate lucencies
- √ irregular focal hyperechoic region within myometrium
- √ bilateral theca lutein cysts, 4 – 8 cm in size

KRUKENBERG TUMOR

= ovarian tumors from GI tract cancer (stomach, colon) now including pancreatic + biliary primaries; 2% of females with gastric cancer develop Krukenberg tumor

Δ Krukenberg tumors antedate the discovery of the primary lesion in up to 20%!

Age: any age, most common in 5th – 6th decade

√ in 80% bilateral hypo- / hyperechoic mass ± cystic degeneration

MACROSOMIA

= FETAL GROWTH ACCELERATION

= fetus large for gestational age (LGA) with EFW >90th percentile for age / >4,000 g at term

√ AC >3 SD above the mean for age (most reliable measurement)

√ estimated fetal weight (EFW) including fetal head, abdomen, femur length >90th percentile (± 15% accuracy)

√ low FL:AC ratio

√ low HC:AC ratio

√ enlarged thigh circumference

√ low FL:thigh circumference ratio

MALIGNANT GERM CELL TUMOR OF OVARY

Age: 14 years on average

- pelvic / abdominal pain
- pelvic / abdominal mass
- elevated alpha-fetoprotein (60% in immature teratoma; 100% in endodermal sinus tumor)
- elevated β-hCG (30% of endodermal sinus tumors)

√ average diameter of 15 cm

√ unilateral, rarely bilateral

√ calcifications (40%)

√ homogeneously solid (3%), predominantly solid (85%), predominantly cystic (12%)

MUCINOUS OVARIAN TUMOR

Incidence: 20% of all ovarian tumors; benign:malignant = 7:1

Histo: nonciliated tall columnar epithelium, cysts lined by mucus-secreting cells (similar to endocervix)

Age: middle adult life, rare before puberty + after menopause

Cx: rupture may lead to pseudomyxoma peritonei

A. MUCINOUS CYSTADENOMA

Age: reproductive years + postmenopause

√ multilocular cyst with thin septa

√ complex cysts with solid elements

√ usually unilateral, bilateral in 5%

Cx: malignant transformation in 12%

B. MUCINOUS CYSTADENOCARCINOMA

difficult to differentiate from benign variety

√ solid tissue areas within cystic septated adnexal mass

√ usually unilateral, bilateral in 20%

√ capsular infiltration with loss of definition + fixation

OMPHALOCELE

= persistence of body stalk = midline defect of anterior abdominal wall secondary to failure of lateral body folds to fuse during 3rd to 4th week of gestation + herniation of intraabdominal contents into base of umbilical cord

Incidence: 1:4,000 to 1:5,500 pregnancies

Age: earliest detection at 12 weeks menstrual age

High incidence of ASSOCIATED ANOMALIES (45 - 72%):

1. Chromosomal (30 – 58%): trisomy 13, 18, 21, Turner syndrome (13% with liver in omphalocele, 77% with bowel in omphalocele)
2. Genitourinary (40%)
3. Cardiac (16 – 47%): VSD, ASD, tetralogy of Fallot, ectopia cordis in pentalogy of Cantrell, DORV
4. Neural tube defects (4 – 39%): holoprosencephaly, encephalocele, cerebellar hypoplasia
5. IUGR (20%)
6. Beckwith-Wiedemann syndrome (10%)
7. GI tract: intestinal atresia (vascular compromise); malrotation; abnormal fixation of liver, esophageal atresia, facial cleft
8. Limb-body wall deficiency; cystic hygroma

- elevated maternal serum AFP in 40%

√ midline defect

  √ defect over entire ventral abdominal wall (mean size 2.5 – 5 cm)

  √ widened cord where it joins the skin of the abdomen

√ cord inserting at apex of defect

√ herniation of abdominal viscera at base of umbilical cord: liver (27%) ± stomach ± bowel

√ hypoechoic Wharton jelly within herniated sac

√ covering peritoneal-amniotic membrane (may rupture in exceedingly rare cases)

√ polyhydramnios (occasionally oligohydramnios)

Cx: (1) Infection, inanition
(2) Immaturity (23%)

Mortality rate: 29 – 55% due to frequency of concurrent malformations + chromosomic abnormalities; 10% mortality if isolated abnormality

DDx: physiologic herniation of midgut into umbilical cord between 8th and 12th week of gestation

PSEUDOOMPHALOCELE
  = deformation of fetal abdomen by transducer pressure
    coupled with an oblique scan orientation may give the
    appearance of an omphalocele

OMPHALOMESENTERIC DUCT CYST
Etiology: persistence + dilatation of a segment of the
              omphalomesenteric / vitelline duct joining the
              embryonic gut and the yolk sac, which is
              formed during the 3rd week and closed by the
              16th week of gestation
Histo: cyst lined by columnar mucin-secreting
           gastrointestinal epithelium
M:F = 3:5
Location: usually in close proximity to fetus
√ umbilical cord cyst up to 6 cm in diameter
Cx: (1)   Compression of umbilical vessels by
              expanding cyst
        (2)   Erosion of umbilical vein from acid-producing
              gastric mucosal lining
DDx: allantoic cyst, umbilical cord hematoma

OVARIAN CANCER
8th leading cause of cancer in women; 3rd most common
gynecologic malignancy = 25% of all gynecologic
malignancies; highest mortality rate of all female cancers
(60%), 4th leading cause of cancer deaths in women,
acounts for 50% of cancer deaths of female genital tract
Incidence: affects 1:70 women; 33 cases per year per
               100,000 women > age 50; 20,500 new
               cases per year with 12,400 deaths
Peak age: 55 – 59 years (80% in women >50 years)
Histo:
    1. Epithelial tumors (70%)
        (a) serous tumor resembling ciliated columnar cells
            of the fallopian tubes (50%)
        (b) endometrioid tumor similar to endometrial
            adenocarcinoma (15 – 30%)
        (c) mucinous tumor similar to endocervical canal
            epithelium (15%)
        (d) mesonephroid tumor similar to clear cell
            carcinoma of kidney (5%)
        (e) undifferentiated tumor (15%)
    2. Germ cell tumors (15%)
        Most common malignant ovarian neoplasm in girls +
        young women
        Age: 4 – 27 years
        (a) mature teratoma (10%) = the only benign variety
        (b) dysgerminoma (1.9%)
        (c) immature teratoma (1.3%)
        (d) endodermal sinus tumor (1%)
        (e) malignant mixed germ cell tumor (0.7%)
        (f) choriocarcinoma (0.1%)
        (g) embryonal carcinoma (0.1%)
    3. Metastases (10%)
    4. Stromal tumors (5%)

Increased risk:
    nulliparity, Caucasian race, higher socioeconomic
    group, history of breast cancer (risk factor of 2)

STAGE I a   limited to one ovary
       I b   limited to both ovaries
       I c   + positive peritoneal lavage / ascites
       II a involvement of uterus / fallopian tubes
       II b extension to other pelvic tissues
       II c + positive peritoneal lavage / ascites
       III   intraabdominal extension outside pelvis /
             retroperitoneal nodes / extension to small
             bowel / omentum
       IV   distant metastases
Δ 60 – 75% of patients have stage III / IV disease at time
  of diagnosis!
• occasional pelvo-abdominal pain
• constipation, urinary frequency
• early satiety
• ascites
• paraneoplastic hypercalcemia
• elevated CA-125 levels (in 50% of stage I disease)
US:
    Δ Screening finds adnexal cysts in 1 – 15% of
      postmenopausal women; only 3% of ovarian cysts <5
      cm are malignant!
    √ ovarian size >1.5 cm, ovarian volume >2 cm^3 (ovaries
      may be larger with multiparity, obesity, hormonal
      replacement); 80% of normal ovaries not visualized
    √ omental / peritoneal masses
    √ pseudomyxoma peritonei
    √ liver metastases
    √ ascites
Prognosis:
    38% overall 5-year survival rate, 5% for stage IV
    disease, 14% for stage III disease, 85% for stage I
    disease

OVARIAN FIBROMA
Incidence: 3 – 4%
Age: usually menopausal / postmenopausal
• usually asymptomatic
√ hypoechoic mass with sound attenuation

OVARIAN HYPERSTIMULATION SYNDROME
Incidence: severe OHSS in 1.5 – 6% under Perganol
               therapy
Etiology:
    (1) Induced by hCG therapy with human menopausal
        gonadotropin (Perganol), occasionally with
        clomiphene (Clomid)
    (2) Hydatidiform mole
    (3) Chorioepithelioma
    (4) Multiple pregnancies
Path: enlarged ovaries with multiple follicular cysts,
          corpora lutea, edematous stroma (fluid shift
          secondary to increased capillary permeability)
• abdominal pain (100%) + distension (100%)
• nausea (100%), vomiting (36%)
• acute abdomen (17%)
• dyspnea (16%)
• thrombophlebitis (11%)
• marked hemoconcentration
• fainting (11%)

- blurred vision (5%)
- anasarca (5%)
- hydrothorax
- enhanced fertility

√ ovary >5 cm in longest dimension containing large geometrically packed follicles

√ ovarian cyst >10 cm (100%): usually disappear after 20 – 40 days

√ ascites (33%)

√ pleural effusion (5%)

√ hydroureter (11%)

Cx: (related to volume depletion)
  (1) Hypovolemia + hemoconcentration
  (2) Oliguria, electrolyte imbalance, azotemia
  (3) Death from intraabdominal hemorrhage / thromboembolic event

PARAOVARIAN CYST

= vestigial remnant of Wolffian body = mesonephric tubules off the mesonephric (= Gartner) duct, paralleling vagina and fallopian tube, usually degenerate into vestigial structures

Location: within the two peritoneal layers of broad ligament, between the tube and hilum of the ovary

Types: (a) mesonephric (Wolffian duct)
  (b) paramesonephric (Müllerian duct)
  (c) mesothelial

1. GARTNER DUCT CYST: inclusion cyst; lateral to vagina + uterine wall
2. PAROÖPHORON: medial location between tube + hilum of ovary
3. EPOÖPHORON: lateral location between tube + hilum of ovary
4. HYDATID OF MORGAGNI: most lateral + outer end of Gartner duct

√ thin-walled unilocular cyst, up to 18 cm in diameter

√ may arise out of pelvis (if pedunculated + mobile)

PELVIC INFLAMMATORY DISEASE

Incidence: 10% of women in reproductive age (17% in blacks); formerly married > married > never married

Risk factors: early age at sexual debut, multiple sexual partners, history of sexual transmitted disease, douching

Predisposed: intrauterine contraceptive device (1.5 – 4-fold increase in risk)

Etiology: (a) bilateral: venereal disease (gonorrhea), IUD, S/P abortion
  (b) unilateral = nongynecologic: rupture of appendix, diverticulum, S/P pelvic surgery

Organisms:
  (1) Chlamydia trachomatis + Neisseria gonorrhea (most common with high prevalence of coinfection) damaging protective barrier of endocervical canal with spread to tubes producing fibrosis + adhesions
  (2) Aerobes: Streptococcus, Escherichia coli, Haemophilus influenzae

  (3) Anaerobes: Bacteroides, Peptostreptococcus, Peptococcus
  (4) Tuberculosis (hematogenous)
  (5) Actinomycosis in IUD users

May be associated with Fitz-Hugh-Curtis syndrome (= gonorrheic perihepatitis)

A. **Endometritis**
  √ endometrial prominence
  √ small amount of fluid within uterine lumen
  √ gas reflection within uterine cavity (most specific)
  √ pain over uterus

B. **Salpingitis**
  not depicted by imaging techniques

C. **Hydro- / pyosalpinx**
  = continued secretion of tubal epithelium into lumen of a fallopian tube obstructed at two sites
  √ funnel-shaped kinked thick-walled cystic structure filled with sterile fluid / debris / pus
  √ free fluid / pus in cul-de-sac
  √ loss of definition of uterine borders
  Cx: tubal torsion

D. **Tuboovarian Abscess**
  - pain, fever
  - vaginal discharge, cervical motion tenderness
  Location: usually in posterior cul-de-sac extending bilaterally
  √ multilocular complex mass often with debris, septations, irregular thick wall
  √ may contain fluid-fluid levels or gas

Cx: infertility, ectopic pregnancy, chronic pelvic pain, pelvic adhesive disease, hydrosalpinx

PENTALOGY OF CANTRELL

= sporadic very rare abnormality
1. Midline supraumbilical abdominal defect
2. Defect of lower sternum
3. Deficiency of diaphragmatic pericardium
4. Deficiency of anterior diaphragm: herniation of intraabdominal organs into thoracic cavity is rare
5. Intracardiac abnormality: atrioventricular septal defect (50%), VSD (18%), tetralogy of Fallot (11%)

√ ectopia cordis

PERITONEAL INCLUSION CYST

Histo: cyst lined by hyperplastic mesothelial cells + fibroglandular tissue with chronic inflammation

Predisposed: patients with active ovaries + extensive pelvic adhesions from previous abdominal surgery / pelvic inflammatory disease / endometriosis

Pathogenesis: impaired peritoneal clearing of fluid normally produced by ovaries

√ single / multiloculated cyst contiguous with ovary

Cx: infertility

DDx: paraovarian cyst, ovarian neoplasm, lymphangioma

PLACENTA ACCRETA

= underdeveloped decidualization with chorionic villi growing into myometrium

Incidence:
1:2,500 – 7,000 deliveries; in 5% of placenta previa patients; in 24% after one cesarean section; in up to 67% after >4 cesarean sections

Predisposed: areas of uterine scarring

Risk for placenta accreta:
0.65% after 1 section, 1.8% after 2 sections, 3% after 3 sections, 10% after 4 sections

Associated with   placenta previa (20%)

Types:
1. PLACENTA ACCRETA = chorionic villi in direct contact with myometrium
2. PLACENTA INCRETA = villi invade myometrium
3. PLACENTA PERCRETA = villi penetrate through uterine serosa

√ thinning to <1 mm / absence of hypoechoic myometrial zone between placenta + echodense uterine serosa / posterior bladder wall

√ thinning / irregularity / focal disruption of linear hyperechoic boundary echo (= uterine serosa-bladder wall interface)

√ focal mass-like elevations / extensions of echogenic placental tissue beyond uterine serosa

√ >6 irregular intraplacental lacunae (= vascular spaces)

Cx: (1) Retention of placental tissue
(2) Persistent postpartum bleeding
(3) Emergent hysterectomy
(4) Maternal death

PLACENTA EXTRACHORIALIS

= attachment of placental membranes to the fetal surface of the placenta rather than to the placental margin
= chorionic plate smaller than basal plate, ie, the transition of membranous to villous chorion occurs at a distance from the placental edge that is smaller than the basal plate radius

1. CIRCUMMARGINATE PLACENTA
   Incidence: up to 20% of placentas
   • No clinical significance
   √ placental margin not deformed

2. CIRCUMVALLATE PLACENTA
   = attachment of fetal membranes form a folded thickened ring with underlying fibrin + often hemorrhage
   Incidence: 1 – 2% of pregnancies
   Cx: premature labor, threatened abortion, increased perinatal mortality, marginal hemorrhage

PLACENTAL ABRUPTION

= ABRUPTIO PLACENTAE
= premature separation of placenta from the myometrium secondary to maternal hemorrhage into decidua basalis between 20th week and birth

Incidence: 0.5 – 1.3% of gestations

Risk factors:
previous history of abruption / perinatal death / premature delivery; hypertension; vascular disease; smoking; drugs (cocaine); fibroids; trauma; fetal malformations

Associated with   intraplacental infarction / hematoma
• vaginal bleeding (80%)
• abdominal pain (50%)
• consumptive coagulopathy = DIC (30%)
• uterine rigidity (15%)

Site:
(a) marginal (most common site)
    low-pressure bleed due to tears of marginal veins; associated with cigarette smoking
(b) retroplacental
    high-pressure bleed due to rupture of spiral arteries; associated with hypertension + vascular disease

√ hyperechoic / isoechoic hematoma (initially difficult to distinguish from placenta)

√ hypoechoic / complex collection between uterine wall + placenta in 50% within 1 week (hematoma / placental infarction)

√ anechoic collection within 2 weeks

√ separation / rounding of placental margin

√ abnormally thick + heterogenous placenta (if blood isoechoic)

√ elevation of chorioamnionic membrane
(DDx: incomplete chorioamnionic fusion during 2nd trimester, blighted twin)

Prognosis:
(1) Only large hematomas (occupying >30 – 40% of the maternal surface) result in fetal hypoxia
(2) Abruptions with contained hematoma have worse prognosis
(3) Responsible for up to 15 – 25% of all perinatal deaths
(4) Normal term deliveries in 27% of hematomas detected >20 weeks GA
(5) Normal delivery in 80% of intrauterine hematomas detected <20 weeks GA

Cx: (1) Perinatal mortality (20 – 60%), up to 15 – 25% of all perinatal deaths
(2) Fetal distress / demise (15 – 27%)
(3) Premature labor + premature delivery (23 – 52%) (3-fold increase)
(4) Threatened abortion during first 20 weeks
(5) Infant small-for-gestational age (6 – 7%)

DDx: (1) Normal draining basal veins
(2) Normal uterine tissue
(3) Retroplacental myoma
(4) Focal contraction
(5) Chorioangioma
(6) Coexistent mole

PLACENTA MEMBRANACEA

= presence of well-vascularized placental villi in the peripheral membranes

Cause: ? endometritis, endometrial hyperplasia, extensive vascularization of decidua capsularis, previous endometrial damage by curettage

• repeated vaginal bleeding extending into 2nd trimester + abortion at 20 – 30 weeks
• postpartum hemorrhage

√ thickened outline over whole gestational sac (0.2 – 3.0 cm)

√ may show additional distinct disc of placenta

PLACENTA PREVIA

= abnormally low implantation of ovum with the placenta covering all / part of internal cervical os

Incidence:

0.5% of all deliveries; in 7 – 11% of women with 2nd + 3rd trimester vaginal bleeding; in 0.26% with unscarred uterus; in 0.65% after one cesarean section; in up to 10% after >4 cesarean sections

Cause:

defective decidual vascularization in areas of endometrial scarring causing compensatory placental thinning; placenta occupies a greater surface of the uterus with increased probability for encroachment upon internal os

Predisposed:

(1) Previous uterine incision (cesarian section, myomectomy)
(2) Older women
(3) Multiparous women

Types on clinical examination:

1. Central / total previa (1/3) = complete covering of internal os
2. Partial previa = internal os partially covered by placenta
3. Low-lying placenta = low placental edge without extension over internal os; palpable by examining finger

• painless vaginal bleeding in 93% (usually 3rd trimester / as early as 20 weeks)

Δ 3 – 5% of all pregnancies are complicated by 3rd trimester bleeding; of these 7 – 11% are due to placenta previa!

US - FALSE POSITIVES (5 – 7%):

1. Placental "migration" / rotation
   = differential growth rates between lower uterine segment + placenta
   Δ 63 – 93% will have normal implantation at term!
   — conversion to normal position: anterior wall > posterior wall of uterus
   — NO conversion if placenta attaches to both posterior + anterior walls
2. Overfilled urinary bladder
   bladder-induced compression leads to apposition of the lower anterior + posterior uterine walls (cervical length >3.5 – 4 cm) simulating a placenta previa
3. Focal myometrial contraction (myometrial thickness >1.5 cm) in the region of the lower uterine segment

US - FALSE NEGATIVES (2%):

1. Obscuring fetal head
   remedied by Trendelenburg position / gentle upward traction on fetal head
2. Lateral position of placenta previa; remedied by obtaining oblique scans
3. Blood in region of internal os mistaken for amniotic fluid

Cx: (secondary to premature detachment of placenta from lower uterine segment)

(1) Maternal hemorrhage (blood from intervillous space)
(2) Premature delivery
(3) IUGR
(4) Perinatal death (5%)

Rx: precludes vaginal delivery + pelvic examination

POSTMATURITY SYNDROME

= inability of aging placenta to support demands of fetus

Incidence: in 15% of all post-term gravidas

• meconium-stained amniotic fluid
√ grade 3 placenta (in 85%), grade 2 (in 15%), grade 1 (in 0%)
√ decreased subcutaneous fat + wrinkling of skin
√ long fingernails
√ decreased vernix

Cx: meconium aspiration, perinatal asphyxia, thermal instability

Post-term fetus

= fetus undelivered by 42nd week MA

Incidence: 7 – 12% of all pregnancies

Risk of perinatal mortality:

2-fold at 43 weeks MA, 4- to 6-fold at 44 weeks MA

PREECLAMPSIA

= TOXEMIA OF PREGNANCY

Incidence: 5% of pregnancies, typically during 3rd trimester

Clinical triad:

• pregnancy-induced / -aggravated hypertension
• proteinuria
• peripheral edema

Cx:

@ CNS
@ Liver: hematoma, infarction
@ Kidney

ECLAMPSIA

• convulsions + coma

PREMATURE RUPTURE OF MEMBRANES

= spontaneous rupture of chorioamniotic membranes before the onset of labor

Types:

(a) Preterm premature rupture of membranes (PPROM) <37 weeks GA
(b) Term premature rupture of membranes (TPROM) >37 weeks GA

Incidence: overall 2.1 – 17.1%; PPROM 0.9 – 4.4%; in 29% of all preterm deliveries; in 18% of all term deliveries

Risk of recurrence: 21% of women with PPROM

Cause: ? infection of membranes

Cx:

(a) TPROM:
    — >24 hours may result in intrapartum fever
    — >72 hours may result in chorioamnionitis + still birth

(b) PPROM: respiratory distress syndrome (9 – 43%),
neonatal sepsis (2 – 19%)

PREPLACENTAL HEMORRHAGE
= BREUS MOLE = SUBCHORIAL HEMORRHAGE
Incidence: in 4% of all placental abruptions
Etiology: massive pooling + stasis due to extensive
venous obstruction
Risk for fetal demise: 67% overall; 100% for hematomas
>60 ml

PRIMARY OVARIAN CHORIOCARCINOMA
= NONGESTATIONAL CHORIOCARCINOMA
Incidence: extremely rare; 50 cases in world literature
Age: <20 years
• elevated serum hCG
√ predominantly solid tumor with areas of hemorrhage +
necrosis
DDx: metastasis to ovary from gestational
choriocarcinoma (reproductive age)

PUERPERAL OVARIAN VEIN THROMBOPHLEBITIS
Etiology: bacterial seeding from puerperal endometritis
with secondary thrombosis (pregnancy +
puerperium are hypercoagulable states)
Incidence: 1:600 – 1:2,000 deliveries
• presents on 2nd / 3rd postpartum day
• lower abdominal / flank pain (>90%)
• palpable thrombosed ovarian vein (50%) *⇒ Echogenic mass*
• fever if diagnosis delayed
Location: R:L = 8–9:1, occasionally bilateral
CT:
√ tubular structure in location of ovarian vein with low-
density center + peripheral enhancement
Cx: IVC thrombosis; pulmonary embolism (25%); left
renal vein thrombosis; septicemia; metastatic
abscess formation
Mortality: 5%
Rx: IV antibiotics + heparin; ligation of involved vessel
at most proximal point of thrombosis after failure to
improve after 3 – 5 days

RETROPLACENTAL HEMATOMA
= accumulation of blood behind placenta, which may
dissect into placenta / myometrium secondary to rupture
of spiral arteries
Incidence: 4.5%; 16% of all placental abruptions
• external bleeding
√ thickened heterogeneous appearing placenta
(hematoma of similar echogenicity as placenta)
√ rounded placental margins + intraplacental
sonolucencies
Cx: (1) Precipitous delivery
(2) Coagulopathy
(3) Fetal demise (accounts for 15 – 25% of all
perinatal deaths);
risk for fetal demise with hematomas >60 ml:
6% before 20 weeks GA; 29% after 20
weeks GA

SEROUS OVARIAN TUMOR
Incidence: 30% of ovarian tumors;
benign:malignant = 1:9
Histo: lined by tall columnar epithelial cells (like
fallopian tubes), filled with serous fluid
Age: 20 – 50 years (malignant variety later)
A. SEROUS CYSTADENOMA
second most common benign tumor of the ovary (20%)
√ uni- / multilocular thin-walled cyst with an
occasional septum
√ up to 20 cm in diameter
√ mostly unilateral, bilateral cysts in 20 – 30%
Cx: malignant transformation in 10%
B. SEROUS CYSTADENOCARCINOMA
= 60% of all ovarian carcinomas
√ solid papillomatous areas within cystic mass
√ loss of capsular definition + tumor fixation
√ mostly bilateral (70%)
√ ascites secondary to peritoneal surface
implantation
√ lymph node enlargement (periaortic, mediastinal,
supraclavicular)

SERTOLI - LEYDIG CELL TUMOR OF OVARY
Origin: from hilar cells of ovary
Incidence: <0.5%
Age: any age; most common in 2nd – 3rd decade
• androgenic
√ hypoechoic mass simulating fibroid
√ may have cystic / hemorrhagic degeneration

SINGLE UMBILICAL ARTERY
Etiology:
(1) Primary agenesis of one umbilical artery (usually
first appears in 5th menstrual week)
(2) Secondary atrophy / atresia of one umbilical artery
(3) Persistence of original single allantoic artery of the
body stalk
Incidence:
0.2 – 1% of singleton births; 5% in dizygotic twins; 2.5%
in abortuses; increased incidence in trisomy D / E,
diabetic mothers, white patients, spontaneous abortions
Associated with:
(a) Congenital anomalies (21%):
1. CHD (most frequent): VSD, conotruncal
anomalies
2. Abdomen: ventral wall defect, diaphragmatic
hernia
3. CNS: hydrocephalus, holoprosencephaly, spina
bifida
4. GU: hydronephrosis, dysplastic kidney
5. Esophageal atresia, cystic hygroma, cleft lip
6. Polydactyly, syndactyly
(b) IUGR
(c) Premature delivery
(d) Perinatal mortality (20%): stillbirth (66%)
(e) Marginal (18%) / velamentous (9%) insertion of
umbilical cord
(f) Chromosomal anomalies (67%): trisomy 18 >
trisomy 13 > Turner syndrome > triploidy

Site: L > R
√ axial view of cord shows 2 vessels
√ single umbilical artery nearly as large as umbilical vein
√ incurvation of distal aorta toward common iliac artery on the side of patent umbilical artery
√ ipsilateral hypoplastic common iliac artery
√ absence of abdominal portion of umbilical artery on ipsilateral side of missing umbilical artery
√ color flow imaging permits earlier (15 – 16 weeks) + more confident diagnosis

Prognosis:
   (1) 4-fold increase in perinatal mortality (14%) with concurrent major abnormality
   (2) Isolated single umbilical artery does not affect clinical outcome
DDx: normal single umbilical artery near placental end (umbilical arteries normally unite with allantoic artery near placental insertion)

STEIN-LEVENTHAL SYNDROME
Incidence: 2.5% of all women
Etiology:
   deficient aromatase activity (catalyst for conversion of androgen into estrogen) resulting in androgen excess; exaggerated pulsatile release of LH stimulates continued ovarian androgen secretion at the expense of estradiol; reduction of local estrogen impairs FSH activity; this results in accumulation of small- + medium-sized atretic follicles without final maturation into graafian follicles
Path:
   pearly white ovaries with multiple cysts below the capsule, which are lined by a hyperplastic theca interna layer showing pronounced luteinization; granulosa cells are absent / degenerating; corpora lutea are absent
Age: late 2nd decade

Associated with: Cushing syndrome, basophilic pituitary adenoma, post-pill amenorrhea, virilizing ovarian / adrenal tumor
• secondary amenorrhea / oligomenorrhea
• reduced infertility / sterility
• periodic abdominal discomfort
• obesity
• mild facial / severe generalized hirsutism
• cystic acne
• cephalic hair loss
• elevated LH levels
• normal / decreased FSH
• increased androstenedione / testosterone
• elevated estrone / estradiol

√ normal ovarian size (in 30%)
√ bilaterally enlarged ovaries (70%), volume of 6 – 30 cm³
√ excessive number of developing follicles
   (a) multiple (over 5) small cysts of 5 – 8 mm in subcapsular location (40%)
   (b) hypoechoic ovaries (25%)
   (c) isoechoic ovaries (5%)

Cx: endometrial cancer <40 years of age (due to unopposed chronic estrogen stimulation)
DDx: ovaries in congenital adrenal hyperplasia
Rx: (1) Ovulation induction with clomiphene (Clomid) / menotropins (Perganol)
   (2) Wedge resection (transient effect only)

STUCK TWIN
= one twin with IUGR residing within an oligo- / anhydramniotic sac of a diamniotic twin pregnancy
√ amnion invisible secondary to close contact with fetal parts
√ fetus fixed relative to the uterine wall without change during shift in maternal position
√ diminished / absent active fetal motion
√ absence of intermingling of fetal parts between twins
Prognosis: fetal death in utero

SUCCENTURIATE LOBE
= ACCESSORY LOBE = separate mass of chorionic villi connected to main placenta by vessels within membrane
Incidence: 0.14 – 3%
Cx: (1) Retained in utero with postpartum hemorrhage
   (2) Placenta previa with intrapartum hemorrhage
   (3) VASA PREVIA = succenturiate vessels traversing internal os, which may rupture resulting in fetal blood loss

SUBCHORIONIC HEMORRHAGE
= separation of chorionic membrane from decidua with accumulation of blood in subchorionic space (placental membranes are more easily stripped from myometrium than from placenta)
Incidence: 81% of all placental abruptions; in 91% before 20 weeks MA
• may lead to vaginal hemorrhage after dissection through decidua
√ detached placental margin from adjacent myometrium (60%)
√ hematoma contiguous with placental margin (100%)
√ predominant hemorrhage often separate from placenta, even on opposite side of placenta
Prognosis: probably no risk for fetal demise

TERATOMA OF NECK
= germ cell tumor of neck
√ polyhydramnios in 30% (from esophageal obstruction)
√ complex mass in cervical region
Cx: airway obstruction
DDx: cystic hygroma, goiter, branchial cleft cyst, cervical meningocele, neuroblastoma of neck, hemangioma of neck

TERATOMA OF OVARY
= immature derivatives of all 3 germ cell layers
Incidence: rare
Age: childhood / adolescence
√ cystic / complex mass (most frequently)
√ usually large solid mass with internal echoes

THECA CELL TUMOR OF OVARY

= THECOMA

Incidence: 1 – 2% of al ovarian neoplasms

ge: >30 years (30%), postmenopausal (70%)

- estrogenic
- √ hypoechoic mass with sound attenuation
- √ unilateral

THECA LUTEIN CYST

- associated with abnormally high levels of hCG secondary to
  - (a) multiple gestations
  - (b) trophoblastic disease (hydatidifom mole, choriocarcinoma)
  - (c) normal pregnancy (uncommon)
- √ multiple bilateral large septated cysts
- √ several cm in size
- √ involution after source of gonadotropin removed

TORSION OF OVARY

= result of rotation of ovary on its axis producing arterial, venous, and lymphatic stasis

Age: usually affects prepubertal girls, may occur prenatally

Cause:
  (1) Enlarged ovary (large cyst / tumor, paraovarian cyst)
  (2) Hypermobility of adnexa (more frequent in younger children), excessively long mesosalpinx, tubal spasm

- severe lower abdominal pain, nausea, vomiting, fever
- palpable mass in 50%

Location: more common on right

US:
- √ markedly enlarged hypo- / hyperechoic midline mass with good sound through transmission (due to vascular engorgement + stromal edema)
- √ multiple peripheral cysts (= transudation of fluid into follicles) measuring 8 – 12 mm in diameter (64 – 74%)
- √ good sound transmission (vascular engorgement + stromal edema)
- √ free fluid in cul-de-sac (32%)
- √ absence of Doppler waveforms (not reliable)
- √ ± complex mass (if secondary to cyst / tumor)

TRISOMY 13

Incidence: 1:5,000 births

@ CNS: holoprosencephaly, posterior encephalocele, neural tube defect

@ Skeleton: postaxial polydactyly

@ Heart: VSD

@ Kidney: polycystic kidney, horseshoe kidney

@ GI: omphalocele

Prognosis: few infants live more than a few days / hours

DDx: Meckel-Gruber syndrome

TRISOMY 18

= EDWARD SYNDROME

Incidence: 3:10,000 births

@ OB: Intrauterine growth retardation, polyhydramnios

@ Skeleton: clubfoot, rocker-bottom foot, clenched hand with overlapping index finger, shortened radial ray

@ Heart: VSD, complete AV canal

@ GI: diaphragmatic hernia, omphalocele

@ Kidney: horseshoe kidney

@ CNS: choroid plexus cyst

TWIN-TWIN TRANSFUSION SYNDROME

= MONOVULAR TWIN TRANSFUSION

= INTRAUTERINE PARABIOTIC SYNDROME

= complication of monozygotic twinning with one placenta / one fused placenta of mono- / dizygotic twins

Incidence: 5 – 18% of twin pregnancies; 15 – 20% of monozygotic twins

Cause: unbalanced intrauterine shunting of blood

Time of onset: 2nd trimester

Path: large subchorionic communications between arterial circulation of one twin and venous circulation of the other twin through arteriovenous shunts (= common villous district)

- √ discrepant amniotic fluid volume (75%)
- √ discordant BPD by >5 mm (57%)
- √ discordant estimated fetal weight >25% (67 – 100%)

A. DONOR TWIN
  = twin that transfuses the recipient twin
  - anemic + hypovolemic
  - high output failure + hydrops (rare)
  - √ oligohydramnios (75 – 80%) / "stuck twin" = severe oligohydramnios (60%)
  - √ growth retardation (common)
  - √ morphologically normal

B. RECIPIENT TWIN
  - polycythemia + plethora (volume overload)
  - √ polyhydramnios (70 – 75%)
  - √ fetal hydrops (10 – 50%)
  - √ fetus papyraceus = macerated dead fetus

Cx: Premature labor with 40 – 70% perinatal mortality

DDx: IUGR of one dizygotic twin (two separate placentas, two different sexes)

UTERINE ANOMALIES

= anomalies of fusion of paramesonephric duct (= müllerian duct) completed by 18th week of fetal life

Incidence: 0.1 – 3%

  Δ Uterine anomalies are found in 9% of women with infertility / repeated spontaneous abortions!

  Δ 25% of women with uterine abnormalities have fertility problems!

Associated with:
  urinary tract anomalies in 20 – 50%; possibly increased familial occurrence of limb reduction

CLASSIFICATION:

(classes in parenthesis refer to the classification of the American Fertility Society)

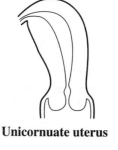

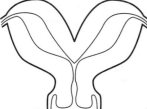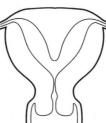

Unicornuate uterus   **Didelphic uterus**

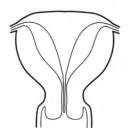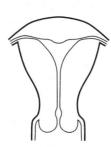

Bicornuate uterus   **Septate uterus (partial)**

Septate uterus (complete)   **Arcuate uterus**

√ separate divergent uterine horns
√ large fundal cleft
√ cervical duplication
√ septation of upper vagina
√ opacification of single deviated horn on HSG
Cx: unilateral hydro- / hematocolpos (if vaginal septum present)
Rx: surgery is rarely performed

2. **Bicornuate uterus** = uterus bicornis (class IV)
   = lack of fusion of corpus
   √ separation of uterine horns with intercornual angle of >105° (demonstrated on luteal-phase US in conjunction with HSG)
   √ fusiform shape of each uterine horn with lateral convex margins
   √ discrepancy in size of the 2 uterine horns
   √ single cervix
   √ elongation + widening of cervical canal + isthmus
   √ bilobed fundal configuration due to a large fundal cleft >1 cm
   Cx: repeated spontaneous abortions (frequently in 2nd – 3rd trimester), premature rupture of membranes, premature labor, persistent malpresentations (transverse lie), SGA infant
   Rx: transabdominal surgery to fuse uterine horns

C. Nonresorption of fibrous sagittal uterine septum
   1. **Septate uterus** (class V)
      Most common anomaly associated with reproductive failure
      √ convex / flat / minimally indented (≤1 cm) fundal contour
      √ distal portion of septum hypoechoic to myometrium (= fibrous tissue)
      √ acute angle of <75° between uterine cavities
      √ duplication of uterine horns on HSG (DDx to bicornuate uterus unreliable)
      √ endometrial canals completely separated by tissue isoechoic to myometrium extending into endocervical canal
      Types:
      (a) Uterus septus
          = complete septum extending into endocervical canal
      (b) Uterus subseptus
          = partial septum involving endometrial canal
   Cx: 90% abortion rate (poor septal vascularity)
   Rx: hysteroscopic metroplasty (= excision of septum)

   2. **Uterus arcuatus** (class VI)
      Most common anomaly unassociated with reproductive failure
      √ NO division of uterine horns
      √ normal fundal contour
      √ smooth indentation of fundal endometrial canal
      √ increased transverse diameter of uterine cavity
      √ single uterine canal with saddle-shaped fundus on HSG

A. Arrested müllerian duct develoment
   1. bilateral: **Uterine agenesis / aplasia** (class I)
   2. unilateral: **Unicornuate uterus** = Uterus unicornis unicollis (class II)
      Incidence: 3 – 6% of uterine anomalies
      ay be associated with ipsilateral renal agenesis
      • infertility in 5 – 20%
      • ? pregnancy wastage
      √ reduced uterine volume
      √ asymmetric ellipsoidal uterine configuration
      √ rudimentary horn may contain endometrium + communicate with main uterine cavity
      √ solitary fusiform "banana-shaped" uterine cavity with lateral deviation within pelvis terminating in a single fallopian tube on HSG

B. Total / partial failure of müllerian duct fusion
   (75% of uterine anomalies)
   1. **Uterus didlphys** (class III)
      = complete duplication with 2 vaginas + 2 cervices + 2 uterine horns
      • usually asymptomatic
      √ two widely spaced uterine corpora, each with a single fallopian tube

D. Inadequate hormonal stimulation during fetal development
1. **Infantile uterus**
2. **Uterine hypoplasia**
   associated with diethylstilbestrol (DES) exposure in utero
   √ mean uterine volume = 50 cm³
3. **T-shaped uterus**
   encountered in 15% of women exposed to DES (diethylstilbestrol) in utero
   √ low uterineolume
   √ uterine fundus thinner than cervix
   √ greater width than depth of corpus + fundus over cervix
   T-shaped lumen on hysterosalpingogram

UTERINE FIBROID

= LEIOMYOMA = benign overgrowth of smooth muscle + connective tissue; commonest cause for uterine enlargement after pregnancy

Hormonal dependency:
   growth secondary to increase in estrogen production in 10 – 20%; shrinkage after menopause

Incidence: in 30 – 40% of women of reproductive age; more prevalent in black women

• palpable mass
• pelvic pain (torsion, infarction, necrosis)
• hypermenorrhea (= heavy prolonged periods)
• infertility

Location: mostly in fundus + corpus; in 3% in cervix
1. intramural (within confines of uterine outline) in 95%
2. subserosal = exophytic
   (a) parasitic fibroid = subserosal fibroid, which has become detached secondary to circulatory occlusion of vessels in pedicle; revitalized through omental / mesenteric blood supply
   (b) intraligamentous fibroid
3. submucosal
   (a) fibroid polyp = partial / complete extrusion of pedunculated submucosal fibroid through cervical canal

√ uterine enlargement
√ lobulated / nodular distortion of uterine outline + indentation of urinary bladder
√ speckled / ringlike / popcorn calcification
√ intramural soft tissue mass, usually multiple, solitary in 2%
√ distortion / obliteration of the contour of the uterine cavity

US (60% sensitivity, 99% specificity, 87% accuracy):
   √ nodular distortion of uterine outline
   √ hypoechoic solid concentric mass (<33%) (= muscle component prevails)
   √ echogenic mass (= fibrous component prevails)
   √ anechoic features (secondary to internal degeneration: atrophic, hyaline, cystic, myxomatous, lipomatous, calcareous, carneous, necrobiotic, hemorrhagic, proteolytic degeneration)

CT:
   √ hypo- / iso- / hyperdense mass containing mixed hyperechoic areas

MRI (86 – 92% sensitivity, 100% specificity, 97% accuracy; desirable for planning myomectomy):
   √ low / medium signal intensity on T1WI
   √ well-circumscribed low signal intensity mass on T2WI with high signal intensity areas (from hemorrhage / hyaline degeneration)

Hysterosalpingography (9% sensitivity, 97% specificity, 76% accuracy)

Cx:
(1) Infertility in 35% (a) if isthmic portion of tube involved (b) from impingement on endometrium interfering with implantation
(2) Increased frequency of spontaneous abortions
(3) Increased frequency of IUGR
(4) Preterm labor in 7% + premature rupture of membranes
(5) Uterine dyskinesia, uterine inertia during labor
(6) Dystocia, obstruction of birth canal during vaginal delivery (if near internal os)
(7) Postpartum hemorrhage
(8) Hydroureteronephrosis
(9) Malignant transformation (in 0.2%)

DDx of necrotic leiomyoma:
(1) Ovarian mass (ovarian cyst, hemorrhagic cyst, endometrioma, cystic dermoid, cystadenoma, malignancy)
(2) Ectopic interstitial pregnancy
(3) Intrauterine gestational sac
(4) Intrauterine fluid collection
(5) Hydatidiform mole
(6) Myometrial contraction (lasts for 15 – 30 minutes)
(7) Cervical tumor
(8) Hematoma of broad ligament
DDx: adnexal mass (if subserosal)

VAGINAL AGENESIS

2nd most common cause of primary amenorrhea
Incidence: 1:4,000 – 5,000 women
• cyclic abdominal pain
May be associated with:
(1) Uterine + partial tubal agenesis (90%)
(2) Unilateral renal agenesis / ectopia (34%)
(3) Skeletal malformations (12%)
(4) McKusick-Kaufman syndrome (hydrometrocolpos + polydactyly + heart defects)
(5) Ellis-van Creveld syndrome

VELAMENTOUS INSERTION

= attachment of cord to chorion laeve
Incidence: 0.09 to 1.8%
Associated with congenital anomalies (in 5.9 – 8.5%):
   esophageal atresia, obstructive uropathy, asymmetrical head shape, spina bifida, VSD, cleft palate
Cx: (1) IUGR
   (2) Preterm labor

NUCLEAR MEDICINE

TABLE OF DOSE, ENERGY, HALF-LIFE, RADIATION DOSE

Organ	Pharmaceutical	Dose	keV	T1/2 phys	(bio)
Brain	Tc-99m pertechnetate	10 – 30 mCi	140	6 h	
	Tc-99m DTPA	10 mCi	140	6 h	
	Tc-99m glucoheptonate	10 mCi	140	6 h	
	Tc-99m Ceretec	20 mCi	140	6 h	
	I-123 Spectamine	3 – 6 mCi	159	13.6 h	
CSF	In-111 DTPA	500 µCi	173, 247	2.8 d	
	Tc-99m DTPA	1 mCi	140	6 h	
Cardiac	Tl-201	1 – 2 mCi	71, 135, 167	73 h	
	Tc-99m pyrophosphate	15 mCi	140	6 h	
	Tc-99m pertechnetate	15 – 25 mCi	140	6 h	
	Tc-99m labeled RBC	10 – 20 mCi	140	6 h	
	Tc-99m sestamibi	25 mCi	140	6 h	
	Tc-99m teboroxime	30 mCi	140	6 h	
Liver	Tc-99m sulfur colloid	3 – 5 mCi	140	6 h	
	Tc-99m DISIDA	4 – 5 mCi	140	6 h	
Lung	Xe-127	5 –10 mCi	172, 203	36.4 d	(13 s)
	Xe-133	10 – 20 mCi	80	5.3 d	(20 s)
	Kr-81m	20 mCi	176, 188, 190	13 s	
	Tc-99m MAA aerosol	3 mCi	140	6 h	(8 h)
Kidney	Tc-99m DTPA	15 - 20 mCi	140	6 h	
	Tc-99m DMSA	2 – 5 mCi	140	6 h	
	Tc-99m glucoheptonate	15 – 20 mCi	140	6 h	
	Tc-99m mercaptoacetyltriglycine	10 mCl	140	6h	
	I-131 Hippuran	250 µCi	364	8 d	(18 min)
	I-123 Hippuran	1 mCi	159	13.6 h	
Thyroid	Tc-99m pertechnetate	5 – 10 mCi	140	6 h	
	I-123	50 – 200 µCi	159	13.6 h	
	I-125	30 – 100 µCi	27, 35	60 d	
	I-131	30 – 100 µCi	364	8 d	
Testes	Tc-99m pertechnetate	10 mCi	140	6 h	
Gastric mucosa	Tc-99m pertechnetate	50 µCi / kg	140	6 h	
Gallium	Ga-67 citrate	3 – 5 mCi	92, 184, 296, 388	78 h	
WBC	In-111 oxine	550 µCi	173, 247	2.8 d	
	Tc-99m Ceretec	10 – 20 mCi	140	6 h	

PEDIATRIC DOSE

Actual doses for pediatric patients may vary in different institutions based on empirical data. As rough guidelines use:

1.   Clark's rule (body weight): $Dose_{Ped}$ = body weight [in lbs.] / 150 x $Dose_{Adult}$

2.   Young's rule (child up to age 12): $Dose_{Ped}$ = Age of child / (Age of child + 12) x $Dose_{Adult}$

3.   Surface area: $Dose_{Ped}$ = (weight [in kg] $^{0.7}$ / 11) / 1.73 x $Dose_{Adult}$

RADIATION DOSE

	Critical organ	rad/mCi
I-131	Thyroid	1,000
I-125	Thyroid	900
In-111 oxine WBC	Spleen	26
I-123	Thyroid	15
In-111 DTPA	Spinal cord	12
Tl-201	Kidney	1.5
Ga-67 citrate	Colon	1.0
Tc-99m MAA	Lung	0.4
Tc-99m albumin microspheres	Lung	0.4
Tc-99m DISIDA	Large bowel	0.39
Tc-99m sulfur colloid	Liver	0.33
Yc-99m pertechnetate	Intestine	0.3
	Thyroid	0.15
Tc-99m glucoheptonate	Kidney	0.2
Tc-99m pertechnetate (+ perchlorate)	Colon	0.2
Tc-99m pyrophosphate	Bladder	0.13
Tc-99m phosphate	Bladder	0.13
Tc-99m DTPA	Bladder	0.12
Tc-99m tagged RBCs	Spleen	0.11
Tc-99m albumin	Blood	0.015
Xe-133	Trachea	

QUALITY CONTROL

Δ Quality control logs should be kept for 3 years!

Radiopharmaceuticals

1. RADIONUCLIDE IMPURITY
   = amount (μCi) of radiocontaminant per amount (μCi/mCi) of desired radionuclide
   Mo-99 breakthrough test:
   (a) allowable contamination of 1:1,000 (= 0.15 μCi Mo-99 per 1 mCi of Tc-99m)
   (b) <5 μCi Mo-99 per administered dose (NRC dropped this requirement, but non-agreement states may still require this)
   Measured after lead shielding of vial (filters 140 keV but permits 452 keV of Mo-99 to pass through)
   Effect of impurity:
   increased radiation dose, poor image quality

2. RADIOCHEMICAL IMPURITY
   Precise registration of different compounds of Tc-99m, eg
   — hydrolyzed reduced Tc [$TcO(OH)_2 \bullet H_2O$]
   — free pertechnetate [TcO^4]$^{-1}$
   can be monitored by paper chromatography
   Effect of impurity with hydrolyzed reduced Tc:
   RES uptake, poor image quality, increased radiation dose

3. CHEMICAL IMPURITY
   Chemicals from elution process are restricted in their amount:
   Tc-99m: <10 μg Al per 1 ml eluate if radionuclide from fission generator;
   <20 μg Al per 1 ml eluate if radionuclide from neutron bombardment
   Aluminum ion breakthrough test:
   One drop of generator eluate placed on one end of special test paper containing aluminum reagent; equal-sized drop of a standard solution of Al $^{3+}$ (10 ppm) is placed on other end of strip; if color at center of drop eluate is lighter than that of standard solution, the eluate has passed the colorimetric test
   Effect of impurity: degradation of image quality

4. PYROGEN TESTING
   (a) **USP XX test**
   Monitor rectal temperature of 3 suitable rabbits after injection of material through ear vein
   Acceptable results: no rabbit shows a rise of >0.6°C; total rise of all three <1.4°C
   (b) **Limulus amoebocyte lysate test** (LAL)
   Highly specific for Gram-negative bacterial endotoxins, sensitivity 10x greater than USP XX test

Amoebocyte = primitive blood cell of horseshoe crab (Limulus polyphebus); lysate formed by hydrolysis of amoebocyte

Positive result: in the presence of minute amounts of endotoxin LAL forms an opaque gel; response to other pyrogens (particulate contaminations, chemicals) doubtful

Calibrators

1. CONSTANCY = PRECISION
   = reproducibility over time
   Test frequency: daily
   Method: measurement of a long-lived source, usually a Cs-137 standard
   Evaluation: measurement must fall within ± 5% of the calculated activity

2. LINEARITY
   = accurate measurement over large range of activity levels
   Test frequency: 4 x per year
   Method: 1 mCi source activity is measured every 4 hours for 10 / more measurements (down to 10 – 100 μCi)
   Evaluation: measurements must fall within ± 5% of the calculated physical decay curve

3. ACCURACY
   Test frequency: annually
   Method: measurements of three different activity standards whose amount is certified by the National Bureau of Standards (NBS); standard values are decayed mathematically to calibrator date
   Co-57:   123 keV, half-life of 270 days
   Ba-133:   354 keV, half-life of 7.2 years
   Cs-137:   662 keV, half-life of 30 years
   Evaluation: measurements must fall within expected range

4. GEOMETRY
   = to assure that measurement is not dependent upon location of tracer within ionization chamber, usually done by manufacturer
   Test frequency: at installation / after factory repair / recalibration
   Method: 0.5 ml of Tc-99m (activity 25 mCi) is measured in a 3-ml syringe; syringe contents are then diluted with water to 1.0 ml, 1.5 ml, and 2.0 ml and each level remeasured; test is repeated with a 10-ml glass vial

Scintillation camera

Field uniformity
= ability of camera to reproduce a uniform radioactive distribution = variability of observed count density with a homogeneous flux
  - (a) Integral uniformity   = maximum deviation
  - (b) Differential uniformity = maximum rate of change over a specified distance (5 pixels)

Causes for nonuniformity:
  - (1) High kilovoltage drift of photomultiplier (PM) tubes
  - (2) Physical damage to collimator
  - (3) Improper photopeak setting
  - (4) Contamination

Frequency of quality control: daily

A. INTRINSIC FIELD UNIFORMITY TEST
  (without collimator)
  1. Remove collimator + replace with lead ring (to eliminate edge packing)
  2. Place a point source at a distance of at least 5 crystal diameters from detector (4 – 5 feet for small, 7 – 9 feet for large crystals)
  3. Point source contains 200 – 400 μCi of Tc-99m for minimal personnel exposure (avoid contamination of crystal)
  4. Set count rate below limit of instrument (<30,000 counts)
  5. Adjust the pulse height selector to normal window settings by centering at 140 keV with a window of 15% (for Tc-99m studies only)
  6. Use the same photographic device
  7. Acquire 1.25 million counts for a 10" field of view, 2.5 million counts for a 15" field of view
  8. Register counts, time, CRT intensity, analyzer settings, initials of controller

B. EXTRINSIC FIELD UNIFORMITY TEST
  (with collimator)
  1. Collimator is kept in place
  2. Sheet source / flood of 2 – 10 mCi activity is placed on collimator
     - (a) fillable floods: mix thoroughly, avoid air bubbles, check for flat surface
     - (b) nonfillable: commercially available Co-57 source
  3. Other steps as described above

Evaluation:
  - (1) Compare uncorrected with corrected images. Note acquisition time!
  - (2) Store correction flood
  - (3) Rerecord image with corrected flood + check for uniformity

Spatial resolution / linearity
A. Spatial resolution
  = parameter of scintillation camera that characterizes its ability to accurately determine the original location of a gamma ray on an X,Y plane; measured in both X and Y directions; expressed as full width at half maximum (FWHM) of the line spread function in mm
  - (a) intrinsic spatial resolution
  - (b) system spatial resolution

B. Intrinsic spatial linearity
  = parameter of a scintillation camera that characterizes the amount of positional distortion caused by the camera with respect to incident gamma events entering the detector
  - (a) differential linearity = standard deviation of line spread function peak separation (in mm)
  - (b) absolute linearity = maximum amount of spatial displacement (in mm)

Frequency of quality control: every week

  1. Mask detector to collimated field of view (lead ring)
  2. Lead phantom is attached to front of crystal
     - (a) Four-quadrant bar pattern (3 pictures each after 90° rotation to test entire crystal)
     - (b) Parallel line equal spacing (PLES) bar pattern (2 pictures)
     - (c) Smith orthogonal hole test pattern (OHP) (1 picture only)
     - (d) Hine-Duley phantom (2 pictures)
  3. Set symmetrical analyzer window to width normally used
  4. Place a point source (1 – 3 mCi) at a fixed distance of at least 5 crystal diameters from detector on central axis (remove all sources from immediate area so that background count rate is low)
  5. Acquire 1.25 million counts for a small field, 2.5 million counts for a large field on the same media used for clinical studies
  6. Record counts, time, CRT intensity, analyzer setting, initials of controller

(All new cameras are equipped with a spatial distortion correction circuit)

Evaluation:
  Visual assessment of
     - (1) Spatial resolution over entire field
     - (2) Linearity

Intrinsic energy resolution
= ability to distinguish between primary gamma events and scattered events; performed without collimator; expressed as ratio of photopeak FWHM to photopeak energy (in %)

CRT-output / photographic device
  - (1) Check for dirt, scratches, burnt spots on CRT face plates

(2)   Adjust grey scale + contrast settings to suit film

Sources of artifacts

A. Attenuator between source and detector
   Materials: cable, lead marker, solder dropped into collimator during repair, belt buckle / watch / key on patient, defective collimator
   (a) at time of correction flood procedure:
      √ hot spot
   (b) after correction flood procedure:
      √ cold spot

B. Cracked crystal
   √   white band with hot edges

C. PMT failure + loss of optical coupling between PMT and crystal
   √   cold defect

D. Problems during film exposure + processing
   1.   Double exposed film
   2.   Light leak in multiformat camera
   3.   Water lines from film processing
   4.   Frozen shutter: √ part of film cut off
   5.   Variations in film processing

E. Improper window setting
   1.   Photopeak window set too high: √ hot tubes
   2.   Photopeak window set too low: √ cold tubes

F. Administration of wrong isotope
   √   atypically imaged organs

G. Excessive amounts of free Tc-99m pertechnetate
   √   too much uptake in choroid plexus, salivary glands, thyroid, stomach

H. Faulty injection technique
   eg, inadvertently labeled blood clot in syringe leading to iatrogenic pulmonary emboli

I. Contamination with radiotracer
   on patient's skin, stretcher, collimator, crystal

J. CRT problems
   1.   Burnt spot on CRT phosphor
   2.   Dirty / scratched CRT face plates

SPECT quality control

Uniformity
1.   64 x 64 word matrix = 30 million count flood with collimator, orientation and magnification same as patient study
2.   Co-57 sheet source with <1% uniformity variance is necessary
3.   128 x 128 word matrix = 120 million count flood with collimator, orientation and magnification same as patient study

Frequency of quality control: weekly

Center of rotation (COR)
1.   Tc-99m filled line source (5 – 8 mCi) positioned 3 – 5 cm off the center of rotation while keeping scanning palette out of field of view
2.   Direction of rotation to be the same as patient study
3.   Number of steps (32, 64 or 128) to be the same as in patient study
4.   Time per step such that at least 100k counts are acquired
5.   COR must be done with same collimator, orientation and magnification as patient study

Frequency of quality control: weekly

Sources of artifacts
1.   Scanning palette in field of view
2.   Collimator shifting + rotation on camera face
3.   Noncircular orbit of camera head
4.   PM tube failure
5.   PM tube uncoupling
6.   Cracked crystal
7.   Improper peaking of camera

POSITRON EMISSION TOMOGRAPHY

= PET = technique that permits non-invasive in vivo examination of metabolism, blood flow, electrical activity, neurochemistry

Physics:
positron matter-antimatter annihilation reaction with an electron results in formation of annihilation photons, which are emitted in exactly opposite directions (511 keV each); detected by coincidence circuitry through simultaneous arrival at detectors (bismuth germanate) on opposite sides of the patient; collimation not necessary; spatial reconstruction similar to transmission CT; resolution of approx. 8 mm

Cyclotron-produced agents:
(1) F-18 fluorodeoxyglucose (FDG): 110 min half-life; for scanning of glucose metabolism
(2) N-13 ammonia (as NH_3): 10 min half-life; information on perfusion
(3) Others
    positron-emitting radionuclides of
    — C-11: 20 minutes half-life
    — O-15 (as O_2, H_2O, CO_2, CO): 2 min half-life
    — Ga-68, Rb-Isotopes

Applications:
@ Brain
1. Focal epilepsy prior to seizure surgery
   √ interictal decreased uptake of FDG of > 20% at seizure focus (70% sensitivity); hypermetabolism within 30 minutes of seizure
   √ measurement of opiate receptor density with C-11-labeled carfentanil (= high-affinity opium agonist) uptake by μ receptors (found in thalamus, striatum, periaqueductal gray matter, amygdala), which mediate analgesia and respiratory depression
2. Glioma grading / recurrence
   √ high-grade gliomas exhibit hypermetabolic FDG uptake; ratio of tumor-to-contralateral cortex uptake >1.4 indicates mean survival of 5 months, of <1.4 indicates mean survival of 19 months

   √ decreased FDG uptake in radiation necrosis
3. Alzheimer disease
   √ decreased global FDG uptake + severely reduced uptake in temporal and parietal lobes; sparing of sensory and motor cortex + basal ganglia + thalamus
4. Huntington disease, senile chorea
   √ hypometabolism of basal ganglia
5. Schizophrenia
   √ abnormally reduced glucose activity in frontal lobes
   √ dopamine receptors in caudate / putamen elevated to 3 x that of normal levels
6. Stroke, cerebral vasospasm
   √ disassociated oxygen metabolism + brain blood flow
@ Heart
1. Coronary artery disease
   sensitivity of > 95%
   √ salvageable myocardium shows decreased perfusion (N-13 ammonia) but enhanced FDG uptake due to glycolysis

A. REGIONAL CEREBRAL BLOOD FLOW
   (a) breathing of carbon monoxide (C-11 and O-15), which concentrates in RBCs
   (b) Xe-133 inhalation / injection into ICA / IV injection after dissolution in saline: volume distribution is in the water space of the brain; no correction for recirculation necessary because all Xe is exhaled during lung passage, but correction for scalp + calvarial activity is required (for inhalation method)
       √ washout rate of grey matter:white matter = 4 – 5:1

B. GLUCOSE METABOLISM
   for measurements of metabolic rate + mapping of functional activity
   (a) C-11 glucose: rapid uptake, metabolization, and excretion by brain
   (b) F-18 fluorodeoxyglucose: metabolically trapped by brain cells

IMMUNOSCINTIGRAPHY

= imaging with monoclonal antibodies [= homogeneous antibody population directed against a single antigen (eg, cancer cell)], which are labeled with a radiotracer

Hybridoma technique:
antibody-producing B lymphocytes are extracted from the spleen of mice that were immunized with a specific type of cancer cell; B lymphocytes are fused with immortal myeloma cells (= hybridoma)

GALLIUM SCINTIGRAPHY

Gallium-67 citrate

Ga-67 acts as an analogue of ferric ion; used as gallium citrate (water-soluble form)

Production: bombardment of zinc targets (Zn-67, Zn-68) with protons (cyclotron); virtually carrier-free after separation process

Decay: by electron capture to ground state of Zn-67

Energy levels:
- (a) used: 93 keV (38%), 184 keV (24%), 300 keV (16%)
- (b) unused: 91 keV (2%), 206 keV (2%), 388 keV (8%)

Physical half-life: 3.3 d (= 78 hours)
Biologic half-life: 2 – 3 weeks
Adult dose: 3 – 6 mCi or 50 μCi/kg

Radiation dose:
0.3 rads/mCi for whole body; 0.9 rads/mCi for distal colon (= critical organ); 0.58 rads/mCi for red marrow; 0.56 rads/mCi for proximal colon; 0.46 rads/mCi for liver; 0.41 rads/mCi for kidney; 0.24 rads/mCi for gonads

Physiology:
Ga-67 is bound to iron-binding sites of various proteins (strongest bond with transferrin in plasma, lactoferrin in tissue); multiexponential + slow plasma disappearance; competitive iron administration (Fe-citrate) enhances target-to-background ratio by increasing Ga-67 excretion
BINDING SITES:
- (a) Fluid spaces
  1. transferrin, haptoglobin, albumin, globulins in blood serum
  2. interstitial fluid space (increased capillary permeability and hyperemia in inflammation + tumor)
  3. lactoferrin in tissue
- (b) Cellular binding
  1. viable PMNs incorporate 10% of Ga-67 (bound to lactoferrin in intracytoplasmic granules)
  2. nonviable PMNs + their protein exudate (deposition of iron-binding proteins occurs extracellularly at sites of inflammation, sequester needed iron from bacteria)
  3. lymphocytes have lactoferrin-binding surface receptors
  4. phagocytic macrophages engulf protein-iron complexes
  5. bacteria + fungi (siderophores = lysosomes) have iron-transporting protein mechanism
  6. tumor cell-associated transferrin receptor + transportation into cells (lymphocytes bind Ga-67 less avidly than PMNs, RBC do not bind Ga-67)

UPTAKE:
at 24 hours: most intense in RES, liver, spleen (4%), bone marrow (lumbar spine, sacroiliac joints), bowel wall (chiefly colonic activity on delayed images), renal cortex, nasal mucosa, lacrimal + salivary glands, blood pool (20%), lung (<3% = equivalent to background activity), breasts

at 72 hours: activity in liver, skeleton, colon, nasal mucosa, occiput; kidney activity no longer detectable; lacrimal + salivary glands may still be prominent

EXCRETION:
- (a) via GI tract (10 – 20%)
  hepatobiliary pathway + colonic mucosal excretion: enemas + laxatives promote clearing of bowel activity
- (b) via urinary tract (10 – 20% within 24 hours)
  no activity in kidneys + urinary bladder after 24 hours
- (c) via various body fluids
  eg, human milk (mandates to stop nursing for 2 weeks)

TIME OF IMAGING: usually 6, 24, 48, 72 hours
Δ Best target-to-background ratio generally at 72 hours
Δ Optimal target-to-background ratio at 6 – 24 hours for abscess
Δ Optimal target-to-background ratio at 24 – 48 hours for tumor

DEGRADING FACTORS OF IMAGING
√ lesions <2 cm are not detectable
√ photon scatter within overlying tissues
√ physiologic high activity of liver, spleen, bones, kidney, GI tract may obscure lesion

NORMAL VARIANTS OF Ga-67 UPTAKE
1. Breasts: increased uptake under stimulus of menarche, estrogens, pregnancy, lactation, phenothiazine medication
2. Liver: suppressed uptake by chemotherapeutic agents / high levels of circulating iron / irradiation / severe acute liver disease
3. Lung: prominent uptake after lymphangiography
4. Spleen: increased uptake in splenomegaly
5. Thymus: uptake in children
6. Salivary glands: uptake within first 6 months after radiation therapy to neck (may persist for years)
7. Epiphyseal plates in children
8. Previous steroid therapy, chemotherapy, and radiation therapy may decrease Ga uptake

INDICATIONS:
A. Infection
   Gallium has been largely replaced with WBC imaging but can be used in chronic infection

1. Inflamed / infarcted bowel (eg, Crohn disease)
    DDx: normal bowel excretions (must be
            cleared by enema; bowel pathology
            shows persistent activity)
2. Diffuse lung uptake
    sarcoidosis, diffuse infections (TB, CMV, PCP),
    lymphangitic metastases, pneumoconioses
    (asbestosis, silicosis), diffuse interstitial fibrosis
    (UIP), drug-induced pneumonitis (bleomycin,
    cyclophosphamide, busulfan), acute radiation
    pneumonitis, recent lymphangiographic contrast
3. Lymph node involvement
    sarcoidosis, TB, MAI, Hodgkin disease
    DDx: NOT seen in Kaposi sarcoma, a useful
          distinction in AIDS patients with hilar
          nodes

B. Tumor:
    Neoplastic uptake is variable; prominent uptake is
    usually seen in:
    1. Non-Hodgkin lymphoma (especially Burkitt)
    2. Hodgkin disease
    3. Hepatoma
    4. Melanoma
    Useful in:
    — detection of tumor recurrence
    — DDx of focal cold liver lesions on Tc-99m
      sulfur colloid scan

NO Ga-67 UPTAKE:
    most benign neoplasms; hemangioma; cirrhosis;
    cystic disease of the breast, liver, thyroid; reactive
    lymphadenopathy; inactive granulomatous disease

Gallium in bone imaging

Increased activity in:
1. Active osteomyelitis (90% sensitivity is higher than
   for Tc-99m MDP)
2. Sarcoma
3. Cellulitis (bone scan followed by gallium scan)
4. Septic arthritis, rheumatoid arthritis
5. Paget disease
6. Metastases (65% sensitivity, less than for bone
   agents)

Gallium in tumor imaging

Particularly useful in evaluating extent of known tumor
disease + in detection of tumor recurrence

A. USEFUL CATEGORY
    1. Lymphoma
       (a) Hodgkin disease: 74 – 88% sensitivity
       (b) NHL: sensitivity varies
          — histiocytic form: 85 – 90% sensitivity
          — lymphocytic well-diff.: 55 – 70% sensitivity
          95% sensitivity for mediastinal disease, 80%
          sensitivity for cervical + superficial lesions; poor
          sensitivity below diaphragm
    2. Burkitt lymphoma: almost 100% sensitivity
    3. Rhabdomyosarcoma: >95% sensitivity
    4. Hepatoma: 85 – 95% sensitivity

5. Melanoma: 69 – 79% sensitivity

B. POSSIBLY USEFUL
    1. NHL: good for large + mediastinal lesions
    2. Nodal metastases from seminoma + embryonal
       cell carcinoma: 87% sensitivity
    3. Non-small cell lung cancer: 85% sensitivity for
       primary of any histologic type, 90% probability for
       uptake in mediastinal nodes, 67% probability
       for uptake in normal mediastinal nodes, 90%
       probability for uptake in extrathoracic metastases

C. NOT USEFUL
    Head & neck tumors, GI tumors (especially
    adenocarcinomas; 35 – 40% sensitivity), breast
    tumor (52 – 65% sensitivity), gynecologic
    tumors (<26% sensitivity), pediatric tumors

Gallium in lung imaging

Δ   Scans obtained at 48 hours, because 50% of
    normals show activity at 24 hours

A. FOCAL UPTAKE
    1. Primary pulmonary malignancy (>90%
       sensitivity)
    2. Benign disorders: granuloma, abscess,
       pneumonia, silicosis

B. MULTIFOCAL / DIFFUSE UPTAKE
    (a) Infection
        1. Tuberculosis
           √ intense uptake in active lesions (97%)
             = parameter of activity
           √ diffuse uptake in miliary TB + rapidly
             progressive TB pneumonia
        2. Pneumocystis carinii
           √ increased uptake at time when physical
             signs, symptoms, and roentgenographic
             changes are unimpressive
        3. Cytomegalovirus
    (b) Inflammation
        1. Sarcoidosis
           70% sensitivity for active parenchymal disease,
           94% sensitivity for hilar adenopathy
           = indicator of therapeutic response to steroids
        2. Interstitial lung disease
           pneumoconiosis, idiopathic pulmonary fibrosis,
           lymphangitic carcinomatosis
        3. Exudative stage of radiation pneumonitis
    (c) Drugs
        1. Bleomycin toxicity
        2. Amiodarone
    (d) Contrast lymphangiography (in 50%)

GALLIUM UPTAKE + NORMAL CHEST FILM
    1. Pulmonary drug toxicity
    2. Tumor infiltration
    3. Sarcoidosis
    4. Pneumocystis carinii

Gallium in renal imaging

Abnormal uptake on delayed images at 48 – 72 hours

(a) <u>Renal tumor</u>
1. Primary renal tumor (variable uptake)
2. Lymphoma / leukemia
3. Metastases (eg, melanoma)

(b) <u>Renal inflammation</u>
1. Acute pyelonephritis (88% sensitivity):
   √ diffuse / focal uptake
2. Lobar nephronia
3. Renal abscess

(c) <u>Others</u>
1. Collagen-vascular disease, vasculitis, Wegener granulomatosis
2. Amyloidosis, hemochromatosis
3. Hepatic failure
4. Administration of antineoplastic drugs

(d) <u>Transplant</u>
1. Acute / chronic rejection
2. Acute tubular necrosis

(e) <u>Urinary bladder</u>: cystitis, tumor

mnemonic: "CHANT An OLD PSALM"
Chemotherapy
Hemochromatosis, **H**epatorenal failure
Acute tubular necrosis, **A**cute lobar nephronia
Neoplasm
Transfusion, **T**uberous sclerosis
Abscess
Obstruction
Lymphoma
Drugs (Fe, drugs causing ATN)
Pyelonephritis, **P**olyarteritis nodosa
Sarcoidosis
Amyloidosis, **A**llograft
Leukemia
Metastasis, **M**yeloma

Gallium imaging in lymphoma

1. Hodgkin disease
   50 – 70% average sensitivity dependent on size, location, technique
2. Non-Hodgkin lymphoma
   30% sensitivity for lymphocytic subtype, 70% sensitivity for histiocytic subtype
   Sensitivity: 90% for mediastinal nodes
   80% for neck nodes
   48% for periaortic nodes
   47% for iliac nodes
   36% for axillary nodes

Gallium imaging in malignant melanoma

TYPES:
1. Lentigo maligna: low invasiveness, low metastatic potential
2. Superficial spreading melanoma: intermediate prognosis
3. Nodular melanoma: most lethal

PROGNOSIS (level of invasion versus 5-year survival):

Level I	(in situ)	100%
Level II	(within papillary dermis)	100%
Level III	(extending to reticular dermis)	88%
Level IV	(invading reticular dermis)	66%
Level V	(subcutaneous infiltration)	15%

<u>Ga-67:</u>
>50% sensitivity for primary + metastatic sites; detectability versus tumor size: 73% sensitivity >2 cm; 17% sensitivity <2 cm

<u>Bone, brain, liver scintigraphy:</u>
show very low yield in detecting metastases at time of preoperative assessment and are not indicated

AGENTS FOR INFLAMMATION

1. **Ga-67 citrate**
   overall 58 – 100% sensitivity; 75 – 100% specificity (lower for abdominal inflammation because of problematic abdominal activity)
   Indication:
   chronic + nonpyogenic inflammation, pulmonary infection + lymphadenitis with HIV-positivity, granulomatous disease (eg, sarcoidosis)
   Pathophysiology:
   leakage of protein-bound Ga-67 into extracellular space secondary to hyperemia + increased capillary permeability; Ga-67 is preferentially bound to nonviable PMNs + macrophages
   1. Leukocyte incorporation (rich in lactoferrin)
   2. Bacterial uptake (iron-chelating siderophores)
   3. Inflammatory tissue stimulates lactoferrin production

   CHRONIC ABDOMINAL INFLAMMATION
   67% sensitivity, 64% specificity, 13% false-negative rate, 5% false-positive rate
   Dose: 5 mCi
   Imaging: routine at 48 – 72 hours (after clearance of high background activity); optional at 6 – 24 hours (prior to renal + gastrointestinal excretion); delayed images as needed
   √ diffuse uptake in peritonitis
   √ localized uptake in acute pyogenic abscess, phlegmon, acute cholecystitis, acute pancreatitis, acute gastritis, diverticulitis, inflammatory bowel disease, surgical wound, pyelonephritis, perinephric abscess

2. **In-111 labeled WBC**
   = In-111-oxine-labeled autologous leukocytes with 80% sensitivity; 97% specificity, 91% accuracy (superior to Ga-67 citrate); no activity in intestinal contents / urine
   Indication:
   occult sepsis, acute pyogenic infection, abdominal + renal abscess, inflammatory bowel disease, non-pulmonary infection with HIV positivity, prosthetic graft infection (bone / cardiovascular graft), acute + chronic + complicated bone / joint infection

Technique:
Harvesting of cells followed by separation from RBCs and platelets + washing off plasma proteins; chelating agents (oxine = 8-hydroxyquinoline / tropolone) used for labeling; lipophilic oxine-indium complex penetrates cell membrane of white cells; intracellular proteins scavenge the indium from oxine; oxine diffuses out from cell; requires 2 hours of preparation time
Recovery rate: 30% at 1 – 4 hours after injection

Limitations: 19 gauge IV access, leukopenia, impaired chemotaxis, abnormal WBCs, children
Dose: 0.5 mCi
Half-life: 67 hours
Useful photopeaks: 173 keV (89%), 247 keV (94%)

Radiation dose:
13 – 18 rad/mCi for spleen; 3.8 rad/mCi for liver; 0.65 rad/mCi for red marrow; 0.45 rad/mCi for whole body; 0.29 rad/mCi for testes; 0.14 rad/mCi for ovaries (compared with Ga-67 higher dose to spleen, but lower dose to all other organs)
Biodistribution: spleen, liver, bone marrow; blood clearance half-time of 6 – 7 hours

Imaging:
best at 18 – 24 hours following injection of cell preparation; optional at 2 – 6 hours (eg, in inflammatory bowel disease); delayed images as needed; bone marrow uptake provides useful landmarks
√ focal activity greater than in spleen is typical for abscess (comparison based on liver, spleen, bone marrow activity)
√ activity equal to liver (significant inflammatory focus)
√ abdominal activity is always abnormal

False positives:
@ Chest: CHF, RDS, embolized cells, cystic fibrosis

@ Abdomen: accessory spleen, colonic accumulation, renal transplant rejection, GI hemorrhage, vasculitis, ischemic bowel disease, following CPR, uremia, postradiation therapy, Wegener granulomatosis, ALL
@ Miscellaneous: IM injection, histiocytic lymphoma, cerebral infarction, arthritis, skeletal metastases, thrombophlebitis, hematoma, hip prosthesis, cecal carcinoma, postsurgical pseudoaneurysm, necrotic tumors that harvest WBCs

False negatives:
Chronic infection, aorto-femoral graft, LUQ abscess, infected pelvic hematoma, splenic abscess, hepatic abscess (occasionally)

3. Tc-99m-labeled WBC
Optimal use: osteomyelitis in extremities

Advantages over In-111 WBC imaging:
(a) improved photon flux
(b) earlier imaging

Disadvantage:
(1) Biliary excretion leads to bowel activity, which may obscure abdominal abscess if not imaged early
(2) Heart and blood pool may obscure disease

Technique:
Tc-99m Ceretec binds with autologous WBCs and is reinjected

Imaging:
30 minutes (optimum for use in abdomen), 60 minutes, 3 – 4 hours, 24 hours (optional)

False positives:
may be due to unusual marrow distribution, correlation with bone marrow (sulphur colloid) scan may be necessary

BONE SCINTIGRAPHY

Bone agents

A. POLYPHOSPHATES = LINEAR PHOSPHATES
   = CONDENSED PHOSPHATES
   First agents described; contain up to 46 phosphate residues; simplest form contains 2 phosphates = pyrophosphate (PYP)

B. DIPHOSPHONATES
   Organic analogs of pyrophosphate characterized by P-C-P bond; chemically more stable; not susceptible to hydrolysis in vivo; most widely used agents:
   1. ethylene hydroxydiphosphonate (EHDP) = ethane-1-hydroxy-1,1-diphosphonate
   2. methylene diphosphonate (MDP)

C. IMIDODIPHOSPHONATES (IDP)
   Characterized by P-N-P bond

Indications:
   1. Imaging of bone, myocardial / cerebral infarct, ectopic calcifications, some tumors (neuroblastoma)
   2. Rx for Paget disease, myositis ossificans progressiva, calcinosis universalis (inhibits formation + dissolution of hydroxyapatite crystals)

Usual dose: 20 mCi
Radiation dose: 0.13 rad/mCi for bladder (critical organ), 0.04 rad/mCi for bone, 0.01 rad/mCi for whole body

Imaging:
   @ Bone: 2 – 3 hours post injection (fractures may not show positive uptake until 3 – 10 days depending on age of patient)
   @ Myocardium: 90 – 120 minutes post injection (ideal imaging time 1 – 3 days post infarction)

Labeling: Tc (VII) is eluted as a pertechnetate ion; chemical reduction with Sn (II) chloride; chelated into a complex of Tc-99m (IV)-tin-phosphate

Quality Control:
   (1) <10% Tc-99m tin colloid / free Tc-99m pertechnetate (a good preparation is 95% bound)
   (2) Agent should not be used prior to 30 minutes after preparation
   (3) Avoid injection of air in preparation of multidose vials (oxidation results in poor Tc bond)
   (4) Kit life is 4 – 5 hours after preparation

Uptake:
   (a) rapid distribution in ECF; blood clearance rate determines ECF (= background) activity (at 4 hours 1% for diphosphonates, 5% for pyrophosphate / polyphosphate secondary to greater degree of protein binding)
   (b) chemisorbs on hydroxyapatite crystals in bone + in calcium crystals in mitochondria; 50 – 60% (58% for MDP, 48% for EHDP, 47% for PYP) are localized in bone by approx. 3 hours depending on blood flow + osteoblastic activity; myocardial uptake depends on at least some revascularization of infarcted muscle

Excretion:
   via urinary tract (forcing fluids + frequent voiding reduces radiation dose to bladder) by 6 hours in 68% of MDP/EHDP, in 50% of PYP, in 46% of polyphosphates

THREE-PHASE BONE SCANNING
   over area of interest
   1. Rapid sequence flow study (2 – 5 seconds/frame)
   2. Immediate postflow images (1 million counts for central body + 0.5 million counts for extremities)
   3. Delayed images (0.5 – 1.0 million counts) between 3 – 4 hours following injection

Bone marrow agents
for assessment of hematopoiesis / phagocytosis by RES

1. Tc-99m sulfur colloid (10% uptake in bone marrow)

2. In-111 chloride

3. Tc-99m MMAA (mini-microaggregated albumin colloid = not FDA approved) for liver, spleen, hematopoietic marrow
   Particle size: 30 - 100 microns
   Dose: 10 mCi
   Marrow dose: 0.55 rad
   Marrow accumulation at 1 hour:
      6 x higher than for sulfur colloid
      3 x higher than for antimony-sulfur colloid

Indications:
   (a) expansion of hematopoietically active bone marrow
      1. Hematologic disorders to reveal presence of peripheral expansion of functional marrow
   (b) focal defect due to displacement by infiltrating disease
      1. Marrow replacement disorders: eg, Gaucher disease
      2. Bone infarction: eg, sickle cell anemia (DDx from osteomyelitis)
      3. Avascular necrosis in children

Superscan
A. Metabolic
   1. Renal osteodystrophy
   2. Osteomalacia
      √ randomly distributed focal sites of intense activity = Looser zones = pseudofractures = Milkman fractures (most characteristic)

3. Hyperparathyroidism
   √ focal intense uptake corresponds to site of brown tumors
4. Hyperthyroidism
   rate of bone resorption more increased than rate of formation (= decrease in bone mass)
   • hypercalcemia (occasionally)
   • elevated alkaline phosphatase
   √ NOT visible on radiographs
   √ susceptible to fractures

B. Widespread bone lesions
   1. Diffuse skeletal metastases (most frequent) from breast, lung, prostate, bladder, lymphoma
   2. Myelofibrosis / myelosclerosis
   3. Aplastic anemia, leukemia
   4. Waldenström macroglobulinemia
   5. Systemic mastocytosis
   6. Widespread Paget disease

√ diffusely increased activity in bones: particularly prominent in axial skeleton, calvarium, mandible, costochondral junctions (= "rosary beading"), sternum (= "tie sternum"), long bones
√ increased metaphyseal + periarticular activity
√ increased bone-to-soft-tissue ratio
√ "absent kidney sign" = little / no activity in kidneys
√ femoral cortices become visible

Soft tissue uptake

A. Physiologic
   1. Breast
   2. Kidney: accentuated uptake with dehydration, antineoplastic drugs, gentamicin
   3. Bowel: surgical diversion of urinary tract
B. Radiochemical impurity
   (a) free pertechnetate
       √ activity in mouth (saliva), thyroid, stomach (mucus-producing cells), GI tract (direct secretion + intestinal transport from gastric juices)
   (b) excess technetium colloid
       Cause: excess aluminum ions in eluate, hydrolysis of stannous chloride to stannous hydroxide, excess hydrolized technetium
       √ liver uptake
C. Tumor
   (a) Primary tumors
       1. Osteosarcoma: bone foming
       2. Neuroblastoma (35 – 74%): calcifying tumor
       3. Breast carcinoma
       4. Meningioma
       5. Bronchogenic carcinoma (rare)
       6. Pericardial tumor
   (b) Metastases
       1. to liver: mucinous carcinoma of colon, breast carcinoma, lung cancer, osteosarcoma
       2. to lung: osteosarcoma
       3. Malignant pleural effusion

D. Inflammation
   1. Inflammatory process (abscess, pyogenic / fungal infection):
      (a) adsorption onto calcium deposits
      (b) binding to denatured proteins, iron deposits, immature collagen
      (c) hyperemia
   2. Myositis ossificans, polymyositis
   3. Dermatomyositis, scleroderma
   4. Radiation: eg, radiation pneumonitis
   5. Necrotizing enterocolitis
   6. Diffuse pericarditis
E. Trauma
   1. Healing soft tissue wounds
   2. Rhabdomyolysis: crush injury, surgical trauma, electrical burns, frostbite, severe exercise, alcohol abuse
   3. Intramuscular injection sites:
      especially Imferon (= iron dextran) injections with resultant chemisorption; meperidine
   4. Ischemic bowel infarction (late uptake)
   5. Subdural hematoma
   6. Myocardial contusion, defibrillation, unstable angina pectoris
E. Metabolic
   1. Hypercalcemia: uptake in stomach, lung, kidneys, myocardium
   2. Diffuse interstitial pulmonary calcifications: hyperparathyroidism, mitral stenosis
   3. Amyloid deposits
F. Dystrophic soft-tissue calcifications
   Necrotic tumor with dystrophic calcification
   @ Spleen: infarct (sickle cell anemia in 50%), microcalcification secondary to lymphoma, thalassemia major, hemosiderosis, glucose-6-phosphate-dehydrogenase deficiency
   @ Liver: massive hepatic necrosis
   @ Heart: transmural myocardial infarction, valvular calcification, amyloid deposition
   @ Muscle: traumatic / ischemic skeletal muscle injury
   @ Brain: cerebral infarction (damage of blood-brain barrier)
   @ Kidney: nephrocalcinosis

Incidental urinary tract abnormalities

A. Bilateral diffuse increased uptake
   = uptake greater than that of lumbar spine
   (a) excess tissue calcium
       1. Hyperparathyroidism
       2. Hypercalcemia
       3. Osteosarcoma metastatic to kidney
   (b) tissue damage
       1. Chemotherapy (eg, cyclophosphamide, vincristine, doxorubicin, bleomycin, mytomycin-C, S-6-mercaptopurine, mitoxantrone)
       2. Treatment with aminoglyosides / amphotericin B
       3. Radiation therapy
       4. Necrotic renal cell carcinoma (rare)
       5. Renal metastasis (rare)
       6. Acute pyelonephritis

7. Acute tubular necrosis
8. Multiple myeloma
(c) iron overload
   1. Sickle cell anemia
   2. Thalassemia major
B. Bilateral decreased renal uptake
(a) loss of renal function
   1. End-stage renal disease
(b) increased osteoblastic activity (= superscan)
C. Focally decreased renal uptake
(a) space-occupying lesion replacing normal renal parenchyma
   1. Abscess
   2. Cyst
   3. Primary / metastatic renal neoplasm
(b) Scar
   1. Infarct
   2. Chronic pyelonephritis
   3. Partial nephrectomy
D. Uni- / bilateral focally increased GU uptake
(a) urine accumulation
   1. normal upper pole calices (supine position)
   2. Urinary tract diversion / ileal conduit
   3. Urinoma

Photon-deficient bone lesion
= decreased radiotracer uptake
(a) Interruption in local bone blood flow
= vessel trauma or vascular obstruction by thrombus / tumor
   1. Early osteomyelitis
   2. Radiation therapy
   3. Posttraumatic aseptic necrosis
   4. Sickle cell crisis
(b) Replacement of bone by destructive process
   1. Metastases (most common cause): central axis skeleton > extremity, most commonly in carcinoma of kidney + lung + breast + multiple myeloma
   2. Primary bone tumor (exceptional)

Long segmental diaphyseal uptake
A. BILATERALLY SYMMETRIC
   1. Hypertrophic pulmonary osteoarthropathy
   2. "Shin splints"
   3. Ribbing disease
   4. Engelmann disease = progressive diaphyseal dysplasia
B. UNILATERAL
   1. Inadvertent arterial injection
   2. Melorheostosis
   3. Chronic venous stasis
   4. Osteogenesis imperfecta
   5. Vitamin A toxicity
   6. Osteomyelitis
   7. Paget disease
   8. Fibrous dysplasia

Pediatric indications for bone scan
A. Back pain
   1. Discitis
   2. Pars interarticularis defect: SPECT imaging adds sensitivity
   3. Osteoid osteoma: can be used intraoperatively to assure removal of nidus
   4. Sacroiliac infection
B. Nonaccidental trauma

Benign bone lesions
A. NO TRACER UPTAKE
   1. Bone island
   2. Osteopoikilosis
   3. Osteopathia striata
   4. Fibrous cortical defect
   5. Nonossifying fibroma
B. INCREASED TRACER UPTAKE
   1. Fibrous dysplasia
   2. Eosinophilic granuloma
   3. Melorheostosis
   4. Osteoid osteoma

Fractures
TYPICAL TIME COURSE
   1. Acute phase (3 – 4 weeks)
abnormal in 80% <24 hours, in 95% <72 hours; Elderly patients show delayed appearance of positive scan (as much as 5 – 14 days), positive within 1 day in children
√ broad area of increased tracer uptake (wider than fracture line)
   2. Subacute phase (2 – 3 months)
time of most intense tracer accumulation
√ focally increased tracer uptake corresponding to fracture line
   3. Chronic phase (1 – 2 years)
√ slow decline in tracer accumulation
√ in 65% normal after 1 year; in >95% normal after 3 years

RETURN TO NORMAL
Rib fractures return to normal most rapidly; delayed in weight-bearing extremities; complicated fractures with orthopedic fixation devices take longest to return to normal
1. Simple fractures: 90% normal by 2 years
2. Open reduction / fixation: <50% normal by 3 years
3. Delayed union: slower than normal for type of fracture
4. Nonunion: persistent intense uptake in 80%
5. Complicated union (true pseudarthrosis, soft tissue interposition, impaired blood supply, presence of infection)
√ intense uptake at fracture ends
√ decreased uptake at fracture site

VERTEBRAL COMPRESSION FRACTURES
return to normal   in 60% by 1 year
   in 90% by 2 years
   in 97% by 3 years

BRAIN SCINTIGRAPHY

Radionuclide angiography

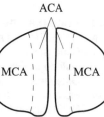

anterior view   posterior view

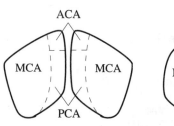
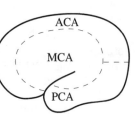

high axial view   left lateral view

Mechanism of accumulation:
disruption of blood-brain barrier

Agents:
A. Tc-99m glucoheptonate
   15 – 20 mCi bolus injection in <2 ml saline; 30 flow images of 2 seconds duration; static image of 1 million counts after 4 hours; delayed image after 24 hours (higher target-to-background ratio than DTPA)
B. Tc-99m DTPA
C. Thallium-201: best predictor for tumor burden

√ increased perfusion in
1. primary / metastatic brain tumor
2. AVM, large aneurysm, tumor shunting
3. luxury perfusion after infarction
4. infections (eg, herpes simplex encephalitis)
5. extracranial lesions: bone metastasis, fibrous dysplasia, Paget disease, eosinophilic granuloma, fractures, burr holes, craniotomy defects
√ asymmetrical decreased perfusion in acute / chronic cerebrovascular disease + mass lesions (tumor, hemorrhage, subdural hematoma)
√ "flip-flop" phenomenon (= decreased perfusion in arterial phase, equalization of activity in capillary phase, increased activity in venous phase) in CVA secondary to late arrival of blood via collaterals + slow washout
√ bilateral absent flow in brain death

Ceretec brain imaging
Pharmacokinetics:
lipophilic radiopharmaceutical distributing across a functioning blood-brain barrier proportional to cerebral blood flow; no redistribution
Indication:
acute cerebral infarct imaging before evidence of CT / MRI pathology; positive findings within 1 hour of event

I-123 spectamine brain imaging
Pharmacokinetics:
initally distributes proportional to regional cerebral blood flow with increased flow to basal ganglia and cerebellum; homogeneous uptake in gray matter; decreased activity in white matter; redistribution over time
√ activity in an area of inital deficit on reimaging (after 4 hours) implies improved prognosis

Seizures
Abnormal cerebral radionuclide angiography within 1 week of seizure activity even without underlying organic lesion
Etiology:
(1) 35% cerebral tumors (meningioma in 34%, metastases in 17%)
(2) Cerebral vascular disease (more common in age >50 years)
(3) Trauma, inflammation, CNS effects of systemic disease
√ transient hyperperfusion of involved hemisphere

Brain tumor
Good correlation between hyperperfusion and enlarged supplying vessels
Etiology:
(1) Meningioma (increased activity in 60 – 80%);
(2) Metastases (increased activity in 11 – 23%);
(3) Vascular metastases: thyroid, renal cell, melanoma, anaplastic tumors from lung / breast

Cerebral death
Increased intracranial pressure results in markedly decreased cerebral perfusion, thrombosis, total cerebral infarction
Path: severe brain edema, diffuse liquefactive necrosis

√ carotid arteries visualized (= confirmation of good bolus)
√ activity stops abruptly at the skull base
√ sagittal sinus not visualized
√ activity in arteries of face + scalp with "hot nose" sign
DDx by EEG:
severe barbiturate intoxication may produce a flat EEG response in the absence of brain death

Arterial stenosis

Δ Radionuclide angiography of limited value!
   (1) Complete occlusion / >80% stenosis of ICA:
       53 – 80% sensitivity
   (2) 50 – 80% stenosis of ICA: 50% sensitivity
   (3) <50% stenosis of ICA: 10% sensitivity

Problematic lesions:
   (1) Bilaterally similar degree of stenosis
   (2) Occlusion of MCA + unilateral ACA
   (3) Vertebrobasilar occlusive disease (20%
       sensitivity)

Radionuclide cisternography

Indications:
   1. Suspected normal pressure hydrocephalus
   2. Occult CSF rhinorrhea / otorrhea
   3. Ventricular shunt
   4. Porencephalic cyst, leptomeningeal cyst, posterior
      fossa cyst

Technique:
   1. Measurement of spinal subarachnoid pressure
   2. Sample of CSF for analysis
   3. Subarachnoid injection of radiotracer

Normal study (completed within 48 hours):
   symmetrical activity sequentially from basal cisterns, up
   the sylvian fissures + anterior commissure, eventual
   ascent over cortices with parasagittal concentration
   √ image lumbar region immediately after injection to
     assure subarachnoid injection
   √ activity in basal cistern by 2 – 4 hours
   √ activity at vertex by 24 – 48 hours
   √ no / minimal lateral ventricular activity (may be
     transient in older patients)

Agents:
   1. Indium-111 DTPA
      Physical half-life: 2.8 days
      Gamma photons: 173 keV (90%), 247 keV (94%)
         detected with dual pulse height analyzer
      Dose: 250 – 500 µCi
      Radiation dose: 9 rads/500 µCi for brain + spinal
                          cord (in normal patients)
      Imaging: at 10-minute intervals / 500,000 counts up
                   to 4 – 6 hours; repeat scans at 24, 48, 72
                   hours

   2. Technetium-99m DTPA
      Not entirely suitable for imaging up to 48 – 72 hours;
      DTPA tends to have faster flow rate than CSF; used
      for shunt evaluation + CSF leak study since leak
      increases CSF flow
      Dose: 4 – 10 mCi

Radiation dose: 4 rads for brain + spinal cord

   3. Iodine-131 serum albumin (RISA)
      prototype agent; beta emitter
      Physical half-life:
         8 days; high radiation dose of 7.1 rads/100 µCi;
         no longer used secondary to pyrogenic reactions

   4. Ytterbium-169 DTPA
      Physical half-life: 32 days
      Gamma decay: 63 keV; 177 keV (17%); 198 keV
                        (25%); 308 keV
         dual pulse height analyzer set for 177 + 198 keV
      Dose: 500 µCi
      Radiation dose: 9 rads/500 mCi for brain + spinal
                          cord (in normal patients)

CSF leak study

Purpose: localization of origin of CSF leak in patient with
             CSF rhinorrhea / otorrhea
Causes of dural fistula:
   (a) traumatic: in 30% of basilar skull fractures
   (b) nontraumatic: brain, pituitary and skull tumors;
                       skull infections; congenital defects

Location of dural fistula:
   cribriform plate > ethmoid cells > frontal sinus

Method:
   1. Weigh cotton pledgets
   2. Pledgets placed by ENT surgeon in the anterior and
      posterior turbinates bilaterally
   3. Radiopharmaceutical injected intrathecally via
      lumbar puncture; immediate post-injection view of
      lumbar region to assure intrathecal placement
   4. Pledgets removed and weighed 4 – 6 hours after
      lumbar injection
   5. Pledget activity counted + indexed to weight
   6. Results compared to 0.5 ml serum specimens drawn
      a the time of pledget removal
   7. Pledget to serum count ratio of >1.5 is evidence of
      CSF leak
   8. With active leak patient should be placed in various
      positions with various maneuvers to accentuate leak

Hydrocephalus

A. Normal-pressure hydrocephalus:
   √ reversal of normal CSF flow dynamic = tracer moves
     from basal cisterns into 4th, 3rd + lateral ventricles
   √ loss of ω sign

B. Obstructive hydrocephalus:
   √ delay (up to 48 hours) for tracer to surround
     convexities + reach arachnoid villae
   √ positive ω sign

THYROID AND PARATHYROID SCINTIGRAPHY

SUPPRESSION SCAN
  = to define autonomy of a nodule
  √ suppression of a hot nodule following T_3/T_4 administration is proof that autonomy does not exist
STIMULATION SCAN
  = to demonstrate thyroid tissue suppressed by hyperfunctioning nodule
  √ administration of TSH documents functioning thyroid tissue (rarely done)
PERCHLORATE WASHOUT TEST
  = to demonstrate organification defect
  √ repeat measurement of radioiodine uptake following oral potassium perchlorate shows lower values if organification defect present

Tc-99m pertechnetate

Physical decay: 10 mCi Tc-99m decays to 2.7×10^{-7} mCi Tc-99
Physical half-life: 2×10^5 years
Biologic half-life: 6 hours
Decay: by photon emission of 140 keV

Quality control:
  (1) <0.1% Mo-99 (= 1μCi/mCi), maximum of Mo-99 at 5 μCi
  (2) <0.5 mg aluminum/10 mCi Tc-99m
  (3) <0.01% radionuclide impurities

Administration: oral / IV
Dose: 3 – 5 mCi administered IV 20 minutes prior to imaging (100 – 300 mrad/mCi)

Pharmacokinetics:
  Uptake: in thyroid, salivary glands, gastric mucosa, choroid plexus
  Excretion: mostly in feces, some in urine

Uptake in thyroid:
  0.5 – 3.7% at 20 minutes (time of maximum uptake) assessment of trapping function only; NO organification; may be almost completely discharged by perchlorate
Comparison to iodine:
  (a) target-to-background ratio less favorable than with iodine
  (b) greater photon flux than iodine = detectability of small thyroid lesions (>8 mm) is improved
  (c) lesions with pertechnetate-iodine discordance (= hot on Tc-99m pertechnetate + cold on radioiodine) are very rare + due to Tc-99m avid cancer

Imaging:
  (a) Collimator: usually with pinhole collimator for image magnification (5-mm hole)
  (b) Distance: selected so that organ makes up 2/3 of field of view, significant distortion of organ periphery occurs if detector too close

  (c) Counts: 200,000 – 300,000 counts are usually acquired within 5 minutes after a dose of 5 – 10 mCi of Tc-99m pertechnetate
  (d) Image must include markers for scale + anatomic landmarks + palpatory findings

Iodine-123

Δ Agent of choice for thyroid imaging!
Production:
  in accelerator; contamination with I-124 dependent on source (Te-122 in ~ 5%, Xe-123 in ~ 0.5%); contamination with I-125 increases with time elapsed after production

Physical half-life: 13.3 hours
Decay: by electron capture with photon emission at 159 keV (83% abundance) + X-ray of 28 keV (87% abundance)
Dose: 200 – 400 μCi orally 24 hours prior to imaging (radiation dose of 7.5 mrads/μCi)

Uptake: iodine readily absorbed from GI tract (10 – 30% by 24 hours), distributed primarily in extracellular fluid spaces; trapped + organified by thyroid gland; trapped by stomach + salivary glands
Excretion: via kidneys in 35 – 75% during first 24 hours + GI tract

Disadvantage compared to Tc-99m pertechnetate:
  (1) More expensive
  (2) Less available
  (3) More time-consuming
  (4) Higher dose to thyroid (but less to whole body)

Iodine-131

Indication: thyroid uptake study, thyroid imaging, treatment of hyperthyroidism, treatment of functioning thyroid cancer, imaging of functioning metastases

Production: by fission decay
Physical half-life: 8.05 days (allows storing for long periods)
Decay: principal gamma energy of 364 keV (82% abundance) + significant beta decay fraction of a mean energy of 192 keV (92% abundance)

Dose: 30 – 50 μCi (1.2 rad/μCi = 50 rad for thyroid)
Radiation dose:
  (90% from beta decay, 10% from gamma radiation) 0.6 mrad/mCi for whole body; 1.2 mrad/μCi for thyroid (critical organ)
Pharmacokinetics: identical to I-123

Disadvantage:
  (1) Too energetic for gamma camera, well suited for rectilinear scanner with limited resolution

(b) High radiation dose prohibits use for diagnostic purposes

(c) Ectopic thyroid tissue just as well detectable with I-123 or Tc-99m pertechnetate

Iodine fluorescence imaging

Technique:
collimated beam of 60 keV gamma photons from an Am-241 source is directed at thyroid, which results in production of K-characteristic x-rays of 28.5 keV; x-rays are detected by semiconductor detector

Advantage:
(1) No interference with flooded iodine pool / thyroid medication
(2) Measures total iodine content
(3) Low radiation exposure (15 mrad) acceptable for children + pregnant women

Disadvantage: dedicated equipment necessary

Thyroid uptake measurements

Agents: I-123 / I-131 (easier to use), Tc-99m pertechnetate (requires calibration)

Uptake:
measuements at both 4 and 24 hours prevents missing the occasional rapid turnover hyperthyroid patient returning to normal by 24 hours; uptake values distinguish different causes of hyperthyroidism

(a) normal: >25% at 4 hours, >35% at 24 hours
(b) increased: in Graves disease
(c) decreased: in subacute thyroiditis

N.B.:
Uptake values do not diagnose hyperthyroidism, which is done with laboratory values (T_4, T_3, TSH) and clinical history

Parathyroid scintigraphy

= Technetium-thallium subtraction imaging

Sensitivity: 72 – 92% (depending on size, smallest adenoma was 60 mg)

Specificity: 43% (benign thyroid adenomas, carcinomas, lymph nodes also concentrate thallium)

Method:
(1) IV injection of 1 – 3 mCi Tl-201 chloride; images recorded for 15 minutes with 2-mm pinhole collimator
    √ concentrates in normal thyroid + enlarged parathyroid glands
(2) IV injection of 1 – 10 mCi Tc-99m pertechnetate; images recorded at 1-minute intervals for 20 minutes
    √ pertechnetate concentrates only in thyroid
(3) Computerized subtraction

Indication:
Localization of one / more parathyroid adenoma (hyperplasia not visualized), may be more sensitive than CT / MRI in detection of ectopic mediastinal parathyroid tissue and in post-operative context

LUNG SCINTIGRAPHY

Perfusion agents

Tc-99m macroaggregated albumin

Preparation:

human serum albumin (HSA) is heat-denatured + pH adjusted; added stannous chloride precipitates albumin into tin-containing macroaggregates; lyophilization prolongs stability; added Tc-99m pertechnetate is reduced by $SnCl_2$ and tagged onto the MAA particles

Quality Control (USP guidelines):
(1) 90% of particles should have a diameter between 10 – 90 μ
(2) No particle should exceed 150 μ
(3) Should be at least 90% pure (by ascending chromatography)
(4) A batch of Tc-99m MAA should not be used >8 hours after preparation
(5) Preparation should not be backflushed with blood into syringe, causes "hot spots" on lungs

Physical half-life: 6 hours
Biological half-life: 6 hours

Dose:

approximately 4 mCi + >60,000 particles (recommended number of 200,000 – 500,000 particles for adequate spatial distribution + good image quality)
CAVE:
(1) Critically ill patients with pulmonary arterial hypertension / left-to-right cardiac shunts need reduction in number of particles but not tagged activity!
(2) Children up to age 5 need reduction in number of particles + tagged activity!

Radiation dose (rads/mCi):
0.013 for whole body, 0.25 for lung (critical organ), 0.01 for gonads

PHYSIOLOGY

90% of MAA particles will be trapped in lung capillaries on first pass; 0.22% (= 2 of 1000) capillaries become occluded; protein is lysed within 6 – 8 hours and taken up by RES; particles <1 μ are trapped by RES in liver + spleen

IMAGING

Large field view scintillation camera + parallel hole low-energy collimator
Views: anterior, posterior, lateral, posterior oblique (additional information in 50%), anterior oblique (additional information in 15%); oblique views reduce equivocal findings from 30% to 15%; recording times should be identical for corresponding views

Tc-99m human albumin microspheres
Particle size: 20 – 30 μ
Biological half-life: 8 hours

Ventilation agents

Xenon-133

Fission product of U-235
Decay:

to stable Cs-133 under emission of beta particle (374 keV), gamma ray (81 keV), X-ray (31 keV); beta-component responsible for high radiation dose of 1 rad to lung)

Physical half-life: 5.2 days
Biological half-life: 2 – 3 minutes
Physical properties: highly soluble in oil + grease, absorbed by plastic syringe
Administration: via mouth piece with a disposable breathing unit
Dose: 15 mCi

TECHNIQUE

Ventilation study preferably done before perfusion scan to avoid interference with higher-energetic Tc-99m (Compton scatter from Tc-99m into lower Xe-133 photopeak); feasible however if dose of Tc-99m MAA is kept below 2 mCi + concentration of Xe-133 is above 10 mCi/l of air and if Xe-133 acquisition times for wash-in, equilibrium, wash-out images are kept to about 30 seconds. Posterior imaging routine.
1. Phase
   = single breath phase = inhalation of 10 – 20 mCi Xe-133 to vital capacity in supine position over 10 – 20 seconds (65% sensitivity for abnormalities)
2. Phase
   = tidal breathing = closed loop rebreathing of Xe-133 + oxygen for 3 – 5 minutes = equilibrium phase for tracer to enter poorly ventilated areas; also functions as internal control for air leaks; posterior oblique images improve correlation with perfusion scan.
3. Phase
   = washout / clearance phase; tracer retention at 3 minutes reveals areas of air-trapping; exhaled Xe-133 is stored in charcoal trap

√ poor image quality secondary to significant scatter
√ abnormal scan:
   (a) delayed wash-in (initial 30 seconds of tidal breathing)
   (b) tracer accumulation on equilibrium views (partial obstruction with collateral air drift + diffusion into affected area via bloodstream)
   (c) delayed washout = retention >3 minutes
   (d) tracer retention in regions not seen on initial single breath view

Xenon-127

Cyclotron-produced with high cost
Physical half-life: 36.4 days
Photon energies: 172 keV (22%), 203 keV (65%)

Advantages:
   (1) High photon energy allows ventilation study following perfusion study
   (2) Decreased radiation dose (0.3 rad)
   (3) Storage capability because of long physical half-life

Krypton-81m

Eluted from Rb-81 generator (half-life of 4.7 hours)

Physical half-life: 13 seconds
Biological half-life: <1 minute
Principal photon energy: 190 keV (65% abundance)

Advantages:
   (1) Higher photon energy than Tc-99m so that ventilation scan can be performed following perfusion study
   (2) Each ventilation scan can be matched to perfusion scan without moving patient
   (3) Can be used in patients on respirator (no contamination due to short half-life)
   (4) Low radiation dose (during continuous inhalation for 6 – 8 views 100 mrad are delivered)

   Disadvantages:
   (1) High cost
   (2) Limited availability (generator good only for one day, so weekend availability may not be possible)
   (3) No washout images due to short half-life

√ lack of activity = abnormal area (tracer activity is proportional to regional distribution of tidal volume because of short biological half-life, washout phase not available)

Tc-99m DTPA aerosol

Delivery through a nebulizer during inspiration; less physiological indicator of ventilation + subject to nebulization technique

Carbon dioxide tracer

O-15-labeled carbon dioxide
Physical half-life: 2 minutes (requires on-site cyclotron)
PHYSIOLOGY:
   inhalation of carbon dioxide; rapid diffusion across alveolar-capillary membrane; clearance from lung within seconds

√ cold spot due to failure of tracer entry into airway = airway disease
√ hot spot due to delayed / absent tracer clearance = perfusion defect
87% sensitivity, 92% specificity

Indications:
   1. Emboli can be detected in preexisting cardiopulmonary disease
   2. Equivocal / indeterminate V/Q studies

Quantitative lung perfusion imaging
Indication:
   Determination of post-resection pulmonary function when combined with pulmonary function testing (FEV$_1$)

Technique:
   1. Acquire posterior and anterior perfusion (MAA) image and calculate geometric mean
   2. Separate into right + left and into 2 equal lung zones from top to bottom, which yields 4 segments (upper left, bottom right, etc)

Result:
   Activity in each segment is compared to total activity which yields % perfusion to each lung field

Unilateral lung perfusion
Incidence: 2%

A. PULMONARY EMBOLISM (23%)
B. AIRWAY DISEASE
   (a) Unilateral pleural / parenchymal disease (23%)
   (b) Bronchial obstruction
      1. Bronchogenic carcinoma (23%)
      2. Bronchial adenoma
      3. Aspirated endobronchial foreign body
C. CONGENITAL HEART DISEASE (15%)
D. ARTERIAL DISEASE
   1. Swyer-James syndrome (8%)
   2. Congenital pulmonary artery hypoplasia / stenosis
   3. Shunt procedure to pulmonary artery (eg, Blalock-Taussig)
E. ABSENT LUNG
   1. Pneumonectomy (8%)
   2. Unilateral pulmonary agenesis

Perfusion defects
A. VASCULAR DISEASE
   (a) <u>Acute / previous pulmonary embolus</u>
      1. Pulmonary thromboembolic disease
      2. Fat embolism
         √ nonsegmental perfusion defect
      3. Air embolism
         √ characteristic decortication appearance in uppermost portion on perfusion scintigraphy
      4. Embolus of tumor / cotton wool / balloon for occlusion of AVM / obstruction by Swan-Ganz catheter, other foreign body
      5. Dirofilaria (dog heart worm): clumps of heart worms break off cardiac wall + embolize pulmonary arterial tree
   (b) <u>Vasculitis</u>
      1. Collagen vascular disease
      2. IV drug abuse

3. Previous radiation therapy:
   √ defect localized to radiation port
4. Tuberculosis
(c) Vascular compression
   1. Bronchogenic carcinoma:
      √ perfusion defect depending on tumor size + location
   2. Lymphoma / lymph node enlargement
   3. Fibrosing mediastinitis
   4. Idiopathic pulmonary fibrosis:
      √ small subsegmental defects in both lungs
   5. Aortic aneurysm
(d) Altered pulmonary circulation
   1. Absence / hypoplasia of pulmonary artery
   2. Peripheral pulmonary artery stenosis
   3. Bronchopulmonary sequestration
   4. Primary pulmonary hypertension
      √ upward redistribution + large hilar defects
      √ multiple small peripheral perfusion defects
   5. Pulmonary venoocclusive disease
   6. Mitral valve disease
      √ predilection for right middle lobe + superior segments of lower lobes
   7. Congestive heart failure
      √ diffuse nonsegmental VQ mismatch
      √ enlargement of cardiac silhouette + perihilar regions

√ reversed distribution: more activity anteriorly than posteriorly
√ accentuation of fissures
√ flattening of posterior margins of lung (lateral view)
√ pleural effusion

B. AIRWAY DISEASE
1. Asthma, chronic bronchitis, bronchospasm, mucous plugging
2. Bronchiectasis (bronchiolar destruction)
3. Emphysema (bulla / cyst)
4. Pneumonia / lung abscess
5. Lymphangitic carcinomatosis
√ perfusion defects in area of hypoxia (reflex vasoconstriction)
√ abnormal ventilation to a similar / more severe degree
√ mostly nonanatomic multiple defects (in 20%)

PULMONARY EMBOLIC DISEASE

Segmental defect = involves >75% of a known bronchopulmonary segment
Subsegmental defect = involves 25 – 75% of a known bronchopulmonary segment

Perfusion images will detect:
(a) 90% of emboli that completely occlude a vessel >1 mm in diameter

Interpretation criteria for V/Q lung scans

Probability of PE	Biello criteria	PIOPED criteria
Normal	√ normal perfusion	√ normal perfusion
Low	√ small V/Q mismatches √ focal V/Q matches without corresponding CXR abnormality √ perfusion defects substantially smaller than CXR abnormality	√ small perfusion defects regardless of number / ventilation scan finding / CXR finding √ perfusion defect substantially smaller than CXR abnormality; ventilation findings irrelevant √ V/Q match in ≤50% of one lung / ≤75% of upper / mid / lower lung zone; CXR normal / nearly normal √ single moderate perfusion defect with normal CXR; ventilation findings irrelevant √ nonsegmental perfusion defects
Indeterminate	√ diffuse severe airway obstruction √ matched perfusion defects + CXR abnormalities √ single moderate V/Q mismatch without corresponding CXR abnormality	abnormality not defined by low / high probability
High	√ perfusion defects substantially larger than CXR abnormalities √ ≥2 moderate / ≥1 large V/Q mismatches; no corresponding CXR abnormality	√ ≥2 large perfusion defects; ventilation scan + CXR findings normal √ >2 large perfusion defects substantially larger than matching ventilation / CXR abnormality √ ≥2 moderate + 1 large perfusion defect; ventilation + CXR findings normal √ ≥4 moderate perfusion defects; ventilation + CXR findings normal

Lung Segments

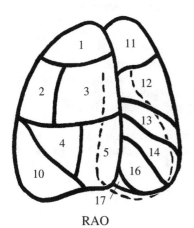

RAO

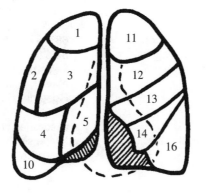

ANT

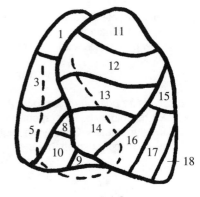

LAO

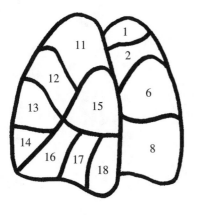

LPO

POST

RPO

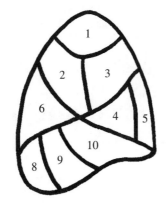

R LAT

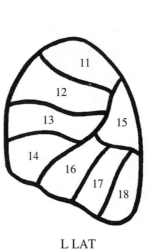

L LAT

RUL		**RML**		**RLL**		**LUL**		**LLL**	
1	apical	4	lateral	6	superior	11	apicoposterior	15	superior
2	posterior	5	medial	7	mediobasal	12	anterior	16	anteromedial basal
3	anterior			8	posterobasal	13	superior lingual	17	laterobasal
				9	laterobasal	14	inferior lingual	18	posterobasal
				10	anterobasal				

(b) 90% of surface perfusion defects that are larger than 2 x 2 cm

Therapeutic implications:
   (a) high probability scan : treat for PE
   (b) indeterminate scan   : pulmonary angiogram
   (c) low probability scan : consider other diagnosis, unless clinical suspicion very high

Indications for pulmonary angiography:
1. Embolectomy is a therapeutic option
2. Indeterminate V/Q scan with high clinical suspicion + risky anticoagulation therapy

3. Specific diagnosis necessary for proper management (vasculitis, drug induced, lung cancer with predominant vascular involvement)

Overall accuracy:
68% for perfusion scan only,
84% for ventilation-perfusion scan
<u>False-positive scans:</u>   nonthrombotic emboli, IV drug abuser, vasculitis, redistribution of flow
<u>False-negative scans:</u>   saddle embolus

√ associated with normal ventilation scan in >90%
√ "stripe sign" = peripheral rim of activity indicates nonembolic cause

HEART SCINTIGRAPHY

Imaging choices:

1. PLANAR imaging
2. SPECT imaging
   improves object contrast by removing overlying tissues
3. QUANTITATIVE analysis
   = circumferential profiles = plotting of average counts along equally spaced radii emanating from center of LV makes interpretation more objective + reproducible

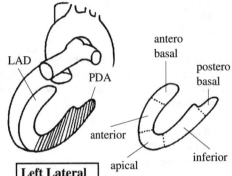

Anterior

Left ventricular anatomy and projections

A. AP
   √ displays anterolateral wall, apex, inferior wall
   √ decreased activity at apex of LV due to thinning in 50%
B. LEFT LATERAL
   displays inferior wall, anterior wall
C. LAO 40° / LAO 70°
   Δ Most often used projection; for all exercise studies
   √ displays interventricular septum, posterior wall, inferior wall
   √ best projection to separate right + left ventricles
   √ best projection to evaluate septal + posterior LV wall motion
D. RAO 45°
   √ displays anterior + inferior ventricular wall
   √ useful during 1st-pass studies with temporal separation of ventricles
E. LPO 45° (rarely used)
   10° caudal tilt minimizes LA contamination of LV region
   √ displays anterior + inferior ventricular wall
   √ preferred over RAO 45° because LV is closer to camera
F. Angled LAO (slant-hole collimator / caudal tilt)
   √ separates ventricular from atrial activity
   √ highlights apical dyskinesis

Left Lateral

Ejection fraction

Ejection fraction (EF) = stroke volume (SV) divided by end-diastolic volume (EDV)

stroke volume = end-diastolic volume (EDV) minus end-systolic volume (ESV)

EF = [EDV - ESV] / [EDV]

$$= [ED_{counts} - ES_{counts}] / [ED_{counts} - BKG_{counts}]$$

sensitive indicator of left ventricular function

Accuracy in detection of coronary artery disease:
   (a) Exercise EF: 87% sensitivity; 92% specificity
   (b) Exercise ECG: 60% sensitivity; 81% specificity

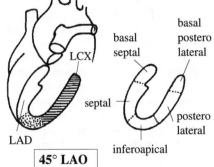

45° LAO

LAD supplies:	upper 2/3 of interventricular septum
	anterior wall
	part of lateral wall
	apex of left ventricle (in most patients)
LCX supplies:	posterior portion of left ventricle
	lateral portion of left ventricle
RCA supplies:	lower 1/3 of interventricular septum
	inferior wall of right + left ventricle

Interpretation:

@   Left ventricle
Mean normal value = 67 ± 8%
   (increase under stress normally >5 – 7%)
Probably abnormal ≤ 55%
Definitely abnormal <50%
Peak exercise LVEF is an independent predictor of
coronary artery disease

@   Right ventricle
mean normal value >45%
   (RV ejection fraction is smaller than for LV
   because RV has greater EDV than LV but the
   same stroke volume)
False-positive with   (a) inadequate exercise
                      (b) recent ingestion of meal

√ EF unchanged / decreased in coronary artery disease
√ new regional wall motion abnormality under exercise in
   coronary artery disease
√ correlates well with clinical severity of myocardial
   infarction

Shortcoming:
   poor study in patients with atrial fibrillation because of
   inability to achieve adequate cardiac gating (exercise
   MUGA can yield more sensitive assessment of coronary
   artery disease)

Blood pool agents
Tc-99m-labeled RBCs
= agent of choice because of good heart-to-lung ratio
Technique:
(1) IN VITRO LABELING
   } 50 ml drawn blood incubated with Tc-99m
      reduced by stannous ion; RBCs washed and
      reinjected
   Δ Recently developed labeling kit allows
      excellent in-vivtro labeling with only 3 ml of
      blood and is no longer time consuming and
      expensive
(2) IN VIVO LABELING
   } IV injection of stannous pyrophosphate (1 vial
      PYP diluted with 2 ml sterile saline = 15 mg
      sodium pyrophosphate containing 3.4 mg
      anhydrous stannous chloride)
   } 15 – 30 minutes later injection of Tc-99m
      pertechnetate (+7), which binds to "pretinned"
      RBCs (reduction to Tc-99m [+4])
   Δ Least time consuming + easiest method!
   Δ Worst labeling efficiency (30% not tagged to
      RBCs + excreted in urine)!
(3) IN VIVTRO LABELING
   = MODIFIED IN VIVO METHOD
   } 10 minutes after IV injection of 1 mg stannous
      pyrophosphate 10 ml of blood are drawn +
      incubated with Tc-99m pertechnetate for 10 –
      20 minutes with small amount of heparin added
      + reinjected (3-way stopcock technique)
   Δ Preferred method because of high labeling
      efficiency with little free pertechnetate!

NOTA BENE: poor tagging in
(1) Heparinized patient
(2) Injection through IV line (adherence to wall)
(3) Syringe flushed with dextrose instead of saline

Dose: 15 – 30 mCi (larger dose required for stress
             MUGA + obese patients);
             for children: 200 μCi / kg (minimum dose of
             2 – 3 mCi)
Radiation dose: 1.5 rad for heart, 1.0 rad for blood,
                    0.4 rad for whole body

Tc-99m HSA
HSA = human serum albumin
Indication: drug interference with RBC labeling (eg,
                heparinized patient)
Physiology: (a) albumin slowly equilibrates throughout
                     extracellular space
                (b) poorer heart-to-lung ratio than with
                     labeled RBCs

Myocardial perfusion imaging agents
Potassium-43
Not suitable for clinical use because of its high energy

Thallium-201 chloride
= cation produced in cyclotron from Tl-203
Decay: by electron capture to Hg-201
Energy spectrum: 71 keV of Hg-K X-rays (98%
                        abundance); 135 keV (3%) +
                        167 keV (10%) gamma-rays
Physical half-life: 73 hours
Biological half-life: 10 ± 2.5 days
Dose: 1.5 – 3 mCi (the larger dose for SPECT)
Radiation dose:
   3 rad for kidneys (critical organ) (1.2 rad/mCi); 1.2 rad
   for gonads (0.6 rad/mCi); 0.7 rad for heart + marrow
   (0.34 rad/mCi); 0.5 rad for whole body (0.24 rad/mCi)

Quality control: should contain <0.25% Pb-203,
                     <0.5% Tl-202 (439 keV)
Indications:
1. ACUTE MYOCARDIAL INFARCTION
2. CORONARY ARTERY DISEASE
   particularly useful over ECG in:
   (a) conduction disturbances (eg, bundle branch
        block, preexitation syndrome)
   (b) previous infarction
   (c) under drug influence (eg, digitalis)
   (d) left ventricular hypertrophy
   (e) hyperventilation
   (f) ST depression without symptoms
   (g) if stress ECG impossible to obtain

Sensitivity: overall 82 – 84% for stress Tl-201
                 (60 – 62% for exercise ECG)
(a) increased with:
   (1) Severity of stenosis (>50%)
   (2) Greater number of involved arteries
   (3) Stenosis of left main > LAD > RCA > LXC

(b) decreased with:
  (1) Presence of collateral
  (2) Beta blockers
  (3) Time delay for poststress images
Specificity: overall 91 – 94% for stress Tl-201
  (81 – 83% for exercise ECG)

IMAGING
1. FIRST-PASS EXTRACTION = exercise image
   = stress thallium image
   = map of regional perfusion obtained within minutes after injection at peak exercise; initial distribution proportional to myocardial blood flow, arterial concentration of radioisotope, and muscle mass; 300,000 – 400,000 counts / view (approximately 5 – 8 minutes sampling time), should be completed by 30 minutes
2. REDISTRIBUTION IMAGE = delayed image
   = equilibrium between tracer uptake and efflux dependent on blood flow + mass of viable tissue + concentration gradients
   = map of ischemic viable myocardium obtained at rest after 2 – 6 hours; washout half-life from myocardium is 54 minutes
3. RESTING REINJECTION TECHNIQUE
   = late reversibility predicts scintigraphic improvement post intervention
   = reinjection of thallium followed by imaging after 18 – 72 hours provides evidence of regional myocardial ischemia + viability not appreciated even on very delayed (24 – 72 hours) redistribution images; the booster dose augments blood concentration of isotope
   Reasoning: 50% of irreversible persistent defects improve significantly after reinjection

INTERPRETATION OF STRESS THALLIUM IMAGES

Immediate Image	Delayed Image	Diagnosis
normal	normal	normal
defect	fill-in	exertional ischemia
defect	persistent	myocardial scar
defect	partial fill-in	scar + ischemia / persistent ischemia

1. Initial phase = first-pass extraction
   √ temporary defect accentuated by exercise
   √ defect >15% of ventricular surface suggests >50% stenosis of coronary artery

2. Redistribution phase (on 2 – 4-hour images)
   √ wash out in normal areas + increased uptake in viable ischemic zones
   √ permanent defect = myocardial infarction / fibrosis
   √ increased lung activity (= >50% of myocardial count) indicative of
     (a) left ventricular failure due to severe LCA disease / myocardial infarction

(b) pulmonary venous hypertension due to cardiomyopathy / mitral valve disease
√ activity in right ventricle due to
  (a) increase in ventricular systolic pressure
  (b) increase in mean pulmonary artery pressure
  (c) increase in total pulmonary vascular resistance

FALSE-POSITIVE THALLIUM TEST (37 – 58%)
  A. Infiltrating myocardial disease:
    1. Sarcoidosis
    2. Amyloidosis
  B. Cardiac dysfunction:
    1. Cardiomyopathy
    2. IHSS
    3. Valvular aortic stenosis
    4. Mitral valve prolapse (rare)
  C. Decreased cardiac perfusion other than myocardial infarction:
    1. Cardiac contusion
    2. Myocardial fibrosis
    3. Coronary artery spasm (severe unstable angina may cause defect after stress + on redistribution images, but will be normal at rest!)
  D. Normal variant:
    1. Apical myocardial thinning
    2. Attenuation due to diaphragm, breast, implant, pacemaker

FALSE-NEGATIVE THALLIUM TEST
  1. Under influence of beta-blocker (eg, propranolol)
  2. "Balanced ischemia" = symmetric 3-vessel disease
  3. Insignificant obstruction
  4. Inadequate stress
  5. Failure to perform delayed imaging
  6. Poor technique

Disadvantages:
  (1) Low energy makes resolution difficult (improved success with SPECT)
  (2) Imaging must be completed by 45 minutes post injection or redistribution occurs

Thallium uptake & distribution
Intracellular uptake via Na/K-ATPase analogue to ionic potassium, but less readily released from cells than potassium; distribution is proportional to regional blood flow; uptake depends on quality of regional perfusion + integrity of sodium-potassium pump

@ Blood pool
  } <5% remain in blood pool 15 minutes post injection
@ Myocardium:
  } uptake depends on (a) myocardial perfusion (b) myocardial mass (c) myocardial cellular integrity
  Δ Frst-pass extraction efficiency is 88%!
    REMEMBER: 90% in 90 seconds!

} 4% of total dose localizes in myocardium (myocardial blood flow = 4% of cardiac output)
} peak myocardial activity at 5 – 15 minutes after injection
} uptake can be increased by 1 – 2% through exercise / myocardial hypertrophy
} right heart faintly visualized during rest (15% of perfusion to right side); well seen during stress test, tachycardia, volume / pressure overload

@ Skeletal muscle + splanchnicus:
} first-pass extraction efficiency is 65%
} accumulate 40% of injected dose
} 4 – 6 hours fast + exercise decreases flow to splanchnicus and increases cardiac uptake

@ Lung:
} 10% of total dose localizes in lung
} <5% activity over lung is normal
} augmented pulmonary extraction with left ventricular dysfunction, bronchogenic carcinoma, lymphoma of lung

@ Kidney:
} accumulates 4% of injected dose
} excretion of 4 – 8% within 24 hours

@ Thyroid:
} increased uptake >1% in Graves disease + thyroid carcinoma

@ Brain:
} uptake only after disruption of blood-brain barrier

Tc-99m sestamibi
Pharmacokinetics:
— relatively rapid clearance from circulation with high myocardial uptake proportional to myocardial blood flow
— long retention time in myocardium with little recirculation

Excretion:
through biliary tree (give milk after injection and before imaging to decrease GB activity)
Dose: 25 mCi (Cardiolite®)
Imaging: optimum images 1 hour after injection (may be imaged up until 3 hours)

Advantages over thallium:
(1) Improved dosimetry related to shorter half-life allows larger doses with less patient radiation
(2) Improved photon flux means faster imaging + allows cardiac gating
(3) Higher photon energy means less attenuation artifact from breast tissue / diaphragm + less scatter
(4) NO redistribution
(5) Temporal separation of injection and imaging allows injection during acute myocardial infarct when patient may not be stable for imaging; after stabilization + intervention (angioplasty / urokinase) imaging can demonstrate the pre-intervention defect

Technique:
1-day protocol:
Improved detection of reversibility compared to stress-rest protocol
1. Rest images 60 – 90 minutes after injection of 8 mCi Tc-99m sestamibi
2. Wait 0 – 4 hours
3. Stress patient followed by injection of 25 mCi Tc-99m sestamibi at peak stress (increased myocardial blood flow means increased myocardial uptake)
4. Image 30 – 60 minutes later (optimum imaging time of stress-induced defects)
2-day protocol (stress-rest protocol):
1. Stress images on 1st day: Tc-99m sestamibi given at peak stress; imaging after 30 – 60 minutes delay to allow liver activity to decrease
2. Repeat on 2nd day if stress views abnormal

Tc-99m teboroxime
Pharmacokinetics:
— very rapid clearance time from circulation (rapid uptake by myocardium with high extraction efficiency)
— distribution proportional to cardiac blood flow EVEN at high blood flow levels (sestamibi + thallium plateau at high levels of flow)
Dose: 25 – 30 mCi (Cardiotec®)
Imaging: must begin immediately post injection due to rapid washout; rest image can immediately follow stress image

Stress test
Rationale:
increased heart rate will unveil insufficient regional perfusion secondary to coronary artery disease
Technique:
} exercise in erect position (peak heart rate lower if supine) on treadmill or bicycle; isometric handgrip exercise raises blood pressure less (but adequate for evaluation)
} starting point of workload selected according to preliminary exercise results (at an average of 200 kilowatt pounds)
} workload increments by 200 kilowatt pounds up to 85% of predicted maximum heart rate (= 220 - age) / exercise limited by symptoms of chest pain, dyspnea, fatigue, arrhythmia, ischemic ECG (cardiologist with crash cart should be available)
} Pharmacologic stress test = stress test substitute (in patients who cannot exercise because of severe peripheral vascular disease / arthritis / pain):
(1) IV infusion of 0.15 ml/kg/min dipyridamole (= Persantine® = vasodilator with 3 – 5-fold increase in coronary artery blood flow) for 4 minutes (effect reversible by administration of aminophylline)
(2) IV infusion of 0.14 gm/kg/min adenosine (= Adenocard®, Adenoscan®) for 6 minutes (drug half-life of 15 seconds)

End-points for discontinuing exercise:
  a. Symptoms: chest pain, dyspnea, fatigue, leg cramps, dizziness
  b. Signs: fall in BP >10 mm Hg below previous stage, ventricular tachycardia, run of 3 successive ventricular premature beats

Problems with exercise imaging:
  (1) Sensitivity to detect ischemic lesions decreases with suboptimal exercise (in particular for older population)
  (2) Higher false-positive tests in women (artifacts from overlying breast tissue)
  (3) Propranolol (beta blocker) interferes with stress test, should be discontinued 24 – 48 hours prior to testing

Applied to:
  1. <u>Thallium imaging</u> (redistribution images after stress test):
    } injection of 1.5 – 2 mCi of Tl-201 during peak exercise, continuation of exercise for additional 60 seconds before imaging commences
    Clues for stress images:
    √ RV myocardium well visualized
    √ little pulmonary background activity
    √ little activity in liver, stomach, spleen
    √ distribution more uniform after stress than during rest
    Δ Degree of liver uptake useful as direct measure of level of exercise!
  2. <u>Gated blood pool imaging</u> (response of EF)
    √ increase in ejection fraction from 63 – 93% in normals
    √ increase in ventricular wall motion (anterolateral > posterolateral > septal)

Ventricular function
First-pass ventriculography
= FIRST TRANSIT = recording of initial transit time of an intravenously administered tight Tc-99m bolus through heart + lungs; limited number of cardiac cycles available for interpretation; additional projections / serial studies require additional bolus injection

Accuracy: good correlation with contrast ventriculography

Agents: pertechnetate, pyrophosphate, albumin, DTPA, sulfur colloid (almost any Tc-99m-labeled compound except lung scanning particles), Tc-99m-labeled autologous RBCs most commonly

Indication:
  (1) Only 15 seconds of patient cooperation required
  (2) Calculation of cardiac output + ejection fraction (RBCs)
  (3) Subsequent first-pass studies within 15 – 20 minutes of initial study possible (DTPA)

  (4) Separate assessment of individual cardiac chambers in RAO projection (temporal separation without overlying atria, pulmonary artery, aortic outflow tract), eg, for right ventricular EF and intracardiac shunts

Gating:
  Improved images obtained by selection of time interval corresponding only to RV passage of bolus averaged over several (3 – 5) individual beats; gating may be done intrinsically or with ECG guidance

Imaging:
  Region of interest (ROI) over RV silhouette in RAO projection; background activity taken over horseshoe-shaped ventricular wall; counts in ROI displayed as function of time; 25 frames/second for 20 – 30 seconds

Evaluation of:
  1. Obstruction in SVC region
  2. Reflux from RA in IVC region
  3. Stenosis in pulmonary outflow tract
  4. R-L shunt
  5. Contractility of RV
  6. Sequential beating of RA and RV

Equilibrium images
= "blood pool" radionuclide angiography = imaging after thorough mixing of Tc-99m-labeled radiopharmaceutical (HSA / RBCs) throughout vascular space
} acquisition of images during selected portions of cardiac cycle gated by R-wave; each image is composed of >200,000 counts (2 – 10 minutes) obtained over several hundred cycles after equilibrium has been reached; high quality images can be obtained in different projections
} gated acquisition from 16 – 24 equal subdivisions of the R-R cycle allows display of synchronized cinematic images (assembled to composite single-image sequence) of entire cardiac cycle
  √ may be displayed as time activity curves reflecting changes in ventricular counts throughout R-R interval
    — measured functional indices: preejection period (PEP), left ventricular ejection time (LVET), left ventricular fast filling time (LVFT$_1$), left ventricular slow filling time (LVFT$_2$), PEP/ LVET ratio, rate of ejection + filling of LV
} at rest: count density 200 – 250 counts/pixel requires generally 7 – 10 minutes acquisition time for 200,000 – 250,000 counts / frame
} during exercise: 100,000 – 150,000 counts/frame requires an acquisition time of 2 minutes

Evaluation of:
  1. LV ejection fraction
  2. Regional wall motion
  3. Valvular regurgitation

Interpretation:
1. Heart failure: decreased EF, prolongation of PEP, shortening of LVET, decreased rate of ejection
2. Hypertensive heart: normal systolic indices, normal EF, prolonged LVT_1
3. Hypothyroidism: prolonged PEP, normal EF
4. Aortic stenosis: mild reduction of EF, prolonged LV emptying time, decreased rate of ejection, normal rate of filling

√ area of decreased periventricular uptake secondary to
(a) pleural effusion >100 ml
(b) ventricular hypertrophy

Gated blood pool imaging
= MULTIPLE GATED ACQUISITION (MUGA)
Recording of:
(1) Ejection fraction (EF) of left ventricle before + after exercise (>6 million counts, 32 frames)
(2) Regional wall motion of ventricular chambers (>4.5 million counts, 24 frames)
(a) at rest : myocardial infarction, aneurysm, contusion
(b) during exercise : ischemic dyskinesia (detectable in 63%)
(3) Regurgitant index

Projection:
(a) best septal view (usually LAO 45°) for EF; often requires some cephalad tilting of detector head
(b) two additional views for evaluation of wall motion (usually anterior + left lateral views)

Imaging:
Physiologic trigger provided by R-R interval of ECG ("bad beat" rejection program desirable)
(a) gated images obtained for 5 minutes
(b) 2-minute image acquisition time for each stage of exercise

PROs: (1) Higher information density than 1st-pass method
(2) Assessment of pharmacologic effect possible
(3) "Bad beat" rejection possible
CONs: (1) Significant background activity
(2) Inability to monitor individual chambers in other than LAO 45° projection
(3) Plane of AV valve difficult to identify

Radiation dose: 1.5 rad for heart; 1.0 rad for blood; 0.4 rad for whole body

MYOCARDIAL INFARCT
Hot Spot Imaging
= INFARCT-AVID IMAGING
Agent: Tc-99m pyrophosphate (standard), Hg-203 chlormerodrin, Tc-99m tetracycline, Tc-99m glucoheptonate, F-18 sodium fluoride, indium-111 antimyosin (murine monoclonal antibodies to myosin)

Pathophysiology in MYOCARDIAL INFARCTION:
Pyrophosphate uptake into myocardial necrosis through complexation with calcium deposits >10 – 12 hours post infarction, requires presence of residual collateral blood flow; 30 – 40% maximum accumulation in hypoxic cells under conditions of diminished blood flow

Uptake post infarction:
— earliest uptake by 12 – 24 hours;
— peak uptake by 48 – 72 hours;
— persistent uptake seen up to 5 – 7 days with return to normal by 10 -14 days

Sensitivity:
90% for transmural infarction, 40 – 50% for subendocardial (nontransmural) infarction
Specificity:
as low as 64%

Dose: 15 – 20 mCi IV (minimal count requirement of 500,000/view)
Imaging: at 3 – 6 hours (60% absorbed by skeleton within 3 hours)

Indications:
1. Lost enzyme pattern = patient admitted 24 – 48 hours after infarction
2. Equivocal ECG + atypical angina:
(a) left ventricular bundle branch block
(b) left ventricular hypertrophy
(c) impossibility to perform stress test
(d) patient on digitalis
3. ST depression without symptoms
4. Equivocal enzyme pattern + equivocal symptoms
5. S/P cardiac surgery (perioperative infarction in 10%, enzymes routinely elevated, ECG always abnormal), requires preoperative baseline study as 40% are preoperatively abnormal
6. for detection of right ventricular infarction
NOT HELPFUL:
1. In differentiating multiple- from single-vessel disease
2. Typical angina
3. Normal ECG stress test + NO symptoms

SCAN INTERPRETATION
Grade 2+ and above are positive
Grade 0   no activity
Grade 1+   faint uptake
Grade 2+   slightly less than sternum, equal to ribs
Grade 3+   equal to sternum
Grade 4+   greater than sternum
√ "doughnut" pattern = central cold defect (necrosis in large infarct) usually in cases of large anterior + anterolateral wall infarctions
√ uptake in inferior wall extending behind sternum (anterior projection) suggests RV infarction
√ SPECT imaging improves sensitivity (eliminates rib overlap)

√ diffuse uptake can be seen in angina, cardiomyopathy, subendocardial infarct, pericarditis and normal blood pool (normal blood pool can be eliminated with delayed imaging)

FALSE POSITIVES (10%)
A. Cardiac causes
   1. Recent injury: myocardial contusion, resuscitation, cardioversion, radiation injury, adriamycin cardiotoxicity, myocarditis, acute pericarditis
   2. Previous injury: left ventricular aneurysm, mural thrombus, unstable angina, previous infarction with persistent uptake
   3. Calcified heart valves / coronaries (rare) / chronic pericarditis
   4. Amyloidosis
B. Extracardiac causes:
   1. Soft tissue uptake: breast tumor / inflammation, chest wall injury, paddle burns from cardioversion, surgical drain, lung tumor
   2. Osseous: calcified costal cartilage (most common), lesions in rib / sternum
   3. Increased blood pool activity secondary to renal dysfunction / poor labeling technique (improvement on delayed images)

FALSE NEGATIVES (5%)
Myocardial metastasis

PERSISTENTLY POSITIVE SCAN (>2 weeks)
= ongoing myocardial necrosis indicating poor prognosis, may continue on to cardiac aneurysm, repeat infarction, cardiac death
— in 77% of persistent / unstable angina pectoris
— in 41% of compensated congestive heart failure
— in 51% of ECG evidence of ventricular dyssynergy
Prognosis: the larger the area the worse the mortality + morbidity

Cold spot imaging
= NONAVID IMAGING = myocardial perfusion study for acute myocardial infarction

Agent: Tl-201 (at rest)

Sensitivity   after onset of symptoms:
96% within 6-12 hours, 79% after 48 hours, 59% in remote infarction; sensitivity for SPECT (seven pin-hole tomography) 94% > planar scintigraphy 75%

√ fixed permanent defect in acute infarction
√ fixed permanent defect at rest + on stress thallium + redistribution images in old infarction
√ "cold defect" at rest may represent transient ischemia in unstable angina

N.B.:   Tl-201 cannot distinguish between recent + remote infarction!

MYOCARDIAL ISCHEMIA
can be assessed
(a) directly with stress Tl-201 imaging
(b) indirectly with gated blood pool imaging (wall motion, ejection fraction)

LOCATION OF PERFUSION DEFECTS
(1) Right coronary artery (RCA) best seen on left LAT / AP projections
     √ inferior + posteroseptal segments
(2) Circumflex branch of left coronary artery (LCX) best seen on LAO projection
     √ posterolateral segment
(3) Anterior descending branch of left coronary artery (LAD)
     √ anteroseptal, anterior, anterolateral segments

N.B.:   decreased activity in apical + posterior segments is not reliably correlated with disease of any vessel!

Intracardiac shunts
Agents administered by peripheral IV injection:
Tc-99m macroaggregated albumin, Tc-99m pertechnetate, DTPA, sulfur colloid, labeled RBCs
Method:
C2/C1-method = measures hemodynamic significance of a shunt; raw data obtained from pulmonary activity curve (gamma variate method, two-area ratio method, count method); accuracy depends on the shape of the input bolus (single peak of <2 seconds duration); measuring C1, C2, T1, T2

A. NORMAL
    C2/C1 is <32%
B. L-R SHUNT
    Indication: ASD, VSD, AV canal, aortopulmonic window, rupture of sinus of Valsalva aneurysm
    √ C2/C1 >35% (area A = primary pulmonary circulation; area B = L-R shunt; area (A - B) = systemic circulation; Q_P / Q_S = area A / area (A - B) = 0.91)
C. R-L SHUNT
    Indication: Tetralogy of Fallot, transposition, truncus, Ebstein anomaly
    √ early arrival of tracer in left side of heart + aorta (first-pass method) prior to arrival of activity from lungs to LV
    √ quantification possible only by registration of sum of activity of trapped macroaggregate / microspheres in brain + kidneys

Causes of abnormal non-shunt-related activity:
(1) Radiopharmaceutical breakdown
     √ free pertechnetate activity in salivary glands, gastric mucosa, thyroid, kidney
(2) Hepatic cirrhosis abnormal pulmonary vascular channels bypassing the lung (in 10 – 70%)
(3) Pulmonary AVM

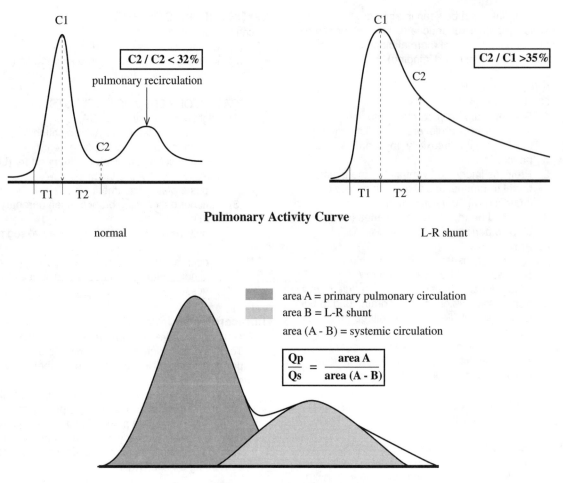

Pulmonary Activity Curve

normal   L-R shunt

Two-Area Ratio Method

LIVER AND GASTROINTESTINAL TRACT SCINTIGRAPHY

Tc-99m IDA analogs

= Tc-99m acetanilide iminodiacetic acid analogs (IDA)

Dependent on the substance's lipophility, there is a trade-off between renal excretion + hepatic uptake (BIDA is the most lipophilic, HIDA the least lipophilic)

1. HIDA (2,6-dimethyl derivative): [H = hepatic] bilirubin threshold of <18 mg/dl; 15% renal excretion
2. BIDA (parabutyl derivative): bilirubin threshold of <20 mg/dl
3. PIPIDA (paraisopropyl derivative): 2% renal excretion
4. DIDA (diethyl derivative)
5. DISIDA (diisopropyl derivative) = Disida®, Disofen®, Hepatolite®: bilirubin threshold of <30 mg/dl
6. TMB-IDA (m-bromotrimethyl IDA) = Mebrofenin®, Choletec®: $T_{1/2}$ uptake is 6 minutes, $T_{1/2}$ excretion is 14 minutes in normals

Quality control: the final compound should contain
— 90 – 100% Tc-99m IDA
— <10% Tc-99m tin colloid
— <10% Tc-99m sodium pertechnetate

Pharmacokinetics:
Bloodstream: tracer bound predominantly to albumin, which decreases renal excretion (renal excretion seen in most normals); dissociation of albumin + Tc-99m-IDA takes place at space of Disse
Liver: peak liver activity 5 – 10 minutes post injection = hepatic phase; 85% extracted by hepatocytes; tracer enters anion pathway of bilirubin
Δ Delayed liver uptake implies hepatocyte dysfunction / CHF (less likely)
Δ Look for liver lesions on early images
Bile: secretion by hepatocytes without conjugation; CBD + cystic duct visualized within 15 minutes (not always visualized in normals); GB visualized by 20 minutes
Δ Activity in right paracolic gutter / intraperitoneal space implies post-operative bile leak
Bowel: excretion into duodenum by 30 minutes; bowel visualized within 1 hour; no enterohepatic recirculation

Dose: 3 – 7 mCi for adults (higher dose may be needed for high bilirubin level + for tracer with lower bilirubin threshold)
Radiation dose: 2 rad for upper large bowel; 0.55 rad for gallbladder; 3 rad/mCi for small bowel; 0.01 rad/mCi for whole body

Patient preparation:
1. Narcotics (opiates) + sedatives which increase tone of sphincter of Oddi are stopped 6 – 12 hours before exam
2. Fasting of at least 2 – 4 hours but <24 hours

3. Cholecystokinin-C-terminal octapeptide = Sincalide (slow IV injection of 0.02 µg/kg Kinevac®) may be used to empty gallbladder about 30 minutes before tracer injection in patients on prolonged fasting (gallbladder atony + retained bile and sludge secondary to absence of endogenously produced CCK)
Useful in: (a) patient fasting >24 hours / on total parenteral nutrition
(b) acalculous cholecystitis
Side effect: increase in biliary-to-bowel transit time

Equipment:
Large field-of-view scintillation camera fitted with LEAP collimator; spectrometer set at 140 keV with 20% window
Computer software for deconvolutional analysis allows determination of percent of hepatic arterial and percent of portal venous blood flow to liver (helpful in assessment of liver transplants)

Imaging:
at 5 – 10-minute intervals for 60 minutes; if gallbladder not visualized at least up to 4 hours; RLAT, RAO, LAO projections to confirm gallbladder position
Δ Look for enterogastric reflux as a cause of biliary gastritis!

IV morphine sulfate (0.04 µg/kg):
contracts sphincter of Oddi + raises intrabiliary pressure with retrograde filling of gallbladder; maximal effect 5 minutes post injection; shortens study time to 1 hour in cases of nonvisualization of gallbladder when injected 30 – 40 minutes into study; increases accuracy from 88% to 98% and specificity from 83% to 100%

Normals:
gallbladder appearance within 60 minutes (90% within 30 minutes); gallbladder visualization within 30 minutes after administration of morphine; small bowel activity within 90 minutes (80% within 60 minutes)

Gallbladder ejection fraction (GBEF)

$$GBEF = GB_{initial} - GB_{post} / GB_{initial}$$

Indication:
(1) to increase sensitivity of study for acute (acalculous) cholecystitis
(2) in patients with atypical GB pain and no cholelithiasis

Technique:
1. Select ROI about GB
2. Administer Sincalide in a dose of 0.02 µg/kg body weight IV over 30 minutes (with infusion pump)
Normal result: >30% GBEF

Technetium-99m sulfur colloid
= LIVER-SPLEEN SCAN

Indications: liver, spleen, bone marrow, acute rejection in renal transplant, lower GI bleeding, gastric emptying

Preparation:
Tc-99m pertechnetate and sodium trisulphate are heated in a water bath (95 ± 5°C) for 10 ± 2 minutes; sulfur atoms aggregate to form a "colloid" (average particle size 0.1 – 1 μ with a range of 0.001 – 1 μ; true colloid has a particle size of 0.001 – 0.5 μ); gelatin is added to prevent further growth of particles

Quality control:
- (a) >92% remain at origin of ascending chromatography
- (b) upper limit for particle size is 1 μ
- — Usual cause for poor preparation are excessive / prolonged heating or a pH >7
- — Preparation should not be used >6 hours (agglomeration of particles with aging)

Dose: usually 3 – 6 mCi (8 mCi for SPECT)
Radiation dose: 0.3 rad/mCi for liver (critical organ);
0.02 rad/mCi for whole body;
0.025 rad/mCi for bone marrow

Imaging: 15 – 30 minutes post IV injection

Pharmacokinetics:
accumulation in liver (85%), spleen (10%), bone marrow (5%); lung localization is rare (presumably secondary to circulating endotoxins + macrophage infiltration)

A. RETICULOENDOTHELIAL LOCALIZATION
√ colloid shift away from liver in diffuse hepatic dysfunction / decreased hepatic perfusion
√ increased bone marrow activity in hemolytic anemia
√ increased splenic activity in hypersplenism of splenomegaly / cancer / systemic illness

B. BONE MARROW LOCALIZATION
Hematopoietic system extends into long bones in children; recedes to axial skeleton, femora, and humeri with age
Δ Bone marrow distribution cannot be used to determine sites of erythropoiesis!

C. ABSCESS LOCALIZATION
Sulfur colloid phagocytized by PMNs + monocytes
Labeling:
- (a) in vivo: small labeling yield
- (b) in vitro: 40% labeling efficiency, but difficult + time-consuming preparation

Colloid shift
A. Hepatic dysfunction
1. Cirrhosis
2. Hepatitis
3. Chronic passive congestion

B. Augmented perfusion of spleen + bone marrow
1. Hematopoietic disorders
2. Long-term corticosteroid therapy

Focal hot liver lesion
1. IVC / SVC obstruction
√ increased perfusion of quadrate lobe located at posterior aspect of medial segment left hepatic lobe (collateral pathway via umbilical vein)
2. Budd-Chiari syndrome
√ "increased" perfusion of caudate lobe (actually decrease of activity elsewhere in liver)
3. FNH (varying amount of Kupffer cells)
√ hot / cold / isoactive with surrounding parenchyma
4. Regenerating nodules of cirrhosis

Defects in porta hepatis
1. Normal variant (thinning of hepatic tissue overlying portal veins + gallbladder)
2. Biliary causes: dilatation of bile ducts, gallbladder hydrops
3. Enlarged portal lymph nodes
4. Metastases
5. Hepatic cyst
6. Hepatic parenchymal disease (pseudotumor)
7. Hepatic compression by adjacent extrinsic mass
8. Postsurgical changes following cholecystectomy

Focal liver defects
A. Neoplastic
(a) primary liver tumor: hepatoma, hemangioma, hepatic adenoma, FNH
(b) metastases: 85% sensitivity, 75 – 80% specificity (for lesion >1 - 2 cm)
B. Infectious disease / abscess
C. Benign cyst
D. Trauma
E. Pseudotumor = normal variant

Mottled hepatic uptake
1. Cirrhosis
2. Acute hepatitis
3. Lymphoma
4. Amyloidosis
5. Granulomatous disease (sarcoid, fungal, viral, parasitic)
6. Chemo- / radiation therapy

SPLENIC SCINTIGRAPHY
1. Tc-99m sulfur colloid: 3 – 5 mCi
2. Tc-99m heat-denatured erythrocytes

Indication:
(1) Splenic trauma (2) Accessory + ectopic spleen
Technique:
20 – 30 minutes after injection of pyrophosphate IV 15 – 20 ml of blood are drawn + incubated with 2 mCi of pertechnetate; blood is heated to 49.5°C for 35 minutes and reinjected

Δ Fragmentation of RBCs from overheating increases hepatic uptake!
Imaging: 20 minutes post injection

Radionuclide esophagram
Preparation: 4 – 12 hours fasting; imaging in supine / erect position
Dose: 250 – 500 μCi Tc-99m sulfur colloid in 10 ml of water taken through straw
Imaging: when swallowing begins

√ normal transit time: 15 seconds with 3 distinct sequential peaks progressing aborally
√ prolonged transit time: achalasia, progressive systemic sclerosis, diffuse esophageal spasm, nonspecific motor disorders, "nutcracker" esophagus, Zenker diverticulum, esophageal stricture + obstruction
Difficult interpretation in: hiatal hernia, GE reflux, Nissen fundoplication

Gatroesophageal reflux
89% correlation with acid reflux test
Cause:
(1) Decreased pressure of lower esophageal sphincter
  (a) transient-complete relaxation of LES
  (b) low resting pressure of LES
(2) Transient increase in intraabdominal pressure
(3) Short intraabdominal esophageal segment
Age of population: usually 6 – 9 months, up to 2 years
• poor weight gain
• vomiting, aspiration, choking
• asthmatic episodes, stridor, apnea

Detection: upper GI examination with barium, distal esophageal sphincter pressure measurements, 24-hour pH probe measurement in distal esophagus (gold standard), radionuclide examination
Preparation: 4 hours / overnight fasting; abdominal sphygmomanometer (for adults)
Dose: 0.5 – 1.0 mCi Tc-99m sulfur colloid in 300 ml of acidified orange juice (150 ml juice + 150 ml 0.1 N hydrochloric acid) followed by "cold" acidified orange juice
Imaging: at 30 – 60-second intervals for 30 – 60 minutes, images taken in supine position from anterior; sphygmomanometer inflated at 20, 40, 60, 80, 100 mm Hg
Interpretation:
Reflux (in %) = ([esophageal counts - background] / gastric counts) x 100
√ up to 3% magnitude reflux is normal
√ evidence of pulmonary aspiration (valuable in pediatric age group)

Cx: reflux esophagitis secondary to
(a) delayed clearance time of esophageal acid load: tertiary / repetitive esophageal contractions, supine position of refluxor, aspiration of saliva, stimulation of salivary flow, stretched phrenoesophageal membrane in hiatal hernia

(b) delayed gastric emptying: increased intragastric pressure (gastric outlet obstruction), viral gastropathy, diabetes
Prognosis:
(1) Self-limiting process with spontaneous resolution by end of infancy (in majority of patients)
(2) Persistent symptoms until age 4 (1/3 of patients)
(3) Death from inanition / recurrent pneumonia (5%)
(4) Cause of recurrent respiratory infections, asthma, failure to thrive, esophagitis, esophageal stricture, chronic blood loss, sudden infant death syndrome (SIDS)
Rx:
(1) Conservative therapy: avoidance of food + drugs that decrease pressure in LES, elevation of head during sleep, acid neutralization, cimetidine / ranitidine (reduction of acid production), metoclopramide / domperidone (increase sphincter pressure + promote gastric emptying)
(2) Antireflux surgery

Gastric emptying
Dose: 0.5 – 1 mCi
  (a) Tc-99m sulfur colloid cooked with egg white / liver pâté as solid food
  (b) In-111 DTPA for simultaneous measurement of liquid phase
Imaging: one-minute anterior abdominal images obtained at 0, 10, 30, 60, 90 minutes in erect position if dual-head camera available; anterior and posterior imaging performed with geometric mean activity calculated
Pharmacokinetics:
79% tracer activity in stomach for solid phase at 10 minutes; 65% at 30 minutes; 33% at 60 minutes; 10% at 90 minutes
Normal result: 50% of activity in stomach at time zero should empty by 60 ± 30 minutes
√ acutely delayed emptying in stress (pain, cold), drugs (morphine, anticholinergics, levo-dopa, nicotine, β-adrenergic antagonists), postoperative ileus, acute viral gastroenteritis, hyperglycemia, hypokalemia
√ chronically delayed gastric emptying in gastric outlet obstruction, postvagotomy, gastric ulcer, chronic idiopathic intestinal pseudoobstruction, GE reflux, progressive systemic sclerosis, dermatomyositis, spinal cord injury, myotonia dystrophica, familial dysautonomia, anorexia nervosa, hypothyroidism, diabetes mellitus, amyloidosis, uremia
√ abnormally rapid gastric emptying in gastric surgery, ZE syndrome, duodenal ulcer disease, malabsorption (pancreatic exocrine insufficiency / celiac sprue)

Gastrointestinal bleeding
Detection depends on:
(1) Rate of hemorrhage (≥ 0.05 ml/minute); NUC more sensitive than angiogram
(2) Continuous versus intermittent bleeding (most GI hemorrhages are intermittent)

(3) Site of hemorrhage
(4) Characteristics of radionuclide agent

ANGIOGRAPHY:
requires a bleeding rate of approximately 0.5 ml/min;
63% sensitivity for upper GI bleed;
39% sensitivity for lower GI bleed

1. Tc-99m sulfur colloid
Indication: bleeding must be active at time of tracer
administration; length of active imaging
can be increased by fractionating dose
— Disappearance half-life of 2.5 – 3.5 minutes (rapidly
cleared from blood by RES + low background
activity)
— Active bleeding sites detected with rates as low as
0.05 – 0.1 ml/min
— Not useful for upper GI bleeding (interference from
high activity in liver + spleen) or bleeding near
hepatic / splenic flexure
Dose: 10 mCi (370 MBq)
Imaging:
every image should be for 500,000 – 1,000,000
counts with oblique + lateral images as necessary
(a) every 5 seconds for 1 minute ("flow study" =
radionuclide angiogram)
(b) 60-second images at 2, 5, 10, 15, 20, 30, 40, 60
minutes; study terminated if no abnormality up to
30 minutes
(c) delayed images at 2, 4, 6, 12 hours
√ extravasation of tracer seen in active bleeding
Specificity: almost 100% (rare false-positives due to
ectopic RES tissue)
False positives:
Transplanted kidney, ectopic splenic tissue, modified
marrow uptake, male genitalia, arterial graft, aortic
aneurysm

2. Tc-99m-labeled RBCs (in vivtro labeling preferred)
Indications: acute / intermittent bleeding (0.35 ml/
minute)
— Remains in vascular system for prolonged period
— Liver + spleen activity are low allowing detection of
upper GI tract hemorrhage
— Low target-to-background ratio (high activity in great
vessels, liver, spleen, kidneys, stomach, colon;
probably related to free pertechnetate fraction)
Dose: 10 – 20 mCi
Imaging:
(a) every 2 seconds for 64 seconds
(b) static images for 500,000 – 1,000,000 counts at
2, 5 and every consecutive 5 minutes up to 30
minutes + every 10 minutes until 90 minutes
(c) delayed images at 2, 4, 6, 12 hours up to 36
hours
Localization of bleeding site:
may be difficult secondary to rapid transit time
(reduced bowel motility with 1 mg glucagon IV) or too
widely spaced time intervals; overall 83% correlation
with angiography

√ increase in tracer accumulation over time in abnormal
location
√ bleeding site conforms to bowel anatomy
√ change in appearance with time consistent with bowel
peristalsis
Sensitivity: in 83 – 93% correctly identified bleeding
site (50 – 85% within 1st hour, may become positive
in 33% only after 12 – 24 hours); collection as small
as 5 ml may be detected; superior to sulfur colloid
— 50% sensitivity for blood loss <500 ml/24 hours
— >90% sensitivity for blood loss >500 ml/24 hours
False positives (5%): physiologic uptake in stomach +
intestine, renal pelvis uptake, hepatic hemangioma,
varices, inflammation, isolated vascular process
(AVM, venous / arterial graft)
False negatives: 9% for bleeding of <500 ml/24 hours

3. Tc-99m pertechnetate
Indication: bleeding from functioning gastric mucosa
in Meckel diverticulum / intestinal duplication; consider
in adults up to age 25; independent of bleeding rate
Pathophysiology: tracer accumulation in mucus-
secreting cells
Δ Avoid barium GI studies + endoscopy + irritating
bowel preparation prior to study!
Dose: 5 – 10 mCi (185 – 370 MBq)
Imaging:
(a) radionuclide angiogram 2 – 3 seconds/frame for
1st minute
(b) sequential 5-minute images up to 20 minutes with
5,000 – 1,000,000 counts per image
Sensitivity: >80%
enhanced by
— fasting for 3 – 6 hours to reduce gastric
secretions passing through bowel
— nasogastric tube suction to remove gastric
secretions
— premedication with pentagastrin (6 μg/kg SC 15
minutes before study) to stimulate gastric
secretion of pertechnetate
— premedication with cimetidine (300 mg qid x 48
hours) to reduce release of pertechnetate from
mucosa
— voiding just prior to injection
False positives:
Barrett esophagus, duodenal ulcer, ulcerative colitis,
Crohn disease, enteric duplication, small bowel,
hemangioma, AV malformation, aneurysm, volvulus,
intussusception, urinary obstruction, uterine blush
False negatives:
Ulcerated epithelium

Levine / Denver shunt patency
Technique:
sterile injection of 0.5 – 1 mCi Tc99m MAA / sulfur
colloid via paracentesis
Imaging:
over abdomen (or chest) to detect uptake in liver (or
lung), which confirms patency

RENAL AND ADRENAL SCINTIGRAPHY

Renal agents
1. Agents for renal function: Tc-99m DTPA,
  I-131 Hippuran
2. Renal cortical agents: Tc-99m DMSA
3. Renal combination agent: Tc-99m glucoheptonate

Tc-99m DTPA
= Tc-99m diethylenetriamine pentaacetic acid
= agent of choice for assessment of
  (1) Perfusion
  (2) Glomerular filtration = relative GFR
  (3) Obstructive uropathy
  (4) Vesicoureteral reflux

Pharmacokinetics:
chelating agent; 5 – 10% bound to plasma protein; extracted with 20% efficiency on each pass through kidney (= filtration fraction); excreted exclusively by glomerular filtration (similar to inulin) without reabsorption / tubular excretion / metabolism
Time-activity behavior:
— abdominal aorta (15 – 20 seconds)
— kidneys + spleen (17 – 24 seconds); liver appears later because of portal venous supply
— renal cortical activity (2 – 4 minutes): mean transit time of 3.0 ± 0.5 minutes; static images of cortex taken at 3 – 5 minutes
— renal pelvic activity (3 – 5 minutes): peak at 10 minutes; asymmetric clearance of renal pelvis in 50%; accelerated by furosemide

Biologic half-life: 20 minutes
Dose: 10 – 20 mCi

Radiation dose: 0.85 rads/mCi for renal cortex; 0.6 rads/mCi for kidney; 0.5 rads/mCi for bladder; 0.15 rads/mCi for gonads; 0.15 rads/mCi for whole body

Adjunct:
Lasix administration (20 – 40 mg IV) 20 minutes into exam allows to assess renal pelvic clearance with accuracy equal to Whitaker test (DDx of obstructed from dilated but non-obstructed pelvocalyceal system)

[Tc-99m glucoheptonate]
largely replaced by Tc-99m MAG3

Pharmacokinetics:
rapid plasma clearance + urinary excretion with excellent definition of pelvocalyceal system during 1st hour; extracted by (a) glomerular filtration and (b) tubular excretion (30 – 45% within 1st hour); 5 – 15% of dose accumulate in tubular cells by 1 hour; cortical accumulation remains for 24 hours

Imaging:
(a) collecting system within first 30 minutes
(b) renal parenchyma after 1 – 2 hours (interference of activity in collecting system)

Biologic half-life: 2 hours
Dose: 15 (range 10 – 20) mCi
Radiation dose: 0.17 rads/mCi for kidney;
0.008 rads/mCi for whole body;
0.015 rads/mCi for gonads

Tc-99m DMSA
= Tc-99m dimercaptosuccinic acid
= suitable for imaging of functioning cortical mass: pseudotumor versus lesion

Pharmacokinetics:
high protein-binding + slow plasma clearance; 4% extracted per renal passage; 4 – 8% glomerular filtration within 1 hour and 30% by 14 hours; 50% of dose accumulates in proximal + distal renal tubular cells by 1 hour (= cortical agent)

Imaging: after 1 – 24 hours (optimal at 34 hours); improved sensitivity to structural defects with SPECT

Biologic half-life: >30 hours
Dose: 5 – 10 mCi
Radiation dose: 0.014 rads/mCi for gonads;
0.015 rads/mCi for whole body

[I-131 OIH]
largely replaced by Tc-99m MAG3
= I-131 orthoiodohippurate (Hippuran®)
= good for evaluation of renal tubular function / effective renal plasma flow; agent with highest extraction ratio without binding to renal parenchyma; visualizes kidney even in severe renal failure

Pharmacokinetics:
80% secreted by proximal tubules; 20% filtered by glomeruli; maximal renal concentration within 5 minutes; normal transit time of 2 – 3 minutes; approximately 2% free iodine (Lugol's solution administered to protect thyroid)

Imaging:
in 15 – 60-second intervals for 20 minutes; renal uptake determined from images obtained by 1 – 2 minutes (patient in supine position for equidistance of kidneys to camera)

Biologic half-life: 10 minutes (with normal renal function)
Dose: 200 (range 150 – 300) µCi

Radiation dose: 0.06 rads/200 µCi for bladder;
0.02 rads/200 µCi for kidney;
0.02 rads/200 µCi for whole body;
0.02 rads/200 µCi for gonads

Tc-99m mercaptoacetyltriglycine (MAG3)

= renal plasma flow agent similar to OIH but with imaging benefits of Tc-99m label (improved dosimetry)

Pharmacokinetics:
correlates with renal plasma flow; clearance is less than Hippuran
Dose: 10 mCi
Evaluation:
true renal plasma flow = MAG3 flow (obtained off renogram curve) multiplied by a constant (varies between 1.4 and 1.8)

Differential renal function

Agents:
(1) Tc-99m DTPA:
measurements prior to excretion within first 1 – 3 minutes; images taken at 1.5-second intervals for 30 seconds followed by serial images for next 30 minutes
(2) I-131 Hippuran:
measurements prior to excretion within first 1 – 2 minutes

Evaluation: generation of time-activity curves

√ increased hepatic + soft tissue uptake with impaired renal function
√ measurements usually not significantly affected with differences in renal depth
√ measurements are accurate in renal obstruction if obtained within 1 – 3 minutes
√ prediction about functional recovery not possible following surgical relief of obstruction

Radionuclide cystogram

Technique:
Infusion of 0.5 – 1 mCi Tc-99m pertechnetate-saline mixture into bladder

Imaging:
posterior upright views throughout filling and voiding phases; review on cinematic loop helpful; residual bladder volume can be calculated

Advantage:
lower radiation dose to child than comparable contrast study

ADRENAL SCINTIGRAPHY

A. ADRENOCORTICAL IMAGING AGENTS
1. NP-59
2. Selenium-75 6-β-selenomethylnorcholesterol (Scintadrin®)

B. SYMPATHOADRENAL IMAGING AGENTS
1. I-131 / I-123 metaiodobenzylguanidine (MIBG)

I-131 metaiodobenzylguanidine (MIBG)

Indications:
Apudomas = tumors of neural crest origin (C cells of thyroid, melanocytes of skin, chromaffin cells of adrenal medulla, pancreatic cells, Kulchitsky cells), which share the presence of neurosecretory granules capable of accumulating I-131 MIBG
(1) Pheochromocytoma (80 – 90% sensitivity, >90% specificity); tumors as small as 0.2 g have been detected
(2) Neuroblastoma, carcinoid, medullary thyroid carcinoma, nonfunctioning retroperitoneal neuroendocrine tumor, middle mediastinal paraganglioma, adrenal metastasis of choriocarcinoma, Merkel (skin) tumor

Pharmacokinetics:
Chemically similar to norepinephrine, which is synthesized by adrenergic neurons + cells of the adrenal medulla; localizes in storage granules of adrenergic tissue by means of energy- and sodium-dependent uptake mechanism; not metabolized to any appreciable extent;
Normal activity is seen in liver, spleen, bladder, salivary glands, myocardium, lungs; 85% of injected dose is excreted unchanged by kidneys

Method:
Lugol solution administered orally (50 mg of iodine per day) for 4 – 5 days starting the day before injection (to block thyroid uptake of free iodine)

Dose: 0.4 mCi (14.8 MBq) or maximally 0.5 mCi/1.73 square meters of body surface MIBG

Radiation dose: 35 rad/mCi for adrenal medulla, 1.0 rad/mCi for ovaries, 0.4 rad/mCi for liver, 0.22 rad/mCi for whole body

Imaging: 24, 48, (72) hours after injection

False-negative scan:
uptake blocked by reserpine, imipramine, other tricyclic depressants, amphetamine-like drugs

I-123 metaiodobenzylguanidine

also allows SPECT imaging
Dose: 10 mCi
Radiation dose:
2.76 rad/mCi for adrenals, 0.07 rad/mCi for ovaries, 0.05 rad/mCi for liver, 0.02 rad/mCi for whole body
Imaging: at 6 and 24 hours

Iodocholesterol

Agent: I-131 6-beta-iodomethyl-19-norcholesterol (NP-59); NO FDA approval (available as investigational new drug)

Indications: adrenocortical imaging
(1) ACTH-independent Cushing syndrome (adenoma, cortical nodular hyperplasia)
(2) Adrenocortical carcinoma
√ spectrum from nonfunctioning to functioning
(3) Primary aldosteronism (adenoma, bilateral adrenal hyperplasia)
improved scintigraphic discrimination requires dexamethasone suppression before + during imaging
(4) Hyperandrogenism (adrenal adenoma, zona reticularis hyperplasia, polycystic ovary disease, ovarian stromal hyperplasia, androgen-secreting ovarian neoplasm)
(5) Incidentaloma = euadrenal mass
√ localization to side of CT-depicted adrenal mass (= concordant uptake) suggests hyperfunctioning adenoma
√ markedly diminished / absent uptake (= discordant uptake) or symmetric uptake (= nonlateralization) suggests space-occupying mass (eg, cyst) / malignant adrenal mass

Pharmacokinetics:
NP-59 is incorporated into low-density lipoproteins (LDL), circulates to adrenal cortex, absorbed from LDL complex by low-density lipoprotein receptors, esterified in adrenal cortex; adrenocortical uptake affected by adrenocortical secretagogues (corticotropin, angiotensin II);
Enterohepatic excretion may obscure adrenals (prior laxative administration beneficial)

Dose: 1 mCi (37 MBq) with slow IV injection
Radiation dose:
26 rad/mCi for adrenals, 8.0 rad/mCi for ovaries, 2.4 rad/mCi for liver, 2.3 rad/mCi for testes, 1.2 rad/mCi for whole body

Method:
Lugol solution administered orally (50 mg of iodine per day) for 4 – 5 days starting the day before injection (to block thyroid uptake of free iodine); mild laxative administered to decrease bowel activity

Imaging:
(a) 5 – 7-day interval between injection + imaging;
(b) 3 – 5-day interval between injection + imaging in case of dexamethasone suppression (1 mg four times daily for 7 days prior to and throughout 4 – 5 days of postinjection imaging interval)

STATISTICS

Incidence = number of diseased people per 100,000 population per year

Prevalence = number of existing cases per 100,000 population at a target date

Mortality = number of deaths per 100,000 population per year

Fatality = number of deaths per number of diseased

Decision Matrix:

		GOLD STANDARD			
T		normal	abnormal	subtotal	
E	normal	TN	FN	T-	npV
S	abnormal	FP	TP	T+	ppV
T					
	subtotal	D-	D+		total
		spec	sens		acc

TP = test positive in diseased subject
FP = test positive in nondiseased subject
FN = test negative in diseased subject
TN = test negative in nondiseased subject
T+ = abnormal test result
T- = normal test result
D+ = diseased subjects
D- = nondiseased subjects

Sensitivity
= ability to detect disease
= probability of having an abnormal test given disease
= number of correct positive tests / number with disease
= true positive ratio = TP / (TP + FN) = TP / D+
• D+ column in decision matrix
Δ independent of prevalence

Specificity
= ability to identify absence of disease
= probability of having a negative test given no disease
= number of correct negative tests / number without disease
= true negative ratio = TN / (TN + FP) = TN / D-
• D- column in decision matrix
Δ independent of prevalence

Accuracy
= number of correct results in all tests
= number of correct tests / total number of tests
= (TP + TN) / (TP + TN + FP + FN) = (TP + TN) / total
Δ depends much on the proportion of diseased + nondiseased subjects in studied population

Δ Not valuable for comparison of tests
Example: same test accuracy of 90% for two tests

Test A: 90% sensitivity, 90% specificity

		GOLD STANDARD		
T		normal	abnormal	subtotal
E	normal	90	10	100
S	abnormal	10	90	100
T				
	subtotal	100	100	200

Test B: 33% sensitivity, 100% specificity

		GOLD STANDARD		
T		normal	abnormal	subtotal
E	normal	170	20	190
S	abnormal	0	10	10
T				
	subtotal	170	30	200

Positive predictive value
= positive test accuracy
= likelihood that a positive test result actually identifies presence of disease
= number of correct positive tests / number of positive tests
= TP / (TP + FP) = TP / T+
• T+ row in decision matrix
Δ dependent on prevalence
Δ PPV increases with increasing prevalence for given sensitivity + specificity
Δ PPV increases with increasing specificity for given prevalence

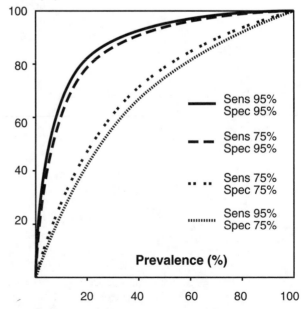

PPV (%)

Prevalence (%)

Sens 95%
Spec 95%

Sens 75%
Spec 95%

Sens 75%
Spec 75%

Sens 95%
Spec 75%

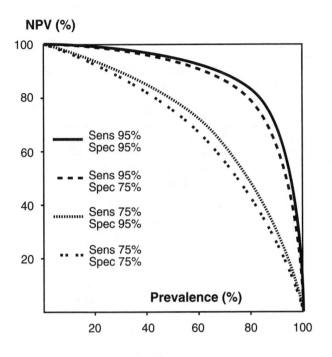

NPV (%)

Legend:
— Sens 95% Spec 95%
- - - Sens 95% Spec 75%
.... Sens 75% Spec 95%
· · · Sens 75% Spec 75%

Prevalence (%)

Negative predictive value
= negative test accuracy
= likelihood that a negative test result actually identifies absence of disease
= number of correct negative tests / number of negative tests
= TN / (TN + FN) = TN / T-
• T- row in decision matrix
Δ dependent on prevalence
Δ NPV increases with decreasing prevalence for given sensitivity + specificity
Δ NPV increases with increasing sensitivity for given prevalence

False-positive ratio
= proportion of nondiseased patients with an abnormal test result
• D- column in decision matrix
= FP / (FP + TN) = FP / D-
= 1 - specificity = (TN + FP - TN) / (TN + FP)

False-negative ratio
= proportion of diseased patients with a normal test result
• D+ column in decision matrix
= FN / (TP + FN) = FN / D+
= 1 - sensitivity = (TP + FN - TP) / (TP + FN)

Disease prevalence
= proportion of diseased subjects to total population
= (TP + FN) / (TP + TN + FP + FN) = D+ / total
Δ Sensitivity + specificity are independent of prevalence
Δ Affects predictive values + accuracy of a test result

Example:

Test A: sensitivity + specificity of 90%

GOLD STANDARD

T		normal	abnormal	subtotal
E	*normal*	90	10	100
S	*abnormal*	10	90	100
T				
	subtotal	100	100	200

NPV = 90%
PPV = 90%

Test B: prevalence of 10%, 90% sensitivity + specificity

GOLD STANDARD

T		normal	abnormal	subtotal
E	*normal*	162	2	164
S	*abnormal*	18	18	36
T				
	subtotal	180	20	200

NPV = 99%
PPV = 50%

Test C: prevalence of 90%, 90% sensitivity + specificity

GOLD STANDARD

T		normal	abnormal	subtotal
E	*normal*	18	18	36
S	*abnormal*	2	162	164
T				
	subtotal	20	180	200

NPV = 50%
PPV = 99%

Receiver operating characteristics (ROC)
= curvilinear graph generated by plotting TP ratio as a function of FP ratio for a number of different diagnostic criteria (ranging from definitely normal to definitely abnormal)
Y-axis: true-positive ratio = sensitivity
X-axis: false-positive ratio = 1 - specificity; reversing the values on the X-axis results in an identical "sensitivity-specificity curve"

Use:
variations in diagnostic criteria are reported as a continuum of responses ranging from definitely abnormal to equivocal to definitely normal due to subjectivity + bias of individual radiologist

Interpretation:
Δ Increase in sensitivity leads to decrease in specificity!
Δ Increase in specificity leads to decrease in sensitivity!
Δ The most sensitive point is the point with the highest TP ratio
— equivalent to "overreading" by using less stringent diagnostic criteria (all findings read as abnormal)
Δ The most specific point is the point with the lowest FP ratio

— equivalent to "underreading" by using more strict diagnostic criteria (all findings read as normal)
Δ The ROC curve closest to the Y-axis represents the best diagnostic test
Δ Does not consider disease prevalence in the population

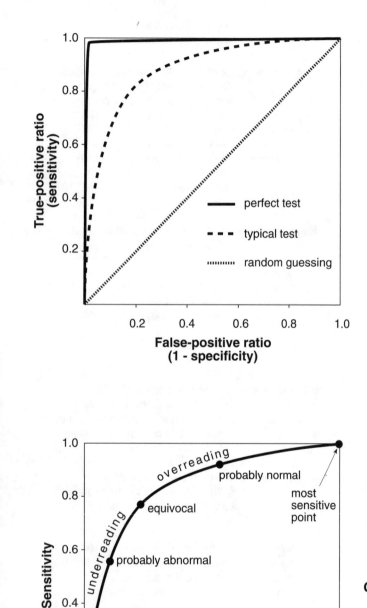

Kappa (κ)

measures concordance between test results and gold standard
Δ Analogous to Pearson correlation coefficient (r) for continuous data!

GOLD STANDARD

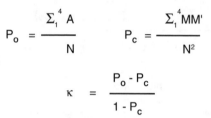

T	A_1	$M_2M'_2$	$M_3M'_3$	$M_4M'_4$	M_1
E	$M_2M'_1$	A_2	$M_2M'_3$	$M_2M'_4$	M_2
S	$M_3M'_1$	$M_3M'_2$	A_3	$M_3M'_4$	M_3
T	$M_4M'_1$	$M_4M'_2$	$M_4M'_3$	A_4	M_4
	M'_1	M'_2	M'_3	M'_4	N

$$P_o = \frac{\Sigma_1^4 A}{N} \qquad P_c = \frac{\Sigma_1^4 MM'}{N^2}$$

$$\kappa = \frac{P_o - P_c}{1 - P_c}$$

Example: $\kappa = 0.743$

GOLD STANDARD

T	18	3	0	0	21
E	2	20	5	2	29
S	1	4	20	3	28
T	0	0	5	17	22
	21	27	30	22	100

Predictive value of κ:
0.00 — 0.20	little or none
0.20 — 0.40	slight
0.40 — 0.60	group
0.60 — 0.80	some individual
0.80 — 1.0	individual

Confidence Limit

= degree of certainty that the proportion calculated from a sample of a particular size lies within a specific range (binomial theorem)
Δ Analogous to the mean ± 2 SD

Complete, Current Coverage...In One Volume

Fundamentals of Diagnostic Radiology
Edited by *William E. Brant, MD* and
Clyde A. Helms, MD

The new standard source on the subject, Brant & Helms' **Fundamentals of Diagnostic Radiology**, provides the complete and current coverage you need of the basics of diagnostic imaging. Designed specifically for the radiology resident, this text is also a first class review tool for Board certification exams, and the perfect starting point for specialists in other disciplines who are interested in diagnostic imaging techniques.

You'll find features such as these...
- [ ] emphasis on current modalities and their most appropriate uses
- [ ] high quality illustrations
- [ ] insights on differential diagnosis and diagnostic problem solving
- [ ] a clear focus on commonly-encountered conditions
- [ ] discussion of AIDS in each section, as appropriate
- [ ] separate sections on breast, pediatric, and nuclear radiology

Reserve your copy of the new standard today!

November 1993/about 1136 pages/1005 illustrations

Please send me ___ copy(ies) of **Fundamentals of Diagnostic Radiology** (#1011-5) at $135.00 each.

This book is available with our 90 Day Extended Guarantee. If you're not completely satisfied, return within 90 days for full credit or refund (U.S. only).

Payment options:
- [ ] Check enclosed [ ] MasterCard [ ] VISA [ ] AMEX [ ] Bill me

CARD #   EXP. DATE

SIGNATURE/P.O. #

NAME

ADDRESS

CITY   STATE   ZIP

PHONE #

- •CA, PA and MD residents please add state sales tax. Prices subject to change without notice.
- •Postage and a $4.00 handling charge will be added. No postage charge for orders paid by check.

Credit card orders call:
Toll Free **1-800-638-0672**
Refer to #B3123l when you order.
Fax   1-800-447-8438

Williams & Wilkins
A Waverly Company

Printed in U.S. - 3/93   B3 0141   BRANTIN B3 1231 0